Neuroscience in Medicine

NEUROSCIENCE IN MEDICINE

SECOND EDITION

Edited by

P. MICHAEL CONN

Oregon National Primate Research Center
Oregon Health and Science University
Beaverton, OR

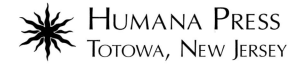
HUMANA PRESS
TOTOWA, NEW JERSEY

For additional copies, pricing for bulk purchases, and/or information about other Humana titles, contact Humana at the above address or at any of the following numbers: Tel.: 973-256-1699; Fax: 973-256-8341; E-mail:humana@humanapr.com; Website: http://humanapress.com

Production Editor: Kim Hoather-Potter.

Cover Illustration: (First image) Fetal monkey cortex stained for GFAP (red) and calcium-binding protein (green). Cornea A., Kirigitti M., and Simerly R. (Second image) Transfected cell expressing GnRH receptor (green) and agonist ligand (red). Cornea A., Janovick J., Lin A., and Conn P.M. Oregon National Primate Research Center, Oregon Health and Science University, Beaverton, Oregon, USA.

Cover design by Patricia F. Cleary.

This publication is printed on acid-free paper. ∞
ANSI Z39.48-1984 (American National Standards Institute) Permanence of Paper for Printed Library Materials.

Printed in the United States of America.   10 9 8 7 6 5 4 3 2 1

Library of Congress Cataloging-in-Publication Data

Neuroscience in Medicine/edited by P. Michael Conn.--2nd ed.
    p.;cm.
    Includes bibliographical references and index.
    ISBN 1-58829-016-6 (alk. paper)   EISBN 1-59259-371-2
    1. Neurobiology. 2. Neurophysiology. 3. Nervous system--Pathophysiology. I. Conn, P. Michael.
    [DNLM: 1. Nervous System Physiology. WL 102 N50594 2003]
QP355.2.N53 2003
612.8--dc21

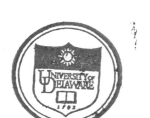

2003047769

PREFACE

The preface to the first edition of *Neuroscience in Medicine* began with a simple statement: "Neuroscience is a fascinating discipline." The interest that provoked the preparation of a second edition means that statement still rings true. The challenge remained to define the core material. I have attempted to restrict certain peripheral topics—the generalities of biosynthesis and gene expression, for example—in order to allow the remaining topics to include new material and, in some cases, to showcase developing areas—neuroimmunology, for example—in the hope that this will pique the interests of the reader and keep the volume fresh.

As in the first edition of *Neuroscience in Medicine*, the authors are selected from leaders in research on their chosen topics who also hold credentials as excellent teachers. Such individuals are rare and, not surprisingly, are very careful with their time. Happily, the authors involved here recognize the significance of their project and have generously made the necessary time commitments to it. Once the manuscripts were in hand, it was the editor's job to make the writing uniform, remove duplicative materials except where essential for ease of understanding, and incorporate additional critical material.

Neuroscience in Medicine is designed to reveal the basic science underlying disease and treatments for neural disorders. Though the chapters are intended to interdigitate, each chapter can be read as a stand alone—that is, each contains a complete discussion of the topic.

I am pleased that the "Clinical Correlations," a popular feature of the first edition, are again included. We have also been aided in our task by the art and editorial staff at Humana, whose help I gratefully acknowledge.

Two participants from the first edition of *Neuroscience in Medicine,* Dr. David K. Sundberg and Dr. Robert F. Spencer, passed away during the ten years since it was published. Their intellectual contribution, collegiality, and helpfulness was missed.

P. Michael Conn

CONTENTS

Contents

CONTRIBUTORS

JOHN D. BOUGHTER, JR., PhD • *Department of Anatomy and Neurobiology, University of Tennessee Health Science Center, Memphis, TN*

KEVIN J. CANNING, PhD • *Department of Physiology, University of Toronto, Toronto, Ontario, Canada*

SONIA L. CARLSON, PhD • *Department of Anatomy and Neurobiology, University of Kentucky College of Medicine, Lexington, KY*

RAFAEL C. CARUSO, MD, PhD • *OGVFB, National Institutes of Health, Bethesda, MD*

MARIE-FRANCOISE CHESSELET, MD, PhD • *Department of Neurology, Reed Neurological Research Center, UCLA School of Medicine, Los Angeles, CA*

ROCHELLE S. COHEN, PhD • *Department of Anatomy and Cell Biology, University of Illinois at Chicago, College of Medicine, Chicago, IL*

P. MICHAEL CONN, PhD • *Oregon National Primate Research Center, Beaverton; and Oregon Health and Science University, Portland, OR*

GREGORY COOPER, MD • *Department of Neurology, The University of Iowa College of Medicine, Iowa City, IA*

MATTHEW ENNIS, PhD • *Department of Anatomy and Neurobiology, School of Medicine, University of Maryland, Baltimore, MD*

MARC E. FREEMAN, PhD • *Department of Biological Science, Florida State University, Tallahassee, FL*

JOHN B. GELDERD, PhD • *Department of Human Anatomy and Medical Neurobiology, Texas A&M University System Health Science Center, College of Medicine, College Station, TX*

A. TUCKER GLEASON, PhD • *Division of Balance Disorders, Department of Otolaryngology – Head and Neck Surgery, University of Virginia, Charlottesville, VA*

ROBERT D. GRUBBS, PhD • *Department of Pharmacology and Toxicology, Wright State University School of Medicine, Dayton, OH*

C. J. HECKMAN, PhD • *Departments of Physiology and Physical Medicine and Rehabilitation, Northwestern University Feinberg School of Medicine, Chicago, IL*

MARY M. HEINRICHER, PhD • *Department of Neurological Surgery, Oregon Health Sciences University, Portland, OR*

J. FIELDING HEJTMANCIK, MD, PhD • *OGVFB, National Institutes of Health, Bethesda, MD*

THOMAS A. HOUPT, PhD • *Department of Biological Science, Florida State University, Tallahassee, FL*

COURT HULL, BS • *Oregon Health and Science University, Portland, OR*

CONRAD E. JOHANSON, PhD • *Department of Clinical Neurosciences, Brown University School of Medicine, Rhode Island Hospital, Providence, RI*

MICHAEL D. LUMPKIN, PhD • *Department of Physiology and Biophysics, Georgetown University Medical School, Washington, D.C.*

BRUCE E. MALEY, PhD • *Department of Anatomy and Neurobiology, University of Kentucky College of Medicine, Lexington, KY*

ROBERT W. MCCARLEY, PhD • *Department of Psychiatry, Harvard Medical School / VA Boston Health Care System, Brockton, MA*

MICHAEL W. MILLER, PhD • *Department of Neuroscience and Physiology, SUNY Upstate Medical University, and Veterans Affairs Medical Center, Syracuse, NY*

MARION MURRAY, PhD • *Department of Anatomy and Neurobiology, MCP Hahnemann University, Philadelphia, PA*

SURESH C. PATEL, MD • *Division of Neuroradiology, Henry Ford Hospital and Health Science Centers, Detroit, MI; Case Western University School of Medicine, Cleveland, OH*

DONALD W. PFAFF, PhD • *Laboratory of Neurobiology and Behavior, The Rockefeller University, New York, NY*

JOHN D. PORTER, PhD • *Department of Ophthalmology, University Hospitals of Cleveland, Case Western Reserve University, Cleveland, OH*

ADAM C. PUCHE, PhD • *Department of Anatomy and Neurobiology, School of Medicine, University of Maryland, Baltimore, MD*

PAUL J. REIER, PhD • *Department of Neuroscience, University of Florida College of Medicine and McKnight Brain Institute, Gainesville, FL*

ROBERT L. RODNITZKY, MD • *Department of Neurology, The University of Iowa College of Medicine, Iowa City, IA*

W. ZEV RYMER, MD, PhD • *Sensory Motor Performance Program, Rehabilitation Institute of Chicago at Northwestern University, Chicago, IL*

MICHAEL T. SHIPLEY, PhD • *Department of Anatomy and Neurobiology, University of Maryland School of Medicine, Baltimore, MD*

MAMADOU SIDIBE, PhD • *Yerkes National Primate Research Center, Emory University, Atlanta, GA*

DAVID V. SMITH, PhD • *Department of Anatomy and Neurobiology, University of Tennessee Health Science Center, Memphis, TN*

YOLAND SMITH, PhD • *Yerkes National Primate Research Center, Emory University, Atlanta, GA*

ROBERT F. SPENCER, PhD • *Deceased. Department of Anatomy, Medical College of Virginia, Virginia Commonwealth University, Richmond, VA*

STEVEN J. ST. JOHN, PhD • *Department of Psychology, Reed College, Portland, OR*

STANKO S. STOJILKOVIC, PhD • *Section on Cellular Signaling, ERRB/NICHD, NIH, Bethesda, MD*

DAVID K. SUNDBERG, PhD • *Deceased. Department of Physiology and Pharmacology, Bowman Gray School of Medicine, Wake Forest University, Winston-Salem, NC*

CHING SUNG TENG, PhD • *Department of Molecular Biomedical Sciences, North Carolina State University, Raleigh, NC*

CHRISTINA T. TENG, PhD • *Laboratory of Reproductive and Developmental Toxicology (LRDT), National Institute of Environmental Health Services (NIEHS), NIH, Research Triangle Park, NC*

DANIEL TRANEL, PhD • *Department of Neurology and Psychology, Benton Neuropsychology Laboratory, The University of Iowa Hospitals and Clinics, Iowa City, IA*

HAROLD H. TRAURIG, PhD • *Department of Anatomy and Neurobiology, University of Kentucky College of Medicine, Lexington, KY*

THOMAS VAN GROEN, PhD • *Department of Neuroscience and Neurology, University of Kuopio, Kuopio, Finland*

MARGARET J. VELARDO, PA, PhD • *Department of Neuroscience, University of Florida College of Medicine and McKnight Brain Institute, Gainesville, FL*

BRENT A. VOGT, PhD • *Department of Neuroscience and Physiology, State University of New York, SUNY Upstate Medical University, Syracuse, NY*

HENRIQUE VON GERSDORFF, PhD • *The Vollum Institute, Oregon Health and Science University, Portland, OR*

SIMONE WAGNER, MD • *Department of Neurology, University of Heidelberg, Germany*

JAMES R. WEST, PhD • *Department of Human Anatomy and Neurobiology, Texas A&M University System Health Science Center, College of Medicine, College Station, TX*

J. MICHAEL WYSS, PhD • *Department of Cell Biology, University of Alabama at Birmingham, Birmingham, AL*

TOM C. T. YIN, PhD • *Department of Physiology, University of Wisconsin Medical School, Madison, WI*

1

Cytology and Organization of Cell Types
Light and Electron Microscopy

Rochelle S. Cohen and Donald W. Pfaff

1. NEURONAL RESPONSE TO A CHANGING ENVIRONMENT

Although neurons are cells that conform to fundamental cellular and molecular principles, they are differentiated from other cells in ways that reflect their unique ability to receive, integrate, store, and send information. Signals received from the internal and external environment are processed by neurons, resulting in the generation of a response that can be communicated to other neurons or tissues. In this way, the organism can successfully adapt to rapidly changing events, ensuring its survival.

All organisms possess stimulus-response systems that permit them to sense environmental fluctuations. In bacteria, for example, intracellular regulatory molecules couple the stimulus to the proper response. Multicellular organisms must communicate information to other cells, some of which may be local, but others are positioned some distance away. Communication may be accomplished by the release of chemical messengers that bind to specific complementary proteins called receptors, located on the surface of other cells. For local communication, diffusion can deliver the messenger to the receptive surface. Mes-

sengers such as hormones, secreted by endocrine cells in response to changes in the internal milieu, may have to travel long distances through the bloodstream to reach their targets. This voyage takes time-seconds, hours, or even days-and hormones are considered slow-acting agents. Because hormones are diluted in the bloodstream, they must be very potent and act at low concentrations to be effective. These properties are sufficient for endocrine functions necessary to keep the organism in a homeostatic state, but more immediate challenges require a rapid coupling of stimulus and response and a faster rate of communication among relevant cells. Rapid communication is achieved exquisitely by the neuron, whose form and function are designed to meet such demands.

The rapidity with which neurons can conduct signals (i.e., time is measured in less than 1 ms) is primarily a function of certain basic features common to all neurons: polarization of their form, unique associations with their neighboring neurons, and special properties of their plasma membranes. Information is conveyed within and between neurons in the form of electrical and chemical signals, respectively. Neurons are organized into complex networks, or functional circuits, which translate these signals into the myriad responses that constitute an organism's behavioral repertoire. Neural circuits develop in a predictable

From: *Neuroscience in Medicine, 2nd ed.* (P. Michael Conn, ed.), © 2003 Humana Press Inc., Totowa, NJ.

manner, achieving organizational specificity at functional sites of contact called synapses. At the synapses, neurons transmit signals with a great degree of fidelity, allowing some behaviors, particularly those necessary for survival, to be stereotyped. Neurons also possess a remarkable ability to modify the way messages are received, processed, and transmitted and may exert profound changes in behavioral patterns. This special property is called plasticity and depends on the molecular and structural properties of the neuron.

In addition to forming specific contacts with other nerve cells, neurons exist in relation to a group of cells collectively known as glia. Some glial cells envelop neurons and their processes and appear to provide them with mechanical and metabolic support. Others are arranged along specific neuronal processes so as to increase the rate of conduction of electrical signals. Glia are considered later in this chapter. We first focus on the neuron, which is the fundamental structural and functional unit of the nervous system.

1.1. Synapses Are the Sites of Directed Communication Between Neurons

The polarization of neuronal shape permits its functioning within a simple or complex circuit. Like other cells, neurons possess a cell body, or perikaryon, which is the metabolic hub of the cell. However, cellular processes extend from this center and give the neuron its unique form and ability to receive and rapidly send signals often over long distances (Fig. 1).

Signals are communicated between neurons at synapses. One neuron forms the presynaptic element, and the subsequent neuron forms the postsynaptic element. Chemical signals, in the form of neurotransmitters or neuropeptides, are concentrated at the presynaptic site. The postsynaptic site contains a high concentration of receptor molecules that are specific for each messenger. Presynaptic and postsynaptic elements are separated by a space of only 20 to 40 µm, ensuring precise and directed transmission of signals.

1.2. Neuronal Polarity Is a Function of Axons and Dendrites

The two main types of cellular processes are called dendrites and axons (see Fig. 1). Dendrites are usually postsynaptic and form an enormous receptive surface, which branches extensively. In some neurons, such as cerebellar Purkinje cells, the dendritic branches form a characteristic elaborate arborization; others are less distinctive. In addition to their growth during normal development, some of these processes remain plastic and can change in length dramatically in the adult. For example, the extent of arborization of the dendritic tree of male rat motor neurons that innervate penile muscles and mediate copulatory behavior appears to he under steroid hormone (i.e., androgen) regulation. In some dendrites, the membranous surfaces are further elaborated to form protrusions called dendritic spines. Chemical signals received by dendrites and their spines are integrated and transduced into an electrical signal, known as the synaptic potential.

The signal triggers the action potential, which is propagated along the neuron's plasma membrane down an elongated process called the axon. Although axons are not as expansive as dendrites, they branch and may innervate more than one effector. The terminal end of an axon is modified to form a bulbous structure, the presynaptic terminal (see Fig. 1). The incoming action potentials cause the release of neurotransmitter molecules that bind to complementary postsynaptic receptors. This binding initiates the other type of electrical signal, the synaptic potential at the postsynaptic site.

The unidirectional or polarized how of information consists of action potentials at the axonal level eliciting synaptic potentials in the postsynaptic cell, which triggers an action potential in that cell and so on. Axons may be as long as 2 meters, permitting long-distance and rapid communication within the circuit.

1.3. Diversity in Form Is a Distinctive Property of Neurons

Although neuronal form follows the basic plan described above, nerve cells show a tremendous diversity in size, shape, and function, which allows them to discriminate the multitude of different types of incoming signals. The detection of commands for muscle contraction is under the control of motor neurons. Information in the form of light, mechanical force, or chemical substances is distinguished by sensory neurons highly specialized for each particular type of sensation. It is perhaps in this group of neurons that structural and functional diversity is most apparent. The rigorous demands of sensory discrimination have imposed on these neurons the requirement to develop specific, highly sensitive detection systems that are able to perceive various degrees of stimulus intensities.

A classic example is the olfactory cell of the male gypsy moth, which can detect a molecule of the female's sex attractant or pheromone released a mile away Equally impressive is the ability of the

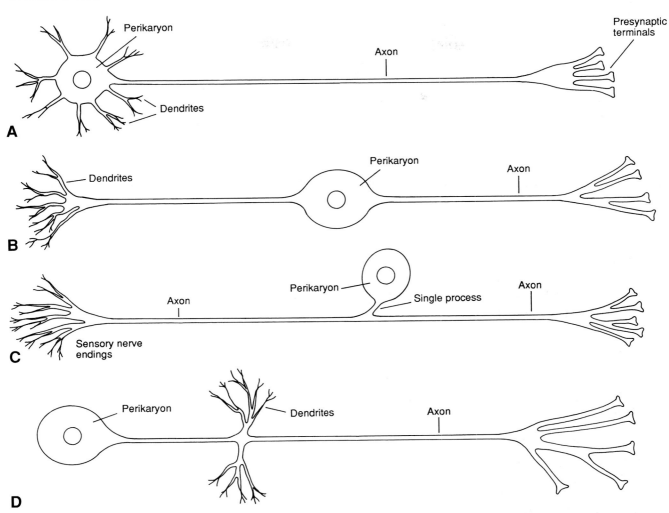

Fig. 1. Polarization of the neuronal form. Nerve cells conduct impulses in a directed manner, although the position of axons and dendrites relative to the cell body and to each other may vary. (**A**) The multipolar neuron is the most prevalent type and shows extensive branching of the dendrites that emanate from the cell body. The axons emerge from the opposite end. (**B**) Bipolar neurons have sensory functions and transmit information received by dendrites along two processes that emerge from the cell body. (**C**) Pseudounipolar neurons are found in the dorsal root ganglion. These neurons are bipolar during early development. Later, the two processes fuse to form a stalk, which subsequently bifurcates into two axons. The action potentials are conducted from sensory nerve endings in skin and muscle to the spinal cord. The action potential usually bypasses the cell body, but in conditions such as a prolapsed vertebral disc, in which the dorsal nerve roots are put under pressure, the cell bodies may also generate impulses. (**D**) Unipolar neurons are found in invertebrates. Axons arise from the dendrites, which emerge from the cell body.

mammalian nasal epithelium to detect and discriminate more than 10,000 different odiferous substances. In terms of the ability to recognize diverse molecules, olfactory neurons are second only to the cells of the immune system. The olfactory neuron, however, is markedly different in form and receptor locale from, for example, the retinal photoreceptor cell. Receptive surfaces consisting of specialized cilia on olfactory neurons contain the receptors and are the primary sites of sensory transduction. In retinal photoreceptor neu-

rons, visual transduction occurs within special cylindrical cellular domains containing stacks of about 1000 membranous discs in which the photon receptors called rhodopsin are embedded.

Sensory and other types of information enter the nervous system by means of a particular neuron, but those signals are rarely sent to the effector neuron directly. Rather, the initial signal is sent to a third class of nerve cell, the interneurons. Interneurons integrate various inputs from other neurons before the information, often in a modified form, reaches its final destination. In this way, various types of inputs (e.g., sensory, hormonal) can be integrated and relayed to other parts of the central nervous system or to motor or endocrine targets. Interneurons contribute to the formation of neural circuits and are to a great extent responsible for the relatively large size and extraordinary complexity of the mammalian nervous system.

1.4. Neuronal Polarity Allows the Directed Flow of Electrical and Chemical Signals

A single neuron may receive a multitude of different inputs from a variety of sources. A motor neuron, for example, receives thousands of presynaptic terminals from many different neurons on its dendritic surface and on its somal and, to some extent, axonal membranes, which may also bear postsynaptic receptors. This input has to be organized into a cohesive message that can be transmitted to its postsynaptic neighbor.

The neuronal plasma membrane plays a key role in integrating and relaying the information in a directed manner and with exceptional speed. Information is conducted within neurons in the form of electrical signals, which are actually changes in the distribution of electrical charges across the neuronal membrane. Charge distribution is highly regulated in neurons by specific and selective proteins called ion channels embedded in the plasma membrane. These transmembrane proteins control the flow of ions and, consequently the distribution of positive and negative charges across the membrane. In resting neurons, the membrane potential is about -60 to -70 mV (i.e., an excess of positive charges outside and negative charges inside). When this potential becomes less negative or depolarized, electrical excitation occurs in the membrane. In axons, this excitation is known as the action potential. The action potential is generated when the membrane potential of the axonal membrane is decreased beyond a threshold value.

2. MECHANISMS OF NEURONAL FUNCTION

Compared with other cells, neurons are unsurpassed in their complexity of form and ability to communicate with lightning speed over long distances. Nevertheless, as eukaryotic cells, they adhere to basic laws that govern cellular function. In many ways, neurons are not so different from other cells, and qualities once ascribed only to neurons may he found elsewhere. Egg

membranes, for example, can depolarize during fertilization and release granules in response to Ca^{2+} entry through specific channels, although the process takes much longer than comparable signaling mechanisms in neurons. Sites of ribosomal RNA synthesis, called nucleoli, are found in all eukaryotic cells but are especially, prominent in neurons, because there is a constant need for ribosomes for new protein synthesis. It appears that basic cellular mechanisms are present in nerve cells but that some of these are amplified to meet the rigorous demands of neuronal form and function.

2.1. The Nucleus is the Command Center of the Neuron

The molecular and cellular diversity within and among neurons reflects a highly controlled differential expression of genes. Gene regulation also determines nerve cell connectivity, which dictates patterns of stereotyped behaviors. It is also becoming evident that more complex behaviors, such as memory and learning, may require the synthesis of new proteins, which ultimately depends on the expression of particular genes.

As eukaryotic cells, neurons sequester their genome in the nucleus, the largest and most conspicuous feature of the perikaryon (Fig. 2). The nucleus contains chromosomal DNA and the machinery for synthesizing and processing RNA, which is subsequently transported to the cytoplasm, where information encoded in the DNA is expressed as specific proteins. The nucleus is separated from the rest of the cytoplasm by a porous double membrane, the nuclear envelope. The nuclear envelope protects the DNA molecules from mechanical perturbations caused by cytoplasmic filaments. Moreover, it separates the process of RNA synthesis (i.e., transcription) from that of protein synthesis (i.e., translation). This segregation of function has an important advantage over the situation in prokaryotes, in which transcription and translation occur simultaneously. In these organisms, protein synthesis begins before the completion of transcription, limiting the opportunity for modifying the RNA. Translation in eukaryotes does not begin until the RNA is transported into the cytoplasm. In the nucleus, the RNA may be modified in such a way that specific portions of the RNA molecule are removed (i.e., RNA splicing) or altered. These complex changes have important implications for cell function. Mechanisms that control variability at the level of transcribed RNA allow a single gene to code for several different proteins, resulting in the rich diversity seen, especially in

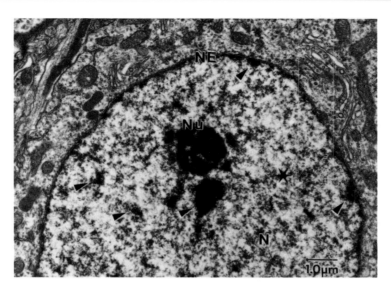

Fig. 2. The nucleus of a hypothalamic neuron. The nucleus (N) is separated from the cytoplasm by a nuclear envelope (NE). A conspicuous nucleolus (Nu) signifies a great demand for ribosomal RNA by the neuron. Proteins called histones associate with DNA to form chromatin, which may appear extended (i.e., euchromatin) or condensed (i.e., heterochromatin), depending on the translational activity of specific regions of the genome. Most of the nucleus contains fine fibers of euchromatin (*asterisk*). Heterochromatin (*arrowheads*) is seen as clumps within the nucleus, on the inner surface of the nuclear envelope, or associated with the nucleolus.

neurons, in the form of neuropeptides, receptors, ion channels and cytoskeletal proteins.

2.1.1. Chromatin Structure in the Regulation of Gene Activity

The degree of complexity of gene expression is further multiplied at another, even more fundamental level of gene regulation: the DNA. Genes are turned on by complexes of proteins called transcription factors. Each of these proteins possesses special DNA-binding domains and requires direct contact with the DNA to function.

However, the long stretch of DNA, which in humans measures about 3 cm long, is folded thousands of times to fit into a nucleus only a few micrometers in diameter. Such compaction creates a potential problem for factors that must gain free access to corresponding binding sites and other regulatory regions on the DNA strand. Another group of proteins, called histones, packs the DNA so that it is folded, coiled, and compressed many times over to form fibers called chromatin, visible as fine threads in the interphase nucleus (*see* Fig. 2) and, in an even more contracted form, as chromosomes in the dividing cell.

In the mature neuron, the nucleus remains in interphase. DNA is segregated into morphologically distinct areas, reflecting the degree of chromatin condensation, which is a function of nuclear activity (*see*

Fig. 2). Ribosomal DNA genes and their products are separately packed into a structurally defined compartment called the nucleolus that is specialized for ribosomal RNA synthesis. Highly coiled regions for the genome appear as dense, irregularly shaped clumps known as heterochromatin. These areas of condensed chromatin are situated within the nucleus along the inner nuclear membrane, in association with the nucleolus or dispersed within the nucleus proper. Other regions of the genome readily available for transcription into messenger RNA appear as fine filaments and are known as euchromatin.

2.1.2. Nucleolus as the Site of Ribosomal RNA Synthesis

The nucleolus is a prominent spherical region of the nucleus (*see* Fig. 2) containing that portion of the genome dedicated to the transcription of ribosomal DNA and the mechanisms for the assembly of ribosomal subunits, the precursors of mature ribosomes. Large precursor ribosomal RNA molecules are processed in the nucleus, resulting in the degradation of almost half of the nucleotide sequences. The remaining ribonucleoprotein molecules form two subunits that are independently transported into the cytoplasm, where the mature ribosomes are assembled. The nucleolus is evident only in the interphase nucleus; in other cells that undergo mitosis, it decondenses, ribo-

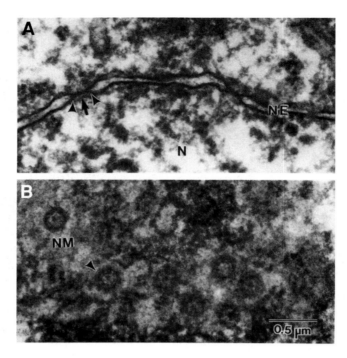

Fig. 3. Electron micrographs of nuclear pores. (**A**) The perpendicular section of the nuclear envelope (NE) shows the continuity of the inner and outer nuclear membranes (*arrowheads*) around a nuclear pore (*arrow*) of the nucleus (N). (**B**) A surface view shows the arrangement of nuclear pores in the nuclear membrane (NM). One of the nuclear pores (*arrowhead*) shows the octagonal configuration of proteins comprising the nuclear pore complex.

somal RNA synthesis stops, and ribosomal DNA genes associate with specific regions of the chromosomes called nucleolar organizing regions.

2.1.3. Nuclear Pore Complex Controls Traffic Between the Nucleus and Cytoplasm

The double membrane comprising the nuclear envelope presents a formidable barrier between the nucleus and cytoplasm. Macromolecular traffic into and out of the nucleus is achieved by perforations in the nuclear envelope. At various points along the envelope, the inner and outer membranes are in continuity around the edges of each pore (Fig. 3). The nuclear pore is not a simple opening. A complex of eight large proteins surround the aperture on the external surface of the inner and outer membranes. These proteins form the nuclear pore complex (*see* Fig. 3), central to which is the actual orifice through which particles are transported. Some particles, such as the assembled mature ribosomes, are too large to gain entrance through these passageways, ensuring that protein synthesis is restricted to the cytoplasm. Other particles, such as ribosomal subunits, may be larger than the channel but

can be actively transported through the pores, although they may be distorted along the way.

2.1.4. Dynamic Nuclear Morphology Reflects Alterations in the Genome

Although nuclear events occur on a molecular scale, they may be detected by gross adjustments in nuclear morphology. The overall size and shape of nuclei and nucleoli can change with the metabolic and physiologic demands of the neuron. Depending on transcriptional activity, various segments of the chromatin can condense or decondense, resulting in a relative change in the disposition of heterochromatin and euchromatin and altering the general appearance of the nucleus. For example, in the hypothalamus, a brain area controlling female reproductive behavior, the gonadal steroid hormone estrogen exerts a profound influence on nuclear morphology, altering its size, shape, and position of heterochromatic regions. Nucleolar size is also subject to the physiologic conditions of the cell. Estrogen treatment has a pronounced effect on precursor ribosomal RNA levels, which are accompanied by a significant increase in nucleolar area in the hypothalamus of ovariectomized animals. Nucleolar hypertrophy is followed by a massive increase in rough endoplasmic reticulum in these neurons.

2.2. Neurons Are Actively Engaged in Protein Synthesis

Information contained within the genome is expressed as biologically active peptides in the cell body or perikaryon of the neuron. Some peptides are neuron specific, such as some of the neurosecretory peptides, cytoskeletal proteins, ion channels and receptors. Others are common to all cells and are involved in increasing the efficiency of transcriptional and translational events related to the production, transport, and release of these proteins.

2.2.1. PROTEINS SYNTHESIZED BY NEURONS FOR EXPORT

Appreciation of the tremendous protein synthetic activity of the nerve cell and its functional implications is relatively recent. Neuronal form and membrane properties were the main focus of earlier neurobiologists. However, the compelling discovery of glandular cells in the spinal cord of fish by Carl Speidel in 1919 and of neurosecretory cells in the hypothalamus by Ernst Scharrer in 1928 directed attention to the great degree of biosynthetic activity in the perikaryon. Ernst Scharrer noticed that the secretory activity of diencephalic neurons was comparable to that seen in endocrine cells. This observation stimulated further interest in finding structural counterparts of the secretory process in neurons. The mechanisms involved in peptide biosynthesis and posttranslational processing are now well known. The related molecular and biochemical events have been detailed in the previous chapters. In this chapter, we describe the structural correlates of these functions as they occur in various parts of the nerve cell.

2.2.1.1. Synthesis of Exportable Neuropeptides on the Rough Endoplasmic Reticulum. Neurons must transmit chemical information and electrical signals over very long distances. Proteins are synthesized, packaged, processed, stored, and released in different domains of the neuron. The synthesis of exportable proteins begins in the perikaryon. Preribosomal subunits produced in the nucleolus enter the cytoplasm, where they are assembled and activated to form functional ribosomes. In some cases, they attach to membranous cisternae comprising the rough endoplasmic reticulum (Fig. 4). The outer nuclear membrane ramifies within the cytoplasm as it encircles the nucleus

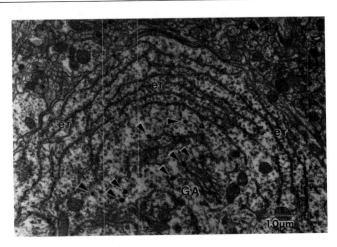

Fig. 4. Electron micrograph of a hypothalamic neuron actively engaged in the synthesis and packaging of exportable proteins. Many cisternae of rough endoplasmic reticulum (er) are arranged in parallel stacks. The Golgi apparatus (GA) and associated dense-cored vesicles (*arrowheads*) are also visible. (Cohen RS, Pfaff DW. Ultrastructure of neurons in the ventromedial nucleus of the hypothalamus with or without estrogen treatment. Cell Tissue Res 1981; 217:463.)

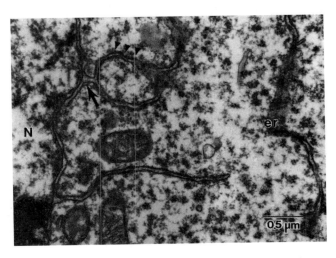

Fig. 5. Electron micrograph of the outer nuclear membrane ramifying within the cytoplasm. Portions of the outer nuclear membrane (*arrow*) extend into the cytoplasm and, together with associated ribosomes (*arrowheads*), become part of the protein synthetic machinery of the neuron. A cisterna of the rough endoplasmic reticulum (er) is seen to the right of the micrograph. *N*, nucleus.

and, studded with ribosomes, also becomes part of the protein synthetic apparatus (Fig. 5).

Messenger RNAs associated with ribosomes are translated into precursor proteins. The precursors are

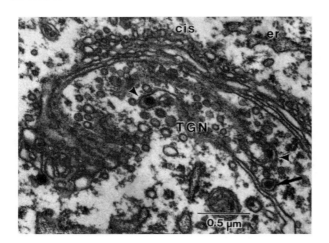

Fig. 6. Electron micrograph of a Golgi apparatus of a hypothalamic neuron. Small vesicles surround the Golgi apparatus on all sides. The cis face is located near the rough endoplasmic reticulum (er); the opposite side is designated as the *trans* Golgi network (TGN). Secretory material is detected within the peripheral portions of the cisternae (*arrowheads*) of the TGN. A dense-cored vesicle (*arrow*) containing material of similar density is seen at the periphery of the TGN.

larger than the biologically active peptides and must he enzymatically cleaved and modified to attain their final form. Instructions about whether a given protein is destined for export are also encoded in the DNA of its precursor. A portion of the complementary messenger RNA is translated into a signal peptide, which directs ribosomes to the cisternae of the rough endoplasmic reticulum. Peptides lacking a signal sequence can not gain entry to the cisternae.

The disposition and extent of rough endoplasmic reticulum vary and appear to depend on the prevailing demands for secretory protein synthesis in a functional group of neurons. In nerve cells that are quiescent in regard to the production of exportable proteins, cisternae of the rough endoplasmic reticulum appear as discrete sacs and seem to occupy only a small fraction of the cellular space. Neurons actively engaged in secretory protein synthesis contain large stacks of elongated cisternae that fill a considerable portion of the perikaryon.

2.2.1.2. Packaging and Modification of Exportable Neuropeptides in the Golgi Apparatus.
The Golgi apparatus is composed of a series of flattened, smooth-surfaced, membranous sacs and a variety of associated small vesicles, which encom-pass the Golgi apparatus on all sides (Fig. 6). The Golgi cisternae are arranged in a polarized fashion, reflecting their

morphology and function. The forming or cis face approaches the rough endoplasmic reticulum; the opposite side is designated as the maturing or trans face or trans-Golgi network. Vesicles bud off from the smooth transitional portion of the rough endoplasmic reticulum and transport their contents to Golgi sacs on the cis face. Here, they deliver the newly synthesized precursor protein by fusion of the vesicle membrane with the Golgi membrane. The secretory material is later detected within the cisternae occupying the trans-Golgi network. Often, at the periphery of the sacs, the membranes appear to constrict around a dense granule that is the concentrated precursor protein (*see* Fig. 6). The granule-containing membranous compartment is pinched off, forming a dense-cored vesicle. Although the details of protein processing within the Golgi apparatus have not yet been elucidated, its overall function is known: the preparation and packaging of the secretory protein, still in its precursor form for transport to the axon terminal for storage or release.

2.2.1.3. Formation of the Active Neuropeptide Within the Neurosecretory Vesicle.
The actual enzymatic processing of the precursor and generation of individual biologically active peptides appears to occur distal to the Golgi apparatus as the secretory vesicle makes its way down the axon. Conditions, such as pH, necessary for the maximal activity of the processing enzymes are optimal. The relatively simple structure of the secretory vesicle—a dense core surrounded by a single membrane—belies its dynamic role in generating active neuropeptides. Various enzymatic activities have been located in neurosecretory vesicles, and some have been purified and characterized. The vesicle membrane contains proteins that regulate the internal vesicular environment. On the appropriate signal, active neuropeptides are released by exocytosis, which is fusion of the vesicle membrane with the plasma membrane at the presynaptic site.

2.2.2. Proteins Synthesized for Use Within the Neuron

The synthesis of exportable proteins represents only a portion of the total protein synthetic effort by the neuron. The elaboration of the cytoskeletal framework and the synthesis of other proteins including ion channels, receptors, second messenger systems, and other proteins destined for maintenance and renewal of the cytoplasm and its organelles, also depend on translation of messenger RNAs. These proteins are synthesized on free ribosomes that are plentiful in all nerve cells.

Axons possess a highly organized transport system to convey proteins to presynaptic terminals or back to the cell body. Dendrites, their postsynaptic specializations, and dendritic spines also require proteins for growth, maintenance, and function. Although there is an indication of molecular transport to these sites, the identities of the molecules and the nature of the transport mechanism has just begun to be explored. Moreover, evidence for local protein synthesis suggests that not all dendritic and postsynaptic proteins arrive from the cell body. The presence of polyribosomes beneath postsynaptic membrane specializations and at the base of dendritic spines provides the machinery for local protein synthesis. The existence of local protein synthetic mechanisms is further supported by the presence of some messenger RNAs in distant dendritic arbors, suggesting that growth-dependent and activity-dependent synaptic alterations, including changes in morphology, may be regulated partially by the local synthesis of key synaptic proteins.

2.3. Smooth Membrane Compartments in Neurons Serve as Reservoirs for Calcium

In addition to the intramembranous compartments that directly participate in the synthesis, packaging and transport of secretory peptides, other cisternal and vesicular structures are evident within the various domains of the neuron. The membranous sacs are visible as smooth-surfaced compartments in a variety of configurations. Some appear as relatively short sacs, but others are longer and anastomose within neuronal processes. In the cell body, smooth membrane profiles are arranged in stacks or emanate from cisternae of the rough endoplasmic reticulum. One of the most morphologically complex variations of these structures resides in the dendritic spine, where parallel, smooth-surfaced cisternae alternate with electron-dense bands of unknown composition.

All of the diverse structures are thought to function in the release and sequestration of calcium within the neuron. Calcium is central to most aspects of neuronal function, including membrane permeability; mediation of the effects of neurotransmitters, hormones, and growth factors; cytoskeletal function; and vesicle release. In neurons, calcium mobilization is achieved, at least in part, by the binding of inositol 1,4,5-triphosphate (IP_3) to intracellular receptors located on the aforementioned membranous cisternae. IP_3 is a sec-ond messenger generated on receptor-stimulated hydrolysis of phosphatidylinositol 4,5-biphosphate by phospholi1pase C, an enzyme activated by signal transduction mechanisms.

3. CYTOSKELETON DETERMINATION OF NEURONAL FORM

A singular feature of neurons is their overall extraordinary length, enabling them to transmit signals over great distances. This property is reflected in the polarity of neuronal form and function, which is governed by regional specialization of the plasma membrane and by differences in the cytoskeletal composition of dendritic and axonal processes emerging from the cell body. Although the neuronal cytoskeleton provides a structural framework on which various organelles and cellular events are organized, it is by no means a static configuration. Throughout the neuron, molecular alterations in cytoskeletal proteins reverberate as microscopically visible changes in movement of the cytoskeleton, its associated organelles, and the shape and extent of some of the processes. Although the cytoskeleton permits the general pattern of individual neurons to remain constant and identifiable, alterations in cytoskeletal dynamics enable the neuron to respond to environmental-dependent or activity-dependent fluctuations. This apparent contradiction is resolved by the inherent nature of cytoskeletal elements that exist in different structural and functional states of assembly and disassembly. Moreover, these structures may be stabilized and destabilized, providing yet another dimension to the number of possible conformations of ct skeletal form.

The interactions of various cytoskeletal elements with their associated proteins or with each other contribute to the unique structural and functional identity of axons and dendrites and their associated dendritic spines. The cytoskeleton also interacts with the neuronal plasma membrane at specific sites, including the initial segment of the axon, special loci along the axon called nodes of Ranvier, and presynaptic and postsynaptic membranes, forming complex submembrane filamentous arrays. Such membranous-cytoskeletal associations may restrict the movement of important membrane proteins, such as receptors, at that site or communicate events occurring at the membrane to underlying areas. In this section, we describe components of the neuronal cytoskeleton and how they contribute to the architecture of the neuron and confer specificity to each structural domain.

3.1. The Neuronal Cytoskeleton Provides Internal Support

Axons and dendrites emerge from the perikaryon as delicate strands. Axons may be as much as a million times longer than wide. Consequently, these fragile processes require internal support. The rigidity of the cytoskeletal network is apparent after removal of the neuronal membrane with detergents that selectively extract membrane lipids and proteins. In experiments using detergent-treated cultured nerve cells, isolated neuronal processes, and isolated submembranous cytoskeletal patches, the cytoskeleton remains intact, and its shape is virtually identical to its original conformation. The cylindrical form of the axonal cytoskeleton is so cohesive that investigators, using the classic model of the squid giant axon to study axonal transport mechanisms, equate the extrusion of its contents, the axoplasm, to that of toothpaste being squeezed out of its tube. Even isolated submembrane filamentous arrays, such as those found beneath the postsynaptic membrane, appear to retain their curvature after the rigorous processes of homogenization of brain and centrifugation, lysis, and detergent treatment of isolated synaptic compartments; only after sonication or extremely acidic conditions do these tenacious structures dissociate into their component parts.

3.2. The Components of the Neuronal Cytoskeleton Include Microtubules, Neurofilaments, and Microfilaments and Their Associated Proteins

The dual nature of the neuronal cytoskeleton, reflected in its rigidity and plasticity, is a function of three filament types: microtubules, neurofilaments, and microfilaments or actin filaments. Each cytoskeletal element acts in conjunction with a specific set of associated or binding proteins. Some of these crosslink the filaments to each other, the plasma membrane, and other intracellular organelles and are responsible for the gelatinous and relatively stiff consistency of the cytoskeleton. Other associated and binding proteins affect the rate and extent of filament polymerization, providing a mechanism for localized plastic changes.

Microfilaments consisting of the protein actin are 6 nm in diameter and are prominent in cortical regions, particularly in the highly specialized submembrane filamentous structures, such as the presynaptic and postsynaptic membrane specializations. Microtubules

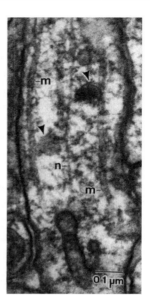

Fig. 7. Electron micrograph of the axonal cytoskeleton. The two prominent cytoskeletal elements in this region are microtubules (m) and neurofilaments (n). The microtubules are 25 nm in diameter and form tracks for the transport of various organelles, such as vesicles (*arrowheads*). The neurofilaments belong to the ubiquitous class of intermediate filaments and are 10 nm in diameter. Neurofilaments are relatively stable polymers that may contribute to the resiliency and caliber of axons.

are long, tubular structures that are 25 nm in diameter and form tracks for the transport of various organelles and molecules, although the microtubules are themselves also capable of movement (Fig. 7). The microtubules and actin consist of globular subunits that can assemble and disassemble with relative ease. Neurofilaments that are 10 nm in diameter are a subdivision of the ubiquitous class of intermediate filaments found in all cells (*see* Fig. 7). Mammalian neurofilaments consist of three fibrous subunits that have a very high affinity for each other, and polymers composed of these subunits are very stable. Neurofilament subunits are synthesized and assembled in the cell body and then directed down the axon, where they contribute to its resiliency and its caliber. Neurofilaments are degraded at the entrance to the nerve terminal by Ca^{2+} activated proteases located at that site.

3.2.1. ACTIN AND TUBULIN POLYMERS

Subunits of actin, a 43-kd globular protein, and microtubules, a heterodimer of two 50-kd globular proteins called α-tubulin and β-tubulin, assemble into polymers that bind to identical subunits at each end of

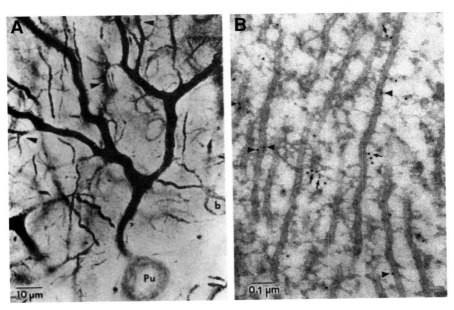

Fig. 8. Dendrites labeled with antibodies to microtubule-associated protein (MAP) 2. The technique of immnunocytochemistry uses antibodies to localize specific proteins in neurons. These antibodies are detected by secondary antibodies tagged with an enzyme or gold particle. (**A**) The enzyme, such as peroxidase, catalyzes a reaction that results in an electron-dense precipitate, as seen in the light micrograph, in which antibodies to MAP 2 label the dendritic tree (*arrowheads*) of a Purkinje cell. (**B**) Alternatively, the secondary antibody can be tagged with gold particles, seen as black dots in the electron micrograph, in which they localize MAP 2 to microtubules (*arrowheads*) and cross-bridges (*arrows*) between them. *Pu*, Purkinje cell; *b*, basket cell. ([**A**] Is reprinted from Bernhardt R, Matus A. J Comp Neurol 1984; 226:207, with permission of Wiley-Liss, a division of John Wiley and Sons, Inc New York.)

a preexisting polymer. The lengths of the polymer are determined by cellular mechanisms that control the rates of association and disassociation at the ends of each rod. In some polymers, there is a constant flux of monomers at each end. In more stable polymers, dissociation of the subunits at each end-is slow or does not occur at all. Stability can be achieved by blocking the dissociation reaction at either end. Both tubulin and actin monomers are asymmetric so that they can only link up with each other in a specific orientation. Consequently, the resultant polymer is polarized and has plus and minus ends, a feature permitting polymers to grow in a directed manner.

3.2.2. Cytoskeletal-Associated Proteins

Cytoskeletal-associated proteins regulate cytoskeletal structure and function and characterize specific neuronal domains. Purified tubulin monomers can spontaneously assemble into microtubules in the presence of GTP. However, polymerization is greatly enhanced in impure preparations. The impurities are actually a group of accessory proteins that are subdivided into two categories: microtubule-associated pro-

teins (MAPs) and tau proteins. These proteins induce the assembly and stabilization of microtubules by binding to them. The tau proteins facilitate polymerization by binding to more than one tubulin dimer at the same time. MAPs have two domains, one of which binds to the microtubule and the other to an adjacent MAP molecule, filament, or cell organelle. MAPs provide the neuron with a mechanism for structural plasticity and variability. About 10 kinds of MAPs have been identified, and they appear to be differentially expressed during brain development. Specific MAPs appear to be restricted to different neuronal processes. MAP 2, for example, is expressed in dendrites but not axons (Fig. 8); conversely, MAP 3 is present in axons but not in dendrites.

Although microtubules appear in parallel array, actin filaments in neurons are usually visible as a tangled meshwork. The network sometimes appears as a dense submembranous array, as in the postsynaptic density (PSD) immediately beneath the postsynaptic membrane. However, the network may be less dense, as in the subsynaptic web immediately beneath the PSD and extending throughout the dendritic spine.

Actin filaments are also associated with a group of accessory proteins, the actin-binding proteins, which bundle them or cross-link them to form a gel. Some binding proteins join the filament ends to obstruct further polymerization, and others link actin to the membrane. Actin-binding proteins are regulated by second messengers, such as calcium or cyclic nucleotides.

3.2.3. MOLECULAR MOTORS

Other proteins associated with the cytoskeleton are the molecular motors, which harness energy to propel themselves along filaments. These proteins are enzymes that hydrolyze ATP and GTP and use the liberated energy to move themselves along the polymer. Motion is achieved because each of the steps of nucleotide binding, hydrolysis, and release of ADP or GDP plus phosphate causes a concomitant change in the conformation of the motor protein such that it is directed forward. Myosin motors walk along actin filaments, which are pulled along in the process. This action is important in the motility of growth cones, the pioneering tip of developing nerve cell processes. Motor proteins are also associated with microtubules, where they are involved in organelle transport in neuronal processes.

3.2.4. CYTOSKELETAL-BASED TRANSPORT SYSTEM OF NEURONS

Neuronal processes span great distances to reach their presynaptic and postsynaptic targets, which can be meters away from the cell body in large organisms. Neuropeptides synthesized and packaged in the perikaryon must embark on long journeys to far-removed nerve terminals. Although some synaptic components can be synthesized and recycled locally, others must be imported from the cell body or returned there for degradation by lysosomes, for example. Molecular and organelle traffic to and from these remote areas requires active mechanisms, because diffusion alone would take an inordinate amount of time.

Bidirectional traffic in axons delivers proteins and organelles to and from the nerve terminal by anterograde and retrograde transport, respectively Anterograde transport delivers neuropeptide-containing vesicles and cytoskeletal proteins; retrograde transport returns endocytotic and other vesicles. Axonal transport has two components: a fast component, traveling at rates of 200 to 400 mm/day, and slow component, which consists of a slow component a (SC$_a$) and a slow component b (SC$_b$), moving at rates of 0.2–1 mm/d and 2–8 mm/d, respectively. The fast component carries membranous vesicles, and the slow compartment carries cytoskeletal proteins.

Fast transport involves movement of vesicles along tracks composed of microtubules. Microtubule motors generate the force required to propel organelles along the path. Two of these motors, kinesin and dynein, are ATPases that are activated on binding to the microtubule. Kinesin directs movement toward the plus end of the microtubule and dynein toward the minus end. In axons, most microtubules have their positive end toward the terminal and can guide movement in either direction. In dendrites, about half of the microtubules are oriented with their plus ends toward the dendritic tip, and the other half have their minus ends toward the tip. Differences in microtubule orientation in axons and dendrites may be one of the mechanisms underlying the selective transport of organelles into dendrites or axons.

4. NEURONAL SYNAPSES

Electrical signals can be conveyed directly from cell to cell at special sites called gap junctions (Fig. 9). Ions pass from one cell to another through relatively large channels that connect the cytoplasm of the two cells while isolating the flow from the intracellular space. In neurons, these electrical synapses permit rapid and direct electrical transmission and may also play a role in synchronizing neuronal activity. However, their invariant form and paucity of regulatory molecules preclude any major involvement in plastic events. Gap junctions are also found elsewhere in the nervous system between supportive cells, called astrocytes, where they participate in buffering the extracellular ionic milieu.

Chemical synapses are the main sites of interactions of nerve cells (Fig. 10). All synaptic junctions share common features that guarantee precise and directed transmission of signals. Although the general scheme remains relatively constant, variability in some of the molecular components, such as neurotransmitter, ion channels, receptors, and second messengers, and the dynamic properties of the supporting cytoskeleton enable each synapse to maintain its individuality, record past experiences, and vary responses to new signals.

4.1. Synaptic Structure Follows a Basic Plan

Chemical synapses conform to a basic architectural plane despite their location along the neuron or within the nervous system itself, but during the past two decades, it has become apparent that the morphology

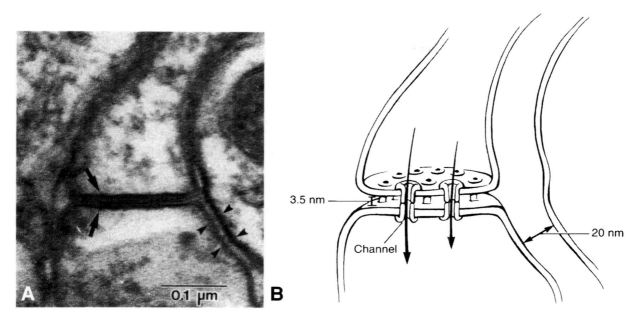

Fig. 9. Structure of the gap junction. (**A**) In the electron micrograph, the membranes of two glial cell processes in close apposition form a gap junction (*arrows*). Notice the wider extrajunctional space (*arrowheads*) to the right of the gap junction. (**B**) The diagram shows a section of the half channels in each membrane that join to form a pore, which allows communication between the cytoplasm of the two cells. The space between the two membranes of the gap junction is only 3.5 nm, much smaller than the extrajunctional space of 20 nm.

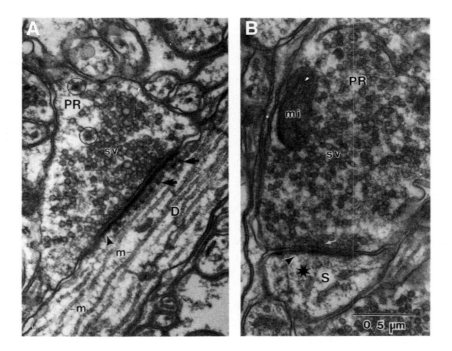

Fig. 10. Basic features of synaptic junctions in the central nervous system. (**A**) The presynaptic terminal (PR) ends on a dendrite (D) characterized by microtubules (m), and (**B**) another that ends on a spine (S) characterized by an actin filament network (*asterisk*). In both cases, synaptic vesicles (sv) are seen in the presynaptic terminal, and a prominent postsynaptic density (*arrowhead*) is located behind the postsynaptic membrane. In (**A**), the presynaptic terminal also contains dense-cored vesicles (circled), and in (**B**), the terminal contains a mitochondrion (mi). Some of the synaptic vesicles (*white arrow*) in (**B**) are located or docked near the presynaptic membrane. In the dendrite in (**A**), specializations called subsynaptic bodies (*black arrows*) are located on the cytoplasmic face of the postsynaptic density.

of synaptic connections in the adult mammalian brain is not static. Synapses display structural plasticity, undergoing alterations in size, shape, and number. These changes have important implications in synaptic transmission, because they may modify the way in which incoming signals are received. Because morphologic alterations may reflect marked rearrangements of the molecular structure of synapses, these changes may be long lasting and signify the generation or maintenance of long-term processes, such as memory.

All synaptic junctions consist of presynaptic and postsynaptic elements (*see* Fig. 10). In synapses in the central nervous system, very fine filamentous material extends between the two processes in the cleft region. The most conspicuous feature of the presynaptic terminal are the small (40 nm in diameter), clear synaptic vesicles containing acetylcholine or amino acid neurotransmitters. Mitochondria are also visible, as are dense-cored vesicles, some containing neuropeptides imported from the perikaryon and others containing catecholamines synthesized in the terminal. The portion of presynaptic membrane directly apposing the postsynaptic membrane is called the active zone. Sometimes, this area is marked by a dense submembranous array. The presynaptic nerve terminal contacts a postsynaptic element. In the central nervous system, this may be a cell body, dendrite (*see* Fig. 10A), dendritic spine (*see* Fig. 10B), another axon, or axon terminal.

The most striking postsynaptic feature is the dense, submembrane filamentous array beneath the postsynaptic membrane called the PSD (*see* Fig. 10). Extending from this area is a fine meshwork of actin filaments and their binding proteins. In dendrites, this network is contiguous with microtubules; in dendritic spines, the filamentous web fills the head and neck region of this process. Some postsynaptic membranes lack a well-developed PSD.

Synapses also form between nerves and muscles (Fig. 11). With the light microscope, axons can be seen to approach the muscle. At a specific site on the muscle, called the end-plate region, the axons give rise to several branches that display multiple swellings, each of which represents a presynaptic terminal. Ultrastructural examination reveals that the nerve terminal is closely apposed to the sarcolemma of skeletal muscle with a basal lamina lying in between the two components. The sarcolemma is thrown into distinctive folds. Acetylcholine receptors are located on the portions of the membrane directly opposing the active zones. A

dense microfilamentous network extends from the membrane on the cytoplasmic face of the postsynaptic membrane and holds the receptors in place.

4.2. The Presynaptic Nerve Terminal Is the Site of Transmitter Release

Information transfer between neurons occurs in a matter of milliseconds. During this time, action potentials speed along the axonal membrane at rates between 1 and 100 m/second to the presynaptic nerve terminal, where the frequency of their firing is translated into specific quantities of neurotransmitter release. The rapidity of signal conduction over long distances demands that the nerve be ready to respond to a barrage of incoming action potentials at all times. Although axonal transport replenishes the terminal with some needed molecules, organelles, and neuropeptide-containing vesicles, the rates of delivery are not fast enough to prepare the terminal with the small molecules (i.e., acetylcholine, amino acids, catecholamines) comprising the bulk of chemical messengers that mediate neurotransmission. Even fast anterograde transport can only convey membranous vesicles at a rate of 200 to 400 mm ($\approx$1 fl) each day. Consequently, the nerve terminal comes equipped with mechanisms for neurotransmitter synthesis, storage, and release and mechanisms for membrane recycling. Presynaptic terminals, however, lack the elaborate protein synthetic and packaging machinery found in the perikaryon. Even free polyribosomes are difficult to detect, although there is some evidence for presynaptic protein synthesis. Most of the synthetic enzymes and some membrane proteins required to construct synaptic vesicles must be imported from the cell body.

Neurotransmitters are primarily released from synaptic vesicles, although there is compelling evidence for additional nonvesicular release of acetylcholine from a cytoplasmic pool. Knowledge that synaptic vesicles mediate neurotransmitter release comes from the important discovery in 1952 by Paul Fatt and Bernard Katz that acetylcholine is released from terminals at the neuromuscular junction in quanta. A relatively constant number (about 10,000) of neurotransmitter molecules are released simultaneously. Since that time, neuroscientists have been actively engaged in experiments supporting this finding. Electron microscopic studies of nerve terminals revealed the presence of synaptic vesicles. When these vesicles were isolated, they were shown to contain acetylcholine. It was then proposed that the number of transmitter

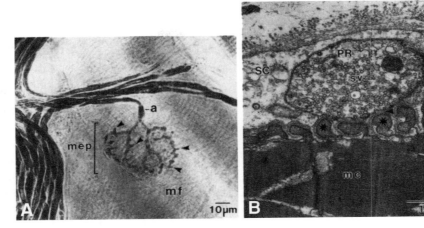

Fig. 11. Neuromuscular junction seen by **(A)** light and **(B)** electron microscopy. In **(A)** an axon (a) gives rise to a motor end plate (mep) on the muscle fiber (mf). The motor end plate exhibits many swellings (*arrowheads*). These represent the presynaptic terminals, one of which is seen it higher magnification in **(B)**. The presynaptic terminal (PR), filled with synaptic vesicles (sv), contacts the sarcolemma folds (*asterisks*) of the muscle cell (mc). A basal lamina (*arrowhead*) is found in between the terminal and sarcolemma. A portion of glial cell, known as a Schwann cell (SC), surrounds the terminal. ([B] Courtesy of Virginia Kriho, University of Illinois at Chicago, Chicago, IL.)

molecules in each quanta is equivalent to the number of acetylcholine molecules in each vesicle.

Synaptic vesicles occupy precise locales within the terminal; they are clustered and then docked near the active zone (*see* Fig. 10B). They appear to be held in place there by actin, which is connected to the vesicle by a neuron-specific protein, synapsin. However, vesicles that have already released transmitter must be replaced by those next in line, necessitating a transient depolymerization of actin filaments so that the vesicles are free to approach the membrane. Phosphorylation of synapsin releases vesicles from the cytoskeleton, permitting them to proceed to the docking site at the presynaptic membrane. Specific proteins within the vesicle membrane and presynaptic membrane interact to hold the vesicle in place. Vesicle fusion occurs so fast that it is thought to involve a conformational change in a specific protein—perhaps a change in a preassembled calcium-dependent pore from a closed to an open state. The extra vesicle membrane, now a part of the presynaptic membrane, is internalized by a clathrin-dependent mechanism and brought to an endosomal sac, where membrane proteins are sorted and new vesicles pinch off the cisternae.

It is thought that there are two release pathways: one for clear vesicles and mother for neurosecretory vesicles.

The latter are not concentrated near the active zone and require a lower calcium concentration and a higher frequency of stimulation for release at other sites along the terminal membrane. Dense-cored vesicle release may represent a basal secretion, in contrast to the phasic release of clear vesicles.

4.3. The Postsynaptic Element Is the Site of Signal Transduction

Neurotransmitters bind to specific sites called receptors on the postsynaptic membrane. This interaction is the initial step in a cascade of events that transduce the chemical message into an intracellular signal that affects the behavior of the postsynaptic neuron. Neuronal responses to incoming signals may include immediate alterations in membrane permeability or more long-lasting modifications in synaptic or neuronal architecture, which may modify the nature of the postsynaptic response. Signal transduction pathways in neurons attain an extraordinary level of complexity, increasing the number of adaptive responses by logarithmic proportions.

4.3.1. POSTSYNAPTIC DENSITY

Beneath the postsynaptic membrane is a dense filamentous array, the PSD (*see* Fig. 10). The intimacy of its association with the overlying membrane suggests that it restricts receptors at that site, similar to the way acetylcholine receptors are clustered at the sarcolemmal membrane of the neuromuscular junction by actin and its binding proteins. However, several properties of the PSD suggest a more dynamic role in nerve transmission. Although the PSD usually is a saucer-shaped structure, there are variations of this basic form, including differences in length, curvature, and the presence or absence of perforations. Moreover, quantitative electron microscopic analyses reveal that these parameters change in specific brain areas with various physiologic and behavioral inputs. The PSD contains actin that, together with its binding proteins also found here, may mediate dynamic changes in shape.

The major protein in cerebral cortex PSDs, for example, is the 51-kd, autophosphorylatable, Ca^{2+}/calmodulin-dependent protein kinase II, which comprises 30% to 50% of this structure. Mutant mice lacking one of the isoforms of this enzyme are also deficient in their ability to produce long-term potentiation (LTP). LTP is an electrophysiologic correlate of memory; after a given input, a synapse gets stronger and retains this new strength for a long period.

4.3.2. Dendritic Spines

Approximately 100 yr ago, Santiago Ramón Cajal wrote that cortical dendrites seem to "bristle with teeth." He called these protuberances collateral spines, and it is only recently that we have gained some insight into their precise function. Dendritic spines are protrusions of the dendritic surface that receive synapses, almost all of which are excitatory. They consist of spine heads of various diameters that are connected to the parent dendrite by necks, which also vary in length and thickness (Fig. 12). The spine shape is often categorized as thin, stubby, or mushroom shaped. Cortical neurons have thousands of dendritic spines, each located every few micrometers along the dendritic shaft.

The cytoskeletal network comprising the interior of the spine includes actin and its binding proteins, myosin, Ca^{2+}-ATPase, calmodulin, and spectrin. Several reports suggest a role for actin and myosin in spine contractility that may lead to changes in the shape or number of spines. Among the inputs that appear to result in changes in spine shape or number are hormonal manipulations, long-term potentiation, dietary factors, and chronic ethanol consumption. The importance of proper dendritic spine structure is underscored by observed aberrations in the shape of dendritic spines in mental retardation. Recent studies implicate spines as calcium isolation compartments that decouple calcium changes in the spine head from those in the dendritic shaft and from neighboring spines. These experiments have important implications for explain-

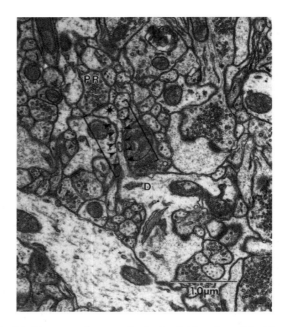

Fig. 12. Electron micrograph of a dendritic spine of the hippocampus. A presynaptic terminal (PR) contacts a thin dendritic spine (*brackets*) that emanates from a dendrite (D). The dendritic spine is characterized by a head (*asterisk*) and neck (*arrowheads*) region. Notice the complexity of the surrounding nervous tissue, known as the neuropil. (Modified from Stiller RJ. Neuronal Ca^{2+}: getting it up and keeping it up. Trends Neurosci 1992; 15:317, and from Harris KM, Jensen FF, Tsao B, Dendritic spines of CA1 pyramidal cells in the rat hippocampus serial electron microscopy with reference to their biophysical characteristics, J Neurosci 1992; 12:2685. Courtesy of Dr. Kristen M. Harris, Children's Hospital and Harvard Medical School, Boston, MA, and with permission from Richard Miller, University of Chicago, Chicago, IL.)

ing LTP. LTP may be synapse specific; its expression is a function of activation of calcium-dependent processes at the synapse, such as the activity of the Ca^{2+} and calmodulin-dependent protein kinase II described previously, which is also implicated in long-term processes. Calcium levels may be regulated by a unique membranous structure called the spine apparatus, because Ca^{2+}-ATPase, the IP_3 receptor, and calcium are localized there.

5. GLIAL CELLS

Neuronal form is largely a function of the internal cytoskeletal framework. However, neurons are also supported externally by a second type of cell in the nervous system, the glial cell. Glial cells are present in the central and peripheral nervous systems. Glia fill in all spaces not occupied by neurons and blood vessels,

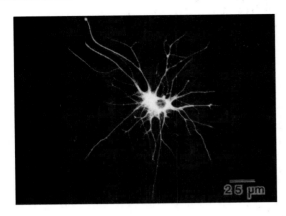

Fig. 13. Light micrograph of an astrocyte in a primary culture prepared from neonatal rat brain. The cell was incubated with antibodies to glial fibrillary acidic protein, which was detected by a fluorescein-labeled secondary antibody. Many processes emerge from the cell body, giving the cell its star-shaped appearance. (Courtesy of Dr. Harry Yang, University of Illinois at Chicago, Chicago, IL.)

surrounding and investing virtually all exposed surfaces in the central nervous system and axons in the peripheral nervous system. Glia vary in morphology, and their function is not restricted to mechanical support. In the central nervous system, glia are subdivided into four main types: astrocytes, oligodendrocytes, ependymal cells, and microglia. In the peripheral nervous system, Schwann cells function in a manner similar to that of oligodendrocytes, forming insulating myelin sheaths around axons that facilitate conduction.

5.1. Glia Play a Variety of Roles in the Nervous System

Astrocytes are stellate-shaped cells with a multitude of processes that radiate from the cell. These processes are supported internally by a glial-specific intermediate filament protein, glial fibrillarv acidic protein (Fig. 13).

Some astrocytic processes may terminate as swellings called end-feet on neurons and blood vessels. Astrocytes may accumulate extracellular potassium resulting from the repeated bring of neurons. The potassium may then be released by astrocytic end-feet onto blood vessels to increase their diameter. In this way, increased neuronal activity may be supported by a concomitant increase in blood flow and oxygen consumption. Astrocytes may provide structural and metabolic support for neurons and regulate the ionic composition of the milieu around the nerve cell.

Because of the emphasis on these supportive roles, astrocyte structure was historically viewed as being subservient to that of the neuron, with the form of the neuron dictating the shape of particular astrocytic processes. This view has evolved into a more dynamic one for the astrocyte, which may regulate neuronal shape, synaptic connectivity, and some aspects of neuronal function.

Morphologic analyses indicate that astrocytic processes preferentially contact neuronal surfaces over those of other glia, despite a ratio of glia to neurons of at least ten to one. Other evidence suggests that associations between neurons and glia are constantly in flux throughout the life of the organism. Glia may promote or inhibit the outgrowth of neuronal processes during development by synthesizing and secreting various adhesion molecules. In some parts of the developing nervous system, such as the cerebellum and neural tube, radial glial cells form a transient scaffold that guides the migration of immature neurons to their final destinations. The migrating neurons wrap around these pole-shaped cells and crawl along them. After completion of the trip, the radial glia disappear and may be transformed into astrocytes.

In the central nervous system, astrocytes and macrophages, called microglia, remove the cellular debris resulting from degenerative processes. Ependymal cells form the ciliated lining of the central canal system of the brain and spinal cord; processes on the opposite surface may terminate on blood vessels.

5.2. Glia Form Myelin Sheaths that Increase the Speed and Efficiency of Conduction in Axons

Oligodendrocytes and Schwann cells form myelin sheaths around axons. These sheaths are formed by the attenuation of the glial cytoplasm to such an extent that most of the sheath is composed of concentric layers of plasma membrane wrapping around the axon (Fig. 14). In oligodendrocytes, several processes extend out from the cell, tapering as they encounter an axon, and wrap around a portion of its length. One oligodendrocyte can ensheathe many axons, all of different neuronal origins. Individual Schwann cells dedicate themselves to a single axon. The exposed patch of axon in between adjacent segments of the myelin sheath is called the node of Ranvier (Fig. 15). Most of the Na^+ ion channels of the axon are confined to this site. Because of the lack of channels between the nodes and great insulating action of the myelin sheath, there

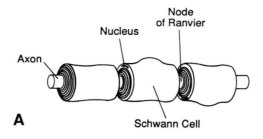

A

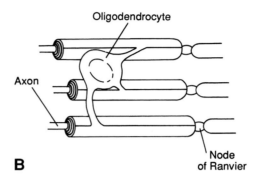

B

Fig. 14. Diagrams of myelinated axons of the peripheral and central nervous systems. **(A)** In the peripheral axon, several Schwann cells wrap their plasma membrane concentrically around a single axon. The stretch of axonal membrane, called the axolemma, between adjacent Schwann cells is known as the node of Ranvier. **(B)** In the central axon, several glial processes emerge from one oligodendrocyte and ensheathe several axons of different origins.

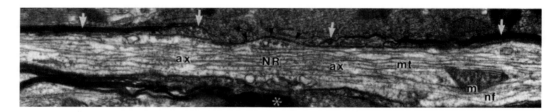

Fig. 15. An electron micrograph of the myelin sheath of an axon (ax). The sheath is interrupted at regular intervals, called nodes of Ranvier (NR), where portions of the axonal membrane, called the axolemma (*arrowheads*), are exposed. Sodium ion channels are concentrated in the axolemma at the nodes. Mt, microtubules; m, mitochondron.

is virtually no current flow across these segments. The action potential bypasses these stretches of membrane by jumping from node to node. This type of rapid propagation is known as saltatory conduction. An added advantage is that energy is conserved; fewer ions enter and leave the axon so less energy is expended in returning the membrane to its original polarized state by active transport mechanisms.

SELECTED READINGS

Alberts B, Bray D, Lewis J, Raff M, Roberts K. Watson JD. Molecular biology of the cell, 2nd ed. New York: Garland Publishing, 1989.

Firestein S. A noseful of odor receptors. Trends Neurosci 1991; 14:270.

FitzGerald MJT. Neuroanatomy basic and applied. London: Bailliere Tindall, 1985.

Hall ZW. 1992. An introduction to molecular neurobiology. Sunderland, MA: Sinauer Associates, 1992.

Kandel ER, Schwartz JH, Jessell TM. Principles of neuroscience, 3rd ed. New York: Elsevier, 1991.

Kurs EM, Sengelaub DR, Arnold AP. Androgens regulate be dendritic length of mammalian motoneurons in adulthood. Science 1986; 232:395.

Linstedt AD, Kelly RB. Molecular architecture of the nerve terminal. Curr Opin Neurobiol 1991; 1:382.

Pomeroy SL, Purves D. Neuron/glia relationships observed over intervals of several months in living mice. J Cell Biol 1988; 107:1167.

Rasmussen AT. Some trends in neuroanatomy. Dubuque, IA: William C. Brown, 1947.

Rodriguez FM. Design and perspectives of peptide secreting neurons. In Nemeroff CB, Dunn AJ (eds). Peptides, hormones and behavior. New York: Spectrum Publications, 1984; 1.

Silva AJ, Stevens CF, Tonegawa S, Wang Y. Deficient hippocampal long-term potentiation in α-calcium-calmodulin kinase II mutant mice. Science 1992; 257:201.

Stevens CF. Bristling with teeth. Curr Biol 1991; 1:369.

Steward O, Banker GA. Getting the message from the gene to the synapse: sorting and intracellular transport of RNA in neurons. Trends Neurosci 1992; 15:180.

Wolff JR. Quantitative aspects of astroglia. Comptes Rendu du VIe Congres International de Neuropathologic 1970; 31:327.

2   Anatomy of the Spinal Cord and Brain

Bruce E. Maley

CONTENTS

1. INTRODUCTION

The central nervous system (CNS) is divided into a rostral *brain* and a caudal *spinal cord*. The brain is contained in the cranial cavity, and the spinal cord is located in the vertebral canal that is formed by the 31 vertebral foramina from the individual vertebra. The two are continuous with one another at the foramen magnum of the occipital bone. The twelve pairs of cranial nerves—which arise from the brain and the thirty-one pairs of spinal nerves originating from the spinal cord with their associated ganglia—are, by convention, part of the peripheral nervous system. Both the brain and spinal cord are organized into *gray matter* in which the neuronal cell bodies are located and *white matter*, which contains the long myelinated tracts of the CNS.

2. SPINAL CORD

The spinal cord, continuous with the brain's medulla oblongata, is a long cylinder beginning at the foramen magnum and extending to the second lumbar vertebra. It is divided into thirty-one segments composed of eight cervical, twelve thoracic, five lumbar, five sacral, and one coccygeal segment. Each spinal cord segment has an associated pair of spinal nerves that arise as a series of fine rootlets. Each spinal nerve is formed from *dorsal root fibers*,

which are sensory fibers whose cell bodies are in spinal ganglia located outside the CNS and *ventral root fibers*, which are motor fibers originating from ventral horn cells in the spinal cord gray matter (Figs. 1,2). At cervical levels C1–C4, fibers from the accessory nerve (cranial nerve XI) originate from the lateral side of the spinal cord intermediate between the dorsal root fibers and ventral root fibers. In contrast, the vertebra column, which surrounds and protects the spinal cord, has seven cervical vertebra, twelve thoracic vertebra, five lumbar vertebra, five sacral vertebra typically fused into a single sacrum, and three to four coccygeal vertebra also fused into a common coccyx. Although the number of spinal cord segments is roughly equivalent to the thirty-three vertebra, each of its segments is relatively shorter than the corresponding vertebra. As a result, the spinal cord ends at the level of the second lumbar vertebra in adults. In infants, the spinal cord ends more caudally at the third lumbar vertebra. The remainder of the vertebral canal below the level of the second lumbar vertebra is composed of the obliquely oriented dorsal roots and ventral roots traveling to their proper point of exit from the vertebral canal at the appropriate intervertebral foramina.

The spinal has two noticeable swellings along its length—a *cervical enlargement* at lower cervical to upper thoracic levels to accommodate the increase of neurons for innervation of the upper limb and a *lumbar enlargement* at lumbar to upper sacral levels for innervation of the lower limb. At its termina-

From: *Neuroscience in Medicine, 2nd ed.* (P. Michael Conn, ed.), © 2003 Humana Press Inc., Totowa, NJ.

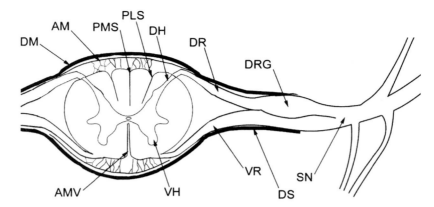

Fig. 1. Schematic diagram of a cross-section of the spinal cord. The gray matter occupies the central region of the spinal cord, and is composed of the ventral horn (VH) and dorsal horn (DH). The anterior median fissure (AMF) extends through the white matter to the gray matter. The posterior median sulcus (PMS) and posterolateral sulcus (PLS) are located on the posterior side of the white matter. The dorsal root (DR) originates from cell bodies in the dorsal-root ganglion (DRG) to enter the dorsal horn, and the ventral root (VR) begins as axons of the ventral horn. Dorsal-root fibers and ventral-root fibers unite distal to the dorsal-root ganglion to form the spinal nerve (SN). The dura mater (DM) covers the spinal cord and extends to the intervertebral foramen as a dura sleeve (DS). The arachnoid membrane (AM) lies deep to the dura mater and has fibrous strands that extend to the pia mater on the surface of the spinal cord.

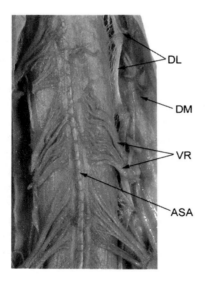

Fig. 2. Anterior surface of the spinal cord. The dura mater (DM) has been cut to reveal the ventral rootlets (VR) that comprise one ventral root of the spinal cord. The anterior spinal artery (ASA) lies in the anterior median fissure. Posterior to the ventral roots, the denticulate ligament (DL) is visible as a tooth-like extension from the surface of the spinal cord to the dura mater. Anterior surface of the brainstem. Midbrain, pons, and medulla are visible, as are the origin of cranial nerve III through XII.

tion, the spinal cord narrows into the *conus medullaris*, representing a reduction in neuronal cell bodies and myelinated tracts.

The spinal cord's anterior (ventral) surface has a deep *anterior median fissure* along its entire length, which typically contains the anterior spinal artery. The anterior median fissure extends deeply to the central gray matter, dividing the anterior half of the spinal cord into two separate cylinders. On its posterior (dorsal) side, several longitudinal depressions are visible—a midline *posterior median sulcus* and two *posterolateral sulci*, where the dorsal roots of the individual spinal nerves originate, on either side of the posterior median sulcus. A *posterior intermediate sulcus*, intermediate between the dorsal median sulcus and the posterolateral sulcus, is present beginning at upper thoracic levels. Its formation results from the location of two separate ascending sensory tracts, the fasciculus gracilis and fasciculus cuneatus, from the lower limb and upper limb, respectively (Figs. 1,3).

The spinal cord is divided into an outer layer of white matter and an inner core of gray matter. The *white matter* is composed of longitudinally oriented myelinated fiber tracts that ascend and descend the length of the spinal cord. The *gray matter* takes the shape of an "H" and is composed of paired dorsal horns and ventral horns. Between the first thoracic level and the second lumbar spinal cord level, the gray matter contains an additional horn (cell column), known as the intermediolateral cell column, intermediate between the ventral horn and dorsal

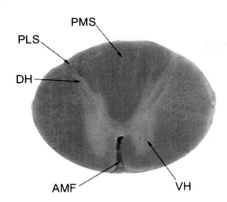

Fig. 3. Cross-section of the cervical spinal cord. The gray matter occupies the central region in the form of an "H." The ventral horn (VH) forms the legs of the "H," and the dorsal horn (DH) forms the arms of the "H." The white matter surrounds the gray matter. It has an anterior median fissure (VMH) and a posterior median fissure (PMF) that divide the white matter into left and right sides. The dorsolateral sulcus (DLS) is located at the entrance of dorsal-root fibers into the dorsal horn.

horn. Contained within the horizontal, interconnecting gray matter is the *central canal*, a part of the ventricular system of the CNS. The central canal is usually not patent its entire length.

2.1. Blood Supply of the Spinal Cord

The spinal cord receives its blood supply from three longitudinal arteries, which are supplemented from segmental vessels along the length of the spinal cord. Extensive anastomoses occur between the longitudinal arteries and the segmental arteries. The *anterior spinal artery* (Fig. 2) is the principal artery of the anterior two-thirds of the spinal cord, and the paired *posterior spinal arteries* are responsible for the posterior third of the spinal cord. The anterior spinal artery originates as a common trunk from the union of the paired vertebral arteries as they pass through the foramen magnum into the cranial cavity. The posterior spinal arteries arise either from the vertebral arteries or the posterior inferior cerebellar arteries, which are typically branches of the vertebral arteries. The anterior spinal artery runs the entire length of the anterior median fissure, although it reaches its largest diameter in the cervical and upper thoracic level and then begins to diminish in size as it descends further down the spinal cord. The posterior spinal arteries run the entire length of the spinal cord and are located in the posterolateral sulci. The vascular supply to the spinal cord is most

attenuated between T3 and T9 levels, and this level of the spinal cord is most vulnerable to ischemia. The anterior spinal artery throughout its length receives anastomotic branches from segmental vessels that enter intervertebral foramina with the ventral and dorsal-root fibers. In cervical levels segmental arteries arise from vertebral arteries, the ascending cervical branch of the inferior thyroid artery and the deep cervical branch of the costocervical trunk. At thoracic levels, posterior intercostal arteries arising from the descending aorta supply segmental arteries to the spinal cord. At lumbar levels, lumbar arteries originating from the abdominal aorta supply blood, and sacral arteries from internal iliac arteries supply the lowest levels of the spinal cord. Each segmental artery at every level enters an intervertebral foramen to give origin to dorsal radicular and anterior radicular arteries that follow and supply the dorsal roots and ventral roots. Periodically, these give rise to *anterior medullary artery* and *posterior medullary arteries*, which anastomose with the anterior spinal artery and the posterior spinal artery. Typically, there are three medullary arteries supplying cervical spinal cord levels, two supplying thoracic levels and two for the lumbar spinal cord. The *great anterior medullary artery (of Adamkiewicz)*, located around the 8th to 11th thoracic level, is noticeable because of its large size and is responsible for supplementing the blood supply to the lumbar enlargement. Posterior medullary arteries are smaller and more numerous than the anterior medullary arteries, with an average of 3–5 for each spinal cord region. The anterior spinal artery and the two posterior spinal arteries supply the majority of the gray matter and white matter of the spinal cord, although occasional medullary branches arise from radicular arteries located on the surface of the spinal cord.

2.2. Venous Drainage of the Spinal Cord

The veins that drain the spinal cord begin as capillaries within it—as *intramedullary veins*, which drain into the more superficial *intradural (pial) veins* located external to the spinal cord in the pia mater. The *anterior median vein*, located in the anterior median fissure, is the most consistent of the intradural veins. Several less consistent veins may also be present, including the posterior median vein located in the posterior median sulcus, anterolateral veins located in the region of exit of the ventral roots, and posterior lateral veins located in or near the entrance of the dorsal roots. Each of these veins freely communicates with its neighbors, forming large anastomotic channels along the surface of the spinal cord. At the base of the skull the intradural veins unite to form several trunks that also drain into the posterior inferior cerebellar veins and vertebral veins of the cranial cavity. The intradural veins communicate with the *internal vertebral venous plexus* located in the epidural space of the vertebral canal along its entire length. The internal vertebral plexus can be divided into an *anterior internal vertebra venous plexus* located between the vertebral body and the spinal cord and a *posterior internal vertebral venous plexus* between the vertebral arch and the spinal cord. The internal vertebral venous plexus in turn drains more superficially into the *external vertebral venous plexus* surrounding the vertebral column. The external vertebral plexus consists of an *anterior external vertebral plexus* around the vertebral bodies and the *posterior external vertebral plexus* lying on the surface of the vertebral arch. Both the anterior and posterior external vertebral plexi anastomose with one another and drain into the systemic segmental veins, including the deep cervical veins, intercostal veins, lumbar veins, and lateral sacral veins.

2.3. Meninges of the Spinal Cord

The spinal cord is covered by three connective tissue layers known as the *meninges*. The most superficial layer is the *dura mater* (Fig. 2). The spinal dura mater begins at the foramen magnum and extends caudally as a sac to the second sacral vertebra. At each intervertebral foramen, the dura mater extends as a *dural sleeve* to cover the dorsal roots, ventral roots, and spinal ganglia. It ends at the external edge of the intervertebral foramen, where it becomes continuous with the epineurum of the spinal nerve. At the caudal end of the vertebral canal, the dura mater ends as the *dural sac*, a blind end sac. The *arachnoid membrane* (spider-like), the second meningeal layer, is deep to the dura mater and consists of a fine network of connective tissue fibers that extend to the surface of the spinal cord. It follows the contours of the dura mater and is present in the dural sleeves and the dural sac. The *pia mater* (delicate mother) is the deepest and thinnest meningeal layer, and is typically adherent to the surface of the spinal cord, following its fissures and sulci. It is a vascular layer containing arteries

supplying the spinal cord and veins that drain the spinal cord. The *denticulate ligaments* are irregularly found, sawtooth-like lateral extensions of the pia mater that extend laterally from the side of the spinal cord between the dorsal roots and ventral roots to the overlying dura mater/arachnoid membrane. The pia mater extends beyond the spinal cord caudally as a fine filament, the *filum terminale* from the conus medullaris. It passes through the dural sac in the midst of the *cauda equina* to anchor to the coccyx. In the dural sac it is known as the filum terminale interna, and once it passes through the dura sac it is the filum terminale externa.

Several spaces are associated with the meninges of the spinal cord. The *epidural space* is superficial to the dura mater and contains significant amounts of fat that protect the spinal cord and the internal vertebral plexus of veins, which drain blood from the spinal cord to the more superficial external vertebral venous plexus. The *subdural space*, which is a potential space only under normal conditions, lies deep to the dura mater but superficial to the arachnoid membrane. The *subarachnoid space* separates the arachnoid membrane from the deeper pia mater. Cerebrospinal fluid (CSF), produced by the choroid plexus of the brain's ventricular system, is contained within the subarachnoid space, and allows the spinal cord to float within this space.

3. BRAIN

The brain is divided into a forebrain (prosencephalon), consisting of the cerebral cortex and thalamus, midbrain (mesencephalon), and hindbrain (rhombencephalon), composed of the pons, cerebellum, and medulla oblongata. The medulla oblongata, pons, and midbrain are collectively described as the brainstem. The brain is located in the cranial cavity. Its floor is divided into three horizontal shelves or fossae, from rostral to caudal, which are successively lower (Fig. 4). The anterior cranial fossa is composed of the crista galli and cribriform plate of the ethmoid, the greater wing of the sphenoid and frontal bones. The orbital surface, so named because it forms the roof of the orbit, supports the orbital surface of the frontal cortex. The ethmoid bone on either side of the midline crista galli is perforated (cribriform plate) to allow the olfactory nerves to pass from the nasal cavity into the paired olfactory bulbs, which are connected to the cortex by the posteriorly running olfactory tracts. Posterior to the greater wing of the sphenoid

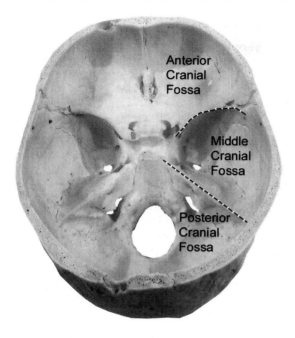

Fig. 4. Floor of the cranial cavity demonstrating the anterior cranial fossa, middle cranial fossa, and posterior cranial fossa.

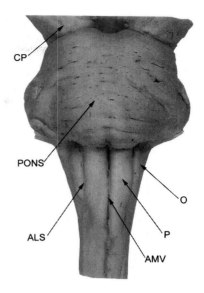

Fig. 5. Anterior surface of the brainstem. The cerebral peduncles (CP) of the midbrain are rostral to the pons. The medulla contains the pyramids (P), separated from the olive (O) by the anterior lateral sulcus (VLS). The pyramids are located on either side of the anterior median fissure (AMF).

is the middle cranial fossa. It extends to the petrous ridge of the temporal bone. The temporal cortex's inferior surface rests on the tegmen tympani of the temporal bones, and in the midline the depression of the sella turcica of the sphenoid bone houses the pituitary and infundibulum of the hypothalamus. The posterior cranial fossa is located posterior to the petrous ridge of the temporal bone and is bounded by the mastoid process of the temporal bone laterally and the clivus of the occipital bone medially. Its floor posteriorly contains the foramen magnum that allows continuation of the brainstem to the spinal cord. The brainstem and the cerebellum are contained in the posterior cranial fossa. Its roof is formed by the tentorium cerebelli of the dura mater.

3.1. Medulla Oblongata

The medulla oblongata, located in the posterior cranial fossa, is the most caudal portion of the brainstem and is continuous with the spinal cord at the foramen magnum (Fig. 5). Its anterior surface contains two prominent ridges along its length. The most medial pair of ridges is the *pyramids* formed by the corticospinal tracts, and the more lateral ridges are the *olives*, formed by the inferior olivary nuclei. Each pyramid is separated from the other by

an *anterior median fissure* and from the more lateral olive by the *anterior lateral sulcus*. The anterior lateral sulcus contains the hypoglossal nerve (CN XII) fibers. The olive is bounded laterally by the *posterior lateral sulcus*, which contains the fibers of the glossopharyngeal nerve (CN IX), the vagus nerve (CN X) and the bulbar portion of the accessory nerve (CN XI). The posterior surface of the medulla contains the tubercle of the nucleus gracilis medially and the tubercle of the nucleus cuneatus laterally (Fig. 6). It opens into a diamond-shaped region known as the *rhomboid fossa*, which forms the floor of the fourth ventricle. The medulla oblongata is continuous rostrally with the pons. At the junction of the pons with the medulla, the abducens nerve (CN VI) arises medially, and both the facial nerve (CN VII) and vestibulocochlear nerve (CN VIII) originate in the lateral groove formed at the pons-medulla junction.

3.2. Pons

The pons, located in the posterior cranial fossa, lies against the basilar portion of the occipital bone (Fig. 5). It is continuous with the medulla oblongata caudally and the midbrain rostrally. Its anterior region contains pontine nuclei scattered among major descending tracts, and the posterior region

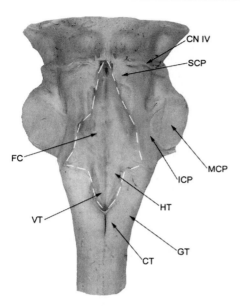

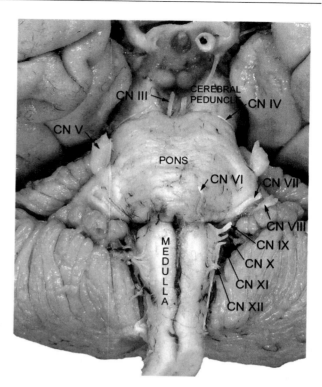

Fig. 6. Posterior surface of the brainstem, demonstrating the rhomboid. The rhomboid fossa (*outlined by dashed lines*) is visible after removal of the cerebellum. The facial colliculus (FC), hypoglossal trigone (HT), and vagal trigone (HT) are located on the floor of the rhomboid fossa. The cuneate tubercle (CT) and gracile tubercle (GC) are located caudal to the rhomboid fossa. Rostral to the rhomboid fossa cranial nerve IV is seen originating from the posterior surface of the brainstem. The inferior cerebellar peduncle (ICP), middle cerebellar peduncle (MCP), and superior cerebellar peduncle (SCP) are visible.

Fig. 7. Anterior surface of the brainstem. The medulla, pons, and cerebral peduncles (anterior representation of the midbrain) are labeled. The individual cranial nerves arising from each region of the brainstem are labeled. The midline oculomotor nerve (CN III) arises in the interpeduncular fossa (between the cerebral peduncles) rostral to the pons. The trochlear nerve (CN IV) wraps around the cerebral peduncle from the posterior surface of the midbrain. The trigeminal nerve (CN V) is a large nerve arising from the middle cerebellar peduncle of the pons. The abducens nerve (CN VI) arises from the midline of the pontomedullary junction, and the facial nerve (CN VII) and vestibulocochlear nerve (CN VIII) originate from the lateral region of the pontomedullary junction. The glossopharyngeal nerve (CN IX), vagus nerve (CN X), and accessory nerve (CN XI) arise lateral to the pyramid. The hypoglossal nerve (CN XII) arises in the ventrolateral sulcus between the pyramid and olive.

contains nuclei for CN VI, CN VII, and CN VIII (Fig. 7). The pons is expanded along its lateral sides for passage of fibers to the cerebellum in the *middle cerebellar peduncles*. The trigeminal nerve (CN V) arises from the anterior surface of the middle cerebellar peduncle. The pons' posterior surface contributes to the rostral half of the rhomboid fossa of the fourth ventricle (Fig. 6).

3.3. Midbrain

The midbrain, contained in the posterior cerebral fossa, is located between the pons caudally and the thalamus and hypothalamus superiorly. The cerebral aqueduct of the ventricular system passes through it. The anterior region is characterized by the prominent *cerebral peduncles* that define a depression described as the *interpeduncular fossa* (Figs. 5,7). The oculomotor nerves (CN III) arise from the midbrain medial to the cerebral peduncles in the interpeduncular fossa (Fig. 7). The posterior region of the midbrain, also known as the tectum, is composed of the *corpora quadrigemina*, four prominent tubercles consisting of the rostral *superior colliculi* (colliculus, singular), and the more caudal *inferior colliculi* (Fig. 8). The trochlear nerve (CN IV) is the only cranial nerve to arise posteriorly from the brainstem.

3.4. Cerebellum

The cerebellum is located in the posterior cranial fossa, immediately anterior to the tentorium cerebelli and posterior to the pons and medulla, where

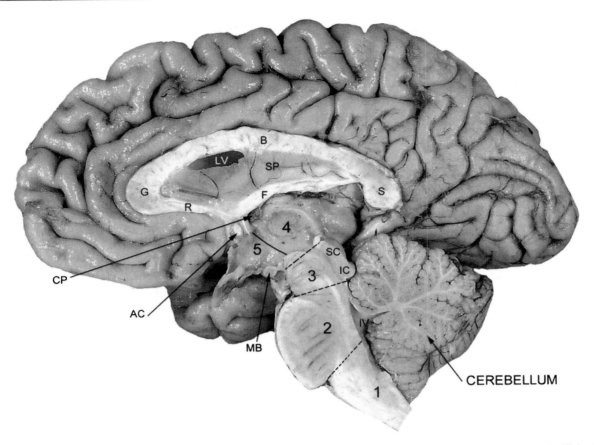

Fig. 8. Midsagittal section of the brain. The brainstem composed of the medulla oblongata (**1**), pons (**2**) and midbrain (**3**) is visible. The cerebellum lies posterior to the caudal brainstem and forms the roof of the fourth ventricle (IV). The corpora quadragemina, made up of the superior colliculus (SC) and inferior colliculus (IC), is located posterior to the cerebra aqueduct. The diencephalons, containing the thalamus (**4**) and hypothalamus (**5**), is rostral to the midbrain. The mammilary bodies (MB) are anterior prominences of the hypothalamus. The anterior commissure (AC) is rostral to the hypothalamus, and the fornix (F) arches over the thalamus. The corpus callosum is composed of the rostrum (R), genu (G), body (B), and splenium (S). The septum pellucidum (SP) separates the lateral ventricle (LV) of each cerebral hemisphere.

it completes the roof of the fourth ventricle along with its extensions, the superior medullary velum and inferior medullary velum (Figs. 8,9). The best way to visualize the physical arrangement of the cerebellum is to view it as a planar structure folded upon itself as a piece of paper is folded upon itself, so that its inferior edge is brought up in contact with its superior edge. The cerebellum is notable for its extensive, transversely oriented *folia* (Figs. 8,9). It is composed of two lateral *cerebellar hemispheres* that are continuous with the midline *vermis* (Figs. 9A,B). The separation of vermis from cerebellar hemispheres is less obvious on the superior surface than on the inferior surface of the cerebellum. Many fissures separate the cerebellum into its major lobes. The two most important fissures—the primary fis-

sure and the posterolateral fissures—divide the cerebellum into three major lobes, anterior, posterior, and flocculonodular (Figs. 8,9). The *primary fissure* separates the anterior lobe from the posterior lobe and, the *posterolateral fissure* separates the posterior lobe from the flocculonodular lobe. The remaining fissures, such as the horizontal fissure and prepyramidal fissure, help to separate the cerebellum into additional lobules. The cerebellar hemisphere's lobules from its rostral to caudal edges are the anterior quadrangular, posterior quadrangular, superior semilunar, inferior semilunar, gracile, biventar, tonsil, and flocculus. The vermis lobules from its rostral to caudal edges are the lingula, central, culmen, declive, folium, tuber, pyramis, uvula, and nodulus.

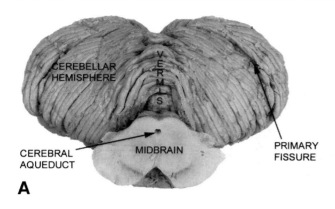

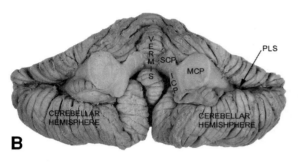

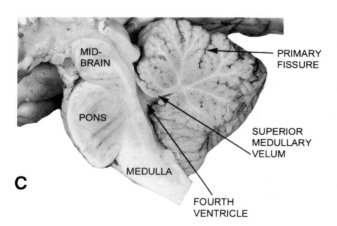

Fig. 9. (A) Anterior view of the cerebellum. The cerebellum, with its cerebellar hemispheres and vermis, lies posterior to the midbrain. The primary fissure separates the anterior lobe from the posterior lobe. The cerebral aqueduct is located in the midbrain. **(B)** Inferior view of the cerebellum. The two cerebellar hemispheres are present laterally, and the vermis is located in the midline. The posterolateral sulcus separates the posterior lobe from the flocculonodular lobe. The inferior cerebellar peduncle (ICP), middle cerebellar peduncle (MCP), and superior cerebellar peduncle (SCP) are visible. **(C)** Sagittal view of the cerebellum. The cerebellum lies posterior to the pons and medulla, and helps to define the roof of the fourth ventricle by its superior medullary velum and inferior medullary velum. The primary fissure separates the anterior lobe from the posterior lobe. The midbrain lies rostral to the pons.

3.5. Forebrain

The diencephalon and telencephalon comprise the forebrain (prosencephalon). The diencephalon is composed of the thalamus and hypothalamus, and is located between the midbrain caudally and the cerebral cortex rostrally (Fig. 8). The thalamus is located posterior to the hypothalamus. Posterior to the thalamus, the midline pineal body is connected to it by the habenular commissure. The third ventricle separates the two sides of the thalamus, and it extends ventrally down into the hypothalamus. Its separation from the thalamus is best visible from the midline, where the hypothalamic sulcus separates the two regions (Fig. 8). The hypothalamus, located on the anterior surface, connects to the pituitary through its tuberal (infundibular) region, which is located immediately posterior to the optic chiasm. Posterior to the tuberal region a pair of small swellings, known as mammillary bodies are formed by the mammillary nuclei of the hypothalamus (Fig. 8).

The two cerebral cortices comprise the majority of the brain, and each cortex is characterized by prominent folds, gyri (gyrus, singular) separated from each other by sulci (sulcus, singular), which invaginate into the depth of the cortex (Figs. 10,11). The cerebral cortex on each side is composed of an outer layer of gray matter, where the majority of neuronal cell bodies are located and a deeper layer of white matter formed by myelinated and unmyelinated axons from the neuronal cell bodies. The two cerebral cortices, are separated from one another on its superior side by the longitudinal fissure containing the falx cerebri of the dura mater, yet are connected deep in the longitudinal fissure by the corpus callosum. The corpus callosum is composed of myelinated axons that connect the two cortices and more caudal regions.

The cerebral cortex is divided by sulci or fissures into five lobes—the frontal, parietal, temporal, occipital, and insular cortices (Figs. 10–12). Several major sulci separate the major lobes from one another. The frontal cortex is separated from the parietal lobe by the central sulcus, a vertically running sulcus that begins at the longitudinal fissure in the midline and ends just short of the lateral sulcus on the lateral surface of the brain (Fig. 10). The lateral sulcus separates the temporal lobe from the frontal cortex and parietal cortex (Fig. 10). The parietal cortex on the lateral surface of the cerebral cortex is bounded by the central sulcus rostrally and

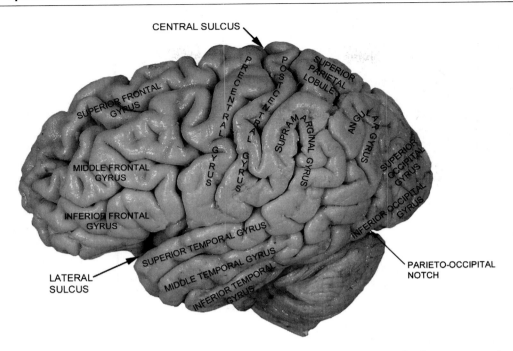

Fig. 10. Lateral surface of the cerebral hemispheres demonstrating the major gyri. The central sulcus separates the frontal cortex from the parietal cortex. The lateral sulcus separates the temporal cortex from the frontal and parietal cortices. An imaginary vertical line drawn from the parieto-occipital notch separates the parietal cortex from the occipital cortex.

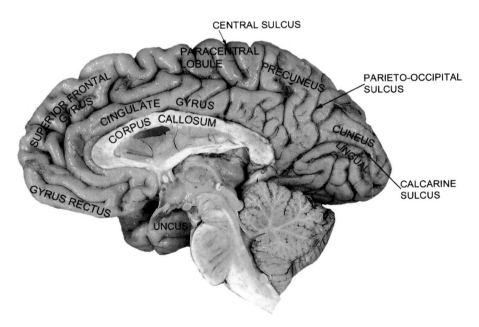

Fig. 11. Midsagittal section of the brain with cortical gyri labeled. The central sulcus extends medially into the longitudinal fissure. The parieto-occipital sulcus separates the parietal cortex from the occipital cortex. The calcarine sulcus separates the cuneus from the lingual gyrus.

is poorly delineated from the occipital lobe by a shallow indentation, parieto-occipital notch, just superior to the cerebellum (Fig. 10). On the medial surface, the separation between the parietal lobe and occipital lobe is more clearly defined by the vertically oriented parieto-occipital sulcus (Fig. 11). The

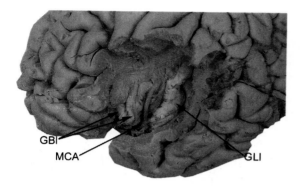

Fig. 12. Lateral surface of the cerebral cortex. The frontal operculum, parietal operculum, and temporal operculum have been removed to reveal the deeply located insula in the lateral sulcus. The middle cerebral artery (MCA) is located on the surface of the insula. Both gyrus longus insulae (GLI) and gyri brevi insulae (GBI) are present in the insula.

insular cortex lies deep inside the lateral sulcus and is most easily seen when the temporal cortex is pulled away from the frontal and parietal cortices (Fig. 12).

The frontal cortex is the most rostral portion of the cerebral cortices, and extends posteriorly to the central sulcus. It contains four prominent gyri on its lateral surface separated by corresponding sulci (Fig. 10). Three of its gyri (superior frontal gyrus, middle frontal gyrus, and inferior frontal gyrus) are horizontally oriented at the rostral end of the frontal cortex, and the fourth gyrus (precentral gyrus) is vertically oriented caudal to the first three gyri. The superior frontal gyrus begins anterior to the precentral gyrus and ends at the rostral pole of the brain. It is separated from the wide middle frontal gyrus by the superior frontal sulcus. The middle frontal cortex that is immediately inferior to the superior frontal gyrus is the broadest of the frontal gyri and also begins at the anterior border of the precentral gyrus. The inferior frontal sulcus is its inferior border, separating it from the inferior frontal gyrus. The inferior frontal gyrus is continuous inferiorly with the lateral orbital gyrus on the floor of the anterior cranial fossa. The frontal cortex on its inferior (orbital) surface is many times composed of four gyri that form an "H." These four gyri are the lateral orbital gyrus, anterior orbital gyrus, posterior orbital gyrus, and the medial orbital gyrus. The gyrus rectus is most medial, lying immediately lateral to the longitudinal fissure. Upon it lie the olfactory bulb and its centrally located olfactory tract.

The temporal cortex on its lateral surface lies inferior to the lateral sulcus, separating it from the frontal and parietal cortices (Fig. 10). Posteriorly, it is continuous with the parietal cortex. The temporal cortex contains three horizontally oriented gyri: superior temporal gyrus, middle temporal gyrus, and inferior temporal gyrus. The posterior surface of the superior temporal gyrus in the lateral sulcus is the transverse gyrus, which is associated with the auditory system. The superior temporal sulcus separates the superior temporal gyrus from the middle temporal gyrus, and the inferior temporal sulcus separates the middle temporal gyrus from the inferior temporal gyrus. The temporal cortex continues inferiorly and medially as a lateral occipitotemporal gyrus, a medial occipitotemporal gyrus, and the most medial parahippocampal gyrus, which has the uncus at its most anteromedial extent (Fig. 11).

The parietal cortex is located between the frontal cortex anteriorly and the occipital cortex posteriorly (Figs, 10,11). It is separated from the frontal cortex by the central sulcus and from the occipital cortex by the parieto-occipital sulcus. The most prominent gyrus is the vertically oriented postcentral gyrus immediately posterior to the central sulcus. The remainder of the parietal cortex lies posterior to the postcentral gyrus and is divided into a superior parietal lobule and an inferior parietal lobule. They are separated from each other by the intraparietal sulcus. On the lateral surface, the inferior parietal lobule can be divided into the supramarginal gyrus that arches over the posterior end of the lateral fissure, and the angular gyrus that arches over the superior temporal sulcus (Fig. 11).

On the superolateral surface, the occipital cortex appears as a continuation of the parietal cortex (Fig. 10). Only on the anterior edge of the cortex can a separation be discerned, where a slight indentation, parieto-occipital notch or pre-occipital notch, is present (Fig. 10). The remainder of the lateral surface of the occipital cortex has poorly defined gyri, although a superior occipital gyrus and an inferior occipital gyrus are often described. On its medial surface the vertically oriented parieto-occipital sulcus clearly separates it from the more anterior parietal cortex (Fig. 11). The horizontal calcarine sulcus separates several small gyri superior to it, collectively known as the cuneus, from the more inferior lingual gyrus.

The insula is located deep within the lateral sulcus. It is composed of two or more gyri brevi insulae and two or more gyri longus insulae (Fig. 12). The middle cerebral artery passes into the lateral sulcus on the surface of the insula. The portions of the frontal cortex, temporal cortex, and parietal cortex that form the border of the lateral sulcus and therefore cover the insula are described as the operculum. Thus, the frontal operculum is the part of the frontal cortex that helps to form the superior border of the lateral sulcus, and also participates in covering more rostral regions of the insula.

3.6. Arterial Supply of the Brain

The brain receives its blood supply from two paired arterial sources, the vertebra arteries and the internal carotid arteries (Fig. 13). The *vertebral arteries*, arising from the subclavian arteries at the base of the neck, ascend through the transverse foramina of the upper six cervical vertebral to enter the foramen magnum at the base of the skull. Once inside the cranial cavity, the two vertebral arteries unite on the anterior surface of the brainstem to form a single *basilar artery*. Prior to their union they each give rise to an arterial branch that joins with its opposite member to form the anterior spinal artery, which descends back through the foramen magnum to run along the anterior surface of the spinal cord. Each vertebral artery gives rise to the posterior inferior cerebellar artery that supplies the posterior surface of the cerebellum.

The *basilar artery* begins at the pontomedullary junction and courses along the anterior surface of the pons and midbrain until it terminates as the posterior cerebral arteries just rostral to the oculomotor nerve (Fig. 13). Before its termination it gives off several branches. Its first branch is typically the *anterior inferior cerebellar artery* which supplies the medial and lateral surface of the cerebellum. Multiple *pontine branches* arise from the basilar artery, supplying the pons as well as the midbrain. The *labyrinthine artery* arises in the midst of the pontine branches. It follows the facial nerve and vestibulocochlear nerve into the internal auditory meatus to supply the internal ear. The *superior cerebellar artery* arises from the basilar artery prior to the oculomotor nerve's origin, and is responsible for suppling the more superior surface of the cerebellum. The *posterior cerebral arteries*, which course around the cerebral peduncles to reach the posterior surface of the brainstem and caudal surface of the cerebrum, are the final pair of branches from the basilar artery. The posterior cerebral arter-

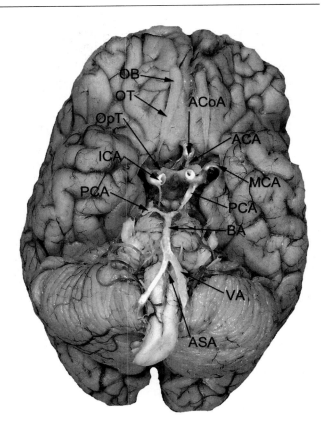

Fig. 13. Anterior surface of the brain, demonstrating circle of Willis and its associated arterial supply. The two vertebral arteries (VA) unite to form the basilar artery (BA). The anterior spinal artery (ASA) arises from the individual vertebral arteries prior to their union. The basilar artery terminates as the posterior cerebral arteries (PCA) It communicates with the internal carotid artery (ICA) via the posterior communicating artery (PCoA). The middle cerebral artery (MCA) originates from the internal carotid artery and enters the lateral sulcus, and the anterior cerebral artery (ACA) also arises from the internal carotid artery to enter the longitudinal fissure. A short vessel, the anterior communicating artery (AcoA), connects the two anterior cerebral arteries in the longitudinal fissure. In addition to the vascular supply on the anterior surface of the brain, the olfactory bulb (OB), olfactory tract (OT), and optic nerves (ON) are identified.

ies communicate via posterior communicating arteries with the internal carotid artery.

The *internal carotid artery*, one of two terminal branches of the common carotid artery, begins at the C4 level of the neck. It ascends through the neck without forming any branches and enters the skull through the serpentine-shaped carotid canal of the temporal bone to enter the cranial cavity. In the cranial cavity it is first located in the cavernous sinus of the sella turcica. Its first branch is the ophthalmic artery, which supplies the orbit. The internal carotid artery passes through the diaphragma sellae and immediately terminates as three branches to supply the cerebrum and diencephalon. The *posterior communicating artery* courses posteriorly to anastomose with the posterior cerebral arteries (Fig. 13). The *middle cerebral artery* arises from the lateral side of the internal carotid artery and courses laterally and posteriorly to enter the lateral fissure. It major branches can be divided into striate branches and cortical branches. The striate arteries are numerous, and are responsible for blood supply to the striatum. Cortical branches supply lateral surfaces of the cerebral cortex, including the orbital surface, precentral gyrus, middle frontal gyrus, inferior frontal gyrus, superior parietal gyrus, inferior, parietal gyrus, supramarginal gyrus, angular gyrus, superior temporal gyrus, middle temporal gyrus and inferior temporal gyrus. The *anterior cerebral artery* follows the corpus callosum—first anteriorly and superiorly and then posteriorly in the longitudinal fissure to supply medial surfaces of the cerebral cortex. In the first part of longitudinal fissure along the anterior surface, the two anterior cerebral arteries are connected by a very short *anterior communicating artery*. Central branches of the anterior cerebral artery supply the septum pellucidum, corpus callosum, and rostral portions of the basal ganglia. Cortical branches supply olfactory-bulb medial surfaces of the frontal and parietal cortex (gyrus rectus, medial orbital gyrus, superior frontal gyrus, middle frontal gyrus, cingulate gyrus, and the precuneate gyrus).

An anastomotic channel known as the circle of Willis is formed from branches of the internal carotid artery and the vertebral artery system. The arteries that contribute to the circle of Willis are the internal carotid artery anterior cerebral artery, anterior communicating artery, posterior communicating artery, and the posterior cerebral artery.

3.7. Venous Drainage of the Brain

Veins that drain the brain are tributaries of dural sinuses that ultimately empty into the internal jugular vein. They begin deep within the parenchyma of the brain and drain superficially, and can be divided into cerebral veins, cerebellar veins, and veins of the brainstem. The cerebral veins are composed of internal cerebral veins that drain the deep regions of the cerebrum and external cerebral veins located in the sulci and gyri. The superficial cerebral veins, located within the pia mater, are further divided into superior cerebral veins, middle cerebral veins, and inferior cerebral veins. The superior cerebral veins are located on the superolateral and medial surfaces of the cerebral cortex within their sulci, and drain directly into the superior sagittal sinus. The middle cerebral vein drains the lateral surface of the cerebral cortex, where they empty into the superior sagittal sinus via the superior anastomotic vein (Trolard's vein), or into the transverse sinus by way of the inferior anastomotic vein (Labbe's vein). The inferior cerebral veins are located on the anterior surface of the cerebral cortex. The more anterior branches drain into the superior cerebral veins, and the more posterior branches empty into the middle cerebral vein. The internal venous drainage of the cerebral cortex is conducted by the great cerebral vein (Galen's vein), and begins by its tributaries—the internal cerebral veins that drain the deep regions of the cerebral cortex. These in turn are formed by the thalamostriate and choroid veins. The great cerebral vein joins with the inferior sagittal sinus to empty into the straight sinus of the dural sinuses. The cerebellum is drained by the superior cerebellar veins and the inferior cerebellar veins on its surface. The superior cerebellar veins pass anteriorly and medially to enter the straight sinus, and the inferior cerebellar vein drains into the superior petrosal sinuses or transverse sinuses. The brainstem is drained by a venous plexus composed of anterior vessels that drain into the vertebral venous plexus, lateral venous plexus that drains into the inferior petrosal sinus, and a posterior plexus that drains into the great cerebral vein or straight sinus.

3.8. Ventricular System

The ventricular system of the brain is a series of cavities and passages connected to one another throughout the different brain regions. It contains cerebrospinal fluid (CSF), which is produced by the choroid plexus that is also located in the ventricles (Fig. 14). The ventricular system opens into the subarachnoid space, allowing CSF to surround the brain and spinal cord for support and protection. A *lateral ventricle* is contained within each cerebral hemisphere, and is separated by the septum pellucidum. Each lateral ventricle is in the form of a "C" and is subdivided into four interconnected regions. Its *frontal horn*, located in the frontal cortex, is continuous with the *body* located in both the frontal cortex and parietal cortex. Posteriorly, the body curves anterolaterally into the temporal cortex as

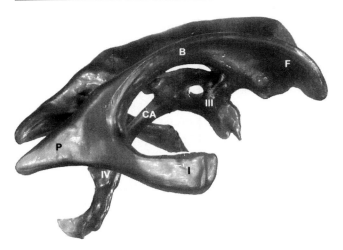

Fig. 14. Cast of the ventricular system of the human brain. The ventricular system of the brain was filled with latex, and the brain tissue was then removed to reveal the arrangement of the ventricular system. The two lateral ventricles are each composed of the frontal pole (F), body (B), posterior pole (P), and inferior pole (I). The lateral ventricles communicate with the midline third ventricle (III) via the interventricular foramen (InVF). The cerebral aqueduct (CA) allows communication between the third ventricle and the fourth ventricle (IV).

the *inferior horn*. The *posterior horn* extends from the body into the occipital cortex as it begins to curve into the inferior horn. The lateral ventricles communicate with the remainder of the ventricular system by the *interventricular foramen (of Monro)*, which is located at the midrostral end of the lateral ventricles anterior to the fornix. It connects each lateral ventricle to the midline thin, *third ventricle* between the two sides of the diencephalon. The *cerebral aqueduct*, located in the tectum of the midbrain, connects the third ventricle posteriorly with the fourth ventricle. The *fourth ventricle* is located between the cerebellum dorsally and the pons and medulla oblongata anteriorly. It is continuous with the central canal of the spinal cord. More importantly, the fourth ventricle opens into the subarachnoid space by the median foramen (of Majendie) and the lateral foramina (of Lushka), which are located in its roof. These foramina allow the CSF to move from the ventricular system into the subarachnoid space.

The subarachnoid space is enlarged in places, allowing accumulations of CSF between the arachnoid membrane and pia mater that help to cushion and protect the brain from the surrounding skull. The posterior *cerebellomedullary cistern*, the site

of drainage of the lateral and median foramina openings from the fourth ventricle, is the largest of the subarachnoid spaces. It is located between the medulla and cerebellum posteriorly and is continuous with the subarachnoid space surrounding the dorsal side of the spinal cord. The *quadrigeminal cistern* (cistern of the great cerebral vein) is located posteriorly, but is located in the interval between the splenium of the corpus callosum and the superior surface of the cerebellum. It is continuous with the cerebellomedullary cistern caudally. The *pontine cistern* is located on the anterior surface of the pons between it and the more caudal medulla oblongata. It is continuous caudally with the subarachnoid space surrounding the ventral side of the spinal cord and the interpeduncular cistern more rostrally. The *interpeduncular cistern*, located between the cerebral peduncles, contains the origin of the oculomotor nerve (CNIII). This region is also described as the interpeduncular fossa on specimens that have had their meninges removed. The *chiasmatic cistern* is the rostral continuation of the interpeduncular cistern. It is located anterior and inferior to the optic chiasm on the anterior surface of the brain. This cistern is in turn continuous laterally with the subarachnoid space in the cranial fossa.

The CSF located in the ventricular system is produced by the *choroid plexus* found in the roof of the lateral ventricles, third ventricles, and fourth ventricles. The choroid plexus is a complex vascular system composed of pia mater covered by ependymal cells. Production of CSF by the choroid plexus results in circulation beginning in the lateral ventricle, through the third ventricle into the fourth ventricle, and out from the median and lateral foramina into the subarachnoid space. Once in the subarachnoid space, the CSF circulates throughout the subarachnoid space surrounding the brain and spinal cord, and is then reabsorbed into the venous system from the subarachnoid space at the superior sagittal sinus by tuft-like protrusions, the *arachnoid granulations* of the arachnoid membrane.

3.9. Meninges of the Brain

The dura mater of the cranial cavity is composed of a superficial *periosteal layer* and a deeper *meningeal layer*. The meningeal layer is continuous with the meningeal layer of the spinal cord in the vertebral canal at the foramen magnum, and the periosteal layer ends at the foramen magnum. Both layers in the cranial cavity are adherent to one another except in regions where the venous dural sinuses force them apart. The arachnoid membrane lies deep to the dura mater and is continuous with the arachnoid membrane of the vertebral canal. Like the arachnoid membrane in the vertebral canal, it has fibrous extensions down to the pia mater. The pia mater in the cranial cavity follows the surface of the brain and is found in sulci of the cerebral cortex, cerebellum, and the fissures of the brain. Along the posterior surface of the third ventricle and the rostral end of the fourth ventricle the pia mater invaginates into the ventricular spaces to contribute to the formation of the choroid plexus of these regions. Epidural and subdural spaces that are associated with the spinal cord are not present in the cranial cavity. The subarachnoid space is filled with CSF and surrounds the brain and allows it to float in the cranial cavity. It is continuous with the subarachnoid space of the vertebral canal surrounding the spinal cord. A number of enlarged regions of the subarachnoid space are present on the anterior and posterior sides of the brain, and have already been described.

Extensions of the meningeal layer of the dura mater are located in specific regions of the brain, and contain some dural sinuses used to drain blood away from the brain. The first is the vertically oriented *falx cerebri*, which extends into the longitudinal fissure between the two halves of the cerebral cortex. The second is the horizontally oriented *tentorium cerebelli*, attached from the occipital bone posteriorly to the petrosal ridge of the temporal bone anterolaterally. It is located between the anterior surface of the occipital cortex and the superior surface of the cerebellum. In the midline the tentorium cerebelli does not attach to any bony structure, forming the tentorial incisure which allows the brainstem to continue from the posterior cranial fossa into the middle cranial fossa. The third is the vertically oriented *falx cerebelli* located between the two cerebelli cortices. The fourth is the horizontal *diaphragma sellae* that covers the sella turcica. The falx cerebelli has the occipital sinus along is posterior free edge. The diaphragma sellae contains the cavernous sinus. Dural sinuses are modified venous structures contained within the dura mater of the cranial cavity. The *superior sagittal sinus* is present along the superior edge of the falx cerebri, where it is bounded by both the periosteal dura mater

and the meningeal dural mater. It begins rostrally at the crista galli of the ethmoid bone and continues posteriorly to empty into the confluens of the sinuses. The superior sagittal sinus receives the CSF drainage by way of arachnoid villi that extend into its lumen. It also communicates with superficial veins of the scalp and emissary veins that drain the overlying bone of the skull. Along the inferior free edge of the falx cerebri the *inferior sagittal sinus* is contained entirely within the meningeal layer of the dural mater. It also begins at the crista galli and empties into the straight sinus at the anterior border of the junction of the falx cerebri and tentorium cerebelli. The *straight sinus* begins at the anterior border of the tentorium cerebelli, where it receives blood from the great cerebral vein (of Galen) and the straight sinus and empties posteriorly into the confluens of the sinuses. The *confluens of the sinuses*, located on the internal occipital protuberance of the occipital bone communicates with the superior sagittal sinus, straight sinus, occipital sinus, and transverse sinuses. The *transverse sinuses*, formed between the periosteal and meningeal layers of dura mater, is located along the posterior edges of the tentorium cerebelli, where it is in contact with the occipital and parietal bones. These drain blood from the confluens of the sinuses and the superior sagittal sinus anteriorly. The *sigmoid sinuses* are continuations of the transverse sinuses as they leave the tentorium cerebelli, and take a medial and inferior serpentine course along the surface of the occipital bone to help form the internal jugular vein. The *cavernous sinuses* are located deep to the diaphragma sellae on either side of the sella turcica of the sphenoid bone. They communicate with one another by *intercavernous branches*. The cavernous sinuses are unique to other dural sinuses because they contain the internal carotid artery and abducens nerve (CN VI) within their lumen, and the ophthalmic and maxillary divisions of the trigeminal nerve (CN V) and the oculomotor nerve (CN III) in its wall. Anteriorly, the cavernous sinus communicates with superficial veins of the face, the ophthalmic veins, and the pterygoid plexus. Posteriorly, the cavernous sinus communicates with the inferior petrosal sinus, superior petrosal sinus and the basilar plexus of veins. The *superior petrosal sinus*, located within the anterolateral border of the tentorium cerebelli, is located along the superior border of the petrous ridge of the temporal bone. It begins at the cavernous sinus and joins with the transverse sinus to empty into the sagittal sinus. The *inferior petrosal sinus* begins at the cavernous sinus and follows the temporo-occipital suture to the jugular foramen, where it forms the internal jugular vein with the sigmoid sinus.

SELECTED READINGS

Carpenter MB. Human Neuroanatomy, 7th ed., Baltimore, MD: Williams and Wilkins, 1976.

Clemente C. Gray's Anatomy, 30th ed., Philadelphia, PA: Lea & Febiger, 1996.

Noback CR. The Human Nervous System. New York: McGraw-Hill Publishing Co., 1981.

Peters A, Jones EG, (eds). Cerebral Cortex. New York: Plenum Press, 1994.

3

Ion Channels and Electrical Signaling

Stanko S. Stojilkovic

CONTENTS

1. ELECTROPHYSIOLOGICAL CHARACTERISTICS OF CELL MEMBRANES

1.1. Introduction

Membranes in all cell types regulate the extra- and intracellular ionic environment. In neurons and other excitable cells, regulation of the ionic environment is also crucial for the development and maintenance of the specific signaling pathway for these cells, known as the *electrical signaling system*. This system is composed of two basic elements: i) a lipid bimolecular diffusion barrier, termed *lipid bilayer*, that separates cells from their environment, and ii) two classes of macromolecule proteins, known as *ion channels* and

From: *Neuroscience in Medicine, 2nd ed.* (P. Michael Conn, ed.),
© 2003 Humana Press Inc., Totowa, NJ.

ion carriers, that regulate the movement and distribution of ions across the lipid barrier in the plasma membrane, as well as in the endoplasmic reticulum (ER) and nuclear membranes (Fig. 1). Neurons, like other cell types, also signal through nonelectrical plasma membrane-dependent mechanisms, independently of ions and proteins responsible for ion transport, and this *receptor-mediated signaling* frequently interacts with the electrical signaling system. This chapter focuses on electrical signaling in neurons. For receptor-mediated signaling in neurons, *see* Chapter 5.

1.2. Lipid Bilayer Separates Cells from Their Environment

Phospholipids and several other types of lipids contribute to the membrane structure. The major cell-membrane lipids consist of a hydrophylic head,

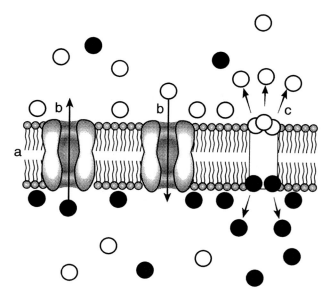

Fig. 1. Two essential components of neuronal-cell membrane responsible for electrical signaling are: the phospholipid bilayer (**a**) and two classes of macromolecular proteins, ion channels (**b**) and ion transporters (**c**). A difference in concentration of an ion across the plasma membrane will result in a net movement through channels away from the side of higher concentration to the side of lower concentration by passive transport known as diffusion (**b**). An ion pump is working in the opposite direction of the concentration gradient (**c**).

commonly a glycerophosphorylester, and a hydrocarbon tail, usually containing two hydrophobic fatty acids. When exposed to water, phospholipid molecules usually orient with their two hydrophobic hydrocarbon tails to one another and their hydrophylic polar or charged head groups adjacent to the water molecules. In the cell membrane, tails orient back-to-back so that the hydrophobic lipid tails of one layer face the hydrophobic tails of the other, whereas the hydrophilic heads point outward away from the middle of the membrane. Such a double-layered structure is known as a *lipid bilayer* (Fig. 1). Detergents transform lipid bilayers into water-soluble micelles, whereas cholesterol stabilizes bilayers.

The bilayer structure serves several important functions in intracellular and intercellular signaling. i) The hydrophobic tails of the lipid molecules tend to be chemically incompatible with water-soluble substances containing inorganic ions. As a result, the lipid bilayer serves as a barrier to the movement of ions across the membrane, effectively separating the intracellular and extracellular ionic compartments. One class of bilayer lipids provides substrates for signal transduction enzymes, leading to the generation of

several intracellular signaling molecules. ii) Separation of intracellular and extracellular conducting solutions is provided by an extremely thin hydrophobic, insulating layer (1.5–3 nm). This forms a significant electrical capacitor, or storage of electrochemical energy that drives the signaling process. iii) The protein components of the membranes, including carriers and ion channels, are embedded in the lipid bilayer and are oriented and grouped in a manner that serves their respective functions. Lipid membranes are also critical in forming organelles, such as the endoplasmic reticulum (ER), which is composed of rough ER, in neurons called Nissl substance, and smooth ER. The latter contains ion transporters and channels, and provides an additional mechanism for intracellular signaling in neurons.

1.3. Ion Pumps and Ion Channels Transport Ions in Opposite Directions

The lipid bilayer retains vital cell compartments, but also prevents the exchange of ionized substrates between the cell and its environment, which is critical not only for electrical signaling but also for cell metabolism in general. This function is mediated by specific ion-transporter mechanisms. Ion carriers, including the Na^+-K^+ pump, the Ca^{2+} pump, Na^+-Ca^{2+} exchanger, Cl^--HCO_3^- exchanger, and glucose transporters, are macromolecules fixed in the membrane and their transporter-binding sites are exposed alternatively to the intracellular and extracellular media or luminal and intracellular face of the ER membrane. Ion pumps require adenosine triphosphate (ATP) as the source of energy to move ions from a side of low concentration to a side of high concentration. For example, Na^+ and K^+ are moved across the membrane by the Na^+-K^+ exchange pump in opposite directions. In every pump cycle, three Na^+ are moved from cytosol to the extracellular fluid, two K^+ are moved from the extracellular fluid into the cytosol, and one ATP is required to make this movement (Fig. 2). This process has been observed in nearly all cell types that have been studied. The ATP-dependent Ca^{2+} transporters are expressed in both plasma membrane and ER membrane and pump Ca^{2+} from cytosol to the extarcellular fluid and the ER fluid, respectively. Together with Na^+-Ca^{2+} antiporters, these pumps maintain low concentrations of intracellular free Ca^{2+} (about 100 nm). Thus, by working against the concentration gradient, an ion pump is building up a high concentration of ions on one side of the membrane, and such ion gradients are required for the most basic neuronal functions.

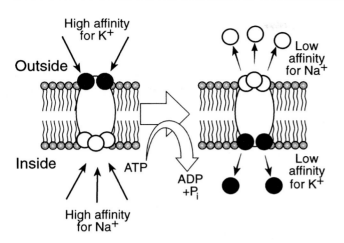

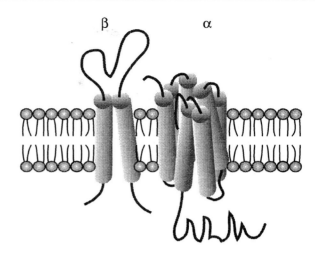

Fig. 2. A schematic representation of the sodium-potassium pump transporting Na^+ and K^+ across the membrane against their electrochemical gradient. In one conformation state, the carrier binds $3Na^+$ on the intracellular surface and $2K^+$ on the extracellular surfice, both with high affinity (*left panel*). Following a series of conformation changes driven by ATP hydrolysis, the carrier releases Na^+ to the extracellular fluid and K^+ on the cytoplasmic surface (*right panel*). In that conformation stage, the carrier has a low affinity for Na^+ and K^+, limiting the reverse transports of ions. The activity of the sodium-potassium pump is critical in establishing and maintaining the resting potential.

Fig. 3. Ion channels are expressed in all living cells, and have numerous functions. This includes establishing a resting membrane potential, generating action potentials and action potential-dependent intracellular calcium signals, and controlling cell volume and net flow of ions and fluids. Voltage-gated Ca^{2+} influx can regulate contraction, secreting, gating, and control activity of various intracellular enzymes. Ion channels can have different TM topologies and are usually composed of several subunits. Subunits have different number of TM domains connected by intracellular and extracellular chains.

However, excitation and electrical signaling *per se* are carrier-independent and are dependent on movements of ions through ion channels. This movement is determined by ion gradient across the cell membrane and does not require energy. Ion channels have water-filled pores through the membrane, which are permeable for ions, and in some cases for small molecules as well. An ion channel is usually built of several subunits, each of which is composed of helical strands that form transmembrane (TM) domains. These domains are connected by extracellular and intracellular chains of amino acids (Fig. 3). The role of ion channels is to set the permeability of the membrane. One group of channels passes cations (positively charged ions), and the other group passes anions (negatively charged ions). Some channels are nonspecific for cations, but most channels are ion-selective—e.g., they allow the passage of a specific ion. This property had been used to name the channels—e.g., Na^+, K^+, Ca^{2+} channels. Some channels are continuously open to the flow of ions and are termed *leakage channels*. Others are transiently open to ion fluxes and are known as *gated channels*. Closing the channel is a conformation change that may involve a decrease in diameter of the pore, or the movement of terminal parts of protein to block the pore to the flow of ions. A part of the molecule that moves to occlude or open the channel is termed a *gate*. There are five major groups of channels. i) *Voltage-gated channels* open or close in response to changes in electrical potential across the cell membrane. ii) *Ligand-gated channels* require a binding of a particular signaling molecule to open or close. iii) *The stretch-sensitive channels* opens or closes in response to a mechanical force. iv) *Intracellular channels* are expressed in ER and nuclear membranes. v) Connexins form gap junctions, which operate as *intercellular channels*.

1.4. Signaling Proteins Other Than Channels and Carriers

Signaling proteins of the cell membrane include three groups of proteins. i) *Adhesion* and *anchor* proteins help bind one cell to another and fasten the membrane to an internal network of proteins, respectively. ii) *Receptors* are proteins that bind the extracellular messengers and respond to this by generating intracellular messengers. Each receptor is specific for only one type of signaling molecule, as well as to its close chemical analogs. In neuronal cells they are usually concentrated on the postsynaptic membranes. iii) Receptors transduce signaling by activating a chain

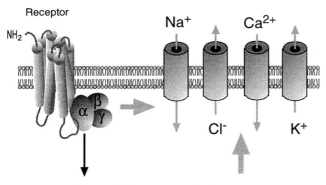

Second Messenger Pathways

Fig. 4. Seven TM-domain receptors are coupled to hetero-trimeric G proteins, leading to the activation of several intracellular signaling pathways, including phospholipase C and adenylyl cyclase-dependent pathways. Receptor-induced dissociation of α and β/γ dimers provides a mechanism for regulation of ion-channel gating by these subunits (membrane-delimited pathway). The gating of channels is also controlled in a second-messenger-dependent manner.

reaction or a cascade of events, usually by activating membrane-bound enzymes. The first protein in the cascade is G protein, which in turn activates other membrane-bound proteins, including adenylyl cyclase, phospholipases C and D, and phosphodiesterases. This also leads to the generation of *intracellular messengers*, such as cyclic adenosine monophosphate (cAMP), cyclic guanosine monophosphate (cGMP), $InsP_3$, diacylzglycerol, and phosphaditic acid, as well as activation of kinases, including protein kinase A (PKA), protein kinase C (PKC), and protein kinase G (PKG) (*see* Chapter 5). These intracellular messengers have numerous functions, including the control of ion-channel conductivity (Fig. 4).

1.5. Ion Concentrations Differ Across the Cell Membrane

The concentrations of various ions in the two conducting solutions, the intracellular and extracellular, are different. All living cells maintain differential ion concentrations across the cell membrane. Table 1 lists the concentrations of major ions in a mammalian cell-model. Na^+, Ca^{2+}, and Cl^- are predominantly found extracellularly, whereas K^+ and organic ions are concentrated intracellularly. The concentration gradient across the membrane has two major functional consequences for excitable cells: i) It provides the electrochemical energy to drive signaling. Na^+ and K^+ are essential for this process, and Ca^{2+} concentration gra-

dient also helps to drive the signaling. ii) Ca^{2+} influx through plasma-membrane channels also serves as an intracellular messenger to activate many intracellular biochemical processes, including synaptic transmission. The concentration gradient for Ca^{2+} across the ER membrane resembles that of the plasma membrane, and the release of this ion from the luminal side plays a critical role in intracellular signaling of excitable and nonexcitable cells.

1.6. Every Neuron Has a Membrane Potential

There is a balance of electrical charge within the cytosol and extracellular fluid compartment, termed *macroscopic electroneutrality*. On the other hand, there is a difference in electrical potential across the membrane of each cell. Experimentally, this difference can be measured by placing a glass microelectrode into the cytoplasm and the other electrode in external fluid (Fig. 5). In excitable cells, a steady electrical potential difference of about –50 to –70 mV is detected. In nonexcitable cells, the potential difference is smaller. By convention, the sign of potential difference indicates that the inside of the cell is electrically negative with respect to the outside. The membrane potential is always given as that of intracellular compartment relative to the extracellular compartment. This difference is termed the *membrane potential*. Nearly every aspect of electrical signaling in excitable cells depends in some way on the membrane potential. Signals that decrease membrane potential are *depolarizing* and those that increase the membrane potential are *hyperpolarizing*.

1.7. The Membrane Potential as Cellular Force

Separation of charges of opposite sign, like those by plasma membrane, provides the basis for electrical phenomena. As in physics, we can talk about the *potential difference*, measured in volts (V), *current*, measured in amperes (A), *conductance*, measured in siemens (S), and *resistance*, which is measured in ohms (Ω). As stated previously, in cells the potential difference is generated by unequal cations and anions on two sides of the membrane. When positive and negative electrodes are placed in an ion solution, cations will flow toward the negative pole and anions toward the positive pole, and both carry electrical current toward the negative pole. The size of current is determined by the potential difference between the

Table 1
Distribution of Free Ion Concentrations and Equilibrium Potentials
For a Mammalian Cell Model

Ion	Extracellular concentration (mM)	Intracellular concentration (mM)	Equilibrium potential (mV)
Sodium	145	12	+67
Potassium	5	150	−91
Calcium	1.5	0.0001	+128
Chloride	125	5	−86

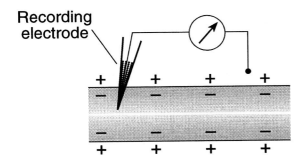

Fig. 5. The intracellular recording of membrane potential in an axon using a fine glass microelectrode. The *circle with arrow* indicates a combined amplifier and voltage-measuring device.

electrodes and the electrical conductance of the solutions between electrodes. The conductance in salt water depends on salt concentrations and mobility of ions. Resistance is the reciprocal of conductance. Furthermore, capacitance (C) is a measure of how much charge must be transferred from one conductor to another, and is defined as:

$$C = Q/E \qquad (1)$$

where Q is the charge and E is voltage difference across the conductor. The unit of capacitance is farad (F). Because electrical capacitance is inversely related to the thickness of the insulating region separating two conductors, the 1.5–3-nm lipid barrier makes a very efficient capacitator, in the order of 1 $\mu F/cm^2$ of membrane surface.

The resistance of the cell membrane indicates how difficult it is for ions to move through. If there are few open channels for an ion, the membrane has a high resistance and a low conductance for that ion. In general, the conductance of a particular membrane depends on several factors: i) the density of the channels; ii) the number of channels that are open; and iii) the maintenance of ion concentrations. The first two factors are the most significant for conductance across

the membrane, whereas the relevance of ion concentrations depends on the volume of the cells and myelination of the membrane. For example, in a nonmelinated cell of 25 μm in diameter, the amount of charge required to be move across cell membranes to support physiologic changes in membrane potential is usually accompanied with negligible changes in the ion concentrations across the membrane (1 of about 200,000). However, in small cells and in axons, depletion and recovery of ions in cytoplasm during electrical signaling compared to the stored-up ions is much higher, and could affect electrical signaling during the sustained activation.

1.8. Membrane Potential and Ion Movements

In neurons that are electrically inactive (quiescent), membrane potential is in a steady state and is termed *resting potential*. This potential results from a separation of positive and negative charges across the plasma membrane. This means that the movement of ions across the membrane in one direction is balanced by the movement of the same number of ions in the opposite direction. In general, three factors contribute to the movement of ions: concentration gradient, electrical gradient, and carrier activity. i) A concentration of the ion on the two sides of the membrane should result in *diffusion*, a net movement of ions away from a region of greater concentrations toward a region of lesser concentration. Thus, if the membrane is permeable for ions, they will move down its concentration. The net transfer is proportional to the concentration difference across the cell membrane, does not require energy, and is termed a *passive transport*. ii) Electrical potential differences across the cell membrane also influence ion movement. Cations in the pore of channels will be moved toward the negative interior of cells, whereas anions will be moved toward the positive exterior of cells, and this transport does not require energy. iii) Pumps also participate in the transport of ions across the membrane, but the energy stored in ATP is required and ions are moved against their concentration gradients (*active transport*).

The intact membrane is essential for the maintenance of resting potential. In cells with a damaged membrane, a resting potential rapidly declines to zero. Also, if channels are continuously open and conduct all ions, passive transports will bring the resting potential to zero because of diffusion of ions. Furthermore, cells have to be bathed in medium containing ion concentrations comparable to that of in vivo extracellular medium. For example, with an increase in external concentrations of K$^+$ from the physiological 5 mM to 50 mM by adding KCl, the resting potential, will decline. In other word, the cell will depolarized. This simple experimental procedure indicates that concentration gradient for K$^+$ is important in controlling resting potential, and is frequently used to activate voltage-gated Ca^{2+} entry. Finally, inhibition of metabolic activity attenuates the carrier activity, leading to gradual (over hours) decline of resting potential to zero. These observations indicate that the generation and maintenance of resting potential requires: i) unequal distribution of ions across the membrane; ii) the selective permeability of ion channels and their ability to close; iii) the energy-dependent transport, which is not critical in rapid responses, but is required to maintain a resting potential over a long period of time.

1.9. Single-Ion Electrochemical Equilibrium

To understand the generation of negative membrane potential in cells, we will first discuss a hypothetical cell-model that contains sodium chloride extracellularly, potassium aspartate intracellularly, and a plasma membrane expressing K$^+$ channels only. Initially, both intracellular and extracellular sides will be electrically neutral, because of the equal numbers of cations and anions. If the cell contains open channels that are selective only for K$^+$, this ion will move through the channels down its concentration gradient until the concentrations are equal on both sites. Since K$^+$ is charged, however, the diffusion of each K$^+$ makes the inside slightly more negative relative to outside, leading to the generation of a potential difference, as well as the generation of an electrical field across the plasma membrane. Initially the efflux of K$^+$ will dominate, followed by greater influx. At equilibrium, a steady state in which the tendency for further changes disap-

pears, a membrane potential has been established based on a single ion and the selective permeability of the channels in membrane. The potential difference at which the equal movements occur is called the *equilibrium potential*, also known as Nernst potential. Thus, equilibrium potential is the membrane potential at which there are no net ion movements and the ion gradients and membrane potential will remain stable indefinitely. The equilibrium potential for four major ions can be calculated using the Nernst equation:

$$E_K = RT/zF \ln [K]_o/[K]_i \qquad (2)$$

$$E_{Na} = RT/zF \ln [Na]_o/[Na]_i \qquad (3)$$

$$E_{Ca} = RT/zF \ln [Ca]_o/[Ca]_i \qquad (4)$$

$$E_{Cl} = RT/zF \ln [Cl]_i/[Ca]_o \qquad (5)$$

where R is the gas constant, T is temperature (in degrees Kelvin), z is valence of the ion, and F is the Faraday constant.

1.10. Real Cells Are Not at Equilibrium

The balance of efflux and influx of K$^+$ in a mammalian cell-model (Table 1) would be reached at a membrane potential of –91 mV, for Na$^+$ the balance would be at +67 mV, and for Cl$^-$ at –86 mV. The sign of the equilibrium potential reflects the polarity of the intracellular site of the cell. However, the resting potential of cells (about –60 mV) is different from the equilibrium potential for all four ions, indicating that in the physiological-like situation none of them is in equilibrium and that the steady status of the resting potential is reached by other forces. The magnitudes and direction of these forces became obvious by comparing the resting potential with the equilibrium potential for a particular ion. For example, +67-mV equilibrium potential for Na$^+$ and –60-mV resting potential indicate that concentration and electrical gradient will favor entry of Na$^+$, if channels are permeable for this ion. In a case of K$^+$ ion, the actual resting potential is not large enough to counter the force of diffusion forcing a small but constant K$^+$ efflux. As shown in Fig. 6, there is more force moving Na$^+$ into the cells than there is moving K$^+$ out. At a membrane potential of –60 mV, the sum of diffusion and electrical forces (net driving force) for K$^+$ is 31 mV and for Na$^+$, it is 127 mV. However, at resting potential only a few Na$^+$-conducting channels are open. In other words, the permeability of membrane for Na$^+$ at resting potential is very low. There is also a small but constant K$^+$ efflux.

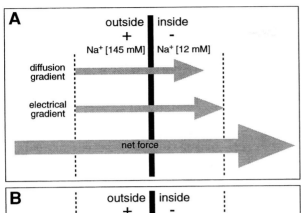

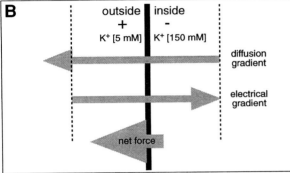

Fig. 6. Schematic representation of the magnitude and directions of passive forces acting on Na$^+$ and K$^+$ in a mammalian cell-model. The algebraic difference between the diffusion gradient and electrical gradient indicates the direction and magnitude of the net force in a resting cell.

Finally, the passive influx of Na$^+$ and efflux of K$^+$ is balanced by the action of the Na$^+$-K$^+$ pump, which brings two K$^+$ for three Na$^+$ that are expelled.

1.11. Multi-Ion Electrochemical Equilibrium

An ion electrochemical gradient illustrates the forces on ion movement through a single channel-type, but real cells express more than one ion channel-type. Furthermore, the dissociation between the resting potentials and equilibrium potentials introduces a need to integrate the permeability of the membrane for ions (in addition to the concentration of the ions in two conductors), which is not a factor in the Nernst equation. Thus, in order to calculate membrane potential in a multi-ion system, we need to know the equilibrium potential for each permeant ion and the permeability for each ion. This new equation was derived by Goldman (1943) and Hodgkin and Katz (1949):

$$E_m = \frac{RT/F \ln P_K[K^+]_o + P_{Na}[Na^+]_o + P_{Cl}[Cl^-]_i}{P_K[K^+]_i + P_{Na}[Na^+]_i + P_{Cl}[Cl^-]_o} \quad (6)$$

in which R, T, F, and z are as defined in Nernst equation and P$_{Na}$, P$_K$, and P$_{Cl}$ are the permeabilities of the membranes to Na$^+$, K$^+$, and Cl$^-$, respectively. Since absolute permeabilities are difficult to measure, the equation can be also expressed in terms of relative permeabilities:

$$E_m = \frac{RT/F \ln [K^+]_o + (P_{Na}/P_K)[Na^+]_o + (P_{Cl}/P_K)[Cl^-]_i}{[K^+]_i + (P_{Na}/P_K)[Na^+]_i + (P_{Cl}/P_K)[Cl^-]_o} \quad (7)$$

The frequently used permeability ratios for P$_K$: P$_{Na}$: P$_{Cl}$ are 1 : 0.04 : 0.45.

Two important conclusions are derived from ion concentrations and permeabilities. i) The resting potential most closely approximates the calculated Nernst equilibrium potential for the most permeable ion. ii) The membrane potential is most influenced by changes in concentrations of the permeable ion. For example, if a membrane is equally permeable to Na$^+$ and K$^+$, the membrane potential would be about −15 mV. However, because the measured resting potentials in neurons closely approximate the calculated equilibrium potential for K$^+$, it is likely that the membrane is more permeable to K$^+$ than to Na$^+$ at rest.

2. ELECTRICAL EXCITABILITY OF THE CELL MEMBRANE

2.1. Excitable Cells Fire Action Potentials

The properties of the cell membrane and ion channels expressed in membrane provide a rationale for the development of resting potential, as well as the development of *nerve impulses*, technically termed *action potentials*. The main distinction between these two processes is that the membrane potential is generated by channels that are active at rest, whereas nerve impulses are generated by channels that open when the cell is electrically active. Action potential is a brief transient reversal of membrane potential that speeds along the axons of nerve cells, but also over the membranes of many muscle and endocrine cells. It propagates regeneratively as an electrical wave without decrement and at high and constant velocity. Action potential provides an effective mechanism for rapid signaling over the long distance. As shown in Fig. 7, in response to an electrical shock, the membrane potential changes from its resting value toward zero; thus, a rapid *depolarization* of the membrane occurs. This is followed by *reverse polarization*, with the interior of cells being positive relative to the outside.

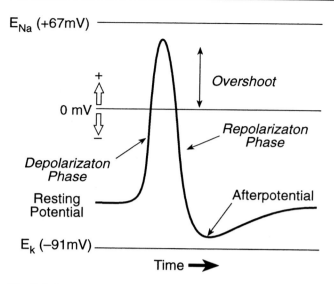

E_{Na} (+67mV)

0 mV

+

Overshoot

Repolarizaton Phase

Depolarizaton Phase

Resting Potential

Afterpotential

E_k (−91mV)

Time ➜

Fig. 7. Schematic representation of a neuronal action-potential. The action potential waveform is composed of several components. A rapid depolarization from a resting potential of about −60 mV leads to the reverse polarization, which peaks below the Na^+ equilibrium potential. The peak value above 0 mV is known as overshoot. The repolarization phase is usually cell-type-specific; in some cells it occurs rapidly, whereas in others it occurs with delays. During the repolarization phase, the membrane potential can briefly become more negative than the resting potential, and is known as a hyperpolarizing afterpotential. The repolarization value usually does not exceed the K^+ equilibrium potential.

The membrane is then seen to *repolarize*. Typically, a short *hyperpolarization* follows the initial return of membrane to resting potential. Cells that can make action potentials spontaneously or in response to an electrical shock are known as *electrically excitable*.

2.2. Neurons Also Generate a Variety of Slow Potentials

Only when neurons were exposed to levels beyond the threshold stimuli did they respond with firing of action potentials; the subthreshold stimuli produce only *localized responses*. These experimentally induced responses resemble slow potentials recorded from neurons, especially on the synaptic site of actions of neurotransmitter molecules and sensory endings. Localized responses are slow potentials that may take a depolarizing or hyperpolarizing form. At post-synaptical membranes these responses are called *postsynaptic potentials* and in sensory endings they are called receptor potentials (*see* Chapter 5).

2.3. Action Potential and Ion Movements

The electrochemical energy of membrane potential and the sequence of the permeability change to ions account for the generation of action potential. In a series of elegant experiments with voltage-clamped cells, Hodgkin and Huxley were able to precisely calculate the changes in the conductance of Na^+ and K^+ during action potential. The voltage-clamp method provides the direct measurements of ion conductivity as electrical current across the cell membrane. Furthermore, by changing the solutions, it is possible to resolve the individual ionic components. These experiments revealed that the opening and closing of Na^+ and K^+ channels is controlled by membrane potential. Hodgkin and Huxley made a kinetic model of the opening and closing for these two channels; the simplified version of this is shown in Fig. 8A. They were able to calculate the theoretical shape of the action potential from these conductance changes, and to find a remarkable similarity with the recorded action potentials. Fig. 8B shows the temporal relationship between channel opening and action-potential waveform.

The initiation of action potential in axons depends on Na^+ influx, and in some cells on Ca^{2+} influx. Depolarization of neurons induced by an electrical shock, or generated at synapses—if sufficient strong and occuring in the region of membrane expressing Na^+/Ca^{2+} and K^+ channels—triggers an increase in the probabilities of these channels to open. Na^+ channels respond more rapidly compared to K^+ channels, and the membrane permeability to Na^+ rises relative to that of K^+. If a few Na^+ channels are open, they have a minimal effect on membrane potential. As a result, the membrane potential will return to normal. A stronger depolarization, however, will activate more Na^+ channels. Both the concentration gradient for Na^+ and the negative intracellular potential facilitate Na^+ influx, which further depolarizes the cell and activates more Na^+ channels to open and more Na^+ entry, further depolarization, and an action potential. At the peak membrane potential, the membrane is about 20 to 50 times more permeable to Na^+ than to K^+—the reverse situation of the relative permeabilities for these two channels at resting membrane potential. Such a massive influx of positive charge makes the inside of cells positive for a short period, and the polarity of membrane reverses.

The repolarization phase of action potential that returns membrane to the resting level results from

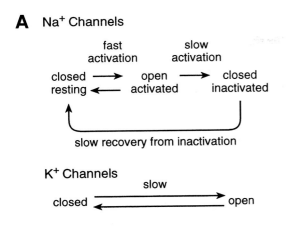

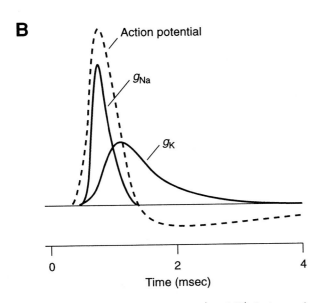

Fig. 8. Changes in conductance of Na⁺ and K⁺ during action potentials. **(A)** Simplified diagram illustrating the voltage-dependent opening and closing of Na⁺ and K⁺ channels. **(B)** Time-course of changes in membrane potential and conductance for Na⁺ and K⁺ channels calculated from voltage-clamped experiments. (Adapted from Hodgkin and Huxley, J Physiol 1952;117:500.)

changes in the permeability of both K⁺ and Na⁺ channels. The initial depolarization of cells mediated by Na⁺ also increases the opening probability of K⁺ channels, but slightly later than the gates of Na⁺ channels. This results in a delay of the peak flow of K⁺ current, which is known as delayed rectifier K⁺ current. Although the membrane is depolarized, Na⁺ channels became nonconducting because of a phenomenon called *channel inactivation*. Sodium-channel inactivation kinetics are rapid. This leaves the activated K⁺

channels to dominate the membrane permeability and to repolarize membrane to resting level. The continuous opening of K⁺ channels at that time-point accounts for development of afterhyperpolarization. Eventually, K⁺ channels close at more negative potentials, and the resting potential is restored. The peak of action potentials is always less than the equilibrium potential for Na⁺, and the hyperpolarization that follows an action potential is never more negative than equilibrium potential for K⁺. Also, the generation of typical action potentials is not affected by abolition of carrier activities, consistent with the hypothesis that changes in the permeabilities of channels and passive movement of ions are sufficient for the generation of action potential.

2.4. Action Potentials Are All or None

The explosive depolarization is preceded by a small decrease in the membrane potential initiated by Na⁺ influx. This decrease in membrane potential must be sufficient to depolarize the cell to a certain *threshold voltage*. If reached, action potential will be generated independently of further strength of the depolarizing stimulus. Also, the peak amplitude of action potential is not related to the strength of depolarizing stimulus; once it is triggered, action potential is a self-driving phenomenon. This is known as *all-or-none* feature of action potential, in contrast to the graded nature of the voltage changes in synapses (*see* Chapter 4).

2.5. How Does the Action Potential Propagate?

Long-distance communication in the nervous system is possible because action potentials propagate smoothly down an axon maintaining the same amplitude. The general principles by which action potentials propagate are similar in nonmyelinated and myelinated axons and are dependent on localized currents. The action-potential-induced depolarization of cell membrane spreads a small distance in either direction inside the axon. This occurs because the intracellular and extracellular media are better conductors than the cell membrane. Thus, an action-potential-affected area smoothly depolarizes the region ahead of the action potential. Once this depolarization reaches the threshold, opening of Na⁺ channels further advances the wave of excitation. Although localized current also flows into the area behind the advancing action potential, it does not develop into an action potential. Na⁺ channels in this region are inactivated, and channels

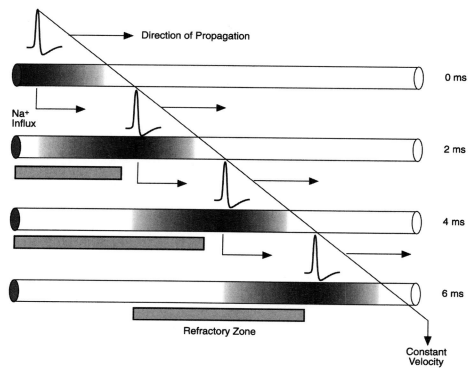

Fig. 9. The propagation of action potential along axons occurs at a constant velocity. The scheme illustrates four time-points during the propagation of an action potential. The gray areas indicate the intensity of changes in membrane potential, with the darkest area corresponding to the peak of the action potential. The localized currents flow in the front of action potential, but also into the area behind the advancing action potential. Because Na⁺ channels remain in an inactivated state following action-potential depolarization, however, a refractory zone occurs, forcing action potential to travel in only one direction.

are in a nonconducting mode. This is known as the *refractory period*, an important feature that forces action potential to travel in only one direction (Fig. 9).

2.6. Myelin Enhances the Speed of Action Potential

The speed of action-potential propagation depends on the density of Na⁺ channels and the diameter of axon. For example, the squid axons have a diameter of approx 1 mm and conduction velocity of almost 100 m/s, whereas mammalian C-fibers have a diameter of <2 μm and conduct with a speed of 1–2 m/s. Thus, the more channels are expressed per unit area and the larger diameter of axon, the more rapidly the propagation of action potential occurs. Neither of these two features is physiologically attractive, because of the energy cost and because a single nerve would be packed with only a few axons. Still the majority of mammalian nerves are packed with hundreds of axons, with diameters of only 10–20 μm, but their conductance velocity is approx 50 m/s. This has been achieved by the expression of myelin around axons, which increases the velocity of action-potential propagation.

In myelinated neurons, the majority of the axon is covered by myelin. However, the myelin wrap surrounding an individual axon is interrupted at 1–1.5 mm intervals, and these regions are known as *nodes of Ranvier* (about 20 μm long). A single glial cell, known as a Schwann cell covers one *internodal area* with myelin. In such axons, depolarization also spreads from an excitable to a nonexcitable patch by localized currents, but the action potential develops only at the nodes of Ranvier (Fig. 10). The area under myelin wrap is practically nonconducting and almost entirely without Na⁺ channels, and the insulating properties of myelin restrict the currents on the nodes of Ranvier. The nodal membrane expresses a high density of channel per unit compared to the nonmyelinated axons and dendrites, which helps to depolarize the long internodal myelin. The local current flow from one node to the next causes a new action potential to be generated there, skipping the myelinated area—a phenomenon known as *salutatory conduction*, which involves the jump of action potential from node to node. This in turn speeds the progression of action potential and saves on the expression of channels and

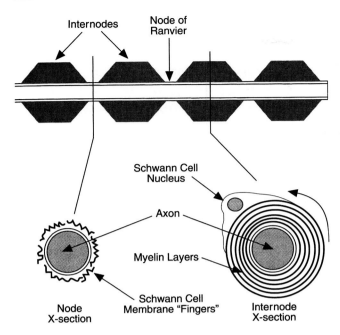

Fig. 10. Myelination of axons enhances the speed of action-potential signaling. Concentric layers of glial cell membranes known as myelin frequently envelop the nerve axons. The myelin wrap is interrupted at regular intervals, known as nodes of Ranvier. Only at these nodes, axon membrane is excitable, because the myelin sheath prevents the movement of ions away from the outside of the axon. The myelinated regions between nodes are known as internodes.

carriers and energy needed for the propagation of action potentials.

2.7. Neurons Do Not Require Energy to Conduct Action Potential

The Na^+-K^+ pump is needed to account for the leak of Na^+ and K^+ at rest and the small amount of these two ions transferred during the action potential. However, inhibition of ATP production does not block the action potential firing. Such cells can conduct several action potentials without difficulty, indicating that immediate metabolic energy is not required for this process. In unmyelinated neurons, the gain of Na^+ and the lost of K^+ per action potential depend on the axon diameter. For example, in the absence of ATP, squid axon of approx 1 mm diameter can generate about 10^5 action potentials, whereas mammalian axon of 0.2 μM diameter can only fire 10–15 action potentials before the intracellular Na^+ concentration would be doubled. The intracellular gain of Na^+ and the lost of K^+ per action potential in myelinated neurons are dramatically reduced because of the low-capacitance properties of myelin.

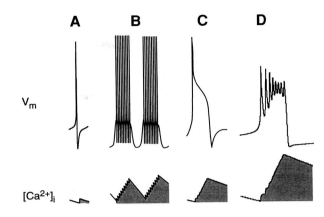

Fig. 11. Cell type-specific action-potential waveforms and calcium signals. Schematic representation of (A) a rapid single-action potential (axonal-type); (B) periodic bursting baseline firing of action potentials followed by quiescent periods; (C) plateau-type of action potentials (cardiac-type); and (D) plateau-bursting-type of action potentials (endocrine cell-type).

2.8. Action Potentials Can Have Different Shapes and Functions

Excitable cells differ in the pattern of action potentials and the frequency of spiking. The action potential in axons is sharp, and short in duration (Fig. 11A). Many neurons, including mollusk neurons, exhibit the periodic bursting activity followed by quiescent phases (Fig. 11B). Other cells, such as cardiac, fire a long-lasting plateau-type of action potentials (Fig. 11C), whereas pituitary somatotrophs, lactotrophs, and beta panceratic cells generate the plateau-bursting type of action potentials (Fig. 11D). The pattern of action potential is determined by the types and density of channels expressed in a particular cell type. The relevance of Na^+ and K^+ channels in generating action potential in axons has been previously described. In some cells, voltage-gated Ca^{2+} channels substitute for Na^+ channels in the depolarization phase of action potential. The delayed rectifier K^+ channels and ether a-go-go (erg) channels are the key players in shaping the action potential. Other K^+ channels can influence the pattern of action potential. For example, Ca^{2+}-activated K^+ channels in interactions with delayed rectifier K^+ channels can facilitate hyperpolarization of cells and delay the spike activity for several seconds. In cells that exhibit spontaneous firing of action potentials, variable channels can play a role in pacemaking (such as T-type Ca^{2+} channels and cyclic nucleotide-regulated cation channels) or oppose pacemaking (including M and inward rectifier K^+ channels).

Action potential is a signaling element in excitable cells. Both the frequency and the shape of action potential encode the signal. In cells or in regions of cells expressing voltage-gated Ca^{2+} channels, action potentials promote Ca^{2+} influx. In such cells, the shape of action-potential waveform and the pattern of firing determine the pattern of calcium signals. In general, rapid single-action potentials generate *localized Ca^2 signals*, known also as *domain Ca^{2+}*, which can be detected by nearby Ca^{2+}-activated K^+ channels, but not by fluorescent dyes. On the other hand, plateau and plateau-bursting action potentials can generate *global Ca^{2+} signals*. Periodic bursting activity followed by quiescent periods can also result in global, oscillatory Ca^{2+} signaling (Fig. 11, *bottom panels*).

3. VOLTAGE-GATED CHANNELS

Voltage-gated channels are macromolecular complexes in the lipid membrane containing the *aqueous pores* and *voltage-sensors*. The part of the pore, known as the *ionic selectivity filter* is narrow enough to distinguish among Na^+, K^+, Ca^{2+}, and Cl^-. The voltage-sensor is the charged component that senses the electrical field in the membrane and drives conformation changes, leading to opening and closing of the gates near the mouth of the pore. The voltage-dependent opening of ionic channels is known as activation. After only a few milliseconds, or in as much as several hundred milliseconds, the channel closes and the flow of ion is again blocked, in a process known as *inactivation*. Following inactivation, the channel returns to its resting state until the next membrane depolarization triggers the whole process again.

The first evidence that voltage-gated channels are discrete entities came from experiments with different drugs and toxins. Initially, tetrodotoxin (TTX) and saxitoxin were found to inhibit Na^+ current. Experiments with tetraethylammonium (TEA) ion in the presence and absence of TTX helped to identify K^+ channels. With time, the list of useful blockers of K^+ channels increased progressively, and included Cs^+, Ba^{2+}, 4-aminopyridine, apamin, and charybdotoxin. The identification and development of drugs and toxins useful for the characterization of voltage-gated Ca^{2+} channels also progressed, and included dihydropyridines, verapamin, Cd^{2+}, Ni^{2+}, and ω-conotoxin GVIA. The part of ion channel molecule operates as receptor, binding a drug in a specific and reversible manner. In many cases, this has been used to quantify channels in specific tissues. Binding of drugs also affects the conductivity of channels. Two sister compounds may have opposite effects on conductivity.

For example, nifedipine acts as an antagonist and Bay K 8644 acts as an agonist for L-type voltage-gated Ca^{2+} channels.

Combined pharmacological and electrophysiological experiments have revealed that there is a high diversity of K^+ channels, whereas voltage-gated Ca^{2+} and Na^+ channels are less diverse. The same combination of tools, as well as the use of fluorescent antibodies for specific ion channels, has also confirmed that ion channels can be highly localized. In addition to the nodes of Ranvier, these include dendrites, synaptic boutons, and nerve terminals. Finally, recent molecular biology- and protein chemistry-based techniques have provided a great deal of information about the structure of ion channels. A remarkable finding was that that the α-subunit of Na^+ channels and $α_1$-subunit of Ca^{2+} channels have similar amino acid sequences and folding. The K^+-channel α subunit is smaller, but with obvious homology to Na^+ and Ca^{2+} channels, indicating that these three families of channels form a homologous gene superfamily. In rodents, 9 genes for Na^+-channel family, 10 genes for Ca^{2+}-channel-family, and over 75 genes for the K^+-channel family have been identified.

3.1. Gigaseal and Patch-Clamp Methods

Earlier studies by Hodgkin, Huxley, and Katz suggested the presence of discrete ion-channel proteins with an aqueous pore permeable to ions. Neher and Sakmann confirmed this hypothesis. They developed the patch-clamp method for single-channel recording, which uses glass electrodes with the tip opening of several micrometers in diameter and with a smooth surface achieved by heat polishing. By pressing the pipet against the living cells, they recorded a single-channel current with an acetylcholine-activated channel for the first time. Hamill and collaborators further developed this technique by showing that the pipet can fuse with membrane to form a high-resistance seal. As shown in Fig. 12, this can be achieved by application of gentle suction, drawing a small patch of membrane into the electrode opening. After a few seconds, an unexpectedly high resistance and mechanical stability is achieved between the membrane and the glass surface, with a negligible flow of ions between the two surfaces. This seal is known as a *gigaseal* because electrical resistances between the inside of the electrode and the extracellular fluid are in tens of gigaohms. If the patch of membrane contains an individual ion channel, most of the current passes from the electrode

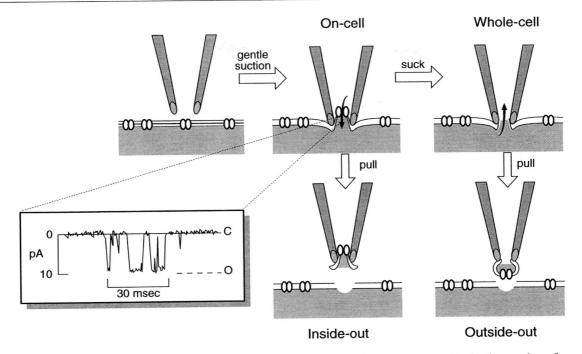

Fig. 12. The patch-clamp recording methods. All patch-clamp methods use glass electrodes with the tip opening of several μm in diameter and with a smooth polished surface. The methods start with placing the electrode against an intact cell and application of gentle suction. After establishing a strong bond, the voltage of the electrode interior can be clamped at any level, and single channels can be recorded in this on-cell mode. The inset illustrates the sporadic opening of Ca^{2+}-activated K^+ channels; o, open, conducting state; c, closed state. As indicated in the figure, the same electrode can be used to obtain the additional patch-clamp configurations.

flow through the single channel. This model of recording is known as *on-cell* or *cell-attached patch* mode, and Inset in Fig. 12 illustrates K^+-current movement through Ca^{2+}-controlled K^+ channels recorded by this method.

The gigaseal permits three additional modes of recording. The seal between the membrane and pipet is so tight that its withdrawal frequently rips the patch of membrane from the cell. The patch is sealed to the pipet and can be bathed in variety of solutions. This configuration is termed *inside-out* or *excised-patch* mode (Fig. 12). The cell-attached patch can be ruptured by suction without affecting the seal to the cell, or the permeabilization of the patch membrane can be achieved by antibiotics, including nystatin and amphotericin. These configurations are known as *whole-cell* and *perforated-cell* modes, respectively. In the first model, the interior of cells is dialyzed in a short time by the recording pipet solution. The perforated patch membrane is semipermeable; thus, it is permeable only for monovalent ions. Finally, from the whole-cell mode one can achieve the *outside-out patch* mode by pulling the pipet away from the cell (Fig. 12).

3.2. Voltage-Gated Na⁺ Channels Depolarize Cells

The family of Na^+ channels is a relatively homogenous with respect to their molecular structures and functions. Na^+ channels can be classified into two general groups, TTX-sensitive and -insensitive. The sensitivity of channels to TTX varies, depending on tissue; nerve and skeletal-muscle Na^+ channels are more sensitive to TTX than the cardiac channel. Mammalian TTX-sensitive Na^+ channels expressed in the brain are composed of large (260,000) α subunit associated with $β_1$ (36,000) and $β_2$ (32,000) polypeptides, whereas Na^+ channels in skeletal muscle are composed only of α and $β_1$ subunit. The probable arrangement of these subunits is shown in Fig. 13. The four repeated domains of α subunit have greater than 50% internal sequence identity. Each domain contains six segments that make TM α helices, whereas $β_1$ and $β_2$ subunits have a single TM domain. When expressed, α subunit of skeletal muscle accounts for TTX binding site, pore, voltage gate and sensor, and contains the sites for phosphorylation by protein kinases on the intracellular surface. Mammals express nine genes for α subunit,

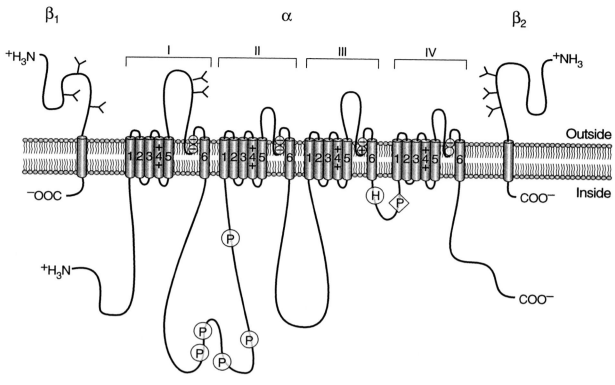

Fig. 13. Structural transmembrane folding model of voltage-gated Na⁺ channels. In this and Figs. 17 and 19, α-helices are illustrated as cylinders, and extracellular and intracellular chains of amino acids as full lines. Positively charged 4TM domain illustrates voltage-sensor. P illustrate sites for phosphorylation by protein kinases A and C, respectively.

and the dendrogram shown in Fig. 14 indicates the similarity in their structure.

As discussed earlier, the main function of these channels is to depolarize cells and generate the upstroke of the action potential, and to control the firing amplitude. In many excitable cell-types, these channels are solely responsible for the rapid regenerative upstroke of an action potential. In others, they act in conjunction with voltage-gated Ca^{2+} channels to depolarize cells. The channels from this family can also control pacemaking. There are significant kinetic differences between the fast TTX-sensitive and the slower TTX-insensitive Na⁺ channels, as well as the differences in the pattern of action-potential waveforms in cells expressing these channels. TTX-sensitive Na⁺ channels inactivate almost completely with depolarization to 0 mV and beyond (Fig. 15). A subtype of these channels, however, does not show complete inactivation. TTX-sensitive channels are

permeable for Na⁺, but also for K⁺, but less well (7–10% of that for Na⁺), and to several other ions with order $Na^+ = Li+ > Tl > K^+ > Rb > Cs^+$.

The direct evidence in favor of the hypothesis that S4 segment serves as a voltage-sensor comes from mutagenesis studies with Na⁺ and K⁺ channels. These segments are highly conserved among voltage-gated channels and consist of repeated triplets of two hydrophobic residues followed by a positively charged amino acid. Neutralization of positive charges leads to progressive reduction of the steepness of voltage-dependent gating, as expected for a voltage-sensor. However, a single cluster of three hydrophobic amino acids in the intracellular loop connecting 3TM and 4TM domain is required for inactivation of Na⁺ channels. The substitution of these residues with hydrophilic ones leads to generation of a non-inactivating channel. It appears that Phe[1489] is a critical residue. A *"hinged-lead model"* was proposed to explain the

Channel Name	Human Gene Name	Human Chromosome
Na$_V$1.1	SCN1A	2q24
Na$_V$1.2	SCN2A	2q23-24
Na$_V$1.3	SCN3A	2q24
Na$_V$1.7	SCN9A	2q24
Na$_V$1.4	SCN4A	17q23-25
Na$_V$1.6	SCN8A	12q13
Na$_V$1.5	SCN5A	3p21
Na$_V$1.8	SCN10A	3p22-24
Na$_V$1.9	SCN11A	3p21-24

Fig. 14. Classification of Na$^+$ channels. Figure was adapted from Hille, 2001, Sinauer Associates, Inc. For information about the percentage of amino acid identity among the members of this family, *see* Goldin et al. Neuron 2000; 28:365.

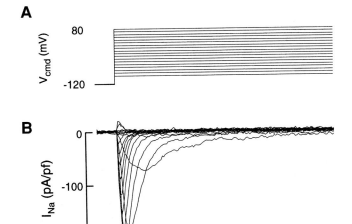

Fig. 15. Activation and inactivation properties of voltage-gated Na$^+$ channels in pituitary gonadotrophs. Voltage-gated I_{Na} were elicited by 100-ms voltage step from –90 mV to 80 mV in 10-mV steps from a holding potential of –120 mV. (Derived from Van Goor et al., Mol Endocrinol 2001; 15:1222.)

mechanism of inactivation of this channel. According to this model, a cluster of hydrophobic residues together with Phe[1489] enters the intracellular mouth of the pore, providing an effective latch to keep the channel inactivated in depolarized cells.

3.3. Voltage-Gated Calcium Channels Have Dual Functions in Excitable Cells

The Ca^{2+}-selectivity and voltage-sensitivity of these channels are common features between two major groups of voltage-gated Ca^{2+} channels, which are separated by their sensitivity to changes in membrane potential. The first group of channels requires only weak membrane depolarization to open. Consequently, they are activated at relatively hyperpolarized membrane potentials and are known as *low-voltage activated* (LVA) Ca^{2+} channels. Activation of these channels is followed by their rapid and complete inactivation, and a strong membrane hyperpolarization is required to bring them out of steady inactivation. Because of such inactivation properties, these channels are often referred to as transient or T-type Ca^{2+} channels. The second group of voltage-gated Ca^{2+}

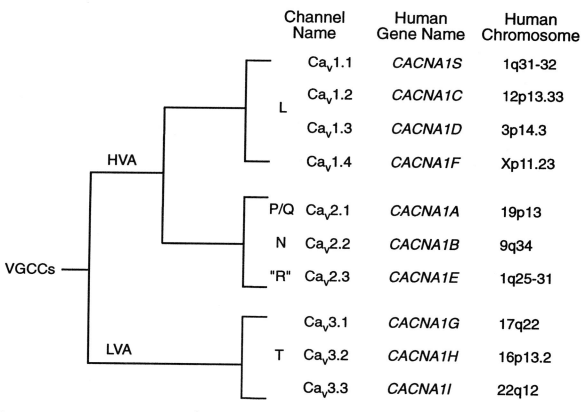

	Channel Name	Human Gene Name	Human Chromosome
L	Ca$_V$1.1	CACNA1S	1q31-32
	Ca$_V$1.2	CACNA1C	12p13.33
	Ca$_V$1.3	CACNA1D	3p14.3
	Ca$_V$1.4	CACNA1F	Xp11.23
P/Q	Ca$_V$2.1	CACNA1A	19p13
N	Ca$_V$2.2	CACNA1B	9q34
"R"	Ca$_V$2.3	CACNA1E	1q25-31
T	Ca$_V$3.1	CACNA1G	17q22
	Ca$_V$3.2	CACNA1H	16p13.2
	Ca$_V$3.3	CACNA1I	22q12

Fig. 16. Classification of voltage-gated Ca^{2+} channels. Figure was derived from Hille, 2001 Sinauer Associates, Inc. For information about percentage of amino acid identity among members of this family of channels, *see* Erlet et al., Neuron 2000; 25:533.

channels requires moderate to strong membrane depolarization to open, and are known as *high-voltage activated* (HVA) Ca^{2+} channels. Among this group, biophysical and pharmacological studies have identified multiple subtypes that can be distinguished by their single-channel conductance, pharmacology, and metabolic regulation: L-, N-, P/Q-, and R-type Ca^{2+} channels (Fig. 16). The L-type calcium channels are sensitive to dihydropyridines and exhibit slow inactivation. N, P/Q, and R-type channels inactivate rapidly but incomplete and are dihydropyridine-insensitive. N-type channels are sensitive to w-conotoxin GVIA, P/Q channels are sensitive to w-Aga- IVA, and R-type channels are resistant to both toxins.

Consistent with the functional studies, molecular cloning has identified several genes that encode different VGCC subtypes. The first Ca^{2+} channel was purified from skeletal muscle, as it is a highly enriched source of L-type Ca^{2+} channels. Purification of the channel has identified five subunits, including a large α_1 (200–260 Kd) subunit and four smaller ancillary subunits: α_2, β, γ, and δ. Since the first α_1 subunit was

cloned from skeletal muscle, several other isoforms have been identified. The α_1 subunit consists of four homologous repeats, each one composed of six TM segments (Fig. 17). Located within the α_1 subunit are: the voltage sensor, gating machinery, channel pore, and multiple PKA phosphorylation sites. Sequence comparison indicates three subfamilies: L-, N-, and T-like channels. As shown in Fig. 16, the L-group is composed of at least four genes, and N- and T-groups of three genes. The complexity of these channels is further increased by alternative splicing and generation of heteropolymers with wild-type channels. In general, voltage-gated calcium channels have diverged much more from each other than Na$^+$ channels.

Voltage-gated Ca^{2+} channels serve two major functions in cells. One function is to generate and/or shape action potentials and to control the gating of several channels (*electrogenic functions*). The other is to allow Ca^{2+} influx during the transient depolarization, which acts as an intracellular second messenger controlling a variety of cellular functions, and this *regulatory func-*

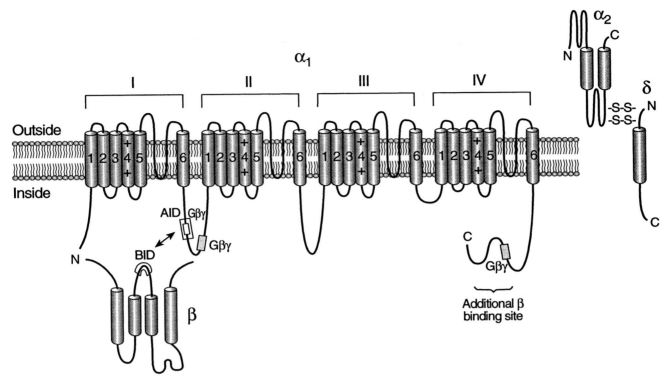

Fig. 17. Structural TM folding model of voltage-gated calcium-channel complex. Diagram indicates the putative TM topologies of α_1 subunit, as well as α_2, β, and δ subunits. The biding sites for $G_{\beta/\gamma}$ dimer are also shown. (Derived from AC Dolphin, J Physiol 1998; 506:3.)

tion is comparable to the actions of membrane receptors. LVA Ca^{2+} channels exhibit rapid and complete voltage-dependent inactivation and are unlikely candidates to promote sufficient Ca^{2+} influx. The major function of these channels is electrogenic; at the resting potential, T-type channels depolarize cells to the threshold level for Na^+ or Ca^{2+} spike. However, HVA channels, inactivate incompletely and are solely responsible to keeping the cells depolarized for a prolonged period. Such action potentials drive Ca^{2+} to generate intracellular Ca^{2+} signals of sufficient amplitude to trigger Ca^{2+}-dependent processes such as neurotransmission. In accordance with this, HVA channels are found at synaptic endings, and Na^+ channels in axons.

Pituitary cells also provide a good example of excitable cells translating their electricity into the intracellular actions of Ca^{2+}. Although three secretory anterior pituitary cells—lactotrophs, somatotrophs, and gonadotrophs—fire extracellular Ca^{2+}-dependent action potentials, voltage-gated Ca^{2+} influx triggers secretion only in lactotrophs and somatotrophs. These two cell-types fire a long-lasting (1–2 s) plateau-bursting-type of action potential spontaneously which generates high-amplitude Ca^{2+} signals. In contrast, gonadotrophs fire single (10–20 ms) action potentials that have a limited capacity to promote Ca^{2+} influx (Fig. 18A). When clamped at –90 mV and depolarized to –10 mV for variable times, the increase in intracellular calcium concentrations was comparable in all three cell-types (Fig. 18C). These observations indicate that the capacity of voltage-gated Ca^{2+} channels to promote Ca^{2+} influx is comparable in three cell types, but that duration of spontaneous action potentials in gonadotrophs is not sufficient to drive threshold Ca^{2+} signals needed for exocytosis.

Co-expression of several Ca^{2+}-channel subtypes in a single cell is common in neurons and endocrine cells. For example, both T- and L-type Ca^{2+} channels are expressed in excitable endocrine cells. In sensory neurons, T-type and L-type Ca^{2+} channels are co-expressed with N-type Ca^{2+} channels. In other neurons, P/Q-type Ca^{2+} channels are also found in conjunction with other VGCC subtypes. Although multiple Ca^{2+}-channel subtypes may be co-expressed in the same cell, they are often distributed nonuniformly in different regions. In inferior olivary neurons, HVA Ca^{2+} channels are found mostly, but not exclusively, in the

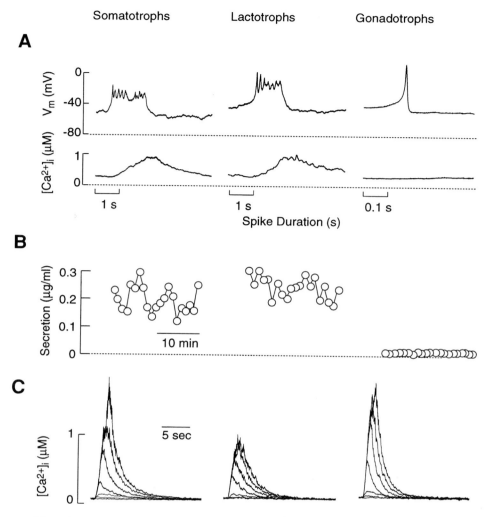

Fig. 18. Cell type-specific action-potential-secretion coupling in spontaneously active pituitary cells. (**A**) The pattern of action potentials and intracellular Ca^{2+} in single cells. Electrical activity and intracellular Ca^{2+} were simultaneously measured in spontaneously active cells. (**B**) Action potential-dependent hormone secretion. Secretion was measured from perifused pituitary cells and normalized to account for a difference in the size of somatotroph, lactotroph, and gonadotroph populations. (**C**) Depolarization-induced rise in intracellular Ca^{2+}. Cells were clamped at –90 mV and depolarized to –10 mV for 25 ms to 2 s. (From Van Goor et al., J Biol Chem 2001; 276:33,840.)

dendrites, whereas LVA Ca^{2+} channels are usually found in the cell body. The distribution of HVA Ca^{2+}-channel subtypes within the same cell may also be nonuniform. In neurons, extensive expression of the α_1 subunits of the N- and P/Q-type Ca^{2+} channels has been found in the dendritic shafts and presynaptic nerve terminals, but not the cell body. Conversely, the α_1 subunits of L-type Ca^{2+} channels were found predominantly in the soma and proximal dendrites, whereas the α_1 subunit of the R-type Ca^{2+} channel was found predominantly in the cell body of central nervous system (CNS) neurons. The nonuniform distribution of Ca^{2+}-channel subtypes likely reflects their different functional roles.

3.4. Potassium and Chloride Channels Tend to Dampen Excitation

The common characteristic of K^+ and Cl^- ions in neurons is their negative equilibrium potential; thus, activation of channels conducting these ions draws the membrane potential closer to their equilibrium potentials and farther from the threshold for firing. These channels tend to stabilize the membrane potential by setting the resting potential, repolarize and hyperpolarize cells after a depolarizing event, and control the interspike interval.

There is an impressive structural and functional diversity of K^+ channels. Over 100 related mammalian genes for K^+-channel subunits have been identified.

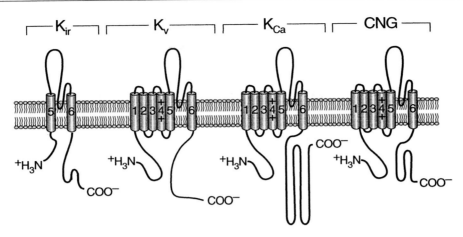

Fig. 19. Structural transmembrane folding model of voltage-gated K^+ channels. K_{ir}, inward rectifier k^+ channels; K_v, voltage-gated K^+ channels; K_{Ca}, Ca^{2+}-activated K^+ channels; CNG, cyclic nucleotide-gated channels.

They occur in several major architectural forms (shown in Fig. 19). The principal element of all K^+ channels is 2TM core, which is found in the bacterial K^+ channel known as KcsA and inwardly rectifying K^+ channels (K_{ir}). Voltage-gated K^+ channels have four additional TM segments, and the S4 segment endows them with voltage-sensitivity. Both 2TM and 6TM channels are homo- or heterotetramers of principal subunits, frequently associated with auxiliary β subunits. There are also 4TM- and 8TM-type of K^+ channels. The simplified dendrogram of major classes of K^+ channels is shown in Fig. 20.

Potassium channels have a similar permeability mechanism. They contain the K^+-channel signature sequence in the selectivity filter and show comparable ion selectivity order ($Tl+ > K^+ > Rb > NH_4$) and are usually blocked by Cs^+. Their permeability for Na^+ and Li^+ is low. In addition to Cs^+, these channels are blocked by TEA from the inside and outside, and some of them by Ba^{2+}. Their opening is frequently modulated by receptors—through G-protein action directly as well as indirectly—through intracellular messengers and kinases. Intracellular Ca^{2+} controls the activity of two K^+ channels, large-conductance voltage-gated (BK) channels and small-conductance voltage-insensitive (SK) channels. BK channels may be blocked by charybdotoxin, iberiotoxin, and paxilline, whereas the SK channel is blocked by apamin. Cyclic nucleotides control activity of two nonselective cation channels from this family, hypeprolarization-activated I_h, and cyclic-nucleotide-gated (CNG) chan-nels. *Cis*-L-diltiazem blocks CNG channels intracellularly. ATP controls an inward rectifier K^+ ($K_{ir}6$) channel. Extracellular $Cs+$ and Ba^{2+} block K_{ir} and erg channels, whereas E4301 specifically inhibits erg channels.

Potassium channels are easily distinguishable by their gating characteristics. There are two classes of *delayed rectifiers*, fast and slow, which serve different functions in neurons. Rapidly activated, delayed-rectifier K^+ (I_K) channels belong to the K_v class of channels. This channel is expressed in unmyelinated axons, motoneurons, and fast skeletal muscle, and is responsible for very short action potentials. Slow delayed rectifiers expressed in cardiac tissue are from erg and KCNQ classes, and are also involved in repolarization of cells. As indicated by their name, the gating kinetics of these channels is slow, which is reflected on the shape of action potential. Erg channels are also expressed in pituitary cells, and play a role in control of spontaneous and TRH-induced electrical activity. Neuronal and endocrine slow-gating KCNQ channels cannot be activated by a single action potential because they gate too slow, but play an important role in control of resting potential. These channels do not inactivate, and are partially open at the resting potential. The best-known member of these channels is *M channel*, which is made up of several subunits from the KCNQ family. The voltage-dependent activity of this channel is modulated by Ca^{2+}-mobilizing receptors. A single cell frequently expresses several types of delayed rectifiers.

Another group of voltage-gated K^+ channels is known by several names: *fast transient, transient outward, rapidly inactivating*, and *A (IA) channels*. These channels are activated when cells are depolarized after prolonged hyperpolarization. A heterogeneous variety of gene products from the K_v family accounts for their formation. Fig. 21 (*right panels*), illustrates a separation of I_A from total K^+ current in an excitable cell. In steady state, this channel conducts in narrow (–65

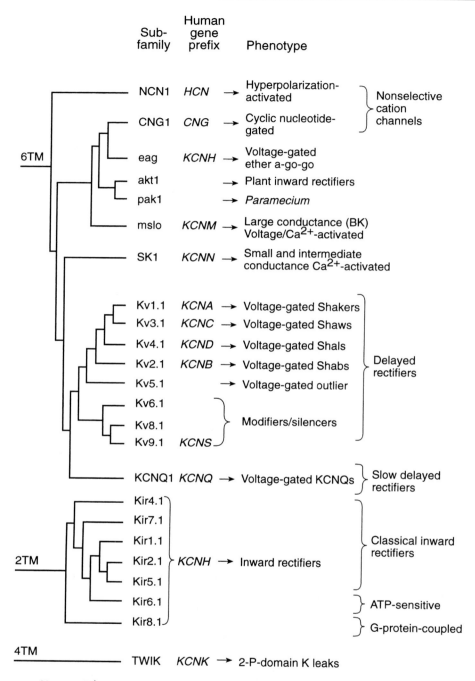

Fig. 20. A dendrogram of known K⁺-channel genes sorted by similarity of amino acid sequence. The alignment was made using a short amino acid sequence in the P-regions of the predominantly mammalian sequences. (Diagram was prepared by WJ Joiner and AM Quinn, and adapted from Hille, 2001.)

to –40 mV) negative voltage range. Because of their rapid inactivation, these channels play important roles in repetitive firing, by opposing the developing interspike depolarization. A single action potential is sufficient to inactivate these channels, and repolarization/hypeprolarization of membrane results from the activity of other K⁺ channels. During a hyperpolarizing period, I_A channels recover from inactivation, whereas other K⁺ channels are shut off. This allows activation of depolarizing currents, which are for some time controlled by I_A. However, because of their progressive depolarization, a balance is lost, and cells fire

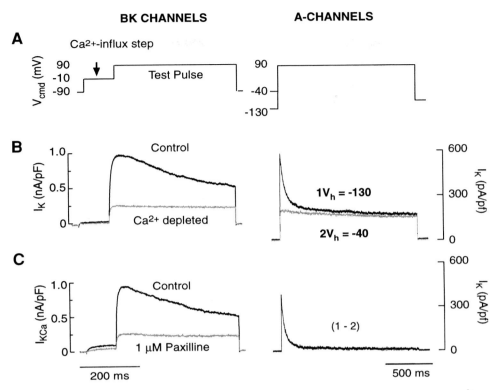

Fig. 21. Characterization of voltage-gated K$^+$ channels in pituitary cells. (**A**) (*Left panel*) Voltage-gated Ca^{2+} influx is required to activate BK channels in pituitary somatotrophs. Two-pulse protocol was used to monitor K$^+$ current. Cells were clamped at –90 mV and depolarized to –10 mV for 100 ms to activated voltage-gated Ca^{2+} channels, followed by 500-ms test pulse to 90 mV. Current was recorded in cells bathed in Ca^{2+}-containing and Ca^{2+}-deficient medium (**B**) and in Ca^{2+}-containing medium in the presence or absence of paxiline (**C**), a specific blocker of BK channels. (Derived from Van Goor et al., J Neurosci 2001; 21:5902.) (*Right panel*) Isolation of transient A current from voltage-gated K$^+$ currents in lactotrophs. Currents were elicited by 1.5-s voltage-steps from –90 to 90 mV from a holding potential of –130 mV (black lines) and –40 mV (gray lines). A-current was isolated by a point-by-point subtraction of two currents. (Derived from Van Goor et al., Mol Endocrinol 2001; 15:1222.)

another action potential. Thus, in such neurons I$_A$ channels control the frequency of firing.

I$_A$ channels are the first K$^+$ channels to be cloned, and the first to be mutated in order to clarify the gating mechanism. The N-terminus of these channels serves as an inactive particle, and all four N-terminus are involved in this process known as "*a ball-and-chain*" mechanism. According to this model of inactivation, the N-terminal segment serves as a tethered ball that binds to the intracellular mouth of the pore. In an intact channel, any of four balls can do it. The mutant channel with deleted N terminus does not inactivate, whereas inactivation is restored by injection of synthetic peptides with the identical amino acid sequence as native N-termini. In contrast to Na$^+$ channels, where the critical residue for inactivation is located just 12 amino acids away from the membrane, the inactivation particle of I$_A$ is located over 200 residues from the plasma membrane.

Calcium influx and agonist-induced release of Ca^{2+} from the endoplasmic reticulum (ER) opens *Ca^{2+}-activated K$^+$ channels* (I$_{K-Ca}$) that hyperpolarize the membrane. The structure of SK-type of I$_{K-Ca}$ is highly comparable to intermediate I$_{K-Ca}$, and both channels are only distantly related to BK I$_{K-Ca}$. SK/IK channels have little voltage-dependence, whereas BK channels have steep voltage-sensitivity. Figure 21 (*left panels*) illustrates a procedure for identification of BK channels in an excitable cell. In GnRH-secreting neurons, pituitary lactotrophs, and GH cells, the spike increase in intracellular Ca^{2+} activates apamin-sensitive SK channels to induce transient membrane hyperpolarization. Similarly, the repetitive membrane hyperpolarization in pituitary gonadotrophs is mediated by the transient activation of SK I$_{K-Ca}$ channels by the oscillatory Ca^{2+} release. There are at least three reasons why I$_{K-Ca}$ channels are incorporated into the Ca^{2+} signaling pathway. First, activation of these channels may relieve the

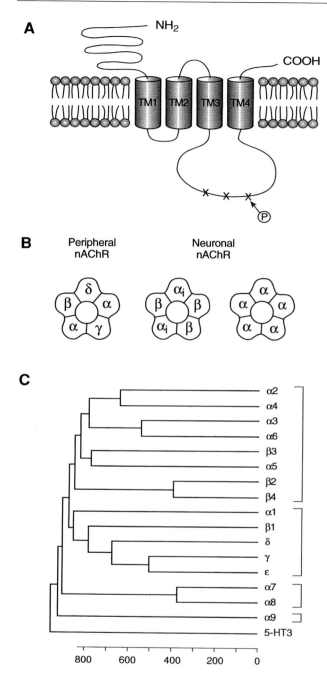

Fig. 22. Structural organization of muscle and neuronal nicotinic channels (nAChRs). **(A)** Putative transmembrane organization of nAChRs. TM, transmembrane domain; X, the potential phosphorylation sites. **(B)** Front view of the models of muscle and neuronal nAChRs. **(C)** Simplified dendrograms of the members of the nicotinic-receptor-channel family. (Derived from JP Changeux Brain Res Rev 1998; 26:198.)

steady inactivation of voltage-gated Na^+ and Ca^{2+} channels, which stimulates or enhances AP generation in some cells. Second, activation of I_{K-Ca} channels may

prevent a lethal increase in intracellular Ca^{2+} concentration by limiting voltage-gated Ca^{2+} influx. Finally, activation of I_{K-Ca} channels and the resulting membrane hyperpolarization may serve to synchronize electrical activity and secretion in cell networks.

Inward rectifier K^+ (K_{ir}) channels are known as *anomalous rectifier*, because their conductance increases under hyperpolarization and decreases under depolarization. The term "inward rectifier" describes their activation of inward current under hyperpolarization, leading to K^+ influx, and almost no K^+ efflux under depolarization. However, this small K^+ efflux carries their usual physiological function. The α subunit of these channels has 2TM domains and functional channel is a tetramer, sometimes with auxiliary subunits. These channels participate to the control of resting potential, and a strong depolarization closes them. The majority of channels are controlled by intracellular messengers. For example, the members of Kir1 and Kir2 are regulated by PKA and PKC, Kir3 by G proteins, and Kir6 by intracellular ATP.

Electrophysiological studies indicate the presence of many types of chloride channels. However, their structural identification is in progress. So-called *Torpedo channels* were the first chloride channels to be cloned. The mammalian version of this channel, called *CCC-1*, is expressed in skeletal muscle and has 11TM segments. Another cloned chloride channel is *cystic fibrosis transmembrane conductance regulator* (CFTR). For its activation, this channel requires phosphorylation by PKA and hydrolysis of ATP. Two members of these channels, GABA and glycine, are also cloned and operate as ligand-gated channels. Like I_{K-Ca}, there are *Ca^{2+}-activated Cl^- channels* (I_{Cl-Ca}). This channel is voltage-dependent, and intracellular Ca^{2+} lowers the depolarization required for their opening. *Maxi-Cl^--channels* are so named because of their large (over 400 pS) single-channel conductance. Finally, *background Cl^- channels* are found in many tissues and participate to the stabilization of membrane potential. Chloride channels are not specific for Cl^-, but conduct many small anions as well as small organic acids, and it is appropriate to refer to them as anion channels.

3.5. Cyclic Nucleotide-Gated Channels are Nonselective Cation Channels

Figure 20 shows that the family of K^+ channels has two members, I_h and CNG channels, which functionally dissociate from other members. Their activation does not dump excitation, but it increases the firing of action potential. Such a paradoxical role for channels that structurally belong to the K^+-channel family comes from their permeability properties; both channels are cation-nonselective. These channels are activated by voltage and by cyclic nucleotides. The intracellular actions of cAMP and cGMP are usually mediated by their PKA and PKG, respectively. However, I_h and CNG channels are directly activated by cAMP and/or cGMP.

Like K_{ir} channels, I_h *channels* are activated by hyperpolarization beyond –60 mV (h stands for hyperpolarization), do not inactivate, and conduct Na^+ and K^+. In cells expressing these channels, their activation leads to slow depolarization, an action consistent with their equilibrium potential of about –30 mV. I_h channels were first identified in cardiac sinoatrial node cells, and subsequently in a variety of peripheral and central neurons. Their voltage-sensitivity is modulated by cAMP. I_h channels serve three principal functions in excitable cells: they determine the resting potential in cells, generate or contribute to the pacemaker depolarization that controls rhythmic activity in spontaneously firing cells, and compensate for inhibitory postsynaptic potentials. A small fraction of I_h is tonically activated at rest and determines the first two functions of these channels. In accordance with this, inhibition of spontaneously active I_h by low extracellular Cs^+ results in hyperpolarization of cells and abolition of spontaneous firing. Also, hyperpolarization of cells by inhibitory postsynaptic potential will increase I_h. Furthermore, in sinoatrial node cells, the hyperpolarization that follows action potential activates these channels, leading to slow depolarization toward the threshold for new action potential. β-adrenergic receptor-mediated stimulation of adenylyl cyclase, and increase in cAMP enhance the size and speed of I_h, resulting in an increase in the firing frequency and heart rate. In thamalic neurons, these channels are crucial in generating the rhythmic bursts of action potentials.

Molecular cloning has revealed over 20 genes that encode different subtypes of CNG α subunits in invertebrates and vertebrates. The subtypes cloned to date are defined as *rod*, *cone*, and *olfactory* CNG channels. These channels are heterotetramers. β subunits do not form functional channels, but modulate the channel properties of α sununits. As with other channels, differential splicing of primary transcripts yields channels of altered structure and behavior. The channels are permeable to Na^+, K^+, and Ca^{2+}, but not to Cl^- and other anions. Rod channels are activated by cGMP and are practically insensitive to cAMP, whereas olfactory CNG channels are activated by cAMP nearly as well as by cGMP. The channels are also expressed in a surprising array of nonsensory cells.

CNG channels are not voltage-sensitive, but their current-voltage curves show an outward rectification. This is a result of activation of Ca^{2+} binding sites in the pore of the channel. In physiological extracellular concentrations, Ca^{2+} binds to this site, resulting in a decrease in conductivity. Other divalent cations mimic the action of Ca^{2+}. In the presence of divalent cations, the unitary conductance of rod channels is less than 100 fS, and in their absence the conductance is approx 30 pS. Calcium also modulates the activity of CNG channels in a calmodulin-dependent manner, leading to a decrease in the sensitivity of CNG channels to cyclic nucleotides. The blockade of conductivity by Ca^{2+} is incomplete, and this ion passes through CNG channels. For example, about 15% of the current by rod CNG channels is carried by Ca^{2+}, and such an influx is a crucial signal for biochemical events that terminate light response. Channels in cones and olfactory neurons allow more Ca^{2+} influx.

4. EXTRACELLULAR LIGAND-GATED CATION CHANNELS

The activation of ligand-gated receptor channels depends on the delivery and binding of a ligand to the extracellular domain of these receptor channels, and termination of their activities requires removal of the ligand, which is usually mediated by a specific pathway for ligand degradation and/or uptake. Because ligand-gated channels are generally activated by neurotransmitters, they are also known as *neurotransmitter-controlled channels*. There are two classes of ligand-gated channels, the *excitatory cation-selective-receptor channels*, operated by acetylcholine, glutamate, 5-hydroxytryptamine (5-HT), and adenosine 5'-triphosphate (ATP), and the *inhibitory anion-selective-receptor channels*, activated by γ-aminobutyic acid (GABA) and glycine. Structural information obtained by cDNA cloning of ligand-gated receptor-channels has led to the identification of several families of evolutionary related proteins. Interestingly, many ligand-gated channels share common agonists with G-protein-coupled receptors (*see* Chapters 4 and 5).

The $5-HT_3$, GABA, and glycine-receptor channels possess structural features similar to the *nicotinic acetylcholine-receptor channel* (nAChR), thus, these receptors can be grouped as one family. These channels are composed of five subunits (pentamers), each of which contributes to the ionic pore. All subunits have a large extracellular amino-terminal region followed by four hydrophobic putative membrane-spanning segments and an extracellular carboxyl terminus (Fig. 22A). *Glutamate-receptor channels* are composed of four TM segments, but their M2 segment forms a pore-loop structure, entering and exiting the cell membrane from the intracellular side. Thus, the N terminus is extracellularly located, whereas the C terminus is intracellularly located, and is regulated by signaling molecules, including the kinases (Fig. 23A). A detailed analysis of the intra-subunit interactions that govern glutamate-receptor assembly indicates that these channels are dimmers of dimmers. The ATP-gated *purinergic-receptor channels*, termed P2X, have only two putative TM domains with the N- and C-terminus facing the cytoplasm (Fig. 24A). As with nicotinic and glutamate channels, the functional diversity of P2X channels is generated by subunit multimerization. It is not clear whether the functional channels are composed of three or four subunits.

During prolonged stimulations with neurotransmitters, the conductance through ligand-gated receptor channels decreases in a process called *desensitization*. At the single-channel-level recordings, desensitization corresponds to the closure of channels during steady agonist application. Desensitized channels are unable to respond to added neurotransmitter, but recover their sensitivity after the agonist is removed. The rates of desensitization and recovery are receptor-specific. Desensitization is analogous to inactivation of voltage-gated channels. The molecular mechanism and physiological importance of desensitization are not fully characterized.

4.1. Neuronal Nicotinic Acetylcholine Receptor Channels Conduct Ca²⁺

The native nAChR was initially identified as a pentamer protein of about 300,000 MW from the fish electrical organ. Recombinant DNA studies revealed close homologies between nAChR subunit sequences derived from electrical organ and skeletal muscle tissue, as well as between muscle and neuronal nAChRs. Five peripheral nAChR subunits, labeled as α_1, β_1, δ, γ, and ϵ, and ten neuronal nAChR subunits, labeled as α_2 to α_9 and β_2-β_4, were identified (Fig. 22A). In both muscle and neuronal nAChRs, the large N-terminal domain contains the ligand-binding sites. The TM segment M2 forms the wall of ion channel, and the variable C-terminal domain faces the cytoplasm and is

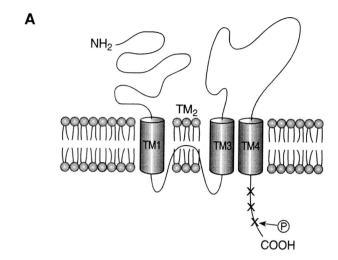

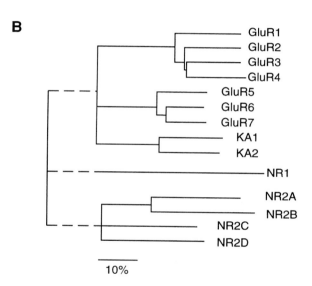

Fig. 23. Structural organization of glutamate-receptor channels. (**A**) TM topology of glutamate ion channels. TM, transmembrane domain. TM$_2$ does not cross the membrane, although it contributes to the lining of the pore. X, the potential phosphorylation sites. (**B**) Simplified dendrograms of the members of the glutamate-receptor channel family. (Derived from S Ozawa, Prog Neurobiol 1998; 54:581.)

subject to regulation by phosphorylation (Fig. 22A). Both peripheral and neuronal receptors form heteropentamers that form barrel-like structures. In muscle and electrical organs, nAChRs are composed of four subunits: α, β, γ or ϵ, and δ. The neuronal AchRs assemble according to the general 2α, 3β stoichiometry, with possibly more than one α-subunit class within a pentamer. Fig. 22B illustrates the models for periph-

A

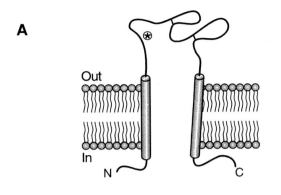

B

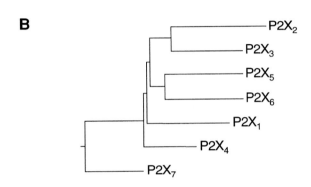

C

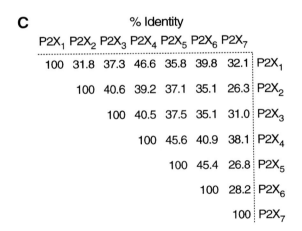

Fig. 24. Structural organization of cation-conducting purinergic-receptor channels. (A) Topological model of purinergic-receptor channels. (B) The relationship among seven P2X subunits. (C) Percentage identity of 7 rat P2X subunits. (Derived from Khakh et al., Pharmacol Rev 2001; 53:107.)

eral and neuronal nAChRs. In reconstitution experiments, neuronal subunits also form functional homo-oligomeric channels. In addition, multiple combinations of both α and β subunits from two or more different

subtypes form a wide range of functional hetero-oligomers. These multiple combinations of nAChR subunits possess distinct pharmacological and physiological properties. Also, the subunit composition determines the rate of desensitization. Furthermore, the distribution of neuronal nAChR subunits within the brain of adult animals varies. The expression of these subunits during embryonic and postnatal development is highly specific for a particular subunit.

Neuronal nAChRs exhibit a higher permeability to Ca^{2+} than muscle and electrical organ receptors. This is because of the multiple combinatorial possibilities available for the assembly of the various subunits into hetero-oligomers. For example, the α_7/α_8 subunit-based homo-ologomers are highly permeable for Ca^{2+} compared to Na^+, whereas subunits α_2 to α_6 and β_2 to β_4 from hetero-oligomeric channels have similar permeabilities for Ca^{2+} and Na^+. The specific amino acids important for Ca^{2+} permeability and selectivity of neuronal nAChRs are located in the M2 domain. The muscle nAChRs are the least permeable to Ca^{2+}, and the estimated percentage of the inward current carried by Ca^{2+} is only 2%. For these channels, receptor activation and plasma-membrane depolarization are the primary initiator for excitation-contraction coupling. Upon binding of acetylcholine, nAchR channels open to allow Na^+ to flow through the channel. The resulting depolarization opens voltage-gated Ca^{2+} channels and initiates Ca^{2+} release from SR through RyRs. In skeletal muscle, activation of voltage-gated Ca^{2+} influx in the T-tubule plasma membrane is the primary signal that activates intracellular Ca^{2+} release channels and ultimately stimulates muscular contraction.

The role of nAChRs in neuromuscular coupling is well-established. In contrast, although the nAchRs are found in most parts of the brain, their functional significance is not well-characterized. Both Ca^{2+} influxes through activated nAChRs and Ca^{2+} potentiation account for the physiological actions of these channels. Calcium potentiation is a process in which Ca^{2+} influx through one channel regulates the efficacy of other ligand-gated channels, leading to the modulation of membrane excitability in neurons, as well as their ability to integrate synaptic and paracrine signals. Furthermore, nAChR-dependent Ca^{2+} signals enhance protein-kinase activity in myotubes, leading to phosphorylation of the nAChR γ subunit. Since this process is dependent on Ca^{2+} influx, it can be considered as autoregulation of phosphorylation by nAChRs. Recent results indicate that point mutation in this receptor may abolish desensitization, increase the affinity for agonists, and convert the effects of competitive antagonists into the agonist responses. Such mutations also occur spontaneously in humans and may be involved in diseases such as congenital myasthenia or frontal-lobe epilepsy.

4.2. GABA and Glycine Receptors Are Anion-Permeable Channels

GABA is a major inhibitory transmitter in the vertebrate CNS that acts through three different receptor classes: *GABA_A*, *GABA_B*, and *GABA_C receptors* (*see* Chapter 5). GABA_A and GABA_C receptors are ligand-gated Cl⁻ channels. GABA_A receptor subunits show 20–30% sequence identity with AchR, glycine receptor, and 5-HT3 receptor. Several subunit classes and isoforms within each class of the GABA_A receptor have been cloned, including $\alpha 1–\alpha 6$, $\beta 1–\beta 3$, $\gamma 1–\gamma 3$, δ, ϵ, π, $\rho 1–\rho 3$. Various isoforms of the ρ-subunits are the major molecular components of GABA_C receptors. Within these families, additional variants arise through alternative splicing. The expression of these subunits varies within the brain. GABA_A receptor is a pentameric assembly derived from a combination of various subunits. The preferred combination includes two α, two γ and one β subunit. However, the co-localization of these three types of subunits is not an absolute requirement for the formation of functional channel. The great diversity of receptor subunits leads to profound differences in tissue distribution, ontogeny, pharmacology, and regulation of GABA_A receptors. GABA_A receptors are targets for many drugs in wide clinical use, including benzodiazepines, barbiturates, neurosteroids, ethanol, and general anesthetics, which increase the conductance through GABA channels. Bicuculline inhibits GABA_A but not GABA_C channels. At the single-channel level, barbiturates increase the opening time of channels, whereas benzodiazepines increase the number of channel openings.

Glycine is the other main inhibitory neurotransmitter in the CNS, particularly in the spinal cord and in the brainstem, whereas GABA is more abundant in rostal parts of the CNS. The *glycine receptors (GlyRs)* are also pentameric proteins composed of three α and two β subunits. There are four isoforms of α subunits, which have highly homologous sequences but different pharmacological and functional properties. GlyRs heterogeneity is further increased by alternative splicing of α subunits. The α subunit contains the ligand-binding site and is sufficient to form functional homomeric channel, whereas β subunit modulates the pharmacological and conductance properties of the GlyRs. The TM2 segment generates an ion-permeable pore. Both α and β subunits contain recognition motifs for various protein kinases, including PKA and PKC and tyrosine kinases. At synapses, GlyRs are clustered at the postsynaptic membrane directly opposite to the presynaptic release sites, and are linked to the subsynaptic cytoskeleton by a membrane protein named gephyrin. There are many similarities between GABA_A and GlyRs, including ion selectivity, which arise from their close and conservative evolutionary relationship, and both channels are more distantly related to nAChRs and 5-HT3 receptors.

4.3. Some Glutamate-Receptor Channels Are Voltage- and Ligand-Gated

Glutamate-receptor channels (GluRs) are traditionally divided into three major subtypes: the α-amino-3-hydroxy-5-methyl-4-isoxazole propionic acid (*AMPA*); *kainite*; and *N*-methyl-D-asparate- (NMDA) receptor channels. Molecular cloning has revealed numerous subunits for each receptor group. For NMDA-receptor channels, NR1 and NR2A to NR2D subunits have been established. For the non-NMDA-receptor channels, GluR1-GluR4 denote the AMPA-sensitive family, whereas GluR5-GluR7, KA1, and KA2 denote the kinate subclass. The phylogenic trees of these subunits are shown in Fig. 23B. In addition to these 14 subunits, two cDNAs for β subunits have been cloned. A single δ subunit also exists and belongs to the GluR-type subunit, but the function of this particular subunit is unknown. Finally, the molecular diversity of NR1 and GluRs is further increased by variants created by alternative splicing and RNA editing. The M2 amino acids line the inner-channel pore, and specific residues in this segment determine the ion selectivity of the channel.

In addition to the specific structure and pharmacology, NMDA channels exhibit a different excitation behavior than those not activated by NMDA. These channels are both ligand- and voltage-gated. Full activation of the NMDA receptor requires application of two ligands, L-glutamate and glycine. The NMDA receptors only become fully activated by glutamate after their Mg^{2+} block has been relieved by membrane depolarization. The NMDA receptor exhibits low-binding-affinity sites for Ca^{2+}, which results in a low selectivity among cations. However, because of the lower-affinity binding, Ca^{2+} moves through the pore rapidly. Their kinetics is much slower, resulting in a large Ca^{2+} influx and long-term metabolic or structural changes. The importance of Ca^{2+} signals generated by NMDA-receptor channel activity is also well-established. Some of the most important functions of the nervous system, such as synaptic plasticity, are dependent on the behavior of NMDA-receptor channels and Ca^{2+} influx through these channels.

Kainate and AMPA-receptor subunits do not form mixed channel complexes, but both types of receptors can be expressed in the same neuron. Native AMPA receptors are either homomeric or heteromeric oligomers composed of these multiple subunits. AMPA receptors in mammalian CNS differ considerably with respect to gating kinetics and Ca^{2+} permeability. Although AMPA channels were generally considered to be permeable only to Na^+ and K^+, some native AMPA receptors display a substantial permeability to Ca^{2+}, and a weaker selectivity among the divalent cations compared to NMDA channels. The rapid kinetics of AMPA receptors are suitable for rapid neurotransmission. The Ca^{2+} permeable AMPA receptors are involved in the excitatory synaptic transmission in hippocampal and neocortical nonpyramidal neurons. It is believed that Ca^{2+} influx through these channels plays a significant role in modulating the long-term synaptic functions. A number of recent studies have also indicated the role of kinate receptors at neuronal synapses. Both presynaptic and postsynaptic localization of these receptors has been suggested. Depending on the subtype of receptors and the localization, these channels may exhibit stimulatory or inhibitory action.

4.4. Purinergic-Receptor Channels Are Expressed in Excitable and Nonexcitable Cells

With the use of molecular cloning techniques, seven P2XR subtypes have been identified to date—denoted as $P2X_1R$ through $P2X_7R$—and several spliced forms have been observed. P2XR subtypes differ with respect to their ligand-selectivity profiles, antagonist sensitivity, and cation selectivity. Their activation leads to an increase in intracellular Ca^{2+} concentration, with Ca^{2+} influx occurring through the pores of these channels and through voltage-gated Ca^{2+} channels, following the initial depolarization of cells by P2XR-generated currents. They can form ion permeable pores through homo- and heteropolymerization. Each subunit is proposed to have two TM helices (M1 and M2) connected by a large extracellular loop, with both N- and C-termini located in the cytoplasm (Fig. 24A). From the N-termini through the second TM domain, the cloned subunits exhibit a relatively high level of amino acid sequence homology (Fig. 24B,C). In contrast, the C-termini vary in length and show no apparent sequence homology, except for the region nearest to the second TM domain.

In addition to ligand-selectivity profiles and antagonist sensitivity of P2XRs, they also differ with respect to their desensitization rates. Based on the observed differences in their current and calcium desensitization kinetics, homomeric P2XRs are generally divided into three groups: $P2X_1R$ and $P2X_3R$ desensitize very rapidly, $P2X_4$ and $P2X_6$ desensitize at a moderate rate, whereas $P2X_2R$, $P2X_5R$, and $P2X_7R$ show little or no desensitization (Fig. 25). Heteropolymerization results in channels that desensitize with a pattern different from those seen in cells expressing homomeric channels. Native P2XRs also desensitize with different kinetics, which reflect their structure. The differences in desensitization rates of P2XRs are reminiscent of those seen among subtypes of other ligand-gated receptor channels. The site-directed mutagenesis experiments indicated the relevance of C-terminus structure on P2XR desensitization patterns and have identified the region around Arg^{371} as important in this process. Calcium and PKC may also play a role in control of receptor desensitization and recovery from desensitization through still uncharacterized pathway(s). A dual control of receptor-channel function resembles that of voltage-gated channels.

In contrast to the well-characterized structure and pharmacology of P2XRs, their physiological significance is not well-understood. In general, Ca^{2+} is a charge carrier through these channels, although the permeability of Ca^{2+} vs. Na^+ varies widely among different cell types. Thus, these channels can serve as Ca^{2+} influx channels. These channels also facilitate Ca^{2+} influx indirectly, by depolarizing cells and activating voltage-gated Ca^{2+} channels. In addition to stimulating intracellular Ca^{2+} signals, the paracrine actions of ATP on purinergic receptors can generate the cell-to-cell spread of Ca^{2+} signals in glial cells in the absence of gap-junctional communication. The best-characterized agonist role of ATP is in synaptic transmission from sympathetic nerves, where ATP acts as a co-transmitter with noradrenaline. ATP has also been implicated in parasympathetic-, sensory-, and somatic-neuromuscular transmission. About 40% of hypothalamic neurons in culture respond to ATP by a

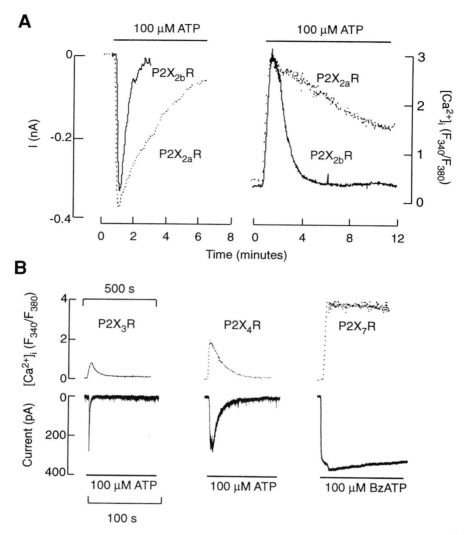

Fig. 25. Characterization of recombinant ion-conducting purinergic receptors (P2XRs) expressed in GT1 neurons. Patterns of current (*left panel*) and Ca^{2+} signals (*right panel*) by P2X$_{2a}$R and its splice form P2X$_{2b}$R (**A**), as well as by P2X$_3$R, P2X$_4$R, and P2X$_7$R (**B**). (Derived from Koshimizu et al., Mol Pharmacol 2000; 58:936.)

rapid increase in intracellular Ca^{2+} because of Ca^{2+} entry through P2XRs. Purinergic receptor-channels are expressed in neurons, as well as in other excitable cells, including pituitary cells, and nonexcitable cells, including gonadal cells and limphocytes.

5. INTRACELLULAR AND INTERCELLULAR CHANNELS

The expression of ion channels is not limited to the plasma membrane. Two types of channels, *ryanodine-receptor channels* (RyRs) and *inositol 1,4,5-trisphosphate-receptor channels* (IP$_3$Rs) are expressed in the ER/sarcoplasmic reticulum membrane and nuclear

membrane. RyRs provide an effective mechanism for transduction and translation of electrical signals inside of cells, whereas IP$_3$Rs are activated by two classes of plasma-membrane receptors known as *Ca^{2+}-mobilizing receptors*. Their activation is independent of the electrical status of cells and represents the major pathway for Ca^{2+} signaling in nonexcitable cells. However, this signaling pathway is also operative in excitable cells, including neurons. Activation of IP$_3$Rs leads to stimulation of voltage-insensitive Ca^{2+} channels expressed on the plasma membrane, and this process is known as *capacitative Ca^{2+} entry*. Channels that accommodate capacitative Ca^{2+} entry are also expressed in both excitable and nonexcitable cells.

5.1. Voltage-Gated Ca^{2+} Influx Activates Ryanodine Receptors

RyRs were originally identified as Ca^{2+} release channels expressed in the SR of skeletal muscle fibers and cardiac myocytes, where they play a central role in excitation-contraction coupling. These channels are also expressed in neurons, chromaffin cells, sea urchin eggs, and several nonexcitable cell types. Mammalian tissues express three isoforms: RyR_1 is expressed predominantly in skeletal muscle, RyR_2 is expressed in cardiac muscle, and RyR_3 has a wide tissue distribution, including the nonexcitable cells. RyR_1 and RyR_2 channels display a 66% identity, whereas the RyR_3 channel is much shorter. RyRs are tetramers, with a large N-terminal region forming heads, and a C-terminal region that forms the Ca^{2+}-selective channel. Although these channels are frequently co-expressed with IP_3Rs, the physiological importance of their co-expression and their variable density within the cells are still largely unknown.

RyRs are the largest known ion channels and are susceptible to many different modulators, including cytosolic calcium, membrane potential, and several intracellular messengers. As in the regulation of IP_3Rs, intracellular Ca^{2+} is a major regulator of RyRs; at low concentrations, Ca^{2+} promotes release, whereas higher concentrations are inhibitory. However, the inhibition of RyRs by high intracellular Ca^{2+} concentration is somewhat controversial, because it requires intracellular Ca^{2+} to be in the millimolar concentration range, which is not reached under physiological conditions. The ability of Ca^{2+} to stimulate its release from the endoplasmic/sarcoplasmic reticulum via RyRs is known as *Ca^{2+}-induced Ca^{2+} release*. This process is of fundamental importance for coordinating the elementary Ca^{2+}-release events into Ca^{2+} spikes and waves. Unlike IP_3Rs, RyRs can release Ca^{2+} in response to an increase in intracellular Ca^{2+} concentration with no other change in the concentration of second messengers. This is crucial for excitation-contraction coupling. For example, in cardiac cells, Ca^{2+} entry through dihydropyridine-sensitive channels activates RyRs to induce a further increase in intracellular Ca^{2+}. In skeletal-muscle cells, the dihydropyridine receptors act primarily as voltage sensors to directly activate RyRs in response to membrane depolarization.

In addition to Ca^{2+}, there are numerous other endogenous modulators of RyRs. The best-known is ryanodine, which activates and inhibits RyRs, depend-

ing on its concentrations. At $1–10$ μM concentration, ryanodine locks the channel in a sub-conductance stage that slows the opening and closing of the channel. At higher concentrations, ryanodine inhibits RyRs, and this action is mimicked by ruthenium red. Other modulators are endoplasmic/sarcoplasmic reticulum Ca^{2+}, cytosolic pH, Mg^{2+} and other cations, Cl^- and other anions, nucleotides, cyclic adenosine 5'-diphosphate ribose, several protein kinases, calmodulin, and other Ca^{2+}-binding proteins. Caffeine is a standard pharmacological tool for the activation of RyRs. It acts on RyRs in both intact cells and isolated channels. Another pharmacological agent, dantrolene, has biphasic effects on RyR_1; in nanomolar concentrations it increases the open probability of these channels and in micromolar concentrations it inactivates the channel.

5.2. IP_3 Receptors Are Intracellular Ligand-Gated Channels

Activation of IP_3Rs is triggered by seven membrane-domain receptors coupled to G proteins and tyrosine kinase plasma-membrane receptors. Calcium-mobilizing receptors that are coupled to G_q/G_{11}, as well as several receptors coupled to G_s and G_i activate phospholipase C-β, whereas tyrosine kinase receptors activate phospholipase C-γ. Both enzymes hydrolyze the membrane-associated phosphatidylinositol 4,5-bisphosphate to increase the production of IP_3 and diacylglycerol. IP_3 rapidly diffuses into the cytosol to activate IP_3Rs. In contrast, diacylglycerol (DAG) remains in the plasma membrane, where it acts on PKC.

IP_3Rs are composed of four similar subunits that are noncovalently associated to form a four-leaf clover-like structure, the center of which makes the Ca^{2+}-selective channel. The IP_3 binding sites are located within the first 788 residues of the N terminus of each subunit. Complete cDNA sequences of three distinct IP_3R encoding genes have been determined. Most cells express multiple isoforms of IP_3Rs, indicating that they have different functions. Analysis of the single-channel function of type-1, type-2, and type-3 IP_3R revealed isoform-specific properties in terms of their sensitivity to IP_3 and Ca^{2+}. IP_3Rs are present in almost all cells and are localized in the ER membrane, nuclear membrane, and possibly the plasma membrane in some cell types. Functionally reconstituted purified IP_3Rs respond to IP_3, with an increase in the open probability resulting from a large conformational change. The release of Ca^{2+} is electrically compensated by an inward potassium flux.

Cytosolic Ca^{2+} is the major messenger that controls IP_3R gating. In the presence of stimulatory concentrations of IP_3, type-1 and type-2 IP_3Rs respond to increases in intracellular calcium in a biphasic manner; Ca^{2+} increases IP_3R activity at low concentrations and inhibits it at higher concentrations. Conversely, the type-3 IP_3R open probability increases monotonically as the concentration of cytosolic Ca^{2+} increases. In both cases, the binding of IP_3 to residues within the N-terminal domain of IP_3Rs is required for cytosolic Ca^{2+} to exhibit its messenger function. Like voltage-gated channels, several other factors also modulate the activity of IP_3Rs, including PKA, PKC, calcium/calmodulin-dependent protein kinase II, adenine nucleotides, and pH. Two inhibitors, heparin and decavanadate, competitively inhibit IP_3 binding to IP_3Rs yet neither inhibitor is highly specific. Caffeine, a RyR stimulator, inhibits IP_3Rs. A series of xestospongins have been identified as noncompetitive IP_3R antagonists.

5.3. Calcium Release Is Coupled to Capacitative Ca^{2+} Entry

The term "capacitative Ca^{2+} entry," by analogy with a capacitor in an electrical circuit, implies that intracellular Ca^{2+} stores prevent entry when they are charged (filled by Ca^{2+}), but promote entry as soon as the stored Ca^{2+} is discharged (released). The similarities in the properties of this entry within different cell types, including excitable cells, suggest a common mechanism. In addition to Ca^{2+}-mobilizing agonists, capacitative Ca^{2+} entry can be activated by injection of IP_3 or its nonmetabolized forms into the cell, inhibition of the Ca^{2+} pump by thapsigargin, discharge of the intracellular content by calcium ionophores, or prolonged incubation of cells in Ca^{2+}-deficient medium. Injection of heparin, an IP_3R inhibitor, completely blocks agonist and IP_3-induced Ca^{2+} mobilization and capacitative Ca^{2+} entry. Because depletion of the ER Ca^{2+} stores is followed by the influx of Ca^{2+} into the cell, the channels involved in such influx were termed store-operated Ca^{2+}-selective plasma-membrane channels (SOCCs). At the present time, the nature of these channels and the mechanism of their regulation in response to store depletion are unknown. Several types of channels have been suggested to mediate capacitative Ca^{2+} entry: calcium release-activated (CRAC) channels,

Ca^{2+}-activated nonselective channels, transient-receptor-potential protein (TRP) channels, and CaT1, a member of the "osm" channels.

Until recently, it was believed that neurons do not express SOCCs. However, recent evidence suggests that neurons and other excitable cells also express SOCCs, and that these channels act as a Ca^{2+} influx pathway and as pacemaker channels to modulate action-potential-driven Ca^{2+} entry. For example, depletion of the ER Ca^{2+} stores by the activation of Ca^{2+}-mobilizing receptors or thapsigargin activates SOCCs in N1E-115 neuroblastoma cells and GnRH-secreting neurons. Because of its depolarizing nature, I_{SOCC} functionally operates as a pacemaker current in GnRH neurons, opposing the hyperpolarizing action of I_A. It is likely that SOCCs have dual action in neurons, to conduct Ca^{2+} and to facilitate voltage-gated Ca^{2+} influx.

5.4. Electrical, Ca^{2+}, and Chemical Coupling by Gap-Junction Channels

The cytoplasmic compartments of neighboring cells are frequently connected by *gap junctions*, which are clusters of intercellular channels that form a cytoplasmic bridge between adjacent cells to allow for the cell-to-cell transfer of ions, metabolites and small messenger molecules, including Ca^{2+}, ATP, cAMP, cADP-ribose, and IP_3. Thus, gap-junction channels provide an effective mechanism for electrical, calcium, and metabolic coupling, depending on the size of the pore. Vertebrate intercellular channels are made up of a multigene family of conserved proteins called *connexins*. The invertebrate gap-junction channels have no detectable sequence homology with vertebrate gap junctions, although they exhibit similar functions and membrane topology. These channels are known as *innexins*.

To date, at least 20 connexin genes have been identified. Connexins are made up of four hydrophobic TM domains, with the N- and C-termini located in the cytoplasm. In the plasma membrane, six connexin subunits assemble in a circle to form hemichannels known as *connexons*, which can contain a single type of connexin (homomeric), or multiple connexins (heteromeric) to form the hemichannel pore. When two connexons from adjacent cells come together, they form an intercellular channel that spans the gap between the two cells. Two identical connexons or different connexons can join to form either homotypic or heterotypic intercellular channels, respectively. The presence of heteromeric connexins and heterotypic intercellular channels can produce a diverse group of structurally different intercellular channels, with different permeabilities and/or functions. A variety of other factors, including membrane potential, Ca^{2+}, pH, and phosphorylation of channels, can also alter gap-junction channels. Several neurotransmitters and hormones, such as dopamine, acetylcholine, GABA, and estrogens, have also been found to alter intercellular channel activity.

Initially, gap junctions were detected as an electrical conductance between the presynaptic and postsynaptic elements. This type of synapse is termed *electrical synapse* to distinguish it from typical chemical synapse. Cell-to-cell connection though gap junction can be studied by electrophysiology, or under the fluorescent microscope by injecting the fluorescent dyes (Lucifer yellow for example) into one cell and monitoring the diffusion of dye into its neighbors. The current-voltage relationship of gap junction is usually linear and sometimes asymmetric, rectifying, which provides one-direction flow. In addition to ion conductance, several lines of evidence implicate gap-junction channels in mediating the propagation of intercellular Ca^{2+} waves, leading to the synchronization of cellular function in a particular tissue. Because of the non-selectivity of gap-junctions to ions and small molecules, several diffusible second-messenger molecules are potential candidates for mediating the propagation of intercellular Ca^{2+} waves via gap junctions, including Ca^{2+} and IP_3.

6. A CROSS COMMUNICATION BETWEEN ELECTRICAL AND RECEPTOR-MEDIATED SIGNALING PATHWAYS

Hormones and neurotransmitters acting through their respective receptors can modulate the gating properties of voltage-gated and ligand-gated channels. This modulation is dependent on signal-transduction pathways of receptors. These includes direct action of heteromeric G proteins on channels (termed *membrane-delimited pathway*) and indirect, through intracellular messengers, including Ca^{2+}, cyclic nucleotides, nitric oxide, ATP, and PKA, PKC, and PKG (termed *intracellular-messenger-dependent pathway*) (Fig. 4). The first pathway is limited to the regulation of a few channels, whereas the second pathway represents a common mechanism by which receptors can influence channel activity.

Inhibition of voltage-gated Ca^{2+} channels can occur through the fast membrane-delimited pathway, in which the $\beta\gamma$ dimer of the G_i/G_o proteins is a direct intermediate between the plasma-membrane receptor and channels. This is a time- and voltage-dependent process. As a fraction of the total Ca^{2+} channels open much more slowly and require larger depolarization to open, this produces a slowing of the activation kinetics and a reduction in the current amplitude. In contrast, several G_i/G_o-coupled receptors, including dopamine, somatostatin, and endothelin-A, activate K_{ir} channels in $\beta\gamma$ dimmer-dependent manner, leading to hyperpolarization of the membrane, cessation of action-potential firing, and a decrease in intracellular Ca^{2+} concentration and hormone secretion.

The activity of voltage-gated Ca^{2+} channels can also be modulated in a second-messenger-dependent manner. For example, in cardiac myocytes, activation of PKA augments Ca^{2+} influx through voltage-gated Ca^{2+} channels. The effects of PKA phosphorylation have been attributed to an increase in the probability of the channel being open and to an increase in the mean open time. Also, in rat and human pituitary adenoma cells, pituitary adenylate cyclase-activating polypeptide stimulates TTX-sensitive Na^+ channels via an adenylate cyclase-PKA pathway to increase hormone secretion. Phosphorylation also plays an important role in the modulation of several other channels, including BK, K_{ir}, IP_3Rs, and P2XRs.

Receptors can also modulate the activity of another K^+ channel, the M-type. Inhibition of this current was first observed in response to the activation of muscarinic receptors in bullfrog sympathetic ganglion neurons, as indicated by the name M-type current. Since then, it has been demonstrated that activation of a variety of receptors suppresses this current, including GnRH, bradykinin, opioids, substance P, ATP, adrenergic, TRH, and angiotensin II receptors. Because these receptors are typically coupled to the phospholipase C pathway, it is likely that $InsP_3$-induced Ca^{2+} release accounts for this inhibition. Intra- and extracellular Ca^{2+} is also involved in control of the gating of several other channels. We have already discussed I_{K-Ca} and I_{Cl-Ca} channels. Calcium also activates a nonselective cation channel. L-type Ca^{2+} channels are inhibited in Ca^{2+}-calmodulin-dependent manner. Calcium is a principal factor controlling RyR gating and co-factor in controlling IP$_3$R gating. Calcium also inhibits the conductivity of CNG channels in a dual mechanism, directly and through a calmodulin-dependent mechanism.

Several other intracellular molecules can modulate the gating of channels. As previously discussed, cyclic nucleotides are crucial in the regulation of two channels, CNG and I$_h$. Thus, activation of adenylyl-cyclase pathway by G$_s$-coupled receptors leads to stimulation of both channels, whereas activation of G$_i$/G$_o$-coupled receptors leads to a decrease in cAMP production and a silence of these channels. Nitric oxide provides an additional mechanism for stimulation of cGMP production (through activation of soluble guanylyl cyclase). Nitric oxide itself has been implicated as a messenger in regulating CNG and BK channels. Intracellular ATP and ADP control Kir6 channels.

Electrical activity and the associated Ca^{2+} influx also influence the receptor-mediated intracellular signaling. Voltage-gated Ca^{2+} influx has been shown to play an important role in sustained activation of phospholipases C and D. Spontaneous electrical activity is coupled to the activation and/or inhibition of adenylyl cyclase, nitric oxide synthase, and soluble guanylyl cyclase activities. There is also a cross-communication between plasma membrane and ER channels. For example, voltage-gated Ca^{2+} influx facilitates IP$_3$-mediated Ca^{2+} release during the sustained agonist stimulation. Thus, two pathways for signaling in neurons, electrical and receptor-controlled, are not independent of each other, but interact to provide the synchronized control of cellular functions.

SELECTED READINGS

Catterall WA. Structure and regulation of voltage-gated Ca^{2+} channels. Annu Rev Cell Biol 2000; 16:521–555.

Choe S. Potassium channel structures. Nature Rev Neurosci 2002; 3:115–121.

Dermietzel R. Gap junction wiring: a 'new' principle in cell-to-cell communication in the nervous system. Brain Res Rev 1998; 26:176–183.

Galzi JL, Changeux JP. Neuronal nicotinic receptors: molecular organization and regulations. Neuropharmacology 1995; 6:563–582.

Harvey R, Betz H. Glycine receptors. In Encyclopedia of Life Sciences, Nature Publishing Group, London: www.els.net, 2001: 1–6.

Hille B. Ion Channels of Excitable Membranes. Sunderland, MA: Sinauer Associates, Inc., 2001.

Hille B, Catterall WA. Electrical excitability and ion channels. In Siegel et al., (eds). Basic Neurochemistry Philadelphia-New York: Lippincott-Raven, 1999: 119–137.

Khakh BS, Brunstock G, Kennedy C, King BF, North RA, Seguela P, et al. Current status of the nomenclature and properties of P2X receptors and their subunits. Pharmacol Rev 2001; 53:107–118.

Madden DR. The structure and function of glutamate receptor ion channels. Nature Rev Neurosci 2002; 3:91–101.

Mehta AK, Ticku MK. An update on GABAA receptors. Brain Res Rev 1999; 29:196–217.

Putney Jr JW. Channeling calcium. Nature 2001; 410:648–649.

Taylor CW. Inositol trisphosphate receptors: Ca^{2+}-modulated intracellular Ca^{2+} channels. Biochim Biophys Acta 1998; 1436:19–33.

Zagotta WN, Siegelbaum SA. Structure and function of cyclic nucleotide-gated channels. Annu Rev Neuroci 1996; 19:235–263.

Zucchi R, Ronca-Testoni S. The sarcoplasmic reticulum Ca^{2+} channel/ryanodine receptor: modulation by endogenous effectors, drugs and disease states. Pharmacol Rev 1997; 49:1–51.

Demyelinating Disorders

Gregory Cooper and Robert L. Rodnitzky

Disorders of myelin can be divided into conditions in which there is destruction of myelin—the demyelinating disorders—and those in which there is an abnormality in the makeup of myelin, known as the dysmyelinating disorders. Demyelination can result from a great variety of causes, including autoimmume, toxic, metabolic, infectious, or traumatic conditions. The dysmyelinating disorders are heritable conditions resulting in inborn errors of metabolism that affect myelin. Central or peripheral nervous system myelin can be affected in these conditions, but most clinical syndromes related to disorders of myelin primarily affect the brain and spinal cord.

IMPAIRED OR BLOCKED IMPULSE CONDUCTION

Impaired or blocked impulse conduction is the cause of most clinical symptoms related to myelin disorders. Demyelination prevents saltatory conduction in normal rapidly conducting axons. Instead, impulses are propagated along the axon by continuous conduction, or in the extreme, there is total conduction block. The latter may result from the markedly prolonged refractory period in demyelinated segments, and explains why rapidly arriving, repetitive impulses are especially likely to be blocked.

Demyelination may also affect conduction by rendering axon function more susceptible to changes of the internal milieu, such as alterations of pH or temperature. The enhanced effect of temperature change on the function of demyelinated central nervous system (CNS) pathways is well-known, and can be the cause of prominent and precipitous neurologic symptoms after temperature elevation in multiple sclerosis is known as *Uhthoff's phenomenon*. Persons who experience this phenomenon notice the onset of new symptoms, such as monocular blindness, profound extremity weakness, or severe incoordination, whenever they develop a mildly elevated body temperature. With more profound elevation of body temperature, such as that occurring during a warm bath or as a result of a fever, neurologic dysfunction can be still more severe. Usually, when body temperature reverts to normal, neurologic function returns to baseline. Uhthoff's phenomenon is based on the principle that conduction block supervenes in demyelinated fibers when they reach a critical threshold temperature. This threshold temperature may be just above normal body temperature, explaining why such symptoms may develop after only a slight temperature elevation, such as that seen as part of normal diurnal variation.

DISEASES THAT AFFECT MYELIN

Many different processes can be involved in the etio-pathogenesis of myelin disorders. Adrenoleukodystrophy is an example of a metabolic disorder of myelin. It is an X-linked peroxisomal disorder in which there is impaired oxidation of very-long-chain fatty acids, with resultant abnormalities of myelin.

Progressive multifocal leukoencephalopathy is an infectious condition resulting in demyelination. It is caused by an opportunistic viral infection of oligodendroglial cells in immunosuppressed patients, such as those with acquired immunodeficiency syndrome. Oligodendroglial death leads to widespread demyelination, especially in the posterior portions of the cerebral hemispheres. The resultant severe neurologic dysfunction is ultimately fatal.

Radiation is an example of a form of trauma that can lead to demyelination. For this reason, patients undergoing radiation therapy in which the brain or spinal cord is in the field of treatment may later develop neurologic symptoms. Toxic agents such as cancer chemotherapy drugs can result in demyelination, especially when instilled directly into the cerebrospinal fluid (CSF).

Autoimmune mechanisms can result in demyelination. This process is believed to be important in the pathogenesis of one of the most common demyelinating disorders, multiple sclerosis (MS).

MS HAS A DISTINCT AGE, GENDER, RACE, AND GEOGRAPHIC PROFILE

MS is a relatively common neurologic disorder. The prevalence of MS in the United States and Northern Europe is approximately 100 per 100,000, and almost 300,000 Americans are afflicted with this condition. Women are affected 1.5 times more often than men. The age distribution of MS is distinct in that onset before the age of 15 or after the age of 45 is unusual. The white population, especially persons of northern European ancestry, has a much higher incidence of MS than Asians or African blacks.

Within the United States and to a certain degree throughout the world, there is a distinct geographic distribution of MS, with temperate zones having the highest incidence. In the United States, this distribution results in a strikingly higher prevalence of MS in the upper Midwest than in the deep South. The precise meaning of these geographic variations remains unclear, but some migration studies have suggested that environmental factors, such as a Viral exposure are largely operative in childhood, because emigration from a high prevalence zone before adolescence appears to reduce the risk of developing MS.

MS IS CHARACTERIZED BY THE PRESENCE OF NUMEROUS DISCRETE AREAS OF DEMYELINATION THROUGHOUT THE BRAIN AND SPINAL CORD

In MS, multiple plaques of demyelination are found in the CNS. Within these areas, there is evidence of inflammation, proliferation of glial tissue, and severe destruction of myelin. In these same areas, axons may remain largely intact. Minimal remyelination of fibers may occur in some plaques, resulting in areas with scant myelin known as "shadow plaques." The pathogenesis of demyelination within these plaques is not fully understood, but it is generally agreed that it involves an immune response mediated by T lymphocytes that recognize myelin components of the CNS. Plaques may occur anywhere in the CNS, but they have a predilection for certain parts of the brain and spinal cord, forming the anatomic basis for the most common clinical symptoms of MS. The most common regions of involvement are the optic nerves, the cerebellum, the periventricular white matter of the cerebral hemispheres, the white matter of the spinal cord, the root-entry zones of spinal or cranial nerves, and the brainstem, especially the pons.

THE SYMPTOMS OF MS REMIT AND REAPPEAR IN CHARACTERISTIC FASHION

MS is marked by a wide range of disparate neurologic symptoms that can occur in a single affected person and, in the most common form, a tendency for symptoms to appear, spontaneously improve, and then reappear or be replaced by new symptoms over time. This relapsing-remitting course may give way to a more gradually progressive course over time. This tendency toward spontaneous remittance of neurologic symptoms is highly characteristic of MS. Typically, serious neurologic symptoms appear and disappear over a period ranging from weeks to several months, independent of medical therapy. The variety of symptoms in a particular patient reflects the widespread dissemination of MS plaques throughout the brain and spinal cord. In a typical MS patient, it is not usually possible to attribute all neurologic symptoms to a single anatomic locus of abnormality; instead, multiple areas of demyelination must be invoked.

Certain neurologic symptoms are much more likely to occur in MS, reflecting the predilection for certain anatomic sites of involvement alluded to previously. These include monocular visual loss (the optic nerve is involved), limb incoordination (cerebellum), double vision (brainstem, or medial longitudinal fasciculus), and weakness of the lower extremities (spinal cord). Other common symptoms include vertigo, extremity numbness, slurred speech, and bladder dysfunction. *L'hermitte's sign* is a frequent finding in MS. It consists of a shock-like sensation whenever the neck is flexed forward. This phenomenon is caused by the heightened sensitivity of demyelinated dorsal column axons to the mechanical stimulation of stretch when the spinal cord is flexed by the offending neck motion.

THE DIAGNOSIS OF MS CAN BE AIDED BY IMAGING STUDIES AND LABORATORY TESTS

Although the unique clinical pattern of MS often allows the diagnosis to be made with confidence, several diagnostic tests are extremely useful in equivocal cases. Magnetic resonance imaging of the brain or spinal cord is a sensitive means of demonstrating multiple areas of demyelination, many of which may prove to be clinically silent. In addition, magnetic resonance imaging can determine whether a given area of demyelination is quiescent or in an active state of evolution. Active plaques tend to enhance with gadolinium, indicating a disruption of the blood-brain barrier.

Examination of the CSF is used to screen for CNS immunoglobulin (IgG) abnormalities, which are common in MS. The rate of IgG synthesis within the CNS, which is typically elevated in MS, can be determined, and the makeup of IgG in the CSF can be evaluated. When normal CSF is subjected to immunoelectrophoresis, the IgGs are diffusely represented at the cathodal region. In MS, the electrophoretic pattern demonstrates one or more discrete bands of IgG known as oligoclonal bands. These are presumed to be specific antibodies, but the antigen(s) against which they are directed have not yet been identified. Testing for the presence of oligoclonal IgG is extremely useful in diagnosing MS because as many as 95% of individuals with proven MS have been found to exhibit this abnormality. Another useful CSF study involves myelin basic protein, a breakdown product of myelin. Because it can be detected in the CSF in the presence of active CNS demyelination, it is useful as an indicator of disease activity.

Electrophysiologic studies such as visual and somatosensory evoked potentials are used to detect subtle physiologic abnormalities in MS that are not yet sufficiently advanced to produce clinical symptoms. These tests measure the speed and completeness of conduction in sensory pathways. The technique involves delivery of a sensory stimulus such as a flash of light, and measuring the time required for an evoked response to be reflected in the cortex and recorded by a scalp electrode. In patients with overt sensory symptoms, slowed conduction can often still be demonstrated in the appropriate sensory pathway even after the symptoms remit.

IMMUNOSUPPRESSION IS THE MOST COMMON FORM OF THERAPY USED IN MS

The propensity for MS symptoms to remit spontaneously makes the scientific evaluation of potential therapies difficult. In the past, poorly designed or uncontrolled studies have led to a multitude of false claims of therapeutic efficacy for a variety of therapies, some of which were quite unorthodox. However, a number of agents now exist for the treatment of MS, which presumably act through an immunomodulatory mechanism. The first agents to be approved by the FDA were interferon-beta-1b (Betaseron) and interferon-beta-1a (Avonex). Putative mechanisms for these medications include inhibition of autoreactive T cells, inhibition of MHC class II expression, metalloproteinase inhibition, altered expression of cell-associated adhesion molecules, and induction of immunosuppressive cytokines and inhibition of proinflammatory cytokines. A third agent, glatiramer acetate (Copaxone), is a polypeptide containing random arrangements of four basic amino acids, believed to mimic myelin basic protein. This agent is felt to act by inducing myelin-specific suppressor T cells and inhibiting myelin-specific effector T cells. All of these agents are used in an attempt to slow progression of the disease, or to reduce the frequency of relapses.

For the treatment of acute relapses, the most commonly used treatments are the corticosteroid drugs, prednisone, or methylprednisolone. These agents are usually administered at high doses and are believed to help reduce inflammation and restore the blood-brain barrier, thereby shortening the course of relapse and speeding recovery.

SELECTED READINGS

Fazekas F, Barkhof F, Filippi M, et al. The contribution of magnetic resonance imaging to the diagnosis of multiple sclerosis. Neurology 1999; 53:448–456.

Noseworthy JH. Progress in determining the causes and treatment of multiple sclerosis. Nature 1999; 399(Suppl):A40–A47.

Poser CM, Paty DW, Scheinberg L, et al. New diagnostic criteria for multiple sclerosis: guidelines for research protocols. Ann Neurol 1983; 13:22.

Rudick RA. Disease-modifying drugs for relapsing-remitting multiple sclerosis and future directions for multiple sclerosis therapeutics. Arch Neurol 1999; 56:1079–1084.

4 Synaptic Transmission

Henrique von Gersdorff and Court Hull

CONTENTS

1. OVERVIEW

The nervous system is comprised of specialized cellular circuits that allow an animal to perform tasks essential for survival. Neurons are organized to form these circuits, and they transmit electrical and chemical signals amongst themselves to process sensory input, initiate behavioral responses, and regulate an animal's internal physiology. The critical link between neurons that permits communication and establishes the foundation for neuronal circuitry is called the *synapse*, and this chapter will discuss fundamental synaptic properties.

Synapses are sites of close cellular contact where fast, highly localized transmission of chemical and electrical signals can occur. The human brain has approx 10^{11} neurons that form about 10^{15} synapses. By comparison, the simple nematode worm *C. elegans* has exactly 320 neurons with only about 7600 synapses. Our brain's capacity to form such an astronomical number of synapses has surely contributed to the success of our species and its vast repertoire of behav-

iors. In order to understand how synapses confer such complexity of neuronal circuitry, it is important to explore the details of information transfer at the synapse.

The process of communication between neurons, termed *synaptic transmission*, is a key aspect of medical knowledge for many reasons. The causes of several mental disorders and neuromuscular diseases can be traced to dysfunctional synapses. Synapses are also the locus of action for various neurotoxins and psychoactive drugs (some of which can cause debilitating and life-long addictions). Finally, determining how synapses transmit signals and how neuronal circuits are remodeled and modulated at the synaptic level will eventually allow us to understand the basis of learning and memory.

Synapses vary widely in shape, size, and function. Presumably, such architectural and functional diversities are tailored for the specialized information transfer and processing needs of individual neurons and circuits. For example, many synapses function as high-fidelity relay stations. The connection between motor neurons and muscle fibers (termed the *neuromuscular junction*), the giant synapses in the mammalian auditory systems involved in sound localization, and the

From: *Neuroscience in Medicine, 2nd ed.* (P. Michael Conn, ed.),
© 2003 Humana Press Inc., Totowa, NJ.

squid giant synapse which allows a rapid escape behavior are all examples of high fidelity relays. These are synapses where reliability is at a premium, and the synaptic architecture is designed as a fail-safe mechanism for information transfer. Other synapses, such as the bouton-type synapses of the cortex and hippocampus, often fail to transmit signals and are thus considered to be comparatively unreliable. These bouton synapses, however, have the capacity to become more fail-safe with repetitive use. This type of change in synaptic strength is an example of *plasticity*, and is thought to underlie the long-lasting storage of information acquired through repetitive use of an associated neuronal circuit. In other words, the specific strengthening of a particular set of synaptic connections may form the basis for some types of learning and memory. Equally important may be the weakening of synaptic connections, a process that could either cause the loss of certain synaptic memory or endow the freedom for retasking a particular neuronal circuit. Thus, synapses must be considered as highly dynamic and plastic structures that can adapt their output to match the demands imposed by their current information processing needs. In this sense, the brain is not "hard wired," and differs fundamentally from an electronic computer.

One consequence of evolution that unifies biology and medicine is the cross-species commonality of underlying mechanisms for critical physiological processes such as synaptic transmission. From genomes to protein structure and function, common molecular motifs are homologously conserved across phylogenetically distant species. Neurobiologists have thus been able to use nonhuman animal models as a means to study and understand synaptic function. Due to an unparalleled ease of access, much of the pioneering work in the field of synaptic transmission comes from studies of the frog neuromuscular junction and squid giant synapse. In addition, relatively new preparations such as the giant bipolar cell synapse from goldfish retina and calyx of Held synapse in the mammalian brainstem have shed much new light on our understanding of synaptic function. These, and many other preparations, have yielded a wealth of information about synapses and revealed several general principles that apply directly to synaptic transmission in the human brain. These general principles of synaptic transmission are further reviewed in this chapter.

2. PROPERTIES OF CHEMICAL AND ELECTRICAL SYNAPSES

Neurons communicate using morphologically and functionally specialized sites of close contact called synapses. Synaptic transmission can be electrical or chemical, though the vast majority of synapses in the mammalian brain are chemical. At *chemical synapses*, molecules of neurotransmitter are released from a presynaptic terminal into a narrow extracellular gap (about 20 to 50 nm) called the *synaptic cleft*. The transmitter molecules then diffuse and bind to recognition sites on target receptors at the plasma membrane of a postsynaptic neuron. This type of synaptic transmission is fast, site-specific, and highly plastic.

A different type of synaptic transmission occurs at *electrical synapse*, where proteins form *gap-junctions* to create a conductive pore between two neurons. This pore is an ionotropic transmembrane channel comprised of connexin proteins on the plasma membrane of each neuron that allows ions and small molecules (e.g., cAMP, ATP, Ca^{2+}, IP_3) to cross between cells. The cytoplasm of two neurons connected by a gap junction is thus physically continuous, and the resulting low-resistance channel allows *electrical coupling*. Transmission at electrical synapses is *bi-directional*, although some gap junctions may transmit better in one direction (i.e., they show *rectification*).

Although electrical coupling limits the variety of signaling between neurons (electrical activity in one neuron is identically passed to its connected partner), it allows much faster communication than chemical signaling and can synchronize the activity of a group of cells that must work together. For example, every neighboring cell in the heart is connected via gap junctions, and the resultant electrical coupling allows the tissue wide coordination of cardiac contractions.

Gap junctions are not, however, static structures. Many tissues contain gap junctions during development which are then lost as the nervous system matures. In addition, gap-junction conductances can be modulated by phosphorylation and/or neurotransmitters in order to alter the dynamic state of entire neuronal circuits. In the retina, for example, circadian changes in dopamine levels modulate the opening of gap junctions and allow retinal circuitry to adapt its light sensitivity from day to night.

By contrast, chemical synapses are far more complex than their electrical counterparts. Chemical

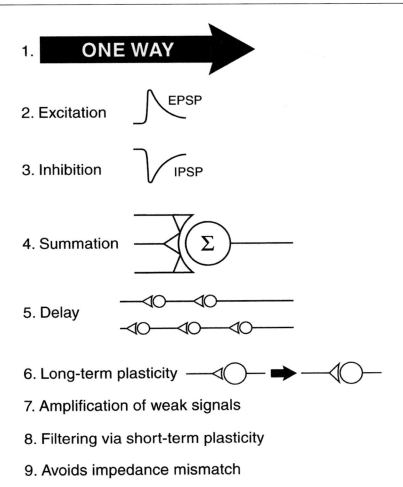

1. ONE WAY

2. Excitation — EPSP

3. Inhibition — IPSP

4. Summation — Σ

5. Delay

6. Long-term plasticity

7. Amplification of weak signals

8. Filtering via short-term plasticity

9. Avoids impedance mismatch

Fig. 1. The multiple advantages of chemical synapses: 1) Chemical synapses are mostly unidirectional and transmit from presynaptic to postsynaptic neurons. Information is thus relayed sequentially to different cells in a neural circuit. 2) Synapses can produce an excitatory postsynaptic potential (EPSP) causing the postsynaptic neuron to fire APs. 3) Synapses can also produce an inhibitory postsynaptic potential (IPSP) suppressing postsynaptic firing of APs. 4) Several small synaptic potentials can be summed by the postsynaptic cell before it fires an AP. This allows the neuron to integrate information from several different sources. 5) Chemical synapses introduce a short synaptic delay in transmission and this can be used for calculating the timing of sensory inputs. In the example shown, information can be routed via a di-synaptic or a tri-synaptic pathway. 6) Synaptic strength or efficacy is plastic and can undergo changes on a long-time scale (hours or days). Synaptic morphology and functional properties can thus change with experience. This is indicated by the larger synaptic connection. 7) Synapses can amplify a weak presynaptic signal. 8) Synaptic strength or efficacy is also plastic on a short-time scale (milliseconds to seconds). This short-term synaptic plasticity can cause synaptic depression or fatigue if the synapse is stimulated at high frequencies. Thus, high-frequency stimulation may be filtered and not transmitted as effectively as low-frequency stimulation. 9) Synaptic transmission avoids impedance mismatch problems that may occur at electrical synapses between neurons of different sizes. (Modified from Gardner, 1995.)

synapses depend on an elaborate cascade of protein–protein and lipid–protein interactions that have only recently been explored at the molecular level. Some of the differences between electrical and chemical synapses are listed in Fig. 1. Chemical synapses occur between axon endings (*presynaptic terminals*) that contain neurotransmitter-filled *synaptic vesicles* and postsynaptic neurons with clusters of neurotransmit-

ter receptors. These two elements are separated by the synaptic cleft (*see* Fig. 2). Chemical synapses are therefore polarized, and primarily mediate synaptic transmission from the presynaptic terminal to the postsynaptic neuron.

Unlike electrical synapses, the synaptic cleft separating pre- and postsynaptic membranes does not permit any direct electrical coupling between neurons (or

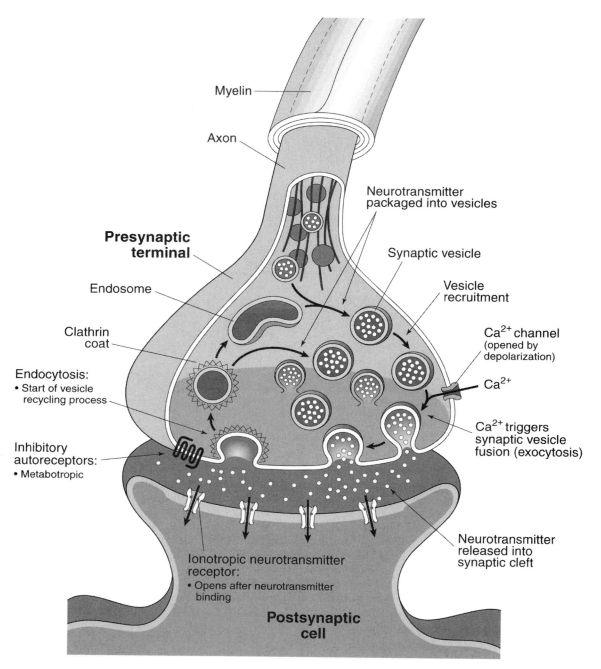

Fig. 2. Chemical synapses and synaptic vesicle recycling. Schematic diagram of the main events involved in chemical synaptic transmission at a typical bouton-type synapse. The presynaptic terminal (or bouton) is filled with neurotransmitter containing synaptic vesicles. Some vesicles are in the cytosol, constituting a reserve pool of vesicles, and some are docked at the presynaptic membrane, constituting a readily releasable pool of vesicles. Reserve vesicles can be recruited to the docked pool. A presynaptic action potential (AP) depolarizes the nerve terminal and opens Ca^{2+} channels located near to the docked pool of vesicles. Ca^{2+} ions trigger synaptic vesicle fusion or exocytosis. Neurotransmitter is thus released into the synaptic cleft where it binds to postsynaptic ionotropic receptors. This binding of neurotransmitter causes ion channels to open, depolarizing or hyperpolarizing the postsynaptic cell. Neurotransmitter can also bind to metabotropic receptors on the presynaptic membrane and these can inhibit further release. Synaptic vesicle membrane that has fused with the presynaptic membrane is retrieved by endocytosis. One common form of endocytosis is clathrin-mediated endocytosis, which forms clathrin coats on endocytosed vesicles. Retrieved vesicles are then recycled via fusion to endosomes or directly back to the reserve vesicle pool where they are refilled with neurotransmitter. (Modified from Neuroscience, edited by Purves et al., 2001.)

any degree of cytoplasmic mixing). The synaptic cleft is spanned by several different kinds of *adhesion molecules* (e.g., cadherins, immunoglobulin cell adhesion molecules, neurexins, neurogligins, integrins, etc.) that provide mechanical stability and align presynaptic vesicle fusion sites (*active zones*) opposite to clusters of postsynaptic neurotransmitter receptors. A hallmark of the active zone that has been revealed by electron microscopy is a set of *docked vesicles* situated close to the plasma membrane (from 2 to 10 vesicles per active zone ideally positioned for immediate release). A second set of synaptic vesicles is commonly found in reserve further from the active zone, and both vesicle clusters are often thought of as discrete pools with functional differences in terms of chemical signaling. In direct apposition to the active zone, the postsynaptic membrane contains an electron dense area called the *postsynaptic density* (PSD). The PSD holds receptors for neurotransmitters, cytoskeletal and scaffolding proteins, and many enzymes localized to trigger signaling cascades.

Chemical transmission is initiated when an action potential (AP) invades the presynaptic terminal. The resulting membrane depolarization opens voltage-gated Ca^{2+} selective ion channels, and Ca^{2+} enters the presynaptic neuron. This Ca^{2+} is the trigger for *exocytosis*, the process by which docked, neurotransmitter-filled synaptic vesicles fuse with the presynaptic membrane to release their contents into the synaptic cleft. The neurotransmitter is then free to diffuse across the synaptic cleft and bind to target receptors on the postsynaptic plasma membrane. These receptors are termed *ligand-gated*, and many of them are ion-selective channels which open in response to neurotransmitter binding. When these ion-selective channels open, extracellular ions flow into the postsynaptic neuron to produce either an *excitatory* or *inhibitory postsynaptic potential* (EPSP or IPSP). The type of postsynaptic potential depends largely on the particular neurotransmitter released from the presynaptic neuron and the specific receptors expressed on the postsynaptic membrane. EPSPs transiently shift the membrane potential toward more positive values, or depolarize the membrane, while IPSPs generally hyperpolarize the membrane. Unlike electrical synapses, chemical synapses can either maintain or invert the sign of a presynaptic signal by transforming a presynaptic excitation to a postsynaptic excitation or inhibition.

Presynaptic terminals are often less than a micron in diameter, and frequently release only a few synaptic vesicles per action potential. The effect of a small

quantity of neurotransmitter on the postsynaptic membrane (the EPSP or IPSP) may therefore be insufficient for triggering a postsynaptic action potential. The postsynaptic neuron, though, can be studded with up to several thousand presynaptic terminals (or boutons), and simultaneous EPSPs and IPSCs are then integrated by the postsynaptic neuron. This process of *summation* allows the postsynaptic neuron to collect input from a variety of synapses before firing its own action potential. Summation of multiple inputs, along with strengthening or weakening of particular synapses, allows the brain a vast computational capacity that would otherwise be impossible with more limited circuitry.

Because chemical synaptic transmission is such an intricate, multi-step process, there is an inherent time lag, or *synaptic delay*, that occurs between a presynaptic depolarization and a postsynaptic response. This delay, which varies between 0.1 and 0.5 ms, depends on the architecture of a particular synapse. Together with other timing cues, such as those introduced by axons of differing length, some neurons are capable of comparing sensory inputs from organ pairs such as the eyes or ears. For example, certain neurons in the auditory brainstem localize sound by comparing inputs from two different synapses carrying signals from each ear. These neurons are *coincidence detectors* for signals arriving from each ear, and the auditory neural circuitry is precisely constructed to accommodate delays introduced by axons of differing length across several synapses.

Synapses are highly dynamic connections that can undergo both short- and long-term changes in their morphology and transmission strength. A brief burst (or tetanus) of neural stimulation can transiently increase or decrease the amplitude of EPSPs or IPSPs. These ubiquitous phenomena are called *short-term facilitation* (increased postsynaptic potentials) or *short-term depression* (synaptic fatigue). Synapses usually recover from short-term facilitation or depression within a few seconds. On the other hand, prolonged high-frequency stimulation of synaptic pairs can sometimes cause a *long-term potentiation* of EPSPs that can last for hours or even days. Conversely, prolonged lower-frequency stimulation of the same synapse pair may induce long-term depression of EPSPs. Two different synaptic inputs can therefore associate to produce what may be a simple, cellular underpin for learning and memory.

Short-term depression may also act as a *frequency-selective filter*. During a tetanus, short-term depression will become increasingly potent as the stimulation frequency increases. Stimulation beyond a certain frequency is therefore filtered out at the synapse level, effectively changing the operational range of an associated neural circuit. Frequency-dependent filters are quite useful in electronics (e.g., to reduce noise and select for particular frequencies), and presumably neural circuits also make use of this synaptic property in analogous ways.

Chemical synapses also have an advantage over electrical synapses in dealing with the problem of *impedance mismatch*. When a small presynaptic cell, which has a proportionally small membrane capacitance, synapses with a larger postsynaptic cell, the smaller cell must be able to evoke a postsynaptic current of sufficient size and speed to bring the larger cell to action potential threshold. If the two cells are connected via gap junctions, the smaller cell would not be able to effectively charge the membrane capacitance of the lager cell via the electronic spread of it's membrane potential. Chemical synapses, however, avoid this problem by using vesicles filled with neurotransmitter which can be released several at a time. Each vesicle contains many thousand molecules of neurotransmitter, which in turn open many thousand postsynaptic ionotropic receptors. A weak presynaptic signal may therefore be amplified chemically to produce a comparatively larger response in the postsynaptic neuron. Such *amplification* is of particular importance at the neuromuscular junction, where the postsynaptic cell is a large muscle fiber (Fig. 3).

One challenge for chemical synaptic transmission involves rapid clearance of neurotransmitter molecules from the cleft. In order to maintain the ability for rapid and discrete signaling, it is important that the neurotransmitter does not linger in the vicinity of postsynaptic receptors causing them to remain active for prolonged periods. Though simple diffusion plays a large role in removing neurotransmitter molecules from the synaptic cleft, complete removal requires specialized enzymes. In most cases, *transporters* accomplish the task of neurotransmitter removal. Transporters are enzymes localized on the plasma membrane of neurons and glial cells, which use existing electrochemical gradients to shuttle molecules of neurotransmitter back into the cell. Pharmacologically, transporters are the locus of action for several drugs, both addictive and therapeutic. Cocaine is a specific blocker of the dopamine transporter, and the anti-depressant drug Prozac™ inhibits the seratonin transporter. At the neuromuscular junction, a different tactic is used for clearing neurotransmitter molecules. Here, an enzyme called *acetylcholinesterase* degrades the transmitter acetylcholine in the synaptic cleft before reuptake. This enzyme is critical, and inhibiting it leads to rapid and profound paralysis. Acetylcholinesterase is the target for some insecticides, the nerve gas sarin, and the crippling autoimmune disorder myasthenia gravis.

Finally, we point out that neurotransmitters released at chemical synapses may also bind *metabotropic receptors* located on both the presynaptic and postsynaptic membranes. Unlike ligand-gated ionotropic receptors, metabotropic receptors have a higher affinity for their ligand and do not directly gate an ion channel. When located on the presynaptic terminal inside or near the synaptic cleft, they are known as *autoreceptors* because neurotransmitter released from the same cell feeds back to affect presynaptic function. Metabotropic receptors interact with G-proteins which couple to other effector proteins (like phosphodiesterases or ion channels), and metabotropic ligand binding is responsible for activating these associated G-protein pathways. Each activated metabotropic receptor can activate several hundred G-proteins, and each activated G-protein can then interact with several hundred effector proteins. This allows for a high degree of signaling amplification.

In summary, the greater flexibility and plasticity available to chemical synapses has made them the favored mode of synaptic transmission in the brains of vertebrates and invertebrates (e.g., the worm *C. elegans* has about 7000 chemical synapses, but only 600 electrical synapses). For the rest of this chapter, the term synapse is synonymous with the chemical synapse.

3. A MODEL SYNAPSE: THE NEUROMUSCULAR JUNCTION

The frog neuromuscular junction (NMJ) was the first synapse to be thoroughly investigated. It has many advantages for the study of synaptic transmission, including its ability for easy access, stimulation, and electrical recording. Figure 3 shows a schematic diagram of the frog NMJ. A single motor nerve axon terminates in several branches on a single muscle fiber. This area of multiple synapses is called the *end-plate region*. A recording electrode that impales the muscle fiber just underneath the end plate region (electrode A in Fig. 3) will record a resting membrane potential of

I *Neuromuscular junction*

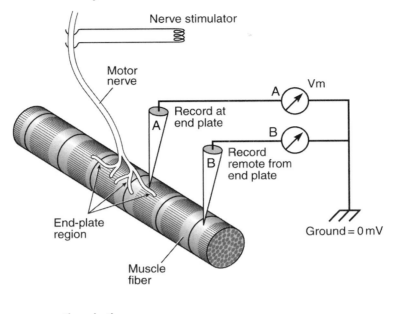

II *No nerve stimulation*

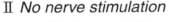

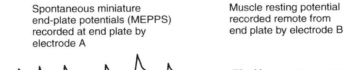

III *Nerve stimulation*

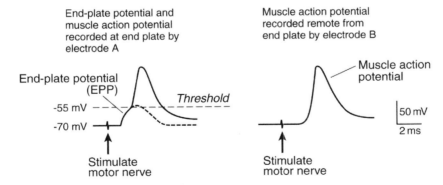

Fig. 3. The Neuromuscular Junction. **(I)** Schematic diagram of electrophysiological recordings from the frog neuromuscular junction. Electrical stimulation of the motor nerve causes APs to invade the nerve terminal where they elicit transmitter release. An intracellular electrode with tip placed inside the muscle and near to the end-plate region (electrode A) can record changes in membrane voltage V_m relative to the ground potential which is set to 0 mV. **(II)** With no nerve stimulation, small and spontaneous miniature end-plate potentials (MEPPS) are recorded by electrode A, but not by the more distantly placed electrode B, which records only the resting membrane potential of −70 mV. MEPPS are caused by the spontaneous fusion or exocytosis of single synaptic vesicles. **(III)** Upon nerve stimulation a large end-plate potential (EPP) is observed in the motor nerve. The EPP depolarizes the nerve above the threshold for triggering a muscle AP. Electrode B also records an AP, since APs actively propagate down the muscle fiber. (Modified from Gardner, 1995.)

about −70 mV. In addition, several spontaneous miniature end-plate potentials (MEPPS or mini-EPSPs) will also be superimposed on the resting membrane potential. These electrical events were first recorded by Fatt and Katz in 1951. A recording electrode placed at some distance from the end-plate (electrode B in Fig. 3) will not detect these MEPPS because *electrotonic attenuation* reduces their already small amplitude (0.5 mV) to levels below the basal noise. Subsequently, in 1954 del Castilho and Katz noticed that the amplitudes of the MEPPS were remarkably consistent and that endplate potentials (EPPs) frequently appeared as multiples of a standard size. The EPP therefore appeared to be composed of discrete units, or *quanta*, corresponding to unitary MEPPs. They called the standard MEPP amplitude the *quantal size* and denoted it with the symbol *q*.

Returning to Fig. 3, when a single action potential was stimulated in the motor nerve, an end-plate potential was recorded by electrode A after a short delay. The shape of the EPP was similar to that of the MEPP, but its size was several-fold larger. The constant scaling factor between the EPP and MEPP was denoted by *m* called the *quantal content* of the EPP. The EPP amplitude invariably exceeded the threshold for action potential generation, so a muscle action potential was also observed first at the end-plate (electrode A) and then further away (electrode B). Del Castilho and Katz further assumed that the end-plate contained several discrete sites for quantal release. Supposing that a number of these release sites, denoted *N*, were functional at any given time and had an average *probability of release* (P_r), they postulated that $m = N \times P_r$. This elegant statistical analysis of neurotransmitter release still shapes our modern quantitative views of synaptic function.

The morphological correlates of *q*, *m*, and *N* are thought to be the synaptic vesicle, the number of vesicle fusions, and the number of functional active zones in the nerve terminal respectively. Synaptic vesicles are homogenous in size (about 50 nm in diameter at the NMJ) and are believed to contain the same amount of neurotransmitter. Interestingly, certain mutants of the fruit fly *Drosophila* (called *lap* mutants) have unusually large synaptic vesicles and correspondingly larger MEPPs. At the frog NMJ, there are about 300 active zones. This redundancy, or high *N* value, allows for a small P_r at individual active zones but a large overall *m* value. In other words, there is a large safety factor at the NMJ so that it can function as a fail-safe relay to trigger muscle action potentials. One caveat to this general rule occurs when stimulation frequency is high. In this case, P_r is drastically reduced and failures in AP transmission can occur.

4. PRESYNAPTIC EXOCYTOSIS IS CA²⁺ DEPENDENT

Neurotransmitter release occurs when synaptic vesicles fuse with the presynaptic plasma membrane. This process of exocytosis is triggered by the influx of free Ca^{2+} ions into the nerve terminal. Depolarization of the nerve terminal opens voltage-gated Ca^{2+} selective channels, and because calcium concentrations are much higher in the extracellular space than in the cytosol, calcium flows into the cell according to its large electrochemical driving force. This flux of ions produces a current that can be measured, for example, using the *two-electrode voltage clamp* technique. This type of Ca^{2+} *current* recording can be performed in the squid giant synapse. When the postsynaptic neuron is impaled by a third electrode for recording EPSPs, it becomes possible to examine the relationship between a presynaptic Ca^{2+} current and a postsynaptic EPSP (*see* Fig. 4). Small step depolarizations of the nerve terminal from −60 to −30 mV elicit a small, slow Ca^{2+} current and relatively small EPSP in the postsynaptic cell. A stronger presynaptic depolarization from −60 to 0 mV will evoke a lager, more rapid Ca^{2+} current and much larger EPSP. Similarly, short depolarizations will produce smaller EPSPs than longer duration depolarizations of the same magnitude. Using this method for comparing pre- and postsynaptic events, the relationship between calcium influx and postsynaptic response was found to be nonlinear.

Results from the squid giant axon synapse confirmed previous experiments in the frog NMJ showing that transmitter release depends exponentially on Ca^{2+} concentration in the extracellular medium (by a 4th power relationship). Physiological Ca^{2+} ion concentrations are about 2 m*M* extracellularly, and intracellular free Ca^{2+} lies in the range of 100 n*M*. This imbalance results in a large electrochemical driving force toward calcium entry when Ca^{2+} channels are open, and local Ca^{2+} concentrations near the cytosolic mouth of these channels can reach levels as high as 100–300 μ*M* for tens to hundreds of microseconds. Upon entry, calcium ions are thought to bind one or more proteins on docked synaptic vesicles, which act as a sensor for initiating the fusion process. The fusion sensor protein is thus activated by calcium for an

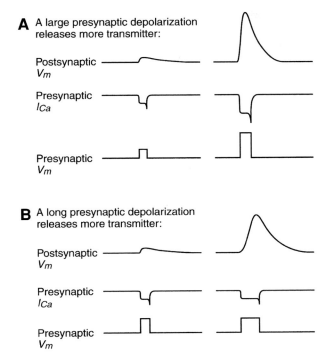

A A large presynaptic depolarization
releases more transmitter:

Postsynaptic
V_m

Presynaptic
I_{Ca}

Presynaptic
V_m

B A long presynaptic depolarization
releases more transmitter:

Postsynaptic
V_m

Presynaptic
I_{Ca}

Presynaptic
V_m

Fig. 4. Ca^{2+} ions and synaptic transmission. Schematic diagram of electrophysiological recordings from the squid giant synapse. Simultaneous pre- and postsynaptic voltage-clamp recordings. **(A)** A step-like depolarization of the presynaptic terminal (bottom trace) causes the opening of voltage-gated Ca^{2+} channels and the activation of a presynaptic Ca^{2+} current. The resulting Ca^{2+} influx triggers transmitter release and a postsynaptic potential change in the postsynaptic cell. A small amplitude presynaptic depolarization elicits a small postsynaptic response, whereas a larger depolarization causes a larger Ca^{2+} current and a larger postsynaptic potential. **(B)** A short depolarization causes a short Ca^{2+} current and a brief and small postsynaptic potential, whereas a longer depolarization causes a longer Ca^{2+} current and a larger postsynaptic potential. (Modified from Gardner, 1995.)

extremely brief period, a fact that may help explain the extremely phasic or transient nature of neurotransmitter release.

One candidate protein for the Ca^{2+} fusion sensor is called *synaptotagmin*. It has two so-called C2 domains (similar to the protein kinase C [PKC] Ca^{2+} binding domain) that bind Ca^{2+}. After binding calcium, synaptotagmin partially inserts itself into phospholipids of the plasma membrane to bind *SNARE-type* proteins crucial for vesicle fusion. SNARE proteins come in two varieties: vesicular (v-SNAREs) and target (t-SNAREs). The v-SNARES are found on synaptic vesicles, while the t-SNARES reside on the plasma membrane. In order for vesicle fusion to occur,

v-SNAREs and t-SNAREs must associate to form a tight *core complex* that is extremely resistant to unbinding. The SNARE core complex is highly, energetically favorable and requires ATP hydrolysis for unbinding. It is believed that this complex serves as a mechanical hair-pin that, when triggered, facilitates mixing of the synaptic vesicle and plasma membrane lipids for vesicle fusion. Evidence that SNARE proteins are essential for vesicle fusion comes from bacterial neurotoxins that selectively degrade SNARE proteins. These toxins are highly potent, and require only a few molecules to completely block synaptic transmission. Botulinum toxin, now routinely used for cosmetic applications, is an example of such a compound.

Free Ca^{2+} may regulate other processes aside from vesicle fusion. For example, the recruitment of synaptic vesicles from reserve pools to the docked or *readily-releasable pool* is accelerated by elevated intracellular Ca^{2+}. Endocytosis, the process of synaptic vesicle reuptake, may also be regulated by Ca^{2+} at some synapses, and short-term facilitation of EPSPs can result from residual Ca^{2+} accumulation during a tetanus. In addition, Ca^{2+} activates different kinases and phosphatases, which regulate several forms of long-term morphological and functional synaptic plasticity.

After synaptic vesicles fuse with the plasma membrane, they are recycled back into the nerve terminal (Fig. 2). The process of vesicular-membrane-reinternalization (or retrieval) from the plasma membrane is called *endocytosis*, and the synapse utilizes several forms of this process. Some types of endocytosis are very fast and occur with a time constant of about 1 s. Other forms are slower (time constant of 10–20 s), and are probably mediated by *clathrin*-coated pits that form on the plasma membrane. Endocytosing vesicles require a GTPase called *dynamin* to 'pinch-off' from the plasma membrane into the intracellular space. Interestingly, the *Drosophila* mutant *shibire* has a temperature-sensitive defect in dynamin and becomes paralyzed at elevated temperatures (e.g., 29°C). Electron microscopy reveals that the nerve terminals of these paralyzed flies are devoid of cytoplasmic synaptic vesicles. Furthermore, the plasma membrane is found to have a string of coated invaginations that cannot pinch off. This observation indicates that the terminals are incapable of completing endocytosis and cannot recycle their vesicular membrane after fusion. Accordingly, the surface area of the terminals is enlarged and there are no vesicles available for continued exocytosis. This dramatic phenotype clearly demonstrates the importance of vesicle recycling for the continuous operation of a synapse. It also illustrates that severe *vesicle-pool depletion* will block synaptic transmission.

5. NEUROTRANSMITTERS AND THEIR RECEPTORS IN THE MAMMALIAN BRAIN

A large proportion of synapses in the mammalian brain are excitatory and use the amino acid *glutamate* as their neurotransmitter. Glutamate is sequestered into vesicles by a *vesicular glutamate transporter* protein in the vesicular membrane. Synaptic vesicles are acidic (pH = 5.7), and the energy from their proton concentration gradient is used to transport neurotransmitter into the vesicle. Synaptic vesicles therefore require a proton ATPase to acidify their interior (or lumen). There are two broad categories of synaptic vesicle proteins: (1) transport proteins (e.g., proton pumps, Na^+/Ca^{2+} exchangers, and Cl^- ion transporters) and (2) trafficking/fusion proteins (e.g., v-SNARES, synaptotagmin, and synapsin). Once glutamate is released into the synaptic cleft, it diffuses away quickly (within milliseconds) and binds to *plasma membrane glutamate transporters* located in pre- and postsynaptic neurons and glia (or astrocytes). These transporters use existing sodium and potassium gradients to drive glutamate back into the cytoplasm. Neurotransmitter is recycled in this manner, and since excessive glutamate is toxic for neurons and can lead to cell-death, the external glutamate concentration is tightly controlled by this reuptake process.

On the postsynaptic cell, glutamate receptors can be classified into two general types: ionotropic and metabotropic receptors. As noted previously, ionotropic receptors gate ion channels directly, whereas metabotropic receptors are coupled to G-proteins. There are three kinds of ionotropic glutamate receptors, each named after the glutamate analog they bind preferentially: AMPA, NMDA and kainate. Glutamate and the synthetic compound AMPA are potent *agonists* for the AMPA-type receptor. The AMPA receptor also has specific *antagonists* such as the compounds CNQX and NBQX. These do not affect the NMDA receptor. Glutamate binding to the AMPA receptor opens a nonselective cation channel permeable to both Na^+ and K^+ ions; an event which tends to bring a negative resting membrane potential towards 0 mV. AMPA receptors have intrinsically fast kinetics and desensitize within

milliseconds when given a continuous pulse of glutamate. The fast EPSPs observed at excitatory synapses are mediated by AMPA-receptor activation. NMDA receptors have slower kinetics, use glycine as a coagonist, and do not desensitize quickly. They are often colocalized at the PSD with AMPA receptors. NMDA and kainite receptors have also been found recently in some CNS presynaptic nerve terminals, but their function is not well understood.

The major inhibitory neurotransmitters in the brain are *GABA* and *glycine*. These transmitters are similarly packaged into vesicles by vesicular GABA/glycine transporters expressed on the membrane of synaptic vesicles. Other neurotransmitters in the mammalian brain include acetylcholine, ATP, adenosine, and several amine transmitters (e.g., dopamine, noradrenaline [or norepinephine], adrenaline (or epinephrine), serotonin, and histamine). The *catecholamine* transmitters (dopamine, noradrenaline, and adrenaline) are all synthesized from the essential amino acid tyrosine in a common biosynthetic pathway. Catecholamines are important in the brain, not only as neurotransmitters, but also as *neuromodulators* that have widespread effects on neuronal circuits. Interestingly, vesicular amine transporters are targets for several pharmacological agents. For example, the antipsychotic drugs 'reserpine' and 'tetrabenazine' inhibit amine transporters, and the psychostimulants 'amphetamine' and 'ecstasy' are thought to dissipate the pH gradient of synaptic vesicles containing amine transmitters.

There are three types of GABA receptors: $GABA_A$, $GABA_B$, and $GABA_C$. The $GABA_A$ and $GABA_C$ receptors are ionotropic, while the $GABA_B$ receptor is metabotropic. The $GABA_A$ receptor is blocked by bicuculine and desensitizes quickly, whereas $GABA_C$ receptors desensitize much more slowly and are insensitive to bicuculine. GABA binding to the $GABA_A$ or $GABA_C$ receptor opens an anion selective Cl^- channel which tends to bring the membrane potential towards the equilibrium potential of Cl^- (about -60 to -80 mV, depending on intracellular Cl^- concentration). This hyperpolarization usually inhibits the postsynaptic neuron from firing action potentials. $GABA_B$ receptors are also known to have an inhibitory function. For example, the $GABA_B$ receptors of some presynaptic terminals inhibit Ca^{2+} channels and cause a reduction of transmitter release. Glycine receptors are ionotropic (anion selective Cl^- channels) and can have very rapid kinetics of activation and deactivation.

6. THE INTERPLAY OF EXCITATION AND INHIBITION

A simple neural circuit that demonstrates how excitatory and inhibitory synapses are combined to produce a functionally significant behavior is the myotatic (or "knee-jerk") spinal reflex (*see* Fig. 5). When a hammer is tapped on the extensor muscle, sensory axons carry the information from the extensor muscle toward the spinal cord. These, or any other axons that carry information to the brain or spinal cord, are called *afferents*. Motor axons, or *efferents*, carry information away from the brain or spinal cord and initiate a behavioral response to the hammer tap (an upward jerk of the leg). Along their path, the sensory afferents branch to make synaptic contact with both motor neurons of the ventral horn and spinal *interneurons* (i.e., neurons that lie entirely in the spinal cord). The sensory axon synaptic terminals release glutamate and are excitatory, whereas the interneurons release inhibitory neurotransmitters (GABA and glycine). The sensory neurons thus excite motor neurons that make synaptic contact with the extensor muscle and cause it to contract. Similarly, the sensory axon terminals excite local inhibitory interneurons that synapse onto the motor neurons innervating the flexor muscle. This causes a relaxation of the flexor and permits the opposing extensor muscle to dominate the behavioral response.

Electrophysiological recordings from the sensory, interneuron, and motor neurons of the myotatic spinal circuit provide insight into how the circuit operates (Fig. 5). There are several types of electrophysiological recordings. *Extracellular recording* with an electrode (usually metal) placed near a neuron measures the all-or-nothing action potentials (APs) produced by the neuron. *Intracellular recordings*, where the electrode (usually a glass micropipet filled with a conducting solution) impales the cell (as in Fig. 3), can detect smaller, sub-threshold synaptic potentials. *Patch-clamp recordings*, where a glass electrode is placed on the membrane of the cell, are very low-noise recordings that can even detect single-channel currents. Examples of extracellular recordings from spinal neurons involved in the myotatic reflex are shown in Fig. 5. Neurons usually have a low level of spontaneous AP firing in the absence of any synaptic or sensory input. The hammer tap to the knee elicits a burst of APs in the sensory neuron, which is followed after a brief delay by a burst of APs in the motor (extensor) neurons and interneurons. The interneurons

then inhibit the firing of the flexor motor neurons. The end result is a leg extension. Recordings of AP onset, duration, and frequency thus provide a real time picture of neuronal activity. By using the complementary intracellular and patch-clamp recording techniques, the mechanisms underlying circuit function can be determined.

7. SYNAPSES ARE HETEROGENEOUS AND CAN BE SPECIALIZED

Synapses can exhibit different functional properties and architectures depending on their specific information transfer and processing needs. We discuss ribbon and calyx type synapses found in the retina and brainstem as examples of highly specialized synapses. We also summarize some of the hallmark properties of the more typical bouton type synapses found in the cortex and other parts of the brain.

Ribbon type synapses are found in the vertebrate retina and the cochlea. Retinal photoreceptors and bipolar cells as well as cochlear hair cells transmit sensory information via this type of synapse. Light and sound stimuli produce tonic and graded membrane depolarizations in these cells which elicits the graded release of neurotransmitter from specialized active zones called *synaptic ribbons*. These synapses are tailored to transmit the large amounts of sensory information involved in vision and hearing.

One technique used to study the synaptic release of neurotransmitter from these cells is time-resolved *membrane capacitance measurements*, which are based on the patch-clamp recording technique. Electrical membrane capacitance is proportional to the surface area of a cell. When there is an increase in cell surface area (e.g., during exocytosis), membrane capacitance increases. Similarly, when surface area decreases (e.g., during endocytosis), membrane capacitance deceases. Net changes in cell surface area of <1% can be detected by this exquisitely sensitive technique. An example of a membrane capacitance (C_m) measurement is shown in Fig. 6. This C_m measurement was obtained from the whole-cell patch-clamp recording of an isolated synaptic terminal of a goldfish retinal bipolar cell. The terminal's baseline C_m value is constant until a step depolarization (from a holding potential of $-60\,mV$ to $-10\,mV$) is given during the gray bar (Fig. 6A). This depolarization opens Ca^{2+} channels and the resulting influx of Ca^{2+} into the terminal triggers the fusion of synaptic vesicles with the plasma

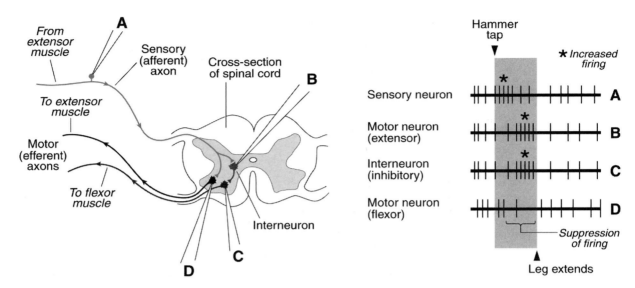

Fig. 5. A reflex circuit in the spinal cord. Schematic diagram of spinal cord circuitry. Extracellular electrophysiological recordings from the four specified neurons are shown on the right hand panel. A gentle hammer tap to the knee causes a burst of APs to travel along the sensory axons (recorded by electrode A) and towards the neurons of the spinal cord. The sensory axon branches into two pathways exciting the motor neurons connected to the extensor muscle (recorded by electrode D) and certain interneurons in the spinal cord (recorded by electrode B). The interneurons then inhibit the firing of the motor neurons connected to the flexor muscle (recorded by electrode C). The hammer tap thus causes the reflex of leg extension. (Modified from Neuroscience, edited by Purves et al., 2001.)

membrane along with an increase in the terminal's surface area. This is detected as a jump in C_m immediately after the depolarization. The size of the jump is 150 femtoF. Since each synaptic vesicle has a diameter of about 30 nm and a capacitance of 26.4 attoF, the C_m jump corresponds to the fusion of about 6000 synaptic vesicles. A strong depolarization can thus elicit the fusion of several thousand vesicles at ribbon synapses. Large vesicle pools that can be released quickly are a characteristic of ribbon-type synapses, and this property allows them to release small or large amounts of transmitter depending on the degree and speed of the presynaptic depolarization. Following the jump in C_m, membrane capacitance decays back to the original baseline following a single exponential time course. The exponential time constant of $\tau = 1.1$ s is a measure of the rate of membrane retrieval (endocytosis). Fused synaptic vesicle membrane can thus be quickly reinternalized and recycled into the terminal.

Figure 6B diagrams the unique architecture of a ribbon-type active zone as seen by electron microscopy. An electron dense "ribbon" sheet has a halo of tethered synaptic vesicles. Vesicles located in the bottom row (black vesicles) are docked to the plasma membrane. They are close to Ca^{2+} channels and presumably poised for rapid exocytosis, constituting an immediately releasable pool of vesicles. The other vesicles (gray vesicles) tethered to the ribbon structure are thought to be next in line for fusion. After these vesicles fuse, the synapse is refractory to subsequent release for a few seconds. The vesicles tethered to the synaptic ribbon may thus be the morphological correlate of a *readily releasable pool* of synaptic vesicles.

A second type of specialized synapse is located in the mammalian auditory brainstem, where *calyx-type synapses* involved in calculating the location of sound sources are found. The morphology of the synapse is shown in Fig. 7. The large calyx- type synaptic terminal has hundreds of small *conventional active zones* in adult animals. Conventional active zones have about 2 to 10 docked vesicles and a cluster of reserve vesicles, as depicted in Fig. 2. Each conventional active zone in the calyx terminal has a different release probability. During a stimulus consisting of a train of presynaptic APs, this heterogeneity of release probabilities means that some active zones (with high release probability) will release transmitter early during the stimulus train, while others (with low release probability) will release late in the stimulus train. This synapse is thus able to faithfully follow a presynaptic train of APs, even when this train occurs at a very high frequency (e.g., 800 Hz). The large number of active zones also ensures

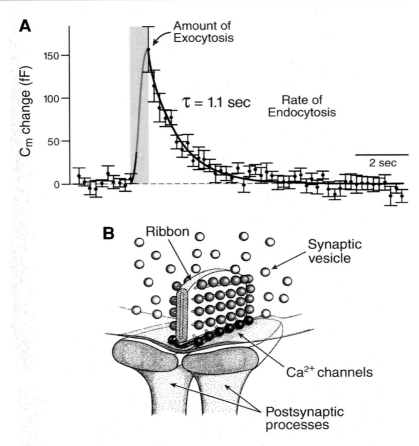

Fig. 6. (*Opposite page*) Synaptic transmission at a ribbon synapse. (**A**) Membrane capacitance (C_m) measurements from the ribbon-type synaptic terminal of bipolar cells in the goldfish retina. A step depolarization (from the a holding potential of –60 mV to –10 mV), given during the period marked by a gray bar, elicits a jump in C_m of about 150 fF. This corresponds to the fusion (or exocytosis) of about 6000 synaptic vesicles with the presynaptic plasma membrane. Following the jump in Cm the capacitance decays back to the original baseline following a single exponential time course. The time constant $\tau = 1.1$ s and is a measure of the rate of membrane retrieval (endocytosis). (**B**) A 3-dimensional schematic drawing of the ribbon-type active zone of bipolar cell synaptic terminals. The electron dense "ribbon" sheet has a halo of tethered synaptic vesicles. Vesicles located in the bottom row (black vesicles) are docked to the plasma membrane and are close to Ca^{2+} channels. They constitute a readily releasable pool of vesicles. The other vesicles (gray vesicles) tethered to the ribbon structure are thought to be next in line for fusion. (Modified from von Gersdorff, 2001.)

a short synaptic delay because the EPSP is very fast and large. This leads to a precise preservation of AP timing. The ability of the postsynaptic neuron to follow presynaptic APs with high fidelity and short synaptic delays are features that help in the processing of sound localization in this auditory pathway synapse.

Some synapses, like the neuromuscular junction, the calyx-type brainstem synapse, and the squid giant synapse are relatively large and guarantee fail-safe transmission. In adult animals, these synapses are relatively fixed in their transmission characteristics. Most synapses in the mammalian brain are, however, physically small (diameter of <1 μm; *see* Fig. 7), produce small EPSPs, and have a low-release probability. This

makes them rather unreliable in transmitting signals. These synapses are called conventional *bouton-type synapses*. Their small EPSPs may, nevertheless, summate on a postsynaptic neuron to help it fire APs (*see* Fig. 8). The relative timing of presynaptic APs and resulting EPSPs is critical for *spatial* or *temporal summation* (Fig. 8). Bouton-type synapses of the CNS can also change their properties dramatically after certain patterns of neuronal activity. This aspect of synaptic plasticity is a way of storing new information acquired by experience in the synaptic strength of a particular synapse. The small size of bouton-type synapses also allows for a large number of synapses to be packed in a small volume, thus increasing the computational

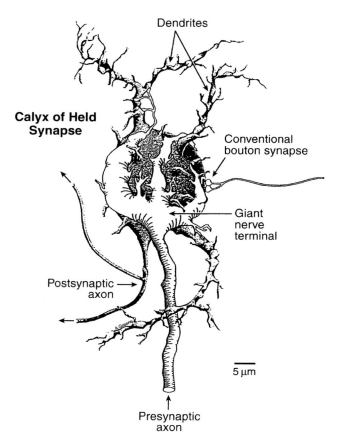

Fig. 7. The calyx of Held synapse. A diagram of the adult calyx of Held, a glutamatergic nerve terminal in the mammalian auditory brainstem. Notice the large caliber axon (4–12 μm) that gives rise to the calyx terminal. The postsynaptic cell has relatively short dendrites and an axon with a collateral branch. A typical bouton-type terminal is indicated for comparison. (Modified from Morest, 1973.)

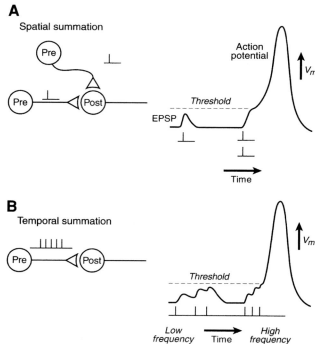

Fig. 8. Spatial and temporal summation at bouton-type synapses. (**A**) Spatial summation. Schematic diagram showing how the input from two small, bouton-type presynaptic terminals can summate to produce a supra-threshold EPSP. The input from just one bouton is not enough to trigger an AP in the postsynaptic cell. However, if the two inputs elicit simultaneous EPSPs in the postsynaptic cell the summed depolarization is enough to trigger an AP. (**B**) Temporal summation. Low-frequency stimulation may not be enough to trigger an AP in the postsynaptic cell. However, high frequency stimulation may cause the individual EPSPs to summate fast enough to trigger an AP. The importance of the relative timing of EPSPs is thus evident from these two examples. (Modified from Gardner, 1995.)

8. SHORT-TERM AND LONG-TERM SYNAPTIC PLASTICITY

capacity of the brain. Often, one presynaptic bouton-type terminal synapses onto one spine-like dendritic structure of a postsynaptic neuron (as depicted in Fig. 2), and a single dendrite can have hundreds to thousands of *postsynaptic spines*. Each bouton-type terminal typically has one conventional active zone with about 2 to 10 docked vesicles and a cluster of reserve vesicles in its cytosol, as depicted in Fig. 2. In total, the whole bouton has about 200 vesicles. Accordingly, these synapses have a small readily releasable pool estimated to be about 10 vesicles. Neuromodulators, such as noradrenaline and dopamine, can also change the output of bouton-type synapses, making them especially flexible transducers of information.

Following a train of presynaptic APs (or a tetanic stimulus) the corresponding postsynaptic potentials can grow in amplitude (a process called *short-term facilitation*) or decrease in amplitude (a process called *short-term depression*). Often, synapses either display short-term facilitation followed by short-term depression or, alternatively, just short-term depression. There are multiple synaptic mechanisms that may underlie these forms of short-term synaptic plasticity. For example, after the first presynaptic AP in a stimulus train, the Ca^{2+} concentration in the terminal decays back to resting levels. However, this decay may take several milliseconds depending on the Ca^{2+}-buffering capacity of the terminal. The second stimuli in the train may thus add upon residual CA^{2+} to elevate Ca^{2+} concentrations to levels higher than the first stimulus. Given the highly nonlinear dependence of transmitter release on Ca^{2+}, short-term facilitation may therefore be due to the high resting Ca^{2+} concentrations reached during a stimulus train.

Short-term depression may be caused by pre- or postsynaptic mechanisms. During a stimulus train the pool of readily releasable vesicles may get depleted at a rate faster than the replenishment rate of newly recruited vesicles. The resulting depletion of the readily releasable pool of vesicles will thus cause synaptic depression. The presynaptic Ca^{2+} current may also become progressively inactivated during a stimulus train leading to decreased release. Alternatively, postsynaptic factors may also lead to reduced EPSPs or IPSPs, since postsynaptic ionotropic receptors may desensitize and/or saturate (i.e.,the receptors may become insensitive to further neurotransmitter release). Stimulation at very high frequencies often leads to short-term depression. Thus, high frequency inputs may be strongly filtered from a neuronal circuit by short-term plasticity.

Some synapses can change their release characteristics for a period of hours to days after receiving a particular stimulus pattern. This form of long-term plasticity may is commonly found in the mammalian hippocampus and cortex. Synaptic strength may thus be increased (a process called *long-term potentiation*) or reduced (a process called *long-term depression*). One mechanism for long-term potentiation involves the properties of the AMPA and NMDA receptors located on postsynaptic dendritic spines. The release of glutamate from bouton-type terminals produces rapid AMPA receptor mediated EPSPs that transiently depolarize the spine. Glutamate also binds to the slower activating and inactivating NMDA receptors colocalized with the AMPA receptors on the spine. However, when the spine is at its initial resting membrane potential, external Mg^{2+} ions block the NMDA channel. Therefore, no current flows through the channel, even though its transmitter-activated gate is opened by glutamate. On the other hand, if the dendritic spine has been previously depolarized by other nearby synaptic inputs, the Mg^{2+} block is removed and the NMDA channel can pass current upon glutamate binding. The NMDA receptor is thus both a voltage-dependent and ligand-gated channel, with the voltage dependence arising from the voltage-dependent Mg^{2+} block of the channel pore. NMDA receptors, unlike most AMPA receptors, are permeable to Ca^{2+} ions. So the NMDA receptor mediated postsynaptic current will increase Ca^{2+} concentrations in the spine, leading to the activation of *Ca^{2+}-dependent kinases* that may phosphorylate the AMPA receptor and thus augment its current. Furthermore, Ca^{2+} ions in the spine may trigger the release of *retrograde messengers* that feedback onto the bouton terminal to increase its release probability. These molecular events can produce long-term changes in synaptic strength. The NMDA receptor can thus operate as a *coincidence detector* for spine depolarization by other synaptic inputs and glutamate release from its own opposing bouton terminal. This association of different synaptic inputs, which are activated at specific times, and the resulting selective strengthening of a particular synapse may constitute a cellular mechanism for learning and memory.

ACKNOWLEDGMENT

We acknowledge with thanks the use of several figures modified from the chapter on synaptic transmission by Daniel Gardner that appeared in the earlier edition of this text.

SELECTED READINGS

Gardner D. Synaptic transmission. Conn MP (ed.): In *Neuroscience in Medicine*, J.B. Lippincott Company, Philadelphia, 1995.

Kandel E, Siegelbaum, SA. Transmitter release. InKandel E., Schwartz JH, Jessell TM (eds): *In Principles of Neural Science*, Fourth Edition. McGraw Hill, New York, 2000.

Morest DK, et al. Stimulus coding at the caudal levels of the cat's auditory nervous system. In *Basic Mechanisms of Hearing*, edited by Möller AR, Academic Press, New York, 1973.

Purves D, Augustine GA Fitzpatrick D, et al.: Synaptic transmission *In Neuroscience* Second Edition. Sinauer, Sunderland, MA, 2001.

von Gersdorff H. Synaptic ribbons: versatile signal transducers. Neuron 2001; 29:7–10.

5 Pre- and Postsynaptic Receptors

Robert D. Grubbs and David K. Sundberg*

1. RECEPTOR STRUCTURE AND FUNCTION

A receptor is a cell component, usually a protein, that combines with a drug, a transmitter, or a hormone to alter the cellular response.

2. RECEPTOR CLASSIFICATION SCHEMES: ANATOMICAL, PHARMACOLOGICAL, AND STRUCTURAL/MECHANISTIC

There are several classifications of receptor systems. These include anatomic, pharmacologic, and since the advent of molecular biologic techniques, mechanistic classifications. The earliest anatomic classification systems were based on the location of specific types of receptors. Examples include somatic or autonomic, parasympathetic or sympathetic, and postsynaptic or presynaptic (e.g., having the receptor on the nerve terminal or dendrite and serving neuromodulatory function) classification systems.

The pharmacologic classification of receptors has been developing since the late 1800s, when the transmitter substances were first isolated and chemically characterized. Receptors are classified according to transmitter groups and their response to drugs. Recep-

*Deceased.

From: *Neuroscience in Medicine, 2nd ed.* (P. Michael Conn, ed.),
© 2003 Humana Press Inc., Totowa, NJ.

tors that respond to the catecholamines (e.g., dopamine, norepinephrine, and epinephrine) are known as catecholaminergic or sometimes "adrenergic" receptors. Because some respond better to norepinephrine than to epinephrine, they have been further subdivided into α- and β-adrenergic receptors. Both of these receptor subtypes have been further characterized into types 1 and 2 (e.g., β_1, β_2). These types can be demonstrated when relatively small chemical differences in the transmitter structures selectively affect only one population of receptors. This extensive system has made it necessary for the student to learn a multitude of receptor subtypes, but the subtypes have been convenient for the purposes of research, therapy, and the pharmaceutical industry. For example, it is possible to develop a drug (e.g., β_2-adrenergic agonist) that dilates bronchial smooth muscle in an asthmatic that does not have significant effects on the β_1 receptor of the heart, which would greatly increase the heart rate and cause cardiac palpitations.

The structural/mechanistic method for the classification of receptors is based on information obtained from the cloning and sequencing of genes for receptors. Cloning of genes refers to the process of inserting copies of the gene for a specific protein (e.g., a receptor) into bacteria and allowing the natural reproduction and growth of the bacteria to produce the gene, mRNA, or protein of interest for harvest in bulk form.

Using this classification scheme of receptors, four groups or "families" of receptors have been revealed, each with a different molecular mechanism that activates the cell to respond after the transmitter has combined with its receptor. One of the major families includes the ion channel-gated receptors. These receptors form a channel or pore in the membrane through which various ions can travel. Transmitter coupling can open or close the membrane pores.

Another structural/mechanistic family of receptors is the G-protein-coupled receptors (GPCRs). The receptor protein, which spans the membrane seven times, activates a G protein, so named because it binds to and eventually hydrolyzes guanosine 5' triphosphate (GTP). This protein initiates a series of events (e.g., second-messenger system) that produces an effect within the cell, such as the opening or closing of an ion channel, the production of another second messenger, such as cyclic AMP, or the stimulation of genetic translation and transcription.

Although it seems logical that a given member of a pharmacologic class of receptors (e.g., cholinergic) would fall within the same gene family of the structural/mechanistic class of receptors, this is not always the case. The nicotinic cholinergic receptor belongs to the ion-gated family of receptors, and the muscarinic cholinergic receptor, which also responds to acetylcholine, belongs to the *GPCR* family. To this extent, the muscarinic cholinergic receptor and the adrenergic receptor that responds to norepinephrine belong to the same family of membrane proteins.

Other receptor families include the membrane receptors that respond to growth factors and the intracellular cytoplasmic receptors that respond to the steroid hormones (e.g., estrogen, testosterone, and cortisone), and thyroxine. The membrane-bound receptors that respond to growth factors have intrinsic enzymatic activity that is responsible for initiating their cellular response. The cytoplasmic portion of these receptors contains a tyrosine kinase domain that autophosphorylates the dimerized receptor, permitting it to activate a signaling cascade through the activation of one of the small G-proteins, such as Ras. Although receptors for several growth factors have been identified in the brain, their precise role has not yet been determined.

In this chapter, specific receptors are discussed within the framework of the pharmacologic method of classification. This method is important in terms of medical practice and is the basis for therapeutics.

However, we further define the receptors in terms of their structural/molecular mechanisms and the major gene families to which they belong.

2.1. Receptors Can Be Mathematically Characterized Using Biochemical Kinetic Parameters Developed to Understand Enzymes

Receptors are like enzymes that bind to a substrate and catalyze a cellular activity. In the case of enzymes, the activity is usually the addition or deletion of an atom or group of atoms to or from the substrate. In the case of the receptor, the transmitter is not chemically changed. These membrane-bound proteins, when activated by their transmitters, catalyze an activity within the membrane, which may be the opening of an ion channel or regulation of an intracellular signaling pathway that alters the biological state of the cell.

The concept of the cellular receptor was developed in the early 1900s by JN Langley, who ascribed the effects of drugs and hormones to an interaction with a receptive substance (now known as receptor). Later, AJ Clark and other scientists, including AV Hill and JH Gaddum, mathematically described these interactions and developed methods for characterizing them pharmacologically.

The attractive forces between the transmitter or drug and its receptor can be chemically mediated by covalent, ionic, hydrogen binding, or Van der Waals forces. High-energy covalent bonding is rare, occurring only with a few drugs such as the α-adrenergic-receptor blocker phenoxybenzamine. This type of binding is irreversible, noncompetitive, and is not utilized by any transmitter. Ionic attractions occur between cationic (e.g., positive) and anionic (e.g., negative) charges of different molecules and provide an attractive force that enables the transmitter to find the receptor. Hydrogen bonding is the attraction between hydrogen atoms and unpaired electrons in nitrogen or oxygen atoms, and is important for attracting the ligand to the receptor. Van der Waals forces are weak dipolar interactions, but because of the number of atomic interactions and the complementarity or "fit" between the ligand and receptor, these forces are important for defining the tightness of binding (e.g., affinity) and specificity of the receptor for its transmitter.

The interactions of most transmitters with their receptors follow Michaelis-Menten kinetics, as do biochemical enzymatic reactions. Fig. 1 shows two curves generated by measuring the binding of a transmitter

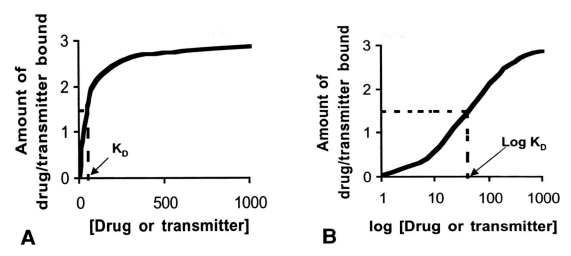

Fig. 1. (A) Graph of a Michaelis-Menten type plot in which the amount of a labeled drug or transmitter bound to receptor is plotted against the concentration of drug or transmitter in the assay. The concentration that produces 50% of the maximal receptor occupancy (B_{max}) represents the dissociation constant (K_d). **(B)** Graph of a typical concentration-dependent binding curve, in which the amount bound is plotted against the log of the concentration. In this case, the concentration that produces half of the B_{max} is the log of the K_d.

such as acetylcholine to its receptor. This could be the effect of increasing concentrations of acetylcholine on the firing rate of a neuronal pathway in the forebrain. In the graph on the left (often called a Michaelis-Menten curve), increasing concentrations of the transmitter lead to an increased response that eventually plateaus. This plateau has been shown by kinetics to represent the maximal number of receptors present in the tissue sample, B_{max}. The transmitter concentration that produces one-half of the maximal binding possible in this preparation yields a number known as the K_d or dissociation constant. This number describes the affinity of the receptor and is defined as the amount of substrate needed to activate or occupy one-half of all the receptors. If this number is low (e.g., in the pM or nM range), the receptor-transmitter interaction is said to be a high-affinity interaction. If the concentration of the transmitter needed to cause one-half of the maximal effect is high (e.g., in the μM or mM range), the receptor is said to have a low affinity for this particular substance.

The graph in Fig. 1B represents the same data shown in Fig. 1A, only with the x-axis modified so that the logarithm of the transmitter concentration is plotted against the amount of transmitter bound to the receptor. This method, commonly called the log dose-response plot, consistently yields a sigmoidal curve and is useful for characterizing pharmacologic interactions, providing the log of the K_d. Although the

Michaelis-Menten or direct plot and the log dose-response plot provide a good first approximation of the affinity of transmitter-receptor interaction, it is difficult to obtain precise estimates of the K_d or the B_{max} directly from these plots because they are nonlinear. To obtain an accurate estimate of these binding parameters, the Scatchard plot and the Hill plot are often used. Fig. 2 shows representative examples of these plots.

In the Scatchard plot, the amount of a radiolabeled transmitter or drug bound to its receptor is measured and plotted, as shown on the left side of Fig. 2. Briefly, the amount of a radioactive ligand that is bound to a membrane preparation (x-axis) is plotted against the ratio of the amount bound to free ligand present in the reaction (y-axis). If this relation is not linear, as shown by the dotted line, it indicates that more than one population of receptors is present with high and low dissociation constants, or that a receptor has multiple binding sites and that there is cooperativity between these binding sites. The x-intercept of this plot provides the number or receptors present in a particular tissue (B_{max}) and the negative reciprocal of the slope gives the K_d of those receptors.

The Hill plot can be used to determine whether a receptor-agonist interaction displays positive or negative cooperativity. Cooperativity means that the binding of one transmitter molecule to a receptor influences the binding and action of another molecule of the same

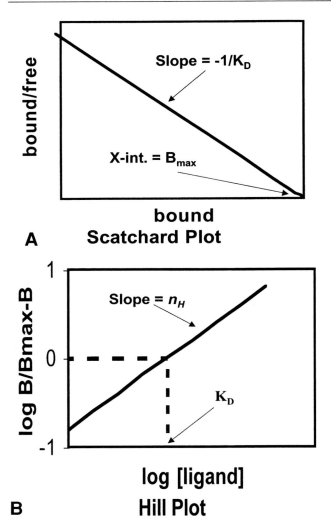

A   Scatchard Plot

B   Hill Plot

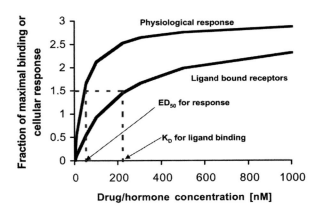

Fig. 3. Comparison of binding and response parameters typically observed in response to increasing amounts of a ligand (transmitter or drug agonist).

Fig. 2. (A) The graph represents a typical Scatchard plot. The ratio of the amount of a labeled ligand or transmitter bound to a membrane preparation over the total free amount of radiolabeled ligand added is plotted against the amount of ligand bound. This plot provides the total number of receptors (B_{max}) and their dissociation constant (K_d), which is determined from the slope. If the response is curvilinear (*dotted line*), it indicates that there are two or more populations of receptors with different K_d values. **(B)** The Hill plot compares the log of the amount bound corrected for the maximal possible binding (B_{max}) to the log of the ligand or transmitter concentration. The slope of this plot reveals if there is positive or negative cooperativity between the binding sites on a given receptor. If the slope is equal to 1, there is no cooperativity.

transmitter. The log of the ratio is the amount of a drug that is bound at a given dose of that drug over B_{max}—the amount bound is plotted against the log of the dose (*see* Fig. 2). This relationship generally produces a linear plot, and the slope of this line is usually referred to as the Hill coeffcient, *nH*. If the slope is 1, there is

no cooperativity. If the slope is greater than 1, there is more than one binding site for the drug causing positive cooperative interaction. The point at which the abscissa value equals zero also represents the apparent K_d for this binding interaction.

These same analytical approaches are applied to the characterization of dose-response relationships for drugs and transmitters in isolated tissue or in vivo, but yield different parameters, E_{max} and ED_{50} for in vivo or EC_{50} for in vitro studies (*see* Fig. 3). If the ED_{50} of the physiologic effect produced by a drug is compared with the K_d measured by the binding of this drug to its receptor, a discrepancy usually arises that results in the production of the maximal physiological effect at a concentration well below that required to saturate the available receptor population in this tissue. This discrepancy led R.P. Stephenson to propose the concept of spare receptors—that the theory it is not necessary to occupy all of the available receptors to elicit the maximal response possible for a cell or tissue. Stephenson also attempted to explain differences in the ability of drugs to produce the same effect in a given tissue by proposing that the drugs had different efficacies. Efficacy is a pharmacologic term that refers to the intrinsic ability of a drug to produce a response.

2.2. Receptors Can Be Multi-Subunit Ion Channels in the Membrane or Single Polypeptides That Modulate an Effector System Through Phosphorylation and Second Messengers

Much of our current knowledge regarding the appearance of cellular receptors and how they work has come from studies in which the receptors were

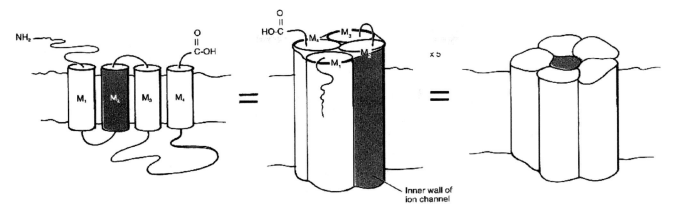

Fig. 4. The structural components of a ligand-gated ionic-channel receptor. The graph shows the subunit protein with the four membrane-spanning domains (*left*). This protein clusters to form a single subunit of the receptor (*center*). Five of these subunits fit together to form a ligand-gated ion channel (*right*). The M2 subunit (*shaded*) has repeating sequences of charged amino acids and makes up the inner wall of the ionic channel.

solubilized from the plasma membrane, chromatographically purified, and then reconstituted into lipid vesicles called liposomes. This work was tedious but crucial to our understanding of the receptor complex. The second major scientific approach that has helped us understand receptors has been the molecular biologic methods needed to "clone" receptor genes and sequence them to determine the amino acids of the expressed proteins. The use of "homology" cloning and sequencing (e.g., isolating unknown genes by using molecular probes for known genes or proteins) has revealed a wide variety of receptors, sometimes for totally unrelated transmitter systems. Such was the case for the muscarinic receptor, which was found to have a high degree of homology (e.g., degree of structural similarity) to the adrenergic-type, single-subunit receptors. Two receptors that received much of the early interest fall into each of the major classes of receptor families. The nicotinic acetylcholine receptor is a ligand-gated (e.g., directly triggered) ion-channel receptor type, and the β-adrenergic receptor is a G-protein-coupled (e.g., second-messenger) receptor type.

2.3. Ligand-Gated Ion Channel Receptors

Ligand-gated ion-channel receptors are composed of five protein subunits, each of which has four membrane-spanning domains. The nicotinic cholinergic receptor was studied largely because of its accessibility. The electric organ of the eel and ray is a tissue that is rich in cholinergic nicotinic receptors. Much effort has gone into isolating and characterizing the receptor from the membrane of this tissue. The isolated recep-

tor appeared to be "oligomeric" because it had several protein subunits. The receptor subunits were isolated and purified, and part of the amino acid sequence was determined. The possible DNA sequences (e.g., DNA probe) coding part of the receptor protein were synthesized. Using these small DNA probes, known as oligoprobes, a library of genes was screened for homologous sequences. A messenger RNA was isolated and sequenced that was similar to the isolated protein. Surprisingly, many of the cloned subunits demonstrated a great deal of homology. This was particularly true in the hydrophobic segments that are believed to span the lipid membrane. These methods have confirmed that the nicotinic receptor contains several protein subunits that together surround an ionic channel through the membrane. These subunits exhibit many differences. An α subunit contains an extracellular sequence on the amino-terminal end that binds the transmitter acetylcholine. Two of these α subunits are contained in each of the muscle-type nicotinic receptors.

In all of the ligand-gated receptor proteins (e.g., nicotinic, γ-aminobutyric acid [GABA], glycine, and glutamate receptors), one of the membrane-spanning domains of each subunit contains a repeating sequence of the polar amino acids, threonine, and serine. These are believed to line the channel surface itself and serve as the lipid-water interface within the channel. Each receptor has five of these channel-lining domains, α-helical sections known as the M2 domains, one contributed by each of the five subunits. Our concept of the receptor subunits that combine to make up the pentameric nicotinic receptor is shown in Fig. 4.

Table 1
Attributes of Ligand-Gated Ion-Channel Receptors

Receptor	Subtype	Comment	Effector[§]
GABA	A		Cl^-
Glutamate	NMDA	Glycine[*]	$Na^+/K^+/Ca^{2+}$
	AMPA		$Na^+/K^+/Ca^{2+}$
	Kainate		$Na^+/K^+/Ca^{2+}$
Glycine		Strychnine[†]	Cl^-
Serotonin	5-HT$_3$		
Nicotinic	Muscle	50 ps[‡]	$Na^+/K^+/Ca^{2+}$
	Neural	15–40 ps[‡]	$Na^+/K^+/Ca^{2+}$

[*]The NMDA glutamate receptor has a glycine-binding site.
[†]The glycine receptor is strychnine-sensitive.
[‡]The muscle nicotinic receptor is open longer than the neural receptor; time is given in picoseconds.
[§]The effector pathways represent the opening of ionic channels.

The M2-spanning domain that lines the channel is shaded.

Since the elucidation of the nicotinic-receptor structure, several other ligand-gated ionic-channel systems have been described. These include γ-aminobutyric acid (GABA), A-type and the glycine receptors, which form channels for chloride ion and function to hyperpolarize or inhibit nerve cells; several subtypes of the glutamate receptor that comprise a channel for calcium, sodium, and potassium ions, similar to the nicotinic receptor; and the serotonin (5-HT$_3$) receptor that is an intrinsic channel for cations. Table 1 lists the known ligand-gated ion channels and some characteristics of these receptors. All of these receptors except the NMDA receptor are related in that they are pentameric, have four membrane-spanning domains per subunit, and have an M2-spanning domain that lines the ion channel.

When the receptive subunit of these receptors is occupied by a neurotransmitter, a conformational change of the five-subunit complex allows the channel to open and the appropriately sized ion to enter the cell (Fig. 5). The type of ion that can traverse the channel seems to depend on the molecular radius of the ion, how tightly it combines with water molecules (free energy of hydration), and the strength of polar sites within or just outside the channel. For example, the sodium ion is smaller than the potassium ion, but is excluded from the potassium channel. This is probably because it has a higher free energy of hydration and affinity for water molecules and cannot be dehydrated by the relatively weak ionic charges of the amino acids that make up the potassium channel. All of the cationic (e.g., Na^+, K^+, Ca^{2+}) or positively charged ion

channels have groupings of negatively charged amino acids (e.g., glutamate and aspartate) close to the mouth of the ion channel. These amino acids are probably important in removing the water from the cations (e.g., dehydrating) and producing Na^+ or K^+ channel selectivity.

In the case of the chloride channel for GABA or glycine, positively charged amino acids (e.g., arginine and lysine) are localized near the mouth of the channel. This is important in allowing the anions to enter the channel. The polar serine and threonine residues that line the M2 domain of the channels do not appear to determine the ionic specificity of the channel, but are essential for maintaining the aqueous interface.

2.4. G-Protein-Coupled Receptors

The G-protein-coupled receptors (GPCRs) are composed of a single-protein unit that has seven membrane-spanning domains. The prototypical G-protein receptor is represented by the β$_1$-adrenergic receptor of the heart, which has received much attention because of the development of specific drugs that interact with it and the therapeutic importance of these drugs in treating heart disease, asthma, and hypertension. Studies of the cardiac β receptor indicate that it is associated with a membrane-bound protein that has guanylate nucleotidase activity, hydrolyzing GTP to guanosine 5' diphosphate (GDP). It was painstakingly solubilized from the membrane and partially sequenced. Eventually, this led to the cloning of a gene for a protein that had seven membrane-spanning domains. Fig. 6 shows the current conception of the GPCR. The amino-terminal portion of the protein is

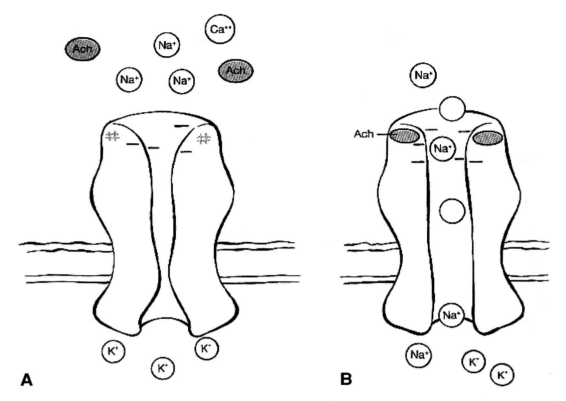

Fig. 5. (A) Resting and **(B)** stimulated nicotinic receptors. Combination of the α subunits of the receptor with acetylcholine causes the channel to open and allows sodium to enter the neuron and depolarize it. This receptor is drawn roughly to scale to show that about two-thirds of the receptor protein is extracellular.

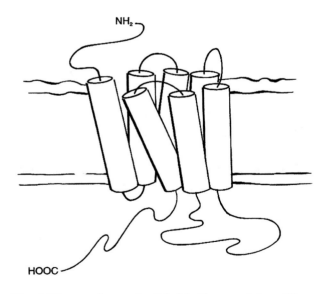

Fig. 6. The guanine nucleotide-binding regulatory (G-protein)-coupled receptor protein (GPCR) is composed of seven hydrophobic membrane-spanning domains with three intracellular and extracellular loops of amino acids. The amino-terminal end of the protein is extracellular, and the carboxyl-terminal end is in the cytoplasm of the postsynaptic neuron. The third intracellular loop is believed to be responsible for activating the appropriate G protein.

found extracellularly, and the carboxyl-terminal end is inside the cell. There is a large intracellular loop of protein between spanning domains five and six. This loop is believed to interact and regulate the G-protein "transducer" that is responsible for initiating the postsynaptic neural event.

Homology cloning of these GPCRs uncovered a wide variety of different receptors. Many of these are shown in Table 2. When genetic probes were made against portions of the known G-protein receptors and compared with a gene library, several previously unrecognized genes for receptor subtypes were revealed. For example, five separate genes were identified for the muscarinic cholinergic receptor. Table 2 lists the most important functional effects of many GPCRs.

2.4.1. G Proteins

A major receptor-transducing element is called the guanine nucleotide (G) protein and is composed of three protein subunits. An integral part of this family of receptors is the G protein, which represents the transduction element between the receptor and the second-messenger system that ultimately induces the cellular response. Much of the functional specificity

Table 2
Characteristics of Selected G-Protein-Coupled Receptors

Receptor type	Subtypes	AA/TMD[*]	Effector pathways[†]
Adenosine	A_1, A_3	h326/7, h318/7	↓cAMP
	A2A, A2B	h412/7, h332/7	↑cAMP
Adrenergic	α_{1A}, α_{1B}, α_{1D}	h466, h519, h572/7	IP$_3$/DAG
	α_{2A}, α_{2B}, α_{2C}	h450, h450, h461/7	↓cAMP
	β_1, β_2, β_3	h477, h413, h408/7	↑cAMP
Cannabinoid	CB_1, CB_2	h472, h360/7	↓cAMP
Dopamine	D_1, D_5	h446, h477/7	↑cAMP
	D_2, D_3, D_4	h443, h400, h387/7	↓cAMP
Glutamate	mglu$_1$, mglu$_5$	h1194, h1212/7	IP$_3$/DAG
	mglu$_2$, mglu$_3$, mglu$_4$,	h872, h877, h912,	↓cAMP
	mglu$_6$, mglu$_7$, mglu$_8$	h877, h915, h908/7	
Histamine	H_1	h487/7	IP$_3$/DAG
	H_2	h359/7	↑cAMP
	H_3	h445/7	↓cAMP
Serotonin	5-HT$_{1A}$, 5-HT$_{1B}$, 5-HT$_{1D}$,	h421, h390, h377, h365,	↓cAMP
	5-ht$_{1E}$, 5-ht$_{1F}$	h366/7	
	5-HT$_{2A}$, 5-HT$_{2B}$, 5-HT$_{2C}$	h471, h481, h458/7	IP$_3$/DAG
	5-HT$_4$, 5-ht$_6$, 5-HT$_7$	h387, h440, h445/7	↑cAMP
	5-ht$_{5A}$, 5-ht$_{5B}$	h357, m370/7	??
Muscarinic	M_1, M_3, M_5	h460, h590, h532/7	IP$_3$/DAG
	M_2, M_4	h466, h479/7	↓cAMP

[*]Number of amino acids (AA) in the receptor/number of transmembrane-spanning domains (TMD).
The letter before the number of amino acids denotes the species; h, human; m, mouse.
[†]The effector pathways produce changes in adenylate cyclase and resulting in changes in cyclic 3'5'-AMP or modulation of phospholipase activity with changes in inositol trisphosphate (IP$_3$) and diacylglycerol (DAG) as second messengers.

of these receptors resides in the type of G-protein to which they preferentially couple. For example, the α_1- and α_2-adrenergic receptors respond to endogenous norepinephrine but initiate entirely different cellular events. The α_1-receptor activation activates a G protein ($G_{q/11}$), which initiates the activity of membrane phospholipase, eventually resulting in increased intracellular calcium. The α_2-receptor, although similar in terms of the ligand-binding unit, activates what is called a G_i protein (i for inhibitory), which inhibits adenylate cyclase activity and generally causes inhibitory neuromodulatory activity. The β receptors couple to G_S proteins (s for stimulatory), which activate adenylate cyclase as well as many cellular processes. A similar picture has emerged for the families of dopamine and muscarinic cholinergic receptors.

Other G proteins are involved in sensory modulation. In the nasal mucosa, odorant molecules bind to GPCRs that activate a G protein, called G_{olf} for olfactory G protein. One of the earliest characterized G proteins was called transducin (G_t). This molecule is responsible for initiating the signal from stimulation of the rhodopsin molecule by light. Rhodopsin is a receptive protein with seven membrane-spanning domains that is covalently bound to 11-*cis*-retinal.

The G-protein complex is actually composed of three protein subunits known as the α, β, and γ subunits. There is an excess of α subunits in the cytoplasm that probably compete for the appropriate β and γ membrane-bound subunits. The β and γ subunits are highly conserved membrane proteins, and they anchor the α subunit near the receptor. The β-γ complex also stabilizes the binding of GDP to the α subunit and inhibits its activation. When the receptor is occupied by a transmitter, the α subunit is released and becomes activated. The α subunit is capable of binding GTP and activating or inhibiting the effector or second-messenger system, such as adenylate cyclase. The G-protein system allows for a high degree of amplification of the signal. Each receptor typically activates 10–20 G proteins.

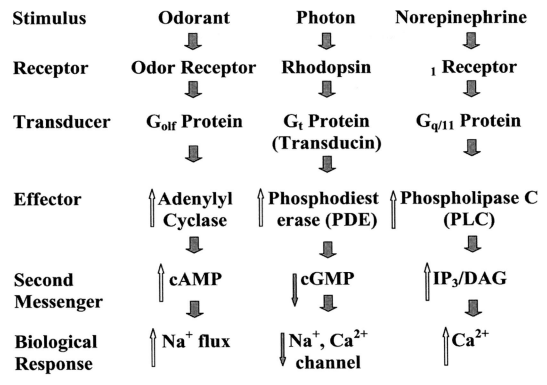

Fig. 7. Representative G-protein-mediated response pathways for stimuli of olfactory, visual, and transmitter origin. PLC, phospholipase C; cAMP cyclic 3'5'-adenosine monophosphate; cGMP, cyclic 3'5'-guanosine monophosphate; IP_3, inositol trisphosphate; DAG, diacylglycerol. The arrows indicate activation ($\uparrow$) or inhibition ($\downarrow$).

Many bacterial toxins interfere with G-protein systems. The agent responsible for cholera—cholera enterotoxin—irreversibly activates the G_S protein, increasing the intracellular cyclic AMP. Pertussis toxin irreversibly inhibits the G_i proteins.

2.4.2. PHOSPHORYLATION

Many effector mechanisms ultimately produce the phosphorylation of a protein that results in the inhibition or excitation of the postsynaptic cellular event. The final steps in the postsynaptic response include the activation of a second-messenger system by the α subunit of the G protein and triggering of a phosphorylation system. Several second-messenger systems are involved, including the cyclic nucleotide system, cyclic AMP, and cyclic GMP, calcium-calmodulin, the production of nitric oxide from arginine, and the phospholipase C products of inositol triphosphate (IP_3) and diacylglycerol (DAG). Fig. 7 shows several G-protein and second-messenger or effector pathways for sensory stimuli such as smell and vision and for neurotransmission by norepinephrine.

2.5. Nitric Oxide

A novel effector system that may also represent a transducer or a transmitter is the simple molecule nitric oxide. Although muscarinic vasodilation had been studied for decades, the exact mechanism of this action of acetylcholine was unknown. The muscarinic receptor in the vasculature is not innervated, but it can be activated by circulating choline esters. In the early 1980s, Furchgott found that the muscarinic receptor of the vasculature occurred on the endothelium rather than vascular smooth muscle. The well-known vasodilation induced by stimulation of this receptor was found to be a secondary effect of the production of nitric oxide by the endothelium. This small, very short-lived molecule easily traverses lipid membranes, enters the smooth muscle, and activates a guanylate cyclase that in turn activates myosin light-chain kinase, which relaxes the muscle. Nitrate vasodilators, such as nitroglycerin, have been used for years to alleviate angina pectoris. This is another example of the body having an endogenous chemical that resembles drugs that have been used for centuries.

Originally called endothelial-derived relaxing factor, nitric oxide is generated by the action of an enzyme that uses the amino acid arginine as a substrate. The enzyme is known as nitric oxide synthetase and is widely distributed in the brain. In the future, it will be interesting to see whether this compound is given transmitter, transducer, or effector status in the overall scheme of how the brain works.

2.6. Receptors as Part of the Effector Pathway

Some receptors are part of a second-messenger-generating system, and directly stimulate the effector pathway. These receptors are themselves the transducers and the generators of the second messengers. Some of these are membrane-bound proteins that include receptors for growth factors, atrial natriuretic peptide, and activin. In the case of growth factors and the polypeptide activin, the receptors themselves are enzymes. Activation by these molecules causes receptor phosphorylation that allows them to function as a protein tyrosine kinase or protein serine-threonine kinase, respectively. The atrial natriuretic peptide receptor is a guanylate cyclase that results in increased intracellular cyclic GMP. Each of these membrane-bound receptors has only one membrane-spanning domain that anchors it to the membrane, unlike the seven spanning domains of the GPCRs. Others, such as the steroids, bind to soluble cytoplasmic receptors that interact with specific promoter regions of genes to initiate or inhibit gene translation. This group of receptors is not discussed in this chapter.

3. NEUROTRANSMITTERS AND THEIR RECEPTORS

Mushrooms, herbs, and bacterial and snake toxins have contributed much to our knowledge of neurotransmitters and their receptors. Early in the development of human civilization, pharmacology was mostly the jurisdiction of herbalists and alchemists. Plant and animal products have provided useful sources of drugs for various ailments and research tools to advance our knowledge of the function of the body and brain. Some of these remedies were quite sophisticated—the plant belladonna, which contains the alkaloid atropine, was burned in an open fire and inhaled by the ancient Hindus for allergies and asthma. Curare, the nicotinic blocker, from the Amazonian jungles, was used to paralyze game; and willow bark

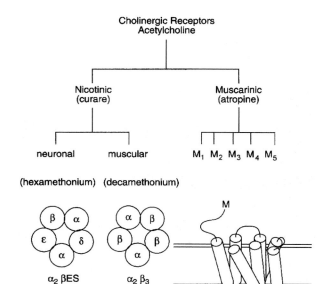

Fig. 8. The family of cholinergic receptors. This flowchart shows the subdivision of cholinergic receptors and the names of their subtypes. The drugs in parentheses are antagonists that block those receptors. The diagram below the chart shows the proposed subunit configuration of the two nicotinic receptors and the structure of the muscarinic receptor.

(e.g., salicylate) was used to cure fever and pain. Bacterial toxins from *Vibrio cholerae* and *Bordetella pertussis*, which causes whooping cough, interact with G proteins. The snake toxin α-bungarotoxin was essential for characterizing and purifying the nicotinic receptor. These natural products have proven to be important for our present understanding of the brain transmitters and receptors that mediate bodily function and cognition.

3.1. Cholinergic Receptors Fall into Both Main Genetic Families of Transmitter Receptors

Cholinergic receptors were the first receptor types to be identified and pharmacologically classified in the early 1900s. The subdivision of these receptors grew out of an interest in herbs that have been used for centuries as medicines or poisons. The major subdivisions of the cholinergic receptor systems are shown in Fig. 8 with a representative drug that selectively acts on that system.

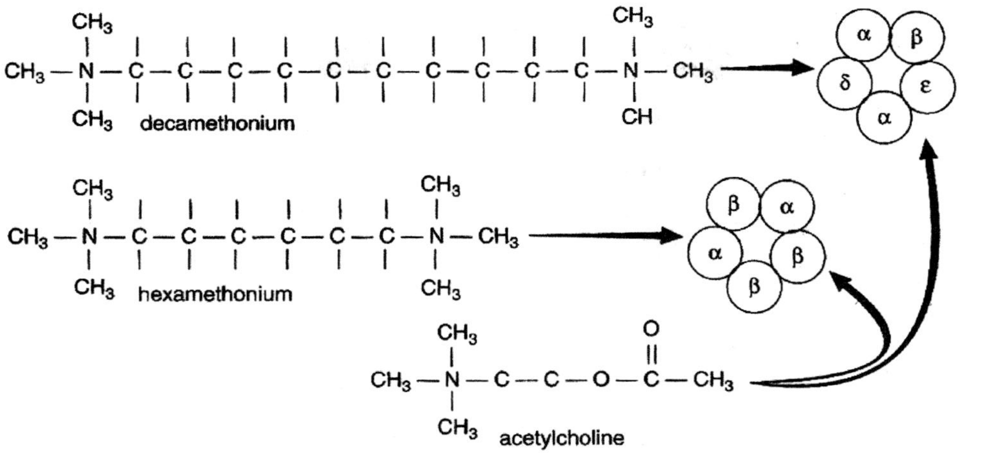

Fig. 9. Structures of the selective neuromuscular and ganglionic (e.g., neural) nicotinic receptor antagonists. Decamethonium selectively blocks the muscle receptor, and hexamethonium blocks the neural receptor. The makeup of the pentameric subunits and the distance between the two subunits may partially explain this specificity. Acetylcholine stimulates both of the receptors.

3.2. Nicotinic Receptors

Nicotinic receptors are ligand-gated ionic channels for sodium, and selectively respond to the active ingredient in tobacco. The first major subdivision of the cholinergic receptor was named after a plant alkaloid, nicotine, that was introduced into western European cultures by Native Americans. Nicotine selectively stimulates cholinergic receptors at the neuromuscular junction and the autonomic ganglia. This receptor is also found in the brain, although it is much less prevalent than the muscarinic cholinergic receptor.

Early studies by Dale and Langley showed that, although semipurified acetylcholine stimulated skeletal muscle and the visceral smooth muscle, nicotine was selective only for the neuromuscular junction and the ganglia. Langley was able to map out the sympathetic and parasympathetic autonomic ganglia by applying a tincture of nicotine to peripheral-nerve ganglia and observing the visceral effects in the frog.

Further subdivisions of the nicotinic receptor were made during the 1930s and 1940s. Paton and Zaimis noticed that the nicotinic receptor of the neuromuscular junction was blocked by a molecule with two quaternary nitrogens separated by 10 carbon atoms (e.g., decamethonium) but that the autonomic ganglia was selectively blocked by a similar molecule with a separation of only six carbon atoms (e.g., hexamethonium). These molecules resembled two acetylcholine molecules linked back to back, but separated by different distances. A second subdivision of the cholinergic

receptor was then postulated: muscle and neuronal or ganglionic nicotinic receptors. Fig. 9 shows the structures of hexamethonium, decamethonium, and acetylcholine and the subunit makeup of the two nicotinic receptors.

Much of the molecular biology of the nicotinic receptor was discussed in the previous section on ligand-gated ion channels. The nicotinic receptor was originally isolated from the electric organ for the eel. To facilitate its purification, the snake-venom toxin, which tightly binds to the a subunit of the nicotine receptor, α-bungarotoxin, was used. By radiolabeling this toxin, the purification of the nicotinic receptor could be followed through various chromatographic steps.

With the help of molecular biologic techniques, we know that the human neuromuscular nicotinic receptor is very similar to the electric eel receptor. It contains five subunits that surround a membrane channel that, when open, allows positively charged ions to flow into the cell. Two of the five protein subunits of the nicotinic receptor have binding sites for acetylcholine (i.e., α subunit). The makeup of the other three subunits may affect the distances between the α subunits of muscle-type and ganglia-type nicotinic receptors, which could explain the pharmacologic specificity of the receptors (*see* Fig. 8). The neuronal or ganglionic receptor appears to have two α and three β subunits rather than the α (2), β (1), γ (1), and δ (1) makeup of the muscle receptor.

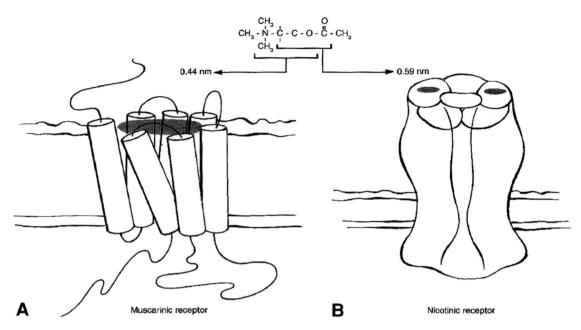

Fig. 10. Diagram of how acetylcholine can interact with the muscarinic (*left*) and nicotinic (*right*) receptor. This theory contends that the distance between the quaternary nitrogen of acetylcholine and an atom capable of donating a pair of electrons is the structural requirement for an agonist. Because acetylcholine has two methyl groups separating the nitrogen and the oxygen, it can exist in both configurations. The muscarinic receptor requires a distance of about 0.44 nm, and the nicotinic receptor requires 0.59 nm.

3.3. Muscarinic Cholinergic Receptors

Muscarinic cholinergic receptors are GPCRs that are activated by muscarine, a substance found in the mushroom, *Amanita muscaria*. Euripides, an ancient Greek, was the first to describe the poisonous effects of *Amanita muscaria*, to which he lost several family members. The general syndrome of mushroom poisoning has become known as the SLUDE syndrome, which is an acronym for salivation, lacrimation, urination, defecation, and emesis. This acronym describes quite accurately the toxicologic effects of parasympathetic overstimulation by acetylcholine-like agonists, muscarine, and acetylcholinesterase inhibitors. This receptor is found on the postganglionic parasympathetic effector organs and in eccrine sweat glands, and is the most common cholinergic receptor found in the brain; it is 10 to 100 times more prevalent than nicotinic receptors.

How can the nicotinic and muscarinic receptors respond to the same neurotransmitter but also possess the capacity to respond selectively to different drugs? One explanation has been that acetylcholine is not a rigid molecule, because the two methyl groups separating the quaternary nitrogen of choline and the acetyl

groups can freely rotate. This conformation allows the quaternary nitrogen and an atom capable of donating a pair of electrons to exist at various distances. When they are in their closest configuration (0.44 nm), they can "fit" into the muscarinic receptor, and when they are in their more distant configuration (0.59 nm), they can fit into the nicotinic receptor (Fig. 10). Examination of the structures of nicotine and muscarine have shown that these rigid molecules have chemical characteristics similar to acetylcholine and are separated by similar intermolecular distances.

Molecular biologic techniques have revealed other important differences between the nicotinic and muscarinic receptor that explain their pharmacologic and physiologic uniqueness. Unlike the ligand-gated ion-channel nicotinic receptor, the muscarinic receptor is a GPCR receptor that uses a second-messenger system to accomplish its actions. Although acetylcholine is a fast transmitter (1–2 ms) when stimulating the nicotinic receptor, it acts like a slow transmitter (100–250 ms) when activating the muscarinic receptor. Like the β-adrenergic receptor, the muscarinic receptor is composed of a single membrane-bound protein that has seven membrane-spanning domains within its structure. Five separate muscarinic-receptor genes have been cloned, two of which have pharmacologic and therapeutic importance.

The *M2* receptor is the most common peripheral muscarinic receptor. It is blocked by the drug atropine and is found in the heart, bronchi, gastrointestinal tract, and bladder smooth muscle. Stimulation of this receptor affect the appropriate G protein, depending on the tissue type. This can lead to a decrease in cyclic AMP or activation of K^+ channels. In the smooth muscle of the bronchi and gastrointestinal tract, the G_i-mediated decrease in cyclic AMP will lead to contraction. In the heart, activation of non-ligand-gated potassium channels decreases the heart rate and automaticity.

The M_1 muscarinic receptor is widely found in the brain, in the autonomic ganglia, and on hydrochloric acid-secreting cells of the stomach. This receptor uses the IP_3-DAG second messenger system and is selectively blocked by the drug pirenzepine. Atropine also blocks this receptor. The pharmacologic differences in these muscarinic receptors may be therapeutically important for the treatment of peptic ulcers.

4. CATECHOLAMINE RECEPTORS

Soon after the discovery of sympathetic transmitters in the early 1900s, it was observed that the postsynaptic actions they produced were extremely variable, stimulating some systems and inhibiting others. Specifically, they stimulated the heart and most vascular smooth muscle, but they inhibited bronchial, some vascular, and gastrointestinal smooth muscle. To explain these differences, Cannon proposed in the early 1920s that there were two sympathetic transmitters: sympathin E excited smooth muscle, and sympathin I inhibited smooth muscle. With the discovery of epinephrine in the adrenal glands and norepinephrine in the sympathetic nerves, this hypothesis held for decades. In 1948, Raymond Alquist proposed that the diversity of physiologic actions of catecholamines could be explained by the existence of distinctly different receptor subtypes. He called these adrenergic receptors the α and β receptors.

Alquist's hypothesis was based on the actions of several adrenergic agents and derivatives on visceral activity; among these agents were norepinephrine, epinephrine, and isoproterenol. The excitatory actions of the catecholamines were ascribed to α-receptor activation. The agents that were most potent in stimulating these actions were norepinephrine and epineph-

rine. α-Adrenergic activation by these agents included vasoconstriction and pupillary dilation. β-receptor stimulation tended to be predominantly inhibitory and included bronchial dilation, decreased gastrointestinal motility and bladder smooth-muscle tone, vasodilation of some vascular beds, and cardio-acceleration. The agents that that stimulated these β-receptor functions tended to have larger substitutions on the amine group of the catecholamine. Isoproterenol and epinephrine were much more potent stimulators of these receptors than norepinephrine, which has no methyl groups on the amine terminal. Many of the β-receptor agonists and antagonists synthesized subsequently share this property, strengthening the hypothesis that β-receptor selectivity is largely based on a bulky amino-terminal substitution of the biogenic amine. Fig. 11 provides a breakdown of the various therapeutically important subtypes of adrenergic receptors.

4.1. α-Adrenergic Receptors

α-adrenergic receptors can stimulate postsynaptic events ($α_1$) and through presynaptic receptors can inhibit neuronal activity ($α_2$). The α-adrenergic receptors were pharmacologically subdivided in the 1970s, when the actions of some drugs were found to interact with presynaptic alpha-like receptors that inhibited neuronal activity. Molecular biological techniques have shown that there are six separate genes for various α receptors. All of these receptors and all of the known β and dopamine receptors belong to the G-protein-coupled family, and each is a single membrane-bound protein that has seven membrane-spanning domains. Fig. 11 describes the shared molecular mechanisms of many of the adrenergic receptors.

The $α_1$ receptor, as described by Alquist, is an excitatory receptor that couples to a G protein that activates the enzyme phospholipase C. This enzyme cleaves the membrane lipid, phosphatidylinositol bisphosphate (PIP_2), into two separate second messengers. DAG remains within the membrane and activates protein kinase C (PKC). This kinase is capable of phosphorylating serine and threonine residues of a number of substrates within the membrane or in the cytoplasm. The other second messenger derived from PIP_2 is inositol trisphosphate (IP_3). This water-soluble molecule is released into the cytoplasm, where it binds to IP_3-sensitive Ca^{2+} channels on the endoplasmic reticulum (ER) to trigger the release of Ca^{2+}. Ca^{2+} then activates tissue-specific secondary-effector systems.

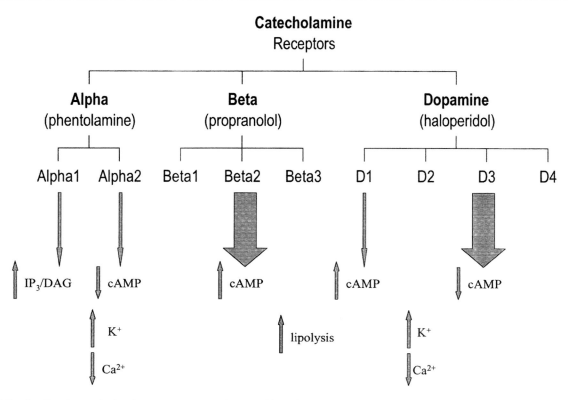

Fig. 11. The family of catecholamine receptors are shown with their subtypes and major effector pathways. The drugs in parentheses are selective blockers for the different receptors.

The ability of the α_1 receptor to stimulate a single-transducer system to activate two second-messenger systems (PKC and cytosolic Ca^{2+}) from the same substrate (PIP_2) provides additional amplification of the original transmitter and α-receptor interaction.

The elucidation of the α_2-adrenergic receptor helped to explain several confusing observations related to the autonomic nervous system and the central nervous system (CNS). Many of the side effects of α-receptor blockade seemed to resemble activation of the sympathetic and the parasympathetic nervous system. For example, the side effects of the nonselective α-blocking drug phentolamine included increased gastrointestinal motility (e.g., diarrhea) and elevated circulating levels of the sympathetic transmitter norepinephrine. This plasma norepinephrine is able to activate the unblocked β receptors. With the development of α_2-type agonists, such as clonidine, the opposite effects were found. This type of drug seemed to turn off sympathetic and parasympathetic activity. Clonidine is useful for high blood pressure because it decreases sympathetic norepinephrine release. However, one of its side effects is decreased gastrointestinal motility.

The α_2-type receptors are found predominantly on neurons within the brain, or presynaptically on sympathetic and parasympathetic nerves. The α_2 receptor is coupled to a G_i protein, which results in a decrease in cyclic AMP, inhibition of Ca^{2+}-channel opening, and increased potassium-channel activity (*see* Fig. 11). The resulting effect is inhibition of neuronal activity. α_2-adrenergic agonists have been found to be useful for opiate and nicotine withdrawal symptoms.

4.2. β-Adrenergic Receptors

Both of the major β-adrenergic receptors are coupled to a G_s protein, which results in an increase in cyclic AMP. β-adrenergic-receptor responses in the peripheral autonomic nervous system include dilation of a variety of smooth muscles, stimulation of metabolic functions such as lipolysis and glycogenolysis, and an increase in heart rate. From a therapeutic standpoint, drugs that are selective for the β receptors of different tissues are important. For example, a drug that selectively stimulates the β receptor of bronchial smooth muscle (causing bronchodilation) could be useful in asthma, and a drug that selectively blocks the cardiac β receptor might be beneficial for angina or

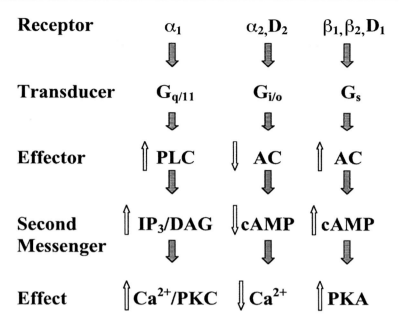

Receptor	α_1	α_2, D_2	β_1, β_2, D_1
⇓	⇓	⇓	⇓
Transducer	$G_{q/11}$	$G_{i/o}$	G_s
⇓	⇓	⇓	⇓
Effector	⇑ PLC	⇓ AC	⇑ AC
⇓	⇓	⇓	⇓
Second Messenger	⇑ IP_3/DAG	⇓ cAMP	⇑ cAMP
⇓	⇓	⇓	⇓
Effect	⇑ Ca^{2+}/PKC	⇓ Ca^{2+}	⇑ PKA

Fig. 12. Catecholamine effector pathways. Some G-protein and effector-pathway mechanisms are shared by different types of catecholamine receptors. PLC, phospholipase C; IP_3, inositol trisphosphate; DAG, diacylglycerol. The arrows indicate activation (*up arrow*) or inhibition (*down arrow*).

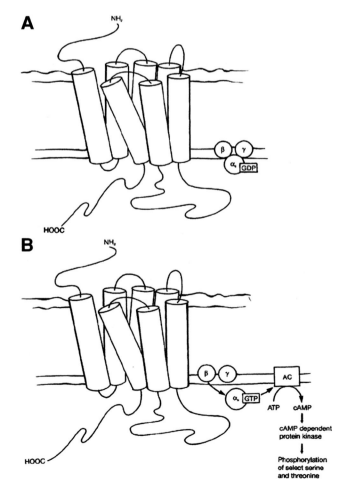

high blood pressure. The search for selective β-adrenergic drugs did lead to the discovery of specific β_1 blockers (e.g., atenolol) and β_2 agonists (e.g., terbutaline) and the cloning of three different β receptors that range in size from 400 to 477 amino acids. All of these β receptors use the same transducer and effector systems. As shown in Fig. 12, they activate a G_s protein that stimulates cyclic AMP formation, leading to phosphorylation of various cellular serine and threonine residues by a cyclic AMP-dependent protein kinase.

The β receptor is the prototypical GPCR that was the first to be isolated and cloned (*see* Fig. 13). The β_1-adrenergic receptor is the subtype responsible for increased heart rate and lipolysis, and most of the other receptors, including those involved in bronchodilation, are defined as β_2. (This can be easily remembered, because there is one heart [β_1] and only two lungs [β_2]). There are also β receptors in the CNS, although the sub-classifications have not been worked out.

Fig. 13. Conceptualized GPCR. The β-adrenergic receptor is coupled to the G-protein complex. (**A**) The G protein is composed of β and γ subunits, which are anchored in the membrane, and an α subunit, which binds GTP and can be released into the cytoplasm to activate the second-messenger system. (**B**) In this case, the second messenger is cyclic AMP, which is generated when adenylate cyclase (AC) is activated by the G protein.

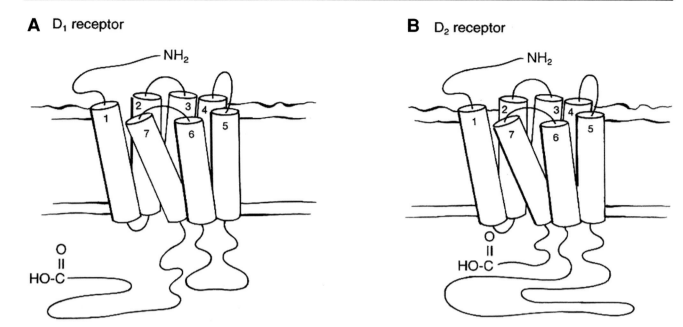

A D₁ receptor

B D₂ receptor

Fig. 14. The dopamine-receptor family subtypes are drawn roughly to scale, showing the structure of two dopamine (D_1 and D_2) receptors. (**A**) The D_1 receptor stimulates adenylate cyclase and has a short third cytoplasmic loop between TM domains 5 and 6. It also has a longer carboxyl-terminal end. (**B**) The D_2 receptor, which inhibits adenylate cyclase, has a long third cytoplasmic loop and short carboxy-terminal end. The seven membrane-spanning domains exhibit a high degree of homology.

4.3. Dopamine Receptors

Central dopamine receptors are involved in the neuropathologies that underlie movement disorders such as Parkinson's disease and mental illness. Four dopamine receptors have been pharmacologically defined, and five have been cloned. Most of the actions of dopamine receptors occur in the CNS, although some do mediate peripheral functions. The central actions include vasodilation in the kidney vasculature (D_1 receptor), inhibition of sympathetic ganglionic activity (D_2), and inhibition of prolactin secretion by the anterior lobe of the pituitary (D_2). The D_2 receptor also inhibits acetylcholine release from the striatum. This is the transmitter function that is deranged in Parkinson's disease, and demonstrates why L-DOPA, the precursor of dopamine, and trihexyphenidyl, the cholinergic muscarinic blocker, are effective in alleviating the tremors associated with this disorder. Antipsychotic drugs, such as chlorpromazine and haloperidol, produce their therapeutic effects primarily through binding to D_2 receptors in the CNS. The D_1 and D_5 receptors stimulate cyclic AMP formation, and the D_2, D_3, and D_4 receptors inhibit the formation of this second messenger. These receptors are also capable of altering phosphoinositide turnover, inhibiting Ca^{2+} channels, and enhancing K^+ conductances in some brain regions.

The dopamine D_2-receptor gene was the first to be cloned using a probe against the β-adrenergic receptor. The D_1 and D_2 receptors are both found in the caudate/putamen, nucleus accumbens, and olfactory tubercle. In contrast, D_3 receptors are found in the olfactory tubercle, nucleus accumbens, and the islands of Calleja, and the D_4 receptors are found in the frontal cortex, the midbrain, and the amygdala. D_5 receptors are expressed in the hippocampus, thalamus, and hypothalamus. The structures of the D_1 and D_2 receptors is shown in Fig. 14. The major differences are found in the size of the cytoplasmic loop between the membrane-spanning domains 5 and 6 and the size of the cytoplasmic carboxyl terminal. The D_2 receptor that inhibits adenylate cyclase has a long loop between the transmembrane (TM)-spanning domains 5 and 6 and a short carboxyl terminal. The opposite is true for the D_1 receptor. These cytoplasmic, intracellular loops of the protein are believed to interact with their specific G protein to mediate the appropriate effector mechanisms.

4.4. Serotonin Receptors are Diverse

Serotonin receptors are a diverse family in structure and function, including 13 G-protein-coupled subtypes and one multi-subunit, ligand-gated ion channel. Figure 15 shows the cloned serotonin receptors and

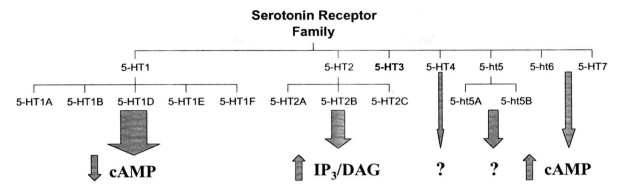

Fig. 15. The serotonin (5-HT) family of receptors, giving the breakdown of receptor subtypes and their effector pathways. Notice that the 5-HT$_3$ receptor is a ligand-gated ion channel, and the rest are GPCRs. IP$_3$, inositol trisphosphate; DAG, diacylglycerol. The effector pathways for the 5-HT$_4$ and 5-HT$_5$ subtypes are presently unknown. The lower-case (5-ht) denotes a cloned receptor with no physiological correlate at present.

their second-messenger systems. The GPCR subtypes can be grouped in families on the basis of which G proteins they preferentially interact with: 5-HT$_{1A}$, 5-HT$_{1B}$, 5-HT$_{1E}$, 5-HT$_{1D}$ and 5-HT$_{1F}$ couple to a G$_{i/o}$ transducer and inhibit cyclic AMP production; 5-HT$_{2A}$, 5-HT$_{2B}$, and 5-HT$_{2C}$ couple to G$_{q/11}$ and stimulate phosphoinositide turnover; 5-HT$_4$, 5-HT$_6$, and 5-HT$_7$ couple to Gs and stimulate cyclic AMP production. These receptors are important in sleep–wake cycles, cognitive function, and mental health problems such as schizophrenia and depression.

Only a small percentage of the total body serotonin is found in the brain; high concentrations are found in the periphery, particularly in the gastrointestinal tract and platelets. Nonetheless, brain serotonin is widely distributed and serves a wide range of functions. Physiological studies have shown that the 5-HT$_1$ receptors tend to be inhibitory, and 5-HT$_2$ receptors are excitatory. The 5-HT$_{1A}$ receptor is found in highest concentrations in the hippocampus and the raphe nucleus, where it appears to be an autoreceptor and inhibits the intrinsic pacemaker activity of the serotonergic neurons. The 5-HT$_{1D}$ receptor also inhibits cyclic AMP formation and is most prevalent in the basal ganglia, globus pallidus, and the substantia nigra, where it may be involved in control of voluntary muscle. The 5-HT$_2$ receptor activates phosphoinositol metabolism and causes depolarization of neurons in the cortex. All of these 5-HT receptors have extensive homology with the other GPCRs. They show the greatest amount of variability in the third cytoplasmic loop, between the fifth and sixth membrane-spanning domains, which is an area believed to initiate the G-protein response.

The 5-HT$_3$ receptor is a ligand-gated ion channel that causes depolarization and excitation of neurons in the peripheral nervous system, entorhinal cortex, and the area postrema. Like other ligand-gated channels, the 5HT$_3$ receptor is composed of five protein subunits each with four transmembrane domains that coalesce to form an ionic channel.

4.5. Histamine Receptors

Specific histamine-receptor-blocking drugs are therapeutically useful in motion sickness, as sedatives, and for allergic disorders. Receptor binding and molecular biologic techniques have demonstrated the existence of three histamine receptors that are each coupled to a different type of G-protein, and therefore to completely different effector pathways. As the case with most transmitters, histamine has peripheral and central actions.

When acting through H$_1$ receptors, histamine is a potent vasodilator, causing a drop in blood pressure with flushing of the face and engorgement of mucosal vasculature. This receptor is coupled to phosphoinositol metabolism, causing an increase in the second messengers IP$_3$ and DAG. The classic antihistamine drugs, such as diphenhydramine, work on this receptor. Blockade of histamine H$_1$ receptors in the brain causes sedation and inhibits motion sickness, which is the basis of a large market for over-the-counter antihistamines. There is also evidence that the histaminergic pathway activates phospholipase A, which cleaves arachidonic acid from membrane phospholipids, activating lipoxygenase and cyclooxygenase pathways.

The histamine H$_2$ receptor increases cyclic AMP, and is the target of drugs used to decrease gastric acidity. In the stomach, an H$_2$ receptor is responsible for stimulating the parietal cell to secrete hydrochloric acid. The selective H$_2$ blockers, such as ranitidine, block this action of histamine and have revolutionized the treatment of peptic ulcers. In the heart, there is an H_2 receptor that causes an increased heart rate that is not blocked by the β-blocking agent propranolol.

The H_3 receptor is widely distributed throughout the CNS and appears to function as an autoreceptor on many neurons. (An autoreceptor is defined as a cell-surface receptor that is sensitive to the neurotransmitter release by the neuron expressing this receptor.) In humans, the H_3 receptor has been shown to modulate the release of histamine and norepinephrine in the cerebral cortex, and it has been implicated in regulating the release of many additional neurotransmitters in the striatum, hypothalamus, hippocampus, substantia nigra, and spinal cord of the rat and other mammals. A variety of H_3-selective agonists and antagonists is now being evaluated for therapeutic potential for a number of disorders including Alzheimer's disease, attention-deficit hyperactivity disorder (ADHD), epilepsy, and obesity.

4.6. Receptors for Amino Acid Neurotransmitters

The amino acids glutamate, glycine, and γ-aminobutyric acid (GABA) occur in concentrations 1000 times higher than the better-characterized biogenic amines and acetylcholine. The fundamental importance of these transmitters in CNS function appears to be reflected in the number and complexity of receptors that have been identified and their widespread distribution. Amino acid receptors fall into the two major receptor structural categories: GPCRs and ligand-gated ion channels.

4.6.1. GABA Receptors

Both classes of GABA receptors are inhibitory, acting as ligand-gated chloride channels (GABA$_A$) or by modifying cyclic AMP and changing potassium and calcium channels (GABA$_B$). GABA serves as the major inhibitory transmitter in the brain and is usually found within interneurons in the cortex and cerebellum. (These neurons have relatively short axons.) The GABA$_A$ receptor is a pentameric complex containing three or four different types of protein subunits (*see* Fig. 16). All of the subunits have four TM domains and, like the glycine receptor, have extensive homology with the nicotinic cholinergic receptor. Many subunits have been cloned, including six α, four β, three γ, three ρ, and one δ, ε, π, and θ. Although the number of possible combinations of these subunits offers a mind-boggling array of putative GABA receptors, the

most common subunit stoichiometry observed contains α-, β-, and γ-subunits. The α and β subunits contribute to the GABA recognition site, and it appears that the α and γ subunits are necessary for benzodiazepine binding.

The GABA$_A$ receptor is pharmacologically interesting, because it has specific binding sites for a number of seemingly unrelated drugs and agents. Benzodiazepine binding facilitates the inhibitory action of GABA on the receptor by augmenting the chloride-channel conductance. This explains much of the sedative and anti-anxiety action of benzodiazepines such as diazepam (Valium™) or chlordiazepoxide (Librium™). The ability of the GABA receptor to bind to benzodiazepines, as determined by affinity chromatography, was used to isolate and characterize these receptors. Other binding sites on the GABA$_A$ receptor exist for the barbiturates, alcohol, and certain anesthetic steroids. All of these agents augment the action of GABA and inhibit of CNS activity to induce sedation and sleep. The GABA$_B$ receptor is structurally and pharmacologically distinct from the GABA$_A$ receptor. As a member or the GPCR family, the GABA$_B$ recepor is unique in being a heterodimer held together by coiled-coil interactions in the C terminus and probably other domains. The receptor is activated when GABA binds to the N terminus of one subunit (GABA$_{B1}$) producing a conformational change in the other subunit (GABA$_{B2}$). The activated receptor then ineracts with G protein to initiate signaling. Pharmacologically, the GABA$_B$ receptor is selectively activated by baclofen, a drug that is used clinically to treat spasticity.

4.6.2. Glycine Receptor

The glycine receptor is found in the spinal cord and brainstem, and is inhibited by the poison strychnine. Although the GABA receptor is the principal inhibitory receptor in the brain and brainstem, the glycine receptor serves this role in the spinal cord. The inhibitory glycine receptor is a pentameric ligand-gated receptor composed of α and β subunits that form a chloride channel. Activation of this channel leads to the entry of chloride ion into the cell, hyperpolarizing the membrane and inhibiting neural activity. One of the best-understood glycine pathways in the spinal cord runs through the Renshaw cell, which inhibits the α motorneuron. When this important feedback inhibition is blocked by strychnine, the resulting seizures can lead to death. This is the basis for using strychnine in rat poison. Sensory information in the spinal cord is

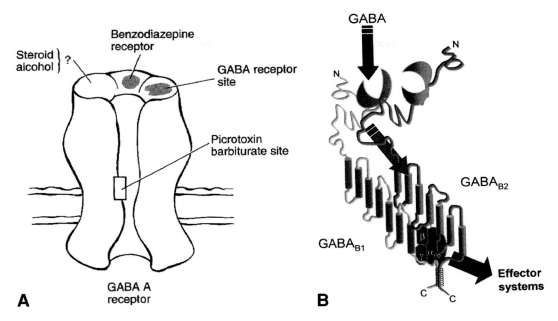

Fig. 16. Diagrams of the GABA receptors. **(A)** The GABA$_A$ receptor is a pentamer of non identical subunits that form a chloride ion channel. It has specific binding sites ofr barbiturates, benzodiazepines, and steroid anesthetics which augment the inhibitory action of GABA. **(B)** The GABA$_B$ receptor is a heterodimeric GPCR in which GABA binds to the N terminus of one subunit (BABA$_{B1}$) and induces a conformation change in the other subunit (GABA$_{B2}$). The activated complex can then interact with a G protein to initiate the biological response. (Figure 16B taken from Robbins, MJ et al. (2001) J Neuroscience 21: 8043–8052; used with permission of the Society for Neuroscience, Copyright 2001.)

also probably filtered through glycine receptors, because low doses of strychnine increase tactile sensations. Although strychnine has a long history of use, there is no rational therapeutic basis for its use.

Glycine plays an important modulatory role through a binding site on one of the glutamate receptors. Glycine binding to this *N*-methyl-D-aspartate (NMDA) subtype of the glutamate receptor increases the frequency of cation-channel opening (e.g., excitation). This effect is not antagonized by strychnine.

4.6.3. GLUTAMATE RECEPTORS

The acidic amino acids glutamate and aspartate stimulate almost all brain neurons. This action is so widespread in the CNS, in contrast to the discrete sites of action for other transmitters, that it was assumed for many years to be a non-physiological, insignificant response to a metabolic intermediate. However, as experimental results mounted that satisfied more of the criteria for a neurotransmitter, acceptance of the transmitter role for these compounds was eventually achieved. Furthermore, at least eleven different excitatory amino acid receptors are now known to exist, and specific neural pathways that use these acidic amino acids as their transmitters have been defined.

Glutamate appears to be the major stimulatory transmitter system in the brain. These pathways seem to have long axonal projections, and communicate information between major brain structures, such as the cortex to midbrain areas.

The eleven known glutamate-receptor subtypes belong to both the ligand-gated ionic-channel family ("ionotropic"—NMDA, AMPA, Kainate subtypes), and the GPCR family ("metabotropic" glutamate receptors—mglu$_{1-8}$). The ionotropic glutamate receptors seem to belong to a different gene family than the nicotinic, GABA, and glycine receptors. In the glutamate receptors that have been cloned, the extracellular amino terminal of the subunit peptides are much longer, containing almost 500 amino acids rather than the 200 found in the nicotinic receptor. Like the other ligand-gated channels, the non-NMDA glutamate receptors are pentameric and have four TM domains within each subunit; the subunit stoichiometry of the NMDA receptor remains unknown (Fig. 17).

Activation of an ionotropic glutamate receptor by an excitatory amino acid opens a cationic channel that depolarizes and stimulates the postsynaptic neuron. In the case of the AMPA- and kainate-receptor subtypes, stimulation by the drugs quisqualate and kainate,

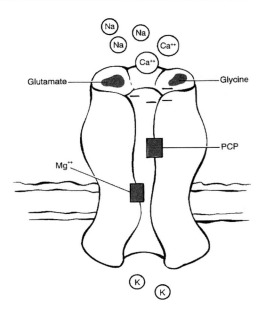

Fig. 17. NMDA subtype of the glutamate receptor. The diagram of the glutamate *N*-methyl-D-aspartate (NMDA) receptor shows ligand-binding sites for glutamate, glycine, magnesium, and the drug phencyclidine (PCP). When the cell becomes depolarized, magnesium is released from the interior of the channel, which allows glutamate to open the receptor channel. A glycine-binding site is also needed for channel activation. The NMDA receptor is unique in that calcium can enter the channel, as do sodium and potassium.

respectively, quickly renders the channel permeable to sodium and potassium. The NMDA receptor is relatively slow and has an unusual form of voltage regulation. The channel has a Mg^{2+}-binding site that inhibits ion flow when occupied. Mg^{2+} binding to this site is voltage-dependent, so that when the neuron is depolarized by other neural mechanisms, the Mg^{2+} can be displaced and the receptor channel opened by glutamate or NMDA. The NMDA-receptor channel is permeable to Ca^{2+} in addition to sodium and potassium. A unique aspect of the NMDA receptor is that it requires the presence of glycine to function adequately.

The NMDA receptor is distributed throughout the brain, particularly in the cortex and hippocampus.

NMDA receptors appear to play an important part in the development of long-term depression (LTD), long-term potentiation (LTP), and synaptic plasticity. (LTD and LTP represent cellular forms of "memory".) The distribution of the AMPA receptor parallels that of the NMDA receptor, and the kainate receptor is localized in specific regions of the brain, including the hippocampus. Overactivation by glutamate and the

application of large concentrations of the selective agonists (e.g., kainate and ibotenic acid) is neurotoxic. It appears that overstimulation of these ligand-gated glutamate channels triggers postsynaptic neuronal death, probably by elevating intracellular Ca^{2+} to toxic levels.

The metabotropic glutamate receptors are currently divided into three groups based on similarities in primary sequence, agonist pharmacology, and G-protein-effector coupling. Group I receptors ($mglu_1$ and $mglu_5$) preferentially couple to $G_{q/11}$, which links them to phospholipase C and the production of DAG and IP_3. Group II receptors ($mglu_2$ and $mglu_3$) have very similar pharmacological profiles and couple to $G_{i/o}$ to inhibit cyclic adenosine monophosphate (cAMP) production. Group III receptors ($mglu_4$, $mglu_6$, $mglu_7$, and $mglu_8$) also couple to $G_{i/o}$, but are pharmacologically distinct from Group II. Structurally, these receptors differ from most GPCRs in that they have a large N-terminal domain, which serves as the glutamate-binding site. Although metabotropic glutamate receptors are widely expressed throughout the brain, specific subtypes appear to be differentially expressed. As a class, the metabotropic glutamate receptors appear to play an important neuromodulatory role in the CNS.

4.7. Peptide Receptors Demonstrate a Diversity of Biologic Activity

Just as there was an explosion in the discovery of neuroactive peptides around 1970, the advent of molecular biologic techniques stimulated the discovery of a vast array of neuropeptide receptors. Almost all of these belong to the GPCR family, but the exceptions are important. Atrial natriuretic peptide is also present in the brain and acts on a protein receptor that has only one membrane-spanning domain. The cytoplasmic extension of this receptor is itself a guanylate cyclase, which is activated when the receptor is occupied by an agonist. Table 3 lists representative neural peptides, their subtypes, their effector pathways, and the number of amino acids and membrane-spanning domains within their structures.

5. CONCLUSION

There are numerous neurotransmitter receptors that belong to only a few major gene families. However, a given transmitter often has several subtypes of receptors that use different G-protein coupling and effector systems. In several cases, transmitters have

Table 3
Representative Neural Peptides

Peptide	Subtype	Effector pathways	AA/TMD[†]
Angiotensin II	AT_1, AT_2		
Atrial Natriuretic	ANP_A, ANP_B	cGMP	1061/1, 1047/1
Bradykinin	B_1, B_2	IP_3/DAG	353/7, 364/7
Corticotropin-releasing factor	CRF_1, CRF_2	cAMP	415/7, 411/7
Neuropeptide Y	Y_1,Y_2,Y_3,Y_4,Y_5	cAMP	384, 381, 375, 445, 290/7
Neurotensin	NTS1, nts2	IP_3/DAG	418/7, 410/7
Opiate receptors	DOP (δ opioid peptide)	cAMP	372/7
	KOP (κ opioid peptide)		380/7
	MOP (μ opioid peptide)	cAMP	400/7
Tachykinins	NK_1, NK_2, NK_3	IP_3/DAG	407, 398, 468/7
Vasopressin	V_{1a}, V_{ib}	IP_3/DAG	418/7, 424/7
	V_2	cAMP	371/7
Oxytocin	OT	IP_3/DAG	389/7
VIP (Vasoactive Intestinal peptide)	$VPAC_1$, $VPAC_2$	cAMP	457/7, 438/7

[†]Number of amino acids (AA) in the receptor/number of transmembrane-spanning domains (TMD). The artrial natriuretic peptide receptor has a single TMD and contains a guanylate cyclase domain.

receptors that belong to entirely different families, such as ligand-gated-channel and GPCR subtypes. The receptor-effector coupling system offers extensive diversity for biologic actions, and remarkable specificity despite its use of a limited number of chemical messages.

SELECTED READINGS

Alexander SPH, Peter JA. (eds) TIPS Receptor and Ion Channel Nomenclature (Vol. 11). Trends Pharmacol Sci 2000; 21: (Suppl).

Caulfield MP, Birdsall NJM. International Union of Pharmacology. XVII. Classification of muscarinic acetylcholine receptors. Pharmacol Rev 1998; 50:279–290.

Cooper JR, Bloom FE, Roth RH. The Biochemical Basis of Neuropharmacology, 7th ed. New York: Oxford University Press, 1996.

Hardman JG, Limbird LE, Molinoff PB, Ruddon RW. (eds) Goodman and Gilman's The Pharmacological Basis of Therapeutics, 9th ed. New York: The McGraw-Hill Companies, 1996.

Hill SJ, Ganellin CR, Timmerman H, Schwartz JC, Shankley NP, Young JM, et al. International Union of Pharmacology. XIII. Classification of Histamine Receptors. Pharmacol Rev 1997; 49:253–278.

Hoyer D, Martin G. 5-HT receptor classification and nomenclature: towards a harmonization with the human genome. Neuropharmacology 1997; 36:419–428.

Kenakin TP, Bond RA, Bonner TI. Definition of pharmacological receptors. Pharmacol Rev 1992; 44:351.

Limbird LE. Cell Surface Receptors: A Short Course on Theory and Methods, 2nd ed. Boston: Kluwer Academic Publishers, 1996.

Strange PG. Antipsychotic drugs: Importance of dopamine receptors for the mechanisms of therapeutic actions and side effects. Pharmacol Rev 2001; 53:119–133.

6 Neuroembryology and Neurogenesis

Ching Sung Teng and Christina T. Teng

CONTENTS

1. INTRODUCTION

This chapter first introduces the embryonic development of the neural plate into the neural tube and then discusses the central nervous system (CNS). The proliferation, differentiation, and migration of the neuronal and neural-crest cells are discussed. Finally, current studies on perinatal neuronal apoptotic death and its prevention by survival factors are introduced.

2. EMBRYONIC DEVELOPMENT OF THE NERVOUS SYSTEM

2.1. Early Development of the Neural Tube

The nervous system is one of the first structures to appear in the human embryo. Starting at the third week of development, the *neural plate* is a thickened dorsal *ectodermal plate*. Initially the lateral edges of the plate elevate to form the *neural folds*, creating a linear groove between them. After constant induction by the adjacent *notochord*, the neural folds become more

From: *Neuroscience in Medicine, 2nd ed.* (P. Michael Conn, ed.),
© 2003 Humana Press Inc., Totowa, NJ.

elevated and fuse with each other in the midline, and the neural groove is gradually transformed into the *neural tube*. This tube becomes separated from the rest of the ectoderm (Fig. 1A–F). The fusion of the tube starts in the cervical region, but is delayed at the cranial and the caudal ends of the embryo. The last parts of the neural tube to close, located cranially and caudally, are known as the anterior and posterior *neuropores* (Fig. 2). These are normally closed by the end of the fourth embryonic week. In the early stage of development, the neural tube has been divided into four regions, and their derivatives are presented in Table 1. The neural tube forms the CNS, with its hundreds of billions of *neurons*, and can be classified into six major divisions: (i) spinal cord, (ii) brainstem, (iii) pons and cerebellum, (iv) mesencephalon, (v) diencephalon, and (vi) cerebral hemispheres.

2.2. Neural Crest

During the fusion of the neural plate, a group of neural-plate cells escape into the space between the tube and the surface of ectoderm (Fig. 1F). These *neural-crest* cells give rise to the sensory ganglia of

111

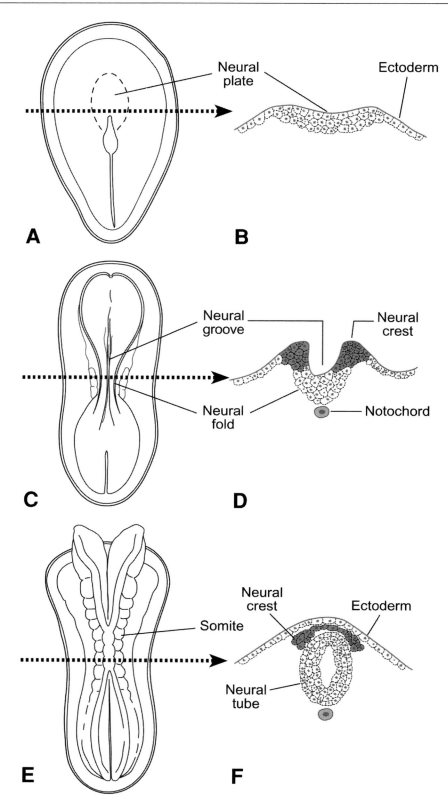

Fig. 1. Stages in the formation of neural tube and neural crest. (**A,B**) The neural plate on the dorsal side of the embryo. (**C–F**) The formation of the neural groove and neural tube. The neural crest forms an intermediate zone between the neural tube and surface ectoderm. The notochord is located on the midline of the embryo just ventral to the developing neural tube.

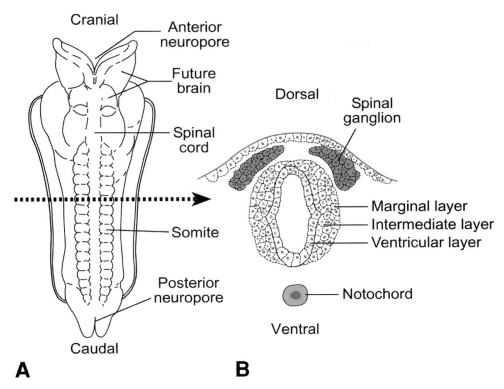

Fig. 2. Formation of neuropores. **(A)** Dorsal view of a human embryo at 3.5 wk. A chain of somites is located on each side of the neural tube. **(B)** Cross-section at the *level of arrow* to show how the neural-crest cells develop into spinal ganglion, and the formation of ventricular, intermediate, and marginal layers in the spinal cord.

Table 1
Derivatives of Regions of the Neural Tube

Region	Derivative
Dorsal plate	Roofs of the third, fourth ventricles.
	Tela choroidea (a vascular plexus over the roof of the ventricle).
Dorsolateral plate	Association neurons (all neurons other than motor neurons and primary sensory neurons).
	This region makes up the bulk of the CNS.
Ventrolateral plate	Motor neurons (neurons whose axons end on skeletal muscle fibers or postganglionic neurons)
	The cranial end of the mesencephalon.
Ventral plate	No significant derivatives.

the spinal and cranial nerves, and to the postganglionic autonomic neurons (Fig. 2B). Other cells derived from the neural-crest cells are the *chromaffin cells* of the adrenal medulla and the *glial cells* in the peripheral nervous system as well as *melanoblasts*. Cells, tissues, and organs that either contain or are constituted of neural crest-derived cells are listed in Table 2.

2.3. Spinal Cord and Brainstem

After the neural tube is closed, the *neuroepithelial cells* in the tube begin to give rise to the primitive nerve cells or *neuroblasts*. The proliferation of neuroblasts in the *mantle layer* and each side of the neural tube develops into ventral and dorsal thickenings. These thickenings are known as the *basal plates* and the *alar plates*, respectively. As a general rule, the basal plate begins its differentiation before the alar plate. The boundary between these two is marked by a longitudinal groove, the *sulcus limitans*. This sulcus runs along the length of the neural tube, and divides the rapidly expanding side wall of the neural tube (Fig. 3A,B). The sulcus limitans remains visible in the lower part of

**Table 2
A List of the Cell Types, Tissues, and Organs that Either Contain
or are Constituted of "Neural Crest-Derived Cells"**

Cell types	Tissues or organs
Adipocytes	Adrenal gland
Adrenergic neurons	Blood vessels
Angioblasts	Cardiac septa
Calcitonin-producing (C) cells	Connective tissue of glands (thyroid, parathyroid, thymus, and pituitary)
Cardiac mesenchyme	Cornea
Cholinergic neurons	Craniofacial bone
Chondroblasts	Dentine
Chondrocytes	Dermis
Fibroblasts	Eye
Mesenchymal cells	Endothelia
Odontoblasts	Heart
Satellite cells	Smooth muscles
Schwann cells	Spinal ganglia
Sensory neurons	Striated muscles
Smooth myoblasts	Sympathetic nervous system

the *brainstem* in the adult. The neuroblasts in the basal plate form the *ventral* and *lateral gray columns*, which contain somatic and autonomic motor neurons, respectively. The alar plates form the sensory area (or dorsal gray column), containing neuroblasts that become *sensory neurons* (Fig. 3C,D).

Spinal nerves are formed by the juncture of a dorsal sensory root made up of processes from neurons located in the dorsal-root ganglia carrying afferent impulses toward the *spinal cord* and a ventral motor root made up of axons carrying efferent nerve impulses away from the spinal cord (Fig. 4). Most of the axons in the ventral roots arise from somatic and autonomic motor neurons in the ventral and lateral gray column of the spinal cord. The axons from the ventral roots will grow and innervate the striated muscle masses that are functionally classified as somatic efferent fibers. Between the dorsal and ventral roots, the lateral column is developed in the thoracic and upper lumbar regions of the spinal cord. The axons from the neurons of the lateral column make up part of the spinal nerves. They grow toward the periphery in the trunk region and synapse with the neural crest-derived neurons in the sympathetic ganglia. The *chain ganglias* of the sympathetic division of *the autonomic nervous system* are connected to the spinal cord by the *gray ramus communicans* and the *white ramus communicans*. The axons of the spinal-cord neurons are known as *preganglionic fibers* and those of the ganglia are termed *postganglionic fibers*. The neurons of the parasympathetic

division of the autonomic nervous system are located in the cervical and sacral regions of the spinal cord. The axons from these neurons grow and synapse with the postganglionic neurons in the wall of the gut (Fig. 4).

In the 3-mo human embryo, the spinal cord extends the entire length of the embryo. After that time, the *vertebral column* and the *dura* grow more rapidly than the spinal cord itself, gradually increasing the length of the vertebae column relative to the cord. The terminal end of the spinal cord will eventually shift to a higher level than the corresponding vertebra (Fig. 5A–C). Consequently, the lower end of the cord is at the level of the third lumbar vertebra at term. This differential growth continues after birth, and the spinal cord eventually terminates at the level of L_2. The dorsal and ventral nerve fibers of the *lumbar* and *sacral segments* that exit from the terminal end of the cord are known as the *cauda equina*. The caudal end of the neural tube remains attached to the *coccygeal* section of the vertebral column, which is a thin filament known as *filum terminale* (Fig. 5D).

2.4. The Primary Brain Vesicles

After the anterior neuropore closes, this region is known as the *lamina terminalis*. This cranial end of the neural tube expands to form the three main divisions of the developing brain, separated by two constrictions. The primary *brain vesicles* are the *prosencephalon* (forebrain), the *mesencephalon* (midbrain), and the *rhombencephalon* (hindbrain) (Fig. 6A). Because

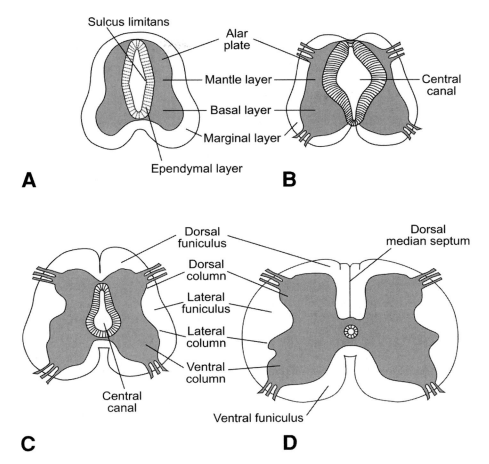

Fig. 3. Development of the human spinal cord. Cross-section of the human spinal cord at various stages of development. (**A**) 4-mm (3.5 wk) embryo. (**B**) 11-mm (5.5 wk) embryo. (**C**) 30-mm (9 wk) embryo. (**D**) 80-mm embryo.

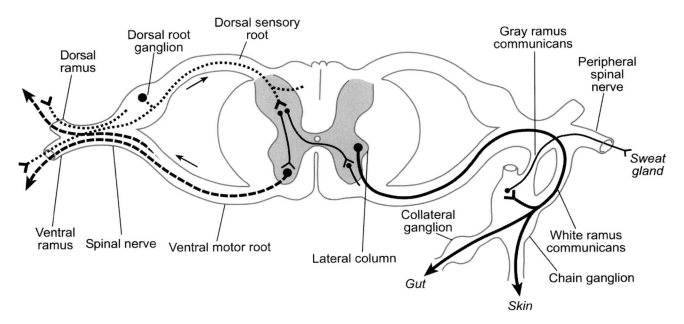

Fig. 4. Components of spinal nerves. A typical pathway of spinal nerve is shown on the *left side* of the figure. The connection of nerve fibers of the sympathetic nervous system is presented in the *right side*.

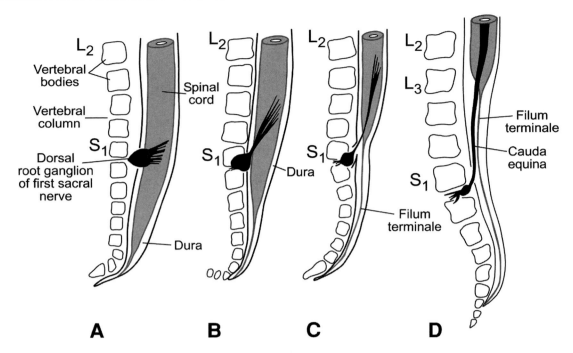

Fig. 5. Formation of the cauda equina. The relationship between the lengths of the spinal cord and the vertebral column at various stages of development. **(A)** Third month. **(B)** Fourth month. **(C)** Fifth month. **(D)** Newborn.

of the continuous growth of the three primary vesicles, the originally straight neural tube shows two external flexures, the *cephalic* and *cervical flexures*, during the third and fourth week of development. A third, known as *pontine flexure*, occurs during week five in the region of the developing *pons*. These flexures divide the midbrain from the hindbrain and the hindbrain from the spinal cord (Fig. 6B,C). The *optic cup* is from an outgrowth of the forebrain, and the brainstem is derived from the midbrain and part of the hindbrain. The *cerebellum* is a hindbrain derivative (*see* Table 3).

2.5. Myelencephalon and Metencephalon

The development of the *myelencephalon* results mainly from the expansion of the *fourth ventricle* into a large cavity that separates the alar plates. As the fourth ventricle continues to expand, its dorsolateral plate moves laterally. This stretches the *roof plate*, and it becomes thin. Consequently, the lateral walls separate the alar and basal plates by a distinct groove, the sulcus limitans (Fig. 7A). Later, three groups of nuclei are derived from each of the alar or basal plates (Fig. 7B). The myelencephalon gives rise to the medulla oblongata, which is continuous with the spinal cord (*see* Table 4).

The *metencephalon* consists of a pair of enlarged areas of the dorsolateral plate, the *rhombic lips*, which join dorsally in a midline segment—the vermis, to form the *cerebellar plate*. The cerebellar plate continues to grow and form the *hemispheres* of the *cerebellum* (Fig. 8). Both the hemispheres and vermis contain a group of intracerebellar nuclei and a folded cortex. The ventral portion of the metencephalon will develop into the pons, which consists of a group of *pontine nuclei* originally derived from the alar plate that have migrated to this location (Fig. 8A). The function of the pontine nuclei is to serve as the center for communication by sending their axons to the cerebellum. Blood vessels invade the dorsal plate and form the *choroid plexus*.

Within the cerebellar cortex, a radial migration of cells takes place during early development. During the eighth week, the cerebellar plates constructed by three cellular layers—the *neuroepithelial, mantle,* and *marginal* layers—is established. Neuroepithelial cells first migrate to the surface of the cerebellum, where they form the *external granular layer*. The daughter cells of this layer migrate inward to pass the *Purkinji cells* and form the *internal granular layer*. After birth, the cortex of the cerebellum consists of a *molecular layer*,

A

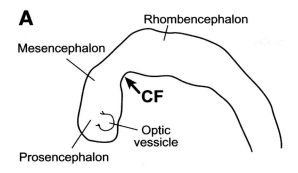

B

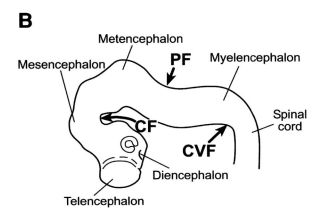

C

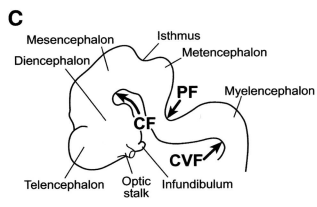

Fig. 6. Changes in the external brain configuration during early development. (**A**) 3.5-wk embryo. (**B**) 5-wk embryo. (**C**) 5.5-wk embryo. CF, cephalic flexure; PF, pontine flexure; CVF, cervical flexure.

which is occupied by the dendrites of the Purkinji cells and *Golgi* neurons, and an internal granular layer beneath the Purkinji cells (Fig. 8B,C). The generation of *neuronal processes* generally occurs after the completion of cellular migration. However, axon growth may precede cell migration in some cases. For example, in the cerebellar cortex, during the internal migration of granule cells, the cells first extrude in a horizontal process and then leave behind a perpendicular process, giving the axon a T-shaped appearance.

2.6. Mesencephalon

In comparison to other developing brain vesicles, the mesencephalon shows no striking structural modification and is soon overshadowed by the cortices of the cerebellum and *cerebrum*. Because of the expansion of the basal and alar plates, the central cavity of the mesencephalon reduces to a narrow channel, the *cerebral aqueduct*, connecting the fourth ventricle of the hindbrain to the *third ventricle* of the *diencephalon*. The *crus cerebri* (or the base of *cerebral peduncle*), a derivative of the basal plate, connects the descending nerve fibers from the cerebral cortex to the metencephalon and spinal cord. The anterior and the posterior *colliculi* found in the *tectum* of the alar plates serve as the centers for the auditory reflexes and visual impulse (Fig. 9).

2.7. Diencephalon

Early in the development of the diencephalon, the roof plate of the third ventricle, formed by *ependymal cells* as a thin layer invaded by blood vessels, to form the choroid plexus. The lateral wall of the third ventricle gives rise to the main structure of the diencephalon: the *epithalamus*, *thalamus*, and *hypothalamus*. However, there are no ventralateral plate derivatives in the diencephalon. In the floor of the third ventricle, three swellings can be identified—the *optic chiasm*, *infundibulum*, and *mammillary* body (Fig. 10A). Later, a pair of *optic vesicles* appears on both sides of the forebrain. They are connected to the ventricle of the diencephalon by the *optic stalk*, and become the major portions of the eye.

The epithalamus is the precursor of the *habenular nuclei* and *pineal gland*. A longitudinal groove, the *sulcus hypothalamicus*, appears in the dorsolateral area, separating the thalamus from the hypothalamus. The thalamic areas undergo rapid proliferation and fuse at the midline, and the central cavity is therefore transformed into a slit-like third ventricle. The development and function of the thalamus and *cerebral cortex* are closely interrelated throughout the stages of prenatal and postnatal life. The cell groups in the hypothalamus are associated with autonomic and endocrine functions.

Table 3
The Adult Derivatives of the Early-Brain Vesicles

Early brain vesicles (3.5 to 4-wk embryo)	Developing brain (4 to 5-wk embryo)	Adult derivatives
Prosencephalon (forebrain)	Telencephalon	Cerebral cortex Basal ganglia
	Diencephalon	Epithalamus Thalamus Hypothalamus Subthalamus
Mesencephalon (midbrain)	Mesencephalon	Mesencephalon
Rhombencephalon (hindbrain)	Metencephalon	Pons Cerebellum
	Myelencephalon	Medulla oblongata

As the neuronal cells continue with proliferation, migration, and differentiation, the three primary brain vesicles develop into the major structures of the adult brain.

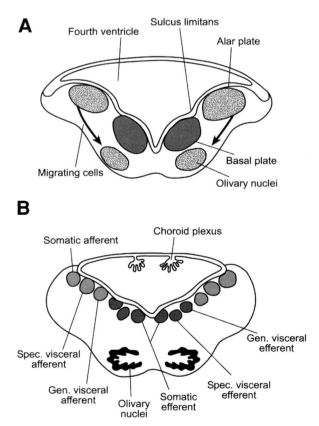

Fig. 7. Differentiation of alar and basal plates of the myelencephalon. (**A**) The 5-wk embryonic myelencephalon shows the lateral expansion of the fourth ventricle. This results in the formation of alar- and basal-plate nuclei. Arrows indicate the path followed by cells of the alar plate to the olivary nuclear complex. (**B**) Three groups of the cranial sensory neurons are derived from the alar plate, whereas cranial motor neurons are differentiated from the basal plate. Note that the olivary nuclei are groups of sensory way station; their function is to make connections with the cerebellum.

Table 4
The Afferent and the Efferent Components of Cranial Nerves
in Conjunction with the Alar and Basal Plates

Origin	Group of nuclei*	Nerves originated
Alar plate	General somatic afferent	V, VII, IX, X
	Special somatic afferent	VIII
	Special visceral afferent	I, VII, IX, X
	General visceral afferent	V, VII, IX, X
Basal plate	General somatic efferent	III, IV, VI, XII
	Special visceral efferent	V, VII
	General visceral efferent	III, VII, IX, X

*In the CNS, an accumulation of nerve-cell bodies are themselves called nuclei (a somewhat confusing terminology in comparison to the nuclei of *eukaryotic cells*).

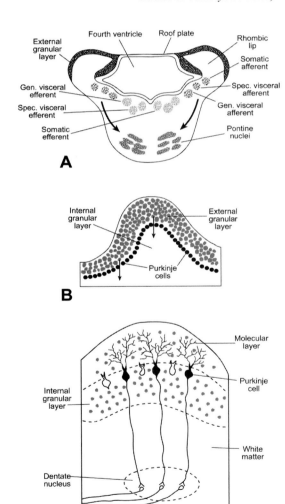

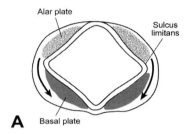

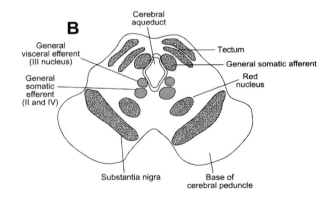

Fig. 9. Differentiation of the mesencephalon. **(A)** Primitive stage of mesencephalon shows the position of the alar and basal plates. The arrows indicate the path followed by the cells of the alar plate to the red nucleus and substantia nigra. **(B)** Fusion of ventral part of the cavity and differentiation of nuclei (e.g., tectum and general somatic [visceral] afferent [efferent] nucleus).

Fig. 8. Development of cerebellum from metencephalon. **(A)** The rhombic lips expand partly into the lumen of the fourth ventricle and partly into the dorsal direction and give rise to the cerebellum. **(B)** External granular layer fully formed, and Purkinji cells are positioned in the cortex. The arrows indicate (*continued*) the inward migration of cells to the internal granular layer. **(C)** Purkinji cells separate the external and internal granular layers. As development proceeds, cells of the external layer migrate inward to the inner layer, leaving an empty layer—the molecular layer.

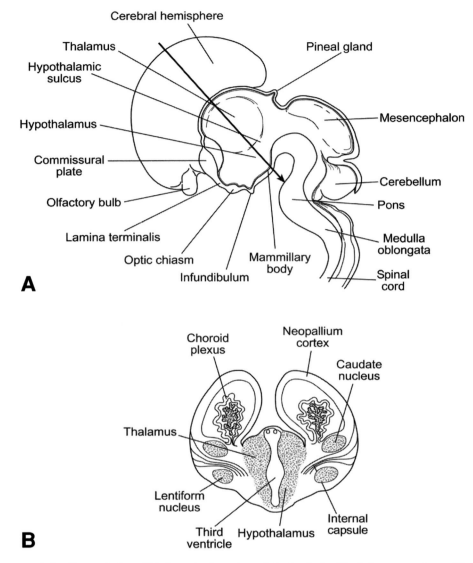

Fig. 10. Development of the diencephalon. **(A)** A sagittal section of the brain in 10-wk human embryo. The thalamus and the hypothalamus are derived from alar plates and separated by the hypothalamic sulcus. The roof plate of the diencephalon develops into the pineal gland (or epiphysis), whereas the infundibulum becomes part of the pituitary gland. **(B)** Cross-section of **A** at the level indicated. The corpus striatum is separated into the caudate nucleus and lentiform nucleus by a bundle of internal capsule.

2.8. Telencephalon

The *telencephalon* consists of two cerebral hemispheres and the lamina terminalis. The cavities of the hemispheres form the lateral ventricles, which communicate with the third ventricle. The mantle zone of the basal part of the hemispheres thickens and bulges into the lumen of the lateral ventricles to form the *corpus striatum*. The corpus striatum is later divided into two parts, the *caudate nucleus* and the *lentiform nucleus*, by a bundle of axon fibers (the *internal capsule*) from the cerebral cortex. As development proceeds, the lentiform nucleus changes into the *putamen* and the *globus pallidus*, which are closely associated with the internal capsule together with the caudate nucleus and the thalamus (Fig. 11A). This complex, derived from the corpus striatum, is the center for correlation of sensory impulses and control of motor activity.

Ependymal cells form a thin layer of the hemisphere well, known as the *pallium*, which becomes the cerebral cortex. Initially, the cerebral cortex is divided into two regions: the *neopallium* and the *palaeopallium*. In

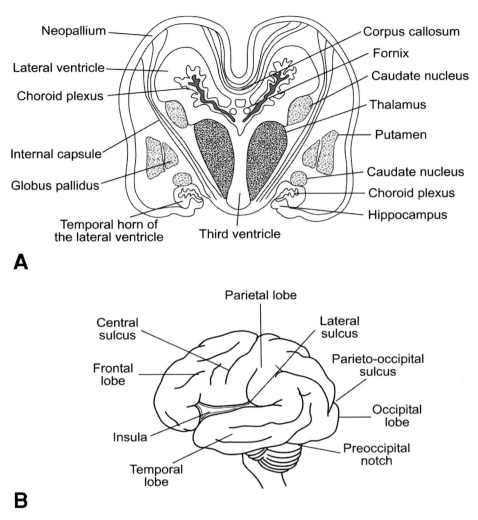

Fig. 11. Development of the telencephalon. **(A)** Cross-section of the brain of 21-wk human embryo. Note that the separation of lentiform nucleus into the putamen and the globus pallidus, and the hippocampus has changed its position as a result of the growth of the hemispheres. **(B)** The development of the cerebral surface. Diagram of a newborn human brain.

the neopallium, the ependymal cells actively divide into a large number of *neuroblasts* that migrate to the mariginal layer and then differentiate into the neurons. Consequently, the wall of the neopallium thickens and its neurons become stratified. The histogenesis of the cortical cells follows a distinctive inside-out pattern. That is, the early formed neuroblasts occupy a deep position and form the deeper layers of the cortex, and those formed at later times move to the surface and displace the older cells deeper into the basal layers of the cortex. At birth, a large number of pyramidal cells appear in the motor cortex, and granular cells are found in the sensory area. The choroid plexus, the *choroidal fissure*, and *hippocampus* of the lateral ventricles are also derived from the thin part and the medial wall of the pallium, respectively.

As a result of rapid growth of cerebral hemispheres in anterior, posterior, and dorsal directions in the telencephalon, the formation of numerous folds (*gyri*) and grooves (*sulci*) are created on the surface. The appearance of these folds and grooves serves as the landmark to divide the cerebral hemispheres into five different lobes: the *frontal, parietal, occipital,* and *temporal lobes,* and the *insula* (Fig. 11B). Three commissures—the *anterior* and *hippocampal commissure*—and *corpus callosum*—are established in the area of the lamina terminalis to provide the connection of the two cerebral hemispheres. Among them, the corpus callosum is one of the most important and largest commissure. It consists of a large bundle of fibers that cross the midline of the brain and connect one side of the CNS to the other. These fibers extend first anteriorly and then posteriorly, thereby covering the dorsal plate of the telencephalon. The plate becomes thicker and serves as the route for the growing callosal fibers. The anterior commissure connects the *olfactory bulb* and the area of the *temporal lobes*. The fibers of the hippocampal commissure arise in the *hippocampus* and form an arching system to connect the mammillary body and the hypothalamus.

3. NEUROGENESIS IN THE EMBRYONIC NERVOUS SYSTEM

3.1. Proliferation and Differentiation of the Neuroepithelial Cells

In vertebrate species, the wall of the newly closed neural tube consists of the neuroepithelial cells—a group of multipotent progenitor cells. They form a thick layer of pseudostratified epithelium over the entire wall of the neural tube and divide rapidly, resulting in the production of a neuroepithelial layer. The cells in this layer give rise to the primitive nerve cells or neuroblasts. Neuroblasts represent the first stage in the differentiation of the neurons, migrate away from the lumen, and settle into other portions of the neural tube. They form the mantle layer that eventually becomes the gray matter of the spinal cord. The neuroblasts pass successively through a-polar, bi-polar, and uni-polar to multi-polar stages. The unipolar cell grows out of the mantle zone to become a part of the marginal layer below the external limiting membrane (Fig. 3A). This process becomes the axon of the nerve cell and may synapse with dendrites of other nerve cells within the spinal cord, or it may leave the neural tube as motor fiber growing peripherally to contact muscle cells and glands. In addition to the neuroblastic cells, the neuroepithelial cells also give rise to the *glioblasts* and *ependymal cells*—the supportive cells of the nervous system. The glioblasts differentiate into both *astrocytes* and *oligodendroglia cells*. Ependymal cells remain in the innermost ventricular layer, and form the epithelial lining of the neural canal.

3.2. The Origin and Formation of Cortical Neurons

In contrast to neuron in the spinal cord, the neurons in the developing cerebellar and cerebral cortices migrate from the mantle zone through the marginal zone and form a layered sheet of gray matter externally. In the cerebral cortex, two neuronal types are generated in distinct proliferative zones. First, the *excitatory pyramidal cells* are also derived from the neuroepithelial cells in the cortical ventricular zone, and use the radial glial fibers to migrate and take their position in the cortex. In the cortical plate they accumulate in an inside-out sequence to form the six-layered structure of the cortex. The mechanism responsible for the disposition of these neurons is still unknown. Second, the *inhibitory nonpyramidal* cells are mainly derived from the *ganglionic eminence* of the ventral telencephalon. Relatively few nonpyramidal cells are derived from the cortical neuroepithelium. These neurons use tangential migratory paths to reach to the cortex. They may follow distinct pathways along axonal bundles of the corticofugal fibers to accumulate in the cortex as a layer of the cortical interneurons. Since the nonpyramidal cells first appear in the marginal zone, some of them form Cajal-Retzius (CR) cells that, through the release of *reelin*, enhance the migration of pyramidal neurons. A recent discovery indicates that in the mouse embryo, CR cells produce EMX2 protein (a product of *Emx2* homeobox gene), which in term stimulates the synthesis and release of reelin in the CR cells.

3.3. Migration of the Neural-Crest Cells

After the formation of the neural tube, the neural crest appears as two longitudinally running bands of cells on either side of the spinal cord. The cells of the neural crest migrate away from their original locations and become widely distributed throughout the body. One stream of the cells migrates dorsolaterally into the superficial ectoderm dorsal to the neural tube and the *somites*. These are the precursors of the pigment cells. The other branch of the neural-crest cells migrates ventrally between the neural tube and the somites. They will develop into the *sensory ganglia* of the cranial nerves and the posterior roots of the spinal nerves, and the ganglia of the *autonomic nervous system*.

In recent years, great attention has been given to the migration of neural-crest cells. Although the factors that initiate the migration of these cells are still unknown, the prerequisites for the initiation of this process are: (i) The migratory routes are predictable from a given species, and yet the pathways of migration can vary from species to species. (ii) The presence of an incomplete *basal lamina* is important for the initiation of cell migration. A fully established basal lamina overlying the cells is impenetrable to the cells. (iii) The components of the *extracellular matrix* (ECM) play important roles in the cell migration.

Fibronectin, laminin, and collagen types I and IV promote migration. On the contrary, collagen types II, V, and IX, aggregan, and versican inhibit migration. Moreover, neural-crest cells are contributing to the synthesis of some ECM components, since it is important for the cells to have sufficient cell-free extracellular space for migration. The cells also produce proteases and plasminogen activator to create a path on ECM through which they migrate. (iv) Five hours prior to the onset of migration, the cell-cell gap-junctions were diminished. The loss of *cellular adhesion molecules* (N-CAM, or N-cadherin) was found after initial migration of the cells. However, specific cadherins are expressed in various subpopulations to provide the interaction in the migrating cells. (v) Factors such as TGFβ 1 and 2 and their related protein Dorsalin-1 were found to sitmulate neural-crest cell migration. A similar effect in this regard has been demonstrated by the transcription factor PAX-3. Any defect in PAX-3 gene (or Splotch mutant) severely delays the onset of neural-crest migration from the neural tube. Other motility-inducing factors, such as hepatocyte growth factor/scatter factor (HGF/SF), are also involved in cell motility.

During the process of migration when the cells run into the physical barriers such as basal laminae, blood vessels, and somitic cells in the head or trunk region, they stop migration and start accumulation. The cessation of migration and the settlement of neural-crest cells in their final sites are determined by factors intrinsic to neural-crest cells, or by the extracellular microenvironments they encounter. For example, in certain final sites, tissues express versican that inhibits the function of the molecules, (e.g., fibronectin, laminin, and collagen type I), and consequently stop the migration. Furthermore, the abnormalities involved in the production of laminin and collagen type IV prevent the colonization of the cells. This is also known as the lethal-spotting (Ls/Ls) mutant in mice.

3.4. Sources of Trophic Support for Developing Neurons

The growth and survival of neurons are determined by the presence of a family of intrinsic factors. These are nerve-growth factor (NGF), brain-derived neurotrophic factor (BDNF), neurotrophin (NT-3, NT-4/5, and NT-6), and epidermal growth-factor-receptor family (ErbB, ErbB2, ErbB3, and ErbB4). These factors mediate their action on responsive neurons by binding to the cell-surface receptors. For example, all neurotrophins bind to the neurotrophin receptor ($p75$), and NGF, BDNF, and NT-3 bind to TrKA, TrKB, and TrkC (receptor tyrosine kinases), respectively. Other extrinsic factors that are outside the CNS are several fibroblast growth factors (FGFs), leukemia inhibitory factor (LIF), insulin-like growth factor (IGF), and platelet-derived growth factor (PDGF). In addition, some extrinsic factors may show dual effects. For instance, the bone morphogenetic proteins (BMPs), which enhance the growth of astrocyte, they suppress the growth of oligodendoglia. Finally, the effects of these factors are not restricted to specific neuronal populations, and each type of neuron is influenced by several growth factors. In general, neurons change their trophic factor requirements throughout development.

4. NEURONAL APOPTOSIS IN THE DEVELOPING NERVOUS SYSTEM

4.1. The Function of Neuronal Apoptosis

During the embryonic proliferation phase, many more neurons are formed than the number present in the mature nervous system, indicating that in the developing nervous system there is widespread death of large numbers of neurons. Evidence shows that this neuronal death is a genetic *programmed cell death* or *apoptosis*. Apoptosis is one of the major events in the process of *neurogenesis* (e.g., cellular proliferation, migration, differentiation, and cell death). In the developing nervous system, certain neurons must be removed in an orderly fashion by apoptosis.

The functions of neuronal apoptosis are predicted: (i) To eliminate the neurons that have made inappropriate synaptic connections with other neurons or their own targets. This is to ensure optimal numerical relationships between neurons and target cells. (ii) To remove the neurons that serve transient developmental functions or those located in the *ectopic sites*. (iii) To facilitate the *pattern formation* and *morphogenesis* of the CNS in early development. Finally, apoptotic death represents a natural innate control mechanism within the neuron that is able to react to the changes in its surrounding environment such as shortage of nutrient, a lack of trophic factors, and an altered endogenous endocrine state. Thus, the apoptotic death of neurons has frequently been interpreted as their failure to compete for limited amounts of population-specific target-derived trophic factors (or the *neurotrophic theory*).

Table 5
Localization of Early Neural Apoptosis

Developmental stage	Location
Neurulation	Neural plate, neural fold, and neural tube
Neural-crest formation	Premigratory and migratory neural-crest cells
Eye induction and formation	Forebrain, optic vesicle, and optic cup
Early neurogenesis	Neural tube and spinal cord
Mid neurogenesis	CNS, cerebral cortex, retina, and PNS ganglia

Neuronal apoptosis is not uniform throughout the nervous system. A higher rate of apoptotic neuronal death was found in the primordial cortex (90%) than in the spinal cord, where approx 50% of the motoneurons die. A similar rate of cell death was found in the interneurons of the retina.

4.2. Apoptosis in Precursor Cells in Early Neural Development

In addition to the previously mentioned common form of apoptosis in the developing nervous system, neurons are involved that are relatively differentiated and have well-established synaptic connections. Other examples of apoptotic cell death are discovered during earlier developmental stages, when the neurons are the proliferating neural precursor cells or recent postmitotic cells (Table 5). These discoveries raise the question of the magnitude and the role of this early neural-cell death. This rare form of cell death may eliminate unwanted precursor cells with inappropriate phenotypes, or may create the environment for pattern formation in the nervous system.

4.3. The Mechanisms of Neuronal Apoptosis

Apoptosis is an important process of neurogenesis in the developing CNS. To understand the functional mechanism behind developmental nerve-cell death, cell culture by removal of survival factors from the culture medium has been well-established for investigation. For instance, the withdrawal of NGF from cultured sympathetic neurons is one good example. Studies utilizing this model system show the characteristic cell death pattern in the dying neurons—e.g., chromatin condensation, cell shrinkage, membrane blebbing, the elevation of caspase-3 activity, a laddering type of DNA fragmentation, and *de novo* protein synthesis. The removal of NGF results in a decrease in the basal activity of the mitogen-activated protein kinase (MAPK), followed by a series of metabolic changes, including the increased production of reactive oxygen species (ROS), decreased glucose uptake, and decreased RNA and protein synthesis.

During the initiation phase of neuronal apoptosis, the c-Jun N-terminal kinase (JNK) and *p*38 MAPK are activated. These kinases consequently induce a sustained activation of c-Jun proteins. Consistently high levels of c-Jun are generally required to serve as a regulator for the *de novo* protein synthesis that is needed for apoptotic cell death. In the late apoptotic phase, some biochemical events converge on mitochondria as a common pathway. These events include the loss of mitochondrial membrane potential, generation of ROS, calcium flux, and the release of cytochrome C for caspase activation. Recently, 14 caspases have been identified as the aspartate-specific cysteine proteases, of which caspase-3 and -9 appear to play significant roles in the developing CNS. Caspase-3, a member of the executioner caspases, can proteolytically cleave a number of cellular proteins, resulting in the morphological feature of apoptosis.

4.4. Factors that Prevent Neuronal Apoptotic Death

In the embryonic stage, the intrinsic neurotrophins are the major factors that regulate neuronal survival during the period of active programmed cell death. Other trophic supports for developing neurons to survive are: (i) the trophic signals obtained from cellular interactions with glia and other non-neuronal cells through gap-junctions; (ii) the exposure to steroid hormones such as sex steroids and adrenal cortical hormones; and (iii) the interaction between the anti- and pro-apoptotic genes' products of the *bcl-2* gene family that determines neuronal susceptibility to apoptosis. During CNS development, Bcl-XL protein appears to be the anti-apoptotic member, whereas Bax protein emerges as the pro-apoptotic member of the Bcl-2 family. They are both capable of forming heterodimers, and therefore through their interaction may determine neuron survival or death.

SELECTED READINGS

Brodal P. (ed) The central nervous system. New York: Oxford University Press, 1998; 54–91.

Burek MJ, Oppenheim RW. Cellular interactions that regulate programmed cell death in the developing vertebrate nervous system. In Koliatsos, VE, Ratan, RR. (eds.) Cell Death and Diseases of the Nervous System. Totowa, NJ: Humana Press, 1999: 145–179.

De la Rosa EJ, de Pablo F. Cell death in early neural development: beyond the neurotrophic theory. Trends Neurosci. 2000; 23: 454–458.

Hall BK. (ed) The Neural Crest in Development and Evolution. New York: Springer-Verlag, 1999; 14–33.

Heimer L. (ed) The Human Brain and Spinal Cord: Functional Neuroanatomy and Dissection Guide. New York: Springer-Verlag, 1983; 9–41.

Hopper AF, Hart NH. (ed) Foundations of animal development, 2nd ed. New York: Oxford University Press, 1985; 479–522.

Langman J. Medical Embryology, 4th ed. Baltimore: Williams and Wilkins, 1981; 320–345.

Le Douarin NM, Kalcheim C. (eds) The neural crest, 2nd ed. Cambridge, UK: Cambridge University Press, 1999; 23–59.

Levison, SW, Nowakowski RS. (eds) Neuroepithelial Stem Cells and Progenitors. Basel: Karger, 2000; 106–138.

Martin JH. (ed) Neuroanatomy: Text and Atlas. Stanford, Connecticut: Appleton and Lange, 1996; 33–59.

Teng CS. Protooncogenes as mediators of apoptosis. In Jeon KW (ed). International Review of Cytology San Diego, CA: Academic Press, 2000; pp. 137–201.

Woodgate AM, Dragunow M. Apoptosis of nerve cells, In Cameron RG, Feuer G (eds). Apoptosis and Its Modulation by Drugs. New York: Springer-Verlag, 2000; 197–233.

Disorders of Neuronal Migration

Gregory Cooper and Robert L. Rodnitzky

Abnormalities in the process of neuronal migration during embryogenesis result in CNS structures that are dysfunctional, architecturally abnormal, or totally absent. Several distinct mechanisms can be operative in the etiopathogenesis of clinical disorders related to disrupted neuronal migration. Some neuronal migrational disorders are heritable, and others are presumed to be the result of ischemic, toxic, or metabolic damage during the perinatal period.

CORTICAL NEURONS IN NEURONAL MIGRATION DISORDERS

The most common neuronal migration abnormalities involve the neocortex. Normal neuronal migration to the cerebral cortex takes place during the 8th to the 24th week of gestation. Neurons originating deep in the brain along the surface of the ventricles migrate to the cortex along a network of extensions of glial cells known as radial glia. The first neurons to arrive populate the deepest layer of the cortex, and successive groups of arriving cells occupy progressively more superficial positions. It has been postulated that some structural abnormalities of the cortex are the result of perinatal insults that have caused the death of radial glia or disruption of the network they normally form. The end result is a group of conditions characterized by abnormal laminar or columnar neuronal cortical architecture. In these conditions, a variety of abnormalities are often apparent on gross inspection of the brain, including decreased overall brain size and weight (e.g., microcephaly), abnormally small cortical gyri (e.g., polymicrogyria), or more commonly, enlarged gyri (e.g., macrogyria). Microscopically, abnormal clusters of misplaced neurons (e.g., heterotopias) can also be seen. When the overall size and weight of the brain is subnormal, it suggests that there may have been an insufficient number of cells migrating rather than merely misguided migration. Abnormal formation of the corpus callosum is commonly associated with disordered neuronal migration and can be readily appreciated on gross inspection of the cut brain.

Many of these gyral and callosal abnormalities can be identified in life through the use of magnetic resonance imaging. This enhanced ability to identify such abnormalities has proven that they are much more common than once believed. Before modern neuroimaging, only patients with severe neurologic dysfunction (e.g., epilepsy, mental retardation, weakness, and incoordination) were identified as being afflicted with a neuronal migration disorder, usually at autopsy. It is now understood that similar, but much milder, clinical syndromes can occur and affect a far greater number of persons.

EPILEPSY AS A SYMPTOM OF ABNORMAL CORTICAL NEURONAL MIGRATION

Neuronal migration abnormalities can be so severe that they are incompatible with life, or so mild that they are asymptomatic. Among those who survive with these disorders, epilepsy is the most common neurologic symptom. Even small foci of abnormally placed cortical neurons can sufficiently disrupt normal interneuronal physiology to result in epilepsy. The convulsive seizures associated with neuronal migration disorders are often relatively refractory to medical therapy. The modern assessment of a newborn infant who demonstrates a failure to thrive and intractable epilepsy includes a neuroimaging evaluation to investigate the possible presence of one of the cortical dysplasias related to abnormal neuronal migration.

KALLMANN'S SYNDROME AS A PROTOTYPE OF THE HERITABLE DISORDERS OF NEURONAL MIGRATION

It is estimated that between 5% and 20% of neuronal migration abnormalities are genetic in origin. Kallmann's syndrome is an inherited condition limited to males, characterized by an inability to smell and underdevelopment of gonadal function. The impaired olfaction is related to lack of development of the olfactory bulbs and tract, and the hypogonadism is caused by deficiency of a hypothalamic hormone, leuteinizing hormone-releasing hormone (LHRH), that is critical to the development of the male gonads. The neurons which ultimately secrete LHRH are formed in the olfactory placode, and then migrate from the placode up the nervous terminalis into the forebrain behind the olfactory bulb, and up the olfactory tract into the hypothalamus. The abnormalities are caused by defective neruonal migration of olfactory neruons and of neurons producing gonadotropin-releasing hormone. Both classes of neurons probably share a common origin in the migration pathway, which explains the linkage of these seemingly disparate anomalies.

The isolation of an X-linked Kallmann's syndrome gene, *KAL1*, may shed considerable light on the pathogenesis of inherited disorders of neuronal migration. The predicted protein of this gene shows similarity to neuronal-cell adhesion and axonal path-finding molecules, which suggests that the gene may influence neruonal migration. This notion has been supported by the discovery that this gene was deleted in a patient with Kallmann's syndrome. Other autosomal recessive and autosomal dominant pedigrees have been identified, but linkage data is not yet available.

Mutations of another gene called *filamin 1 (FLN1)* on the X-chromosome can lead to subependymal heterotopias. The product of this gene is an actin filament crosslinking protein that also links membrane proteins to actin. It is speculated that filamin provides a link between membrane receptors and the actin cytoskeleton of the neuron, allowing proper migration along the radial glia from the germinal matrix to the cortex.

SELECTED READINGS

Barkovich AJ, Kuzniecky RI. Gray matter heterotopia. Neurology 2000; 55:1603–1608.

Duchowny M, Jayakar P, Levin B. Aberrant neural circuits in malformations of cortical development and focal epilepsy. Neurology 2000; 55:423–428.

Franco B, Guioli S, Pragliola A, et al. A gene deleted in Kallmann's syndrome shares homology with neural crest cell adhesion and axonal path-finding molecules. Nature 1991; 353:529.

Walsh CA. Genetic malformations of the human cerebral cortex. Neuron 1999; 23:19–29.

Whiting S, Duchowny M. Clinical spectrum of cortical dysplasia in childhood: diagnosis and treatment issues. J Child Neurology 1999; 14:759–771.

7 The Vasculature of the Human Brain

Suresh C. Patel and Simone Wagner

1. INTRODUCTION

The human brain is a highly metabolic organ with no effective mechanism of storage of oxygen and glucose. The brain needs a constant supply of large amounts of blood, and blood flow is auto-regulated by brain. The brain comprises 2% of total body weight; 15% cardiac output goes to brain, which utilizes 25% of total oxygen consumption. The vasculature of the brain and spinal cord consists of an arterial input, intervening capillaries, and a venous drainage system. There are no lymphatic vessels in the central nervous system (CNS).

The intracranial vasculature differs from that found in the rest of the body in several ways. Arteries and veins of the brain are bathed by cerebrospinal fluid

(CSF) after they pierce the dura mater and arachnoid membranes. All intracranial veins drain into the dural venous sinuses, and these do not exist outside the skull. There are also differences in structure, innervation, and functional responses to injury. For example, subarachnoid hemorrhage may have profound and long-lasting effects on the cerebral arteries. The presence of blood in the spinal fluid may induce sustained vasoconstriction in neighboring arteries, but blood applied to the tunica adventitia of extracranial arteries does not induce sustained vasospasm. Many fine details about these differences are incompletely characterized, partly because most observations on the nature of neurogenic responses in intracranial vessels have been carried out in animals, and vascular responses to pharmacological and electrical stimuli vary widely among species.

Intracranial blood vessels are involved in two types of common diseases of the brain: ischemic lesions;

From: *Neuroscience in Medicine, 2nd ed.* (P. Michael Conn, ed.), © 2003 Humana Press Inc., Totowa, NJ.

Table 1
The Intracranial Arterial System

Intracranial cavity
Tentorium cerebelli divides the intracranial cavity into supratentorial and infratentorial
   compartments.
Falx cerebri subdivides the supratentorial cavity into right and left compartments.

Anterior (Carotid) circulation
Supratentorial intracranial cavity.
Right and left cerebral hemispheres within supratentorial intracranial cavity are supplied
   by internal carotid arteries.

Posterior (Vertebrobasilar) circulation
Brainstem and cerebellum within the infratentorial intracranial cavity are supplied by the
   vertebrobasilar system.
Posterior cerebral arteries are branches of the basilar artery (posterior circulation) and
   supply part of the cerebral hemispheres (supratentorial compartment).

infarcts, which are the sites of brain-tissue destruction caused by insufficient or lack of blood supply; and hemorrhages, which are sites of spontaneous rupture of intracranial vessels resulting in intracranial hemorrhage (subarachnoid, parenchymal, or intraventricular). Epidural hemorrhage is caused by rupture of intracranial meningeal vessels, and subdural hemorrhage is caused by rupture of the bridging cortical veins between the surface of the cerebral hemispheres and the dural venous sinuses.

1.1. Human Vasculature Can Be Visualized In Vivo By Four Different Modalities

The intracranial human vasculature is visualized in vivo by different techniques including conventional arterial digital subtraction catheter angiography (Fig. 1), screen film catheter angiography, magnetic resonance angiography (MRA) (Figs. 2,10), computed tomographic angiography, and by Doppler ultrasound. The older screen film angiography (Fig. 3) and current digital subtraction angiography are the gold standard for visualizing the intracranial vasculature. These are invasive procedures that involve inserting a catheter selectively into the carotid or vertebral arteries with the injection of an iodinated contrast agent. The risk of complications resulting from the invasiveness of the procedure, such as stoke, is less than 1%. Both the magnetic resonance angiography and Doppler sonography are noninvasive methods for visualizing the intracranial vasculature, which do not involve the injection of contrast medium and use the flow within the vessels to visualize the vasculature. The current refinement in the time-of-flight, phase-contrast methods of MRA and contrast enhanced MRA has made

MRA the noninvasive method of choice for evaluating larger intracranial and extracranial arteries and the larger dural venous sinuses. Computed tomographic angiography does involve injection of an iodinated contrast material intravenously for visualizing the major intracranial arteries, such as circle of Willis and larger dural venous sinuses, without inserting an arterial catheter.

The undulating surface of the brain formed by gyri and sulci is responsible for the wavy, undulating appearance of the superficial cortical arteries and veins on cerebral angiography.

2. INTRACRANIAL ARTERIAL SYSTEM (TABLE 1)

The intracranial cavity is divided into the supratentorial compartment and infratentorial compartment by the tentorium cerebelli. The contents of the supratentorial compartment include the two cerebral hemispheres, which are supplied by anterior or carotid circulation. The contents of the infratentorial compartment or the posterior cranial fossa include the brainstem and the cerebellum, which are supplied by the posterior circulation or vertebrobasilar circulation.

The great vessels (branches) of the arch of the aorta supply blood to the head and neck (Fig. 1). The three major branches of the aortic arch are: brachiocephalic trunk (innominate artery), left common carotid, and left subclavian arteries (Figs. 1,2). The brachiocephalic trunk divides into the right subclavian artery and the right common carotid artery. The right and left vertebral arteries are branches of respective subclavian arteries (Fig. 1). Both common carotid arteries termi-

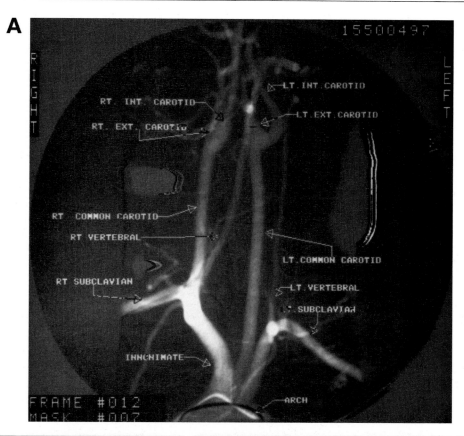

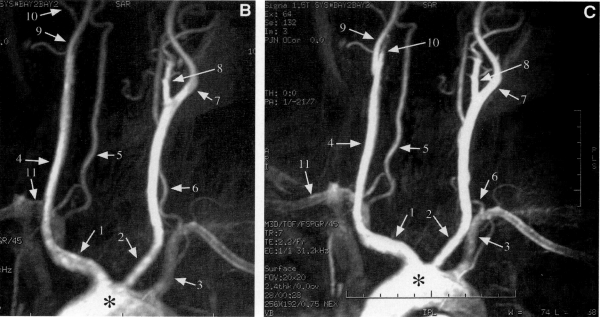

Fig. 1. (A) Left anterior oblique projection of a digital subtraction arch aortogram shows the branches of the arch of the aorta and the arteries in the neck. RT, right; LT, left; Ext, external; Int, internal. **(B,C)** Contrast (Gadolinium) enhanced magnetic resonance angiography of arch of aorta and brachiolephalic arteries *(asterisk) arch of aorta. **1,** Innominati artery. **2,** Left common carotid artery. **3,** Left subclavian artery. **4,** Right common carotid artery. **5,** Right vertebral artery. **6,** Left vertebral artery. **7,** Left internal carotid artery. **8,** Left external carotid artery. **9,** Right internal carotid artery. **10,** Right external carotid artery. **11,** Right subclavian artery.

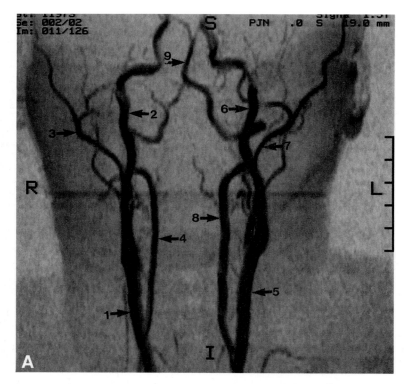

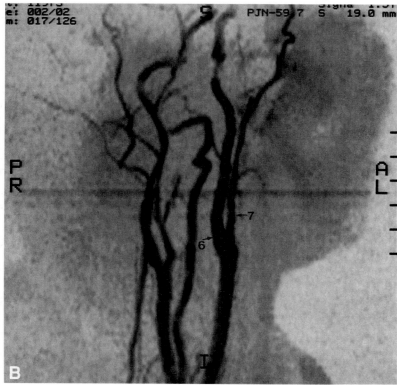

Fig. 2. (A,B) 2D time-of-flight magnetic resonance angiography. The frontal and oblique projections show the vessels in the neck. **1,** Right common carotid artery. **2,** Right internal carotid artery. **3,** Right external carotid artery. **4,** Right vertebral artery. **5,** Left common carotid artery. **6,** Left internal carotid artery. **7,** Left external carotid artery. **8,** Left vertebral artery. **9,** Basilar artery.

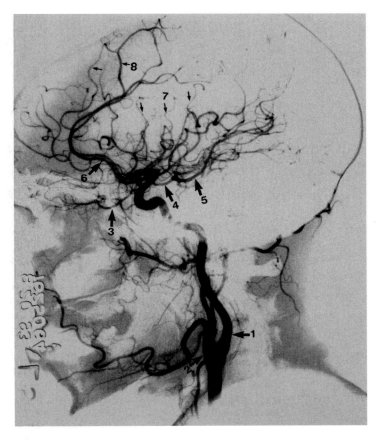

Fig. 3. Selective left common carotid angiogram. Lateral projection: **1,** Internal carotid artery. **2,** External carotid artery. **3,** Ophthalmic artery. **4,** Posterior communicating artery. **5,** Posterior cerebral artery. **6,** Right and left anterior cerebral arteries. **7,** Cortical branches of the middle cerebral artery. **8,** Cortical branches of the anterior cerebral artery.

nate in the mid portion of the neck into the external and internal carotid arteries (Fig. 3). The two internal carotid and two vertebral arteries supply blood to the brain.

The external carotid arteries supply the soft tissues of the neck and face, the sinonasal cavity, the external ear, and the soft tissue of the scalp (Fig. 4). The middle meningeal branch of the external carotid artery enters the intracranial cavity through the foramen spinosum and supplies the meninges of the intracranial cavity.

Intracranial arteries are of two types: extradural or epidural arteries and intradural arteries. The extradural or epidural arteries are also known as meningeal arteries, which are branches of the external carotid artery and supply blood to the meninges and the extradural segments of the intracranial nerves. The intradural arteries, are branches of internal carotid and vertebral arteries, and are present in the subarachnoid space of the intracranial cavity after the internal carotid and vertebral arteries penetrate the dura mater and the arachnoid membrane.

2.1. Anterior (Carotid) Circulation

2.1.1. THE INTERNAL CAROTID ARTERY (TABLE 2)

The internal carotid artery within the neck (cervical segment) has no angiographically visible branches. The internal carotid artery enters the skull base within its own carotid canal located in the petrous portion of the temporal bone (Figs. 3,5). The internal carotid artery emerges from the petrous bone, enters the intracranial cavity and immediately lies within the cavernous sinus (cavernous segment). The intracranial internal carotid artery is subdivided into the cavernous segment (cavernous sinus), clinoid segment (at the level of the anterior clinoid process), ophthalmic segment (at the origin of the ophthalmic artery), and communicating segment (at the origins of the posterior communicating artery and anterior choroidal artery). The ophthalmic artery is the largest branch of the internal carotid artery (Fig. 3) and supplies the eye, the orbit, and adjacent paranasal sinuses.

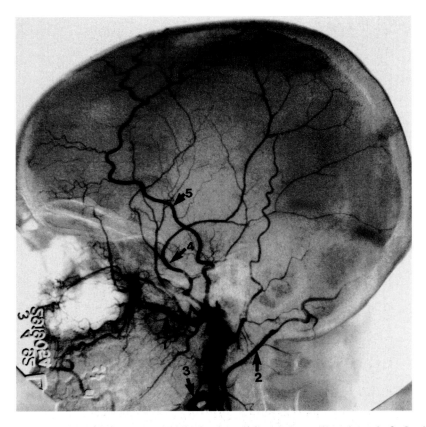

Fig. 4. Selective left external carotid angiogram. Lateral Projection: **1,** Internal maxillary branch. **2,** Occipital branch. **3,** Facial-lingual branch. **4,** Middle meningeal branch. **5,** Superficial temporal artery.

Table 2
The Intracranial Internal Carotid Artery

Branches
Middle cerebral artery
Anterior cerebral artery
Ophthalmic artery
Posterior communicating artery
Anterior choroidal artery
Superior hypophyseal arteries
Meningohypophyseal artery
Inferolateral artery
Capsular arteries

Brain structures supplied
Cerebral hemispheres
The eye, optic nerve, optic chiasm, and optic tracts
Midbrain through interior coroidal artery
Thalamus and internal capsule through posterior communicating artery
Pituitary gland and hypothalamus
Meninges of the skull base

The posterior communicating artery (Figs. 3,6) is an important anastomotic channel for the circle of Willis connecting the anterior (carotid) circulation to the posterior (vertebrobasilar circulation) and connects the internal carotid artery to the ipsilateral posterior cerebral artery. The perforating branches of the posterior communicating artery supply the thalamus, optic tract, and internal capsule. The anterior choroidal artery (Fig. 6) is a small, constant branch of the distal internal carotid artery and supplies blood to the optic tract, posterior limb of the internal capsule, ipsilateral cerebral peduncles, choroid plexus of the ipsilateral lateral ventricle, medial temporal lobe, thalamus, and part of the corpus striatum. The relatively small branches of the intracranial internal carotid artery include the meningohypophyseal artery, inferolateral trunk, and capsular and superior hypophyseal arteries. These numerous small branches supply the meninges of the skull base, the cranial nerves in the cavernous sinus, and the pituitary gland.

The internal carotid artery terminates into the anterior cerebral and middle cerebral arteries (Figs. 5,6).

2.1.2. THE ANTERIOR CEREBRAL ARTERY (TABLE 3)

The anterior cerebral artery is divided into the proximal horizontal segment and distal segment (Figs. 5,6).

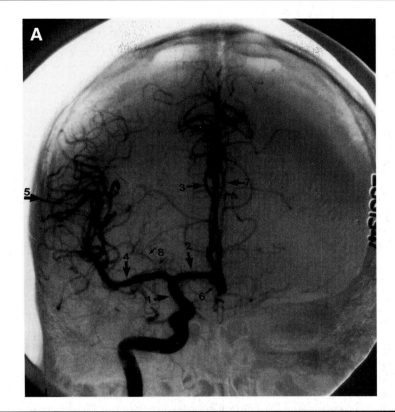

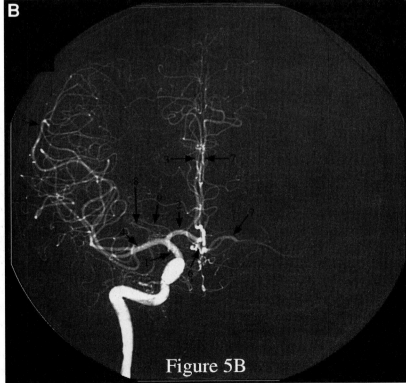

Figure 5B

Fig. 5. (A,B) Selective right internal carotid angiogram. Frontal projection: **1,** Intracranial segment of the internal carotid artery. **2,** Proximal anterior cerebral artery. **3,** Distal right anterior cerebral artery. **4,** Proximal middle cerebral artery. **5,** Distal middle cerebral artery. **6,** Anterior communicating artery. **7,** Left anterior cerebral artery visualized through patent anterior communicating artery or right carotid angiogram. **8,** Lenticulostriate arteries. **9,** Anterior choroidal artery.

Table 3
Anterior Cerebral Artery

Branches

Superficial cortical branches
Orbital frontal
Frontal
Parietal

Callosal branches
Pericallosal
Callosal marginal

Perforating branches
Recurrent artery of Heubner
Medial striate or medial lenticulostriate

Blood supply
Medial surface of cerebral hemispheres
Medial and inferior surface of the frontal lobe and medial
    parietal lobe
Corpus callosum
Caudate nucleus, anteromedial and inferior basal ganglia,
    internal capsule

Anterior communicating artery
Connects the two anterior cerebral arteries

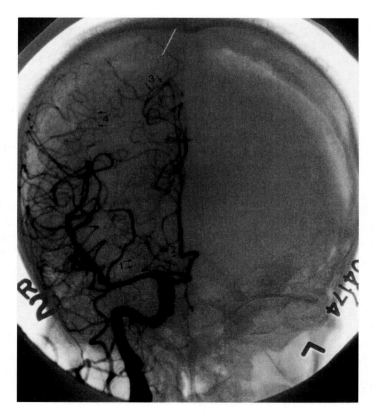

Fig. 6. Right carotid angiogram. Frontal projection: **1,** Lenticulostriate arteries. **2,** Anterior choroidal artery. **3,** Cortical branches of the anterior cerebral artery. **4,** Cortical branches of the middle cerebral artery.

Table 4
The Middle Cerebral Artery

Branches

Superficial cortical branches
Anterior temporal
Orbitofrontal
Prefrontal
Precentral sulcus
Central sulcus
Postcentral sulcus
Parietal, angular, temporal, and occipital

Perforating branches
Lenticulostriate arteries

Blood supply
Basal ganglia
Internal capsule
Anterior temporal lobe and most of the lateral surface of
the cerebral hemisphere

The branches of the proximal segment of the anterior cerebral artery include the medial striate arteries, recurrent artery of Heubner, and callosal perforating arteries. There are two large orbital and frontal cortical branches. The perforating branches of the proximal segment of the anterior cerebral artery supply the head of the caudate nucleus, anteromedial and inferior basal ganglia, inferomedial internal capsule, anterior commissure, and the anterior portion of the corpus callosum. The cortical branches of the proximal segment of the anterior cerebral artery supply the inferior and medial portion of the frontal lobe, gyrus rectus, and olfactory bulb and tract (Figs. 3,5–7).

The branches of the distal segment of the anterior cerebral artery include the pericallosal artery, callosomarginal artery, parietal branches, and terminal cortical branches. The branches of the distal segment of the anterior cerebral artery supply the anterior two-thirds of the medial cerebral hemisphere, the small strip of cortex over the cerebral convexity, and the corpus callosum.

The anterior communicating artery (Figs. 5,10) connects the proximal segments of both the anterior cerebral arteries in the midline and is an important anterior anastomotic channel within the circle of Willis.

2.1.3. THE MIDDLE CEREBRAL ARTERY (TABLE 4)

The middle cerebral artery is the larger of the two terminal branches of the internal carotid artery (Figs. 5,6) and its vascular territory is most commonly involved in the thromboembolic ischemic disease of the brain. The proximal segment of the middle cerebral artery extends laterally to the level of the sylvian fissure and divides into numerous cortical distal branches. The proximal segment of the middle cerebral artery gives off numerous perforating branches known as lenticulostriate arteries (Figs. 5,6) and an anterior cortical temporal branch. The lenticulostriate arteries supply most of the caudate nucleus, the basal ganglia, and the internal capsule. The anterior temporal arteries supply the anterior pole of the temporal lobe.

The distal segment of the middle cerebral artery runs in the insular or sylvian fossa superiorly, and then arches underneath the frontal operculum over the temporal lobe horizontally and emerges from the sylvian fissure and supplies the lateral surface of the cerebral hemisphere. All the branches of the distal segment of the middle cerebral artery are cortical branches. The orbitofrontal and prefrontal cortical branches supply the inferior surface or the orbital surface of the frontal lobe laterally and the frontal pole. The central cortical branches are precentral sulcal, central (rolandic) and postcentral sulcal branches that supply the rolandic area, both anterior and posterior to the central sulcus over the lateral surface of the cerebral hemisphere. The posterior cortical branches of the middle cerebral artery are the posterior parietal, angular, temporal, and occipital branches. All the cortical branches of the middle cerebral artery supply the cortical lateral surface of the frontal, parietal, occipital, and temporal lobes (Figs. 3,5–7).

2.1.4. THE POSTERIOR CEREBRAL ARTERY (TABLE 5)

Posterior cerebral arteries are the two terminal branches of the basilar artery (Fig. 8). Although the posterior cerebral artery is part of the vertebrobasilar circulation, the posterior artery supplies the supratentorial structures of the cerebral hemisphere, mainly the temporal and occipital lobes. The posterior cerebral artery is connected to the internal carotid artery through the posterior communicating artery (Figs. 3,10) establishing the collateral pathway between the anterior (carotid) and posterior (vertebrobasilar circulation), part of the circle of Willis. The distal or the tip of the basilar artery and the two terminal posterior cerebral arteries encircle the midbrain. The branches of the proximal segment of the posterior cerebral artery are: the perforating branches (thalamoperforating, thalamogeniculate), peduncular branches, choroid plexus (medial posterior choroidal artery,

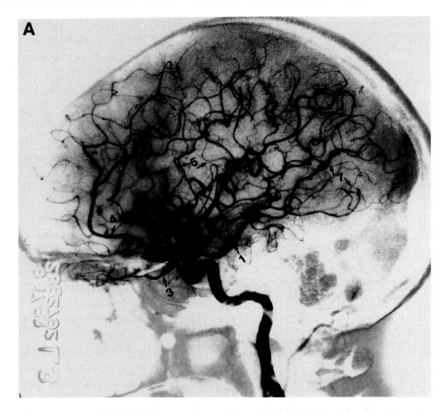

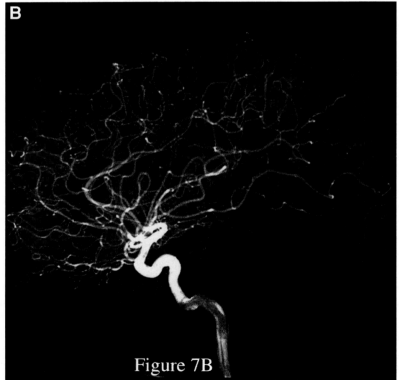

Fig. 7. (A,B) Selective left internal carotid angiogram. Lateral projection: **1,** Posterior cerebral artery is a direct continuation (fetal origin) of the posterior communicating artery. **2,** Anterior choroidal artery. **3,** Ophthalmic artery. **4,** Anterior cerebral artery. **5,** Cortical branches of the middle cerebral artery. **6,** Cortical branches of the anterior cerebral artery. **7,** Cortical branches of the posterior cerebral artery. **8,** Cavernous segment of left internal carotid artery.

Table 5
The Posterior Cerebral Artery

Branches

Superficial cortical branches
Temporal
Parietal occipital
Calcarine

Callosal
Splenial

Choroidal
Posterior medial choroidal
Posterior lateral choroidal

Perforating
Thalamoperforating
Thalamogeniculate
Peduncular

Brain structures supplied
Medial surface of the parietal lobe
Medial and inferior surface of the temporal lobe
Occipital lobe
Splenium of the corpus callosum
Choroid plexus of the third and lateral ventricles
Thalamus migraine
Posterior limb of the internal capsule and midbrain

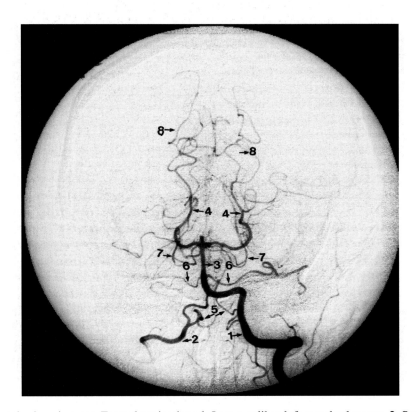

Fig. 8. Selective left vertebral angiogram. Frontal projection: **1,** Large-caliber left vertebral artery. **2,** Smaller caliber (anatomic variant) right vertebral artery. **3,** Basilar artery. **4,** Posterior cerebral arteries. **5,** Posterior inferior cerebellar artery. **6,** Anterior inferior cerebellar artery. **7,** Superior cerebellar artery (duplicated). **8,** Cortical branches of the posterior cerebral arteries.

Table 6
Intracranial Vertebral Artery

Branches
Posterior inferior cerebellar artery
Anterior spinal artery
Posterior spinal arteries
Meningeal arteries
Perforating arteries

Blood supply
Medulla oblongata
Upper cervical spinal cord
Inferior surface of the cerebellar hemisphere
Inferior vermis

lateral posterior choroidal artery), anterior temporal cortical artery, middle temporal cortical artery, posterior temporal cortical artery, and splenial branches (Fig. 9).

The proximal segment of the posterior cerebral arteries supply blood to the posterior thalamus, hypothalamus, internal capsule, midbrain, splenium of the corpus callosum, inferior surface of the temporal lobe, the choroid plexus of the third ventricle (medial posterior choroidal artery), and the choroid plexus of the lateral ventricle (lateral posterior choroidal artery).

The branches of the distal posterior cerebral artery are the parietal occipital branch, calcarine branch, and anterior, middle, and posterior inferior temporal branches. The distal segment of the posterior cerebral artery supplies blood to the medial posterior third portion of the cerebral hemisphere, which includes part of the parietal lobe and most of the occipital and temporal lobes (Figs. 7–9).

2.2. Posterior (Vertebrobasilar) Circulation

2.2.1. THE VERTEBRAL ARTERIES (TABLE 6)

The two vertebral arteries penetrate the dura and the arachnoid membrane at the level of the foramen magnum to enter the intracranial cavity. Both vertebral arteries course over the lateral surface of the lower medulla and come to lie between the clivus and the ventral surface of the medulla. The two vertebral arteries join to form the basilar artery in front of the brainstem at the pontomedullary junction (Figs. 2,8,9).

Anterior and posterior meningeal branches of the vertebral artery supply the meninges of the posterior cranial fossa. The anterior spinal artery (Fig. 8) and the paired posterior spinal arteries begin their courses within the intracranial cavity as branches of the verte-

bral arteries or posterior inferior cerebellar arteries, and supply the spinal cord along with numerous radiculomedullary arteries within the spine. The spinal branches and the small number of perforating branches arising from the vertebral artery supply the lower medulla, upper cervical spinal cord, and the inferior cerebellar peduncles.

The posterior inferior cerebellar artery (PICA) is the largest branch of the vertebral artery (Figs. 8,9) and supplies the lateral and posterior aspect of the medulla, the choroid plexus of the fourth ventricle, the cerebellar tonsils, the inferior cerebellar vermis, and the inferior aspects of the cerebellar hemispheres.

2.2.2. THE BASILAR ARTERY (TABLE 7)

The basilar artery is formed by the union of the two vertebral arteries at the level of the pontomedullary junction and the origin of the sixth cranial nerves (Figs. 2,8,9). The basilar artery courses over the ventral surface of the pons behind the clivus and terminates in front of the midbrain into two posterior cerebral arteries at the level of the origins of the third cranial nerves posterior to the dorsum sella. The branches of the basilar artery are anterior inferior cerebellar arteries (AICA) (Figs. 8,9), superior cerebellar arteries (SCA) (Figs. 8,9), perforating branches, and labyrinthine artery. The median pontine perforating, paramedian pontine perforating, and lateral circumferential branches form the numerous perforating branches of the basilar artery and supply the pons, midbrain, and cerebellar peduncles. The median and paramedian perforating branches are associated with the same disease process as the striate branches of the anterior cerebral and middle cerebral arteries in chronic hypertension with lacunar infarcts.

The anterior inferior cerebellar artery supplies the anterior or ventral surface of the cerebellar hemisphere, pons and cerebellar peduncle (Fig. 8,9).

The superior cerebellar artery arises just proximal to the bifurcation of the basilar artery and supplies the superior and lateral surface of the cerebellar hemispheres, the superior cerebellar peduncle, pons and the superior cerebellar vermis (Fig. 8,9).

The tip of the basilar artery at the level of the bifurcation into the two posterior cerebral arteries also gives rise to small thalamoperforating or thalamogeniculate branches, which supply the thalami and the internal capsules (Fig. 9).

All the arteries of the posterior or the vertebrobasilar circulation supply the contents of the infratentorial posterior cranial fossa, except the two posterior cere-

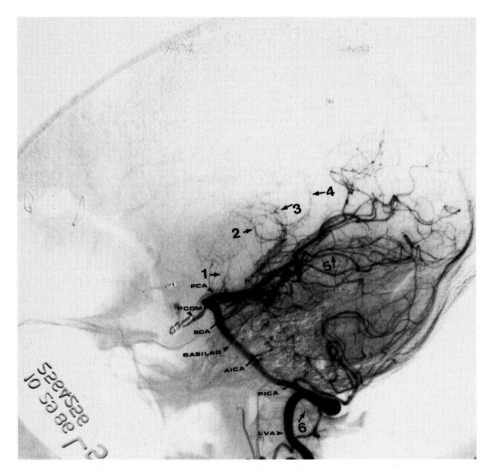

Fig. 9. Selective left vertebral angiogram. Lateral projection: LVA, Left vertebral artery; PICA, Posterior inferior cerebellar artery; AICA, Anterior inferior cerebellar artery; SCA, Superior cerebellar artery; PCOM, Posterior communicating artery; PCA, Posterior cerebral artery. **1,** Thalamogeniculate branches (perforating) of posterior cerebral artery. **2,** Posterior medial choroidal artery. **3,** Posterior lateral choroidal artery. **4,** Splenial branches. **5,** Hemispheric branches of SCA. **6,** Anterior spinal artery.

Table 7
Basilar Artery

Branches
Anterior inferior cerebellar artery
Superior cerebellar arteries
Posterior cerebral arteries
Pontine perforating
Labyrinthine (internal auditory)

Blood supply
Brainstem
Mainly pons
Anterior surface of the cerebellum
Superior surface of the cerebellum
Superior vermis
Midbrain
Part of the thalamus
Labyrinth of inner ear

bral arteries that course through the tentorial incisura into the supratentorial compartment supplying the cerebral hemispheres.

2.2.3. LEPTOMENINGEAL OR PIAL VESSELS

Pial vessels describe the branches of the circle of Willis arteries that course through the surface of the brain for various distances before penetrating into the brain parenchyma. Numerous arterial anastomoses exist among these leptomeningeal or pial branches. Two types are found: large-diameter end-to-end anastomoses that connect branches from two different arterial stems (e.g., branches of the middle and anterior cerebral arteries) and extremely-small-diameter anastomoses connecting branches from the same or a different parent artery. The diameter of the largest anastomoses joining arterioles end-to-end varies from

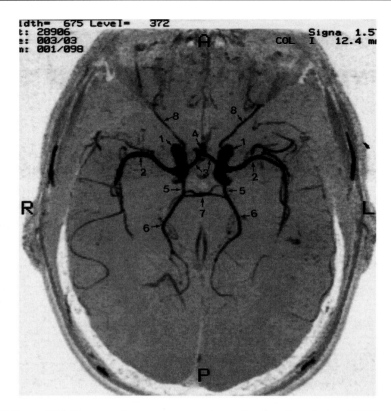

Fig. 10. Axial view of 3D time-of-flight magnetic resonance angiography showing circle of Willis. **1,** Internal carotid artery. **2,** Middle cerebral artery. **3,** Anterior cerebral artery. **4,** Anterior communicating artery. **5,** Posterior communicating artery. **6,** Posterior cerebral artery. **7,** Basilar artery. **8,** Ophthalmic artery.

25 to 90 μm. The average diameter of the small, straight anastomoses is 10 μm.

2.2.4. Intraparenchymal or Penetrating Arteries

Cortical arteries divide into small pial vessels before penetrating the cortex. Each penetrating cortical artery forms a vascular palisade that supplies the respective capillary bed. Major vessels supplying the cortex enter the gyral surface at a perpendicular angle; those with the largest caliber and longest course supply the deepest cortical layers. Anastomoses forming a continuous horizontal layer appear in layer three of the cortex among the large pyramidal cells, but the greatest number of these connecting vessels is visible in layers four and five, and few are visible in layer six of the cortex.

Central arteries at each gyrus always have a large diameter (260–280 μm) at their point of origin. Peripheral arteries have an average diameter of 150–180 μm. On the cortical surface, all arterioles measuring 50 μ or less penetrate the cortex or anastomose with neighboring ones. Penetrating vessels into the cerebral cortex are short arterioles (<100 μm in diameter) devoid of continuous internal elastic lamina and

having a tunica media composed of one or two layers of smooth-muscle cells. Most penetrating arterioles have a diameter of approx 40 μm.

Some of the large *penetrating arteries* are branches that originate directly from the trunk of a large vessel, such as the middle cerebral artery and the basilar artery. These branches supply the basal ganglia and the thalamic nuclei, respectively. Penetrating arteries at these sites are long, muscular vessels (100–400 μm in internal diameter) endowed with internal elastic lamina and three or four layers of smooth-muscle fibers in the tunica media.

One of the few groups of vessels supplying gray-matter structures that lack anatomic anastomoses among themselves are the *lenticulostriate branches* originating from the main trunk of the middle cerebral artery. The lenticulostriate vessels have been implicated as being the source of the most common type of nontraumatic intracerebral hemorrhage-hypertensive hemorrhage.

Forty percent of the total vascular resistance in the CNS can be traced to the penetrating parenchymal arteries that are less than 200 μm in diameter. Chronic arterial hypertension increases the resistance in these small arteries, protecting the microvasculature (e.g., arterioles, capillaries, venules) from the effects of sustained high blood pressure. The vascular resistance in extracranial organs is primarily a function of arterioles.

Blood flow to subcortical white matter fibers, also called U-fibers, is supplied by arteries and arterioles, but the deeper white-matter structures (e.g., centrum semiovale) are supplied only by nonanastomosing, long, radial arteries.

Long, transcortical vessels traverse the cortex without branching and, on entering the subjacent white matter, form a cascade of vessels that terminates in a periventricular plexus. The long, penetrating radial arteries that supply the cerebral hemispheric white matter do not interconnect with one another. The name *terminal arteries* has been applied to these and other nonanastomosing vessels.

2.3. The Structure of Intradural Arteries is Different from that of Other Arteries

The histologic structure of the arteries supplying the brain changes as these vessels penetrate the dura mater. The elastic fibers, which in extracranial arteries are distributed throughout the entire width of the arterial wall, condense into a subendothelial elastic lamina after the arteries penetrate the dura mater (Fig. 11). The thickness of the tunica media is decreased in intracranial vessels compared with arteries of the same caliber located outside the skull.

Intradural arteries and veins are bathed in *CSF*, even after the arteries penetrate the cerebral parenchyma; this is made possible by perivascular sheath-like extensions of the subarachnoid space into the brain parenchyma. The anatomic, perivascular structures within the brain that contain the brain vessels in the subarachnoid space are known as the Virchow-Robin spaces. The arteries and arterioles in the Virchow-Robin spaces lack tunica adventitia; in these vessels, the muscular tunica media is surrounded by a single-cell layer of leptomeningeal origin. The Virchow-Robin space disappears when the *glia limitans*, a subpial structure formed mainly by the endfeet of astrocytes and attached to the pial membrane, fuses with the basal lamina of the smallest arterioles and capillaries.

Intracranial arteries frequently exhibit *medial defects* or interruptions in the continuity of the smooth-muscle layers at bifurcation sites (e.g., distal carina). These are the same sites in which saccular aneurysms

develop in persons with inherited disorders of connective tissue metabolism.

At the branching sites of the intracranial arteries such as proximal carina, there are *intimal cushions* or sites where well-demarcated intraluminal protrusions are formed by subendothelial aggregates of smooth-muscle fibers. These intimal cushions become more apparent with increasing age, but their functional significance has not been elucidated. Normal intracranial arteries in persons younger than 20 yr of age probably lack vasa vasorum; aging and diseases associated with this process, such as atherosclerosis, may induce the development of a few vessels in the tunica adventitia of intradural arteries.

2.4. Three Types of Nerve Fibers Have Endings on the Walls of Large Intracranial Arteries

2.4.1. PAIN-SENSITIVE FIBERS

Pain-sensitive fibers were first demonstrated in humans by electrical stimulation of arteries attached to the dura (e.g., the branches of the external carotid artery) and arterial branches of the internal carotid artery located within the subarachnoid space. Substance P is the main tachykinin involved in the transmission of nociceptive information. Using immunohistochemical methods, substance P has been identified on the tunica adventitia of large intracranial vessels. Many intracranial and extracranial blood vessels that supply the brain are surrounded by axonal terminals originating from the trigeminal and the upper dorsal root ganglia. The densest network of these fibers exists on the tunica adventitia of the major arterial branches as they emerge from the circle of Willis.

The caudal portion of the basilar artery and both vertebral arteries and their tributaries are innervated by fibers originating in the upper cervical dorsal-root ganglia. The central projections of the fibers originating from the trigeminovascular system are not fully understood.

Bleeding in the subarachnoid space is one of the best-known causes of severe headache; this is a unique response limited to the intracranial vessels. The trigeminovascular system of nerve fibers around arteries, which includes substance P-dependent fibers, is believed to be intimately involved in the mechanism of pain and migraine headaches.

2.4.2. SYMPATHETIC FIBERS

Sympathetic fibers supplying large intracranial vessels originate primarily from the superior cervical

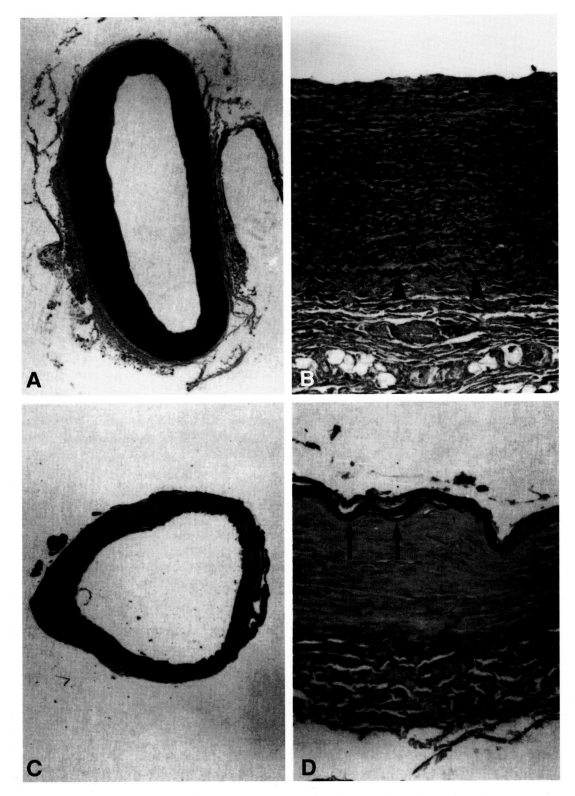

Fig. 11. (A,B) Normal common carotid artery. **(C,D)** Normal intradural portion of the internal carotid artery. The black wavy lines (*arrowheads*) correspond to elastic fibers. The elastic fibers condense into the subendothelial elastic lamina (*arrows*) after the arteries penetrate the dura mater.

Table 8
Collateral Circulation

Circle of Willis
An anastomotic arterial ring at the base of the brain formed by:
Right and left internal carotid arteries
Right and left anterior cerebral arteries
Right and left posterior cerebral arteries
Anterior communicating artery
Posterior communicating arteries

Anterior communicating artery
Connects right and left anterior (carotid) circulation

Posterior communicating artery
Connects the anterior (carotid circulation) to the posterior (vertebrobasilar) circulation

Pial collateral anastomoses
Connect the terminal pial cortical branches of the cerebral arteries across a vulnerable
    water shed or border zone

Pial leptomenigeal anastomoses
Pial Leptomenigeal anastomoses connect pial branches of the cerebral arteries to the
    meningeal branches of the external carotid arteries

Intraorbital anastomoses
Between the branches of the external carotid artery and the branches of the ophthalmic
    artery within orbit

---

ganglion, the middle cervical sympathetic ganglion, and the sympathetic ganglion. In addition to norepinephrine, sympathetic nerve terminals also secrete the vasoconstrictor neuropeptide Y. Sympathetic fibers are not involved in the regulation of the cerebral blood flow, except that sympathetic stimulation blunts anticipated rises in cerebral blood flow during severe arterial hypertension. The most important role of the sympathetic innervation in intracranial arteries is to protect small arteries from the effects of blood pressure surges within the physiologic range.

2.4.3. Parasympathetic Fibers

Parasympathetic fibers to the cerebral blood vessels originate mainly from sphenopalatine, otic, and associated miniganglia. The most dense network of fibers exists around the proximal segments of arteries branching out of the circle of Willis. In addition to cholinergic fibers, parasympathetic nerve endings contain vasoactive intestinal polypeptide (VIP). Nitric oxide synthase (NOS) has been co-localized in the same fibers that contain VIP. NOS may be the same as the endothelium-dependent relaxing factor. Cholinergic mechanisms have a minimal influence in the control of the normal cerebral blood flow.

None of the cerebral perivascular networks of nerve fibers plays a significant role in the normal autoregulation of blood flow to the brain. Autoregulation is primarily the result of myogenic responses to changes in blood pressure or in neuronal metabolism. Sensory, parasympathetic, and sympathetic nerves contribute to the cerebral blood flow regulation and preserve the integrity of the blood-vessel wall only in pathologic conditions such as sustained hypertension and chronic hypotension.

3. COLLATERAL CIRCULATION (TABLE 8)

A system of abundant collateral circulation protects the brain from isolated arterial occlusion or stenosis. Terminal, small pial cortical branches of the cerebral arteries anastomose with each other across a vulnerable watershed or border zone. This abundant end-to-end anastomosis forms an extensive arterial network over the surface of the brain, which facilitates the pial collateral circulation and acts as a protective mechanism against focal disruption of the blood flow to the brain.

This system of collateral or alternate circulation allows distal branches of an occluded artery to fill in a retrograde fashion through the end-to-end anastomoses that connect neighboring vessels and to compensate for the changes in blood flow.

The anterior (e.g., carotid) circulation and the posterior (e.g., vertebrobasilar) circulation are connected by the posterior communicating arteries that connect the internal carotid artery with the ipsilateral posterior cerebral artery. Arterial connection between the right and left anterior (carotid) circulation across the midline is provided by the anterior communicating artery. Credit for the correct description of the arterial anatomic network located at the base of the brain is given to Thomas Willis, and the *circle of Willis* (Fig. 10) designates this arterial network, which provides the best potential collateral flow of blood in vascular occlusive disease.

These anastomotic connections are significant because of the collateral circulation they provide. In many instances, local circulatory abnormalities created by occluding a single artery at points proximal to the circle of Willis can be adequately compensated through the collateral circulation.

The circle of Willis and its feeding branches constitute a symmetric structure in only about 40% of adults examined postmortem. A significant number of anatomic variations, which in most cases reflect the persistence of embryonal or fetal vascular patterns, are found in about 60%. Among the most common variations in the anatomy of the circle of Willis are hypoplasia of one vertebral artery and of the contralateral anterior cerebral artery or a posterior cerebral artery originating from the internal carotid artery instead of the basilar artery.

Anastomoses among branches of the internal and external carotid arteries exist through the ophthalmic artery (e.g., the large branch of the internal carotid artery) and its end-to-end connections with facial branches of the ipsilateral external carotid artery. There are extensive collateral anastomoses between pial meningeal branches of the internal carotid and meningeal branches of the external carotid artery.

4. CAPILLARIES

The perivascular sheath of CSF surrounding penetrating arteries and arterioles disappears where the glia limitans merges with the basal lamina of the brain capillaries. These vessels, which in humans are 4–7 μm in diameter, are composed of one endothelial-cell layer, resting on a basal lamina that completely encircles a pericyte. Pericytes do not form a continuous layer around the endothelial-cell layer; individual pericytes are found at infrequent intervals on the luminal side of the capillary wall. Encircling the basal lamina of the endothelial cell or the pericyte are numerous processes of astrocytes joined to one another by *gap junctions.*

4.1. The Blood–Brain Barrier Refers to a Complex Array of Physical, Metabolic, and Transport Properties of the Capillary Endothelium

Circulating macromolecules, such as globulins and albumin, do not cross the endothelial lining of brain capillaries. This contrasts with the ready escape of circulating macromolecules that normally occurs in most extracranial tissues. The original description of the blood-brain barrier is attributed to Ehrlich who, in 1885 observed that intravenous injections of Evans blue, a dye that circulates bound to albumin, result in the diffuse distribution of the dye to almost every organ and tissue, except the brain and spinal cord.

The concept of a blood–brain barrier describes the inability of circulating macromolecules to enter the extracellular space or interstitial fluid of the brain and spinal cord. The mechanical component of the barrier has been traced primarily to structural characteristics of the endothelial capillary lining of the brain and spinal cord that are lacking in the endothelial lining of capillaries in other organs. A first important feature is that endothelial cells lining capillaries and venules in the CNS are joined at the luminal portion by *zonulae occludentes* or pentalaminar structures that represent the fusion of the outermost layers of two apposing endothelial-cell membranes (Fig. 12). The second factor preventing the escape of circulating macromolecules in the brain is the paucity of endocytotic pits in the endothelium of most vessels in the CNS. In contrast, the endothelial lining of capillaries and venules in extraneural tissues has abundant endocytotic pits and sizable gaps or fenestrae through which circulating particles such as 40-kDa horseradish peroxidase or 445-kDa apoferritin readily escape into the surrounding interstitial fluids.

Cerebral endothelium may become abnormally permeable to circulating macromolecules by several mechanisms: enhanced transcytosis or transport of molecules across the endothelial cytoplasm by means of endothelial vesicles; separation of the endothelial junctions; formation of tubular channels by fusion of endothelial vesicles; and loss of the negative charge on the endothelial surface, particularly loss of the terminal sialic group on the luminal side of the endothelial plasma membrane.

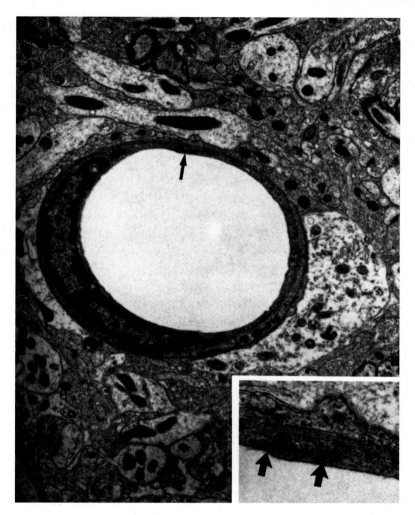

Fig. 12. Normal rat brain capillary (original magnification ×7000). The inset shows a close-up view of the capillary wall to demonstrate a tight junction (*arrows*) (original magnification ×32,200).

4.2. Capillaries at the Circumventricular Organs are Permeable to Circulating Macromolecules

The circumventricular organs are seven small, well-circumscribed areas located at the ependymal border of the third and fourth ventricles (Fig. 13), where capillaries are permeable to hydrophilic solutes. These sites are the pineal body, median eminence, neurohypophysis, subcommisural organ, area postrema, subfornical organ, and organum vasculosum laminae terminalis.

The circumventricular organs are endowed with permeable capillaries that have fenestrated endothelium, with the exception of the subcommisural organ. The functions of the circumventricular organs are uncertain, although some investigators suggest that macromolecular permeability at these sites may be related to the involvement of the respective neuronal groups in the regulation of neuroendocrine functions.

4.3. Immune and Inflammatory Mediators Play an Important Role in a Variety of Pathophysiological Pathways Such as in Cerebral Ischemia

Following cerebral ischemia, leukocytes—through their initial interactions with the microvascular endothelium—play an important role in the development of the infarct. Within hours of the onset of ischemia, polymorphonuclear (PMN) leukocytes accumulate and obstruct the microvasculature, then enter the

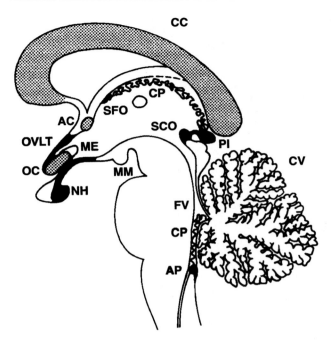

Fig. 13. Midline sagittal schematic drawing of the brain showing circumventricular organs (*dark shaded structures*). NH, Neurohypophysis; ME, Median eminence; OVLT, Organum vasculosum of lamina terminales; SFO, Subfornicial organ; PI, Pineal gland or body; SCO, Subcommisural organ; AP, Area postrema; CP, Choroid plexus; OC, Optic chiasm; AC, Anterior commisure; CC, Corpus callosum (*lightly shaded areas*).

parenchyma, followed by cells of the monocyte/macrophage lineage. Adhesion to the endothelium and transmigration through the vessel wall are influenced by inflammatory mediators, including cytokines. Upon activation, under conditions of ischemia/reperfusion, PMN leukocytes and the endothelium generate free radicals and proteases that contribute to microvascular and tissue injury.

4.3.1. ADHESION RECEPTORS

Adhesion receptors that mediate cell-cell and cell-matrix interactions in the cerebrovasculature belong to three families: selectins, integrins, and immunoglobulin-related receptors. Their inhibition may modulate cellular inflammation and reduce infarction. The access of PMN and other leukocytes to perivascular cells in the developing infarction requires their direct contact with the microvascular endothelium. Following middle cerebral artery (MCA) occlusion (and reperfusion), PMN leukocytes contribute to microvascular obstruction and edema formation during their adherence to the endothelium. Adherence and transmigration of PMN leukocytes through the postcapillary

endothelium involve the sequential interaction of P-selectin, intercellular adhesion molecule (ICAM-1), and E-selectin. The selectin family consists of P-selectin found on platelets and endothelial cells, E-selectin (endothelial cells), and L-selectin (leukocytes). P-selectin on endothelial cells and platelets mediate their interaction with granulocytes and monocytes. Integrins are heterodimeric adhesion molecules with a ubiquitous distribution. The adhesion properties of certain integrins are central to leukocyte transmigration. Firm adhesion is mediated by the interaction of granulocyte β_2-integrins with endothelial cell ICAM-1 (integrin $\alpha_M\beta_2$, MAC-1), or endothelial cell ICAM-1 and ICAM-2 (integrin $\alpha_L\beta_2$, LFA-1).

4.3.2. CYTOKINES

Ischemic cerebral tissues generate cytokines, superoxide free radicals, biogenic amines, and thrombin. These are stimulators for endothelial cells, granulocyte, and platelet activation and adhesion-receptor expression. Cytokines connect the pathophysiologic mechanisms of inflammation and ischemia. Tumor necrosis factor-α (TNF-α), interleukin-1 (IL-1), IL-6, and IL-8, together with monocyte chemoattraction protein-1 (MCP-1) are known protagonists in experimental cerebral ischemia. Cytokine release is important for the transition from focal cerebral ischemia to inflammation.

4.4. Complement Activation

Together with the acute inflammatory response that occurs during cerebral ischemia, complement components are activated, which contribute to cell injury. Activated complement contributes to the extension of the injury by promoting neutrophil accumulation through several mechanisms. In addition, C3a and C5a lead to histamine release, and the C5b-9 complex results in loss of cell-membrane integrity. One possible therapeutic strategy in focal cerebral ischemia would be the blockade of the complement cascade.

5. INTRACRANIAL VENOUS SYSTEM (TABLE 9)

Deep cerebral and superficial cortical veins drain most of the intracranial structures and the brain. The deep and the superficial cerebral veins empty blood into the intracranial dural venous sinuses, which are unique venous channels lined by endothelium and are enclosed between the outer (periosteal) and inner

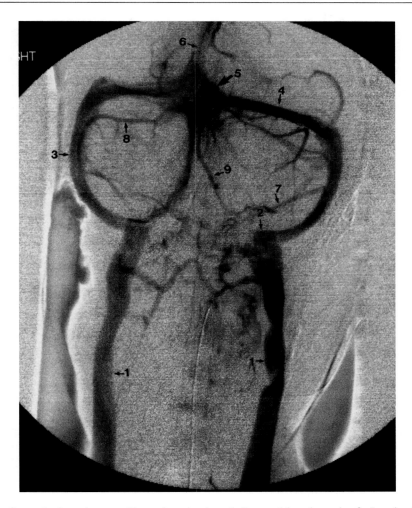

Fig. 14. Venous phase of vertebral angiogram. Frontal projection: **1,** Internal jugular vein. **2,** Jugular bulb. **3,** Sigmoid sinus. **4,** Tansverse sinus. **5,** Confluence of sinus (Torcular Herophili). **6,** Superior sagittal sinus. **7,** Superior petrosal sinus. **8,** Cerebellar hemispheric veins. **9,** Inferior vermian vein.

Table 9
Intracranial Venous System

Deep cerebral venous system
Drains the anastomatic structures of the cerebral hemispheres near the midline, the deep cerebral structures such as the deep white matter, thalamus, basal ganglia, and the upper brainstem.

Superficial venous system
Drains the cerebral cortex and adjacent white matter.

(meningeal) layers of dura. All dural venous sinuses finally converge and drain blood into the right and left internal jugular veins (Figs. 14,15). The internal jugular veins connect with their respective subclavian veins to form innominate veins in the neck. The right and left innominate vein subsequently unite to form the superior vena cava, which drains into the right atrium of the heart. Extensive collateral pathways exist between superficial cortical veins, the deep cerebral veins, and the dural venous sinuses.

5.1. The Deep Venous System (Table 10)

5.1.1. THE DEEP CEREBRAL VENOUS SYSTEM PRIMARILY DRAINS VEINS ORIGINATING IN MIDLINE STRUCTURES

The veins of the deep cerebral white matter, the basal ganglia, and thalami drain centrally and centrifugally into the deep venous system, which ultimately drains into the subependymal veins that are located in the subependymal region around the lateral ventricles. All the subependymal veins drain into the paired internal cerebral veins near the midline and are

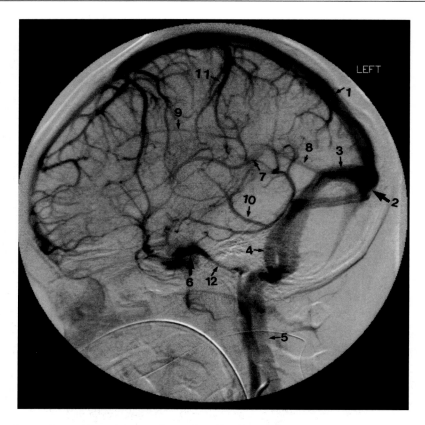

Fig. 15. Early venous phase of carotid angiogram. Lateral projection: **1,** Superior sagittal sinus. **2,** Confluence of sinus or Torcula Herophili. **3,** Tansverse sinus. **4,** Sigmoid sinus. **5,** Internal jugular vein. **6,** Cavernous sinus. **7,** Vein of Galen. **8,** Straight sinus. **9,** Inferior sagittal sinus. **10,** Vein of Labbē. **11,** Superficial cortical veins. **12,** Inferior petrosal sinus.

Table 10
The Deep Venous System

Paired internal cerebral veins
Basal vein of Rosenthal
Great cerebral vein of Galen

Brain structures
Deep white matter of the cerebral hemispheres
Corpus callosum
Thalami
Basal ganglia
Internal capsule
Choroid plexus of the third and lateral ventricles
Subependymal regions of the lateral and upper third ventricles
Medial surface of the temporal lobes
Upper brainstem and superior surface of the cerebellar hemispheres
The medial inferior surface of the parietal and occipital lobes can drain into the deep
    venous system

located in the roof of the third ventricle (Figs. 16,17). The basal veins of Rosenthal (Figs. 16–18) begin near the anterior perforated substance near the sylvian fossa and are formed from confluence of the deep middle cerebral, insular, and striate veins that drain the insular cortex, the corpus striatum, and the deep basal ganglia. The basal vein of Rosenthal courses posteriorly between the cerebral peduncles and the medial surface

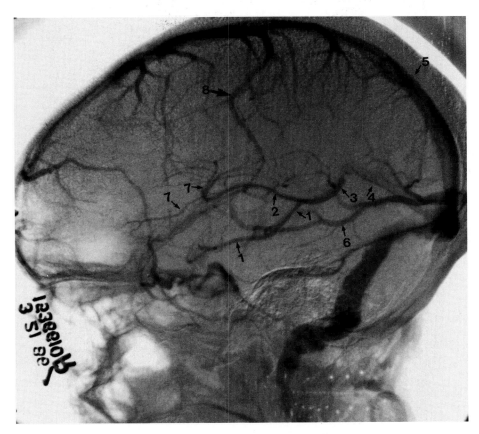

Fig. 16. Late venous phase of the internal carotid angiogram. **1,** Basal vein of Rosenthal. **2,** Internal cerebral vein. **3,** Vein of Galen. **4,** Straight sinus. **5,** Superior sagittal sinus. **6,** Vein of Labbē. **7,** Subependymal tributaries of the internal cerebral vein. **8,** Anastomotic vein of Trolard.

of the temporal lobes and ultimately joins the vein of Galen in the midline (Figs. 16–18). The vein of Galen empties blood into the straight sinus at the junction of the inferior sagittal sinus.

The basal vein of Rosenthal drains blood from the insular cortex, basal ganglia, medial temporal lobe, midbrain, thalamus, choroid plexus of the temporal horn of the lateral ventricle, subependymal region, and the deep white matter of the temporal lobe.

The internal cerebral vein drains blood from the choroid plexus of the third ventricle, choroid plexus of the lateral ventricles, basal ganglia, internal capsule, thalamus, subependymal region of the lateral ventricles, and the deep white matter of the cerebral hemispheres (Figs. 16,17).

The system of the deep cerebral veins includes several veins that drain anatomic structures of the cerebral hemispheres located near the midline; most of these veins converge into the great vein of Galen. The paired midline internal cerebral vein unite to form the great cerebral vein of Galen. Veins from the deep cerebral structures, such as the thalamus, join the subependymal veins that drain into the internal cerebral vein. The basal vein of Rosenthal, the internal occipital vein, and other vessels also contribute to the great vein of Galen. The great vein of Galen, which is 2.0 cm long, is close to the pineal body, quadrigeminal plate, and dorsum of the superior cerebellar vermis. The deep middle cerebral veins drain the insular cortex and portions of the adjacent opercular surface, and these veins usually receive lenticulostriate veins that drain the inferior portion of the basal ganglia. The thalamostriate, anterior caudate, septal, and midatrial veins are tributaries of the internal cerebral vein. Identification of these deep veins with contrast angiography is extremely useful for the localization of lesions, especially tumors, involving midline structures such as the basal ganglia, thalamus, and the pineal body.

The vein of Galen also drains anatomic structures related to the optic chiasm, uncinate gyrus, para-

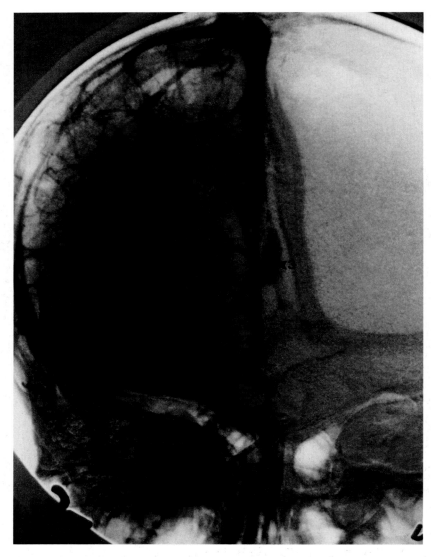

Fig. 17. Frontal projection of the early venous phase of the left carotid angiogram. **1,** Basal vein of Rosenthal. **2,** Thalamostriate tributary (subependymal) of the internal cerebral vein. **3,** Superimposed internal cerebral vein and straight sinus.

hippocampal gyrus, portions of the ventricular temporal horn, and upper brainstem. Venous flow originating from these sites enters the vein of Galen through the basal veins of Rosenthal. The basal vein of Rosenthal originates near the optic chiasm and courses around the cerebral peduncles to terminate into the great vein of Galen. Shortly after its origin, the basal vein is covered by the uncus and the parahippocampal gyrus before it circles around the cerebral peduncle.

The vein of Galen and the inferior sagittal sinus—a venous structure running parallel to the dorsal surface of the corpus callosum within the free edge of Falx cerebri join one another to form the straight sinus, which occupies a midline position in the tentorium

cerebelli. The inferior sagittal sinus courses above the corpus callosum along the free edge of the falx cerebri. This sinus receives numerous veins that drain the roof of the corpus callosum, the cingulate gyrus, and adjacent structures of the cerebral hemisphere; most superior cerebellar veins also drain into the straight sinus. The straight sinus ends in the Torcula Herophili, a dura mater structure located at the site of the internal occipital protuberance. The Torcula Herophili is the site of convergence for the straight sinus and the superior sagittal sinus, which sometimes remain separate from one another. The straight sinus usually drains into the left transverse sinus, and the superior sagittal sinus continues into the right transverse sinus.

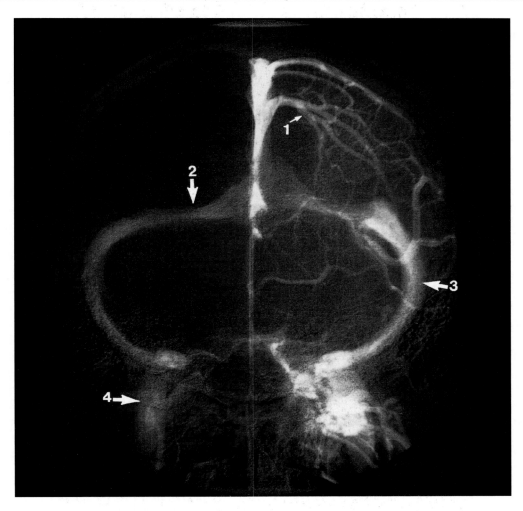

Fig. 18. Frontal projection of the late phase of the left carotid angiogram. **1,** Superficial cortical veins draining into the superior sagittal sinus. **2,** Transverse sinus. **3,** Sigmoid sinus. **4,** Internal jugular vein.

The transverse sinuses drain into the sigmoid sinuses, which originate at the posterior petrous portion of the temporal bone. The sigmoid sinus ends into the jugular bulb within the jugular foramen, where it continues into the internal jugular vein. The superior petrosal sinus usually drains into the proximal portion of the sigmoid sinus. This sinus also receives veins from the cerebellum, the lateral pons, and the medulla. The two internal jugular veins with respective inominate veins converge to form the superior vena cava.

5.2. Superficial Cerebral Veins (Table 11)

5.2.1. SUPERFICIAL CEREBRAL VEINS DRAIN INTO EITHER THE SUPERIOR SAGITTAL SINUS OR TRANSVERSE SINUSES

The numerous superficial cortical veins drain the cortex and the adjacent white matter and lie within the cerebral sulci (Fig. 15–18). Most of the superficial cortical veins are unnamed, because of their variable appearance. The superficial middle cerebral vein, the anastomotic vein of Trolard (Fig. 16) and anastomotic vein of Labbē (Figs. 15,16) are consistently seen. The superficial middle cerebral vein is located along the sylvian fissure. The anastomotic vein of Trolard located along the cortical surface of the anterior parietal lobe, and the vein of Labbē courses over the cortical surface of the temporal lobe. The rich network of collateral anastomosis exists between the numerous superficial cortical veins and between the superficial cortical veins and the deep cerebral veins that become more visible following venous occlusive disease.

Superficial cerebral veins designate the network of venous channels that are visible on the surface of each cerebral hemisphere. Superficial cerebral veins

Table 11
Superficial Venous System

Anastomatic vein of Labbē
Anastomatic vein of Trolard
Superficial middle cerebral vein
Numerous unnamed superficial cortical veins
Brain structures drained
Cortex of the cerebral hemisphere
Rich network of collateral channels exist between the numerous superficial cortical veins

coalesce on the pial surface and convey blood from the outer 1 or 2 cm of the cortex and underlying superficial white matter. The superficial veins are divided into *superior* veins that drain into the superior sagittal sinus, and *inferior* veins whose flow is directed into the transverse sinus; a *middle* group of vessels may drain superiorly or inferiorly. All the superficial veins normally empty into one or more of the major dural sinuses. The inferior superficial veins drain territories located primarily on the ventral surface of the temporal and occipital lobes.

The main draining avenue for most superficial cerebral veins, the superior sagittal sinus, originates at the foramen cecum of the frontal bone, courses anteroposteriorly along the midline of the dura mater, and ends in the Torcula Herophili.

Most superficial veins follow their course through the subarachnoid space over the surface of the various cerebral gyri, and the superior superficial veins usually converge on each side to form 4–6 large veins that, after piercing the arachnoid membrane, terminate in the walls of the superior sagittal sinus. The short segments of these veins located in the subdural space are designated as superficial cortical *bridging* veins. In most instances of subdural bleeding, the hemorrhage is believed to originate from tears in the bridging segment of the superficial cerebral veins.

One of the largest superior superficial veins, which usually runs a course approximately parallel to the central sulcus, is known as the vein of Trolard. Another large superficial vein, running an anteroposterior course over the temporal lobe and establishing connections between the superior and inferior groups of veins, is sometimes designated the anastomotic vein of Labbē which drains into tranverse sinus.

5.3. Posterior Fossa (Infratentorial) Veins (Table 12)

The veins of the posterior fossa are grouped under superior (Galenic) group, anterior (petrosal) group,

and posterior (tentorial) group. The precentral cerebellar vein, superior vermian vein, and anterior ponto mesencephalic veins form the superior Galenic group and drain the superior surface of the cerebellar hemispheres, superior vermis, upper pons, and midbrain (Fig. 19). The anterior (petrosal) group of veins include petrosal veins that drain the ventral surface of the pons, medulla, and ventral surface of the cerebellar hemispheres. The petrosal veins subsequently drain into the superior petrosal sinus. The posterior (tentorial) group of veins includes interior vermian veins that drain the inferior surface of the cerebellar hemispheres and the inferior vermis and dorsal surface of the brainstem (Fig. 20). The inferior vermian veins drain into the tentorial sinus, which subsequently drains blood into either the transverse sinus or the straight sinus (Figs. 14,19,20).

5.4. Dural Venous Sinuses (Table 13)

The major dural venous sinuses are the superior sagittal sinus, transverse sinuses, straight sinus, sigmoid sinuses, and cavernous sinus (Figs. 14,19). Smaller-caliber sinuses are the inferior sagittal sinus, superior petrosal sinus, inferior petrosal sinus, and occipital sinus (Figs. 14,20). The midline superior sagittal sinus and straight sinus join with the right and left transverse sinuses to form the confluence of sinuses known also as Torcula Herophili. The emissary veins connect the extracranial venous system to the dural venous sinuses through the cranium and the skull-base foramina.

Before reaching the right side of the heart through the superior vena cava, the intracranial venous system drains on each side into three or four major sinuses whose flow eventually goes into the internal jugular veins.

All intracranial sinuses are endothelium-lined structures bounded by thick layers of collagenous tissues derived from the dura mater. On the convexity and midline of the brain are the superior and inferior sagittal sinuses and the straight sinus, all of which

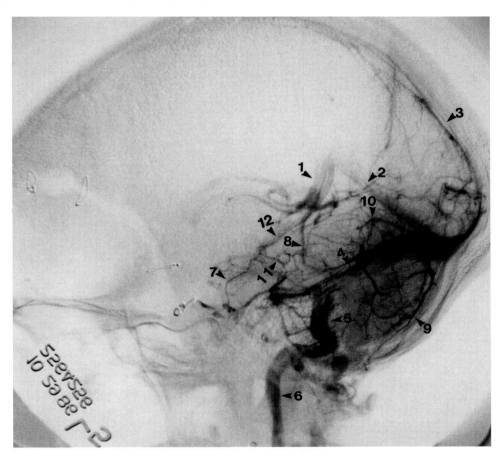

Fig. 19. Lateral protection of the venous phase of the vertebral angiogram showing the veins of the posterior cranial fossa. **1,** Vein of Galen. **2,** Straight sinus. **3,** Superior sagittal sinus. **4,** Transverse sinus. **5,** Sigmoid sinus. **6,** Internal jugular vein. **7,** Anterior pontomesencephalic vein. **8,** Precentral cerebellar vein. **9,** Inferior vermian vein. **10,** Superior vermian vein. **11,** Lateral mesencephalic vein. **12,** Posterior mesencephalic vein (posterior part of basal vein of Rosenthal).

converge into the Torcula Herophili. At the base of the skull, on each side of the pituitary fossa, is a large cavernous sinus that primarily drains veins from the orbit, the pituitary gland, anterior hypothalamic structures, and some of the paranasal sinuses. The cavernous sinuses are located on the lateral surface of the body of the sphenoid bone. The cavernous sinus receives blood from the superior and inferior ophthalmic veins, the sphenoparietal sinus, the inferior petrosal sinus, and the basilar plexus of veins. The basilar veins receive blood from the inferior petrosal sinus, which also drains posteriorly into the marginal sinus and the anterior internal vertebral venous plexus of the spinal cord.

The cavernous sinus drains into the sigmoid sinus through the superior and inferior petrosal sinuses, two structures that run parallel to the petrous portion of the temporal bone. Both the superior and inferior petrosal sinuses communicate anteriorly and medially with the cavernous sinus. The superior petrosal sinus courses along the bone with the attached margin of the cerebellar tentorium, and the inferior petrosal sinus runs inferior and parallel to the superior sinus in the petro-occipital fissure. The superior petrosal sinus drains the ventral surface of the temporal lobe and the dorsal surface of the cerebellum; a few veins from the brainstem may also reach this sinus.

The cavernous sinuses are unique venous structures that contain the cavernous segments of the internal carotid arteries, and the abducens (sixth) cranial nerve, oculomotor (third), trochlear (fourth), and ophthalmic division of the trigeminal (fifth) cranial nerve lie within the lateral wall of the cavernous sinuses. The cavernous sinuses are located on the lateral walls of the body of the sphenoid bone. The superior and inferior ophthalmic veins of the orbits and the sphenoparietal sinus drain into the cavernous sinus. The superior and inferior petrosal sinuses connect the cavernous

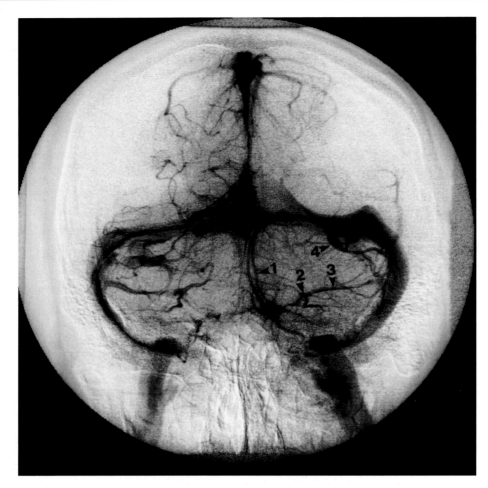

Fig. 20. Frontal projection of the venous phase of the vertebral angiogram: **1,** Inferior vermian vein. **2,** Petrosal vein. **3,** Superior petrosal sinus. **4,** Cerebellar superficial hemispheric veins.

Table 12
Posterior Fossa Venous System

Superior (Galenic) group
Anterior (Petrosal) group
Posterior (Tentorial) group
Brain structures drained
Brainstem
Cerebellar hemispheres
Cerebellar vermis

sinus to the sigmoid sinus and the jugular bulb respectively. The cavernous sinuses also freely communicate with the peterygoid venous plexus in the roof of the nasopharynx through emissary veins and the venous plexus over the clivus.

The major source of disease associated with intracranial veins and sinuses is the occlusion of these draining channels by thrombi or by adjacent structures, such as tumors. Intracranial venous thrombosis is causally related to infectious processes involving structures located near the cavernous sinus, such as the paranasal sinuses, orbits, teeth, skull, and scalp. Infectious processes involving any of the anatomic structures located near the cavernous sinus, such as the intraorbital contents, can lead to the thrombotic occlusion of this sinus.

There are several venous channels connecting extracranial and intracranial veins, known as *emissary veins.* The flow in these and many other cranial venous structures can be easily reversed, because there are no intraluminal valves or structures to ensure unidirectional flow.

Microscopically, the walls of the brain venules are almost indistinguishable from the capillary walls. Venous walls consist of a continuous lining of endothelial cells. The endothelium is nonfenestrated, and the junction of two apposed plasma membranes is

Table 13
Dural Venous Sinuses

Superior sagittal sinus
Transverse sinuses
Straight sinus
Sigmoid sinuses
Cavernous sinuses
Superior petrosal sinuses
Inferior petrosal sinuses
Occipital sinus
Inferior sagittal sinus
Structures drained
Straight sinus
Deep venous system
The superior sagittal sinus, transverse sinus
Sigmoid sinus
The superficial cortical venous system
Cavernous sinus
Pituitary gland
Orbits
Inferior hypothalamus
Part of the posterior paranasal sinuses
Superior and inferior petrosal sinuses
Brainstem
Ventral surface of the cerebellar hemispheres
Torcula Herophili
Confluence of the superior sagittal, transverse sinuses, midline straight, and occipital sinus

Extensive anastamotic collateral channels exist between various dural venous sinuses.

separated only by a narrow cleft, except at the luminal surface, where the membranes form zonulae occludentes. The walls of cerebral veins consist of an endothelium-lined tunica intima surrounded by an adventitial layer. Smooth-muscle cells are not a common component of the venous wall. The wall of dural sinuses consist of an inner lining of endothelium and an outer layer with essentially the same architecture as the dura mater. This outer layer consists chiefly of fibroblasts and large interlaced bundles of collagenous fibers. The arachnoid villi appear shortly after birth, and with advancing age, they form cauliflower-like clusters referred to as pacchionian granulations. They are primarily located along the walls of the superior sagittal sinus and the transverse sinus. The arachnoid villi are intimately involved in the process of transferring spinal fluid from the subarachnoid space to the dural venous sinuses.

Intracranial veins do not collapse, even at transmural pressure of 1.0 mmHg, which contrasts with the process in extracranial veins.

ACKNOWLEDGMENT

This chapter is dedicated to the memory of the late Dr. Julio H. Garcia, whose leadership and enthusiasm was the source of the original chapter and this revision.

SELECTED READINGS

Bohlen und Halbach O. Neurotransmitters and neuromodulators—handbook of receptors and biological effects in Bolen und Halbach O, Dermitzel R (eds). Weinheim, Germany 2002; 1.

Capra NF, Anderson KV. Anatomy of the cerebral venous system. In Kapp JP, Schmidek HH (eds). The Cerebral Venous System and Its Disorders. Orlando: Grune & Stratton, 1984:1.

Damasio H. A CT guide to the identification of cerebral vascular territories. Arch Neurol 1983; 40:138.

De Reuck J. The human periventricular blood supply and the anatomy of cerebral infarctions. Eur Neurol 1968; 5:321.

Edvinsson L. Innervation of the cerebral circulation. Ann NY Acad Sci 1987;529:334.

Goadsby PJ, Sercombe R. Neurogenic regulation of cerebral blood flow: extrinsic neuronal control. In Mraovitch S, Sercombe R. Neurophysiological Basis of Cerebral Blood Flow Control. London, John Libbey, 1996, 285–324.

Gross PM. Capillaries of the circumventricular organs in Ermisch A (ed). Circumventricular Organs. Amsterdam, Elsevier Scientific Publishers, 1992; 219–233.

Lijnen HR, Collen D Endothelium in hemostasis and thrombosis. Prog Cardiovasc Dis 1997; 39:3443–3450.

May AE, Neumann FJ, Preissner KT. The relevance of blood-vessel wall adhesive interactions for vascular thrombotic disease. Thromb Haemost 1999; 82:962–970.

Mraovitch S. Neurogenic regulation of cerebral blood flow: intrinsic control. In Mraovitch S, Sercombe R. Neurophysiological Basis of Cerebral Blood Flow Control. London, John Libbey, 1996; 323–358.

Osborn AG. Diagnostic cerebral angiography. Philadelphia: Lippincott Williams & Wilkins, 1999; 3–217.

Van der Eecken HM. The anastomoses between the leptomeningeal arteries in the brain. Springfield: CC Thomas, 1959.

Weibel J, Fields WS. Atlas of arteriography in occlusive cerebral vascular disease. Philadelphia: WB Saunders, 1969.

Wilkins RH. Cerebral vasospasm. Crit Rev Neurobiol 1990; 6:51.

Young RF. The trigeminal nerve and its central pathways. Physiology of facial sensation and pain. In Rovit RL, Murali R, Jannetta PG (eds). Trigeminal Neuralgia. Baltimore: Williams & Wilkins, 1990; 27–51.

Zhang ET, Inman CBE, Weller RO. Interrelationshilps of the pia mater and the perivascular (Virchow-Robin) spaces in the human cerebrum. J Anat 1990; 170:111–123.

Stroke

Gregory Cooper and Robert L. Rodnitzky

Stroke is the third leading cause of death in the United States, with approx 750,000 new cases and more than 150,000 fatalities each year. Stroke refers to the neurologic dysfunction resulting from a derangement of the blood supply to the brain or spinal cord. The neurologic symptoms of a stroke are often of sudden onset and may be temporary or permanent. Strokes may be ischemic, resulting from impaired blood flow, or hemorrhagic. Cerebral ischemia is a potentially reversible alteration of brain function that results from inadequate delivery of critical blood-borne substrates such as oxygen and glucose. Cerebral infarction occurs if ischemia is severe enough to kill cells. In this circumstance, there is a high likelihood of permanent dysfunction. The brain is particularly sensitive to severe ischemia, with irreversible cell death resulting in 2–3 min in some species and in approx 6–8 min in humans.

PATHOLOGIC MECHANISMS OF STROKE

Cellular Energy Failure is at the Root of Most Neurologic Symptoms that Result from a Stroke

Cell death in stroke results from the failure to synthesize ATP and other nucleoside triphosphates. Without an adequate energy source, cell survival is threatened in several ways. As a result of intracellular acidosis related to enhanced anaerobic glycolysis, mitochondrial respiration is further depressed, free radical formation is enhanced, and lipid peroxidation occurs. Excitotoxicity results from overstimulation of neuronal glutamate receptors. Ion homeostasis is disrupted, with a resultant influx of calcium, sodium, and chloride ions along with water. The enhanced cellular water content further damages individual cells and leads to regional brain swelling, which compresses neighboring blood vessels, further reducing blood supply to the injured area. Cell structure degenerates, because ATP is required to support resynthesis of macromolecules in the normal course of cell maintenance.

Normal Homeostatic Mechanisms in the Cerebral Vascular System May Be Lost Because of Cerebral Ischemia

The process of vascular autoregulation maintains a relatively constant cerebral blood flow despite variations in mean arterial pressure. This system is generally effective as long as the mean arterial pressure does not fall below 60 mmHg or rise above 150 mmHg. As a result of autoregulation, cerebral blood flow increases when there is an elevation of arterial $PaCO_2$. In an area of infarcted brain, autoregulation is typically lost, and the cerebral blood flow passively mirrors changes in systemic blood pressure so that there is virtually no compensation for extremely low or extremely high pressures. The lost ability to respond to increased levels of $PaCO_2$, prevents a normal compensatory increase in blood flow in response to potentially damaging acidosis.

THE NORMAL BLOOD SUPPLY TO THE BRAIN CAN BE DISRUPTED BY SEVERAL MECHANISMS

Blood flow to the brain is diminished by any process that significantly narrows or occludes a nutrient blood vessel. Narrowing of a blood vessel without total occlusion is referred to as stenosis. In a large cerebral blood vessel such as the carotid artery, a substantial stenosis of 50–75% is required before blood flow is seriously diminished. Even under these circumstances, cerebral blood flow can remain relatively normal if collateral circulatory pathways compensate by shunting more blood to the affected region of the brain. Narrowing or occlusion of a cerebral artery is usually the result of lipidladen atherosclerotic deposits attached to the inner surface of the vessel.

If the atherosclerotic deposit does not itself occlude an artery, it may serve as a nidus for the formation of a superimposed occluding blood clot, called a *thrombus*. Occlusion of a critical blood vessel can occur when a blood clot from a distant site, such as the heart, travels through the arterial system and lodges in a blood vessel of smaller caliber within the brain. A clot from a distant origin is referred to as an *embolus*. Cholesterol particles that have broken loose from an area of atherosclerosis and traveled downstream in the vascular system constitute another form of embolus.

A drop in cerebral perfusion pressure can result in diminished blood flow to the brain despite fully patent vessels. Such a drop, usually related to low blood pressure, can be the cause of watershed or border-zone infarctions. The terms watershed and border zone refer to areas of the brain between the terminal distributions of two adjacent arteries, such as the anterior and middle cerebral arteries. Because they are at the end of the pipeline, such regions are subject to low, marginally adequate arterial pressure under normal circumstances. They are therefore the first to fail when blood pressure in the system drops further. If a drop in blood pressure is sufficiently severe and sustained, the entire brain is affected, resulting in *global cerebral ischemia*.

Cerebral hemorrhage, one of the most severe forms of stroke, results from the spontaneous rupture of the wall of a blood vessel that has been weakened by longstanding high blood pressure or from the rupture of a cerebral *aneurysm*, a balloon-like outpouching of the layers of an arterial wall. In the former case, bleeding usually occurs directly into the brain, resulting in an intracerebral hemorrhage. In the latter circumstance, hemorrhage may also occur within the brain substance, but because aneurysms are more typically found on the surface of the brain, hemorrhage into the CSF contained within the subarachnoid space is much more common. Intracerebral and subarachnoid hemorrhages are extremely serious, and either can be fatal, one because of mass effect and compression of adjacent structures within the brain and the other because of associated severe arterial spasm provoked by blood in the CSF.

TRANSIENT ISCHEMIC SYMPTOMS OFTEN PRECEDE CEREBRAL INFARCTION

Under certain circumstances, the symptoms of cerebral ischemia may last only several minutes and then resolve. These episodes are known as *transient ischemic attacks*. By definition, a transient ischemic attack is an episode in which symptoms persist for less than 24 h before resolving, but most last less than 15 min. A common cause of a brief ischemic episode is the passage of an arterial embolus downstream, resulting in the temporary occlusion of a smaller blood vessel until the embolus breaks up and is flushed downstream. These emboli can arise from the heart or from an atherosclerotic lesion in a large blood vessel. The point at which the common carotid artery bifurcates into its internal and external branches is a common site of severe atherosclerosis and often serves as a staging ground for fibrin-platelet or cholesterol emboli. Emboli from this site can travel to the brain, producing sensory, motor, or language dysfunction, or to the arterial supply of one eye, producing the classic syndrome of amaurosis fugax (e.g., fleeting blindness) before they break up. In this condition, the affected person describes a brief episode during which it appears that a fog or a cloud has descended like a window shade over the entire visual field of one eye.

Transient ischemic attacks may also result when a region of the brain being perfused by a severely stenotic artery is temporarily subjected to abnormally low perfusion pressure during an episode of systemic hypotension. This further reduces the already marginal blood supply, resulting in transient neurologic symptoms until the blood pressure returns to normal.

Transient ischemic attacks can be repetitive and stereotypical. Because they are often the forerunner of a subsequent episode which produces a permanent neurologic deficit, a transient ischemic attack mandates immediate investigation to try to identify and correct its underlying cause and prevent a more devastating, irreversible ischemic event.

THE NEUROLOGIC DEFICIT IN ISCHEMIC STROKE DEPENDS ON WHICH BLOOD VESSEL IS INVOLVED

The brain is perfused by the paired carotid arteries and the vertebral basilar system of blood vessels. The neurologic signs and symptoms associated with a stroke depend on which of these blood vessels or their branches are involved.

One of the most common vascular territories to be involved in stroke is that of the *middle cerebral artery*. The middle cerebral artery has deep (e.g., lenticulos-triate) and superficial (e.g., pial) branches. The deep branches perfuse the corona radiata, portions of the internal capsule, and parts of the globus pallidus and caudate nucleus. The pial branches provide blood supply for most of the lateral surface of the frontal, temporal, and parietal lobes. The clinical syndrome resulting from middle cerebral artery stenosis or occlusion depends on which of its branches are most involved. Among the most common clinical findings associated with middle cerebral artery involvement are contralateral limb paralysis and contralateral sensory loss, both involving the arm much more than the leg. The relative sparing of the lower extremity reflects the fact that its representation in the primary motor and sensory cortex is on the medial surface of the frontal and parietal lobes, respectively, areas that are outside the middle cerebral artery perfusion zone. The eyes may become deviated toward the side of the lesion because of destruction of the frontal lobe gaze center responsible for directing rapid eye movements in the horizontal plane to the contralateral side. When this center is damaged, only the intact gaze center in the opposite hemisphere continues to drive gaze, and the eyes are involuntarily directed toward the side of the frontal lobe infarction. Because the speech area is within the middle cerebral artery territory, aphasia is common in dominant hemisphere infarctions. In nondominant hemisphere infarction, especially those involving the parietal lobe, there may be severe disturbances of spatial function, such as *hemispatial neglect*, which is a tendency not to attend to objects or stimuli located in space on the side opposite the infarction. Separate and distinct from hemispatial neglect, there can be contralateral *hemianopia*, which is a loss of half the visual field caused by the involvement of the optic radiations coursing through the temporal and parietal lobes.

The *anterior cerebral artery* perfuses the anterior frontal lobe and the parts of the frontal and parietal lobe on the medial surface of the hemisphere. Because the lower-extremity portions of the motor and sensory homunculus are located on the medial hemispheric surface, anterior cerebral artery infarction preferen-tially produces paralysis and sensory loss in the lower extremity. Aphasia or visual field loss are not typically part of the syndrome.

Occlusion of the *internal carotid artery* can result in infarction of the entire anterior two-thirds of the hemisphere, which constitutes the perfusion area of its two major branches, the anterior cerebral and middle cerebral arteries. Because the anterior cerebral artery often receives significant collateral flow from the opposite anterior cerebral artery through a vessel connecting the two, an internal carotid artery occlusion often results in damage confined largely to areas perfused by the middle cerebral artery.

Occlusion of one *vertebral artery* may go unnoticed if the opposite vertebral artery is patent and allows adequate blood flow into the basilar artery. However, vertebral artery occlusion can result in an infarction of the structures perfused by one of its branches, the *posterior inferior cerebellar artery*. Occlusion of this artery results in infarction of the lateral medulla, and the resultant constellation of neurologic signs, known as *Wallenberg's syndrome*, is one of the most striking examples of predictable clinic-oanatomic correlation in clinical neurology. Structures that are affected in a lateral medullary infarction include the spinal tract of the trigeminal nerve, the spinothalamic tract, the nucleus ambiguous, the inferior cerebellar peduncle, and the sympathetic fibers descending through the brainstem from the hypothalamus.

The neurologic deficit occurring in Wallenberg's syndrome coincides exactly with the function of these structures. Sensory symptoms consist of loss of pain and temperature perception but not touch perception on the ipsilateral side of the face (e.g., uncrossed spinal tract of trigeminal nerve) and loss of pain and temperature sensation on the contralateral side of the body (e.g., crossed spinothalamic tract). There is ipsilateral limb incoordination (e.g., cerebellar peduncle) and a raspy, breathy voice caused by paralysis of the ipsilateral vocal cord (e.g., nucleus ambiguous). In the ipsilateral eye, a small pupil and a drooping eyelid (e.g., Horner's syndrome) are caused by interruption of the descending sympathetic fibers.

Wallenberg's syndrome also illustrates an important principle of clinical neuroanatomic localization. Crossed motor or sensory symptoms, such as involvement of one side of the face and the other side of the body usually imply brainstem pathology when caused by brain infarction.

Occlusion of the *basilar artery* can result in infarction of the entire upper brainstem and both occipital lobes. The massive brainstem dysfunction is often fatal. The paired posterior cerebral arteries originate from the bifurcation of the terminal portion of the basilar artery. Each posterior cerebral artery has a hemispheric branch that supplies the occipital cortex and penetrating branches that perfuse the midbrain in concert with similar branches from the basilar artery. Occlusion of the hemispheric branches on one side causes loss of the opposite half of the visual field (e.g., hemianopia), which is identical (e.g., homonymous) in both eyes. An occlusion of the right posterior cerebral artery resulting in a right occipital infarction causes loss of the left half of the visual field from the right and left eyes.

Occlusion of the hemispheric branches to both occipital cortices results in a form of total visual loss known as *cortical blindness*. Cortically blind persons often deny their visual disability. Each posterior cerebral artery also perfuses the splenium of the corpus callosum. When this structure is infarcted along with the primary visual cortex of the dominant hemisphere, the syndrome of *alexia without agraphia* results. This can be viewed as a disconnection syndrome in which the visual input from the visual cortices are disconnected from the perisylvian cortices, in essence preventing a decoding of the written information. The syndrome of *hemiachromatopsia*, which is an inability to perceive color, occurs when the inferior, medial occipital lobe is infarcted. The cells in this area of the visual cortex are wavelength-selective in response to light and form the basis of color recognition. As is the case with hemianopia, the visual field opposite the side of the lesion is affected.

LACUNAR INFARCTIONS DO NOT CONFORM TO THE DISTRIBUTION OF MAJOR CEREBRAL ARTERIES

Lacunar infarctions are small lesions, usually less than 15 mm in diameter. They are thought to result from occlusion of small, penetrating arteries that have been damaged by chronically elevated arterial blood pressure. Although very small, lacunar infarctions may occur in strategic areas, such as the internal capsule or the pyramidal tract in the pons, where they can cause severe hemiparesis. A lacunar infarction involving the posterior ventral nucleus of the thalamus can cause isolated, severe contralateral sensory loss.

TREATMENT OF STROKE

The treatment of stroke can be divided into the initial and subsequent management of the acute stroke itself, and secondary prevention of further strokes. In ischemic stroke, in addition to basic supportive measures, acute treatment is based on the restoration of normal blood flow. This may be accomplished through the use of thrombolytic agents, such as the tissue plasminogen activator (tPA) given either intravenously or intra-arterially at the site of thrombus. Mechanical recanalization may also be attemtpted at the time of angiography. Patients with large hemorrhagic strokes may require surgical intervention with removal of clot in order to limit the mass effect and damage to other parts of the brain. Early institution of intensive rehabilitation programs after the stroke may improve functional outcome. It has also been shown that admission to an inpatient rehabilitation unit following stroke leads to a better outcome.

Secondary prevention of stroke is, in part, guided by the mechanism of stroke. In ischemic stroke, strategies include prevention of blood-clot formation and improvement of blood-vessel patency. For persons who have experienced an episode of cerebral ischemia, agents such as aspirin, which inhibit platelet aggregation, are of major benefit in preventing recurrent ischemic events. More potent anticoagulant drugs such as warfarin can be used to prevent larger clots in the heart or blood vessels from forming or, once formed, from breaking loose and entering the cerebral circulation. A patient who has had a transient ischemic event or complete stroke as a result of severe carotid artery stenosis often benefits from surgical removal of the atherosclerotic deposit responsible for the arterial narrowing. Experience suggests that stroke patients who have arteries with the highest degree of blockage, in excess of 70%, benefit the most from surgical treatment, with a definite reduction in the risk for future ischemic events. Accessibility considerations limit such surgical procedures largely to the common carotid artery and the extracranial portion of the internal carotid artery, the most common site of surgery. More recently, angioplasty and stenting of stenosed arteries has been employed.

The treatment of intracerebral hemorrhage centers on surgical removal of blood clots that are of sufficient mass to dangerously compress adjacent vital brain structures. A ruptured aneurysm is treated by occluding or tying off the weakened arterial bleb so that it cannot bleed again. Medical therapy is directed at preventing blood vessels from going into spasm in response to the presence of blood in the subarachnoid space. Certain calcium channel-blocking agents are useful for this purpose.

SELECTED READINGS

Biller J. Vascular syndromes of the cerebrum. In Brazis P, Masdeu J, Biller J (eds). Localization in clinical neurology. Boston: Little, Brown and Company, 1996; 535–564.

Brott T, Bogousslavsky J. Treatment of acute ischemic stroke. N Engl J Med 2000; 343:710–722.

Devenport R, Dennis M. Neurological emergencies: acute stroke. J Neurol Neurosurg Psychiatry 2000; 68:277–288.

8

The Choroid Plexus–CSF Nexus
Gateway to the Brain

Conrad E. Johanson

CONTENTS

1. FUNCTIONAL COMPONENTS OF THE CEREBROSPINAL FLUID (CSF) SYSTEM

Cerebrospinal fluid (CSF) has a major impact on the volume and composition of the interstitial fluid that envelops the neurons. Choroid plexus tissue in the four ventricles is the source of up to 80–90% of this actively secreted transcellular CSF, which is derived from the carotid and vertebral blood supplies. As the CSF flows from its choroidal origins to more distal sites, it comes into contact with other membranes that encompass brain tissue: the ependyma, which lines the ventricular system, and the pia-glia and arachnoid membranes which border the subarachnoid space

(SAS). As a result, the composition of the continually flowing CSF, and of the adjacent brain interstitium, is progressively modified by bidirectional exchanges of water, ions, and proteins at these transport interfaces.

The CSF is a dynamic system that works in concert and in parallel with the cerebral capillary transporters to ensure an optimal environment for the neurons. Any disruption in the balance of the transport processes at the blood–CSF barrier (mainly the choroid plexuses) with those at the blood–brain barrier can lead to serious deficits in cerebral function. Although it has long been known that brain water balance, and stability of the extracellular fluid composition, is vitally dependent on choroid plexus function, it has recently become more evident that "downstream" CSF interactions with the brain (at the ependyma, pia/glia, and arachnoid)

From: *Neuroscience in Medicine, 2nd ed.* (P. Michael Conn, ed.), © 2003 Humana Press Inc., Totowa, NJ.

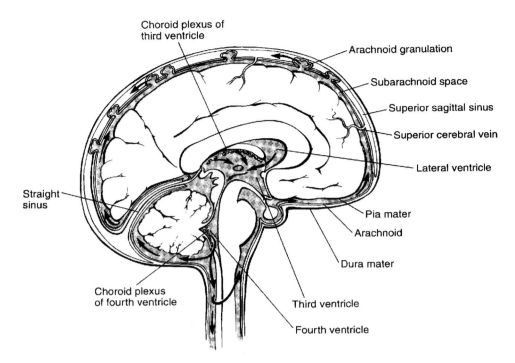

Fig. 1. CSF is formed and secreted by the choroid plexuses in the lateral, third and fourth ventricles. The great vascularity of the plexuses imparts a reddish cast to these tissues. In adult humans, the total weight of the choroid plexus in the four ventricles is about 2–3 g. Choroidal tissue is not present in the subarachnoid CSF space that surrounds the brain hemispheres and spinal cord.

are essential components of a healthy CSF circulatory system.

As the most proximal part of the CSF system, the choroid plexus can be viewed as a "port of entry" for the delivery of many substances to the CNS. The unique array of transporters in the choroid epithelial basolateral (plasma-facing) membrane, compared to the counterpart luminal membrane of the cerebral endothelium, affords opportunities for selectively translocating agents into the CSF–brain domain. Thus, when it is transported from blood to CSF, a substance generally has ready access to neurons and glia because little resistance to diffusion is offered by the permeable gap-junctions between cells lining the interior and exterior surfaces that interface the CSF with the brain. Thus, the choroid plexus–CSF nexus is progressively being viewed as an active gateway for supplying endogenous and exogenous agents to the CNS.

2. WHAT IS THE ROLE OF CSF IN THE TOTAL "ECONOMY" OF THE BRAIN?

CSF is an active secretion into the ventricles by the choroid plexus epithelium, and helps to establish a stable and specialized extracellular fluid environment

for neurons. The anatomical relationship of the choroid plexus–CSF system to the brain and spinal cord is depicted in Fig. 1. The choroidal tissues, suspended in the ventricular cavities, generate a nonvascular, nonlymphatic percolation of fluid that acts like a "third circulation." The continual formation and drainage of CSF allows this unique circulatory system to perform many diverse metabolic and signaling functions for the adult brain. Several physical and biochemical— attributes of CSF are summarized in Table 1.

2.1. Buoyancy Effect

CSF is about 99% water in its composition. Thus, the buoyant properties of the watery CSF help to protect the brain against shearing forces associated with acceleration or deceleration. The comparative specific gravities of the CSF (approx 1.007) and nervous tissue (approx 1.040) are such that the 1400-g human brain weighs only about 45 g, as it is suspended in CSF *in situ*. Thus, injury is avoided because the CSF sufficiently reduces the momentum of the brain in response to stresses and strains inflicted on the head during the course of everyday living. However, the angular acceleration that often occurs in severe trauma may override the normally protective effect of CSF buoyancy, thereby tearing or herniating cerebral tissues.

Table 1
Roles of CSF in Serving the Brain

CSF functions	Examples
Buoyancy effect	Because the brain weight is effectively reduced by more than 95%, shearing and tearing forces on neural tissue are greatly minimized.
Intracranial volume adjustment	CSF volume can be adjusted, increasing or decreasing acutely in response to blood volume changes or chronically in response to tissue atrophy or tumor growth.
Micronutrient transport	Nucleosides, pyrimidines, vitamin C, and other nutrients are transported by the choroid plexus to CSF and eventually to brain cells.
Protein and peptide supply	Macromolecules like transthyretin, insulin-like growth factor, and thyroxine are transported by the choroid plexus into CSF for carriage to target cells in the brain.
Source of osmolytes for brain volume regulation	In acute hypernatremia there is bulk flow of CSF with osmolytes, from ventricles to surrounding tissue. This promotes water retention by shrunken brain, i.e., to restore volume.
Buffer reservoir	When brain interstitial fluid concentration of H^+, K^+, and glucose are altered, the ventricular fluid can help to buffer the extracellular fluid changes.
Sink or drainage action	Anion metabolites or neurotransmitters, protein products of catabolism or tissue breakdown, and xenobiotic substances are cleaned from the CNS by active transporters in the choroid plexus or by bulk CSF drainage pathways to venous blood and the lymphatics.
Immune system mediation	Cells adjacent to ventricles have antigen-presenting capabilities. Some CSF protein drains into cervical lymphatics, with the potential for inducing antibody reactions.
Information transfer	Neurotransmitter agents like amino acids and peptides may be transported by CSF over distances to bind receptors in the parasynaptic mode.
Drug delivery	Some drugs do not readily cross the blood–brain barrier but can be transported into the CSF by endogenous proteins in the choroid plexus epithelial membranes.

2.2. Intracranial Volume Adjustor

Through physiological compensatory mechanisms, CSF volume can be increased or decreased to stabilize intracranial pressure (ICP). A relatively rapid decrease in CSF volume, resultant to enhanced absorption of CSF into venous blood, occurs in response to elevated ICP. However, CSF volume can be increased consequent to slowed absorption of CSF when ICP is reduced. The ability of CSF volume to adjust freely to alterations in ICP is the basis for the Monro-Kellie doctrine. This long-established doctrine recognizes that the brain, together with CSF and blood, is encased in a rigid chamber. Because these tissue and fluid contents are practically incompressible, a change in volume in any single constituent must be balanced by an almost equal and opposite effect in one of the remain-

ing components. Except in pathologic cases when nervous tissue volume is changed (as in Alzheimer's disease), the most common displacements of CSF volume occur in response to acute alterations in blood volume—e.g., those secondary to vasodilation or constriction of the cerebrovascular bed, as with fluctuations in arterial pCO_2.

2.3. Micronutrient Supply System

Secretory mechanisms in choroid epithelial cells transport many water-soluble substances, such as micronutrients, into CSF for eventual transport to target cells in the brain. These substances are needed only in nano- to micromolar concentrations over extended periods of time. Micronutrients transported into CSF include vitamin C, folates, deoxyribonucleosides, vitamin B_6, and certain trace elements. Active transport pump-like carriers in the choroid plexus epithelium pull these micronutrients across the blood-facing basolateral membrane of the plexus. Such substances are subsequently transported from the choroidal cytoplasm into CSF by facilitated diffusion mechanisms in the apical membrane. Thereafter, by both bulk flow and diffusion, these various micronutrients are widely distributed across the ventricular wall (ependymal lining), and more distally in the subarachnoid CSF system across the pia/glial lining, into the brain parenchyma. Ascorbate, or vitamin C, can be considered as a prototype micronutrient that is actively secreted across the blood–CSF barrier (choroid plexus), but not across cerebral capillaries of the blood–brain barrier. Accordingly, the choroid plexus–CSF nexus acts as the primary transport gateway for nourishment of the brain.

2.4. Supplier and Distributor of Peptides and Growth Factors

CSF has a dynamic function as a neuroendocrine pathway for communication and integration within the brain. The choroid plexus is an important factor in the CSF's role in neuroendocrine signaling. Receptors in the choroid plexus for arginine vasopressin, atriopeptin, and angiotensin II indicate that centrally released peptides transported into CSF can act on the plexus to modulate secretion. The choroid plexus also constitutes a pathway for endocrine communication between the periphery and brain. Within the CNS, the choroid plexus is the main site of synthesis of insulin-like growth factor II (IGF-II) and transthyretin (TTR). Following secretion into CSF, IGF-II can reach neurons and glia upon which metabolic and trophic effects are exerted. Transthyretin, known also as the thyroid hormone transport protein, is involved in T_4 transport from blood to choroid plexus to CSF. TTR synthesis occurs early in development, and its transport appears to be vital for life in higher vertebrates. The choroid plexus-CSF distributional system for many hormonal and trophic molecules is critical for brain-cell development and metabolism. Distribution of such CSF-borne signals and growth factors occurs by bulk flow of CSF driven by hydrostatic-pressure gradients between ventriculo-subarachnoid fluid and cerebral (dural) venous blood.

2.5. Source of Osmolytes for Brain

CSF has a relatively high concentration of NaCl—about 20% greater than in serum. Under certain conditions, the Na and Cl in CSF can serve as inorganic osmolytes to help restore brain volume that has been decreased as the result of the net loss of water to blood. In acute hypernatremia, for example, the brain shrinks because there is a net loss of water from the CNS into hypertonic plasma. This initial compensatory phase, involving the movement of CSF (with its inorganic ions) from ventricles into brain parenchyma, precedes the osmotic adjustment phase that occurs several days later when there is net accumulation by brain cells of organic osmolytes such as inositol and taurine.

2.6. Buffering Reservoir

A minimization of increments in ion concentrations in brain interstitial fluid (ISF) is made possible by the ability of ventricular CSF to receive, and consequently to buffer, excessive amounts of ions that can build up in brain interstices. There are pathophysiologic conditions that promote the buildup in ISF of acids (such as ischemia) or K (e.g., seizures). An excess of these ions in brain ISF promotes diffusion, down their respective concentration gradients, into CSF. Thus, the large-cavity CSF reservoir can be viewed as a buffer to accommodate such "spillovers" from brain fluids. By volume dilution, and by transport mechanisms in choroid plexus that actively remove K from CSF or effectively neutralize H in CSF (by choroidal secretion of HCO_3), there is a resultant dampening of oscillations of certain ions in CNS extracellular fluid. CSF [K] is buffered by both the Na-K pump and the NaK2Cl transporters in the apical (CSF-facing) membrane of the plexus epithelium.

2.7. Excretor of Metabolites and Toxic Substances

In addition to supplying substances for brain anabolism and maintenance, the CSF also has the function of excreting various catabolic products of neuronal and glial reactions. For example, there is a drain from brain ISF into CSF of the organic anions 5-OH indoleacetic acid and homovanillic acid—respectively, metabolites of serotonin and dopamine. Once in the CSF, these organic anions are either actively reabsorbed by the choroid plexus into blood or are cleared convectively by bulk flow of CSF through the arachnoid villi into venous blood. Such removal or "sink action" is exerted on numerous organic anions and cations, as well as proteins and other macromolecules. The iodide ion, which is especially toxic to brain tissue, is rapidly transported from the CSF by choroid plexus.

Unfortunately, some antibiotics and other potentially useful agents are actively and efficiently cleared from CSF by the plexus, thereby reducing CSF concentrations to subtherapeutic levels. Organic anion transporters, such as P-glycoprotein and the multidrug-resistant protein (MRP) in the plasma membranes of choroid plexus, actively transport many drugs out of the CNS— from CSF to the venous blood draining the choroid tissue. Pharmacologic manipulation of P-glycoprotein and MRP transporters in CP is a major challenge to pharmaceutical companies that design certain organic anion drugs to attain therapeutic levels in the CSF.

2.8. Mediator of Immune Responses in CNS

The choroid plexus–CSF system plays a role in the immunologic communication between the brain and the periphery. The plexus epithelium is able to present antigen to, and stimulate proliferation of, peripheral helper T-lymphocytes. Moreover, proteins in CSF drain by bulk flow along the SAS that envelops optic and olfactory nerves. Because such CSF drainage routes eventually pass through lymphatic tissue such as cervical nodes, proteinaceous antigenic material in CSF may elicit antibody reactions in the nodes. Such immunologic responses to proteins draining from CSF have implications for interactions between the central and immune systems in pathologic states (e.g., multiple sclerosis or allergic encephalitis), in which certain proteins in CSF display antigenicity.

2.9. Conduit for "Information Transfer"

Transmitters can be moved by CSF over considerable distances to bind to receptors in the parasynaptic mode. Thus, neurotransmitters that escape the microenvironment of the local synapses can be distributed by CSF bulk flow between large cavities and brain interstices. Arterial pulsations generate the forces needed to propel the extracellular fluid, containing the transmitters (e.g., informational molecules), along perivascular and subependymal pathways. Mismatches between receptors and their ligand concentrations, seen at the light microscopic level, support the presence of parasynaptic transmission. Gamma-aminobutyric acid (GABA) is an example of a "mismatched" transmitter that could act at a distance as it is carried via CSF between the ventricles and brain. In this manner, CSF bulk flow along circumscribed routes or channels could serve as the mediator for parasynaptic transmission. Such convective distribution of substances via the CSF-flow pathways is also known as volume transmission.

2.10. Drug Delivery Route to Circumvent Blood–Brain Barrier

In the treatment of brain cancer and other neural disorders, it is difficult to obtain water-soluble drugs

that reach target cells inside the CNS. Many strategies have been employed to facilitate drug delivery to brain parenchyma, with limited success. A particularly promising approach is to promote drug passage across the blood–brain barrier (cerebral capillary endothelium) or blood–CSF barrier (e.g., mainly choroid plexus) by utilizing therapeutic agents that can be transported by endogenous protein carriers in barrier membranes. An important example is azidothymidine (AZT), currently used in treating acquired immunodeficiency syndrome (AIDS). AZT is a nucleoside with affinity for the nuceloside-transport system in choroid plexus. Upon gaining access to CSF, the AZT or other agent is able to easily penetrate the ependymal lining that interfaces the brain ISF (extracellular fluid) with ventricular CSF. Amino acid derivatives may also be therapeutically useful because such drugs are carried by various types of amino acid transporters from plasma, across the cerebral capillary wall, into brain ISF. Once in the ISF, a drug that has penetrated the blood–brain barrier may eventually reach the contiguous CSF of the ventricles or subarachnoid space (if it is not taken up by cells). Chemotherapeutic agents that are transported along the choroid plexus–CSF-ependymal nexus seem to be readily accessible to tumors that grow along the borders of the ventricular system.

3. EARLY DEVELOPMENT OF THE HUMAN CSF SYSTEM

Embryologically, the beginnings of the ventricular system occur when the neural groove closes to form a tube. The earliest fluid within the neural tube precedes the appearance of the choroid plexus, and thus it is not a true CSF. Ciliary action within the fetal ventricles mixes the fluid and thus promotes diffusional exchange of materials across the wall of the neural tube. Early fetal brain fluid is contained within the ventricles because it can not escape into the meningeal (subarachnoid) fluid spaces.

All of the major components of the ventricular systems (e.g., first and second [lateral], third and fourth cavities), are present at early developmental stages of brain growth (Fig. 2A). The lateral ventricles are spherical and close to the middle at 2 mo. During the second trimester, a part of the first and second ventricles expands laterally as the cerebral hemispheres enlarge. Posterior and inferior expansion of the brain forces the cortex into a C shape; thus, several underlying structures (including the lateral ventricles, caudate nucleus, and hippocampal formation of the limbic system), are also molded into a C shape. At birth, the

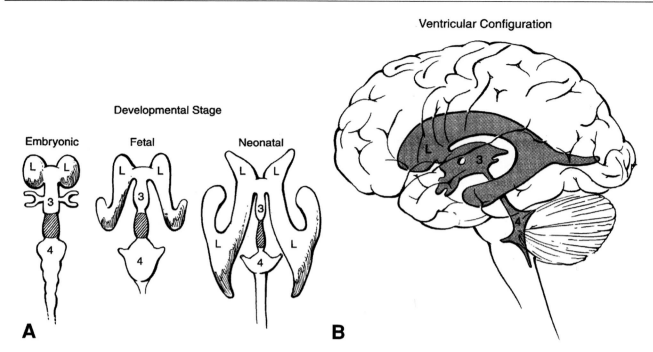

Fig. 2. (A) The shape of the ventricular system at early stages of development. Even by the second month of the first trimester, all of the major components of the human ventricles are present. In the 5-mo fetus, the first and second ventricles grow laterally as the cerebral hemispheres enlarge. By birth, the general configuration of the ventricular system is similar to that of an adult. **(B)** Physical configuration of the cerebroventricular system of the mammalian brain: The right and left lateral ventricles are located in the medial portion of their respective hemispheres. The third ventricle, which is smaller and is situated in the midline, is physically contiguous with the anterior horns of the lateral ventricles above and the fourth ventricle below. The shapes of the four ventricles are discussed in the text, and the interventricular foramina and channels are summarized in Table 2.

general shape of the entire ventricular system is similar to that in adulthood (Fig. 2B).

Choroid plexus tissue first appears in the human ventricles during the second month of intrauterine life. Several stages of differentiation of choroidal tissue have been described. By the third gestational month, the choroid plexuses nearly fill both of the lateral ventricles. Thus, the fetal choroid plexus (relative to brain size) is proportionately larger than that of an adult human being and fills more of the ventricular space. This indicates that the choroid plexus–CSF system (e.g., the ventricular fluid) has a particularly prominent role in providing nutrients to neural tissue during early development, when brain capillary density and blood flow are sparse.

The germinal matrix is contained within the ependymal wall and is the primary source of progenitor cells for the developing fetal brain. Stem cells that give rise to neurons abound in the cell layer just under the ependymal-cell lining. Growth factors of the FGF and TGFβ superfamilies, which regulate the division and differentiation of these primitive cells, are supplied by sites of synthesis such as the choroid plexus epithelium and ependyma. Regulated transport of growth factors, hormones, and other proteins from CSF to the sub-ependymal zone for modulation is an important area of ontogenic neurobiology because of the impact of CSF substances on the developing brain in the fetus.

4. DIMENSIONS OF THE ADULT CSF SYSTEM

A knowledge of the size and shape of the CSF system is essential to understanding phenomena such as the kinetics of drug distribution among CNS regions, neuroendocrine integration of fluid balance within various brain regions, extracellular aspects of the inactivation or promotion of neurotransmitter, and peptide signaling. The interior or proximal portion of the CSF system—the cerebroventricles—is involved mainly with the generation of CSF by the choroid plex-

Table 2
Channels or Narrow Ducts in the CSF

Name of channel	Location and significance
Foramina of Monro	Connect each lateral ventricle to the third ventricle; tissue adhesions may block channels.
Cerebral (sylvian) aqueduct	Connects the third ventricle with the fourth ventricle; narrowest passageway in ventricular CSF flow route and therefore the most likely site of obstruction leading to hydrocephalus.
Foramina of Luschka	Two exits located in the lateral recesses of the fourth ventricle permit access to basal cisterns.
Median foramen of Magendie	Midline at the caudal end of the fourth ventricle; direct access to the cisterna magna.

uses and percolation of the formed fluid down through the ventricles and out into the SAS. The more exterior or distal part of the CSF system—the subarachnoid space—lacks the fluid-generating choroid plexuses, and is therefore involved largely with convection of fluid into drainage sites near the venous sinuses and lymph glands.

The ventricles are linked together by channels or foramina. Ventricular CSF flows from the telencephalon to the rhombencephalon, and it finally mixes with fluid in the SAS at the base of the brain—where CSF flows out of foramina in the fourth ventricle into the cisterna magna and basal cisterns. The cisterna magna results from an arachnoid membrane bridge over the space between the cerebellar hemispheres and the medulla. Table 2 summarizes the channels and pathways that allow communication between large-cavity compartments of CSF.

4.1. Configuration

4.1.1. VENTRICLES

In higher vertebrates, the cerebroventricular system is composed of four interconnected cavities (Fig. 2B), and each contains a choroid plexus. The two lateral ventricles are more or less symmetrical with each other, and are the most prominent in size. The choroid plexus lies as a narrow band of tissue on the floor of each lateral ventricle. A thin layer known as the septum pellucidum separates the lateral ventricles, which are situated in the lower medial portion of the cerebral hemispheres. Thus, the lateral ventricles are not physically contiguous, but both communicate with the third ventricle by way of the interventricular foramina of Monro.

Each lateral ventricle consists of a main body and three horn-shaped recesses. The most rostral part of the lateral ventricle is commonly called the *anterior horn*. It is angled downward into the frontal lobe, and its apex curves around the anterior portion of the caudate nucleus. The *inferior horn* bends around the posterior end of the thalamus, extends backward and then laterally downward within the temporal lobe. The *posterior horn* runs laterally and juts backward into the occipital lobe. The region where the body divides into the inferior and posterior horns is known as the *trigone*.

The third ventricle, a thin cleft in the midline, lies below the body of the lateral ventricles. It houses the smallest choroid plexus tissue, and is located between the two thalami. The third ventricle receives CSF from the lateral ventricle and then passes the fluid downward into the Sylvian aqueduct. Anatomically, the irregularly shaped third ventricle has four prolongations or recesses (Fig. 2B). The front, lower part of this ventricle has adjacent recesses designated as *optic* and *infundibular*. The back, upper part of the third ventricle has recesses named *pineal* and *supra-pineal* because of their proximity to the pineal gland.

The fourth ventricle occupies the most caudal part of the cerebroventricular system. Lying well below the lateral and third ventricles, it is bounded by the pons, medulla oblongata, and cerebellum. The fourth ventricle has the shape of a rhombus. It is convenient to describe this ventricle as having a roof and a floor. The roof is V-shaped, and is composed of thin laminae of white matter situated between the cerebellar peduncles. A medial opening at the caudal end of the roof, known as the foramen of Magendie, is hydrody-

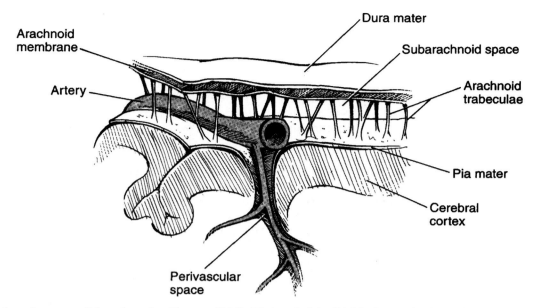

Fig. 3. Meningeal aspects of the subarachnoid space (SAS): The roof of the SAS is the arachnoid membrane, whereas the floor of the SAS is the *intima pia* or the pia-glia (the external limiting membrane of the CNS). The arachnoid and pia-glia, which are ectodermal in origin, are bridged to each other by the arachnoid trabeculae. CSF percolates through the SAS. Blood vessels that enter and leave the nervous tissue carry with them arachnoid and pia-glia, which form a cuff around each major vessel. This cuff is known as the Virchow-Robin space, which serves as a conduit for allowing fluid movement between the brain extracellular space and the SAS proper.

namically significant because CSF flows through this aperture into the SAS. Part of the roof of the fourth ventricle is occupied by the choroid plexus. The fourth ventricular choroid plexus is T-shaped, and the vertical portion lies in the midline.

The floor of the fourth ventricle is divided into symmetrical halves by the *medial sulcus*. Running perpendicular to this sulcus are delicate strands of transverse fibers—the *striae medullares* of the fourth ventricle. Other neuroanatomical features of the floor are the *median eminence* and the *sulcus limitans*. The median eminence is a longitudinal elevation that flanks both sides of the medial sulcus. The *sulcus limitans* lies lateral to this *eminence*.

The analog to the ventricular system in the spinal cord is the spinal (or central) canal. This canal ends within the *filum terminale*. Imaging studies of normal human adults reveal that CSF in the fourth ventricle does not readily exchange with CSF in the central canal.

4.2. Subarachnoid Space

The SAS lies between the arachnoid membrane externally and the *pia mater* internally. In adults, the SAS provides a route by which the fluid can flow to absorptive sites of exit from the CNS. The SAS exten-

sively covers the convexities of the cerebral hemispheres and forms a circumferential sleeve around the spinal cord (*see* overview in Fig. 1). Figure 3 schematizes the architecture of a small section of the SAS.

Because the pia intimately hugs the external contour of nervous tissue, whereas the arachnoid membrane bridges the sulci of the brain and cord, relatively large pockets of SAS are formed in between. The spaces where the bridged-over gaps are large are known as cisterns, and they are found mainly at the base of the brain. One of the largest is the *cisterna magna*, situated between the inferior surface of the cerebellum and the medulla. Because of its readily accessible location at the foramen magnum, the cisterna magna has been widely used in experimental animals as a convenient site for sampling CSF. The *cisterna ambiens* is the pocket of CSF that lies dorsal to the midbrain. Lying between the base of the brain and the floor of the cranial cavity are several other cisternae— those denoted as the pontine, chiasmatic, and interpeduncular.

4.3. Volume of CSF

The total volume of CSF in normal adult humans is about 140 mL. The volume of the ventricular system has been estimated by casting techniques, CAT scans,

Table 3
Extracellular Fluids in the CNS

Fluid	Location and characteristics
ECF	Two main types: CSF in the ventricles and SAS, and the ISF that intimately bathes the parenchymal cells of brain (e.g., neurons, glial cells).
Nascent CSF	Secreted across the apical membrane of the choroid plexuses (i.e., lateral, third, and fourth ventricles) into the ventricular space, referred to as nascent or newly formed CSF; active secretion.
Ventricular CSF	Contained in the four cerebral ventricles and aqueduct; consists mainly of nascent CSF with some exchange of content with the ependymal lining and underlying brain tissue as CSF flows down the ventricular axis.
Subarachnoid CSF	Cranial or spinal SAS; mixture of ventricular fluid that has flowed into the SAS and brain fluid that has gained access to the subarachnoid spaces; subarachnoid and ventricular CSF regarded as large-cavity CSF.
Brain ISF	Actively secreted by endothelial cells in walls of capillaries in brain and spinal cord (e.g., blood–brain barrier), modified by the water and solutes that are exchanged with brain neurons and glia; undergoes transependymal exchange with ventricular fluid; chemical composition similar to that of CSF.
Cerebral endothelial secretion	Endothelium in brain capillaries, in conjunction with astrocyte foot processes on the vascular wall, actively secrete ions and solutes from plasma into the interstices of the brain; fluid-secretory capacity of the blood–brain barrier is less than of the choroid plexuses.

CNS, central nervous system; CSF, cerebrospinal fluid; ECF, extracellular fluid; ISF, interstitial fluid; SAS, subarachnoid space.

and radioisotope distribution. By averaging the data from several techniques, the mean volume of the ventricular system is close to 30 mL. Thus, the composite volume of the four ventricles is about 2% of the brain volume. Studies have found no correlation between ventricular volume (the range of which is 10–60 mL) and brain volume.

Most of the total CSF volume of 140 mL is composed of the 110 mL of CSF in the subarachnoid spaces of the brain and spinal cord. The volume of CSF surrounding the spinal cord is at least 30 mL. Thus, the largest compartment of CSF is the nearly 80 mL in the subarachnoid spaces and cisterns that envelop the cerebral and cerebellar hemispheres.

CSF is only one of the extracellular fluids in the CNS (*see* Table 3). The other major type of extracellular fluid is the ISF that intimately bathes the microenvironment of the neurons and glia in the brain parenchyma. In practice, the CSF and ISF have similar concentrations of many, but not all, substances. Fig. 4 gives the quantitative relationship between the respective volumes of the CSF and ISF. A typical adult brain weighing 1400 g thus has about 280 mL (or g) of ISF and 140 mL of CSF, for a total of 420 mL of extracellular fluid. This can be compared with the approx 800 mL of fluid in the totality of the brain intracellular compartment.

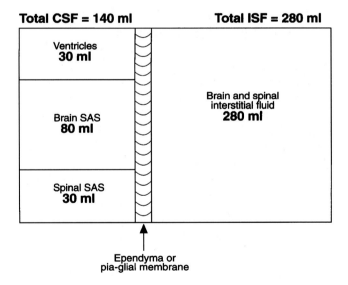

Fig. 4. An analysis of the respective volumes of the fluids in the cerebrospinal compartment and in the interstitial space of the adult human brain: Nearly one-third of the fluid in the CNS lies outside of cells. A typical adult brain weighing 1400 g contains about 140 mL of CSF (10% of its weight) and approx 280 mL of ISF that intimately bathes the neurons and glial cells. The CSF and ISF are in more or less free communication with each other across the permeable interfaces that separate them—e.g., the ependymal lining in the ventricular system and the pia-glial membrane in the subarachnoid system.

5. CELLULAR LININGS THAT DEMARCATE THE CSF SYSTEM

CSF is contained within, and surrounds, the brain and spinal cord. The CSF that bathes both the inside and outside surfaces of the brain is separated from the latter by a membrane composed of a single layer of cells. In the interior of the brain, the thin ependymal lining separates the ventricular CSF from the underlying nervous tissue. On the exterior of the brain, the pia-glial membrane is the interface between CSF in the subarachnoid space and the adjacent cortical tissue. A third membranous interface is the choroidal epithelium, a single layer of epithelial cells (frond-like in shape) that separates ventricular CSF from the blood coursing through the vascular plexus. The epithelial parenchyma of the choroid plexuses have ultrastructural characteristics that are distinct from those of the ependyma and pia-glial cells (Fig. 5).

5.1. Choroid Plexus Epithelial Membrane

The epithelium of the choroid plexus (CP) in all four ventricles consists of tightly-packed cuboidal cells with a finely granular cytoplasm. A distinctive feature of the choroidal epithelium is the *zonula occludens*, or tight junction, located in apical regions between adjacent cells. This tight junction slows down or blocks the blood-to-CSF passage of many hydrophilic molecules and ions. The electrical resistance associated with the CP membrane, however, is not nearly as great as that in the blood–brain barrier or extra-CNS tissues such as the distal tubule or urinary bladder. Consistent with its transporting function, the typical choroid cell has a high density of mitochondria, a rich Golgi apparatus, and an extensive microvilli system on the apical (CSF-facing) membrane. The basal region of the cell is characterized by elaborate infoldings and interdigitations, similar to the ultrastructure of the proximal renal tubule and other fluid-transporting epithelia. In general, the ultrastructure of the choroid cellular organelles reflects the brisk metabolic and transport activity associated with CSF secretion and ion homeostasis.

5.2. Ependymal-Cell Lining

Embryologically, the ependymal lining begins as a layer of spongioblasts lining the neural tube. In late fetal stages the ependyma is multilayered, sometimes attaining a thickness of six to seven layers. In the neonate, the lining has attenuated to two or three layers in depth. In early postnatal development, some ependy-

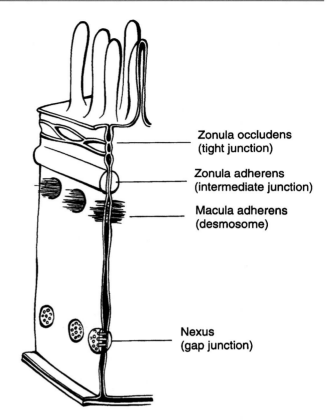

Fig. 5. Ultrastructure of the intercellular junctions in the choroid plexus and in ependymal membranes. An integral part of the blood–CSF barrier is the tight junction or *zonulae occludentes*. These tight junctions are located near the apical (CSF-facing) borders of the choroidal epithelium, where the cells abut each other. The tight junctions are multilayered membranes that completely envelop the cells, thus offering a physical restriction to the diffusion of most solutes between plasma and CSF. On the other hand, gap-junctions are present between the cells of the ependymal and pia-glial linings. The gap-junctions form incomplete belts around the cells, therefore, these intercellular junctions are more "leaky" than their tight-junction counterparts in the choroid plexus. Overall, the composition of CSF resembles brain ISF more than plasma because the gap-junctions in the ependyma permit unrestricted diffusion, whereas the tight junctions in the choroid plexus do not.

mal cells known as tanycytes send long processes that extend from their bases out into the neuropil. By adulthood, the tanycytes have largely disappeared, and the ependymal layer becomes a single layer of cuboidal or columnar cells.

Even within a given species, the ependymal lining in adults is not uniform in structure. Great variations in cellular morphology occur, especially in the third ventricle, where the ependyma are in intimate association with regions such as the hypothalamus and subcommissural organ. Emanation of cilia from the apical surface is common. In a few specialized regions in the ependyma wall, there are tight junctions between ependyma. Most ependymal cells, however, have gap-junction structures in the intercellular regions. The gap junctions do not completely envelop the cells, and thus the intercellular clefts are readily permeable to macro-molecules. Thus, the functional hallmark of the ependyma is its great permeability to virtually all ions and molecules. Therefore, once a drug or endogenous substrate is present in the CSF, it can easily permeate the ependymal wall to reach the neurons and glia.

5.3. The Pia-Glial Membrane and Other Meningeal Tissue

The pia-glial membrane is more like the ependymal lining than the choroid plexus. Discontinuous gap-junctions between the pia-glial elements allow relatively free bidirectional exchange of solutes between cortical ISF and CSF in the subarachnoid space. Large protein markers such as ferritin and horseradish peroxidase move rapidly across the pia-glial membrane, and then penetrate into subpial tissue. The Virchow-Robin spaces—perivascular cuffs of pia-glia and arachnoid that envelop major vessels as they penetrate deeply into the brain—also promote uptake of materials from the subarachnoid fluid, extending down into the brain substance. The facility of passage of large molecules from the subarachnoid CSF into underlying brain gives the impression that the pia-glial membrane, if anything, is more permeable than even the relatively "leaky" ependymal walls that encompass the ventricular CSF.

The pia mater and the arachnoid membrane are known as the leptomeninges. The pia mater, a thin connective tissue membrane, hugs the contours of the brain surface and carries blood vessels that supply nervous tissue. The arachnoid is a thin avascular membrane, located between the pia and dura mater. The arachnoid is separated from the overlying dura by the subdural space and from the underlying pia mater by the SAS, which contains CSF. In the dura mater are venous sinuses, into which CSF is cleared.

6. CIRCUMVENTRICULAR ORGANS

The ventricular wall is the site of several small, individual organs with somewhat similar structures, and distinct yet interrelated functions. These small organs are circumventricular—they surround the ventricles, and they include the area postrema (AP), subfornical organ (SFO), pineal gland (PI), median

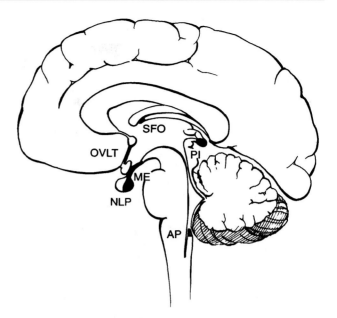

Fig. 6. Sagittal view of the anatomical relationship among the CVOs which are located on the midline of the brain. The CVOs are situated at apparently strategic positions on the surface of the cerebroventricular system to perform neuroendocrine functions. The diminutive CVOs are highly vascular and have a varying number of neurons. The CVOs are generally not protected by a blood–brain barrier and are therefore sites that contain central receptors for peripherally circulating factors (e.g., peptides). Neuronal processes extend into the large perivascular spaces of the CVOs. Each CVO is encompassed by a ring of glial cells (tanycytes) with their tight junctions that help to isolate the CVO from surrounding brain tissue. The area postrema (AP) and subfornical organ (SFO) are attached to choroid plexuses, with which they have vascular shunts. ME, median eminence; PI, pineal gland; OVLT, organum vasculosum of the lamina terminalis.

eminence (ME), organum vasculosum of the lamina terminalis (OVLT), subcommisural organ (SCO), and the neural lobe of the pituitary (NLP) (Fig. 6). The term "neurohypophysis" (NH) refers to both the ME and the NLP. Unlike most regions of the CNS, these so-called circumventricular organs (CVOs) generally have highly permeable capillaries that permit the diffusion of polypeptides and proteins into circumscribed, highly specialized regions of the brain. Thus, most of these CVOs are capable of receiving macromolecular chemical "signals" from blood. Such humoral signals are involved with the integration of neuronal pathways that mediate fluid/electrolyte homeostasis, both inside and outside the CNS.

Most of the CVOs have an ependymal interface as well as a highly permeable capillary interface. Collectively, the ependymal and capillary surface areas of

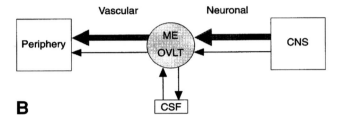

Fig. 7. Schematic diagrams of the vascular, neuronal, and ependymal components of the CVOs. The SFO and AP receive a prominent vascular input (**A**), whereas the ME and OVLT have a substantial vascular output (**B**). Neuronal output is strongest in the SFO and AP, and neuronal input is significant in the ME and OVLT. On the other hand, the SCO has relatively weak vascular and neuronal connectivities, but has substantial secretory and reabsorptive communication with the CSF.

the CVOs are relatively small—about 1% of the ventricles and brain capillary bed, respectively. Despite these diminutive transport interfaces, the CVOs and certain neuropeptide systems such as angiotensin and arginine vasopressin, carry out important functions to maintain fluid balance in the brain and whole organism (Table 4).

CVOs can be categorized in three different ways. The "parenchymal" CVOs such as the SFO and AP have dominant vascular inputs and neuronal outputs (Fig. 7A). Secondly, the "neurohumoral" CVOs or "gates," such as the ME and OVLT, have substantial neuronal inputs and vascular outputs (Fig. 7B). The third classification—the "ependymorgans," as exemplified by the SCO—have an intact blood–brain barrier but extensive communication with the CSF. The major communication of the "ependymorgans" seems to be an active apical release into the ventricular system, and possible absorption from the CSF.

CVOs have structural and functional connectivity. The subfornical organ, which has a major role in integrating water balance via angiotensin signaling, sends and receives input to and from other CVOs. Area

postrema, for example, is physically contiguous with fourth ventricle choroid plexus, and the latter has characteristics of a CVO. Lateral-ventricle choroid plexus blood flow is markedly altered when area postrema is stimulated, suggesting a mechanism by which CVO function can alter CSF formation. In general, the complex anatomical connections of the CVOs with each other, and with the pituitary and autonomic nervous system, enable these tiny CSF-adjacent organs to modulate various endocrine and homeostatic processes that maintain stability of the *internal milieu*.

7. ELABORATION OF CSF

Fluids are generated at multiple sites in the adult CNS. The source of most of the fluid is the choroid plexuses, which elaborate the CSF proper. Extra-choroidal sites of production are a CSF-like secretion by the cerebral capillary wall and the metabolic generation of water resulting from the complete oxidation of glucose by brain parenchyma. Because choroid plexus tissue is the preponderant fluid-production site, representing 75% or more of the total fluid formed, it is customary to regard the true CSF as choroidal in origin.

As an active secretion by the choroidal epithelium, CSF is not simply a passive filtration of fluid across membranes at the blood-CSF barrier. The high rate of secretion of CSF—about 0.5 mL/min/g choroid plexus, is dependent upon a brisk vascular perfusion of the plexus. The blood flow to the plexuses of approx 5 mL/min/g is about 10-fold faster than the average cerebral blood flow. The great vascularity of the plexuses is evident from the reddish cast imparted to the tissue by its relatively large volume (content) of blood.

CSF is continually replenished, and the normal volume of 140 mL turns over about three times every 24 h. Nuclear magnetic resonance studies of humans have provided evidence that CSF production may actually increase at night. However, on average, the net production of approx 0.35 mL of CSF per minute in man indicates a total 24-h formation of at least 500 mL in adults.

The initial step in the CSF secretory process is the filtration of plasma across the choroidal capillaries. The fenestrated endothelium is not a barrier to the movement of macromolecules across the capillary wall into the ISF of the choroid plexus. The interstitium offers minimal restriction to the delivery of ions and other substrates to transporters on the basolateral membrane of the epithelium. Several ion transporters

Table 4
Functions and Anatomic Associations of Some CVOs

Organ	Location	Projections	Functions
Subfornical organ (SFO)	Attached to anterior dorsal wall of third ventricle, between the interventricular foramina of lateral ventricles.	*Afferent:* Central input is poorly characterized, but is probably significant. *Efferent:* Projects into the preoptic area and hypothalamus (e.g., paraventricular and supraoptic nuclei).	Induction of drinking behavior, mediated by angiotensin signals; SFO can modulate fluid homeostasis by many mechanisms through multiple projections to endocrine, autonomic, and behavioral areas of CNS.
Area postrema (AP)	Lies at caudal extent of fourth ventricle on the dorsal medulla in contact with the nucleus of the solitary tract.	*Afferent:* Input from underlying nucleus of the solitary tract and the dorsal motor nuclei of vagus; hypothalamus also innervates AP. *Efferent:* Projections to major relay nuclei for ascending visceral sensory information; major projection to the parabrachial nucleus of the pons.	Modulates interoceptive information that reaches it through visceral sensory neurons or humorally by way of its permeable capillaries; directly affects motor outflow of the dorsal motor nucleus; stimulation of a chemotaxic center causes vomiting.
Organum vasculosum of the lamina terminalis (OVLT)	Lies in the anterior ventral extent of the third ventricle along the lamina terminalis.	Connectivity of the OVLT is poorly understood but seems to have a greater afferent input than efferent outflow.	Implicated in water balance because damage to it and surrounding structures affects drinking behavior and vasopressin release.
Median eminence (ME)	Forms the ependymal floor of the third ventricle in the central portion of the tuber cinereum in the hypothalamus.	*Afferent:* ME receives neuronal input from the arcuate nucleus and medial areas of preoptic hypothalamus. *Efferent:* No efferent projections to the brain; portal circulation carries hormones to anterior pituitary.	Represents the final common pathway for the neural control of hormone production in and secretion from cells of the adenohypophysis (e.g., anterior pituitary).

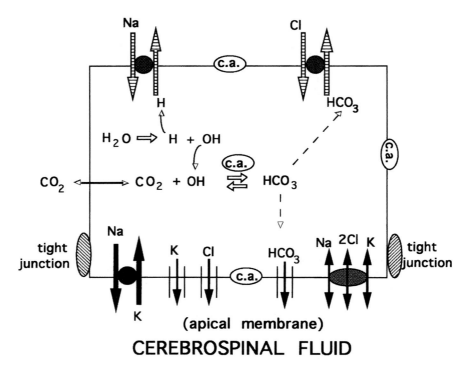

Fig. 8. Schema for ion-transport processes in the choroid plexus that underlie CSF secretion. Coordinated activity of ion transporters and channels in the apical and basolateral membranes of choroid plexus allows the vectorial transport of Na, K, Cl, HCO_3, and water from the epithelium to CSF. Active transporters in the membranes are depicted as circles or an oval. Arrows indicate the direction of the transported ions. Antiporters (exchangers) are *arrows with horizontal lines*. The primary driving force for CSF secretion is Na-K pumping in the apical membrane, which keeps the choroid cell [Na] much lower than extracellular fluid [Na]. As a result, there is a favorable, inwardly directed Na gradient that promotes secondary active transport in the basolateral membrane. For example, Na is taken up by the epithelium in exchange for cellular H ion, and Cl for HCO_3. K, Cl, and HCO_3 (generated in the cell from carbonic anhydrase (c.a.) catalyzed hydration of CO_2) can exit the cell through channels in the apical membrane. Water movement across the apical membrane is intimately associated with the active transport of ions. Na, K, and Cl can also be extruded by a co-transporter (symporter). This unified model has been constructed with transport data obtained from amphibians (E Wright, 1986; T Zeuthen, J Physiol 1991; 444:168) as well as mammals (CE Johanson and VA Murphy. Am J Physiol 1990; 258:F1544).

have been identified, and their vectorial properties are summarized in Fig. 8.

A distinctive feature of mammalian CSF is its relatively low concentration of protein and certain organic substrates. The total protein concentration in adult CSF is 2–3 orders of magnitude lower than in plasma. Glucose and urea concentrations in CSF are held at concentrations 60–70% of those in arterial plasma. Many amino acids are present in CSF at levels only 10–20% of corresponding ones in plasma; this is a result of transporters that actively remove amino acids from CSF. The pH of CSF (7.35) is typically slightly less than arterial blood (7.40), partly because CSF pCO_2, like cerebral venous pCO_2, is higher than arterial pCO2. Interestingly, CSF osmolality is slightly higher than that of plasma (by a few mOsm/L), mainly

because of the relatively high concentrations of Na and Cl in CSF. The appearance of CSF is normally that of a crystal-clear, colorless fluid; any degree of coloration is pathologic. Compositional data obtained from several mammalian species indicate that human CSF is remarkably similar to that of laboratory animals.

7.1. Formation of CSF

Quantitatively, the main constituents of CSF are Na, Cl, and HCO_3. Knowledge of the transport of these ions across the choroid plexus is essential to understanding the key elements of CSF production. The apically-located Na-K pump (ATPase) has a pivotal role (Fig. 8). Primary active pumping of Na from choroid cells to CSF keeps intracellular [Na] low (20–30 mM) compared to the extracellular (interstitial)

[Na] of about 140 mM. Thus, this sets up a substantial inwardly directed transmembrane gradient for Na, which acts as a strong driving force for the secondary active transport of Na into the cell, by Na-H exchange in the basolateral (blood-facing) membrane. Coordinated activity of the basolateral Na uptake and apical Na extrusion systems (Na pump and NaK2Cl cotransport) ensures continual net flux of Na across the choroidal membrane, from blood to CSF. K moves down its electrochemical gradient, choroid cell to CSF, and water accompanies the outward flow of ions across the apical membrane.

With respect to anion transport, Cl uptake by choroid plexus occurs by secondary active transport. Inward transport of Cl across the blood-facing membrane is driven by exchange with intracellular HCO_3. The HCO_3 is amply generated in the cell from the hydration of CO_2, which is catalyzed by carbonic anhydrase. The efflux of Cl and HCO_3, from choroid cell to ventricular CSF, involves anion movement through channels and perhaps also transport proteins like NaK2Cl symport that facilitate extrusion of anions (Fig. 8). Overall, the net transcellular movement of ions in CSF secretion is fueled by ATP—which, when hydrolyzed by its ATPase, provides the energy for creating the essential Na gradient that directly or indirectly drives several transport processes. The obligatory movement of water is intimately coupled to the net transport of anions and cations into the ventricular cavities, likely facilitated by aquaporins. The various transporters depicted in Fig. 8 participate in CSF formation, and concurrently function to help regulate choroid-cell volume and CSF ion homeostasis.

7.2. Composition and Homeostasis of CSF

7.2.1. Nascent Fluid

Newly formed fluid collected directly from the apical surface of the choroid plexus epithelium has a high concentration (mEq/kg H_2O) of Na (158), Cl (138), and HCO_3 (25), and lower concentrations of K (3.3), Ca (1.7), and Mg (1.5). Because of active transport processes in the choroid plexus, the Cl concentration in CSF is consistently greater than in plasma. CSF [K] is normally about 1 to 1.5 mEq/kg H_2O less than in plasma. In addition, the nascent CSF levels of Ca and Mg, respectively, are steadfastly held slightly lower and higher than the corresponding normal concentrations in plasma. The stability of CSF [K] and [Ca] is essential because relatively small deviations in these ion concentrations can alter CNS excitability.

Table 5 relates ionic concentrations in newly formed CSF to those in other fluids.

7.2.2. Mixing of the Choroidal Secretion with Brain Interstitial Fluid

As CSF flows from its site of origin in the CNS interior to more distal regions in the SAS on the exterior surface of the brain and cord, there are small modifications (generally 5–10%) in the ionic composition of CSF (*see* comparison of nascent vs cisternal CSF in Table 5). This occurs because the relatively permeable ependymal and pia-glial linings permit a free exchange of true CSF in the ventricles and SAS with brain ISF. The source of the ISF is presumably a slow but steady secretion by the cerebral capillary wall (the blood–brain barrier) of a fluid similar in composition to CSF. In addition, the exchange of ions and non-electrolytes across the external limiting membranes of the neurons and glia is a contributing element to the ISF composition.

In regard to protein concentration gradients within the CSF system, there is an approximately two-fold difference among regions. Lumbar CSF has about twice as much IgG and albumin as ventricular fluid (Table 6). Such differences reflect regional variations in secretory/reabsorptive phenomena at the blood–CSF barrier. Yet the roughly similar compositions of CSF and ISF ensure that, even after their mixing, the extracellular fluid of the CNS has a characteristic, if not completely uniform, composition. Thus, as the CSF flows down the neuraxis and exchanges with brain tissue, the content of protein and ions in cisternal CSF, spinal fluid, and ISF, although altered, still resembles closely the nascent (ventricular) CSF rather than plasma.

7.2.3. Regional Sampling of CSF and ISF

It is often desirable to sample CSF or brain ISF in order to evaluate the extracellular environment of neurons. Sites of CNS extracellular fluid sampling, for experimental as well as clinical analyses, are: nascent CSF, large-cavity ventricular CSF, cisternal and lumbar fluids, and brain ISF. Nascent or fresh CSF can be collected by pipet as it exudes from the choroid plexus, but complex surgical procedures are necessary to isolate the secreting tissue. CSF sampled from the lateral, third, and fourth ventricles is a mixture of nascent CSF and brain ISF that has percolated across the ependymal lining; it can be sampled by invasive stereotactic procedures that may limit application. The most straightforward and common CSF sampling procedures involve removal of subarachnoid CSF from the

Table 5
Concentrations (mEq/kg H$_2$O) of Ions in Fluids Derived from Plasma

Fluid[a]	Cl$^-$	Na$^+$	K$^+$	Ca^{2+}	Mg^{2+}
Plasma	132	163	4.4	2.62	1.35
Plasma ultrafiltrate[b]	136	151	3.3	1.83	0.95
Choroid plexus fluid (nascent CSF)	138	158	3.28	1.67	1.47
Cisterna magna fluid	144	158	2.69	1.50	1.33

[a]Fluids were collected from cats (Ames A, Sakanoue M, Endo S. J Neurophysiol 1964; 27:674).

[b]Plasma ultrafiltrate data, obtained from dialysis experiments, are values expected if the CSF were formed by passive distribution phenomena rather than by an active secretory process in the choroid plexus.

Table 6
Regional Differences in the Concentrations
of Proteins at Various CSF Sampling Sites

Protein	Ventricular (n = 27)	Cisternal (n = 33)	Lumbar (n = 127)
Total protein	25.6	31.6	42.0
	±1.1	±1.0	±0.5
Albumin	8.3	12.7	18.6
	±0.5	±0.7	±0.6
IgG	0.9	1.4	2.3
	±0.1	±0.1	±0.1

Values are means ± standard errors, given in units of mg/dL. The data demonstrate a gradient of protein concentration from ventricular to spinal fluid. Protein concentrations in CSF are two to three orders of magnitude less than in plasma. Newly secreted CSF has a protein concentration of about 10 mg/dL. A CSF protein content of >500 mg/dL can indicate a lesion that is blocking the SAS.

cisterna magna (mainly in laboratory animals) or the lumbar region (frequently as spinal taps in humans).

Experimental neuroscience has benefited from recent technical advances in microprobe dialysis. With this technique, a tiny probe is inserted into a discrete brain region for the continuous collection of brain ISF as dialysate samples. Microdialysis has been especially useful in evaluating microregional differences in neurotransmitter concentrations. Microprobes have also been placed in the cisterna magna to analyze CSF, by an approach that does not disturb brain tissue or even cause alterations in the normal volume of endogenous CSF.

Whereas relatively small regional differences in CSF or ISF concentrations have been demonstrated for inorganic ions and organic substrates such as urea and glucose, fairly large differences in regional con-

centrations have been observed for neuropeptides secreted by specific cell groups. For example, relatively high concentrations of angiotensin are found in hypothalamus ISF and in nearby third-ventricle CSF. Such concentrations of this peptide dissipate with increasing distances from the hypothalamic source.

7.2.4. HOMEOSTASIS OF CSF COMPOSITION

The hallmark of CSF is its ability to keep a stable composition of solutes in the face of severe excesses or deficiencies in plasma ions and molecules. CSF ion homeostasis is of critical importance because even small alterations in CSF [K], [H], [Mg], and [Ca] can affect respiration, blood pressure, heart rate, muscle tone, and emotional state. CSF composition has been extensively analyzed following acute and chronic perturbations in systemic acid-base parameters and ion concentrations. Analyses of nascent and cisternal CSF samples have revealed the impressive ability of the CSF system to maintain fairly even levels of K, Mg, Ca, and H ions when challenged with wide variations in the concentrations of these ions in plasma. Direct analyses of the choroid plexus indicate that this tissue plays a major role in ensuring that only minor changes occur in the concentrations of various ions in CSF. Even certain organic substrates in CSF, like the water-soluble vitamins B and C, are adequately maintained when the organism is suffering from vitamin-deficient states.

Two factors undergird the ability of the blood–CSF barrier so effectively to buffer changes in CSF composition. First, the choroid plexus, with its tight junctions between epithelial cells, acts as a permeability barrier, thereby thwarting the bidirectional diffusion of substances between blood and ventricular fluid. Secondly, the presence of numerous transporters (for ions as well as organic molecules) enables the plexus to regulate the passage of substances across the barrier. Thus, CSF homeostasis is a function of the finely controlled movement of solutes either by active transport, or by facilitated diffusion (secondary active) systems that do not directly expend energy.

In hypovitaminosis C, for example, the low levels of vitamin C (ascorbate) in plasma are avidly scavenged by an active transporter in the blood-facing membrane of the choroid plexus, for uptake into the epithelium. Once concentrated in the cytoplasm of the plexus, the ascorbate can then move out of the cell by facilitated diffusion across the apical (CSF-facing) membrane. Coordinated transport by these two mechanisms at opposite poles of the cell, working in series, enables the CSF to concentrate vitamin C to a level fourfold greater than plasma. Moreover, the basolateral active transporter for ascorbate is one-way into the cell; thus the vitamin C is not leached from CSF when the plasma level is severely reduced. Comparable mechanisms for other micronutrients, the transport of which is also a function of plasma-substrate concentration and choroid plexus carrier affinity, assure stability of CSF concentration.

7.2.5. Neurohumoral Regulation of CSF Secretion

Neurotransmitters and neuropeptides can modulate the choroidal secretion of ions, water, and proteins. In the choroid plexus, there is a great diversity of receptors for norepinephrine (alpha and beta subtype), serotonin (5-HT_{1c}), angiotensin II (AT_1), vasopressin (V_1), and others. These receptors have been localized to both the vasculature and the choroidal epithelium. An investigation of cultured choroid plexus cells showed that serotonin was able to stimulate the secretion of TTR, a quantitatively important protein involved with transport of hormones such as thyroid T_4 across the blood–CSF barrier. There is currently no evidence for a neurohumoral modulation of choroidal secretion of proteins that can adjust the viscosity of CSF, as in the well-known manner of cholinergic stimulation of salivary glands to secrete protein over wide ranges of concentration in the saliva.

In transport studies of the in vitro choroid plexus (no blood flow), it has been found that several neurohumoral agents (such as serotonin, vasopressin and angiotensin) inhibit the release of Cl from the epithelial cells into an artificial CSF-bathing medium. Because Cl transport from the *in situ* plexus to the ventricular fluid is an integral part of CSF formation, the in vitro studies are consistent with the known effects of serotonin, vasopressin and angiotensin to reduce CSF formation rate in intact animals. Neuropeptides administered in vivo can also curtail CSF formation, by an effect to markedly reduce the rate of blood flow to the choroid plexuses. Thus, substantial reductions in the vascular perfusion of the plexuses cause a rate limitation in the delivery of water and ions to the secreting epithelium.

An important and well-understood aspect of the neurohumoral modulation of CSF secretion is the involvement of the sympathetic nervous system (Fig. 9). The superior cervical ganglia send adrenergic fibers to the choroid plexuses. Upon resection of these sympathetic fibers, there is a significant increase in the rate of CSF formation. This strongly implies that the sympathetic tone on the choroid plexuses is normally inhibitory, and that when this "braking action" is released by blocking sympathetic signals, there is a resultant enhancement of fluid output by the choroidal epithelium. The findings from the denervation experiments have been bolstered by pharmacologic analyses establishing that α and β adrenergic agonists have the ability to inhibit CSF production.

7.2.6. Pharmacologic Manipulation of CSF Formation Rate

The clinical need for selective agents to lower ICP has inspired research to find drugs that can slow down CSF production. Agents from many different pharmacologic classes have been utilized to assess dose-response phenomena in the choroid plexus–CSF

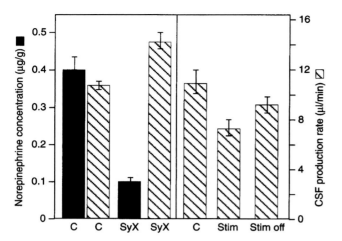

Fig. 9. Regulation of CSF formation by the sympathetic nervous system. The involvement of the sympathetic nerves in rabbit choroid plexus norepinephrine concentration (*bars with solid black fill*) and CSF production (*bars with diagonal lines*) was demonstrated in experiments involving denervation (*left*) and electrical stimulation of nerves (*right*). One week after sympathetic denervation (SyX) of the choroid plexus, there was a substantial decrease in norepinephrine concentration concomitant with a significant increase in the rate of CSF formation, compared with non-denervated controls (C). Electrical stimulation (Stim) of both superior cervical ganglia (which send sympathetic fibers to the choroid plexus) resulted in a statistically significant reduction in CSF production rate. After the stimulation was stopped (Stim off), there was a tendency toward normalization of CSF formation rate. Bars are means ± standard errors. (From C Nilsson et al., 1992.)

system. Acetazolamide, an inhibitor of carbonic anhydrase that is abundantly present in the choroid plexus, consistently reduces CSF formation rate by 50–60%. Acute usage of acetazolamide is therapeutically effective in unloading augmented CSF pressure, but chronic use leads to attenuated efficacy and undesirable systemic acidosis as a side effect. Cardiac glycosides—ouabain for example—markedly reduce CSF production by inhibiting Na-K-ATPase, but have limited therapeutic value because of their poor access to CSF and the ability to raise CSF [K]. Amiloride, by inhibiting the Na-H exchange in the basolateral membrane of the choroid plexus, can decrease CSF formation appreciably if large doses are employed, such as 75–100 mg/kg. Other diuretic-type agents can slow down CSF formation, but they introduce the expected complications resultant to the urinary loss of water and electrolytes. In summary, other agents must be identified to complement the moderately effective use of acetazolamide.

8. INTERACTIONS BETWEEN CP–CSF SYSTEM AND THE BLOOD–BRAIN BARRIER

The blood–CSF barrier (choroid plexus epithelium) and blood–brain barrier (cerebral capillary endothelium) work in concert to impart a relatively stable composition and volume to brain ISF (Fig. 10). Therefore, the microenvironment of neurons is dependent upon transfer of materials at the two barrier interfaces. Each barrier has distinctive transport and permeability characteristics. The integrity of both barriers is essential for the homeostasis of CNS extracellular fluid. Disruption of barrier function, individually or in tandem, can have deleterious effects on brain parenchyma, caused by alterations in fluid composition or pressure. Normally, the integrated flow of solutes and water across the respective barrier interfaces maintains an optimal environment for neurons and glia.

8.1. Biochemical Composition of Brain ISF

CSF formed by the choroid plexus membrane, and brain fluid manufactured at the level of the capillary wall in the cerebrum, cerebellum, and spinal cord, are not simply ultrafiltrates of plasma. Rather, the finely controlled fluids generated across these barriers are the result of active secretory processes. Once secreted into the CNS, the CSF, and the endothelial-derived fluid mix with each other (Fig. 11). Mixing is promoted by bulk flow or diffusion, depending upon the direction and magnitude of hydrostatic pressure or solute concentration gradients, respectively. Fluid mixing occurs mainly at two interfaces, the ependymal lining and the pia-glial membrane. Solute and water movements between CSF and the brain can occur bidirectionally. The vectorial distribution of a substance in a particular direction is a function of a favorable driving force, such as a concentration gradient for diffusion.

With large-cavity CSF as the reference fluid, the CSF can be considered as either a "source" or a "sink" for the brain (Fig. 12). The brisk secretory activity by the choroid plexuses furnishes generous amounts of Na, Cl, Ca, vitamins B and C (and other micronutrients), TTR, IGF-II, leptin, and additional trophic substances to ventricular fluid, allowing the latter to be a "source" of these materials for brain cells. However, nascent CSF is normally low in protein and many metabolites. Consequently, the ventricular fluid as it sweeps down the ventriculo-cisternal axis acts as a drain or "sink" to remove potentially harmful proteina-

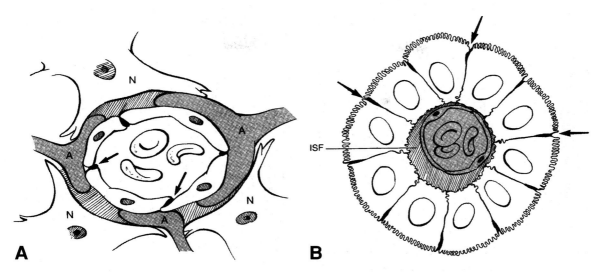

Fig. 10. Parenchymal cells of the blood–brain and blood–CSF barriers. (**A**) Highly idealized schema for the components of the blood–brain barrier. The endothelial cells of the cerebral capillaries lack fenestrations and are tightly joined by *zonulae occludentes* (*see arrows*). Astrocyte foot processes extensively abut the outside surface of the endothelium. The darkened area is the interstitial space surrounding the capillary wall. N = neuron. (**B**) Cross-section of a choroidal villus. A ring of choroid epithelial cells surround the ISF and adjacent vascular core. The basolateral surface of the cells has interdigitations, whereas the outer CSF-facing apical membrane has an extensive microvilli system. Arrows point to the tight junctions between cells at their apical ends.

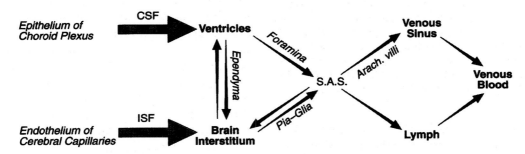

Fig. 11. Schema for fluid formation, exchange, and drainage routes in CNS: CSF is derived from constituents of plasma ultrafiltrate in the plexuses, by an active secretion that occurs in the choroid epithelia. The plexus-generated fluid percolates down the ventricular system, and then out into the SAS in the cisterna magna. From this great cistern, CSF continues to flow in the SAS overlying the hemispheres and cord. Finally, SAS fluid is reabsorped into venous blood by a hydrostatic pressure-dependent mechanism in the arachnoid villi contained within the dura mater, and into the lymphatics via the cranial and spinal nerves. Simultaneous with CSF formation at the blood–CSF barrier (choroid plexus) is the slow production of cerebral ISF by endothelia of the blood–brain barrier. Once formed, ISF undergoes bulk flow exteriorly across the pia-glial membrane into SAS and interiorly into the ventricles, across the ependymal lining. Fluid flow is usually unidirectional through the ventricular foramina and arachnoid villi, but is potentially bidirectional across the ependyma and pia-glia. For example, in pathophysiologic states such as hydrocephalus, when CSF pressure is elevated, fluid can move from the ventricles into the brain tissue. The fluid in the SAS is a mixture of CSF and ISF. Subarachnoid fluid drains into the blood, not only across arachnoid villi but also via lymphatic tissue in the eyes and nose which receive fluid drainage along the nerve roots to these organs. (Adapted from Audus KL, Raub TJ (eds). Pharmaceutical Biotechnology. New York: Plenum Publishing, 1993; 5:467.)

ceous material and various catabolites that have a higher concentration in brain ISF (as a result of brain metabolism and blood–brain barrier leaks) than in CSF. Overall, brain ISF composition is kept within narrow limits by the transependymal fluxes of solutes, the concentration gradients for which are set by transport phenomena at the blood–CSF and blood–brain barriers.

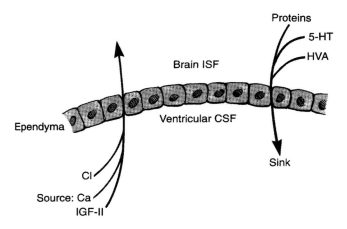

Fig. 12. CSF as a "source" or a "sink" for the brain. Depending upon the prevailing concentration gradient for diffusion across the ependymal wall, the CSF can either supply or remove solutes. The choroid plexus secretes ions, proteins and various micronutrients into the ventricles. These transported solutes are derived from plasma or from the choroidal epithelium, which has the capability to synthesize certain proteins. Once they have gained access to the ventricular system, these solutes are distributed by bulk flow in the CSF, which acts as a supplier (or "source") of materials for target cells in the brain. Conversely, the CSF functions like a drain or "sink" for solutes such as metabolites of neurotransmitters, protein catabolites, or iodide, that are breakdown products of cerebral metabolism, or that leak across barriers from blood. Once in the CSF, these potentially harmful materials are either actively reabsorbed by the choroid plexus or cleared from the CNS by bulk-flow drainage mechanisms. IGF-II, insulin-like growth factor-II; 5-HT, 5-hydroxytryptamine; HVA, homovanillic acid.

8.2. Stability of Brain Volume

Regulation of brain water content, thus the volume, is critical for maintaining ICP within tolerable limits. Brain volume is affected by many physiologic parameters. The influxes of water across the blood–brain and blood–CSF barriers are important determinants of water balance among the CNS compartments. Brain volume must be stabilized at two levels: i) the interstitial (extracellular) fluid, and ii) the neuronal and glial intracellular fluid (ICF).

8.2.1. Interstitial Volume

The ISF volume of the brain is mainly composed of the extracellular water content, and it comprises about 15–20% of the total tissue weight. Water is transported across the relatively impermeable cerebral capillary wall more slowly than it is convected across the more permeable peripheral capillaries (there is low hydraulic conductivity because of the high resistance at inter-endothelial tight junctions in the brain). Therefore, the

Starling Hypothesis, which describes the role of passive hydrostatic and osmotic pressure gradients in driving net filtration in many vascular beds, does not apply to fluid exchange in CNS between cerebral capillaries and the interstitial space that surrounds them. Normally, the water that gains access to brain by slow permeation across cerebral capillaries eventually flows out into the CSF system. As a result, the pressure and volume of ISF are maintained at levels compatible with CNS functions.

Water is also transported into the CNS through the choroid plexuses as an integral part of CSF formation. In fact, most of the water generated in the CNS originates from the four choroid plexuses. Once formed, CSF moves by bulk flow predominantly along pathways of least resistance—e.g., through the ventricular and subarachnoid spaces rather than through the less compliant brain tissue. Consequently, the orderly flow of CSF and ISF along defined pathways normally keeps the extracellular fluid volume, and thus the ICP, relatively constant.

8.2.2. Intracellular Volume

Brain volume is intimately related to water content. The water content of cells is directly dependent upon the total amount of osmotically active solutes. Neurons and glial cells are continually exchanging ions and organic molecules across their external limiting membranes. Cotransporters move solutes such as Na, K, Cl, inositol, and taurine into and out of cells, depending upon concentration gradients and the capacity of the respective transporters. Thus, water follows the net movement of transported solutes. In this manner, cell volume can be stabilized even when extracellular tonicity is altered.

As brain tissue swells or shrinks, e.g., in acute hyponatremia or hypernatremia, the activity of cellular cotransporters is appropriately modified by up- or downregulation. The result is that cell volume is rapidly re-established. Ischemic or pharmacologic disruption of cellular transporters can cause swelling of parenchyma, and thus the whole brain. Various states that alter the size of the intracellular and extracellular compartments in CNS are discussed in the following section.

9. FLUID IMBALANCES: EFFECTS ON BRAIN AND CSF VOLUMES

A consideration of the relative and absolute volumes of the brain and CSF is essential for understanding normal cerebral functions, and those caused by derangements in these fluid systems. Water imbalance in cerebral tissue can affect the tortuosity (degree and geometry of pathway winding) of extracellular channels. Such alterations in the configuration of the interstitial space have implications for excitability phenomena and the transmission of signaling molecules. Moreover, severe contraction of the ventricular volume (as in slit ventricle syndrome) may compromise the ability of the CSF to function as a "sink" for brain metabolites, or even supply trophic substances to neurons. These are examples of how brain and CSF volume changes can affect physiologic functions.

A substantial increase in the brain content of water, such as in edema, can bring about pathologic problems, including tissue herniation and intracranial hypertension. Edema may be generalized or local, e.g., surrounding a tumor or infarct. In severe edematous states, the normal flow of nutrients to brain tissue, and the orderly removal of unwanted catabolic metabolites, can be disrupted. In localized edema, herniation of tissue can involve the cerebellar tonsils through the foramen magnum or the temporal lobe uncus across the tentorium. Edematous states can also be roughly classified as mainly affecting the interstitial or the intracellular compartments of brain water.

9.1. Vasogenic Edema

The most prevalent type of brain edema is the vasogenic disturbance, which commonly occurs in regions bordering ischemia zones. Vasogenic edema is caused by increased permeability of the blood–brain barrier, which allows plasma with its content of proteins and ions to leak across the endothelial wall. The resulting increase in brain ISF volume can raise ICP, slow the electroencephalogram (EEG) and impair consciousness. White matter is particularly affected. Vasogenic edema also frequently appears with head trauma and meningitis, and can be visualized by magnetic resonance imaging (MRI) or computerized tomography (CAT scan). A substantial increase in brain volume from vasogenic edema occurs at the expense of the ventricles, which because of CSF displacement diminish to mere slits on clinical scans.

9.2. Interstitial Edema

Another fluid imbalance, in which the brain extracellular compartment undergoes swelling, is interstitial edema. Elevated intracranial pressure in obstructive hydrocephalus promotes the spread of ventricular water and Na across the ependymal lining into the adjacent white matter. Axial MRI reveals the periventricular edema as a "white rim" around the frontal and occipital horns of the ventricles. Interstitial edema caused by chronic hydrocephalus can be relieved by surgically shunting the CSF to another cavity in the body. Hydrocephalus-induced interstitial edema is associated with ventricular enlargement.

9.3. Cytotoxic Edema

Cytotoxic edema usually involves intracellular swelling of the glia, endothelia, and neurons. As a result of the collecively expanded volume of cells, there is a consequent attenuation of the size of the interstitial space. There are many different causes of cell swelling. They include drug poisoning, water intoxication, hypoxia (from asphyxia), and acute hyponatremia. Under such conditions, there is a net shift of water from the extracellular space to the interior of brain cells. Cytotoxic edema may even coexist with other forms of edema that occur in encephalitis and meningitis. Brain swelling attendant to severe cytotoxic edema leads to marked diminution in the size of the ventricular system and basal cisterns. Such distortion of the ventriculo-subarachnoid spaces can interfere with CSF circulatory dynamics, and thereby disrupt the homeostasis of molecular exchanges normally mediated by the choroid plexus–CSF system.

10. CIRCULATION OF CSF

CSF has been referred to as a "third circulation." CSF is derived from an arterial supply consisting of the anterior and posterior choroidal arteries. Choroidal venous drainage occurs largely by way of the vein of Galen. There are no lymphatic capillaries in the choroid plexuses. However, once secreted into the ventricles, the continuous flow of CSF acts like a quasilymphatic system. This unique anatomical arrangement allows brain extracellular fluid to circulate along circumscribed pathways without the presence of a true lymphatic system.

In addition to serving as clearance conduits, the CSF circulatory pathways provide a means for distributing trophic substances and micronutrients, secreted by choroid plexus, to target cells in the brain. As it heads for multiple venous drainage sites, the human CSF percolates relatively slowly by bulk flow through the ventricular and subarachnoid spaces at a rate of about 0.35 mL per min. CSF flow can be hampered by "upstream" clogging of the choroid plexus (by deposits of Ca, immune complexes, and amyloid) and by "downstream" obstruction in the arachnoid membrane (by fibrosis and amyloid accumulation). When such CSF disruption occurs in certain neurodegenerative states (such as Alzheimer's disease), the kidney-like function of the choroid plexus–CSF system is attenuated, and thus is likely to exacerbate the effects of the primary disease.

10.1. Pressure Gradients

There are several driving forces that propel CSF. Formation of CSF by the choroid plexuses occurs with a hydrostatic pressure head of approx 150 mm of water, thereby providing a force for the forward movement of the newly-formed fluid. Another force that promotes CSF circulation is the strong pulsation of blood coursing through the choroidal vasculature. Moreover, the beating of cilia extending from the apical surface of the choroidal epithelium and some ependymal cells impart an additional thrust on the ventricular CSF. The higher pressure of CSF relative to that in the dural venous sinuses creates a favorable pressure gradient of 70–80 mm water that promotes clearance of CSF by bulk flow from the SAS to the blood.

10.2. Direction of Currents

Ventricular fluid moves from the lateral ventricles through the foramina of Monro, down into the front part of the third ventricle. After leaving the posterior region of the third ventricle, the CSF continues its movement along the aqueduct of Sylvius and eventually empties into the fourth ventricle. Fourth-ventricle CSF seeps into the SAS through three different apertures. Two such exits are the foramina of Luschka, situated at the extreme lateral portions of the fourth ventricle. The third major exit is the foramen of Magendie in the roof of the ventricle, which communicates with the *cisterna magna* or the *cisterna cerebello-medullaris*.

CSF flows from the basal areas of the brain up over the hemispheric convexities until it reaches the arachnoid villi in the walls of the superior sagittal sinus. Thus, CSF from the foramina of Luschka flows forward from the cisterna pontis to the cisterns named *interpeduncularis* and *chiamatis*, from which it sweeps upward over the outer surfaces of both lateral hemispheres. It then progresses anteriorly, upward along the longitudinal fissure and over the corpus callosum, along the Sylvian fissure and over the temporal lobes. At the most distal end of the flow route, the cranial subarachnoid CSF finally encounters the arachnoid villi.

CSF is also directed from the *cisterna magna* down the posterior or dorsal surface of the spinal cord. CSF fills a sleeve of SAS around the spinal cord, and even extends below the end of the cord into the region of the second sacral vertebra. Although the spinal subarachnoid CSF is in effect an anatomical "blind pocket;" nevertheless, there is a slow mixing of spinal CSF with cranial CSF that is induced by changes in posture.

11. DRAINAGE OF CSF

The nature of CSF drainage is of particular interest to neurosurgeons because of the intracranial pressure problems created when CSF is not cleared adequately from the CNS. Normally, the CSF drainage keeps pace with CSF formation, and thus intracranial pressure is stabilized. There are two different bulk flow mechanisms by which CSF leaves the CNS, by drainage directly into the venous blood in the dural sinuses and by drainage via the cranial and spinal nerves into the prelymphatic tissue spaces and then into the lymphatics (*see* Fig. 13).

11.1. Arachnoid Villi

CSF is returned passively—along hydrostatic pressure gradients—across arachnoid villi that separate the SAS from the venous blood in the sinuses of the dura mater. The arachnoid villi have a high degree of hydrodynamic permeability, much more so than in peripheral capillaries. Therefore, if there is a sufficient hydrostatic pressure gradient of at least 30 mm H_2O, and in the right direction (CSF to blood), even large proteins and red blood cells are able to penetrate the one-way valves that regulate CSF flow into the venous sinuses. At about 120 mm H_2O of CSF pressure, the rate of CSF absorption is equal to the rate of CSF production. With additional elevation in CSF pressure, the absorption rate is augmented in proportion to the increment in CSF pressure.

Vacuoles in the mesothelial cells lining the arachnoid villi suggest an additional dynamic process of vacuolation that is pressure-sensitive. Thus, the formation of vacuoles in the valves may constitute transendothelial channels. If venous pressure should exceed that of the CSF, however, then the valves close and prevent reflux of blood back into the subarachnoid CSF system.

11.2. Lymphatics Outside the Brain

With respect to another major CSF drainage pathway, the CSF must first pass through lymphatic tissue before reaching venous blood. Sleeves of subarach-

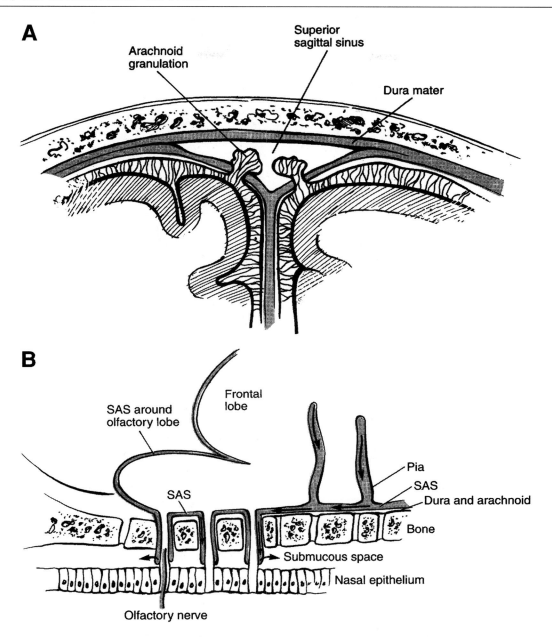

Fig. 13. Drainage of CSF by bulk flow across arachnoid villi in the dura mater and across lymphatic capillaries in the eye and nose. **(A)** A hydrostatic pressure gradient drives the CSF in the SAS across valve-like structures in the arachnoid villi out into the venous sinus. These valves are large enough to allow protein (and even cells) in CSF to pass, but usually only unidirectionally, from CSF to blood. Therefore, once CSF with its macromolecules has flowed into the venous sinus, it has effectively been cleared from the brain. The villi increase in size and number with advancing age. **(B)** Another route for CSF drainage is along the outside of cranial nerves down the submucosal tissue of the nose and eye. CSF can flow via sleeve-like extensions of the SAS around the nerve, through the cribriform plate, and finally reach the submucosal tissue of the nose. Lymphatic capillaries drain the submucous spaces and convey fluid to lymph nodes in the neck. (Adapted from M Bradbury et al. Am J Physiol 1981; 240: F335.)

noid CSF surround both the optic and olfactory nerves in particular as well as the other cranial and spinal nerves. A positive-pressure gradient promotes the flow of CSF along this perineural space that extends into the submucosal tissue of the eye and nose, in which the lymphatic capillaries resorb the CSF and convey it to

the cervical lymph glands. CSF drainage by this route is thus first exposed to the immune system before reaching the venous blood. CSF containing antigenic material (e.g., products of myelin breakdown) can thereby induce antibody reactions that have implications for reactionary immune phenomena in the CNS.

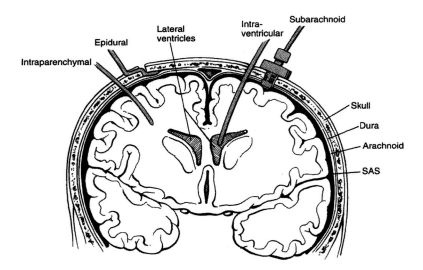

Fig. 14. Various sites for monitoring ICP. The intraventricular catheter is inserted through a burr hole, in the frontal lobe, and down into a lateral ventricle near the foramen of Monro. Placement of a probe in the epidural space carries minimal risk for brain infection because the dura remains intact. The subarachnoid bolt is placed in the SAS, but often needs irrigation with saline to remain patent. Intraparenchymal microtransducers can usually be inserted 2–3 cm into white matter without complications. (From MK Lyons and FB Meyer. Mayo Clinic Proceed 1990; 65:684.)

12. CSF PRESSURE–VOLUME RELATIONSHIPS

The bony skull is virtually incompressible; therefore, intracranial pressure (ICP) will rise when there is a significant increase in any one of the three major constituents of the intracranial space: brain parenchyma, CSF, and vascular tissue. The CSF constituent can be regarded as a potential liability as well as an asset. On the one hand, life-threatening increases in intracranial pressure can ensue when CSF drainage is blocked; on the other hand, CSF can be readily shunted to unload ICP, and the CSF pressure measurement is useful to obtain an objective measure of the response to therapy.

Markedly elevated intracranial or CSF pressure can cause irreversible injury to the CNS. Normally the CSF confers protection against impact pressures and acute changes in arterial and venous pressure. Tumors, infections, neurosurgical procedures, trauma, and diseases, however, can lead to serious elevations in ICP. There are several sites at which ICP can be monitored, and there are numerous treatment modalities available to lower the ICP.

12.1. Normal Ranges of ICP

It is common to evaluate ICP by measuring CSF pressure in the lumbar region. In patients with no pathologic lesions and with normal blood pressure, the average pressure of subarachnoid CSF in the lumbar region of reclining individuals is about 100 mm H_2O. The generally accepted range for lumbar CSF pressure is 50 –150 mm H_2O, which is equivalent to about 4–11 mm Hg. CSF production is relatively constant over the normal range of CSF pressure. However, the production of CSF may decrease when the CSF pressure is substantially elevated, as in severe hydrocephalus. The augmented CSF pressure reduces filtration of plasma across choroidal capillaries, the initial step in CSF formation.

12.2. Measurement of ICP

The pressure on the intracranial contents can be evaluated by placing probes at various depths under the skull bone, either epidurally, or in the SAS, brain parenchyma, or a lateral ventricle. These four sites for monitoring ICP are depicted in Fig. 14. A popular method for measuring ICP has been the intraventricular catheter connected to a manometer by way of a fluid-filled tube. For placement of the catheter, a burr hole is drilled over the frontal lobe. Upon piercing the dura, the catheter is directed into the lateral ventricle with the tip close to the foramen of Monro. Accurate ICP assessments can be made with ventricular probes, but not without occasional complications (Table 7).

Relatively noninvasive pressure probes can be applied epidurally. The epidural pulsations, an indirect measure of ICP, can be monitored by either fiberoptic,

Table 7
Devices and Locations for Monitoring ICP

Location	Advantages	Disadvantages
Intraventricular	Reliable measure of ICP; allows CSF drainage; good pressure waveform.	Invasive; risk of infection, need to enter ventricles; can obstruct.
Epidural	Less invasive, dura remains intact; less risk of infection.	No CSF drainage,; poor measure of ICP; no waveform.
Subarachnoid	Brain theoretically not penetrated, lower risk of infection; ease of placement.	No CSF drainage; brain tissue easily obstructed; fluid-filled system but waveform usually poor.
Intraparenchymal	Non-fluid filled system; fairly reliable measure of ICP.	Invasive; risk of infection; no CSF drainage.

CSF, cerebrospinal fluid; ICP, intracranial pressure. (Adapted from MK Lyons and FB Meyer. Cerebrospinal fluid physiology and the management of increased intracranial pressure. Mayo Clin Proc 190; 65:684; and from JG McComb [personal communication].)

strain gauge or pneumatic systems. However this approach does not have sufficient accuracy to warrant regular usage. Pressure recorded in the SAS, over the convexities, is another way to estimate ICP, but this method lacks reliability. The subarachnoid screw or bolt is a hollow tube that is secured to the calvaria. The device is connected to a fluid-filled system with an externally located pressure transducer. Intraparenchymal pressure recording is useful when a catheter fails to enter the ventricle. The Camino fiber-optic system can be used not only for intra-parenchymal recording, but also for epidural and intraventricular monitorings. Infection rates for any of the pressure-measuring systems are minimal (<1%) if the monitor is left in place for four days or less. Table 7 compares the strengths and limitations of four main approaches (locations) to measure ICP.

12.3. CSF Pulsations and Pressure Waves

Normally, CSF pulsates as the result of continuous changes in both venous and arterial pressures. Intracranial venous pressure decreases and increases, respectively, during respiratory inspiration and expiration. Such alterations in venous pressure during the respiratory cycle are concomitantly transmitted to the CSF pressure. Moreover, arterial systolic pulsations, particularly in the choroid plexus, are normally reflected as synchronous elevations in CSF pressure.

Sustained intracranial hypertension can result in pathologic "plateau waves." Instability of vasomotor control—e.g., loss of cerebrovascular autoregulation and reduction of cerebral blood flow—can trigger a sudden onset of these so-called "plateau waves." Such

clinically-significant plateau waveforms may last 5–20 min and can be associated with an ICP of more than a thousand mm H_2O. The elevated CSF pressure is a result of enhanced cerebral blood volume. "Plateau waves" occur in advanced stages of intracranial hypertension, and may indicate potential damage to the CNS.

12.4. Relationship Between ICP and Cerebrovascular Parameters

Marked elevations in ICP can reduce the arterial blood supply to the brain, causing irreversible damage to nervous tissue. Cerebral perfusion pressure is a critical parameter, and it is defined as the difference between mean systemic arterial blood pressure and the ICP. When the ICP rises to the level of systolic blood pressure, blood flow to the CNS ceases because the perfusion pressure, and thus driving force, becomes negligible. If prolonged, this can result in brain death.

Substantial elevations in ICP are thus capable of compromising the delivery of oxygen and nutrients to the brain. Because of the rigidity of the skull, the relatively fixed volume of the intracranial space cannot accommodate increases in brain-tissue mass, such as those that occur with space-occupying lesions (such as tumors and blood clots) or as the result of edematous fluid accumulation that occurs secondary to trauma. In such cases, the failure to adequately lower the ICP and maintain perfusion can be fatal.

12.5. Management of Elevated ICP

Trauma is a common cause of a rise in ICP. Cerebral edema or bleeding into CSF can markedly elevate

ICP. There are surgical as well as nonsurgical ways to alleviate intracranial hypertension of various origins. Surgical decompression is feasible in many patients such as those with hematomas located epidurally or subdurally, or even in the parenchyma. Drainage of CSF via a ventriculostomy is the prime method of lowering ICP if its elevation is secondary to obstruction of CSF drainage.

When surgery is not indicated, there are postural strategies and several pharmacologic regimens available for unloading ICP. Elevation of the head above the heart facilitates venous drainage in some patients. To minimize cerebral edema from injured cerebral vessels, fluid restriction is useful if the patient does not have *diabetes insipidus*. Extremely high levels of blood glucose should be avoided because hyperglycemia, which often occurs in head injury, can be detrimental to cerebral function if ischemia also occurs. Ventilatory support in the form of hyperventilation can rapidly lower ICP in many patients; this beneficial effect results from constriction of the cerebrovascular bed, which effectively lowers the volume of blood in the brain.

Diuretic administration has been widely used to reduce water content of the CNS, thereby to decrease ICP. Furosemide and acetazolamide curtail the choroid plexus output of CSF into the ventricles, and also function as renal diuretics, eliminating fluid from the body. Mannitol has been widely used as an osmotic diuretic agent because it slowly permeates the blood–brain and blood–CSF barriers. As the result of the osmotic gradient set up between blood and brain, mannitol is thus able to "pull" water from nervous tissue. The dehydrating effect of mannitol may be prolonged by the concurrent use of loop diuretics such as furosemide. Because mannitol may be cleared from blood faster than from CNS, a "rebound" intracranial hypertension can occur if this agent is not carefully administered.

Corticosteroids and barbiturates have limited use in controlling ICP. High doses of glucocorticoids, such as dexamethasone and methylprednisone, decrease ICP in some patients with large brain tumors, by suppression of edema formation and stabilization of cellular membranes in the edematous brain adjacent to the tumor. However, the efficacy of steroid hormones has not been demonstrated in head-injury patients. Barbiturates like pentobarbital have been used when conventional modalities fail to control ICP. The barbi-

turates confer protection by decreasing cerebral blood flow and cellular metabolism, thereby reducing ICP.

12.6. Compression of CSF and the Optic Nerve

The increasing mass of a CNS tumor can occlude drainage of CSF, with a resultant increase in ICP. Tumors distant from the ventricles may not significantly obstruct CSF flow until the mass attains a relatively large size. Tumor growths in the posterior fossa (e.g., in the cerebellum) exert pressure on the roof of the fourth ventricle, thereby obstructing CSF flow into the SAS. Brain tumors that compress the optic nerve can cause papilledema, by a choking of the optic disk caused by the high pressure inside the sleeve of dura mater surrounding the nerve. The sustained papilledema can severely damage the optic nerve and cause blindness. Papilledema can also result from *pseudotumor cerebri* (benign intracranial hypertension), a condition in which there is an increased rate of CSF production and a greater content of water in the brain interstitium. Benign intracranial hypertension, which markedly elevates ICP in young obese women, can be treated with effective resolution in several weeks.

12.7. Hydrocephalus, Ventriculomegaly, and ICP

Hydrocephalus—an increase in CSF volume within the cranial cavity—can occur with or without an elevation in ICP. *Compensatory hydrocephalus* occurs without an increase in ICP, and it represents an increase in CSF volume as a compensation for cerebral atrophy caused by primary CNS disease. Another syndrome, *normal pressure hydrocephalus*, results from impaired CSF absorption into venous blood. CSF composition and pressure are normal. Although ventricles are enlarged, there is no alteration in the size of the cerebral cortex or SAS. In normal-pressure hydrocephalus, the shunting of CSF can relieve the characteristic triad of symptoms: unsteady gait, dementia, and urinary incontinence.

Hydrocephalus with increased ICP can be categorized as either communicating or non-communicating (obstructive). In *communicating hydrocephalus*, there is free communication between ventricular and subarachnoid fluids. Hydrocephalus can be caused by altered CSF dynamics (production or absorption), or by obstruction to the flow of CSF through the SAS. In *obstructive hydrocephalus*, something impedes the percolation of fluid within the ventricles, aqueduct, or fourth-ventricle outlets. Thus, as the result of CSF-flow blockage by developmental abnormalities, inflamed tissue, or tumors, there is a retention of fluid in the ventricles with an attendant rise in ICP.

A continuously elevated ICP in hydrocephalic states with accumulation of CSF causes ventriculomegaly—enlargement of the ventricles, and subsequent compression of cells and their processes. During the early stages of hydrocephalus, there is damage to the ependyma and periventricular white matter. Two to three weeks of severe hydrocephalus can bring about compression of the cortical mantle, sometimes to 25% of its original thickness. Cytological and cytoarchitectural studies of brain cells in animal hydrocephalus models have revealed greatly shrunken somata and an abundance of vacuoles. In severe hypertensive hydrocephalus, there is even a decrease in the number of axons and blood vessels. Surgical shunting of CSF to the peritoneal cavity reduces ventriculomegaly and decompresses the cerebral cortex. If the shunting is done early enough, much of the structural and functional damage to cells can be reversed. Shunting removes many CSF-borne trophic substances from the CNS extracellular fluid, and this effect must be elucidated.

13. CELLULAR COMPOSITION OF CSF

A distinguishing feature of CSF, especially in relationship to blood, is its paucity of cellular elements. CSF usually contains no more than four mononuclear cells or lymphocytes per cubic millimeter. White-cell counts of 5 to 10 per mm^3 can occasionally signify a pathological condition. An elevated cell count in CSF can occur as the result of brain injury, central inflammatory processes, or the spreading of tumor cells. Cytological examination of CSF is becoming more delineative with the application of polyclonal and monoclonal antibodies to identify specific pathologic processes.

13.1. Normal Conditions

The relatively high water content of CSF, e.g., >99%, is reflective of a very low cell count. The only cells routinely observed in normal CSF are a few small lymphocytes (B and T cells) and monocytes. It is even rare to find sloughed choroid epithelial, ependymal, or arachnoidal cells in CSF samples that are otherwise normal in appearance. The relatively impermeable barriers prevent the penetration of formed elements of the blood into the CSF compartment of healthy humans. The occasional appearance of erythrocytes in CSF samples (usually tapped from the lumbar region) indicates contamination of the collected CSF specimen with blood.

13.2. Infective States

CSF pleocytosis is commonly present in acute infections of the CNS. In fungal infections, the predominant type of cell in CSF is the lymphocyte, whereas in bacterial infections it is the neutrophil. In acute bacterial meningitis, 90% or more of the cells in CSF may be neutrophils. With severe infections, especially when a ruptured abscess occurs, CSF cell counts can exceed 20,000 per mm^3 (e.g., μL).

The appearance of ependymal and choroidal cells in CSF, along with the white blood cells, can be a manifestation of neurological diseases and infections. However, the mumps virus is unique in that it causes ependymitis. Such destruction of the ependymal lining can lead to narrowing of the cerebral aqueduct, with resulting hydrocephalus.

The cellular composition of CSF in AIDS patients is highly variable. In one study of HIV-1 infection, only a small percentage of patients developed lymphocytic pleocytosis in CSF, even when the full picture of acquired immunodeficiency syndrome (AIDS) was present. AIDS patients have a high frequency of opportunistic infections. Therefore, their CSF profiles of immune cells will be similar to those caused by the opportunistic invader, although the magnitude of the response may be blunted by the immunodeficient state.

13.3. Neoplastic Diseases

CSF sampling can be used for the management of patients with brain tumors. Primary neoplasms around the brainstem, cerebellum, and spinal cord can abut CSF pathways and shed tumor cells, which appear in the sediment of CSF samples. Medulloblastomas arising from the external germinal layer of the cerebellum may shed many tumorous cells into the CSF. In contrast, meningiomas shed few malignant cells into CSF. Meningiomas are firm, arachnoidal elements that do not readily exfoliate cells; thus, the low frequency of positive CSF specimens.

Metastatic neoplasms (carcinomatosis) have a greater propensity to exfoliate cells than most of the primary tumors. Thus there is a high yield (20–50% positive) from cytologic examination of malignant cells in CSF of patients with cerebral metastases. Carcinomas of the lung, stomach, and breast are among the most common to metastasize into the CSF. The less frequently occurring melanoma usually metastasizes rapidly to the brain and CSF, and is cytologically characterized by pigmentation. Occasionally, the CNS–CSF metastasis is present before the primary peripheral tumor is discovered. Inflammatory cells are often interspersed with tumor cells in the CSF. When the exfoliated tumor cells in CSF are sufficiently characteristic, the primary site of origin outside the CNS can sometimes be identified.

The complete treatment of leukemia is dependent upon CSF cytological analysis. Because many chemotherapeutic agents do not readily penetrate the blood–CSF and blood–brain barriers, malignant cells inside the CNS are often left intact after treatment. Because surviving tumor cells in the subarachnoid CSF can be a reservoir that contributes to a later systemic relapse, it is essential to ascertain the presence of even a small number of leukemic cells in CSF. The technique of flow cytometry combined with monoclonal antibody (MAb) staining enables the detection of small numbers of specific malignant cells. Such CSF examination is important in leukemia management to determine whether radiation or intrathecal treatment is indicated.

14. CLINICAL USAGE OF CSF

Many neurological disorders are associated with changes in the chemical composition of CSF. As metabolic processes in brain tissue are altered by disease or trauma, the numerous cellular metabolites that are released into the surrounding interstitial fluid eventually gain access to the CSF. Thus, CSF biochemical profiles are often altered during illness or injury. Such changes in CSF composition can sometimes mirror modifications in cerebral chemistry. Therefore, clinicians have learned to use CSF findings to guide diagnoses and management. Limitations to this approach have to be recognized. Nevertheless, if CSF sample contents are appropriately interpreted, such biochemical and cellular analyses can be diagnostically valuable.

The SAS in the lumbar spinal cord is a convenient penetration point for sampling CSF, after the potential value and risks of the tapping have been considered. Although computed tomography (CT) has obviated the need for some lumbar punctures (e.g., suspected subarachnoid hemorrhage), there are many indications for procuring CSF samples.

14.1. Diagnostic Aid

Lumbar punctures are done mainly for diagnostic reasons. Analyses of CSF can strengthen the diagnoses of neurosyphilis, multiple sclerosis, and many inflammatory diseases of the brain and its meningeal coverings. Inexplicable seizures should also prompt the analysis of CSF biochemistry. In myelographic procedures, the CSF removed at the initial stage of the procedure should be appropriately characterized to serve as a baseline for future comparisons. Access to the CSF system by way of a lumbar tap also permits the measurement of pressure in clinical assessments of intracranial hypertension.

14.2. Intrathecal/Intraventricular Administration of Drugs

Some drugs that cross the blood–brain and CSF barriers too slowly to be therapeutically useful can be continuously administered intraventricularly (by lateral ventriculostomy) or intrathecally (by infusion into spinal subarachnoid fluid) (see Fig. 15). Injection of drugs directly into human nervous tissue is usually not feasible, but agents infused into the CSF of patients move by bulk flow eventually to spread into the brain and spinal cord by diffusion across permeable interfaces like the ependyma (ventricles) and pia-glia (SAS).

CSF infusion circumvents the barriers and exploits pharmacokinetic factors. Drug metabolism and binding to proteins is usually less of a problem in CSF than in plasma. Central administration of drugs largely avoids renal/hepatic metabolism. Because CSF has a relatively low content of protein, there is much less chance that a drug effect will be diminished by extensive binding to a large reservoir of extracellular albumin or another protein.

There is already an advanced technology of the implantable pump systems to deliver drugs into CSF. Some implanted pumps hold as much as 50 mL and deliver at rates of 75 to 100 µL per min. The variation in delivery rate is about ±5%. Drug dose is regulated by adjusting concentration in the reservoir. Stability of the therapeutic agent is required for many weeks at 37°C in a CSF-like buffer. Diluents (vehicles) are confined to a certain pH and osmolality, and cannot contain a solubilizing agent that is potentially harmful to the exquisitely sensitive brain tissue.

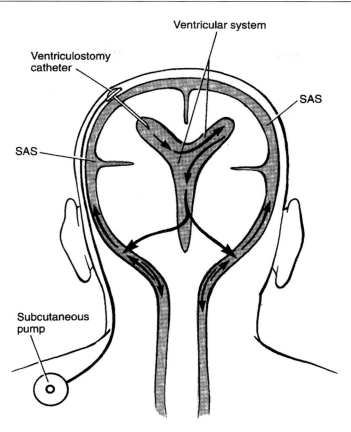

Fig. 15. CSF infusions of drugs through a totally implanted system for constant intraventricular drug infusion. The components of the system include a subcutaneously implanted Infusaid pump, Silastic catheter, and ventriculostomy reservoir and catheter. The amount of drug for the refill is calculated as the product of dose rate times pump capacity, divided by flow rate of pump. SAS, subarachnoid space (From Dakhil S, Ensminger W, Kindt G, et al. Cancer Treatment Reports 1981; 65:405.)

A big plus for the CSF drug-delivery approach is the ability to localize the desired pharmacologic effect. This is significant because many neurologic diseases are circumscribed to a specific region. Drug delivery inside the CNS is most effective when there is an optimal blending of pharmacodynamics and pharmacokinetics. Intrathecal morphine, used successfully in pain control, avoids systemic narcotic effects such as anorexia and oversedation. Intraventricularly administered bethanechol (an acetylcholine agonist) has led to some improvement in Alzheimer's patients. Additional clinical investigations of CNS diseases will reveal how higher brain-center functions can be effectively modified with intraventricular infusions of therapeutic agents.

15. NEW PARADIGMS FOR CSF FUNCTIONS

There is a surge of interest in the CSF concentration and conveyance of neuropeptides, transport proteins and growth factors. The primary sources of these substances, and the kinetics of their distribution throughout the ventricular system and surrounding brain tissue, have numerous implications to developmental neurobiologists and clinicians who treat neurological disorders. As the main transport interface between blood and CSF, the choroid plexuses furnish not only ions and vitamins, but also a wide variety of proteinaceous macromolecules to the CSF-brain system for maintenance as well as reparative purposes.

Peripherally manufactured hormones such as leptin, insulin/IGF-I, and luteinizing hormone are transported from blood to CSF. Although the functional significance of these CSF-borne hormones must be elucidated, it is clear that transport proteins facilitate the passage of hormones from the plexus into the ventricles. One such protein is TTR (or prealbumin), elaborated by choroid plexus for secretion into CSF. The choroid plexus is the only site within the CNS that manufactures and secretes TTR. TTR helps to carry thyroid hormone T4 across the choroid plexuses into ventricular CSF. Schreiber and colleagues have demonstrated mRNA in choroid plexus for other transport proteins, such as ceruloplasmin and transferrin, implicated in the carriage of trace elements like copper and iron, from plasma to CSF. Such a transport path represents an important supply route to the brain, via the CSF.

On the other hand, numerous peptides are synthesized within the CNS for delivery by volume transmission and CSF-flow routes to glia and neurons. The choroid plexus and certain hypothalamic nuclei make and secrete certain peptides into the extracellular *milieu* of the brain. CSF bulk-flow routes through the ventricular and subarachnoid systems then promote the paracrine and endocrine-like distribution of these peptides, including vasopressin, angiotensin, and atriopeptin to various regions in the CNS. Release of these central peptides into brain ISF and CSF is stimulated by alterations in extracellular osmolality or [Na] or by perturbations associated with ischemia and trauma to the brain. Target cells with receptors for these peptides are located in the choroid plexus, CVOs, and at the blood–brain barrier. Vasopressin and angiotensin, which alter the CSF formation rate and blood–brain-barrier permeability, have a modulatory role in fluid and electrolyte balance. Promising vistas for future neuroendocrine research are based on the premise that regulation of brain volume and fluid composition is mediated by diverse physiologic actions induced by these peptides.

In regard to growth factors, the choroid plexus–CSF nexus is of great importance to the brain as it is developing, and again later in life as it is undergoing repair after exposure to stressors. The plexus produces IGF-II, FGF-2, TGF$_\beta$, and HGF as well as binding proteins for growth factors. Research is needed to pinpoint target cells in brain for the many growth factors synthesized/transported by the epithelium of the blood–CSF barrier. During fetal development, cells that form the cerebral cortex arise from a layer of neuroepithelial cells surrounding ventricular CSF. The roles of growth factors and other trophic proteins in modulating stem cells in the subventricular zone, and in the cellular migration processes, are currently the topic of important ontogenetic investigations. For example, brain development is curtailed when hydrocephalus blockage of CSF flow prevents the normal presentation of growth factors and other proteins to proliferative zones near ventricular and subarachnoid

CSF. The ability of the adult brain to repair itself after trauma and stroke is likely dependent, at least in part, upon growth-factor availability from the choroid plexus–CSF system. Ischemia research models have revealed that NGF, IGF, and TGF$_\beta$ administered intraventricularly minimize the development of damage to the adult brain. This indicates the possible therapeutic usefulness of growth factors administered by the CSF route.

Collectively, many studies indicate that a certain complement of proteins, micronutrients and trace elements in CSF is essential for a healthy brain. There is a steadily growing body of evidence that the secretions of the choroid plexus, together with products formed by ependymal and arachnoid cells, produce an extracellular *milieu* that bestows beneficial effects upon neurons. Moreover, in aging/neurodegeneration losses which occur in Alzheimer's disease and cerebrovascular disruptions, the compromised carriage of CSF-borne trophic materials (and reduced clearance of catabolites) may exacerbate disturbances in brain-fluid homeostasis. In treating CNS disorders, it is a worthy goal in gene therapy and pharmacotherapy to employ vectors and antibodies that target choroid and meningeal cells for the purpose of minimizing injury effects and restoring the accommodating functions of the CSF system.

SELECTED READINGS

Aldred AR, Jaworowski A, Nilsson C, Achen MG, Segal MB, et al. Thyroxine transport from blood to brain via transthyretin synthesis in choroid plexus. Am J Physiol. 1990; 258: R338–R345.

Adelman G (ed). Choroid Plexus. Encycl Neurosc, (Vol. I). 1987; 236–239.

Boulton AA, Baker GB, and Walz W (eds). Neuromethods. 9. Neuronal Microenvironment. Clifton, NJ:Humana Press, 1988; 33–104.

Bradbury M. The Concept of a Blood–Brain Barrier. Pitman Press: Bath, England: John Wiley & Sons, 1979; 1–465.

Butler AB. Alteration in CSF outflow in experimental acute subarachnoid hemorrhage. In: Outflow of Cerebrospinal Fluid, Gjerris F, Borgesen SE, and Sorensen PS (eds). Copenhagen:Munksgaard:1989; 69–75.

Chodobski A, Szmydynger-Chodobska J. Choroid plexus: target for polypeptides and site of their synthesis. Microscopy Research and Technique. 2001; 52:65–82.

Cserr HF, Fenstermacher JD, Fencl V (eds). Fluid Environment of the Brain, London:Academic Press, Inc., 1975; 1–289.

Cserr HF, DePasquale M, and Patlak CS. Regulation of brain water and electrolytes during acute hyperosmolality. Am J Physiol 1987; 253:F522–F529.

Davson H, Welch K, Segal MB (eds). The Physiology and Pathophysiology of the Cerebrospinal Fluid. London:Churchill Livingstone: 1987; 1–1013.

Fishman RA. Cerebrospinal Fluid in Diseases of the Nervous System. Philadelphia:W.B. Saunders Co., 1980; 1–325.

Gross PM (ed). Circumventricular Organs and Body Fluids, Vol. 1 Boca Raton, FL: CRC Press, Inc., 1987; 1–203.

Herkenham M. Mismatches between neurotransmitter and receptor localizations in brain: observations and implications. Neuroscience 1987; 23:1–38.

Herndon RM, Brumback RA (eds). The Cerebrospinal Fluid. Amsterdam:Kluwer Academic Publishers, 1989; 1–306.

Johanson C. Biological Barriers to Protein Delivery. Tissue barriers: diffusion, bulk flow and volume transmission of protein within the brain. In Audus KL, Raub TJ (eds). Pharmaceutical Biotechnology, (Vol. 5.) New York:Plenum Pub. Corp., 1993; 467–486.

Johanson CE. Choroid plexus and volume transmission. In Adelman G (ed) Encyclopedia for Neuroscience. (Vol. 1.) 3rd electronic edition, 2003.

Johnson CE, et al. Choroid plexus recovery after transient forebrain ischemia: role of growth factors and other repair mechanisms. Cel Mol Neurobiol 2000; 20:197–216.

Johnston M, Papaiconomou C. Cerebrspinal fluid transport: a lymphatic perspective. News Physiol Sci 2002; 17: 227–230.

Jones HC, Keep RF. The control of potassium concentration in the cerebrospinal fluid and brain interstitial fluid of developing rats. J Physiol 1987; 383:441–453.

Katzman R, Pappius HM (eds). Brain Electrolytes and Fluid Metabolism. Baltimore:The Williams and Wilkins Co., 1973.

Lyons MK, Meyer FB. Cerebrospinal fluid physiology and the management of increased intracranial pressure. Mayo Clinic Proc 1990; 65:684–707.

McAllister J, Cohen K, O'Mara K, Johnson M. Progression of kaolin-induced hydrocephalus in neonatal kittens and decompression with ventriculoperitoneal shunts: correlation of radiologic findings and gross morphology. Neurosurgery 1991; 29: 329–340.

McComb JG, Zlokovic BV. Choroid plexus, cerebrospinal fluid, and the blood-brain interface. In Chick WR (ed). Pediatric Neurosurgery, Imaging of the Developing Nervous System, 3rd ed., Philadelphia:W.B. Saunders;1993.

Milhorat TH. Cerebrospinal Fluid and The Brain Edemas. New York™:Neuroscience Society of New York, 1987; 1–168.

Nathanson JA, Chun LLY. Possible role of the choroid plexus in immunological communication between the brain and periphery. In Johansson BB, Owman C, Widner H (eds). Pathophysiology of the Blood–Brain Barrier. Amsterdam: Elsevier, 1990; 501–507.

Netsky MG, Shuangshoti S. The Choroid Plexus in Health and Disease, Charlottesville:University Press of Virginia, 1975; 1–351.

Neuwelt EA (ed). Implications of the Blood-Brain Barrier and Its Manipulation, Vol. 1. New York: Plenum Medical Book Co.,1989; 1–390.

Nilsson C, Lindvall-Axelsson M, Owman C. Neuroendocrine regulatory mechanisms in the choroid plexus-cerebrospinal fluid system. Brain Res Rev 1992; 17:109–138.

Pollay M. Formation of cerebrospinal fluid. J Neurosurg. 1975; 42:665–673.

Rapoport SI. Blood–Brain Barrier in Physiology and Medicine. New York:Raven Press, 1976; 1–316.

Rennels ML, Gregory TF, Blaumanis OR, Fujimoto K, and Grady PA. Evidence for a 'paravascular' fluid circulation in the mammalian central nervous system, provided by the rapid distribution of tracer protein throughout the brain from the subarachnoid space. Brain Res 1985; 326:47–63.

Spector R. Micronutrient homeostasis in mammalian brain and cerebrospinal fluid. J Neurochem 1989; 53:1667–1674.

Spector R, Johanson CE. The mammalian choroid plexus. Sci American 1989; 260:68–74.

Stopa EG, Berzin TM, Kim S, Song P, Kuo-LeBlanc V, Rodriguez-Wolf M, et al. Human choroid plexus growth factors: What are the implications for CSF dynamics in Alzheimer's disease? Exper Neurol 2001; 167:40–47.

Williams JL, Thebert MM, Schalk KA, Heistad DD. Stimulation of area postrema decreases blood flow to choroid plexus. Am J Physiol 1991; 260: H902–H908.

Wood JH (ed). Neurobiology of Cerebrospinal Fluid, Vol. 1. New York: Plenum Press, 1980; 1–768.

Wright EM. The choroid plexus as a route from blood to brain. Ann NY Acad Sci 1986; 481:214–220.

9 Organization of the Spinal Cord

Marion Murray

1. THE SPINAL CORD

Sensory information from the body is transmitted into the central nervous system (CNS) through the dorsal-root projections into the spinal cord. Motor neurons in the spinal cord project their axons into the periphery to innervate muscles and autonomic ganglia. Somatic perceptions, coordinated movements, and autonomic functions depend on the integrity of the spinal cord and its projections. The neurons and fiber bundles within the spinal cord are organized in a simpler and more uniform way than other parts of the

CNS, but the features of organization and function are similar to those found in more complexly organized regions of the brain.

1.1. Segmental Organization of the Spinal Cord

During early embryonic life, the spinal cord extends almost the whole length of the vertebral canal. As development proceeds, the body and the vertebral column grow at a much greater rate than the spinal cord. As a result, in newborns the spinal cord extends only as far caudally as the mid-lumbar vertebral levels, but in adults only to the level of the first or second lumbar vertebrae (Fig. 1). Dorsal and ventral roots

From: *Neuroscience in Medicine, 2nd ed.* (P. Michael Conn, ed.),
© 2003 Humana Press Inc., Totowa, NJ.

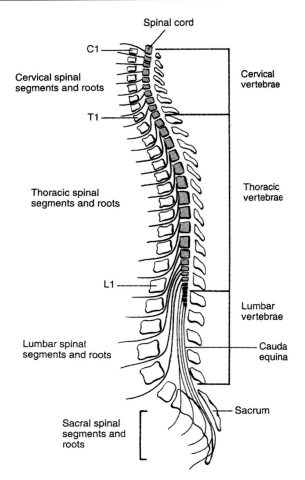

Fig. 1. The organization of the spinal cord into cervical, thoracic, lumbar, and sacral segments. Note the exit of the lumbar and sacral roots through intervertebral foramina located caudal to the spinal segment with which the roots are associated.

enter and leave the vertebral column through intervertebral foramina at vertebral segments corresponding to the spinal segment. Because the vertebral column is longer than the spinal cord in the adult, the caudal roots are longer than the more rostral roots. At its caudal end, the cord tapers markedly to form the *conus medullaris*, and the lumbar, sacral, and coccygeal roots extending to their appropriate vertebral levels form bundles, the *cauda equina* ("horse's tail"), surrounding the *conus*.

The spinal cord is organized into 31 continuous spinal segments. These are divided into cervical (C1–C8) segments, including those that supply the arms, thoracic (T1–T12) segments innervating the trunk and sympathetic ganglia; lumbar (L1–L5) segments supplying the legs, and sacral (S1–S5) and coccygeal (one segment) segments supplying the saddle

region, the buttocks, and pelvic organs, and the parasympathetic ganglia.

A *segment* is defined by dorsal roots that enter and ventral roots that exit the cord (Fig. 2). The axons in the dorsal-roots arise from dorsal root ganglion cells located in the ganglia that are lateral to the vertebral column.

A pair of *dorsal root ganglia* is associated with each segment (except C1, which may have no ganglia). Each dorsal-root ganglion cell gives rise to two *axonal processes*. One axonal process enters a spinal nerve. Some of these peripheral sensory axons receive information from sensory receptors in the skin; the strip of skin supplied by the peripheral process from cells in one dorsal-root ganglion is known as a *dermatome* (Fig. 3). Adjacent dermatomes overlap considerably, so that any portion of the skin is likely to be supplied by sensory axons in several peripheral nerves; damage to a single dorsal-root will therefore result in little sensory loss. The other axonal process arising from the dorsal-root ganglion cell projects through the dorsal root to terminate on neurons within the CNS.

Because sensory information from the body is relayed to the CNS through the dorsal roots, axons originating from dorsal-root ganglion cells are sometimes called *primary afferents*. A small population of dorsal-root axons enters the spinal cord through the ventral-root (ventral root afferents) but their functional significance is unclear. However, most axons in the ventral roots arise from motor neurons in the spinal cord and innervate skeletal muscles or autonomic ganglia. These ventral-root axons join with the peripheral processes of the dorsal-root ganglion cells to form the spinal nerve, which thus contains both sensory and motor axons. Several spinal nerves may join to form a peripheral nerve, which is, of course, also mixed sensory and motor. The axons in the peripheral nerves are classified according to diameter, and this provides a useful correlation with the functions they serve (Table 1).

2. SPINAL NEURONS ORGANIZED INTO NUCLEI AND INTO LAMINAE

In cross-sections, the spinal cord is composed of a butterfly-shaped core of *gray matter* (cell bodies and their processes) surrounded by *white matter* (axons, most of which are myelinated). The gray matter is subdivided into a sensory portion, the *dorsal* (or *posterior*) horn and a motor portion, the *ventral* (or *anterior*) *horn*, separated by an *intermediate zone* (Fig.4).

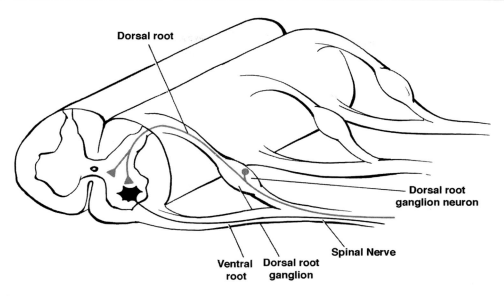

Fig. 2. In the diagram of two segments of spinal cord, three dorsal roots enter the dorsal lateral surface of the cord, and three ventral roots exit. The dorsal-root ganglion contains dorsal-root ganglion cells whose axons bifurcate; one process enters the spinal cord in the dorsal root and the other extends peripherally to supply the skin and muscle of the body. The ventral root is formed by axons from motor neurons located in the spinal cord.

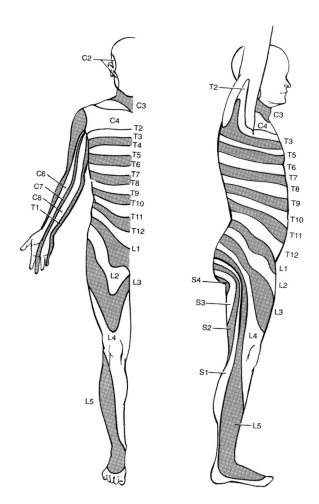

The neurons of the spinal gray matter are also classified according to their projections. These include *sensory relay neurons*, which receive dorsal-root input with axons that project into the ascending pathways, *motor neurons* with axons that exit in the ventral roots, and *propriospinal* cells, spinal interneurons whose axons do not leave the spinal cord. Propriospinal interneurons are by far the most numerous, accounting for about 90% of all spinal neurons.

As in other areas of the nervous system, many of the neurons in the gray matter are organized in functionally related clusters known as *nuclei*. These nuclei may extend the length of the spinal cord, forming columns of functionally related cells. In cross-sections, the neurons in the gray matter can also be seen to have a laminated distribution, particularly in the dorsal horn. Because the histologic differences between laminae reflect functional differences, the spinal gray matter is sometimes also classified into laminae. The various schemes for classifying spinal neurons are compared in Table 2.

The dorsal horn and intermediate zones (laminae I–VII) contain sensory relay nuclei, including the *marginal* (lamina I) and *proprius* (lamina III, IV) nuclei and the *substantia gelatinosa* (lamina II). Motor

Fig. 3. (*Left*) A dermatome is the area of skin supplied by axons from a single dorsal-root ganglion.

Table 1
Axons in Peripheral Nerves

Fibers	Diameters (μm)	Conduction velocity (m/s)	Role or receptors innervated
Sensory			
Ia (A–α)	12–20, myelinated	70–120	Muscle-spindle afferents.
Ib (A–α)	12–20, myelinated	70–120	Golgi tendon organ; touch and pressure receptors.
II (A–β)	5–14, myelinated	25–70	Secondary afferents of muscle spindle; touch, pressure, and vibratory sense receptors.
III (A–δ)	2–7, myelinated	10–30	Crude touch and pressure receptors; pain and temperature receptors; viscera.
IV (C)	5–1, unmyelinated	<2.5	Pain and temperature receptors; viscera.
Motor			
Alpha (A–α)	12–20	15–20	Alpha motor neurons innervating extrafusal muscle fibers.
Gamma (A–γ)	2–10	10–15	Gamma motor neurons innervating intrafusal muscle fibers.
Preganglionic autonomic fibers (B)	>3	3–15	Lightly myelinated preganglionic autonomic fibers.
Postganglionic autonomic fibers (C)	1	2	Unmyelinated postganglionic autonomic fibers.

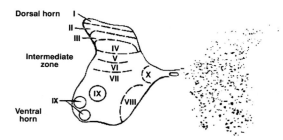

Fig. 4. Composite figure compares the classification schemes for the neurons in the gray matter of the spinal cord. *On the right :* a section stained to show cell distribution and location of nuclei in the lumbar spinal cord, and *on the left,* the related laminar boundaries.

neurons are functionally subdivided into *somatic* and *visceral motor neurons*. Somatic motor neurons are located in the ventral horn (laminae VIII and IX) at all spinal levels, and innervate striated muscle. All visceral motor neurons are located in the intermediate zone (lateral horn, lamina VII) at C8–L3 (sympathetic) or S2–S4 (parasympathetic), and innervate neurons in autonomic ganglia.

3. ASCENDING AND DESCENDING TRACTS IN WHITE MATTER

The white matter is subdivided into dorsal (ascending), lateral (ascending and descending), and ventral (descending)*funiculi*, demarcated by the dorsal medial sulcus, the dorsal-root entry zone, the ventral roots, and the ventral medial sulcus (Fig. 5). The axons in the white matter form pathways that are classified as ascending (sensory), descending (motor), or propriospinal; individual pathways or tracts run in specific funiculi.

Table 2
Classification of Spinal Neurons

Gray matter subdivision	Lamina	Nuclei included in Laminae
Dorsal horn	Lamina I	Marginal nucleus
	Lamina II	Substantia gelatinosa
	Lamina III, IV	Nucleus proprius
Intermediate zone	Lamina V	Reticular nucleus
	Lamina VI	Commisural nuclei
	Lamina VII	Clarke's, intermediolateral nuclei
Ventral horn	Lamina VIII	Medial motor nuclei
	Lamina IX	Lateral motor nuclei
	Lamina X	Central gray

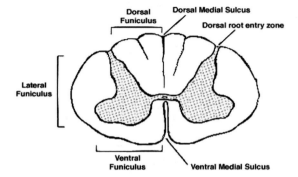

Fig. 5. Cross-section of cervical spinal cord shows major landmarks and divisions of white matter.

Cells in the dorsal-root ganglia and spinal gray matter give rise to the axons that form the pathways that ascend in the dorsal and lateral funiculi. Cell bodies that give rise to the axons in the descending tracts are located in many parts of the brain. Their axons descend in the lateral and ventral funiculi and terminate on motor neurons or on interneurons that project to motor neurons within the spinal gray matter. Descending systems are important in the control of movement and posture. Some descending axons terminate on sensory-relay neurons in the dorsal horn, and can therefore modify sensory input to the CNS.

Propriospinal pathways originate and terminate in the spinal cord itself. These axons may be very short, connecting one cell with its neighbor. They may cross the midline (e.g., commissural fibers) dorsal or ventral to the central canal, or they may ascend or descend in the white matter and connect distant segments of the cord.

3.1. Sensory Tracts Ascend

The input to the CNS from the body must be organized in such a way that information about modality (e.g., type of sensation) and location of peripheral stimulation can be utilized to produce appropriate spinal reflexes and be transmitted to appropriate parts of the brain for sensory processing. Information about a painful stimulus to the skin is distributed in pathways that are different from those that transmit information about nonpainful stimuli, such as light pressure.

Two classes of dorsal-root ganglion cells can be recognized (Table 1): larger cells, whose axons are myelinated (Groups I and II or A α and A β fibers) and smaller cells, whose axons are unmyelinated or thinly myelinated (Groups III and IV or A delta and C fibers). The small dorsal-root ganglion cells are further differentiated by their synthesis of a variety of peptides (e.g., Substance P, somatostatin) which are used as neuromodulators or neurotransmitters.

At the dorsal-root entry zone, the dorsal-root fibers separate into a lateral and a medial division. The lateral division contains finer myelinated and unmyelinated fibers, originating from small dorsal-root ganglion cells, that transmit responses to nociceptive (painful) and thermal stimulation of the skin and viscera. The medial division contains large-caliber fibers from large dorsal-root ganglion cells, whose peripheral receptors lie in muscle, joints, and skin. These fibers relay information about muscle length and tension to interneurons and motor neurons at segmental levels, which provides the basis for spinal reflexes, and information about somesthesis and joint position to the brain, which provides the basis for stereognosis.

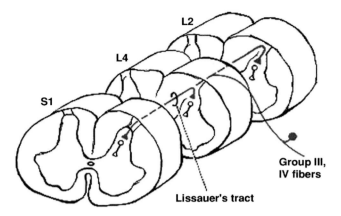

Fig. 6. Entry and central course of axons of the lateral division from one dorsal-root ganglion. These unmyelinated and thinly myelinated axons may branch and ascend or descend several segments in the tract of Lissauer before entering the gray matter and synapsing on second-order neurons in the dorsal horn.

3.1.1. Lateral Division

Axons in the lateral division form a bundle, the tract of *Lissauer* (Fig. 6), at the dorsal-root entry zone. These axons may ascend or descend in Lissauer's tract for several segments before entering into the lateral portion of the dorsal horn to synapse on cells in the dorsal horn (marginal nucleus, substantia gelatinosa, nucleus proprius, Laminae I–IV). This distribution of collaterals rostrally and caudally means that activation of axons in one segment of the lateral division may stimulate dorsal-horn cells over several adjacent segments.

Neurons in the dorsal horn relay sensory information received from dorsal-root axons to nuclei in the brain. These second-order neurons transmit this information through axons that ascend in the lateral funiculus. These sensory-relay neurons receive input from the dorsal roots as well as from various descending (motor) tracts, either directly or via interneurons. In this way, the cell's ability to respond to sensory input is modified by the brain.

The location of an important ascending tract is shown in Fig. 7. Most axons in the *spinothalamic tract* (STT) arise from the marginal cells in lamina I and from the nucleus proprius in lamina III and IV, and transmit nociceptive and thermal information. The axons of these second-order neurons cross to the contralateral spinal cord through the ventral commissure, and ascend in the white matter as the spinothalamic tract to terminate in the thalamus and other targets in the brain. The STT, along with other pathways that

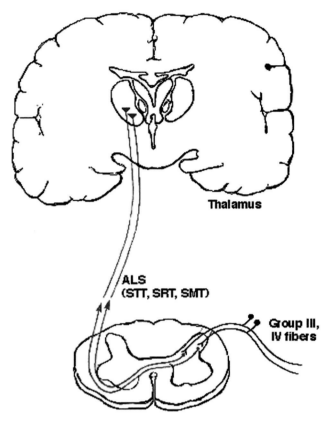

Fig. 7. Formation of the anterolateral system (ALS). Lateral-division axons entering the dorsal-root synapse on second-order neurons, giving rise to axons that cross the spinal cord. Some axons form the spinothalamic tract and ascend to terminate in the thalamus. Some of these axons ascend to terminate in the reticular formation (spinoreticular tract, SRT) or mesencephalon (spinomesencephalic tract, SMT).

ascend to the reticular formation (spinoreticular tract) and mesencephalon, (spinomesencephalic and spinotectal tracts), are located in the ventral (or anterior) lateral portion of the white matter, and are sometimes referred to collectively as the *anterolateral system* (ALS). The function of tracts in the anterolateral system appears to be similar to that of the spinothalamic tract, relaying pain, temperature, and crude touch sensations to the brain.

Axons that contribute to the anterolateral system join the ascending pathways at each spinal segment. As the contribution from one segment enters the white matter, it displaces the fibers from lower segments in a dorsolateral direction. Therefore, these also become laminated and topographically organized. The fibers carrying sensation from the lower limbs are located dorsal and lateral to those representing the upper limbs.

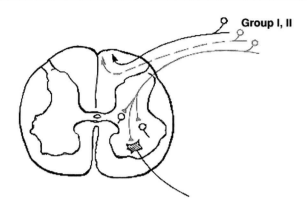

Fig. 8. Axons forming the medial division of the dorsal root enter the spinal cord and then continue into the gray matter at their level of entry, making reflex connections with motor neurons and interneurons at the level of entry, or ascend in the dorsal columns to terminate at more rostral spinal or brainstem levels.

3.1.2. Medial Division

Dorsal-root axons in the medial division have local targets in their segments of entry, as well as collaterals that ascend to terminate in more distant targets in somatosensory relay and cerebellar relay nuclei.

The axons with local segmental targets enter the gray matter at the level of entry of the dorsal root, synapse on interneurons or motor neurons at that segmental level, and subserve reflex organization (Fig. 8). The Ia fibers of the medial division whose peripheral processes innervate stretch receptors in muscle spindles send central processes into the ventral horn, which synapse on the dendrites of motor neurons and on interneurons. This monosynaptic connection between sensory axons and motor neurons is the anatomical basis for the stretch reflex.

Other medial-division axons, including collaterals of axons with segmental targets, enter the white matter in the dorsal funiculus, where they ascend to terminate in relay nuclei for somatosensory or cerebellar pathways. These relay nuclei receive sensory information from the skin, muscles, joints, fascia, and other tissues, then transmit (relay) the information to nuclei in the thalamus. The thalamus relays information to the cortex, where it is consciously appreciated or to the cerebellum, where it contributes to the control of posture and movement without being consciously perceived.

Dorsal-root fibers destined for the somatosensory relay nuclei enter the dorsal funiculus at each segment, medially displacing the fibers originating from more

caudal ganglia. As a result, fibers become laminated (topographically organized). In the cervical region, fibers from sacral dorsal roots are found nearest the midline, and those from cervical roots nearest the dorsal-root entry zone. Fibers representing the lower half of the body (sacral to T_5) ascend in the *gracile fasciculus*; those from the upper half (T_5 to C_2) comprise the *cuneate fasciculus*. Axons in both bundles terminate ipsilaterally in nuclei of the medulla for which they are named (e.g., nucleus gracilis and cuneatus); these nuclei then relay impulses to the thalamus (Fig. 9).

Other dorsal-root axons enter the dorsal funiculus to ascend for several segments before terminating in relay nuclei for cerebellar pathways. The axons arising from dorsal-root ganglion cells in caudal thoracic, lumbar, and sacral regions ascend in the dorsal columns to terminate in *Clarke's nucleus* (Fig. 10), located in segments T1 to L2. Those arising from more rostral ganglia ascend in the dorsal columns to terminate in the *lateral* (or *external* or *accessory*) *cuneate nucleus* in the medulla.

The *dorsal spinocerebellar tract* (DSCT) arises from neurons located in Clarke's nucleus; it ascends in the white matter ipsilaterally and is therefore uncrossed (Fig. 10). The DSCT terminates in the cerebellum. Similarly, the *cuneocerebellar tract* carries information from the lateral cuneate nucleus to the cerebellum. Both nuclei therefore relay sensory information from the periphery to the cerebellum. There is a third pathway to the cerebellum, the ventral spinocerebellar tract (VSCT). Cell bodies whose axons form the VSCT are distributed throughout the dorsal horn and intermediate zone; their axons cross in the ventral commissure to ascend in the contralateral VSCT to the cerebellum, where they cross again before terminating. Although the course of the VSCT differs from that of the DSCT and cuneocerebellar pathways, their functions appear to be similar.

3.2. Central Motor Pathways Descend

The axons that form the central motor pathways arise from cell bodies located at all levels of the brainstem and the cerebral cortex. Many of these tracts undergo partial or complete decussation (crossing) before entering the cord. However, some descend ipsilaterally, enter the gray matter, and then cross in the spinal commissures to terminate on neurons contralateral to their origin. Still other tracts are primarily ipsilateral.

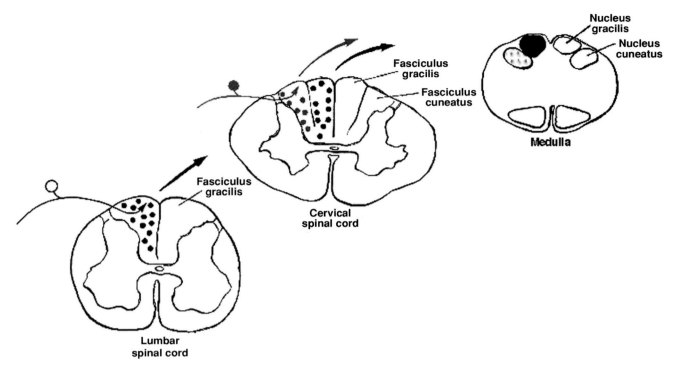

Fig. 9. Axons that mediate fine tactile sensibility form part of the medial division. They ascend in the dorsal columns to the brainstem, where they terminate on second-order neurons in the dorsal-column nuclei. The axons arising from lumbar and low thoracic dorsal-root ganglia ascend in the fasciculus gracilis and terminate in the nucleus gracilis. Axons arising from upper thoracic and cervical ganglia ascend in the more laterally located fasciculus cuneatus and terminate in the nucleus cuneatus located lateral to the nucleus gracilis in the medulla.

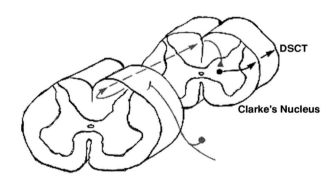

Fig. 10. Axons conveying proprioceptive and muscle information form part of the medial division. Axons from lumbar and caudal thoracic dorsal-root ganglia enter the spinal cord and ascend in the dorsal columns to the thoracic level, where they terminate on second-order neurons in Clarke's nucleus. The axons of Clarke's neurons ascend in the lateral funiculus as the dorsal spinocerebellar tract (DSCT), which terminates on third-order neurons in the cerebellum.

The descending tracts are located in the lateral and ventral funiculi. The location of four important

descending tracts, the *corticospinal, rubrospinal, vestibulospinal,* and *reticulospinal tracts,* is shown in Fig. 11. Most of the axons in these tracts terminate on interneurons , which then project to motor neurons; very few terminate directly on motor neurons. Some descending axons terminate on sensory relay neurons, providing central control over sensory processing.

The *corticospinal tract* arises from the motor, premotor and somatosensory cortex, descends to the spino-medullary junction, where 90% of the axons cross, and then continues to descend as the lateral corticospinal tract in the lateral funiculus contralateral to the cell bodies of origin. The axons that do not cross at the spinal medullary junction descend in the spinal cord as the ventral corticospinal tract but then cross in the spinal cord before their termination. The *rubrospinal tract* arises from neurons in the red nucleus; it is also virtually completely crossed. The *reticulospinal tracts* contains axons that arise from reticular nuclei ipsilaterally and contralaterally. Most of the axons in the vestibulospinal tract are uncrossed.

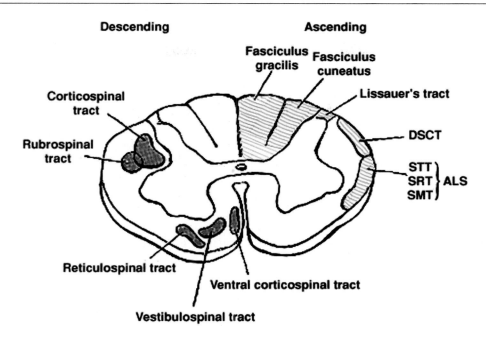

Fig. 11. The approximate location of ascending tracts is shown on the *right* and the location of descending tracts on the *left*.

4. SOMATIC MOTOR NEURONS

4.1. Topographic Organization

Somatic motor neurons express the activity of the CNS. Sherrington called them the final common pathway. Axons from somatic motor neurons exit in the ventral roots and innervate striated muscle. These neurons are located exclusively in the ventral horn (laminae VIII and IX). A medial motor nucleus is present in the ventral horn throughout the length of the cord. These motor neurons innervate axial (trunk) musculature. There are also prominent groups of nuclei located laterally in the ventral horn, which are particularly well-developed in the segments supplying the limbs. The lateral group of nuclei is subdivided functionally into the ventral nuclei, which innervate extensor muscles, and the dorsal nuclei, which innervate flexors. Within these two subdivisions, the nuclei innervating proximal muscles are located medially; those that supply the distal muscles more laterally (Fig. 12).

Motor neurons are among the largest in the spinal cord. Although the motor neuron-cell bodies are localized into discrete nuclei, their dendrites extend into the intermediate zone, the dorsal horn, and even into the white matter. This allows considerable convergence of input onto a motor neuron, and in fact a single motor neuron may receive as many as 10,000 axon terminals from many different sources.

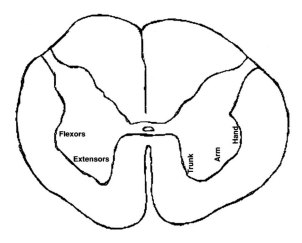

Fig. 12. Somatic motor neurons are organized topographically in the ventral horn. Axial musculature is supplied by motor neurons located medially, and limb musculature by motor neurons located laterally in the ventral horn. Flexor motor neurons are dorsal and lateral to motor neurons innervating extensor muscles.

All motor neurons use the excitatory transmitter acetylcholine. The axons of many motor neurons give off a collateral before exiting in the ventral root. These short *recurrent collaterals* terminate on interneurons. Some of these interneurons are part of a di-synaptic pathway that inhibits motor neurons (motor axon collateral→interneuron→motor neuron). This inter-

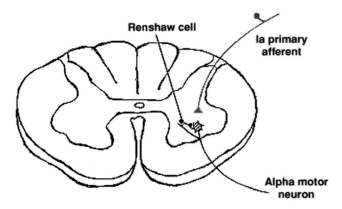

Fig. 13. Renshaw cells. A 1a primary afferent axon makes a monosynaptic contact with an alpha motor neuron whose axon innervates a somatic muscle. The motor neuron also emits a collateral that innervates an interneuron, the Renshaw cell, situated near the alpha motor neuron, which inhibits (recurrent inhibition) the motor neuron.

neuron is called the *Renshaw cell*, and it uses the inhibitory transmitter glycine to inhibit the postsynaptic motor neuron. This feedback circuit permits the regulation of activity in motor neurons by the motor neurons themselves (Fig. 13).

4.2. Visceral Motor Neurons in the Intermediate Zone

Visceral motor neurons innervate neurons in autonomic ganglia; the autonomic ganglion cells innervate viscera. Those preganglionic neurons in the *intermediolateral nucleus* in lamina VII at C8 to L3 send axons to the sympathetic chain and provide central regulation of the sympathetic nervous system. Neurons in the intermediate zone at levels at S2 through S4 form the more poorly defined *sacral parasympathetic nucleus*. Their axons innervate the sacral parasympathetic ganglia, and thus provide central control of the sacral portion of the parasympathetic system that innervates the bowel and bladder. Central control of rostral portions of the parasympathetic system is provided by groups of cranial-nerve nuclei.

4.3. Regional Specializations

At all segmental levels of the spinal cord, the dorsal horn (laminae I through IV), the intermediate zone (laminae V through VII), and the ventral horn (laminae VIII and IX) can be recognized. Regional specializations modify the butterfly shape of the gray matter in characteristic ways. In the spinal segments that innervate the limbs (the cervical and lumbar enlarge-

ments), the number of neurons is greatly increased and the dorsal and ventral horns are concomitantly expanded. Two nuclei located in the intermediate zone, Clarke's and the intermediolateral nuclei, are prominent only in segments that do not innervate the limbs (T1–L2). Therefore, the gray matter has different silhouettes that are characteristic of the particular spinal levels (cervical, thoracic, lumbar, or sacral) (Fig. 14).

The amount of white matter also differs according to segment. Ascending pathways become larger more rostrally because axons from dorsal-root ganglia or from sensory-relay nuclei are added at each segment. Most descending tracts send fibers to terminate in gray matter at all segments. Descending tracts are thus smaller at more caudal levels, because they are continuously depleted of fibers. The circumference of the caudal spinal cord is smaller than at rostral levels, because there is less white matter caudally.

4.4. Spinal Reflexes

The activity of dorsal-root axons is expressed, monosynaptically or polysynaptically, on motor neurons whose axons form the ventral root. This arrangement comprises the *segmental organization* of the spinal cord, and it is this organization that determines the reflex activity of the spinal cord—the reflex activity that persists after a spinal transection that separates the brain from the spinal cord. *Spinal reflexes* are stereotyped responses (contraction, relaxation) made by somatic muscles in response to stimuli that excite receptors in muscle, tendon, or skin. These reflexes may be more readily demonstrable in a spinal transected preparation than in an organism with an intact spinal cord, since they are normally subjected to descending inhibition, but the reflexes make a major contribution in providing muscle tone, posture, and enabling voluntary movement for the organism.

4.4.1. The Stretch Reflex Determines Muscle Tone

When a muscle is passively stretched, it responds by contracting. This is a result of the stimulation of receptors located in muscle spindles. This stretch (or *myotatic*) reflex provides the basis for muscle tone—the slight resistance to stretch found in all healthy innervated muscles.

A striated muscle is composed of two types of fibers: a large number of *extrafusal muscle fibers* and a smaller number of highly specialized sensory structures, the *muscle spindles* (Fig. 15). The muscle spindle is a fusiform structure containing several modified muscle fibers, the *intrafusal* fibers, and the axons that

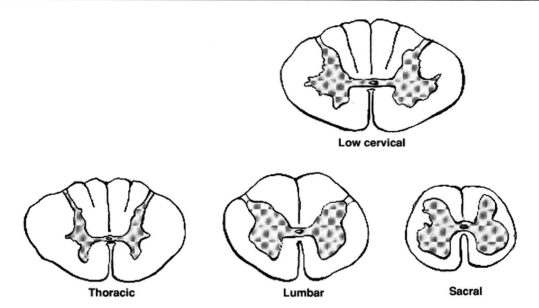

Low cervical

Thoracic   Lumbar   Sacral

Fig. 14. The configuration of gray and white matter at various levels of the spinal cord differs in characteristic ways.

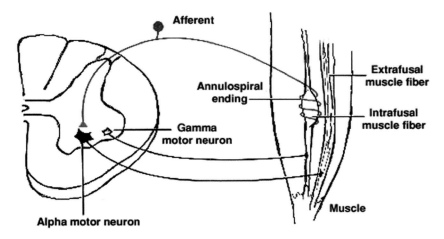

Afferent

Extrafusal
muscle fiber

Annulospiral
ending

Intrafusal
muscle fiber

Gamma
motor neuron

Alpha motor neuron

Muscle

Fig. 15. The gamma loop. A small gamma motor neuron, located near an alpha motor neuron, innervates the poles of intrafusal fibers. The alpha motor neuron innervates extrafusal muscle fibers in the same muscle. Activity in the gamma motor neuron causes contraction of the poles of the intrafusal fiber, which stretches the central zone and activates the peripheral process of the 1a afferent. The 1a afferent is shown innervating the intrafusal fiber peripherally, and the alpha motor neuron centrally (the monosynaptic reflex).

innervate them. Each spindle is encased in a connective tissue capsule.

There are also two types of somatic motor neurons: *alpha* and *gamma motor neurons*. Alpha motor neurons innervate the extrafusal muscle fibers. They are grouped into nuclei that innervate individual muscles. These nuclei also contain small *gamma motor neurons*, which innervate the intrafusal muscle fibers, and control the sensitivity of the muscle spindle to stretch. Gamma motor neurons are located near the alpha

motor neurons, which innervate extrafusal fibers of the same muscle.

The central portion of the intrafusal fiber is noncontractile; this zone is innervated by Ia afferent fibers, which make "annulospiral" endings around the noncontractile central zone. The intrafusal fibers are also innervated by group II afferents, which make another type of ending, the "flower spray" endings, upon them. The polar regions of the intrafusal fiber are contractile. Each pole receives innervation from gamma motor

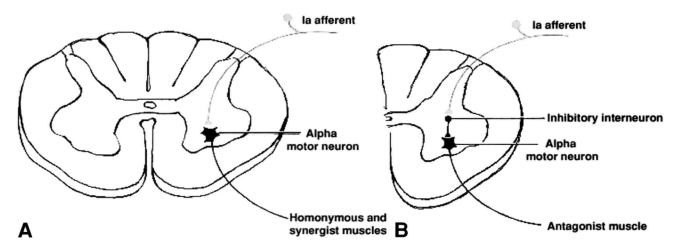

Fig. 16. (A) Monosynaptic reflex pathway. Ia afferents supplying muscle spindles in somatic muscles make monosynaptic excitatory contacts on alpha motor neurons supplying the same muscle and synergistic muscles. Stretch of the muscle produces contraction of that muscle and its agonists. **(B)** Disynaptic inhibitory reflex pathway. Ia afferents also make excitatory contacts on inhibitory interneurons that make synaptic contact with alpha motor neurons that supply muscles that are antagonists to the muscle supplied by the 1a afferent. Stretch of the muscle also produces relaxation of opposing muscles.

neurons. The polar regions of intrafusal fibers respond to gamma efferent stimulation with a slow, maintained "tonic" contraction, thereby stretching the intrafusal fiber that stretches the central region, thus stimulating the Ia and/or II afferent axons.

The central processes of the Ia and II fibers terminate on cells in the spinal gray matter, including the alpha motor neurons supplying the muscle that the peripheral process of the Ia fiber contacts (Fig. 16A). There are also Ia terminals on motor neurons whose muscles are synergists of that muscle. Other important terminations of the Ia fiber are on interneurons, some of which inhibit motor neurons that innervate the muscles that act antagonistically to that of the Ia fiber. There is one synapse in the excitatory path (monosynaptic pathway) and two synapses (disynaptic pathway) or more involved in the inhibitory pathways (Fig. 16B). Passive stretch of a muscle will therefore facilitate contraction of that muscle and its synergists, and with a slight delay, inhibit contraction of the antagonist muscles.

4.4.2. THE INVERSE MYOTATIC REFLEX LIMITS THE STRETCH REFLEX

When a muscle contracts, another type of muscle receptor, the *Golgi tendon organ*, is stimulated. These receptors are located in tendons close to their junctions with muscle, and are stretched during muscle contraction. Golgi tendon organs therefore measure muscle tension. They receive sensory innervation from Ib

dorsal-root axons, but unlike muscle spindles, they do not receive motor innervation. The central process of the Ib fiber terminates on interneurons that inhibit motor neurons of the muscle of origin (e.g., homonymous muscles) and facilitate the antagonists (e.g., heteronymous muscles). This reflex pathway limits (applies "brakes" to) the muscle contractions (Fig. 17).

4.4.3. THE FLEXOR AND CROSSED-EXTENSOR REFLEX CONSTITUTE ANOTHER PROTECTIVE MECHANISM

Noxious or thermal stimulation of the skin or deep tissues excites group III and IV axons in the peripheral nerves. This information is transmitted to motor neurons through interneurons. These polysynaptic pathways permit a divergence of the sensory stimulation so that neurons in many ipsilateral segments and the contralateral side of the cord may be recruited. This type of stimulation produces ipsilateral excitation of flexors and inhibition of extensors, and contralateral inhibition of flexors and excitation of extensors. This reflex pattern is known as the *flexor and crossed-extensor* reflex (Fig. 18).

4.4.4. CENTRAL PATTERN GENERATORS

Not all movement is based on simple reflexes. Within the spinal gray matter there are networks of interneurons distributed bilaterally, which form the *spinal central pattern generators* that activate motor neurons to produce the rhythmic alternating patterns of flexion and extension that comprise the stepping patterns that underlie locomotion. The patterns gen-

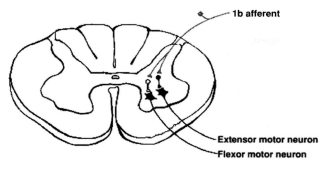

Fig. 17. The inverse myotatic reflex. The Ib afferent innervates a Golgi tendon organ from an extensor muscle peripherally; centrally, this 1b afferent makes excitatory contacts with 2 interneurons. The excitatory interneuron synapses on motor neurons supplying flexor muscles and the inhibitory interneuron synapses on motor neurons supplying extensor motor neurons. Continued stretch of the muscle thus produces relaxation.

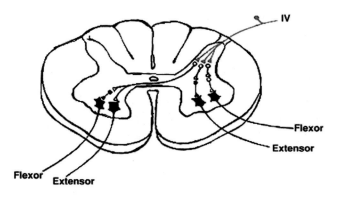

Fig. 18. The flexor-crossed extensor reflex. Painful stimulation activates small-diameter axons that make contacts with interneurons within the gray matter. Through polysynaptic pathways, using interneurons that inhibit and excite flexor and extensor motor neurons on both sides of the spinal cord, the ipsilateral limb flexes—a protective response—and the contralateral limb extends, providing postural support.

erators are normally influenced both by descending and by primary afferent input, but they have the capacity to produce rhythmic activity even when isolated from these inputs. Thus, the basic neuronal machinery for producing stepping is intrinsic to the spinal cord.

5. SPINAL LESIONS

5.1. Spinal Transection Interrupts Neuronal Transmission

Transection of the spinal cord interrupts descending input from the brain to spinal levels below the level of transection, and input to the brain ascending from sensory structures located below the level of transec-

tion. A patient whose spinal cord is transected will undergo a period of "spinal shock", characterized by flaccid paralysis of muscles innervated by motor neurons below the transection. Voluntary control of muscles innervated by motor neurons and perception of sensory events arising below the level of the lesion is permanently lost. Over time, the flaccid paralysis is followed by a bilateral, symmetric spasticity below the level of the lesion. This hyperactivity after recovery from spinal shock is caused by the loss of descending inhibitory influences on spinal neurons.

5.2. Spinal Hemisection Generates Both Ipsilateral and Contralateral Impairment

Hemisection usually results from a slow-growing mass in the spinal cord that deforms the cord compressing descending and ascending axons on one side of the cord and producing functional disorders. Because many ascending systems cross, the sensory impairments arising from hemisection may be referred to the side of the body opposite to the lesion. Important descending pathways cross at supraspinal levels so that the motor impairments are ipsilateral and below the level of the hemisection. Motor function and discriminatory tactile and kinesthetic sense are lost ipsilaterally at levels below the lesion, and pain and thermal sensitivity are lost contralaterally below the lesion. A neurological examination reveals spastic paralysis and diminished touch sensation on the side of the body that is ipsilateral to the lesion, plus a loss of pain and temperature sensation on the other side of the body, the side contralateral to the lesion. The pattern of symptoms resulting from a hemisection is known as the Brown-Sequard syndrome.

5.3. Syringomyelia Produces Bilateral Impairment

Syringomyelia refers to a pathological enlargement (cavitation) of the central canal. As the cavity expands dorsally and ventrally, it interrupts the fibers that cross through the anterior and ventral commissures in the spinal cord, including some ascending sensory pathways, and may involve muscles of the medial motor neuron groups. In the cervical spinal cord, where syringomyelia is prone to occur, interruption of decussating sensory pathways results in bilateral loss of pain and temperature sensation, but with preservation of tactile and kinesthetic sensation. With enlargement of the cavity, wasting and motor dysfunction, particularly of axial muscles innervated by medial motor neurons, indicates encroachment on the ventral horn.

5.4. Pathological Reflexes Have Several Causes

Spasticity is an abnormal increase in muscle tone associated with a loss of descending inhibition of gamma and alpha motor neurons. *Rigidity* is an abnormal increase in muscle tone caused by loss of inhibition of alpha motor neurons. *Flaccidity* is an absence of muscle tone that occurs after loss of peripheral-nerve innervation.

5.4.1. SPASTICITY

Spasticity is a common and severe consequence of spinal injuries in which descending regulation of spinal circuits is impaired. Passive stretch of a muscle evokes a reflex contraction of that muscle. The strength of this monosynaptic stretch reflex is controlled by the gamma motor neurons that innervate that muscle. These gamma motor neurons, in turn, are under excitatory or inhibitory drive from the CNS. Normally, there is a balance of excitation and inhibition, which is reflected in some tension in the polar regions of the intrafusal fibers. This tension stimulates Ia fibers, producing a basal level of excitation of the alpha motor neurons. This balance produces muscle tension or "tone." Increased excitation or decreased inhibition of gamma motor neurons increases tension on the intrafusal fibers, which then become hypersensitive to stretch of the whole muscle, resulting in an abnormal increase contraction in response to stretch, the phenomenon known as "spasticity."

Under such conditions, changes in reflexes are clearly observable clinically. If the stretch is applied continuously to a spastic muscle, the resistance increases but then suddenly gives way, as a result of inhibition by the Golgi tendon organ system. This sudden collapse of resistance is known as the lengthening reaction or clasp-knife effect. The clasp-knife reaction is only revealed when muscle tone is abnormally increased, but its basis, the activation of the Golgi tendon organ, normally contributes to muscle tone.

Spasticity is seen in muscle groups innervated by motor neurons below the level of a spinal transection. An attempt to elicit a tendon reflex produces a greatly increased response. In addition, a mild stimulus provided by stroking the lateral border of the foot will evoke the classic extensor-plantar (e.g., Babinski) response, in which the toes spread and extend instead of flexing as they would normally do.

The exact etiology of spasticity is controversial. A hyperactive stretch reflex has been believed to contribute to spasticity. However, clinical studies show that not all spastic muscles exhibit an increased stretch reflex. The hyperactivity of alpha motor neurons and interneurons, as well as changes in muscle properties resulting from such lesions, undoubtedly also contribute to spasticity.

5.4.2. RIGIDITY

Rigidity is an increased activation of the alpha motor neurons, seen after damage to some descending pathways. Rigidity involves an increased resistance to movements in all directions, and does not depend on the dorsal-root innervation of muscle spindles. This resistance to passive motion felt when examining the patients has been likened to the feeling of bending a lead pipe (lead pipe rigidity). Occasionally, the resistance has a phasic quality, which is known as cogwheel rigidity. Parkinson's disease, which results from degeneration of neurons in the basal ganglia that indirectly project to the spinal cord, produces the purest form of clinical rigidity.

5.4.3. FLACCIDITY

A lesion to motor neurons or their axons produces a flaccid paralysis of the muscle innervated by those neurons. No voluntary movement is possible, there is no resistance to passive movement, and no reflexes can be elicited. If axonal regeneration does not occur, the muscle will atrophy.

6. STRATEGIES TO REPAIR INJURED SPINAL CORD

Injury to the spinal cord produces severe deficits because neurons that are lost are not replaced and axons that are cut do not regenerate. Severe injuries, such as spinal transection, eliminate supraspinal influences and thus eliminate voluntary control of movement. In recent years, several strategies have been developed in animal models with the goal of rescuing injured neurons, promoting regeneration, and thus restoring motor control.

The site of injury is toxic, as a result of release of such substances as glutamate from dying cells or pro-inflammatory cytokines from cells of the immune system that migrate to the injury site. Thus neurons near the site of injury die as an indirect result of the lesion, leading to an enlargement of the injury site (secondary degeneration) and development of additional deficits. Other neurons whose axons have been severed by the lesion may atrophy or die (retrograde degeneration, an apoptotic or programmed-cell-death process). Strategies aimed at countering the toxic environment with anti-inflammatory agents or blocking the apoptotic process with provision of trophic factors or antiapoptotic molecules have been successful in animal models in rescuing neurons destined to die or to atrophy both at the lesion site and distant from it.

Regeneration of CNS axons, long believed to be impossible, is now known to occur in the presence of a permissive environment. This environment can be provided by application of appropriate trophic factors. Provision of trophic factors, either directly by pumps or indirectly by transplantation of cells that produce these factors, has been successful in promoting regeneration in animal models.

Thus, experimental studies have shown that some of the serious consequences of spinal injury can be ameliorated or reversed. The complexity of spinal and supraspinal circuitry will undoubtedly require a combined approach, using several therapeutic interventions to effect the repair of spinal injuries in humans.

SELECTED READINGS

Barbeau H, Fung J. The role of rehabilitation in the recovery of walking in the neurological population. Curr Opin Neurol 2001; 14:735–740.

Grillner S, Zangger P. On the central generation of locomotion in the low spinal cat. Exp Br Res 1979; 34:241–261.

Jankowska E. Spinal interneuronal systems. J Physiol 2001; 533:31–40.

Maynard FM, Brachen MB, Creasey G, Ditunno J, et al. Internal standards for neurological and functional classification of spinal injury. Spinal Cord 1997; 35:266–274.

Rexed B. A cytoarchitectonic atlas on the spinal cord and the cat. J Comp Neurol 1954; 100:297–380.

Sherrington CS. The integrative action of the nervous system. Yale University Press, New Haven, 1906.

Disorders of the Spinal Cord

Gregory Cooper and Robert L. Rodnitzky

Clinical abnormalities of the spinal cord lead to great disability resulting from severe disruption of motor, sensory, and autonomic functions. The distinct longitudinal organization of ascending and descending fiber tracts in the spinal cord, coupled with the segmental groupings of neurons with motor, sensory, and autonomic functions, often allow relatively precise localization of the lesion responsible for a spinal cord syndrome.

CAUSES OF SPINAL CORD DISORDERS

Clinical spinal cord syndromes are more often the result of structural damage than metabolic dysfunction. Although relatively minor aberrations of the metabolic milieu of the brain can result in severe neurologic dysfunction, clinical symptoms related to spinal cord dysfunction are much less likely to be of metabolic origin. Neurologic symptoms can result from spinal cord ischemia, but not as readily as is the case in cerebral ischemia. Spinal cord ischemia severe enough to produce symptoms is commonly the result of atherosclerotic occlusion of the aorta or its branches, embolization to these blood vessels, or vascular malformations within the substance of the spinal cord.

Most clinical spinal cord syndromes result from mechanical disruption or physical degeneration of the constituent cells and fiber tracts of the cord. Typical examples of conditions resulting in mechanical disruption of spinal cord elements include spinal trauma (e.g., spinal column fracture, bullet wound), spinal cord tumors, and intervertebral disc herniation causing spinal cord compression. Degenerative processes causing spinal cord symptoms include demyelination of long tracts (e.g., multiple sclerosis) and neuronal degeneration (e.g., motor neuron disease).

LOCALIZATION OF THE CAUSATIVE LESION

Precise localization of the causative lesion is extremely important in treating spinal cord disorders. Even in the era of modern neuroimaging, a thorough neurologic examination is essential in localizing the abnormality within the spinal cord. Although magnetic resonance imaging or computerized tomography of the spinal cord can be performed in most communities, it is critical to know which part of the spinal cord should be imaged, and it is essential to understand whether the pathology demonstrated by the procedure can explain the patient's symptoms.

The most important clinical finding in attempting to localize spinal cord pathology is the sensory level. A sensory level is a horizontal demarcation of sensory loss on the trunk or a diagonal linear demarcation on an extremity that corresponds to the segmental innervation of skin by the paired spinal nerves leaving the spinal cord. Classically, sensation is lost below the level of a spinal cord lesion, and is intact above it because of the interruption of ascending impulses in sensory spinal pathways such as the spinothalamic tracts or dorsal column pathways by the offending lesion. If the lesion involves the entire spinal cord at a given level, sensation is lost equally on both sides of the body below that level. A sensory level to pain or touch sensation is demonstrated by applying the appropriate stimulus to the skin below the level of the suspected lesion and gradually ascending up the trunk until the stimulus is felt. A sensory level of vibratory perception can be similarly established by applying a vibrating tuning fork at bony landmarks beginning with the toes, proceeding to the ankles, knees, and hips, and ultimately moving up the spinous processes of the vertebrae until a normal sense of vibration is perceived.

SPARING OF SACRAL SENSATION MAY HELP DIFFERENTIATE A LESION IN THE CENTER OF THE SPINAL CORD FROM ONE ON ITS CIRCUMFERENCE

After the fibers that transmit pain and temperature sensations enter the spinal cord, they cross the midline and ascend on the opposite side, where they are progressively displaced laterally by incoming fibers entering and crossing at higher levels. The fibers entering at the lowest (e.g., sacral) level, which are those that are the first to enter, cross, and ascend, come to occupy the most lateral position in the lumbar, thoracic and cervical spinal cord as ascending fibers enter the spinothalamic tracts at higher levels. The extreme lateral position of fibers transmitting sacral sensation protects them from lesions deep within the center of the spinal cord, such as a midline tumor. In such cases, there may be profound loss of sensation below the level of the lesion, with the exception of the saddle or perianal area, subserved by sacral fibers, where sensation is spared. This can be extremely useful to the clinician in determining whether spinal cord pathology is intrinsic to the spinal cord or is causing symptoms by compression from outside.

In cases of external compression, the most laterally placed fibers (those subserving sacral sensation) may be involved first, and the initial sensory level may be considerably below the level of the lesion early in the illness and ascend to the true level with the passage of time as more fibers are compressed. Another clue to the possibility that a lesion may be compressing the spinal cord from the outside is the presence of radicular pain. This is a sharp, stabbing pain that follows the cutaneous distribution of a single dorsal spinal root, caused by irritation of the nerve as it enters the spinal cord. This type of pain is even more likely to occur when the offending lesion is attached to the spinal nerve, as is the case with nerve-sheath tumors. Such tumors are rare, and herniated lumbar or cervical intervertebral discs are by far the most common cause of irritation of a spinal root with resultant radicular pain.

LESIONS INVOLVING HALF THE SPINAL CORD PRODUCE A DISTINCT CLINICAL SYNDROME

The Brown-Sequard syndrome results from interruption of motor and sensory tracts on only one side of the spinal cord. In this condition, the functions of uncrossed fibers are lost on the side of the body ipsilateral to the lesion, and the functions of crossed fibers are lost on the contralateral side. Pain and temperature sensation are lost on the side opposite of the lesion because of the interruption of the crossed lateral spinothalamic tract, and weakness and loss of joint position and vibratory sensation appear on the same side because of interruption of the corticospinal tract and dorsal-column fibers, respectively, which are uncrossed in the spinal cord. Because fibers transmitting pain and temperature sensations may ascend one or two spinal cord segments on the side of entry before crossing the midline to join the contralateral spinothalamic tract, there may be loss of pain and temperature sensation ipsilateral to the side of the lesion over an expanse of skin that correspond to one or two dermatomes at the level of the offending lesion.

A CAPE-LIKE SENSORY LOSS MAY ALSO BE A CLUE TO THE LOCALIZATION OF A SPINAL-CORD LESION

Small lesions involving the region immediately adjacent to the central canal of the spinal cord may involve the anterior white commissure. Because this structure contains fibers that convey pain and temperature sensation from both sides as they cross to join the contralateral spinothalamic tract, these modalities may be preferentially lost in the corresponding dermatomal segments on both sides, often symmetrically. Simple touch, position sense, and vibratory sensation are preserved in the same segments, because fibers that convey these sensations do not pass near the center of the spinal cord. More importantly, all sensory modalities above and below the involved segments remain intact. The most common condition affecting this region of the spinal cord is syringomyelia. The centrally located spinal cord cyst of syringomyelia is commonly found in the lower cervical and upper thoracic spinal cord. In this condition, the area of symmetric sensory loss often includes the arms and upper thorax, giving rise to the term "cape-like sensory loss."

THE ANTERIOR PORTION OF THE SPINAL CORD CAN BE PREFERENTIALLY INVOLVED IN ISCHEMIC LESIONS

The anterior spinal artery perfuses the anterior two-thirds of the spinal cord, excluding the dorsal columns. Occlusion of this artery causes infarction of the anterior spinal cord and results in loss of all sensory and motor functions below the level of the infarction, with the exception of vibratory and proprioceptive sensation and both of which are subserved by the intact dorsal columns. These fiber tracts receive their blood supply instead from the paired posterior spinal arteries.

PATHOLOGY BELOW THE L1–L2 VERTEBRAL LEVEL AFFECTS THE CAUDA EQUINA BUT NOT THE SPINAL CORD

In normal adults, the spinal cord does not extend the entire length of the vertebral column. It does not extend below the second lumbar (L2) vertebral level. Because of this difference in length between the spinal cord and the vertebral column, spinal nerves in the cervical and upper thoracic regions enter or exit at almost right angles, but the lower thoracic, lumbar, and sacral spinal nerves originate at increasingly downward oblique angles. The lumbar and sacral spinal roots originate at the level of the lower thoracic and upper lumbar vertebrae, and then descend in the spinal canal to the corresponding lower lumbar and sacral vertebrae, where they exit. This mass of descending spinal nerves within the spinal canal but below the spinal cord forms the cauda equina. Lesions within the spinal canal below the L2 vertebrae cannot involve the spinal cord; they involve only the cauda equina.

Lesions in this region of the spinal canal do not produce upper motor neuron symptoms or patterns of sensory loss related to interruption of ascending spinal cord fiber tracts. The lesions in this region produce symptoms that are related to involvement of lumbosacral spinal nerves, such as radicular pain, sensory loss involving the lower extremities, or significant bladder and sexual dysfunction. The last two abnormalities reflect involvement of the autonomic fibers contained in the sacral spinal-nerve roots.

At the lower lumbar vertebral level, there is no concern about a spinal needle impaling the spinal cord. The spinal cord does not descend below the L2 level, allowing the removal of cerebrospinal fluid to be accomplished safely with a lumbar puncture of the lower lumbar spinal canal. In this procedure, a sterile needle is passed through the space between adjacent lower lumbar vertebrae into the spinal subarachnoid space (SAS). Although the component roots of the cauda equina are coursing through the SAS within the spinal canal at this vertebral level, an appropriately placed spinal needle nudges them aside without causing damage.

DIAGNOSTIC NEUROIMAGING PROCEDURES AND ELECTROPHYSIOLOGIC TESTS

Myelography had been the premier radiologic diagnostic modality used to investigate spinal cord disorders for several decades until the introduction of computerized tomography (CT) and magnetic resonance imaging (MRI) scanning. Myelography involves the introduction of a radiopaque dye into the spinal fluid through a lumbar puncture so that it outlines the spinal cord, spinal nerves, and cauda equina. CT scanning is sometimes used, but MRI has emerged as the most definitive technique for imaging the spinal cord because of its excellent contrast and its ability to display the cord in axial and sagittal arrays.

Somatosensory evoked potentials (SEPs) are performed by stimulating a peripheral nerve in the leg or arm, typically the tibial or median nerve, and recording the evoked potential over the upper cervical region or scalp. The elapsed time between the application of the stimulus and the arrival of the evoked potential is recorded, as is the amplitude of the response. These potentials reflect passage of the evoked impulse through spinal cord pathways, largely the posterior columns. An abnormality within these pathways may affect the latency of the response or its amplitude. SEPs are useful in identifying subtle pathology of the spinal cord even in the absence of clinical symptoms. They are also used to monitor spinal cord function intraoperatively during procedures that involve significant manipulation of the spinal cord. Scoliosis surgery, during which there may be stretching of the spinal cord, is one example of a procedure during which SEPs are routinely performed.

TREATMENT OF SPINAL-CORD INJURY

Current treatment strategies are aimed at preventing further injury and at subsequent rehabilitation. In cases of trauma, high-dose steroids are given to limit swelling. Compressive lesions may be removed surgically and in cases of fracture or dislocation, the vertebral column may be stabilized surgically. Rehabilitive services focus on optimizing remaining function and at the prevention of complicating illnesses such as bladder infections and skin breakdown from immobility. Although not yet a clinical reality, considerable attention is being focused on the prospects of spinal cord regeneration and restoration of function. Strate-

gies that employ the use of neurotrophic factors such
as NGF, BDNF and NT-3, agents that block inhibitory
factors such as Nogo A, and transplantation of various
tissues including embryonic stem cells, Schwann cells,
and olfactory ensheathing glial cells, are currently
being investigated.

SELECTED READINGS

Behar O, Mizuno K, Neumann S, and Woolf CJ. Putting the spinal
    cord together again. Neuron 2000; 26:291–293.
Brazis PW, Masdeu JC, Biller J. Localization in clinical neurol-
    ogy, 3rd ed. Boston: Little, Brown, 1996; 69.

10 The Cerebellum

James R. West and John B. Gelderd

CONTENTS

1. OVERVIEW

Basically, the cerebellum functions as a comparator and a coordinator. It compares movement intention with performance, and coordinates the equilibrium, posture, and muscle tone needed for smooth, coordinated motor activity. The cerebellum is present in all vertebrates. It receives considerable input from sensory systems, but it functions as a part of the motor system. Despite its motor function, the cerebellum contributes comparatively modest, direct connections to brainstem motor nuclei that give rise to descending spinal pathways (red nucleus, vestibular nuclei). In contrast, the cerebellum projects profusely to all major motor-control regions in the cerebrum via thalamic nuclei. As such, it is a key component for sensorimotor coordination. However, cerebellar damage typically does not produce sensory impairment or decreased muscle strength. In order to influence motor performance, the cerebellum must receive and process a great deal of information on the position and contractile state of muscles, tension within tendons, and the equilibrium of the body. Moreover, it must continuously integrate all of this data with information sent to the muscles from the motor cortex. It should be noted that the cerebellum performs these complex functions automatically, without conscious effort on the part of the individual.

2. THE GENERAL ORGANIZATION OF THE CEREBELLUM

2.1. Gross Morphology of the Cerebellum

The word cerebellum means "little brain," and it is an appropriate name. In the adult human male, the cerebellum weighs about 150 g, comprising about 10% of the total weight of the brain. The cerebellum occupies the posterior cranial fossa, which is separated from the occipital lobes of the cerebral hemispheres by a conspicuous transverse extension of the dura known as the *tentorium cerebelli*. The cerebellum is the largest part of the hindbrain. It overlies a substantial portion of the posterior surface of the pons and medulla oblongata. Developmentally, the cerebellum is derived first from the germinal cells of the alar lamina, and later, toward the end of the embryonic period, from the rhombic lip, and therefore also from sensory precursors.

The cerebellum is a highly convoluted, ovoid-shaped structure that is constricted in the middle. The superior surface is flattened, and the inferior surface is convex. The cerebellum consists of two *cerebellar hemispheres* joined by a narrow, median longitudinal strip, the *vermis* (Fig. 1). On the superior surface of the

From: *Neuroscience in Medicine, 2nd ed.* (P. Michael Conn, ed.),
© 2003 Humana Press Inc., Totowa, NJ.

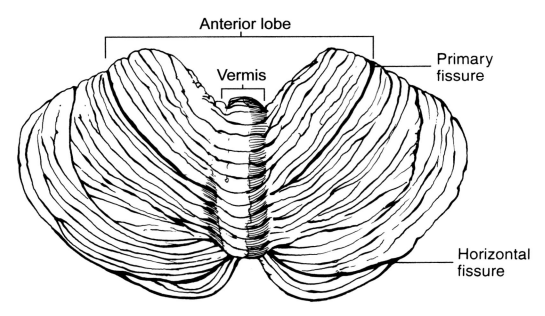

Fig. 1. The superior surface of the cerebellum.

cerebellum, the vermis is seen as an elevated region at the midline, with the cerebellar hemispheres gently sloping in a lateral fashion. In contrast, the inferior surfaces of the hemispheres are convex. Here, the midline vermis is depressed and hidden from view, forming the floor of a deep crevice, the *vallecula. In situ,* the vallecula is occupied by a vertical extension of dura mater known as the *falx cerebelli,* which houses a venous channel for drainage of the cerebellum. Near the midline inferiorly, the cerebellum surrounds the dorsolateral aspect of the medulla with two swellings, the *cerebellar tonsils.* Occasionally, the cerebellar tonsils are useful in diagnosing elevated intracranial pressure (ICP), since they tend to herniate through the foramen magnum as a result of this condition. The region of the hemispheres immediately adjacent to the midline vermis is known as the *paravermis* or *intermediate zone.* With the exception of the flocculonodular lobe, the primary mass of the cerebellum is called the *corpus cerebelli* (Fig. 2).

At the highly convoluted surface of the cerebellum is a distinct, three-layered cortex composed of gray matter. Deep to the cerebellar cortex is an extensive central core of white matter consisting of afferent and efferent axons of the cerebellum. In the midline region, this deep white matter forms the roof of the fourth ventricle. Embedded within the deep white matter near the midline are four pairs of *deep cerebellar nuclei,* which provide the vast majority of the output axons that leave the cerebellum. More laterally and ventrally,

the deep white matter separates into three bilateral pairs of cerebellar peduncles (superior, middle, and inferior), which concomitantly provide both a physical attachment of the cerebellum to the brainstem and a means of communication between the cerebellum and the rest of the central nervous system (CNS). A thin, white lamina, the *superior medullary velum,* stretches between the superior cerebellar peduncles, forming the cranial portion of the roof of the fourth ventricle (Fig. 3). There is also a small *inferior medullary velum,* which stretches between the inferior portion of the cerebellum near the midline and the dorsal aspect of the medulla. This thin membrane forms the caudal extent of the roof of the fourth ventricle, and contains a midline opening known as the *foramen of Magendi.* This opening provides an outlet for the passage of cerebrospinal fluid (CSF) from the fourth ventricle into the subarachnoid space (SAS).

2.2. The Lobes and Fissures of the Cerebellum

The surface of the cerebellum is conspicuously different from the cerebrum, most notably by the appearance of many thin, transversely oriented, leaf-like structures called *folia* and their accompanying parallel fissures. This appearance of the surface of the cerebellum is caused by extensive folding of the cerebellar cortex, resulting in approx 85% of its surface being hidden. Thus, despite the comparatively small size of the cerebellum, its cortex is surprisingly extensive.

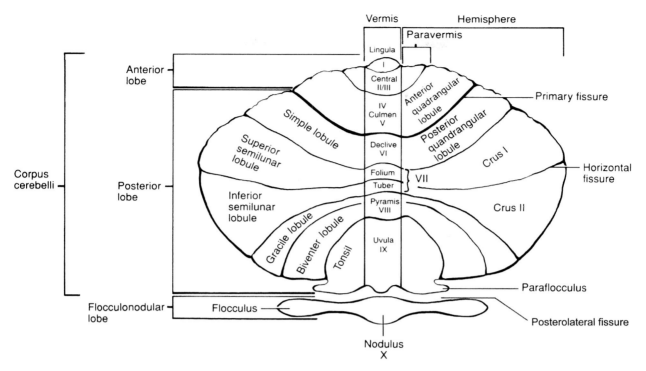

Fig. 2. Schematic of the flattened cerebellum showing the fissures, lobes, and lobules of the cerebellum. The terms on the *left side* of the diagram refer to terminology used for the human cerebellum. Terms on the *right side* refer to terminology used for animals. The Roman numerals designate the ten lobules of the vermis. (The drawing is modified from Larsell, 1951.)

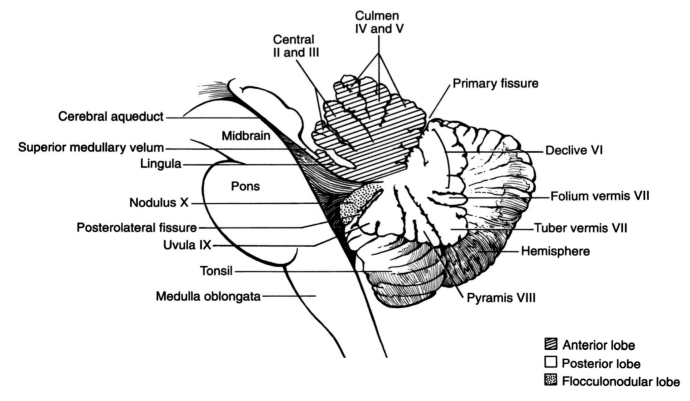

Fig. 3. A midsagittal section through the cerebellar vermis and brainstem.

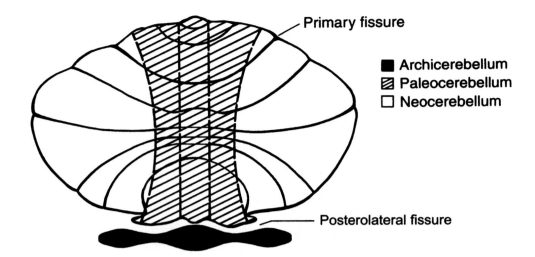

Fig. 4. The functional divisions of the cerebellum are based on phylogenetic development and the termination of afferents to the cerebellar cortex.

For example, if the cerebellar cortex were laid out into a flat sheet, it would extend for almost a meter in length, and have an area of approx 50,000 mm².

Although the cerebellum is divided by many transversely oriented fissures, only the *primary fissure* and the *posterolateral fissure* are significant. They divide the cerebellum into three main lobes—the *anterior lobe*, the *posterior lobe*, and the *flocculonodular lobe* (Figs. 1–5). The anterior lobe is the superior part of the cerebellum, rostral to the V-shaped *primary fissure* (Figs. 1–3). The posterior lobe (sometimes called the middle lobe) is the largest of the three lobes, and is positioned dorsally between the primary fissure and *posterolateral* (prenodular) *fissure* (Fig. 3). Immediately rostral to the posterolateral fissure is the smallest lobe, the flocculonodular lobe (Figs. 2,3,5). The flocculonodular lobe is composed of the midline nodules and the two laterally placed flocculi. The small, semidetached portions of each cerebellar hemisphere that extend medially to merge with the flocculi are nodulus, which forms the rostral pole of the inferior vermis. The deep horizontal fissure (Figs. 1,2) is easily identified, but it *has no apparent functional significance.*

The lobes are divided into lobules, which in turn are further subdivided into many folia. The lobes, lobules, and most of the folia run continuously in a predominantly transverse but somewhat curved direction, from hemisphere to hemisphere so that each has a vermal and two hemispheric components. Traditionally, the lobules are identified by names. In the vermis, the lobules are also identified with Roman numerals (I–X) (Larsell, 1951). The lobular organization can best be distinguished by viewing a midsagittal section through the vermis (Fig. 3), since this is the only region in which all ten lobules are present. For the most part, the separate lobules have no known functional significance; thus, they are of limited use clinically. However, they are often used for descriptive purposes in experimental studies.

2.3. Functional Divisions of the Cerebellum

Based on a combination of criteria, including its phylogenetic development and experimental studies of fiber connections, the cerebellum can be divided into three basic functional divisions (Fig. 4). The *archicerebellum*, or *vestibulocerebellum*, is phylogenetically the oldest division, and as its name implies, it is related functionally to the vestibular system. It receives direct connections from the vestibular nerve, and has reciprocal connections with brainstem vestibular nuclei. It controls balance and coordinates eye movements with movements of the head. The *paleocerebellum*, or *spinocerebellum*, is phylogenetically the next region of the cerebellum to appear. It consists of most of the vermis, paravermis, and anterior lobe. The paleocerebellum receives a variety of sensory inputs from the spinal cord, which it uses for the control of posture, muscle tone, and synergy during stereotyped movements such as walking. The *neocerebellum (cerebrocerebellum, pontocerebellum)*, consists primarily of the large, lateral parts of the posterior lobes. It is the largest and phylogenetically the youngest part of the cerebellum in humans. The neocerebellum receives projections from the pontine nuclei and

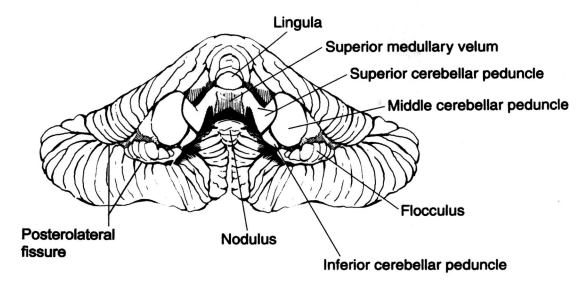

Fig. 5. The anteroinferior surface of the cerebellum, illustrating the cut ends of the three cerebellar peduncles.

Table 1
Principal Inputs to the Cerebellum

Tracts	Origin*	Termination zone*	Peduncle
Ventral spinocerebellar	Spinal cord	V,P	Superior
Tectocerebellar	Sup. and inf. Colliculi	V,P	Superior
Aminergic	LC, RP, VMT	V,P,L	Superior
Corticopontocerebellar	Pontine nuclei	V,P,L	Middle
Dorsal spinocerebellar	Spinal cord	V,P	Inferior
Olivocerebellar	Inf. and access. Olive	V,P,L	Inferior
Cuneocerebellar	Lat. cuneate nucleus	V,P	Inferior
Vestibulocerebellar	Vestibular organ,	F,N,U	Inferior
	Vestibular nuclei	F,V	Inferior
Reticulocerebellar	Reticular formation (RF)	V,P	Inferior
Arcuatocerebellar	Arcuate nucleus	F	Inferior
Trigeminocerebellar	Trigeminal nerve (CN V)	V,P	Inferior

*V, vermal zone; P, paravermal zone; L, lateral zone; F, flocculus; N, nodulus; U, uvula; LC, locus coeruleus; RP, raphe nuclei; VMT, ventral mesencephalic tegmentum; Inf., inferior; Sup., superior; Lat., lateral; Access., accessory; CN V, cranial nerve V.

inferior olivary nuclei that have been relayed from the cerebral cortex. The neocerebellum coordinates the planning of movements, and also functions in the coordination of muscle action required for accurate, nonstereotyped (learned) movements.

2.4. The Cerebellar Peduncles Convey Fibers In and Out of the Cerebellum

The cerebellum is connected to the posterior surface of the lower three segments of the brainstem by three thick pairs of fiber bundles: the *superior, middle,* and *inferior cerebellar peduncles* (Fig 5). All of the inputs and outputs of the cerebellum are routed through these peduncles (Table 1).

The *superior cerebellar peduncle* (*brachium conjunctivum*) physically connects the cerebellum with the lower portion of the midbrain. It contains the principal efferent pathways leaving the cerebellum from the globose, emboliform, and dentate nuclei. The superior cerebellar peduncle also conveys afferent fibers into the cerebellum from the ventral spinocerebellar tract, the tectocerebellar tract, the rubrocerebellar tract, and a small noradrenergic projection from the locus coeruleus.

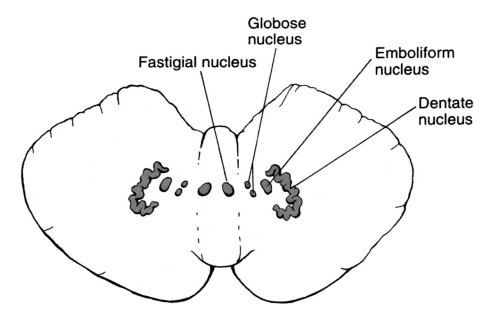

Fig. 6. A diagram demonstrating the four pairs of deep cerebellar nuclei. (Based on Gluhbegovic and Williams, 1980.)

The *middle cerebellar peduncle*, or *brachium pontis*, is the largest of the peduncles, and connects the pons with the cerebellum. It is formed exclusively by afferent fibers provided by the (cortico) pontocerebellar tract. This tract consists of afferent fibers projecting to the cerebellum from the contralateral pontine nuclei. These fibers relay information from all parts of the contralateral cerebral cortex.

The *inferior cerebellar peduncle* is a large bundle of input and output fibers that connects the cerebellum with the medulla oblongata. Seven distinct afferent pathways have been identified that enter the cerebellum through the inferior cerebellar peduncle (Table 1). It is composed of two parts, the larger *restiform body*, which conveys afferent fibers to the cerebellum from spinal cord and brainstem, and the smaller, medially positioned *juxtarestiform body*, which carries a small bundle of vestibular fibers to and from the cerebellum. Important efferent fibers that pass out through the inferior cerebellar peduncle are the cerebellovestibular, cerebello-olivary, and the cerebelloreticular fibers.

2.5. The Deep Cerebellar Nuclei

In humans and the highest primates, there are four pairs of nuclei embedded within the white matter of the cerebellum. From medial to lateral, they are the *fastigial, globose, emboliform,* and *dentate nuclei* (Fig 6). Often, the emboliform and globose nuclei are combined into one cell mass on each side and called the *interposed* or *interpositus nucleus*. Inputs to the

deep cerebellar nuclei are derived from two sources, the Purkinje cells of the cerebellar cortex and extracerebellar sources. Although Purkinje cells provide the output from the cerebellar cortex, the vast majority of Purkinje-cell axons do not leave the cerebellum, but synapse in the deep cerebellar nuclei.

Together with the vestibular nuclei, the deep cerebellar nuclei relay the entire output from the cerebellum to other parts of the CNS. The *fastigial nucleus* is sometimes called the "roof nucleus" because it is located near the midline in the roof of the fourth ventricle. This nucleus receives input from Purkinje cells in the vermis. The fastigial nucleus gives rise to three efferent bundles that project through the juxtarestiform body of the inferior cerebellar peduncle primarily to the vestibular nuclei and reticular formation (RF). The *globose nucleus* actually consists of two or three very small clumps of cells. The *emboliform nucleus* is a small oval nucleus that is lateral to the globose nucleus and medial to the concave hilus of the dentate nucleus. The globose and emboliform nuclei receive inputs from Purkinje cells in the paravermis. The efferent fibers of both the globose and the emboliform nuclei exit the cerebellum through the superior cerebellar peduncle and project to numerous motor control areas in the brainstem, but primarily to the red nucleus on the contralateral side. The *dentate nucleus* is the largest, most laterally placed, and most conspicuous of the deep cerebellar nuclei. In cross-section, it has the appearance of a crumpled band of cells, similar to that

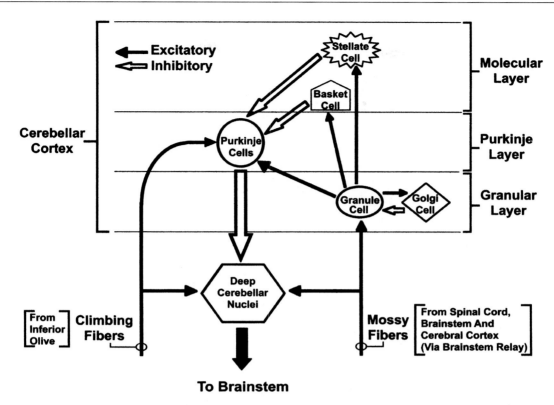

Fig. 7. Simplified diagrammatic representation of the afferent, intracerebellar, and efferent circuitry of the cerebellum, illustrating excitatory and inhibitory components.

of the inferior olive. Careful dissection has shown that it is actually composed of numerous nodules or fingers of gray matter (Gluhbegovic and Williams, 1980). Each dentate nucleus receives input from Purkinje-cell axons from the lateral portions of the ipsilateral cerebellar hemispheres. The efferent fibers from the dentate nucleus represent the primary component of the superior cerebellar peduncle. The main output projects from the hilus of the dentate nucleus to the contralateral ventral lateral (VL) nucleus of the thalamus (with a smaller projection to the ventral anterior (VA) and dorsomedial (DM) nuclei of the thalamus). In addition, there are also small projections to the red nucleus, RF and oculomotor nucleus, all on the contralateral side (Fig. 13).

In addition to distributing cerebellar information to other parts of the brain, collateral axons from all deep cerebellar nuclei project back to the same areas of the cerebellar cortex from which they received Purkinje-cell projections. The deep nuclei also receive collateral inputs from climbing fibers and mossy fibers that project to the cerebellar cortex. Thus, the outputs from the deep cerebellar nuclei represent the main feedback loops from the cerebellum to other areas of

the CNS that are associated with the control of cerebellar function, including the cerebellum itself. A generalized summary of afferent, intracerebellar, and efferent projections of the cerebellum is provided in Fig. 7.

2.6. The Blood Supply to the Cerebellum is Derived from Three Arteries

The cerebellum receives its blood supply from three paired arteries (Fig 8). Two of these arteries supply the inferior surface of the cerebellum. The *posterior inferior cerebellar arteries* (PICA), arise from their respective vertebral arteries just before the latter join to form the basilar artery. The PICAs supply the majority of the inferior surface of the cerebellum, and include branches that supply the inferior vermis, dorsolateral medulla, and restiform body. The *anterior inferior cerebellar arteries* (AICA) typically arise bilaterally near the caudal end of the basilar artery, and supply the more anterior portions of the inferior cerebellum (e.g. the flocculus, the caudal portion of the dentate nucleus, and the middle cerebellar peduncle). The *superior cerebellar arteries* arise bilaterally near the rostral end of the basilar artery. They supply the superior (dorsal) portion of the cerebellum, most of

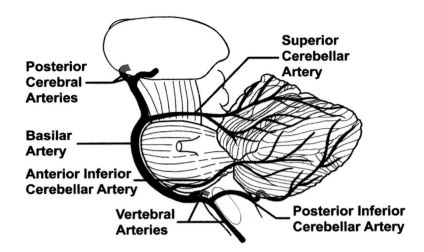

Fig. 8. Lateral view of the cerebellum and brainstem, illustrating the three paired arteries that supply the cerebellum.

the deep cerebellar nuclei, the rostral portion of the middle cerebellar peduncle, and the superior cerebellar peduncle. The venous drainage of the cerebellum is conducted via various venous sinuses and the great cerebral vein.

3. THE CYTOARCHITECTURE OF THE CEREBELLAR CORTEX IS CONSPICUOUSLY UNIFORM

3.1. There Are Three Well-Defined Layers to the Cerebellar Cortex

The cerebellar cortex is a highly convoluted sheet of gray matter about 1 mm thick. Unlike the cerebral cortex, the cerebellar cortex exhibits uniformity both in thickness and in organization. It exhibits a relatively simple but highly organized cytoarchitecture that is remarkably similar in all mammalian species. The cerebellum has three distinct layers, and it contains five major types of neurons. The neurons exhibit a remarkable degree of uniformity in their organization throughout the cortex, both with respect to the transverse and longitudinal axes and to the pial surface (Fig. 9).

The outermost layer (just beneath the pial surface) is known as the *molecular layer*. It is packed with dendrites and axons, but relatively few neurons. Only two neuronal types, *basket cells* and *stellate cells*, have their cell bodies in the molecular layer. During development, there is a transient germinal layer several cells thick between the pial surface and the molecular layer. This is where granule cells are generated; thus, it is called the *external granular layer*. Soon after they are formed, the granule cells migrate through the molecu-

lar and Purkinje-cell layers to reach the granular layer. When granule-cell neurogenesis is complete, the external granular layer disappears. The middle layer, the *Purkinje-cell layer*, is composed of a single layer of Purkinje-cell bodies. The Purkinje cells send their dendrites into the molecular layer and their axons through the granular layer into the medullary white matter. The deepest of the three cerebellar cortical layers is the *granular layer*. It is the thickest layer, densely packed with small *granule cells*. The granular layer also contains a few *Golgi cells* that are located just deep to the Purkinje-cell layer.

3.2. There Are Five Basic Types of Neurons in the Cerebellar Cortex

3.2.1. PURKINJE CELLS

Purkinje cells are highly differentiated neurons, whose cell bodies form a monolayer sandwiched between the molecular and granular layers. The large, flask-shaped cell bodies give rise to large, fan-shaped dendritic arbors that fill the molecular layer in a distinctive pattern that is broad in the transverse plane of the folia and distinctly flattened in the horizontal plane (Figs. 7, 9). Purkinje cells are often called the principal neurons of the cerebellum because they provide the sole output from the cerebellar cortex; all other neurons in the cerebellar cortex are intrinsic neurons. As a Purkinje-cell axon passes through the granule-cell layer it gives off one or more collaterals directed back near the Purkinje-cell layer. Purkinje-cell axons are myelinated, and they synapse on neurons in the deep cerebellar nuclei to be relayed to other regions of the brain. A few Purkinje-cell axons from the vermis

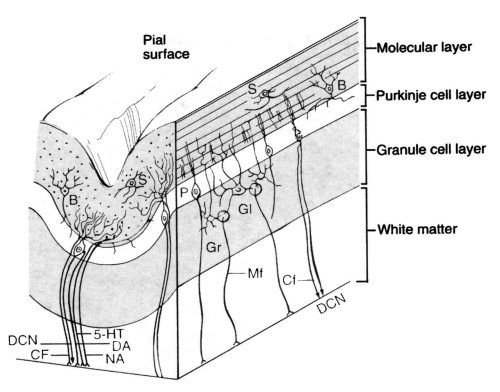

Fig. 9. Schematic of the basic cytoarchitecture of the cerebellar cortex represented by single cerebellar folium. Three types of inputs, climbing fibers (Cf), mossy fibers (Mf), and aminergic fibers (DA, dopaminergic; 5-HT, serotonergic; NA, noradrenergic) are illustrated. Four main types of neurons are identified. P, Purkinje cell; Gr, Granule cell; B, Basket cell; S, Stellate cell. In addition, the glomerulus (Gl) and output to deep cerebellar nuclei (DCN) are illustrated. The orientation of the diagram is such that the surface on the *left side* represents the transverse plane and the *right side* of the diagram represents the longitudinal plane of a folia. (Based in large part on descriptions and drawings from Eccles et al., 1967; and Ito, 1984.)

bypass the deep cerebellar nuclei and synapse directly onto neurons in the lateral vestibular nucleus. Gamma-aminobutyric acid (GABA) is believed to be the inhibitory neurotransmitter of the Purkinje cells.

3.2.2. Granule Cells

There is an immense population of cerebellar granule cells. Cerebellar granule cells are the smallest, most densely packed, and by far the most numerous neuron type in the entire brain. They form the mass of the thick granular layer deep to the Purkinje-cell layer. Granule cells provide the larger of the two principal inputs to the Purkinje cells and contribute the only excitatory input among the intrinsic neurons of the cerebellum. The claw-like terminal branches of granule-cell dendrites act as a functional relay to enable mossy-fiber information to reach the cerebellar cortex. After passing through the Purkinje-cell layer into the molecular layer, each of the small-diameter, nonmyelinated granule-cell axons bifurcate into its characteristic T-shaped junction. The two branches travel 1–1.5 mm in oppo-

site directions horizontally through the molecular layer in the direction of the long axis of the folium, side by side with many thousands of other similar fibers; hence their name, *parallel fibers* (Figs. 7,9,10). There is a geometric relationship between the position of the granule-cell body and the position of the parallel fiber in the molecular layer. The more superficial the granule-cell body is in the granular layer, the more superficial are its parallel fibers in the molecular layer. A single parallel fiber makes multiple synaptic contacts with the dendrites of numerous Purkinje cells. This organization allows each granule cell to synapse with the dendritic spines of several hundred Purkinje cells. Parallel fibers also make synaptic contact with basket, stellate, and Golgi cells. The functional output of granule cells is excitatory, and their neurotransmitter is believed to be glutamate.

3.2.3. Basket Cells

Basket cells are small neurons found in the deeper parts of the molecular layer near the Purkinje-cell

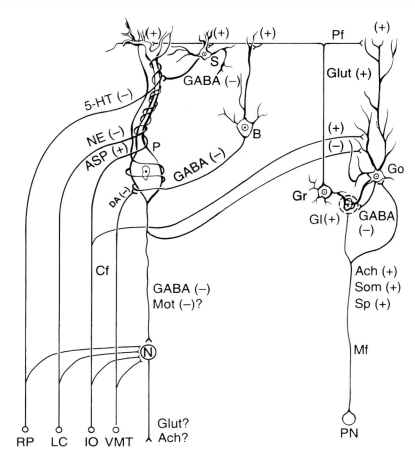

Fig. 10. The essential circuitry of the cerebellar cortex. P, Purkinje cell; Go, Golgi cell; Gr, granule cell; B, basket cell; S, stellate cell; Cf, climbing fiber; Mf, mossy fiber; Pf, parallel fiber; Gl, glomerulus; N, deep cerebellar nuclei; IO, Inferior Olive; LC, locus coeruleus; PN, precerebellar neurons (from various sources); RP, raphe nuclei; VMT, ventral mesencephalic tegmentum; Ach, acetylcholine; Asp, aspartate; DA, dopamine; GABA, gamma-amino butyric acid; Glut, glutamate; Mot, motilin; NE, norepinephrine; Som, somatostatin; SP, substance P; 5-HT, serotonin. (Based in large part on Ito, 1984.)

bodies. Their dendritic trees are unremarkable except that they are oriented as thin wafers; they are broad only in the transverse plane, similar to the orientation of the dendritic trees of Purkinje cells. Basket cells derive their name from the characteristic pericellular basket that their axons form around Purkinje-cell bodies (Fig. 10). The projection field of basket-cell axons is in the transverse plane and is the source of several collateral branches that descend to the cell bodies of Purkinje cells. Each basket-cell primary axon synapses with about a dozen Purkinje cells, but not with the one closest to it. Collateral branches travel in the longitudinal direction, reaching an additional 3–6 rows of Purkinje cells on each side of the primary axon. It is estimated that this allows each basket cell to contact a patch of 100–200 Purkinje cells. The functional output of basket cells is inhibitory, and the available evidence indicates that GABA is the inhibitory neurotransmitter.

3.2.4. Stellate Cells

Stellate cells derive their name from the star-shaped appearance of their dendrites. They are usually located in the outer two-thirds of the molecular layer. Their axons synapse only on Purkinje-cell dendritic shafts (Figs. 9,10). Stellate cells are functionally similar to the basket cells because they receive the same inputs and, like the basket cells, they function to inhibit Purkinje-cell firing. However, since they synapse farther from the Purkinje-cell body than do the basket cells, the influence of stellate cells is less than that of basket cells. It is believed that stellate cells use GABA as their neurotransmitter.

3.2.5. Golgi Cells

Golgi cells are large neurons scattered in the superficial part of the granular layer immediately deep to the Purkinje-cell bodies. Estimates of the size of the

Golgi cell population range from 1:10 Golgi cells to Purkinje cells (Eccles et al., 1967) to a near 1:1 ratio (Ito, 1984). Golgi-cell bodies are approximately the same size as those of Purkinje cells. Although Golgi-cell dendrites are not as elaborate as those of Purkinje cells, their dendritic fields are about three times more extensive (Figs. 9,10). Unlike the dendrites of Purkinje cells, Golgi-cell dendrites are not compressed into the transverse plane of the folia, but instead project both to the molecular and granular layers. The dendrites that enter the molecular layer overlap the dendritic fields of three Purkinje cells in each plane, so that they act as a central point in a functional hexagon that influence about 10 Purkinje cells. Golgi cells receive inputs from mossy fibers. The dendrites that stay in the granular layer contribute to a complex synaptic structure called a *glomerulus*. Golgi-cell axons are conspicuous in appearance. They are short, branch profusely, and also contribute to the formation of the glomerulus. The output from Golgi cells is inhibitory, with GABA as the probable neurotransmitter.

3.3. The Intracortical Circuitry of the Cerebellum Produces a Modulated Inhibitory Output

Based on data from a variety of experimental sources, much of the functional circuitry of the cerebellar cortex has been determined. The connections between mossy fibers and granule cells, granule cells and Purkinje cells, and climbing fibers and Purkinje cells all are excitatory (Figs. 7,10). However, the excitation of Purkinje cells is modulated by several feedback circuits that inhibit Purkinje-cell activity, and therefore suppress transmission from the cerebellar cortex to the deep nuclei. The inhibitory circuits usually limit both the area of the cerebellar cortex that is stimulated and the degree of excitation produced by an incoming signal. Therefore, Purkinje-cell output to the deep cerebellar nuclei is a finely calibrated inhibitory signal (Figs. 7,10).

4. THE INPUT AND OUTPUT SYSTEMS IN THE CEREBELLUM

4.1. There Are Three Basic Categories of Input Fibers to the Cerebellum

Inputs to the cerebellum are directed mainly to the cerebellar cortex (Fig. 7). There are numerous inputs to the cerebellum, but classically they have been combined into two major pathways, *climbing fibers* (olivocerebellar tract) and *mossy fibers* (all other

inputs). More recently, a third small group of *aminergic fibers* that reach the cerebellar cortex has been reported. All of the afferents to the cerebellum arrive through one of the three cerebellar peduncles, but primarily through the inferior and middle peduncles (Table 1).

4.1.1. CLIMBING FIBERS

Classically, climbing fibers have been described as arising from neurons in the inferior olive, which project to the contralateral cerebellar cortex (Figs. 7, 10,13). Although experimental animal studies have challenged that notion (O'Leary et al., 1970), the vast majority clearly do arise from the inferior olive and accessory olivary nuclei. Climbing fibers are named for the manner in which they ascend into the molecular layer to entwine themselves, in ivy fashion, around Purkinje-cell dendritic trees. Each climbing fiber makes several hundred synaptic contacts with the smooth dendritic branches of a single Purkinje cell, so there is no convergence or divergence of the input. Although climbing fibers exert a powerful excitatory influence on individual Purkinje cells, they also provide an excitatory, albeit weaker, input to the Golgi cells and basket and stellate cells, and the deep cerebellar nuclei through collateral branches (Fig. 10). Interestingly, climbing fibers have been postulated to play roles other than influencing motor activity, including a trophic function during development and in plastic reorganization (Ito, 1984). The neurotransmitter of climbing fibers is believed to be aspartate.

4.1.2. MOSSY FIBERS

The mossy-fiber projections to the cerebellum are extensive, and include all of the cerebellar afferents except the climbing fibers and the aminergic projections (Figs. 7,10). They enter the cerebellum through all three peduncles. Myelinated mossy-fiber axons bifurcate many times in the white matter, then lose their myelination as each branch gives off numerous collaterals in the granular layer. Large clump-like swellings, called *rosettes*, are specialized synaptic endings that occur repeatedly along the course of the axon branches. Each mossy-fiber rosette forms the nucleus of a complicated structure called a *glomerulus* (Fig. 10). A glomerulus is a large synaptic complex composed of one mossy-fiber rosette, dendritic contacts from many granule cells, the proximal portions of Golgi-cell dendrites, and terminal branches of Golgi-cell axons. The entire structure is encapsulated in a glial sheath. Each mossy fiber synapses with several hundred granule cells, and each granule cell receives mossy-fiber input from several different mossy fibers, resulting in considerable divergence and convergence of input. Mossy fibers also send collaterals to the deep cerebellar nuclei. In contrast to climbing fibers, mossy fibers activate Purkinje cells indirectly by activating granule cells. In view of the wide variety of their origins, it is not surprising that their neurotransmitters are unknown. However, considering that all mossy fibers are believed to be excitatory, their postulated neurotransmitters include acetylcholine and the neuropeptides, substance P, and somatostatin (Ito, 1984).

4.1.3. Aminergic Fibers

In recent years, experimental studies with animals have identified amine-containing projections to the cerebellum (Fig. 10). A projection of noradrenergic fibers from the locus coeruleus (A_6 cell group) that travels through the superior cerebellar peduncle to synapse with Purkinje-cell dendrites in all parts of the cerebellar cortex has been identified (Bloom, Hoffer and Siggins, 1971). Dopamine-containing fibers from the A10 cell group of the ventral mesencephalic tegmentum project to Purkinje- and granular-cell layers, and also to the interposed and dentate nuclei (Simon et al., 1979). Another input from cell groups B_5 and B_6 in the raphe nuclei in the brainstem is reported to enter the cerebellum through the middle cerebellar peduncle to provide serotonergic fibers to the granular and molecular layers (Takeuchi et al., 1982). Although their existence has been established, little is known about the functional significance of these aminergic inputs.

4.2. There Are Three Primary Sources of Cerebellar Inputs

Although information reaches the cerebellum from a variety of sources (Table 1), the three major sources of afferents are the spinal cord, vestibular system, and the cerebral cortex via brainstem nuclei.

4.2.1. Inputs from the Spinal Cord

Information from the spinal cord reaches the cerebellum through the ventral spinocerebellar tract, dorsal spinocerebellar tract, and the cuneocerebellar tract (Fig. 11). They provide information on the position and condition of muscles, tendons, and joints. The ventral spinocerebellar tract transmits proprioceptive information from all parts of the trunk and limbs, ascending on both sides in the white matter of the spinal cord. The contralateral fibers then recross to the

ipsilateral side, and all of them enter the cerebellum through the superior cerebellar peduncle, terminating as mossy fibers. The dorsal spinocerebellar tract conveys proprioceptive information from the lower trunk and lower limbs. This projection of mossy-fiber inputs ascends in the spinal cord on the ipsilateral side and enters the cerebellum through the inferior cerebellar peduncle. The cuneocerebellar tract transmits proprioceptive information from the upper trunk and upper limbs. Axons arising from the lateral (accessory) cuneate nucleus in the medulla oblongata enter the ipsilateral cerebellum through the inferior cerebellar peduncle to terminate as mossy fibers. It should be noted that all spinal cord afferent pathways to the cerebellum arise and terminate on the ipsilateral side.

Data from experimental studies have demonstrated that the inputs from proprioceptive and tactile stimuli to the cerebellar cortex are organized in two somatotopic maps (homunculi), one centered in the vermis of the anterior lobe and the other (actually a double one consisting of bilateral mirror images) in the posterior lobe. These cerebellar homunculi are considerably less precise than those in the cerebral cortex.

4.2.2. Inputs from the Vestibular System

Primary fibers from the vestibular labyrinth travel via Cranial Nerve VIII to reach the ipsilateral cerebellum through the juxtarestiform body (Fig. 12). A much larger bundle of fibers is directed to the vestibular nuclei in the brainstem, where it is subsequently relayed through the juxtarestiform body to terminate bilaterally in the flocculonodular lobe and most of the remaining vermis as mossy fibers. These vestibular fibers provide important information pertaining to equilibrium.

4.2.3. Inputs from the Cerebral Cortex

Information from multiple regions of the cerebral cortex reaches the cerebellum indirectly from three different pathways, the (cortico) pontocerebellar tract, the (cortico) olivocerebellar tract and the (cortico) reticulocerebellar pathway (Fig. 13)

This information which is destined for the cerebellum, originates from cells in various regions of the cerebral cortex and synapses in the pontine nuclei, the inferior olivary nuclei, and the reticular formation. The (cortico)pontocerebellar pathway continues from neurons in the pontine nuclei that give rise to fibers that cross the midline and enter the cerebellum on the contralateral side through the middle cerebellar peduncle. This huge fiber tract projects to the cerebel-

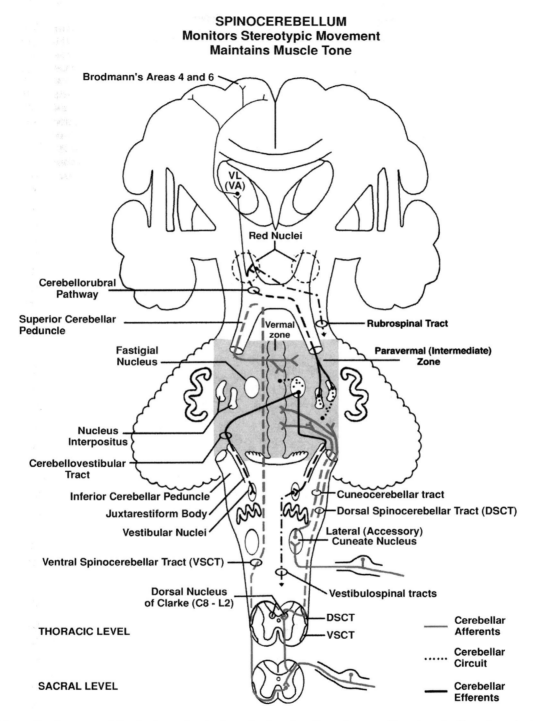

Fig. 11. Schematic diagram of the brain and spinal cord, showing the primary afferent and efferent projections of the spinocerebellum.

lum as mossy fibers. The olivocerebellar pathway relays information from the cerebral cortex that projects to the inferior olive. Inferior olivary fibers cross the midline to enter the cerebellum through the contralateral inferior cerebellar peduncle, where they terminate directly on Purkinje-cell dendrites as climbing fibers. The reticulocerebellar pathway also relays information from the cerebral cortex. Neurons in the

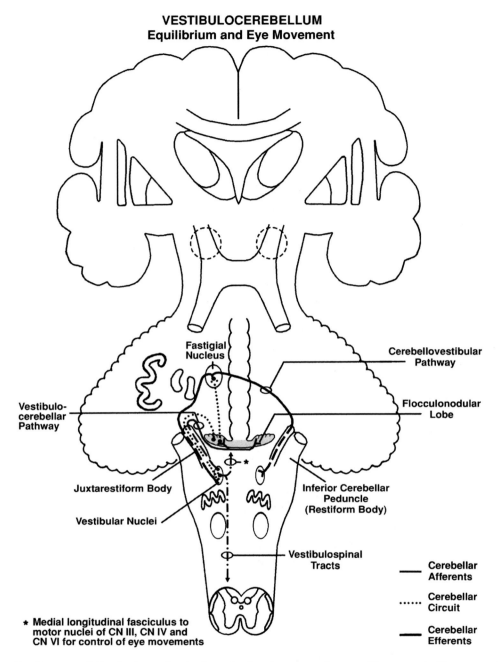

VESTIBULOCEREBELLUM
Equilibrium and Eye Movement

Fastigial Nucleus

Cerebellovestibular Pathway

Vestibulo-cerebellar Pathway

Flocculonodular Lobe

Juxtarestiform Body

Vestibular Nuclei

Inferior Cerebellar Peduncle (Restiform Body)

Vestibulospinal Tracts

Cerebellar Afferents

Cerebellar Circuit

Cerebellar Efferents

★ Medial longitudinal fasciculus to motor nuclei of CN III, CN IV and CN VI for control of eye movements

Fig. 12. Schematic diagram of the brain and spinal cord, showing the primary afferent and efferent projections of the vestibulocerebellum.

brainstem RF give rise to fibers that enter the cerebellum on the ipsilateral side through the inferior cerebellar peduncle to end as mossy fibers.

4.3. The Outputs from the Cerebellum Are Less Complex than the Inputs

There are fewer outputs from the cerebellum than inputs. The sole output from the entire cerebellar cortex is from the axons of Purkinje cells. However, information from most of the Purkinje cells is relayed through neurons in the deep cerebellar nuclei before exiting the cerebellum (Figs. 11–14). All outputs from the cerebellum exit through either the superior or inferior cerebellar peduncles.

The majority of outputs from the cerebellum exit through the superior cerebellar peduncle. The small

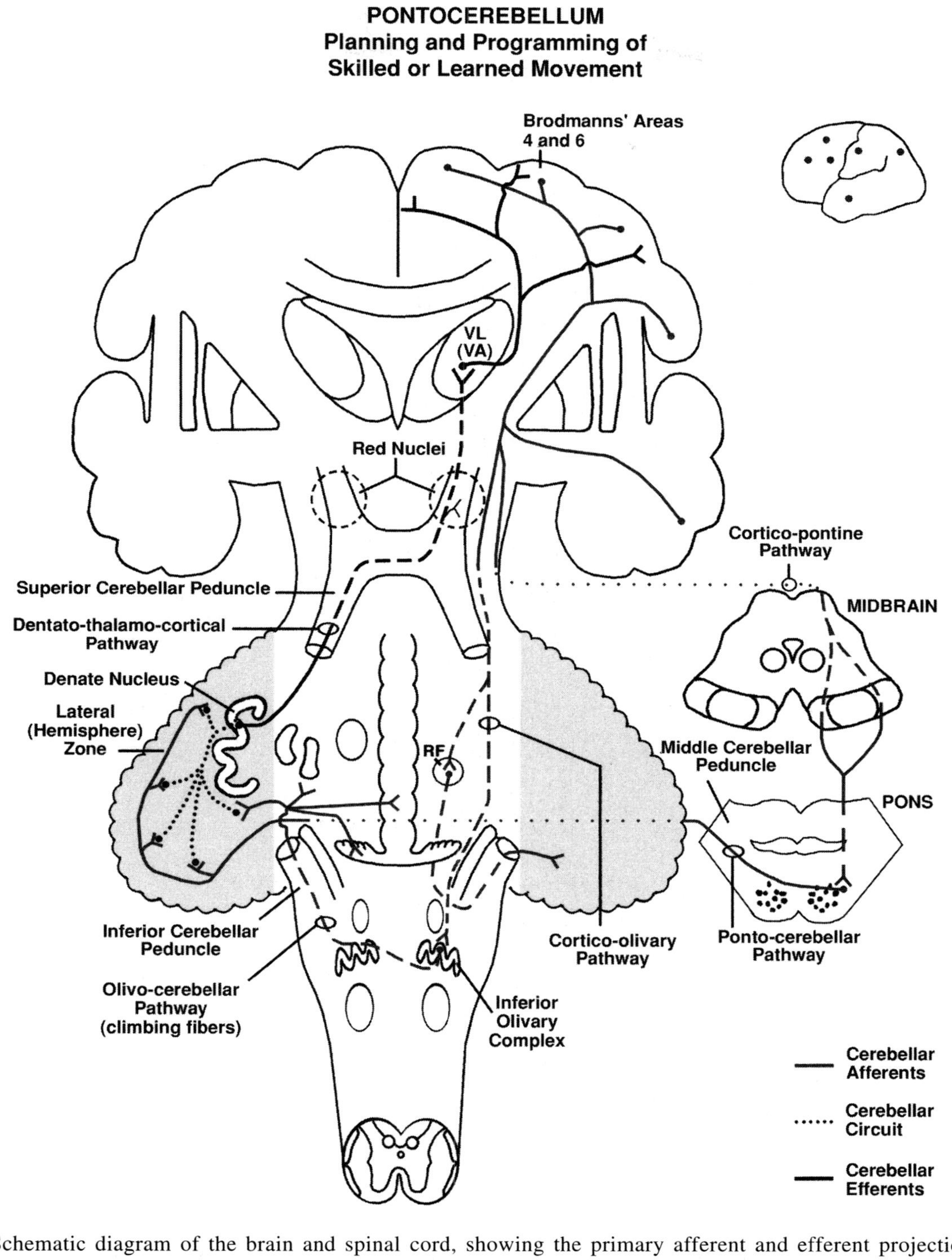

Fig. 13. Schematic diagram of the brain and spinal cord, showing the primary afferent and efferent projections of the pontocerebellum.

projection of Purkinje-cell axons that do leave the cerebellum directly, travel through the juxtarestiform body of the inferior cerebellar peduncle, and synapse in the vestibular nuclei. The output from the other Purkinje cells project to the deep cerebellar nuclei in a specific pattern (Figs. 11–14), and the principal efferents from the cerebellum originate from cells in these deep nuclei. Purkinje cells in the vermis project to the fastigial nucleus, Purkinje cells in the intermediate zone project to the globose and emboliform

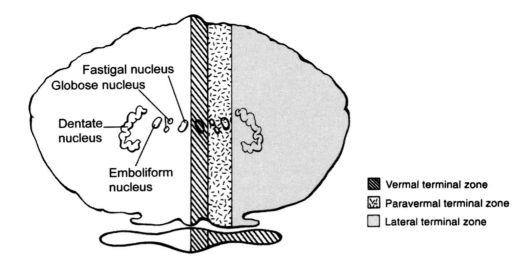

Fig. 14. Diagram illustrating the zones of organization of the cerebellum based on the longitudinal termination of inputs to the cerebellar cortex and their projections to the deep cerebellar nuclei. Compare with Fig. 4.

nuclei, and those in the lateral cerebellar hemispheres project to the dentate nucleus. Some Purkinje cells from the flocculus and nodulus project to both the fastigial and dentate nuclei as well as to the vestibular nuclei.

The outputs from the fastigial nucleus project mainly to the brainstem, where they synapse in the vestibular nuclei bilaterally, and in the reticular formation, where the projection is primarily contralateral. The ipsilateral projections from the fastigial nucleus travel through the juxtarestiform body. The fibers destined for contralateral regions cross the midline while still within the cerebellum, hook around the superior cerebellar peduncle (hence the name *hook bundle* or *uncinate fasciculus*), and then exit through the juxtarestiform body on the contralateral side. Small contralateral projections also reach the cervical spinal cord and the thalamus (Fig. 12).

The largest output from the cerebellum consists of axons passing through the superior cerebellar peduncle (brachium conjunctivum) (Fig. 13). The cells of origin are located in the globose, emboliform, and dentate nuclei. Some of these cells project axons to the inferior olive and RF (the descending limb of the superior cerebellar peduncle). However, the vast majority of the fibers in this peduncle project rostrally to cross to the contralateral side in the midbrain at the level of the inferior colliculus as the decussation of the superior cerebellar peduncle. Many of the axons that originate in the emboliform and globose nuclei, and a few fibers from the dentate nucleus, synapse in the contralateral red nucleus. The majority of the remaining axons from

the dentate nucleus (the *dentatorubrothalamic tract*) continue on to the contralateral thalamus, where they terminate primarily in the VL nucleus, with a smaller contingent terminating in the VA nucleus.

In summary, with the exception of a small bundle of Purkinje-cell axons that project directly to the vestibular nuclei in the brainstem, all outputs of the cerebellum consist of axons with cell bodies located in the deep cerebellar nuclei. Each fastigial nucleus projects bilaterally to the vestibular nuclei. In contrast, the globose and emboliform nuclei on each side project mainly to the contralateral red nucleus, and each dentate nucleus projects primarily to the VL of the contralateral thalamus (Figs. 11–13).

5. CEREBELLAR DYSFUNCTION

In contrast to the detailed knowledge of the specific connections of the relatively simple and uniform cortical organization of the cerebellum, surprisingly little is known about its functions in relation to other regions of the brain. Cerebellar function is best appreciated by considering the effects of lesions on specific parts of the cerebellum. With this goal in mind, two plans of functional organization have been proposed. Although they are similar, they differ somewhat in the resultant functional zones they represent. Various authors use one or the other, or both schemes, to localize cerebellar function.

Based in part on data from both clinical and experimental studies, three so-called "cerebellar syndromes" can be distinguished: (i) Flocculonodular syndrome;

(ii) Anterior-lobe syndrome; and (iii) Neocerebellar syndrome. This distinction has been used by a number of authors to help correlate structural and functional relationships in the cerebellum, and to explain deficits resulting from cerebellar lesions. The flocculonodular syndrome is characterized by problems with maintaining equilibrium, but there is no ataxia of the limbs, hypotonia, or tremor. The anterior-lobe syndrome is characterized by increased postural reflexes. The neocerebellar syndrome is distinguished by ataxia and hypotonia, producing clumsy movements. Although it is possible to demonstrate these syndromes experimentally in animals, pure cerebellar syndromes, especially the anterior-lobe syndrome, are seldom manifested in humans (Brodal, 1981).

It is important to emphasize that since the local circuitry is essentially identical throughout the cerebellar cortex, a strict localization of function does not exist within the cortex itself. Rather, functional localization in the cerebellum is the result of differences in the location of the termination of its afferent and efferent projections. Thus, from a clinical perspective, cerebellar function and dysfunction can best be understood by the organization of three longitudinal zones based on the terminal fields of major inputs to the cerebellar cortex (Fig. 9). These three longitudinal (sagittal) bands are the vermal, paravermal, and lateral zones. This organization represents a crude parcellation of afferent termination zones in the cerebellar cortex, but it should be recognized that it has considerable overlap. The cerebellar cortex continues the longitudinal organization by projecting from the three longitudinal cortical zones to corresponding deep cerebellar nuclei (Fig. 14).

Damage to the cerebellum or its associated afferent and efferent systems produces distinctive symptoms and signs, usually on the same side of the body as the lesion. The remarkable uniformity of the cerebellum suggests that its basic functioning is the same throughout the cerebellar cortex. Therefore, it is not surprising that lesions of deep nuclei and/or superior cerebellar peduncle (e.g., lesions that interrupt cerebellar outflow) produce more severe signs than lesions restricted to parts of the cerebellar cortex. Signs of cerebellar dysfunction in humans are usually the result of lesions that involve more than one specific region of the cerebellum. They manifest themselves as deficits in somatic motor control, with the most common symptoms related to disturbances of gait. For organizational purposes, it is worthwhile to consider separately the results of damage to the vermal, paravermal, and lat-

eral zones. There have been a number of excellent descriptions and reviews of the disorders of cerebellar function (Holmes, 1939; Dow and Moruzzi, 1958; Gilman et al., 1981), to which interested readers are referred.

5.1. Vermal Zone Cerebellar Damage

The vermal or midline longitudinal zone consists of the vermis, the flocculi, the fastigial nuclei, and related input and output fibers. The principal afferents to this zone are from the vestibular organ and nuclei, from the trunk and neck via the spinal cord, and from the reticular formation. Some primary inputs from the vestibular part of the vestibulocochlear nerve (Cranial Nerve VIII) enter the cerebellum as part of the juxtarestiform body and terminate in the flocculus and nodulus—with a small projection to the uvula and lingula of the vermis—as well as sending collaterals to the fastigial nucleus. A larger projection of secondary fibers from the vestibular nuclei also project to most of the vermal zone. Proprioceptive information from the head, particularly from the temporomandibular joint (TMJ) and muscles of mastication, are transmitted through the trigeminocerebellar tract, which originates from the mesencephalic trigeminal nucleus, and projects to parts of the vermis, paravermis, and flocculus via the restiform body.

Functionally, the vermal zone is associated with posture as controlled by trunk (axial) musculature and proximal limb muscles, head position, extraocular movements, equilibrium, and locomotion. Clinical signs resulting from midline cerebellar damage produce disorders of posture and gait, head positions, and eye movements (e.g., nystagmus). Because of its connections with the vestibular system, damage to the flocculus, nodule, and uvula result in a pronounced loss of equilibrium, including truncal ataxia (swaying while standing or staggering while walking with a tendency to fall, usually backwards), and a compensatory, wide-based stance and/or gait. There is an inability to incorporate vestibular information with body and eye movements. When damage is restricted to the vermal zone, these deficits and truncal asynergia are usually present without the disruption of function in individual limbs when tested separately (Gilman, 1986). Midline cerebellar lesions may also result in varying levels of tremor, known as *titubation*, involving the head and/or trunk.

A clinical picture corresponding to the vermal or flocculonodular syndrome seen in children between five and ten years of age occurs as a result of a specific type of tumor known as a medulloblastoma. It usually occurs in the nodulus of the vermis, is characterized by unsteady gait and frequent unexplained falls, and may be accompanied by nystagmus. Medulloblastoma is a neoplasm that is derived from persistent clumps of germinal cells from the external granular layer. This germinal field normally dissipates after about two years of age, which helps to explain why this tumor is the most common type of CNS tumor in children, but never occurs in adults.

5.2. Paravermal Zone Cerebellar Damage

The functional paravermal (or intermediate) zone consists of the cerebellar cortex just lateral to the vermis, together with the emboliform and globose nuclei and interconnected inputs and outputs. The principal source of information to the paravermal zone is the limbs, but afferents are from a variety of sources from spinal cord, brainstem, and cerebral cortex. Outputs project to both rostral and caudal portions of the nervous system. Damage restricted solely to the paravermal zone is found only in experimental animals. In humans, lesions of this region are typically an extension of existing lesions in the vermal or lateral regions of the cerebellum. Functionally, this region seems to be involved in the modulation of velocity, force, and the pattern of muscle movement and changes in muscle tone (either hyper- or hypotonia).

5.3. Lateral Zone Cerebellar Damage

The large lateral zone consists of most of the cerebellar hemispheres (including much of the anterior lobe), the dentate nuclei, and related inputs and outputs. Inputs are from numerous sources, but most important is the projection from the cerebral cortex that is relayed through the pons. Outputs are to the brainstem and thalamus. This region is involved in the planning of voluntary movements in conjunction with the cerebral cortex. Damage to the large lateral hemispheric regions affects the initiation and coordination of volitional movements. The most common type of cerebellar disease involves the hemispheres or some part of their efferent projections. Damage to the lateral zone produces movement disorders of the limbs as well as difficulty in posture and gait. If the lesion is unilateral, the signs are ipsilateral; the patient tends to stagger and deviate to the affected side.

There are a number of common disturbances associated with damage to the lateral cerebellar zone. A lesion of this region can result in any combination of the following signs and symptoms: *Ataxia* is a general term for disturbances or clumsiness of motor activity

related to voluntary movement. *Asynergia*, or limb ataxia, is the reduced ability to execute smooth, coordinated sequential movements. *Hypotonia* is a reduced resistance to passive movement caused by a loss of cerebellar influence. *Asthenia* is an increased propensity for muscle fatigue, which is often associated with hypotonia. *Intention tremor* is an oscillating movement of a limb, which is present only during limb movement. This tremor is particularly pronounced toward the end of a given movement, such as reaching for an object. "Intention" tremor is in contrast to the Parkinson's "resting" tremor, which is manifested while the extremity is at rest. *Adiadochokinesia (dysdiadochokinesia)* refers to uncoordinated, irregular movements that occur during attempted rapid alternating movements, such as pronating and supinating the forearm. In *dysmetria*, the judgement of distance is impaired. This is evident from the inaccurate control of the range and direction of movement, resulting in either undershoot or overshoot of the desired point ("past-pointing"). A related sign is known as "impaired check and rebound." This can be elicited by asking the patient to lean their chest firmly against the examiner's hands, then abruptly removing the examiner's hand. In a patient with normal cerebellar function, their forward movement is quickly checked. The patient with a lateral cerebellar lesion will continue forward, with the patient typically losing their balance or rocking back and forth. There also can be ocular signs, especially *nystagmus*, which is of greatest amplitude when looking to the same side as the lesion. *Decomposition of movement* is a term given to the breaking down of a complex movement into its various components, which appear jerky and uncoordinated, rather than appearing as a smooth, flowing movement. *Dysarthria* refers to disorders in the mechanical component of the articulation of speech resulting from ataxia of the muscles of the larynx. This results in a typical pattern involving explosive, halting speech with garbled words and difficulty in modulating volume.

5.4. General Concepts Related to Cerebellar Damage

Relatively small lesions to the cerebellar cortex produce few discernable deficits. Even the diagnosis of substantial cerebellar damage is often difficult because the effects are often transient, because of the remarkable functional plasticity that can occur. Generally, the onset and spread of pathologic processes is more rapid in older patients, typically resulting in better-defined and more permanent symptoms in this age group. The compensatory plasticity can be so great in response to cerebellar damage in fetal and neonatal life that major signs of cerebellar damage can be lacking, even in cases where an entire cerebellar hemisphere is completely absent (Brodal, 1981).

The cerebellum is vulnerable to damage from a wide variety of sources, including developmental defects, degenerative diseases (both hereditary and nonhereditary), infectious processes, chronic alcoholism, toxic and metabolic effects (including hypoxia), thrombosis of the cerebellar arteries, trauma, and tumors. Damage can occur from either direct or indirect sources. Tonsillar herniation, for instance, causes the cerebellar tonsils to be squeezed out of the base of the skull through the foramen magnum as a result of a tumor or hemorrhaging (Adams et al., 1984). In recent years, considerable experimental data indicate that severe malnutrition during development (Dobbing, 1981) and fetal alcohol exposure (West, 1986) both produce permanent structural damage to the cerebellum.

Lesions restricted to the vermis produce disturbances of the trunk (stance and gait), and lesions of the lateral parts of the cerebellar hemispheres produce disturbances chiefly related to voluntary movements of the limbs. The most prevalent clinical symptoms of cerebellar damage are associated with disruptions of standing and walking. The identification of the loci of damage based on the analysis of cerebellar symptoms is often difficult, since more than one basic cerebellar region is usually affected. Symptoms usually dissipate with time, particularly when the damage occurs in childhood or develops slowly, over a long period of time. Cerebellar damage can have many etiologies. Secondary effects such as pressure, tissue dislocation, or vascular changes caused by associated circulatory disturbances also can produce serious cerebellar damage (Brodal, 1981).

To summarize, there are four important concepts to keep in mind when considering lesions of the cerebellum. These concepts are as follows:

1. Lesions of the cerebellum or its afferent or efferent pathways may disrupt normal coordinated movements, but will not cause paralysis.
2. Because of its internal and external anatomical connections, each cerebellar hemisphere exerts its influence on the muscles of the ipsilateral side of the body.
3. The flocculonodular lobe influences the axial musculature bilaterally.
4. Because of the convergence of the output of the cerebellar hemispheres to the deep cerebellar nuclei and the further subsequent compaction of

efferents through the superior cerebellar peduncle, lesions of the efferent pathway (deep cerebellar nuclei and/or superior cerebellar peduncles) produce more profound and permanent deficits than lesions of the afferent pathways or cerebellar cortex.

6. OTHER FUNCTIONS OF THE CEREBELLUM

In addition to the roles played by the cerebellum in assisting the rest of the brain in controlling and coordinating muscle activity, experimental studies have identified other cerebellar functions. The cerebellum helps to regulate some autonomic functions including respiration, cardiovascular functions and pupillary size. Another function now believed to be influenced by the cerebellum is motor learning. A wide variety of experimental studies have generated convincing data demonstrating that cerebellar circuitry can be altered functionally by experience, and that certain types of motor learning can be prevented or altered by cerebellar lesions. The cerebellum also plays a role in some types of classical conditioning (McCormick and Thompson, 1984). More recent evidence indicates that the cerebellum also may be involved in the early development and retention of cognitive skills in humans (Levisohn et al., 2000; Riva and Giorgi, 2000; Alin et al, 2001). Moreover, new experimental techniques, such as functional MRI, are challenging our current knowledge of cerebellar function (Cui et. al., 2000). Together, these and related studies indicate that despite the voluminous experimental literature focused on the cerebellum, it is clear that cerebellar function is not understood completely. The following recent review articles on cerebellar function are provided in the bibliography for the interested reader: Mauk et al., 2000; Ito, 2000.

ACKNOWLEDGMENTS

The authors would like to express their deep appreciation to Ms. Joan Quarles for her invaluable assistance in the development and rendering of the illustrations for this chapter.

SELECTED READINGS

Adams JH, Corsellis JAN, Duchen LW (eds). Greenfield's Neuropathology. 4t ed., New York:John Wiley & Sons, 1984.

Allin M, Matsumoto H, Santhouse AM, Nosarti C, AIAsady MH, Sterwart A L, Rifkin L, Murray RM. Cognitive and motor function and the size of the cerebellum in adolescents born very preterm. Brain 2001; 124 (Pt 1):60–66.

Bloom FE, Hoffer BJ, and Siggins GR. Studies on norepinehrine-containing afferents to Purkinje cells of rat cerebellum. I. Localization of the fibers and their synapses. Brain Research 1971; 25:501–521.

Brodal A. Neurological Anatomy in Relation to Clinical Medicine, 3rd ed. New York:Oxford University Press, 1981.

Cui CZ, Li EZ, Zang YF, Weng XC, Ivry R, Wang JJ. Both sides of human cerebellum involved in preparation and execution of sequential movements. Neuroreport 2000; 11(17): 3849–3853.

Dobbing J. The later development of the brain. In Davis JA, Dobbing J (eds). Scientific Foundations of Paediatrics, 2nd Ed. London:William Heinemann Medical Books, Ltd., 1981; 744–759.

Dow RS, Moruzzi G. The Physiology and Pathology of the Cerebellum. Minneapolis:University of Minnesota Press, 1958.

Eccles JC, Ito M, Szentágothai J. The Cerebellum as a Neuronal Machine, New York:Springer-Verlag, 1967.

Gilman S. Cerebellum and Motor Dysfunction. In Asbury AK, McKhann GM, McDonals WI (eds). Diseases of the Nervous System, vol. I, London:William Heinemann Medical Books, Ltd., 1986; 401–422.

Gilman S, Bloedel JR, Lechtenberg R. Disorders of the Cerebellum. Philadelphia:Davis, 1981.

Gluhbegovic N, Williams TH. The Human Brain: a photographic guide. Hagerstown, MD:Harper & Row Publishers, Inc., 1980.

Holmes G. The cerebellum of man. Brain 1939; 62:1–30.

Ito M. The Cerebellum and Neural Control. New York, Raven Press, 1984.

Ito M. Mechanisms of motor learning in the cerebellum. Brain Research 2000; 886(1–2): 237–245.

Larsell O. Anatomy of the Nervous System, 2nd ed., New York:Appleton-Century-Crofts, Inc., 1951.

Levisohn L, Cronin-Golomb A, Schmahmann J D. Neuropsychological consequences of cerebellar tumour resection in children: cerebellar cognitive affective syndrome in a paediatric population. Brain 2000; 123(Pt 5): 1041–1050.

Mauk MD, Medina JF, Nores WL, Ohyama T. Cerebellar function: coordination, learning or timing? Curr Biol 2000; 10(14): R522–525.

McCormick DA, Thompson RF. Cerebellum:Essential involvement in the classically conditioned eyelid response. Science 1984; 223:296–299.

O'Leary, Dunsker SB, Smith JM, Inukai J, O'Leary M. Termination of the olivocerebellar system in the cat. Arch Neurol 1970; 22:193–206.

Riva D, Giorgi C. The cerebellum contribures to higher functions during development: evidence from a series of children surgically treated for posterior fossa tumours. Brain 2000; 123 (Pt 5): 1051–1061.

Simon H, Le Moal M, Casal A. Efferents and afferents to the ventral tegmental-A10 region studied after local injection of (^{3}H) leucine and horseradish peroxidase. Brain Res 1979;178:17–40.

Takeuchi Y, Kimura H, Sano Y. Immunohistochemical demonstration of serotonin-containing nerve fibers in the cerebellum. Cell Tissue Res 1982; 226:1–12.

West JR (ed). Alcohol and Brain Development. New York:Oxford University Press, 1986.

11 The Brainstem
An Overview

Harold H. Traurig

CONTENTS

1. EXTERNAL ANATOMY

The brainstem is best viewed when separated from the overlying cerebral hemispheres and cerebellum, and in a midsagittal section of the brain (Figs. 1–3; Chapter 2, Figs. 5–9). The brainstem is continuous with the spinal cord at the foramen magnum of the occipital bone and with the diencephalon at the incisura of the tentorium and the posterior clinoid processes of the sphenoid bone. It consists of the midbrain, pons, and medulla, which lie in close relationship to the cranial surface of the base of the occipital bone. The vertebral and basilar arteries lie between the ventral surface of the brainstem and the occipital bone (Chapter 2, Fig. 13). The paired cranial nerves originate or terminate in the brainstem, except for the olfactory, optic, and spinal portion of the accessory nerve (Fig. 1; Chapter 2, Figs. 5–9). The cerebellum lies posterior to the brainstem and is attached by three pairs of fiber bundles: the inferior, middle, and superior cerebellar peduncles (Fig. 2). The brainstem, cerebellum, roots

of the cranial nerves, and vertebro-basilar arterial system are located in the posterior cranial fossa or infratentorial space (Chapter 2, Fig. 4).

2. VENTRICULAR SYSTEM OF THE BRAINSTEM

The lumen of the embryonic neural tube is represented in the brainstem by the *cerebral aqueduct* and the *fourth ventricle*. The midline *third ventricle*, located between the bilateral components of the *diencephalon*, is continuous caudally with the cerebral aqueduct. The cerebral aqueduct traverses the midbrain to the rostral border of the pons, where it expands as the pyramidal-shaped fourth ventricle, which is located posterior to the pons and medulla (Fig. 2; Chapter 2, Figs. 6,8,9C). Removal of the cerebellum reveals the floor of the fourth ventricle (rhomboid fossa). The fourth ventricle extends into the base of the cerebellum and is bounded by the anterior and posterior medullary veli of the cerebellum. The *anterior medullary velum* becomes continuous with the tectum of the midbrain. The *posterior medullary velum* is a thin membrane consisting of the ependyma, arachnoid, and choroid plexus. The caudal extent of the fourth ventricle continues as the *median aperture (of Magendie)*

From: *Neuroscience in Medicine, 2nd ed.* (P. Michael Conn, ed.),
© 2003 Humana Press Inc., Totowa, NJ.

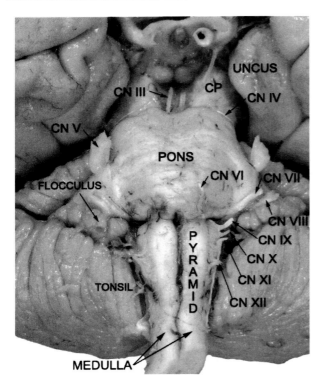

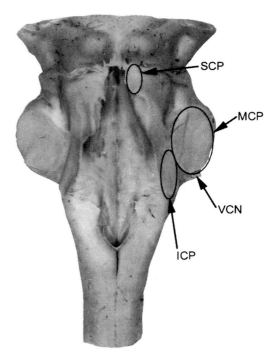

Fig. 1. Anterior view of the brainstem illustrating the cranial-nerve roots. III, oculomotor nerve; IV, trochlear nerve; V, trigeminal nerve; VI, abducens nerve; VII, facial nerve; VIII, vestibulocochlear nerve; IX, glossopharyngeal nerve; X, vagus nerve; XI accessory nerve; XII, hypoglossal nerve. CP, cerebral peduncles of midbrain. The space between the cerebral peduncles is the interpeduncular fossa or cistern; the posterior aspect of this space is the posterior perforated substance of the midbrain (*see* Fig. 6B). Rostral to the midbrain are the mammillary bodies of the hypothalamus. UNCUS, uncus of the parahippocampal gyrus. Note the close relationship to the midbrain. The medulla, pons, and flocculus form the boundaries of the cerebellopontine space (angle); note the close relationships of the facial and vestibulocochlear-nerve roots.

Fig. 2. Posterior view of the brainstem with the cerebellum removed (*see* Chapter 2, Figs. 6,9B). The trochlear nerve arises from the dorsal aspect of the brainstem. The ovals indicate the sectioned cerebellar peduncles. ICP, inferior cerebellar peduncle; MCP, middle cerebellar peduncle; SCP, superior cerebellar peduncle; VCN, vestibulocochlear nerve.

in the posterior medullary velum, which permits the passage of cerebrospinal fluid (CSF) from the fourth ventricle into the *cerebellomedullary cistern (cisterna magna)*. At the pons-medullary boundary, the fourth ventricle extends laterally forming *lateral apertures (of Luschka)*, which permit the passage of CSF into the *pontine cistern*. Each lateral aperture opens into the pontine cistern in close association with the *flocculus* of the cerebellum and the root of the *vestibulocochlear nerve* (Fig. 1). The median and lateral apertures are the only passages for CSF from the ventricular system into the subarachnoid space (SAS) (*see* Chapter 2, Figs. 5–9,14).

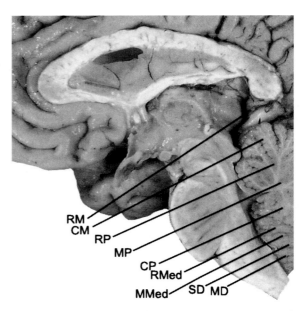

Fig. 3. Midsagittal section of the brain illustrating the diencephalon, brainstem, and cerebellum. (*See* Chapter 2, Fig. 8). The lettered lines correspond to the planes of the axial sections of the brainstem illustrated in Figs. 4–6. RM, rostral midbrain

3. MEDULLA

The anterior aspect of the medulla is composed of paired bundles of fibers, the *pyramids*, which are continuations of the motor pathway from the cortex to the spinal cord (Fig. 1). At the medulla-spinal cord transition, most of the motor-pathway axons cross to the contralateral side forming the *motor* or *pyramidal decussation*, and continue without synapse as the corticospinal tracts into the lateral funiculi of the spinal cord (Fig. 4A).

The *olive*, a prominent swelling on the lateral aspect of the medulla, marks the position of the *inferior olivary nucleus*, a component of the motor system, which projects to the contralateral cerebellum. The *glossopharyngeal* and *vagus nerves* emerge as a series of rootlets just posterior to the olive; the *hypoglossal nerve* rootlets exit the medulla anterior to the olive (Figs. 1,4C).

On the posterior surface of the medulla, the *inferior medullary velum* covers the "V" shaped caudal aspect of the fourth ventricle. This is the location of the *median aperture (of Magendie)* through which CSF passes from the *fourth ventricle* into the SAS. The *cuneate* and *gracilis tubercles* mark the locations of the *nucleus cuneatus* and *nucleus gracilis* (Figs. 4A,B; Chapter 2, Fig. 6). These nuclei are functionally related to the ascending sensory pathways that carry discriminative tactile and proprioceptive sensations.

4. PONS

The base and lateral aspect of the *pons* are formed by a large mass of efferent fibers to the cerebellum, the *middle cerebellar peduncles* (Fig. 1). These axons arise from the *pontine nuclei*, decussate in the base of the pons and project to the contralateral cerebellum. These projections are a component of the pathway that connect motor areas of the cortex to the contralateral cerebellum. The basilar artery in the intact brain occupies the median depression in the base of the pons (Fig. 1; Chapter 2, Fig. 13).

Four pairs of cranial nerves enter and exit the pons. The *trigeminal nerve* roots emerge from the lateral aspect and course forward, crossing the petrous

ridge of the temporal bone to the trigeminal ganglia in the middle cranial fossa. The *abducens, facial* and *vestibulocochlear nerves* are attached to the lateral aspect of the pons-medulla junction (Fig. 1).

The slender *abducens nerve* exits anteriorly from the pons-medullary boundary, courses forward into the middle cranial fossa, then enters the orbit to innervate the lateral rectus muscle (Fig. 1). As it traverses the middle cranial fossa, the abducens nerve accompanies the oculomotor, trochlear, and ophthalmic nerves. All are embedded in the lateral wall of the cavernous sinus and pass through the superior orbital fissure into the orbit.

The *facial* and *vestibulocochlear nerves* are in close relationship to one another, and are attached to the lateral aspect of the brainstem in a space formed by the pons-medulla junction and the overlying cerebellum, the *cerebellopontine space* or *angle*. The facial nerve is slightly more anterior. The facial and vestibulocochlear nerves are in close relationship to the *flocculus* of the cerebellum, the *inferior cerebellar peduncle*, and the *lateral aperture of the fourth ventricle* (Figs. 1,2).

5. MIDBRAIN

The posterior aspect of the *midbrain* is characterized by two pairs of swellings—the *superior* and *inferior colliculi*, which are components of the visual and auditory systems, respectively (Fig. 6A,B). The *pineal gland*, a component of the epithalamus of the diencephalon, rests between the superior colliculi. Just superior to the superior colliculi is the *pretectal area*, which is functionally related to visual reflexes. The *trochlear nerves* emerge from the brainstem immediately inferior to the inferior colliculi (Figs. 1,2). Inferior to the emerging roots of the trochlear nerves the *superior cerebellar peduncles* enter the midbrain. These axons are the principal output pathway from cerebellum to the motor centers in the midbrain and diencephalon.

The anterior surface of the midbrain is composed largely of the paired *cerebral peduncles*. These massive bundles of axons connect cerebral structures associated with motor functions to the motor neurons of the brainstem and spinal cord. The base of the midbrain between the cerebral peduncles is the *posterior perforated substance*, so named because small vessels penetrate the base of the midbrain to supply intrinsic structures. In the intact brain the arachnoid stretches

Fig. 3. (*Continued from opposite page*) Fig. 6B; CM, caudal midbrain Fig. 6A; RP, rostral pons Fig. 5C; MP, mid pons Fig. 5B; CP, caudal pons Fig. 5A; RMed, rostral medulla Fig. 4D; Mmed, mid medulla Fig. 4C; SD, sensory decussation of medulla Fig. 4B; MD, motor decussation of medulla Fig. 4A.

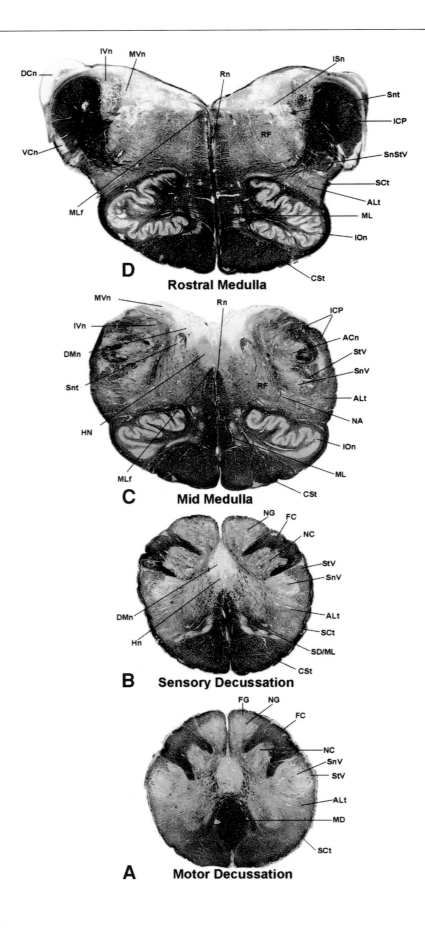

D   Rostral Medulla

C   Mid Medulla

B   Sensory Decussation

A   Motor Decussation

between the cerebral peduncles forming the *interpeduncular cistern* (Fig. 1; Chapter 2, Fig. 7).

The *oculomotor nerve* roots exit the base of the midbrain just medial to the cerebral peduncles (Fig. 1). They pass forward into the middle cranial fossa and enter the orbit carrying motor innervation to extraocular muscles and parasympathetic innervation to the eye.

6. CEREBELLUM

The *cerebellum* lies dorsal to the pons and medulla and is connected to the brainstem by the paired superior, middle, and inferior cerebellar peduncles (Fig. 1; Chapter 2, Figs. 5–9). It consists of *lateral hemispheres* and a midline *vermis*. The midsagittal section reveals the characteristic folia of the cerebellar cortex. On the cortical surface the cerebellum exhibits numerous folds that separate the folia. Superiorly, the cerebellar hemispheres contact the undersurface of the *tentorium cerebelli*. Inferiorly, the cerebellum occupies the intracranial depressions formed by the occipital bone.

The ventral aspect of the cerebellar hemispheres reveals two paired subdivisions, the tonsils and the flocculonodular lobes (Fig. 1).

The *cerebellar tonsils* are inferiorly directed protruberances of the cerebellar hemispheres that overlie the lateral edge of the foramen magnum. In clinical situations that produce increased pressure in the posterior cranial fossa (e.g., a hemorrhage or an expanding tumor), this portion of the cerebellum is wedged between the rim of the foramen magnum and the medulla-spinal cord junction. This situation is termed *"herniation of the cerebellar tonsils."* Cerebellar tonsil herniation can be fatal because it interferes with blood flow to the vital neural centers in the medulla, which regulate cardiovascular and respiratory rhythms.

The *flocculonodular lobes* are formed by the *nodulus*, the most inferior portion of the vermis, and its bilateral extensions, the *flocculi* (singular: flocculus). The flocculonodular lobe serves an important role in vestibular function.

7. CRANIAL NERVES

The *olfactory nerve (I)* is the most rostral of the cranial nerves and consists of several fascicles that are the axons of olfactory neurons located in the mucosa of the superior aspect of the nasal chamber. The olfactory nerve terminates in the olfactory bulb, which lies on the cribriform plate of the ethmoid bone. Axons of olfactory bulb neurons are conveyed by the olfactory tract to the olfactory trigone on the inferior surface of the frontal lobe just anterior to the anterior perforated substance (Chapter 2, Fig. 13). The olfactory bulbs and tracts are actually extensions of the CNS; together with the olfactory nerves, they convey olfactory sensations to the CNS.

The *optic nerve (II)* consists largely of axons of the ganglion neurons of the retina. Those axons originating from the medial (nasal) half of the retina cross in the optic chiasm to join the contralateral optic tract (Chapter 2, Fig. 13). Most axons terminate in the lateral geniculate nuclei of the dorsal thalamus. The axons of the lateral geniculate neurons form the geniculocalcarine tract (optic radiation), which carries visual stimuli to the ipsilateral medial aspect of the occipital lobe (Chapter 2, Fig. 11). Other axons of the retinal ganglion neurons terminate in the superior colliculus and the closely associated *pretectal region* of the midbrain to serve visual and light reflex functions, respectively. The optic nerves and tracts are actually extensions of the brain.

The *oculomotor nerve (III)* emerges into the interpeduncular cistern from the base of the midbrain, medial to the cerebral peduncles and lateral to the posterior perforated substance (Fig. 1). The oculomotor nerve passes anteriorly between the posterior cerebral and superior cerebellar arteries, lateral to the posterior clinoid processes in the middle cranial fossa (Chapter 2, Fig. 4). It is encased in the lateral wall of the cavernous sinus as it continues forward through the superior orbital fissure into the orbit (Chapter 13, Fig. 1). The oculomotor nerve provides motor innervation to the extraocular muscles, except the lateral

---

Fig. 4. (*Opposite page*) Axial sections of the human medulla corresponding to the planes illustrated on Fig. 3. Fourth ventricle is located posterior to Fig. 4C,D. (**A**) motor (pyramidal) decussation; (**B**) sensory (dorsal column) decussation; (**C**) mid medulla; (**D**) rostral medulla. ACn, accessory cuneate nucleus; ALt, anterolateral tracts; CSt, corticospinal tracts; DCn, dorsal cochlear nucleus; DMn, dorsal motor nucleus of vagus; Fc, fasciculus cuneatus; Fg, fasciculus gracilis; Hn, hypoglossal nucleus; ICP, inferior cerebellar peduncle; IOn, inferior olivary nucleus; ISn, inferior salivatory nucleus; IVn, inferior vestibular nucleus; MD, motor (pyramidal) decussation; ML, medial lemniscus; MLf, medial longitudinal fasciculus; MVn, medial vestibular nucleus; NA, nucleus ambiguus; NC, nucleus cuneatus; NG, nucleus gracilis; RF, reticular formation; Rn, raphe of reticular formation; SCt, spinocerebellar tracts; SD, sensory decussation; Snt, solitary nucleus and tract; SnV, spinal nucleus of trigeminal; StV, spinal tract of trigeminal.

rectus and superior oblique muscles. It also carries parasympathetic preganglionic fibers to the ciliary ganglion in the orbit. From this location postganglionic parasympathetic fibers innervate the constrictor of the pupil and the ciliary muscle.

The *trochlear nerve (IV) innervates* only the superior oblique extraocular muscle (Figs. 1,2). It emerges from the brainstem immediately inferior to the inferior colliculus of the midbrain. It is the only cranial nerve to emerge from the posterior aspect of the brainstem. The trochlear nerve then courses anteriorly around the brainstem. Near the posterior clinoid process it becomes encased in the lateral wall of the cavernous sinus, continuing anteriorly, it passes through the superior orbital fissure into the orbit.

The *trigeminal nerve (V)* is the largest of the cranial nerves and supplies sensory innervation to the face, oral, and nasal cavities, and motor innervation to muscles of mastication. The trigeminal nerve consists of a sensory root and a smaller motor root (Fig. 1). Together they exit the lateral aspect of the pons, coursing anteriorly and crossing the petrous ridge of the temporal bone to the trigeminal ganglion in the middle cranial fossa (Chapter 2, Fig. 4; Chapter 13, Fig. 1). The central processes of the trigeminal ganglion neurons form the sensory root of the trigeminal nerve. The peripheral processes form the trigeminal ophthalmic, maxillary, and mandibular divisions, which pass through the superior orbital fissure, foramen rotundum, and foramen ovale respectively, providing sensory innervation to the face and oral structures. (*See* Chapter 13 for details.)

The *abducens nerve (VI)* supplies only the lateral rectus extraocular muscle. It originates from the anterior aspect of the brainstem at the border between the pons-medulla junction (Fig. 1). The abducens nerve crosses the petrous ridge, becomes encased in the lateral wall of the cavernous sinus and passes anteriorly through the superior orbital fissure into the orbit.

The *facial nerve (VII)* emerges as two roots from the lateral aspect of the brainstem at the pons-medulla junction and anterior to the flocculus of the cerebellum (Fig. 1). The larger root provides innervation to muscles of facial expression, the stapedius, and other muscles. The smaller root—the nervus intermedius—conveys parasympathetic preganglionic innervation to the lacrimal, sublingual and submaxillary salivary glands, and sensory fibers carrying taste from the anterior two-thirds of the tongue. The two facial roots course laterally through the internal acoustic meatus

and canal to the geniculate ganglion where the cell bodies for the sensory fibers are located. The motor fibers continue through the facial canal in the temporal bone and emerge from the stylomastoid foramen to distribute motor branches to facial muscles. The parasympathetic fibers follow the great superficial petrosal nerve or the chorda tympani nerve to the pterygopalatine or submandibular parasympathetic ganglia, respectively. Postganglionic fibers provide parasympathetic innervation to the lacrimal, submaxillary, and sublingual glands.

The *vestibulocochlear nerve (VIII)* originates from the sensory neurons in the spiral and vestibular ganglia associated with the auditory and vestibular end organs. The central processes follow the internal acoustic canal, emerge from the internal acoustic meatus, and enter the lateral aspect of the brainstem posterior to the facial nerve and in close relationship to the flocculus of the cerebellum (Figs. 1,2).

The *glossopharyngeal nerve (IX)* originates as several fascicles from the lateral aspect of the brainstem just inferior to the medulla-pons border and posterior to the olive (Fig. 1). The glossopharyngeal nerve provides sensory innervation to the mucosa of the middle ear cavity, oral pharynx, posterior portion of the tongue, and the baroreceptors and chemoreceptors associated with the carotid artery. Parasympathetic preganglionic innervation is provided to the parotid gland through postganglionic relays in the otic ganglion.

The *vagus nerve (X)* originates as eight to ten fascicles inferior to, and in line with, the origin of the glossopharyngeal nerve fascicles (Fig. 1). It provides sensory innervation to part of the skin of the external auditory canal, laryngeal pharynx, larynx, respiratory, and cardiovascular and gastrointestinal tract. The vagus nerve supplies parasympathetic innervation to the glands, mucosae, and smooth muscle of these organ systems. It also supplies voluntary motor innervation to the striated muscles of the pharynx and larynx.

The *accessory nerve (XI)* originates from the brainstem as a few fascicles in line with those of the vagus nerve (cranial portion) and a much larger component from the upper five cervical segments of the spinal cord (spinal portion). The spinal portion courses rostrally along the lateral aspect of the cervical cord, through the foramen magnum and joins the glossopharyngeal and vagus nerves (Fig. 1). Together, they exit the cranial cavity through the jugular foramen. The accessory nerve supplies motor innervation to trapezius and sternocleidomastoid muscles in the neck.

The *hypoglossal nerve (XII)* arises from a line of rootlets anterior to the olive (Fig. 1). It courses through the hypoglossal canal, lateral to the foramen magnum, and provides motor innervation to the intrinsic muscles of the tongue.

7.1. Internal Structure of the Brainstem

Sections of the brainstem reveal the anatomical relationships between the cranial-nerve nuclei and roots, structures associated with cerebellar and motor function circuits and the reticular formation (Figs. 4–6). Figure 3 locates the rostral-caudal plane of these axial sections. In addition, The brainstem is subdivided into the midbrain, pons, and medulla (Fig. 3; Chapter 2, Fig. 8). The *tectum* (L. roof) of the midbrain consists of the superior and inferior colliculi, and the *tegmentum* (L. covering structure) includes the portion of the midbrain anterior to the cerebral aqueduct (Fig. 3), except for the cerebral peduncles (Fig. 1). The pons and medulla do not have components of the tectum; the tegmentum of the pons and medulla includes all areas anterior to the fourth ventricle except the base of the pons and the pyramids (Figs. 4–6; Chapter 2, Figs. 8,9C). Tectum and tegmentum are terms often used to designate locations of brainstem tracts and nuclei.

Ascending sensory pathways from the spinal cord and the voluntary motor pathway descending from the cerebral cortex traverse the brainstem. The motor pathway activates musculature of the contralateral extremities and trunk and the ascending long tracts convey sensations from the contralateral side of the body. Along their courses these long tract axons intersect cranial nerve-root fibers as they emerge from the brainstem, the cranial nerves innervate ipsilateral structures of the head and neck. Lesions at these sites of intersection occur in patients experiencing cerebrovascular accidents (stroke) resulting from diminished blood flow in a branch of the vertebrobasilar system supplying a region of the brainstem. Thus, patients have neurological deficits that reflect one or more cranial nerves ipsilateral to the side of the vascular lesion, but symptoms observable on the contralateral side of the body that reflect involvement of one or more long tracts.

7.2. Spinal Cord Long Tracts Traverse the Brainstem

The *voluntary motor pathway* (pyramidal tract) arises from the motor areas of the cortex. Axons of these cortical neurons traverse the cerebral white matter—the internal capsule—and occupy a central position in the *cerebral peduncle* in the midbrain (Fig. 6). These *corticobulbar* and *corticospinal tracts* innervate cranial nerve motor neurons and the spinal cord motor neurons, respectively. The motor pathway maintains a ventral position as it traverses the brainstem. In the pons, its fibers are separated into groups of fascicles by the intersecting *pontine nuclei* and *pontocerebellar fibers* (Fig. 5). In the medulla the motor fibers, which include the corticospinal tracts, collect in an anteromedial position as the *pyramids* and continue their caudalward course (Figs. 1,4). At the medulla-spinal cord junction, about 90% of the fibers cross to the contralateral side forming the *motor (pyramidal) decussation* (Fig. 4A). The decussating motor fibers loop posterolaterally and continue into the lateral funiculus of the spinal cord as the *lateral corticospinal tract*. Lateral corticospinal fibers terminate on ventralhorn motor neurons that innervate the musculature of the extremities and trunk.

The 10% of motor pathway fibers that do not cross at the motor decussation form the *anterior (ventral) corticospinal tract* in the ventral funiculus of the spinal cord. These fibers decussate in the spinal cord at the level where they synapse on motor neurons that innervate axial musculature.

It is important to note that rostral to the motor decussation, the voluntary motor fibers traversing the brainstem serve the contralateral side of the body. Destruction of the voluntary motor pathway in the brainstem results in *contralateral hemiparalysis*, whereas destruction of the lateral corticospinal tract in the spinal cord results in ipsilateral paralysis of the musculature innervated below the level of the lesion.

Most fibers of the *corticobulbar tract* follow the corticospinal fibers as they traverse the brainstem. Corticobulbar fibers provide innervation to cranial-nerve motor nuclei that innervate skeletal muscles in the head and neck. For most cranial nerve motor nuclei, the corticobulbar innervation is predominantly contralateral. Thus, destruction of one corticobulbar tract results in weakness (paresis) of contralateral muscles innervated by cranial nerves.

One notable exception is corticobulbar innervation of the *facial motor nucleus*. Here, only contralateral corticobulbar fibers terminate on the facial motor neurons that activate facial muscles of the lower half of the face. Facial motor neurons that innervate the upper half of the face receive bilateral corticobulbar innervation. As a result, destruction of one corticobulbar tract

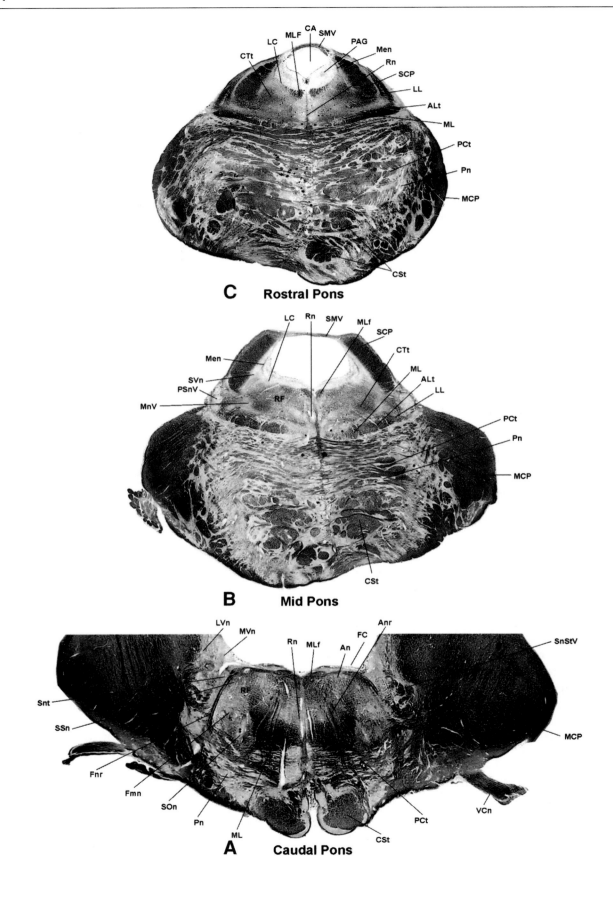

C   Rostral Pons

B   Mid Pons

A   Caudal Pons

rostral to the facial motor nucleus produces facial paralysis of only the contralateral lower half of facial musculature. This observation is termed *central facial paralysis (palsy)* and is observed contralateral to the site of the lesion. In contrast, a lesion destroying the facial-nerve root would result in paralysis of all ipsilateral facial muscles, and is termed a *peripheral facial paralysis*. A peripheral facial paralysis is usually accompanied by loss of all ipsilateral facial-nerve functions.

Other prominent structures in the brainstem play important roles in the regulation of motor function. *Substantia nigra* neurons are located just posterior to the cerebral peduncle, they have reciprocal connections with the ipsilateral putamen and caudate nucleus (Fig. 6). Most of substantia nigra neurons use dopamine as a transmitter and participate in the regulation of body posture and muscle tone.

The *red nucleus* is a prominent feature of the midbrain tegmentum at the level of the superior colliculus (Fig. 6B). Its principal inputs arise from motor areas of the cortex and contralateral cerebellum. Many red nucleus neurons project to thalamic nuclei as a component of the *dentatorubrothalamic tract*. Other red nucleus neurons form contralateral rubrobulbar and rubrospinal tracts, which project to other regulatory neurons and motor neurons of the brainstem and spinal cord.

The *superior cerebellar peduncles* consist mostly of axons arising from the paired dentate nuclei of the cerebellum and are the principal output pathway of the cerebellum (Figs. 2,5B,C). The superior cerebellar peduncles course anteromedially, enter the rostral pons, and decussate in the midbrain tegmentum at the level of the inferior colliculi (Fig. 6A). Some decussated fibers terminate in the contralateral red nuclei; most continue rostrally to terminate in the contralateral thalamus. Collectively, these fibers are the *dentatorubrothalamic tracts*. The dentatorubrothalamic tracts and the related thalamocortical projections to the motor cortex constitute a principal pathway

by which the cerebellum and red nucleus coordinate ongoing motor activities.

The *pontine nuclei* and their axons the *pontocerebellar fibers* together constitute the base of the pons. The pontocerebellar fibers decussate and collect as the *middle cerebellar peduncles*, which project to the cerebellum (Fig. 5). Pontine nuclei receive inputs from all areas of the ipsilateral cerebral cortex; most arise from areas associated with motor functions. The corticopontine fibers follow the cerebral peduncles to terminate on the pontine nuclei.

The *inferior olivary nucleus* is the largest of several similar structures located in the rostral medulla (Fig. 4C,D). It receives input from the cortex, red nucleus, vestibular nuclei, reticular formation, and spinal cord. Its neurons provide a massive projection to the contralateral cerebellum by way of the *inferior cerebellar peduncle* (Figs. 2,4C,D). Inferior olive and pontocerebellar projections are components of motor pathways whereby the activities of cortical and subcortical structures can be integrated with cerebellar functions.

The *lateral* and *anterior spinothalamic (anterolateral) tracts* convey pain, thermal, and general tactile sensations from the contralateral surface of the body. They ascend the lateral funiculus of the spinal cord, traverse the brainstem, and terminate in the thalamus for integration and relay (Figs. 4–6). The thalamocortical fibers project these sensory modalities to the parietal cortex for conscious appreciation of their character and location on the body surface.

Fasciculus gracilis and *fasciculus cuneatus*, the dorsal columns of the spinal cord, carry discriminative tactile, proprioceptive (position) sense and vibratory sense from all levels of the ipsilateral half of the body (Chapter 2, Fig. 6). Axons carrying sensations from the distal parts of the lower extremity are located most medial in the fasciculus gracilis. Axons from progressively more rostral body levels accumulate in a medial to lateral arrangement so that those axons from cervical body levels are located most lateral in the fasciculus

---

Fig. 5. (*Opposite page*) Axial sections of the human pons corresponding to the planes illustrated in Fig. 3. Fourth ventricle is located posterior to Figs. 5A,B. (**A**) caudal pons; (**B**) mid pons; (**C**) rostral pons. ALt, anterolateral tracts; An, abducens nucleus; Anr, root of abducens nerve; CA, cerebral aqueduct; CSt, corticospinal tracts; CTt, central tegmental tract; FC, facial colliculus; Fmn, facial nerve motor nucleus; Fnr, facial nerve root; LC, locus ceruleus; LL, lateral lemniscus; MCP, middle cerebellar peduncle; Men, mesencephalic nucleus of trigeminal; ML, medial lemniscus; MLf, medial longitudinal fasciculus; MnV, motor nucleus of trigeminal; MVn, medial vestibular nucleus; PAG, periaqueductal gray; PCt, pontocerebellar tract; Pn, pontine nuclei; PSnV, principal nucleus of trigeminal; RF, reticular formation; Rn, raphe nuclei; SCP, superior cerebellar peduncle; SMV, superior medullary velum; Sn, spinal nucleus of trigeminal; Snt, solitary nucleus and tract; SOn, superior olivary nucleus; SSn, superior salivatory nucleus; StV, spinal tract of trigeminal; SVn, superior vestibular nuclei; VCn, vestibulocochlear nerve.

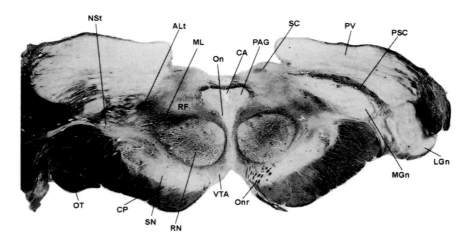

B   **Rostral Midbrain**

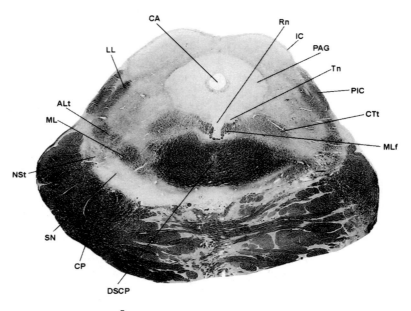

A   **Caudal Midbrain**

Fig. 6. Axial sections of the human midbrain corresponding to the planes illustrated in Fig. 3. V-shaped space between the cerebral peduncles (CP) corresponds to the interpeduncular space (cistern). (**A**) Caudal midbrain, level of the inferior colliculus (IC); (**B**) rostral midbrain, level of the superior colliculus (SC). ALt, anterolateral tracts; CA, cerebral aqueduct; CP, cerebral peduncle; CTt, central tegmental tract; DSCP, decussation of superior cerebellar peduncles; IC, inferior colliculus; LGn, lateral geniculate nucleus; LL, lateral lemniscus; MGn, medial geniculate nucleus; ML, medial lemniscus; MLf, medial longitudinal fasciculus; NSt, nigrostriate tract; On, oculomotor nucleus; Onr, oculomotor nerve root; OT, optic tract; PAG, periaqueductal gray; PIC, peduncle of inferior colliculus of thalamus; PSC, peduncle of superior colliculus; PV, pulvinar of thalamus; RF, reticular formation; RN, red nucleus; Rn, raphe nuclei; SC, superior colliculus; SN, substantia nigra; VTA, ventral tegmental area.

cuneatus. This arrangement is retained as fasciculus gracilis and cuneatus fibers terminate in the caudal medulla as the *nucleus gracilis* and *cuneatus*, respectively (Fig. 4A,B). Axons of nucleus gracilis and

nucleus cuneatus loop ventrally and decussate in the tegmentum of the caudal medulla forming the *sensory decussation* (Fig. 4B). The decussating axons collect as the *medial lemniscus*, which follows a rostral course conveying discriminative tactile and proprioceptive modalities to the thalamus for integration and relay to the parietal cortex (Figs. 4–6).

It is important to note that in the brainstem the sensory tracts are arranged medial to lateral: medial lemnicus most medial, anterolateral (spinothalamic) tracts are intermediate, and the lateral lemniscus is most lateral in position. Medial lemniscus and the anterolateral tracts convey sensory modalities from the contralateral side of the body, the lateral lemniscus carries auditory sensations from both cochleae.

Nonconscious (reflex) proprioceptive sensations are conveyed from mechanoreceptors in the lower extremities and trunk by the *posterior (dorsal)* and *anterior (ventral) spinocerebellar tracts*. These tracts are located along the anterolateral edge of the medulla (Fig. 4). The posterior spinocerebellar tract, projecting from the ipsilateral side of the body, enters the cerebellum by way of the inferior cerebellar peduncle (Figs. 2,4). The anterior spinocerebellar tract carries information from the contralateral side of the body, follows the superior cerebellar peduncle and crosses back to its side of origin in the white matter of the cerebellum (Figs. 2,5B,C).

7.3. Nuclear Components of the Brainstem Cranial Nerves

The *oculomotor nerve* arises predominantly from the ipsilateral *oculomotor nucleus* at the level of the *superior colliculus* of the midbrain (Fig. 6B). The oculomotor nerve consists of axons that innervate all ipsilateral extraocular muscles, except for the lateral rectus and superior oblique. Neurons of the oculomotor nucleus also innervate the levator palpebrae superioris muscle in the orbit, which elevates the upper eyelid. Additionally, a subnucleus of the oculomotor nucleus, the *visceral nucleus* or *Edinger-Westphal nucleus*, contributes parasympathetic preganglionic fibers to the oculomotor nerve, which synapse in the ciliary ganglion in the orbit. The postganglionic branches of the ciliary ganglion innervate the ciliary muscle and constrictor of the pupil. Collectively, the emerging axons of the oculomotor nucleus pass ventrally through the red nucleus and accumulate at the medial border of the cerebral peduncle (Fig. 1).

The *trochlear nucleus* consists of a small bilateral cluster of motor neurons embedded in the *medial longitudinal fasciculus* at the level of the *inferior colliculus* in the tegmentum of the midbrain (Fig. 6A). Trochlear axons course posterolaterally and inferiorly, follow-

ing the boundary of the *periaquaductal grey*. They decussate posterior to the *cerebral aqueduct* and emerge on the posterior aspect of the brainstem just inferior to the inferior colliculi (Figs. 1,2). The trochlear nerves are the only cranial-nerve roots to decussate. Consequently, the trochlear nuclei innervate the contralateral superior oblique muscle, but the trochlear nerve innervates the ipsilateral superior oblique.

The *trigeminal nerve*, which consists of motor fibers of the mandibular division and sensory fibers from all three trigeminal divisions, enters the lateral aspect of the pons, and distributes to the nuclei of the trigeminal system (Fig. 1; Chapter 13, Fig. 2). Root fibers conveying discriminatory tactile sensations synapse in the *principal*, or *chief, sensory nucleus* (Fig. 5B). Other entering sensory fibers carrying nociceptive, thermal, and general tactile sensations turn inferiorly, forming the *spinal tract of the trigeminal* in the lateral tegmentum of the pons and medulla (Figs. 4,5A,B). The spinal tract of the trigeminal continues into the upper cervical cord and along its course, its fibers terminate on the *spinal nucleus of the trigeminal* located just medial to the tract. Neurons of the principal sensory nucleus and spinal nucleus give origin to the trigeminothalamic tract, which project predominantly to the contralateral thalamus The trigeminothalamic tracts follow the medial lemniscus to the thalamus. Thalamocortical fibers project trigeminal sensory modalities to the parietal cortex (Chapter 13, Fig. 6) .

The *mesencephalic nucleus of the trigeminal* consists of a thin column of primary sensory neuron somas located along the border of the *central gray of the fourth ventricle* (Fig. 5B,C). The peripheral axons of these neurons form the *mesencephalic tract of the trigeminal*; together, the tract and nucleus extend superiorly to midbrain levels lying just medial to the *superior cerebellar peduncle*. The peripheral fibers— the mesencephalic tract—and the mesencephalic nucleus convey proprioceptive impulses from the musculoskeletal and oral structures innervated by the trigeminal nerve and project to the cerebellum and brainstem.

The *motor nucleus of the trigeminal* lies just medial to the principal sensory nucleus (Fig. 5B). The axons of these neurons follow the mandibular division of the trigeminal in its peripheral distribution and terminate on skeletal muscles innervated by the trigeminal nerve.

The *abducens nucleus* is located in the tegmentum of the caudal pons (Fig. 5A). The abducens axons course ventrally through the pontine tegmentum, intersecting fibers of the ascending *medial lemniscus.* They incline somewhat inferiorly as they traverse the base of the pons, intersecting the crossing *pontocerebellar fibers* and the descending *corticospinal (pyramidal) tracts.* The abducens root exits ventrally at the pons-medulla boundary and courses forward to the orbit (Fig. 1).

A subgroup of reticular formation neurons near the abducens nucleus provide axons for internuclear circuits. Most of these join the contralateral *medial longitudinal fasciculus* and project principally to the oculomotor nuclei (Figs. 5,6). They are the *paramedial pontine reticular formation (PPRF).* The *vestibular nuclei* and visual centers in the cerebral cortex project to the abducens nucleus. Collectively, the abducens neurons and the PPRF are the *lateral gaze center* because they regulate conjugate eye movements in the horizontal plane (Fig. 5A).

The *facial-nerve root* emerges from the lateral aspect of the brainstem at the pons-medulla boundary and contains motor, sensory, and parasympathetic fibers (Fig. 1). The *facial-motor nucleus* is located in the tegmentum of the caudal pons, and consists of motor neurons destined to innervate the ipsilateral muscles of facial expression, the stapedius and other muscles (Fig. 5A). Its axons course posteromedially, looping posterior to the abducens nucleus, then collecting to pass between the spinal nucleus of the trigeminal and the facial nucleus. They follow an inferior and anterolateral course to exit the brainstem at the pons-medulla boundary.

The facial root also conveys fibers carrying taste sensations from the anterior two-thirds of the ipsilateral tongue. The taste fibers have their cell bodies in the geniculate ganglion, located in the temporal bone, and their central processes join the *solitary tract* and synapse on neurons of the *solitary nucleus* (Fig. 5A). Axons of the solitary nucleus provide brainstem connections for visceral reflexes. Other solitary neurons project taste sensations to the thalamus.

Parasympathetic preganglionic fibers of the facial nerve originate from the small *superior salivatory nucleus* in the lateral tegmentum (Fig. 5A). Their axons terminate on pterygopalatine and submandibular ganglia neurons in the face and floor of the oral cavity, respectively. The postganglionic parasympathetic fibers innervate the lacrimal gland, mucosa of the oral and nasal cavities, and the submandibular and sublingual salivary glands.

Two distinct components form the *vestibulocochlear nerve:* the *cochlear nerve* and the *vestibular nerve* (Figs. 1,2,5A). Both components are the central processes of sensory neurons located in the spiral ganglia of the cochlea or the vestibular ganglia associated with the labyrinth.

The larger cochlear nerve terminates on neurons of the *dorsal* and *ventral cochlear nuclei* located on the lateral aspect of the *inferior cerebellar peduncle* (Fig. 4D). There is a considerable mixture of crossed and uncrossed rostral projections from the cochlear nuclei of the two sides. The crossing axons form the *trapezoid fibers (body),* which interdigitate with the ascending fibers of the *medial lemniscus* and *anterolateral tracts* (5A). The ascending axons collect as the *lateral lemniscus* just lateral to the prominent *superior olivary nucleus* (Fig. 5A). The superior olivary nucleus integrates auditory impulses from the two ears, and therefore plays an important role in localizing sound in the environment. The lateral lemniscus conveys auditory sensations from both ears to the *inferior colliculus* for reflex connections and for relay to the medial geniculate nucleus of the thalamus (Figs. 5C,6A).

The *vestibular nerve* terminals synapse on neurons in the vestibular nuclei, which occupy a considerable area in the lateral tegmentum of the medulla and pons. *Superior, lateral, medial* and *inferior vestibular nuclei* are recognized based on their neuron morphology and connections (Figs. 4C,D,5A,B). The semicircular canals project predominantly to the more rostral components of the vestibular nuclear complex and the utricle and saccule project more prominently to the caudal components. The vestibular nuclei project to the *flocculonodular lobe* (Fig. 1) of the cerebellum by way of the *inferior cerebellar peduncle* and to the abducens, trochlear, and oculomotor nuclei by way of the *medial longitudinal fasciculus* (Fig. 5). Vestibular connections provide the input necessary to coordinate head and body posture with conjugate eye movements. Other projections—for example, from the lateral vestibular nucleus—project vestibulospinal tracts to the spinal cord and play important roles in the regulation of body posture.

The *glossopharyngeal nerve* enters the lateral aspect of the rostral medulla as a series of rootlets consisting of motor and sensory fibers (Fig. 1). Parasympathetic preganglionic fibers of the glossopharyngeal nerve originate from the indistinct *inferior salivatory nucleus* located near the floor of the *fourth ventricle* (Fig. 4D). They synapse on postganglionic parasympathetic neurons in the otic ganglion, which provides secromotor innervation to the ipsilateral parotid gland. The *nucleus ambiguus* in the tegmentum of the medulla gives origin to the small component of glossopharyngeal motor fibers that innervate the stylopharyngeus muscle (Fig. 4C). Sensory neurons are located in small ganglia associated with the proximal end of the glossopharyngeal nerve. They serve taste and other sensations for the posterior third of the ipsilateral tongue and the oral pharynx. The sensory fibers from the oral pharynx constitute the *afferent limb of the gag (palatal) reflex*. A subgroup of glossopharyngeal sensory fibers—the carotid nerve—carries *baroreceptor impulses* from the ipsilateral carotid sinus, thereby participating in the regulation of vital cardiovascular functions. These sensory fibers join the solitary fasciculus and terminate on the *solitary nucleus* (Figs. 4C,D,5A). Solitary neurons project to the brainstem for visceral reflexes such as swallowing and salivation, other solitary neurons project taste sensations to the thalamus. An important subgroup of solitary neurons that project to the vagal neurons diminish heart rate and blood pressure.

The motor fibers of the *vagus nerve* originate from neurons in the *nucleus ambiguus* and from the *dorsal motor nucleus of the vagus* (Fig. 4C). The dorsal motor nucleus is located ventral to the floor of the *fourth ventricle* and lateral to the *hypoglossal nucleus*. Axons from the parasympathetic preganglionic dorsal motor nucleus terminate on ganglionic neurons associated with thoracic and most abdominal organs. Postganglionic parasympathetic fibers innervate mucosae, glands, and smooth muscle. The heart is also innervated by parasympathetic preganglionic neurons located in the region of the *nucleus ambiguus*. In addition, motor neurons in nucleus ambiguus innervate striated muscles of the larynx, pharynx, and palate. They provide voluntary innervation to the vocal muscles and the *efferent limb of the gag (palatal) reflex*. The *vagus nerve* contains sensory fibers whose cell bodies are located in small ganglia associated with the proximal end of the nerve near the jugular foramen. The visceral sensory fibers convey sensations from the organs innervated by the vagus and join the *solitary tract*. Vagal sensory fibers in the solitary tract terminate on the solitary nucleus, which projects throughout the brainstem, serving visceral reflexes.

It should be noted that the facial, glossopharyngeal and vagus nerves contain small components of sensory fibers that innervate skin associated with the auricle and external auditory canal. These fibers join the trigeminal system in the brainstem (*see* Chapter 13).

The *accessory nerve* consists of a cranial portion and a larger spinal component. The *cranial portion* rises from the nucleus ambiguus, and its motor fibers join the vagus nerve to innervate laryngeal muscles. The *spinal accessory nerve* provides voluntary motor innervation to the ipsilateral sternocleidomastoid and trapezius muscles (Fig. 1). The spinal accessory motor neurons reside in the accessory nucleus in the ventral horn of the cervical spinal cord. Spinal accessory rootlets emerge from the lateral aspect of the cervical cord, and coalesce as a well-defined nerve as they ascend superiorly. The spinal accessory nerve passes through the foramen magnum into the posterior cranial fossa, where it joins the vagus and glossopharyngeal nerves. Together, the three nerves exit through the jugular foramen into the neck. As a result of this circuitous course, spinal accessory-nerve function can be diminished or lost as a result of lesions affecting the cervical cord, structures in the posterior cranial fossa or trauma to the lateral aspect of the neck. Symptoms include weakness in turning the head to the contralateral side and lifting the ipsilateral shoulder.

The *hypoglossal nucleus* is a prominent group of motor neurons extending throughout the dorsal aspect of the caudal medulla between the midline and the dorsal motor nucleus of the vagus (Figs. 4B,C). Hypoglossal axons course ventrally just lateral to the *medial lemnincus* and emerge from the medulla between the *pyramids* and the *inferior olivary nucleus* (Fig. 1). Several rootlets combine as the *hypoglossal nerve*, which passes through the hypoglossal foramen to innervate the ipsilateral intrinsic skeletal muscles of the tongue. Destruction of the hypoglossal nucleus, its root, or the hypoglossal nerve results in paralysis of the ipsilateral half of the tongue, when protruded, the tongue deviates to the side of the lesion because of the paralysis of the ipsilateral genoglossus muscle.

The *reticular formation* is a group of nuclei, diverse in morphology, connectivity, and neurochemistry that is present throughout the tegmentum of the brainstem. The *raphe nuclei* constitutes a major subgroup of reticular nuclei, they are located along the midline of the brainstem (Figs. 4C,D,5,6A). Other reticular nuclei are located in the medial and lateral regions of the tegmentum (Figs. 4,5). These nuclei participate in the regulation of visceral homeostasis, muscle tone and other functions (*see* Chapter 12).

ACKNOWLEDGMENTS

The invaluable assistance of Ms. Mary Gail Engle and Dr. Bruce Maley, University of Kentucky, in the preparation of illustrations for this chapter is greatly appreciated.

The Weigert-stained sections of the human brainstem were photographed from the Yakovlev Collec- tion housed at the Armed Forces Institute of Pathology, Washington, DC.

SELECTED READINGS

Duus P. The brainstem and cranial nerves, in *Topical Diagnosis in Neurolog*, Georg Thiem Velag, Stuttgard (3rd ed), 1998; 70–163.

Lindsay KW, Bone I. Raised intracranial pressure, in *Neurology and Neurosurgery Illustrated*, Churchill-Livingstone, New York (3rd ed), 1997; 73–80.

Slaby FJ, McCune SK, Summers RW. The cranial cavity, in *Gross Anatomy in the Practice of Medicine*, Lea and Febiger, Philadelphia, 1994; 581–596.

12 The Brainstem Reticular Formation and the Monoamine System

Harold H. Traurig

CONTENTS

CLINICAL CORRELATION: **DISORDERS OF THE AUTONOMIC NERVOUS SYSTEM**
GREGORY COOPER AND ROBERT L. RODNITZKY

1. INTRODUCTION

The reticular formation (RF) consists of an extensive aggregation of several subtypes of interconnected neurons that extends throughout the brainstem tegmentum. The reticular pathways integrate sensory, visceral, limbic, and motor functions, and project throughout the central nervous system (CNS). Reticular circuits exert important influences on autonomic regulation of vital organ systems, behavior, somatic motor activities, sleep cycles, alertness, and pain modulation.

2. THE RF INTEGRATES NEURAL FUNCTIONS

The term "reticular formation" was adopted by early anatomists to distinguish what appeared to be diffusely interconnected neurons in the brainstem tegmentum from the anatomically more distinct nuclei associated with the cranial nerves. This characterization of the RF suggested that it was poorly organized and served only primitive functions. However, some early investigators, notably Cajal, recognized organization and specificity in the RF based on neuron morphology, location in the brainstem and connectivity. Despite Cajal's work, the RF evoked little research interest until the electrophysiological studies by Moruzzi and Magoun in the 1940s and 1950s demonstrated that the maintenance of consciousness and alertness depended on input from sensory pathways through the brainstem RF to the thalamus and cerebral cortex.

Later studies demonstrate that inputs to specific components of the RF also originate from the cerebral cortex, striatum, limbic system, hypothalamus, cerebellum, and other central neural structures. Certain components of the RF project to these same structures,

From: *Neuroscience in Medicine, 2nd ed.* (P. Michael Conn, ed.),
© 2003 Humana Press Inc., Totowa, NJ.

often through the dorsal thalamus, as well as to the somatic and visceral motor nuclei of the brainstem and spinal cord.

Subgroups of reticular neurons and nerve terminals contain specific combinations of transmitters and peptides, such as serotonin, norepinephrine, acetylcholine, and enkephalin, suggesting that RF functions depend on complex neurochemical interactions.

The RF provides an important matrix for neural integration. Ascending RF projections play key roles in alertness, behavior, and affect. Brainstem RF circuits, together with limbic and hypothalamic input, regulate cardiovascular and respiratory rhythms and other visceral responses through influences on cranial-nerve nuclei and descending connections with autonomic centers in the spinal cord. Reticulospinal tracts also influence the transmission of sensory modalities by dorsal-horn neurons and the activities of alpha and gamma motor neurons, thereby modulating pain transmission, skeletal muscle tone, and somatic reflexes.

3. ANATOMIC CHARACTERISTICS OF RF NEURONS

The RF has been subdivided into a number of nuclei based on their anatomic locations. The more prominent of the reticular nuclei are described here. It is convenient to characterize the RF as three columns of neurons that extend throughout most of the brainstem tegmentum (Fig. 1). Although these columns of neurons are not separated by clearly defined anatomic boundaries, they are distinct from one another based on neuron morphology, neurochemical phenotype, circuitry, and location in the mediolateral plane. The unpaired *raphe nuclei* (e.g., median column) lie in the midline of the brainstem tegmentum (Raphe means seam and refers to the midline of the brainstem.) (Fig. 3). The paired medial and lateral columns of nuclei are found in the central (immediately lateral to the midline) and lateral portions of the tegmentum, respectively (Fig. 1).

RF neurons possess an aggregate of characteristics that distinguish them from most other brainstem neurons. Many have extensive dendritic arborizations that are oriented in a plane perpendicular to the long axis of the brainstem and to the ascending sensory and descending motor tracts. Other brainstem neurons have restricted dendritic fields. RF neuron dendrites typically intermingle with the axons of motor and sensory tracts, suggesting functional interactions. Axons

of many RF neurons are long, form numerous collaterals, and may have ascending and descending branches. Therefore, a single reticular neuron could influence brainstem and spinal-cord neurons associated with several different somatic and visceral functions. Inputs to reticular neurons typically originate from many varied sources. Taken together, these anatomical arrangements reflect the modulatory and integrative roles of the RF.

3.1. Raphe (Median Column) of the RF Lies in the Midline of the Brainstem Tegmentum

Several subgroups of decussating axons traverse the raphe of the brainstem. The most prominent of these are the medial lemniscus, olivocerebellar tract, and trapezoid body (fibers). Raphe neurons are scattered among these decussating axons most prominently in the medulla and pons but they also extend into the midbrain (squares in Fig. 1; Chapter 11, Figs. 4–6). The following raphe nuclei have been described based on neuron morphology: *raphe obscurus* and *raphe pallidus* in the medulla (Fig. 1A,B); *raphe magnus*, *raphe pontis* and *superior central* in the pons (Fig. 1C,D); *dorsal tegmental nucleus* and *nucleus linearis* (Fig. 1E,F) in the midbrain. Many of the raphe neurons contain *serotonin (5-hydroxytryptamine)*, and probably use this indoleamine as a transmitter (Fig. 2).

Raphe serotonergic neurons of the caudal brainstem, such as *raphe magnus*, *raphe pallidus*, and *raphe obscurus*, project prominently to the spinal cord (Fig. 4); those ending in substantia gelatinosa of the dorsal horn are believed to play a key role in modulation of pain transmission to conscious centers. Many pontine and midbrain serotonergic raphe neurons, such as *raphe pontis*, *superior central*, and *dorsal tegmental nucleus*, have rostral projections, directly and indirectly through the diencephalon, to the cerebral cortex and the limbic system. They also project to the noradrenergic neurons of the *locus ceruleus*, thereby participating in the regulation of alertness and sleep cycles (Figs. 3,4; Chapter 11, Fig. 5B,C).

The *mesolimbic region (of Tsai)*, which is located in the posterior perforated substance of the ventromedial aspect of the midbrain, (Fig. 1F; Chapter 11, Figs. 1, 6B) receives serotonergic terminals from raphe and other reticular neurons. Mesolimbic neurons are dopaminergic and project to the mediobasal frontal cortex, hippocampus, amygdala, nucleus accumbens, and other limbic and cortical regions. Evidence indicates that schizophrenic symptoms may result from

■ Raphe (median column)

▲ Precerebellar nuclei

◆ Medial column

● Lateral column

▩ Central tegmental tract

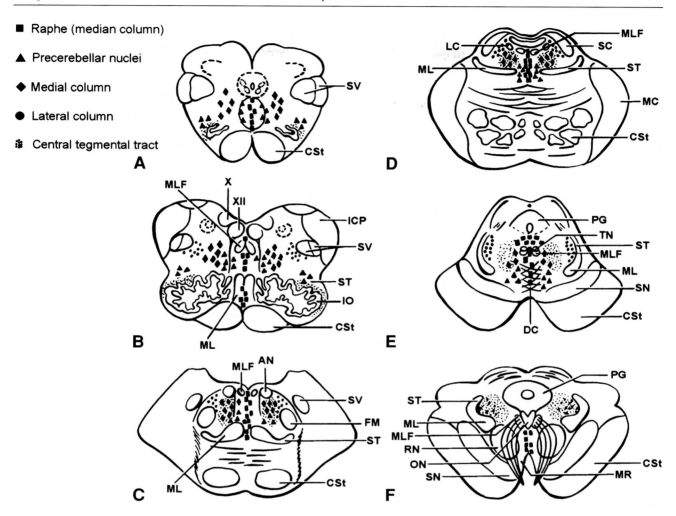

Fig. 1. Representations of the major nuclei of the RF in the brainstem. Anatomic boundaries of these nuclei are indistinct. Numerous subnuclei have been identified based on neuron morphology and neurochemical characteristics. Central tegmental tract (*stippled*) includes ascending and descending axons of the RF. (**A**) Caudal medulla—level of the sensory decussation (medial lemniscus). (**B**) Mid medulla—level of the vagal and hypoglossal nuclei. (**C**) Caudal pons—level of the facial and abducens nuclei; (**D**). Rostral pons—level of the locus ceruleus. (**E**) Midbrain—level of the inferior colliculus. (**F**) Midbrain —level of the superior colliculus. Median Column or raphe of reticular nuclei (*squares*) includes: nucleus raphe obscurus and nucleus raphe pallidus (medulla, **A** and **B**), nucleus raphe magnus, nucleus raphe pontis and central superior central nucleus (pons, **C** and **D**), and nucleus linearis and dorsal tegmental nucleus (midbrain, **E** and **F**). Medial column of reticular nuclei (*diamonds*) includes: ventral reticular nucleus (medulla, **A** and B), gigantocellular nucleus and pontine reticular nuclei (pons, **C** and **D**), and pontine reticular nucleus, pars oralis (midbrain, **E**). Lateral column of reticular nuclei (*large dots*) includes: parvocellular nucleus (medulla and pons, **B** and **C**), parabrachial nucleus (medulla and pons **D** and **E**), and pedunculopontine nucleus and cuneform nucleus (midbrain, **E** and **F**). Precerebellar nuclei (*triangles*) include: paramedian reticular nuclei (medulla and pons, **A**, **B**, and **C**), lateral reticular nucleus (medulla, **A** and **B**) and pontine reticulotegmental nuclei (**D** and **E**). Other relevant structures: AN, abducens nucleus; DC, decussation of superior cerebellar peduncles; ON, oculomotor nucleus; PG, periaqueductal gray; FM, facial motor nucleus; RN, red nucleus; IC, inferior cerebellar peduncle; SP, superior cerebellar peduncle; SN, substantia nigra; IO, inferior olivary nucleus; ST, spinothalamic tracts (anterolateral tracts); LC, locus ceruleus; MC, middle cerebellar peduncle; SV, spinal nucleus and tract of the trigeminal; ML, medial lemniscus; TN, trochlear nucleus; MLF, medial longitudinal fasciculus; X, dorsal motor nucleus of the vagus; XII, hypoglossal nucleus; MR, mesolimbic region.

inappropriate activation of the mesolimbic dopamine projections. Because activities of some dopaminergic neurons are facilitated by serotonin, it is likely that

serotonergic raphe neurons are an important component of the circuitry that regulates limbic-system functions. In this regard, one action of certain antipsychotic

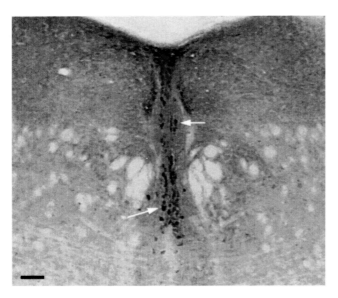

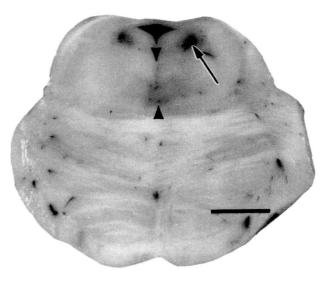

Fig. 2. Serotonergic neurons of the raphe. Immunocytochemical localization of a marker for serotonin in the cell bodies of neurons (*arrows*) in the brainstem raphe of the mouse. Bar = 100 μ. (The author is grateful to Dr. Melissa Zwick, University of Kentucky, who generously provided this illustration.)

Fig. 3. Locus ceruleus, raphe, and central tegmental tract. Unstained section of human rostral pons demonstrating the pigmented, noradrenergic neurons of the locus ceruleus (*arrow*). The shaft of the arrow overlies the central tegmental tract. *Arrowheads* indicate the raphe region of the pons. Bar = 5 mm.

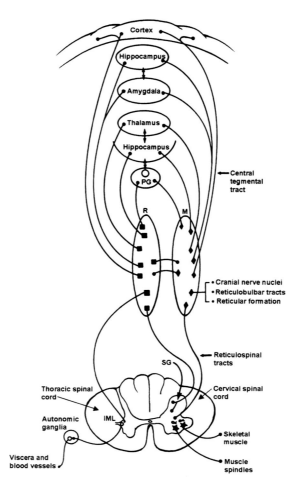

drugs is to downregulate serotonin receptors on dopamine neurons.

3.2. Medial Columns Are the "Effector" Components of the RF

The bilateral medial columns of the RF occupy the central portion of the medullary and pontine tegmentum just lateral to the raphe nuclei (*see* diamond in Fig. 1). The medial columns are subdivided into the *ventral reticular* (Fig. 1A,B), *gigantocellular*, and *pontine reticular nuclei* (Fig. 1C,D). Most of these neurons are large, and have extensive dendritic arborizations oriented perpendicular to the long axis of the brainstem. Long ascending and descending axons with numerous collateral branches originate from medial-column neurons, which terminate on other regions of the RF, the thalamus (e.g., interlaminar nuclei), cranial-nerve nuclei, and the spinal cord (Fig. 4). These ascending and descending axons of the medial columns, or "effector" neurons, collect as reticulocortical, reticulobulbar, and reticulospinal tracts, and convey RF influences throughout the CNS.

3.3. Lateral Columns Are the "Afferent" Components of the RF

The principal lateral column nuclei (*see* dots in Fig. 1) are composed mostly of small neurons, and include the *parvocellular nucleus* in the medulla and pons (Fig. 1B,C), *parabrachial nucleus* in the pons and midbrain (Fig. 1D,E), and *pedunculopontine* and *cuneiform nuclei* in the midbrain (Fig. 1E,F). Lateral-column components in the caudal brainstem are located between the medial reticular column medially and the spinal trigeminal system laterally. Rostrally, the lateral column is ventromedial to the superior cerebellar peduncle.

The neurons of the lateral columns are characterized by prominent inputs from axon collaterals of sensory tracts such as the *trigeminothalamic* and *anterolateral*, *spinoreticular*, and *other tracts*. The sensory input to lateral-column neurons is relayed medially to the medial-column neurons (Fig. 5). For example, the parvocellular nucleus in the medulla and

Fig. 4. (*Bottom opposite page*) Principal efferent projections of the RF. Raphe nuclei (R), e.g., median column, neurons are represented by *squares*. Neurons of the medial column (M) nuclei are represented by *diamonds*. *Dots* represent neuron terminals. IM, intermediolateral nucleus (e.g., preganglionic sympathetic neurons) of the thoracolumbar spinal cord; PG, periaqueductal gray; SG, substantia gelatinosa of the dorsal horn.

pons relay inputs from the ascending spinothalamic, trigeminothalamic, and auditory pathways to the medial column and raphe nuclei. Functionally, these nuclei form descending *reticulospinal* and *reticulo-bulbar tract* projections which provide regulatory influences that modulate sensory transmissions from the periphery (Fig. 4). For example, many of these terminals modulate nociceptive transmissions by activating enkephalinergic interneurons in the substantia gelatinosa of the dorsal horn and in the spinal trigeminal nucleus. They also activate ascending pathways following the *central tegmental tract*, which relay in the thalamus. Related thalamocortical fibers project throughout the cerebral cortex to facilitate alertness (Fig. 4).

Connections of the *parabrachial nucleus* in the pons and midbrain suggest roles in visceral and limbic functions. The midbrain components of the lateral column—the *pedunculopontine* and *cuneiform nuclei*—project to the motor cortex, subthalamus, striatum, substantia nigra, precerebellar, and raphe nuclei, implying roles in motor functions.

The *locus ceruleus* is a compact group of pigmented neurons located in the rostral pons ventrolateral to the fourth ventricle and dorsolateral to the *pontine reticular nucleus* (Fig. 1D,3; Chapter 11, Fig. 5B,C). Locus ceruleus neurons express *norepinephrine*, a catecholamine transmitter. Afferents to locus ceruleus arise from reticular nuclei in the lateral tegmentum of the medulla and pons. One subgroup of these afferents exerts inhibitory influences and another facilitates locus ceruleus activity. Other afferents arise from the cerebral cortex, amygdala, hippocampus, periaqueductal gray, and hypothalamus. The major efferents of the locus ceruleus are to these same structures and to other RF nuclei. These circuits allow the locus ceruleus to respond to new sensory stimuli, and through its widely disseminated noradrenergic projections exert an activating influence throughout the brain.

4. OTHER RELATED BRAINSTEM NUCLEI

There are many other named brainstem nuclei that have some RF characteristics or are functionally closely related to the RF. A few are briefly described below and are considered in detail elsewhere.

The *substantia nigra* of the midbrain consists of neurons that express the catecholamine neurotransmitter *dopamine* (Fig. 1E,F; Chapter 11, Fig. 6). Locus ceruleus (Fig. 3) and substantia nigra neurons contain a melanin-like pigment, which permits the identifica-

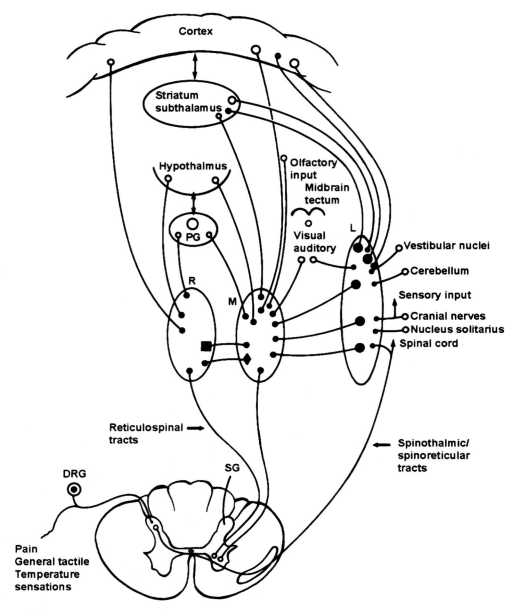

Fig. 5. Principal afferent projections to the RF. The raphe (**R**), e.g., median column, neuron-cell bodies are represented by the *square*. The medial column (**M**) neuron-cell bodies are represented by the *diamond*. Neurons of the lateral column (**L**) nuclei are represented by *large dots*. The *open dots* indicate other neural systems that project to the RF. *Small dots* represent neuron terminals. DRG, dorsal root ganglia; PG, periaqueductal gray; SG, substantia gelatinosa of the dorsal horn.

tion of these nuclei with the unaided eye in unstained brainstem sections.

The *red nucleus* occupies the central midbrain tegmentum (Fig. 1F; Chapter 11, Fig. 6B). Its functional role is exclusively related to contralateral motor regulation; it receives inputs predominantly from the ipsilateral motor cortex, spinal cord, and contralateral cerebellum. In addition, it is reciprocally connected with the lateral reticular nucleus, which projects to the cerebellum. It gives rise to contralateral *rubrobulbar* and *rubrospinal tracts*, which terminate on brainstem reticular neurons, cranial-nerve motor nuclei, and spinal cord motor neurons. Another major projection of the red nucleus follows the *central tegmental tract* (*see* stippling in Fig. 1) to the ipsilateral *inferior olivary nucleus* (Fig. 1A,B; Chapter 11, Fig. 4C,D). The *inferior olivary nucleus* is a prominent structure in the ventral tegmentum of the medulla. It receives indirect input from the RF and directly from the red nucleus by way of the central tegmental tract (Figs. 1,3). Olivocerebellar axons cross through the raphe nuclei in the RF of the medulla, but virtually all terminate in the contralateral cerebellum. These circuits provide a basis for interactions between the RF and structures that regulate motor functions.

Three RF nuclei in the caudal brainstem, collectively termed the *precerebellar reticular nuclei* (triangles in Fig. 1), also have restricted functional roles related to the motor system because they project almost exclusively to the cerebellum. Two of these—the *paramedian reticular* (Fig. 1A–C) and the *pontine reticulotegmental nuclei* (Fig. 1D,E)—form a parallel column of neurons located between the medial column of the RF and the brainstem raphe. The third precerebellar reticular nucleus, the *lateral reticular nucleus* (Fig. 1A,B), is a conspicuous cluster of large neurons in the lateral tegmentum of the medulla, lying between the spinal trigeminal system and the inferior olivary nucleus. Together, these precerebellar nuclei provide integrating circuits between cerebellum, red nucleus, inferior olivary nucleus, and RF that participate in regulating motor functions such as posture, equilibrium, and muscle tone.

The *periaqueductal gray* (Fig. 1E,F; Chapter 11, Fig. 6) surrounds the cerebral aqueduct, and consists of numerous axonal terminals and subgroups of neurons containing many different transmitters and peptides (Chapter 2, Fig. 9A; Chapter 11, Figs. 5C,6). Many of these neurons have extensive dendrites, which intermingle with the midbrain RF. Periaqueductal gray receives its most prominent inputs from the hypothalamus, frontal cortex, and limbic structures (Fig. 4); afferents also originate from the parabrachial and other reticular nuclei, solitary nucleus, and the ascending sensory pathways. Periaqueductal gray provides reciprocal projections to all of the above structures and to the serotonergic raphe nuclei of the medulla. Specifically, it projects to the nucleus raphe magnus in the pons and medulla (Fig. 1C). The nucleus raphe magnus—among others—projects serotonergic terminals to the substantia gelatinosa of the spinal cord (Fig. 4), which activate enkephalinergic interneurons. The enkephalinergic neurons modulate nociceptive stimuli by diminishing activities in the transmission neurons whose axons form the spinothalamic and trigeminothalamic tracts. Thus, the periaqueductal gray, together with the RF, plays a key role in integrating limbic and autonomic functions and in modulating pain perceptions.

5. CLINICAL IMPLICATIONS OF THE FUNCTIONAL INTERACTIONS OF THE RF

RF morphology, circuitry, and chemical transmission characteristics provide an important matrix for the integration of nervous-system activities. The control of vital functions such as regulation of blood pressure depends on integrated circuitry between the cortex, diencephalon, RF, spinal cord, and peripheral tissues. Consequently, inputs converge on the RF from almost all somatic and visceral sensory pathways and from the cortex, hypothalamus, striatum, limbic structures, and spinal cord (Fig. 5). Moreover, the RF provides prominent projections to these same structures (Fig. 4). Because of this integrated circuitry, particular components of the RF influence many neural functions and certain RF regions or nuclei are closely associated with important neural responses, which are described in the following section.

5.1. The RF Participates in the Altering Response

Early studies demonstrated that stimulation of the RF evoked changes in cortical activity characteristic of the arousal induced by sensory stimulation. Later studies revealed that the ascending spinothalamic and trigeminothalamic tracts provided collateral input to the lateral columns of the RF (*see* the parvocellular nucleus, Fig. 1B,C). The lateral column neurons project to the medial columns in the medulla and pons (e.g., ventral reticular, gigantocellular, pontine reticular nuclei; *see* Fig. 1A–D). The medial columns form prominent ascending projections that follow the *central tegmental tracts* (*see* stippling in Figs. 1,3) terminating in the locus ceruleus, hypothalamus, and the intralaminar (e.g., centromedian) nuclei of the dorsal thalamus. Related thalamocortical fibers relay activation throughout the cerebral cortex. Additionally, activation of the locus ceruleus noradrenergic projections to the cortex facilitates the attentional state. Collectively, these rostral projections constitute the *ascending reticular activating system (ARAS)* that supports several important functions. The flow of sensory stimuli through ARAS activates the hypothalamic and limbic structures, which regulate emotional and behavioral responses (i.e., responses to pain). More important, the flow of sensory stimuli facilitates cortical activity. For example, activation of the widely disseminated locus ceruleus noradrenergic projections to the cortex is important in facilitating the attentional state and in generating sleep/wake cycles. Other examples of ARAS activities include the alerting responses to a sudden loud sound, a flash of light, smelling salts, or a splash of cold water in the face. Without cortical activation by ARAS, the individual is less able to detect new specific stimuli and the level of consciousness is diminished.

This discussion should not suggest that the RF is the "center for consciousness." Experimental and clinical observations imply that consciousness, which is a person's ability to be aware of self and environment and to orient toward new stimuli, results from the integrated activities of a number of neural structures, including the RF.

There are important clinical implications related to ARAS function. The RF projections in the ARAS traverse the midbrain tegmentum, and some of these projections follow the central tegmental tract (Fig. 1). Lesions of the midbrain can interrupt the ARAS, leading to *altered levels of consciousness* or *coma* caused by the diminished facilitation of cortical neurons. Lesions that frequently affect the midbrain include cerebrovascular accidents (e.g., stroke) and head trauma. Cerebrovascular accidents interfere with the blood supply to the brainstem, and therefore alter consciousness because of diminished oxygen supply to reticular neurons and ascending pathways.

Head trauma can induce increased intracranial pressure (ICP) as a result of the collection of blood (e.g., hematoma) between the skull and the brain or accumulation of edema fluid in the injured brain. Because the brain is encased in the skull, the increased ICP causes the medial aspect of the temporal lobe (e.g., the uncus of the hippocampal gyrus) to herniate through the incisura of the tentorium, compressing the midbrain (Chapter 11, Fig. 1). This situation is a medical emergency because the herniating temporal lobe can exert pressure directly on the lateral aspect of the midbrain and interfere with its blood supply. These lesions can destroy ARAS pathways in the midbrain, resulting in permanent coma or *persistent vegetative state*.

Certain drugs and metabolic imbalances are believed to induce altered states of consciousness through actions on the RF. Some anesthetics alter consciousness through actions on the RF, while conduction of sensations by the somatic pain pathways to the cortex remains unaffected. The molecular structure of *lysergic acid diethylamide (LSD)* is similar to serotonin. Available evidence suggests that LSD exerts its hallucinogenic effects by inhibition of raphe serotonergic projections to the cortex and limbic system (Figs. 2,4).

5.2. Sleep Is an Active Neural Process that Requires Participation of the RF

The RF plays a prominent role in the elaboration of normal sleep-cycle stages through its circuitry with the cortex and diencephalon. Lesions or stimulations of certain regions of the hypothalamus and frontal lobes also affect sleep cycles.

The *slow-wave component* of the sleep cycle is characterized by synchronized cortical activity. Data demonstrate that pontine raphe serotonergic neuron activities diminish as *slow-wave sleep* progresses. Serotonergic neurons (Fig. 2) also activate the *paradoxical sleep* component, which is characterized by *rapid eye movements* (REM), diminished muscle tone, and a desynchronized electroencephalogram (EEG) similar to that of the waking state. This activation involves the locus ceruleus (Fig. 3; Chapter 11, Fig. 5B,C) whose norepinephrine-containing terminals are distributed to the RF and all parts of the cerebral cortex. Cholinergic mechanisms are also involved in the activation of paradoxical sleep.

Destruction of the serotonergic neurons or inhibition of serotonin synthesis, produces *insomnia*. Lesions of the locus ceruleus and surrounding RF alter the induction of the paradoxical or REM stage of the sleep cycle. The slow-wave and paradoxical stages recur several times during a sleep period. Thus, the sleep cycle depends on a complex neurochemical circuitry linking cholinergic, adrenergic, and serotonergic neurons of the RF with other neural structures.

5.3. The Raphe Nuclei of the Medulla Modulate Pain Transmission

Axons of the ascending spinothalamic and trigeminothalamic tracts convey pain sensations from the viscera and body surface. These tracts also provide collaterals to the lateral columns of the RF (Fig. 5). This input contributes to the ARAS described previously. Also activated by nociceptive input are the serotonergic neurons of raphe and medial column nuclei in the caudal brainstem. Specifically, these nuclei include *raphe magnus* and *gigantocellular nuclei* (Fig. 1C,D). The axons of some of these serotonergic neurons distribute to the spinal trigeminal nucleus by means of reticulobulbar tracts, and others descend in the dorsolateral aspect of the spinal cord white matter by means of reticulospinal tracts to terminate in the dorsal horn (Fig. 4). The serotonin released in the dorsal horn and spinal trigeminal nuclei modulates pain transmission by activating *enkephalinergic inter-*

neurons. Enkephalin inhibits transmission of nociceptive stimuli by pain-pathway neurons. Available evidence suggests that a descending noradrenergic pathway and GABAergic interneurons may also play roles in pain modulation.

Stimulation of the *periaqueductal gray* or the caudal brainstem raphe nuclei induces analgesia. Periaqueductal gray neurons project to the serotonergic neurons of the caudal brainstem, probably involving opiate and non-opiate mechanisms (Fig. 5). In certain patients with intractable pain, brief activation of electrodes implanted in the periaqueductal gray can provide an analgesic effect that lasts for hours or longer.

5.4. RF Participated in Regulation of Skeletal Muscle Tone, Reflexes, and Bony Posture

The RF influences motor activities through its reciprocal connections with the red nucleus, substantia nigra, subthalamus, striatum, motor cortex, and cerebellum (Fig. 5). Midbrain reticular nuclei and the lateral reticular nucleus of the medulla project to the inferior olivary nucleus, as does the red nucleus. The inferior olivary nucleus sends massive projections to the contralateral cerebellum. Through these circuits, the RF participates with other motor- and vestibular-system components in providing a continuously integrated regulation of body posture and muscle tone, which facilitates voluntary motor actions. This regulation is conveyed to the alpha and gamma lower motor neurons by reticulospinal and reticulobulbar tracts, which take origin primarily in the medial columns of the RF. Specifically, midbrain and pontine reticular nuclei (Fig. 1C–F) provide ipsilateral projections to spinal cord via the pontine reticulospinal tracts and exert facilitory effects on axial and limb extensors. Bilateral projections arise from pontine and medullary reticular nuclei (Fig. 1A–C) inhibit lower motor neurons innervating axial extensors but facilitate motor neurons that innervate limb flexors (Fig. 4).

5.5. The RF Participated in the Integration of Conjugative Eye Movements

A portion of the medial columns of the RF in the pons is termed the *paramedian pontine RF* or *PPRF*. The PPRF overlaps the pontine reticular nucleus and integrates horizontal eye movements (Fig. 1C). PPRF receives inputs from the superior colliculus, vestibular nuclei, RF and the frontal eye fields of the cerebral cortex. It projects primarily to the ipsilateral abducens nucleus, and by following the medial longitudinal fasciculus, to the portion of the contralateral oculomotor nucleus that innervates the medial rectus muscle. Through these circuits, the PPRF integrates horizontal, conjugate eye movements in response to head and body position, reflex responses to light, and cortical activity. A group of neurons that regulates conjugate eye movements in the vertical plane has been located in the rostral midbrain.

5.6. The RF Regulated Vital Visceral Responses

RF neurons that participate in regulation of cardiovascular, respiratory, and other visceral functions are intermingled with those serving other functions described earlier. Terms such as *"inspiratory center"* refer to observations of particular physiological responses following stimulation of a region of the RF rather than an anatomically defined cluster of neurons serving only inspiration. Nonetheless, certain areas of the caudal brainstem RF have been shown to influence particular visceral functions.

The evidence suggests that visceral sensory input to the RF is relayed in a polysynaptic manner through collaterals from ascending spinal cord sensory pathways and from the solitary nucleus. Other afferents related to visceral functions reach the RF via descending fibers from the hypothalamus and limbic system— specifically, *dorsal longitudinal fasciculus, medial forebrain bundle* and *mammillotegmental tract.*

RF neurons influencing *cardiovascular responses* are located primarily in the medulla and caudal pons. Cardiac rhythm and blood pressure are diminished after stimulation of raphe and medial column nuclei, primarily gigantocellular nucleus—a *cardiac depressor area* (Fig. 1C,D). Stimulation of the parvocellular nucleus (Fig. 1B,C) in the lateral column of the medullary tegmentum yields opposite effects—a *cardiac accelerator area.* Axons from these "cardiovascular" neurons are believed to provide facilitory or inhibitory influences on parasympathetic preganglionic neurons in the medulla associated with the vagus nerve (e.g., dorsal motor nucleus and nucleus ambiguus) and on the sympathetic preganglionic neurons of the thoracic spinal cord (e.g., intermediolateral nuclei).

RF neurons influencing *respiratory rhythms* are widely distributed in the brainstem. Inspiratory responses are obtained following stimulation of gigantocellular nucleus (Fig. 1C,D), and expiratory responses are activated from the parvocellular nucleus (Fig. 1C,D). These *"respiratory centers"* overlap the "cardiovascular centers" described previously. Another cluster of neurons influencing respiratory rhythms is located in the region of the *parabrachial nucleus* (Fig. 1D,E) in the pons. Efferent fibers from these "respiratory" neurons directly or indirectly influence activities of preganglionic sympathetic and parasympathetic nuclei in the brainstem and spinal cord, as well as motor neurons associated with the *phrenic* and *intercostal nerves*. In some newborn infants, immaturity of these respiratory circuits may alter neural control of respiratory rhythms, placing the child at risk for *sudden infant death syndrome (SIDS)*.

Caudal brainstem lesions that destroy neurons that integrate cardiovascular and respiratory functions present life-threatening situations. For example, cerebrovascular accidents involving the intrinsic vasculature of the medulla or pons can destroy these neurons, resulting in distortions of cardiac and respiratory rhythms and death of the individual.

Increased ICP in the posterior cranial fossa can result in *herniation of the cerebellar tonsils* through the foramen magnum (Chapter 11, Fig. 1; Chapter 2, Fig. 4). In this situation, the pressure exerted on the medulla diminishes its blood supply and interrupts the reticulospinal fibers that link the RF with autonomic nuclei in the spinal cord. In the case of patients with high cervical spinal cord lesions, survival during the acute stages of their injury requires prompt external support to maintain cardiac and respiratory functions. In addition, certain drugs, including anesthetics, can depress activity in these neurons, altering or interrupting cardiovascular and respiratory rhythms.

The hypothalamus plays a major role in maintaining *homeostasis* through integration of somatic, visceral, and endocrine functions. It forms prominent functional connections with cortical areas, olfactory-system and limbic-system structures that generate emotions, and behavioral patterns. The cortex, limbic system and hypothalamus have prominent reciprocal connections with the RF (Figs. 4,5). These anatomical and functional interactions imply that some aspects of emotional display and elaboration of behavior are conveyed through RF influences on autonomic nuclei in the brainstem and spinal cord. It is likely that RF interactions with the striatum and motor neurons influence neurons that elaborate the body postures and muscle tone that accompany emotional expressions and behaviors.

ACKNOWLEDGMENT

Ms. Mary Gail Engle provided invaluable assistance in the preparation of the illustrations for this chapter. Her contributions are greatly appreciated.

SELECTED READINGS

Brodal A. 1981. "The reticular formation and some related nuclei." In Neurological Anatomy in Relation to Clinical Medicine (3rd ed). New York: Oxford University Press, 1981; 394–447.

Carpenter MB, Sutin J. Human Neuroanatomy, 8th ed. Baltimore: Williams and Wilkins, 1983; 315–453.

Garcia-Rill E. Disorders of reticular activating system. Medical Hypothesis 1997; 49:379–387.

Garcia-Rill E, Bittermann JA, Chambers T, Skinner RD, Mrak RE, Husain M, et al. Mesopontine neurons in schizophrenia. Neuroscience 1995; 66:321–335.

Hobson JA, Brazier MA. "The reticular formation revisited: specifying function for a non-specific system". In International Brain Research Organization Monograph Series, vol. 6, New York: Raven Press, 1980.

Kinney H, Burger PC, Harrell FE, Hudson RP. Reactive gliosis in the medulla oblongata of victims of sudden infant death syndrome. Pediatrics 1983; 72:181–187.

Martin G, Holstege G, Mehler WR. "Reticular formation of the pons and medulla". In Paxinos G. (ed). The Human Nervous System, New York: Academic Press Inc., 1990; 203–220.

Monti JM, Monti D. Role of dorsal raphe nucleus serotonin 5-HT1A receptor in the regulation of REM sleep. Life science 2000; 66:1999–2012.

Paxinos G, Törk I, Halliday G, Mehler WR. "Human homologs to brainstem nuclei identified in other animals as revealed by acetylcholinesterase activity". In Pxinos G. (ed). The Human Nervous System New York: Academic Press Inc., 1990; 149–202.

Quattrochi J, Baba N, Liss L, Adrion W. Sudden infant death syndrome (SIDS): a preliminary study of reticular dendritic spines in infants with SIDS. Brain Res 1980; 181:245–249.

Scheibel AB. "The brainstem reticular core and sensory function". In Smith D. (ed). Handbook of Physiology: The Nervous System III, vol. 1 Bethesda: American Physiological Society, 1984; 213–256.

Scheibel ME. Scheibel AB. On circuit patterns of the brainstem reticular core. Ann NY Acad Sci 1961; 89:857–865.

Disorders of the Autonomic Nervous System

Gregory Cooper and Robert L. Rodnitzky

Clinical symptoms of autonomic dysfunction can arise from abnormalities of autonomic pathways within the central or peripheral nervous systems. Mild autonomic dysfunction can occur in otherwise normal persons with advancing age. More substantial autonomic symptoms arise when there is structural disruption of autonomic pathways or when they are involved in degenerative or metabolic conditions.

PERIPHERAL-NERVE DYSFUNCTION

Nerve fibers subserving autonomic function are easily damaged in diseases of the peripheral nerves. The peripheral neuropathies that are most likely to result in autonomic symptoms are those that cause acute demyelination or involve small myelinated or unmyelinated fibers. Among the most common neuropathies in this category are those caused by diabetes, amyloidosis, or porphyria and the Guillian-Barre syndrome. In a neuropathy such as that associated with Friedreich's ataxia, in which the large fibers are reduced in number but small fibers are preserved, there are virtually no autonomic symptoms. Between these two extremes are a variety of neuropathies in which autonomic symptoms are present but which do not constitute the primary disability. Examples include those caused by alcohol abuse, nutritional deficiency, leprosy, chronic kidney failure, and acquired immunodeficiency syndrome.

CENTRAL NERVOUS SYSTEM DISORDERS

Abnormalities of the brain or spinal cord can result in autonomic dysfunction. The autonomic dysfunction can be the primary clinical abnormality or part of a wider syndrome affecting many parts of the nervous system. *Progressive autonomic failure* is a primary autonomic disorder in which there is gradual development of symptoms such as bladder dysfunction, decreased tear production, erectile dysfunction, reduced sweating, and orthostatic hypotension (e.g., decreased blood pressure on standing). The primary pathologic finding is a loss of sympathetic preganglionic cell bodies in the intermediolateral column of the spinal cord. This same syndrome may occur with more diffuse involvement of the central nervous system (CNS) and other nonautonomic symptoms. If autonomic failure is associated with signs of Parkinson's disease, it is assumed that nigrostriatal degeneration has also occurred, and the condition is called the *Shy-Drager syndrome*. If, in addition, other nervous system structures are involved, such as the cerebellum, the entire conglomerate of autonomic, parkinsonian, and cerebellar symptoms is referred to as the *syndrome of multiple system atrophy*.

Among spinal cord disorders, prominent autonomic dysfunction is most likely to be associated with severe transverse lesions. Such lesions at or above the midthoracic spinal cord level typically result in severe orthostatic hypotension. In such cases, there is inadequate control of the sympathetic outflow from the spinal cord below the lesion. This results in inadequate reflex constriction of blood vessels in response to the normal drop in blood pressure associated with assuming the standing position. Persons with transverse spinal cord lesions are typically paraplegic and unable to stand on their own, but caution must be exercised in moving them passively to the upright position because of the risk of severe hypotension.

Bladder function can also be affected by a variety of spinal cord lesions. A lesion involving the conus medullaris or the cauda equina results in an autonomic neurogenic bladder characterized by inability to initiate micturition and marked urinary retention. In this circumstance, the afferent or efferent arc of the micturition reflex, both of which travel through cauda equina parasympathetic nerves, or the center for micturition located in the second, third, or fourth segments of the sacral spinal cord, have been involved by the offending lesion. With spinal cord lesions above the sacral parasympathetic center for bladder control, the bladder reflex remains intact but cannot be controlled by descending inhibitory influences from supraspinal centers. In this situation, the voiding reflex goes unchecked, and there is frequent, spontaneous, and precipitous micturition. Patients with spinal cord lesions of this type can be taught to precipitate this reflex voluntarily by stroking the skin in sacral-innervated areas or by gently compressing the bladder through the abdomen. Using this technique, they regain some control over the timing of voiding.

ABNORMALITIES OF NEUROTRANSMITTER METABOLISM

A deficiency or an excess of neurotransmitters subserving autonomic function can occur. A deficiency of dopamine β-hydroxylase, the enzyme responsible for the final reaction in the synthesis of norepinephrine, has been documented in some persons and appears to be inherited as an autosomal recessive trait. Marked reduction in plasma and cerebrospinal fluid (CSF) norepinephrine levels can be documented in these patients, who often suffer from symptoms of sympathetic autonomic dysfunction, especially orthostatic hypotension. The opposite circumstance prevails in patients with a catecholamine-producing tumor of the adrenal gland known as a pheochromocytoma. In this condition, excessive production of norepinephrine results in hypertension.

Plasma norepinephrine levels can be measured. In the case of pheochromocytoma, the levels of norepinephrine and several other catecholamines measured over a 24-h period are typically elevated. Plasma norepinephrine levels can be useful for other purposes. The response of plasma norepinephrine levels to standing has been used as a means of differentiating preganglionic from postganglionic sympathetic failure. Because most plasma norepinephrine is believed to be derived from sympathetic postganglionic nerve terminals, resting levels of plasma norepinephrine are expected to be normal in a preganglionic sympathetic lesion. When these persons stand, the otherwise normal postganglionic neuron cannot be activated to produce the normal rise in norepinephrine with the expected spillover into the plasma. In postganglionic sympathetic lesions, even the resting level is diminished because of inadequate numbers of norepinephrine-releasing nerve terminals. In this circumstance, the elevation in plasma norepinephrine levels after standing is also less than normal, depending on how widespread the postganglionic dysfunction is.

CLINICAL TESTS USEFUL IN DOCUMENTING AUTONOMIC DYSFUNCTION

Recording the blood pressure in the supine and standing positions while determining the concurrent heart rate is a simple and extremely useful test for sympathetic autonomic dysfunction. If after two minutes of standing the systolic blood pressure has fallen by 30 mmHg or more, a diagnosis of orthostatic hypotension is justified. Absence of acceleration in the heart rate in the face of this hypotension further confirms the presence of autonomic dysfunction.

A variety of provocative tests can be performed to assess the sympathetic mechanisms that control heart rate and blood pressure. These include measuring the extent to which a sustained hand grip, immersing a hand in ice water, or performing difficult mental arithmetic stimulate the sympathetic outflow and elevate the heart rate and blood pressure. One mechanism of evaluating parasympathetic control of heart rate is to have the patient briefly execute the Valsalva maneuver (e.g., forcefully attempt to expel breath against a closed glottis). This results in a transient increase in intrathoracic pressure; with resultant decreased cardiac filling and a lowering of blood pressure. The normal baroreflex response to lower blood pressure should be an elevation in heart rate. On release, there should be an overshoot of the normal blood pressure and slowing of the heart rate. Absence of these reactions is a sign of parasympathetic dysfunction. The response to the Valsalva maneuver is actually much more complex than this and can be divided into three or four component phases, but in its simplest form, it can be a useful screening test for parasympathetic function.

Sweating or sudomotor function is a sympathetic function that can be evaluated by applying Alizarin-red powder to the skin. When the body temperature is elevated, the powder, which is initially white, becomes red wherever it is in contact with perspiration. This can be particularly striking in conditions such as loss of sweating (e.g., anhidrosis) on one side of the face.

Extremely localized autonomic functions can be measured. A classic example is the assessment of sympathetic innervation of the pupil and eyelid. When this innervation is interrupted by a lesion in the sympathetic chain, a syndrome consisting of ptosis (e.g., drooping) of the eyelid, meiosis (e.g., a smaller than normal pupil), and anhidrosis on the same side of the face may occur. Collectively, these neurologic signs are known as *Horner's syndrome*. A series of pharmacologic tests can determine whether Horner's syndrome is present, and if so, whether it is caused by involvement of the first- or second-order neuron in the sympathetic chain (i.e., preganglionic lesion) or the third-order neuron (e.g., postganglionic lesion). An initial test that can determine if Horner's syndrome is present involves the instillation of a dilute solution of cocaine into the conjunctival sac of the involved eye and the opposite normal eye. Cocaine inhibits re-uptake of synaptic norepinephrine. In the normal eye, this causes enhanced sympathetic stimulation of the iris dilator muscle, resulting in enlargement of the pupil. On the side with sympathetic dysfunction, there has been little or no synaptic norepinephrine elaborated, and the pupil dilates considerably less than that on the normal side. This effect occurs regardless of the location of the lesion within the sympathetic pathway.

The next step differentiates a preganglionic lesion from a postganglionic lesion. Paredrine, an amphetamine derivative, is instilled into both eyes. Because amphetamine enhances the release of norepinephrine from sympathetic terminals, the expected normal response is pupillary dilatation, but this only occurs if there is a healthy third-order (postganglionic) neuron. A normal response to Paredrine in a patient with Horner's syndrome suggests that the causative sympathetic lesion is located in the first- or second-order neuron. An abnormal response to Paredrine indicates that the pathology is in the postganglionic neuron.

SELECTED READINGS

Benarroch EE, Chang FLF. Central Autonomic Disorders. J Clin Neurophys 1993; 10:39–50.

Low PA. Autonomic nervous system function. J Clin Neurophys 1993; 10:14–27.

McLeod JG. Autonomic dysfunction in peripheral nerve disease. J Clin Neurophys 1993; 10:51–60.

Shields Jr RW. Functional anatomy of the autonomic nervous system. J Clin Neurophys 1993; 10:2–13.

13 The Trigeminal System

Harold H. Traurig

1. SYNOPSIS

The trigeminal nerve—cranial nerve V—provides sensory innervation to the face and the structures of the oral and nasal cavities. In addition, its motor component innervates the muscles of mastication. Fine (discriminatory) tactile, general (light) tactile, proprioceptive, thermal, and pain sensory modalities are conveyed to the trigeminal nuclei in the brainstem. Axons from the sensory trigeminal nuclei contribute to important reflex circuits and relay sensory information to the thalamus for further integration. Thalamocortical projections relay sensations to the face area of the contralateral postcentral gyrus of the cerebral hemispheres.

The trigeminal system is frequently involved in important clinical conditions because its peripheral and central components have extensive anatomic distributions in the face, cranial cavity, and brainstem.

2. PERIPHERIAL DISTRIBUTION OF THE TRIGEMINAL SYSTEM

2.1. The Trigeminal Nerve Root and Its Three Divisions Course Through the Posterior and Middle Cranial Fossae

From: *Neuroscience in Medicine, 2nd ed.* (P. Michael Conn, ed.),
© 2003 Humana Press Inc., Totowa, NJ.

Trigeminal-nerve-root axons form a large sensory component and a smaller, superiorly positioned motor portion (Figs. 1,3; Chapter 11, Fig. 1). The trigeminal root exits laterally from the mid-pons, interdigitating with the fibers of the middle cerebellar peduncle, and then courses obliquely and superiorly through the *posterior cranial fossa* to the apex of the petrous portion of the temporal bone. The root then crosses the petrous ridge, passing inferior to a ligamentous (attached) portion of the tentorium cerebelli and the superior petrosal sinus into the middle cranial fossa, and enters the trigeminal ganglion. The *trigeminal ganglion* and the origins of the *three divisions of the trigeminal nerve—ophthalmic (V_1), maxillary (V_2), and mandibular (V_3)*—are located in a dural pocket (Meckel's cave) on the anterior slope of the petrous bone (Fig. 1; Chapter 2, Fig. 4).

The sensory axons of the mandibular division are located posterolateral in the trigeminal root. The ophthalmic division sensory axons are in a anteromedial position, and those of the maxillary division are intermediate in position. They originate from several subgroups of unipolar neurons in the trigeminal ganglion.

Near its exit point from the brainstem, the location of the trigeminal root is closely related to arterial branches of the vertebrobasilar system (Chapter 2, Fig. 13) and superior petrosal vein (of Dandy). Compression or irritation of the trigeminal root by these

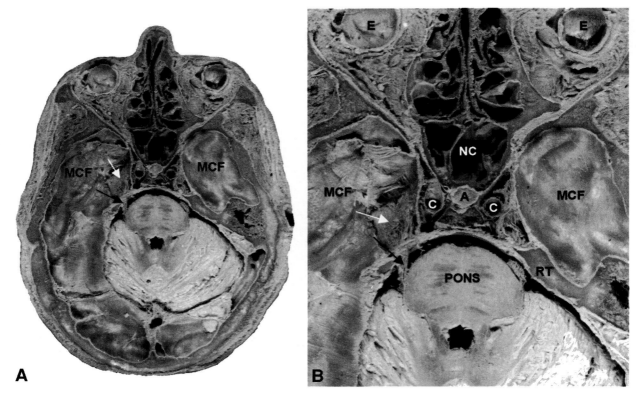

Fig. 1. (A,B) Axial section of the head showing the position of the trigeminal ganglion (*white arrow*) on the anterior slope of the petrous portion of the temporal bone (RT) in the middle cranial fossa (MCF). The root of the trigeminal nerve courses posteriorly into the posterior cranial fossa and enters the pons (*black arrow*). Anterior direction is toward the top of the figures. The plane of the section is inclined superiorly, approx 1 cm on the left side of the specimen. The section passes through the apex of the tentorium cerebelli and reveals the pons and cerebellum in the posterior cranial fossa. **(B)** central portion of **(A)**. Trigeminal ganglion is encased in a dural sleeve, which is reflected anteriorly to reveal the ganglion (*white arrow*). The trigeminal ganglion lies inferior and medial to the temporal lobe, which has been removed in the specimen. In its course, the trigeminal root (*black arrow*) crosses the RT and passes inferior to the superior petrosal venous sinus. A, adenohypophysis in the sella turcica. C, the internal carotid arteries, which are evident just lateral to the sella turcica as they course through the cavernous sinuses; E, eye; NC, nasal cavity.

vessels could evoke the pain syndrome known as *trigeminal neuralgia (tic douloureux).*

The *trigeminal ophthalmic division* passes forward from the trigeminal ganglion embedded in the lateral wall of the cavernous sinus (Fig. 1). It passes through the superior orbital fissure to enter the orbit, where it divides into its peripheral branches. The ophthalmic division conveys sensory innervation from the supratentorial dura, globe, cornea, upper eyelid, regions of the face and scalp, and the mucosa of the ethmoidal, sphenoidal, and frontal sinuses (Fig. 2).

The *trigeminal maxillary division* passes forward from the trigeminal ganglion on the floor of the middle cranial fossa (Chapter 2, Fig. 4) and exits the cranial cavity through the foramen rotundum. It courses through the pterygopalatine fossa, which is bounded

by the palatine bone medially, the pterygoid process posteriorly, and the maxilla anteriorly. Two other important contents of the pterygopalatine fossa are the terminal branches of the maxillary artery and the parasympathetic pterygopalatine ganglion. Trigeminal maxillary branches pass through the pterygopalatine ganglion, and probably provide some sensory collateral terminals to the autonomic neurons that innervate visceral and vascular structures of the nasal and maxillary regions. Peripheral sensory fibers supply the maxillary teeth, gingiva, and mucosae of the maxillary sinus, nasal cavity, and palate. Cutaneous fibers follow the infraorbital nerve to innervate skin of the midface, including the lower eyelid and upper lip (Fig. 2).

The *trigeminal mandibular division* consists of sensory and motor fibers. It courses inferiorly from the

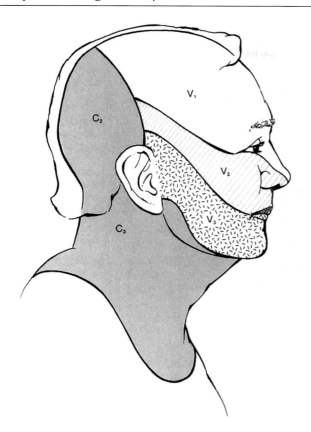

Fig 2. Sensory fields of the ophthalmic (V$_1$), maxillary (V$_2$), and mandibular (V$_3$) divisions of the trigeminal nerve. The sensory fields of the upper cervical spinal nerves are shown (C$_2$, C$_3$). *See* text for description of innervation of the auricle and external auditory canal.

trigeminal ganglion, then exits the cranial cavity through the foramen ovale in the middle cranial fossa (Fig. 1; Chapter 2, Fig. 13). Near the base of the skull, the parasympathetic otic ganglion is attached to the medial aspect of the mandibular division. Sensory innervation is conveyed from the dura, mandibular teeth, and gingiva, the mucosae of the floor of the oral cavity and the anterior two-thirds of the tongue (except taste). Cutaneous branches innervate the skin of the lower lip and cheek (Fig. 2). In conducting an examination of the sensory function of the mandibular division, it is important to remember that the *skin covering the angle of the jaw is innervated by spinal nerve C$_2$.*

The trigeminal nerve provides sensory innervation for the *auricle (pinna)*, *tympanic membrane* and *external auditory canal*. Cutaneous branches of the mandibular division innervate the anterior aspect of the auricle (tragus) and external auditory canal, as well as the anterolateral (external) aspect of the tympanic

membrane. The posterior aspect of the external auditory canal and tympanic membrane and the adjoining part of the auricle (concha) are innervated by cutaneous branches of the facial and vagus nerves. The rim of the auricle (helix) and its posterior surface are innervated by spinal nerves C$_2$ and C$_3$.

The *dura mater* of the anterior and middle cranial fossae, including the superior aspect of the tentorium, receives sensory innervation from the intracranial branches of all three divisions of the trigeminal nerve. Branches of the vagus and upper three cervical spinal nerves provide sensory innervation to the dura of the posterior cranial fossa.

The *trigeminal motor root* innervates the following muscles of mastication: lateral and medial pterygoid, temporalis, masseter, mylohyoid, and the anterior belly of the digastric muscles. It also innervates the tensor veli palatini and tensor tympani. It is important to note that the facial and hypoglossal nerves innervate skeletal muscles of facial expression and the tongue, respectively.

The *trigeminal (gasserian* or *semilunar) ganglion* contains most of the primary sensory cell bodies associated with the sensory trigeminal nerve (Fig. 3). The unipolar sensory neurons vary in size. Unmyelinated axons originate from the small neurons, whereas larger neurons give rise to myelinated axons. Several subsets of neurons have been described based on their expressions of peptides such as substance P (SP), calcitonin gene-related peptide CGRP), galanin, and others (Fig. 4A,B). Approximately 50% of trigeminal ganglion neurons express CGRP and 17% express SP. CGRP and SP are co-expressed by some trigeminal neurons, thus providing three subsets of neurons based on their content of these peptides. For example, one subset expresses CGRP but not SP and another subset expresses SP but not CGRP. A third subset expresses both peptides; specifically, one-fourth of CGRP neurons also express SP and one-half of the SP neurons co-express CGRP (*see* Quartu et al., 1992). The physiological significance of these complex trigeminal neuron chemical phenotypes is not well-understood. Many studies have demonstrated that CGRP and SP satisfy neurotransmitter criteria. These peptides have been implicated in the propagation of nociceptive signaling, inflammatory responses, and other functions. Other primary sensory trigeminal neurons, associated with nonconscious proprioception, are located in the trigeminal mesencephalic nucleus in the pons (Figs. 3,5D).

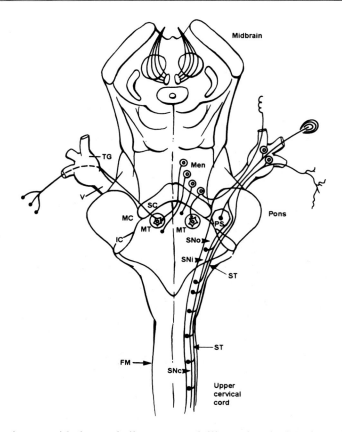

Fig. 3. Posterior view of the brainstem with the cerebellum removed, illustrating the locations of the major components of the trigeminal system. Motor components are represented on the left and sensory components on the right. The trigeminal ganglion (TG) has three divisions (*see* text). The central processes of some trigeminal neurons form the spinal tract of the trigeminal (ST), which lies just lateral to the spinal nucleus (SN) and passes inferiorly through the pons and medulla into the upper cervical spinal cord. FM, level of the foramen magnum; IC, inferior cerebellar peduncle; MC, middle cerebellar peduncle; Men, mesencephalic nucleus; MT, motor nucleus; PS, principal sensory nucleus; SC, superior cerebellar peduncle; SNc, spinal nucleus—subnucleus caudalis; SNi, spinal nucleus—subnucleus; interpolaris; SNo, spinal nucleus—subnucleus oralis; ST, spinal tract; TG, trigeminal ganglion; V, root of trigeminal nerve.

3. CENTRAL CONNECTIONS OF THE TRIGEMINAL SYSTEM

3.1. Spinal Trigeminal Tract in the Brainstem Consists of a Subset of Central Axons of Trigeminal Ganglion Primary Sensory Neurons

A large component of trigeminal sensory A-delta and C-fibers enter the pons with the trigeminal root and turn caudally, forming the *spinal tract of the trigeminal* (Figs. 3,5A,B). The spinal tract courses through the lateral tegmentum of the pons and medulla into the upper cervical cord, where it interdigitates with the dorsolateral fasciculus. Along its caudal course the spinal trigeminal-tract terminals synapse on neurons of the spinal trigeminal nucleus, which lies just medial to the tract throughout its course. These fibers carry nociceptive and mechanoreceptor stimuli from the face and oral cavity peripheral fields, including gingiva and tooth pulp. Many terminals, especially

Fig. 4. (*Opposite page*) Trigeminal ganglion neurons and spinal nucleus and tract of the trigeminal. Immunohistochemical demonstrations of markers for substance P (SP) (**A,C**) and calcitonin gene-related peptide (CGRP) (**B,D**) in human trigeminal ganglia neurons (**A and B**) and spinal tract of the trigeminal in the human medulla (**C,D**). (**A,B**) Note that a subset of small and medium-sized trigeminal neurons are intensely immunoreactive for SP (**A**) or CGRP (**B**) (*arrows*). Most large trigeminal neurons are immunonegative (*arrowheads*). Many SP- or CGRP-immunoreactive peripheral and central processes are evident in the background (×140). (**C,D**) Note that the central processes and terminals of the trigeminal primary afferent neurons, which form the spinal tract of the trigeminal in the medulla, are intensely immunoreactive for SP (**C**) or CGRP, (**D**) (*arrows*). The terminals

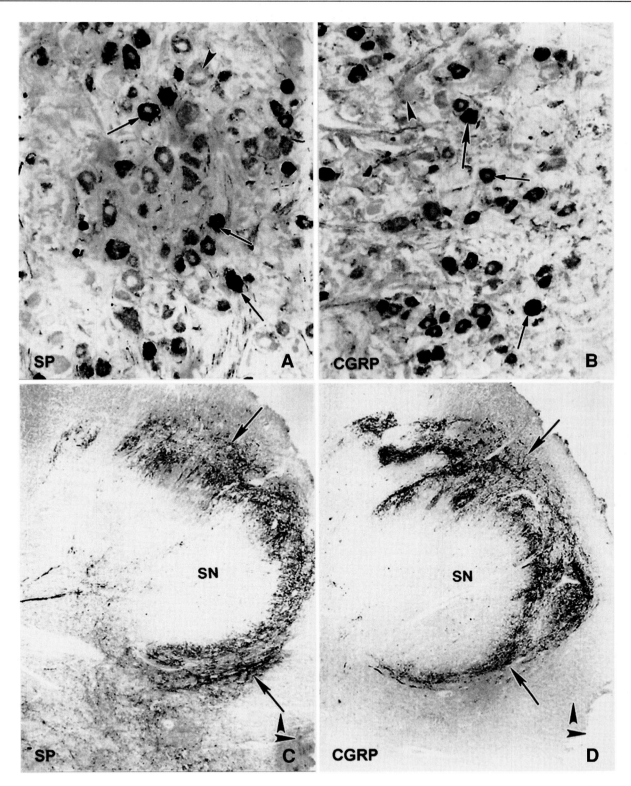

(**Fig. 4.** *Continued from opposite page*) of these primary afferent fibers will synapse on neurons of the spinal nucleus of the trigeminal (SN). The neurons of the SN do not contain SP or CGRP and are thus, immunonegative. The axons of the SN neurons will project to the thalamus as the trigeminothalamic tracts and to other targets (×25). (Illustrations of these preparations were provided by Professor Doctor Marina Del Fiacco, Anatomy, University of Cagliari, Monserrato, Italy. Her generosity is greatly appreciated [*see* Quartu, et al., 1992].)

those containing such peptides as substance P, CGRP, and other peptides associated with thermal and nociceptive transmission, terminate in the *subnucleus caudalis* of the spinal trigeminal nucleus (*see* Figs. 3, 4A,B,5A,B).

Primary sensory axons, which are distributed with peripheral branches of the facial, glossopharyngeal, and vagus nerves also join the spinal trigeminal tract and terminate in the spinal trigeminal nucleus. Sensory fibers following these cranial nerves provide sensory innervation of the skin of the external auditory canal, tympanic membrane, and mucosa of the middle ear cavity.

Axons in the spinal trigeminal tract maintain a precise arrangement in their descending course. The ipsilateral face and head are represented in an inverted orientation—those fibers originating from the ophthalmic division (upper face) are located most ventral in the tract; maxillary division axons are intermediate; and mandibular division axons, along with those from the facial, glossopharyngeal, and vagus nerves, are positioned dorsally in the tract.

Some axons entering with the trigeminal-root bifurcate sending synaptic terminals to spinal trigeminal and principal sensory trigeminal nuclei. These fibers are probably associated with mechanoreceptors and tactile sensations.

3.2. Trigeminal Nuclei Extend from Midbrain Through the Upper Levels of the Cervical Spinal Cord

The *spinal trigeminal nucleus* is the largest of the trigeminal nuclear components extending as a continuous column of neurons from mid-pons to the upper cervical spinal cord (Figs. 3,5A–C). It is composed mostly of small neurons, which receive primary sensory terminals from the spinal trigeminal tract (Fig. 4C,D). Three subnuclei are recognized: the *sub-nucleus oralis* (Fig. 5C), which is anatomically continuous with the principal sensory trigeminal nucleus (Fig. 5D); the *subnucleus interpolaris* (Fig. 5B) in the mid-medulla; and the *subnucleus caudalis* (Fig. 5A) in the caudal medulla, and which overlaps the substantia gelatinosa in the dorsal horn of the upper cervical spinal cord. The detailed cytomorphology, circuitry, and functions of the trigeminal spinal nucleus, especially the subnucleus caudalis, are very similar to those of the substantia gelatinosa in the dorsal horn of the cervical spinal cord.

The rostral portion of the spinal trigeminal nucleus—the subnucleus oralis (Figs. 3,5C)—receives stimuli originating predominantly in the nasal and oral cavities. The caudal component of the spinal trigeminal nuclear complex, the subnucleus caudalis (Figs. 3,5A), is functionally related primarily to nociception from the surface of the face. Specifically, axons innervating the skin around the mouth terminate in the more rostral region of the subnucleus caudalis and progressively more posterior parts of the face terminate on progressively more caudal portions of the nucleus (e.g., in the upper cervical cord). This anatomical arrangement explains the *onion-skin pattern* of sensory loss occasionally seen as a result of lesions that affect the caudal medulla and upper cervical spinal cord. For example, a tumor exerting pressure on dorsolateral aspect of the upper cervical cord may interrupt pain and thermal sensations from the posterior portions of the ipsilateral face, but may spare these sensations in the perioral region.

The *principal sensory trigeminal nucleus* (also known as the chief or superior sensory nucleus of the trigeminal or pontine trigeminal nucleus) receives most of its afferent input from Aβ primary sensory axons, which convey discriminative tactile sensations from the sensory fields innervated by all three trigeminal-nerve divisions (Figs. 3,5D). Other fibers serving

Fig. 5. (*Opposite page*) Axial sections of the human brainstem, demonstrating the components of the trigeminal system. Nerve fibers stain dark; areas containing mostly neuron-cell bodies are relatively unstained. *See* Chapter 11 for rostral-caudal orientation and more complete labeling of structures. (**A**) Medulla—Motor Decussation. ALt, anterolateral tracts; CSt, corticospinal tracts; FC, fasciculus cuneatus ; FG, fasciculus gracilis; MD, motor decussation; NC, nucleus cuneatus; NG, nucleus gracilis; SNc, spinal nucleus—subnucleus caudalis; ST, spinal tract; VTt, ventral trigeminothalamic tract. (**B**) Mid-Medulla. ALt, anterolateral tracts; CSt, corticospinal tracts; DMn, dorsal motor nucleus of vagus; Hn, hypoglossal nucleus; ICP, inferior cerebellar peduncle; IOn, inferior olivary nucleus; ML, medial lemniscus; SNi, spinal nucleus—interpolaris; ST, spinal tract; VTt ventral trigeminothalamic. tract. (**C**) Caudal Pons. An, abducens nucleus; CSt, corticospinal tracts; Fmn, facial motor nucleus; Fnr facial nerve root; MCP, middle cerebellar peduncle; ML, medial lemniscus; MLf, medial longitudinal fasciculus; SNo, spinal nucleus—oralis; ST, spinal tract; VTt, ventral trigeminothalamic tract; VCn, vestibulocochlear nerve. (**D**) Mid Pons. Alt, anterolateral tracts; CSt, corticospinal tracts; DTt, dorsal trigeminothalamic tract; LL, lateral lemniscus; MCP, middle cerebellar peduncle; ML, medial lemniscus; MLf, medial longitudinal fasciculus; Men, mesencephalic nucleus; Mnv, motor nucleus; PSnV, principal nucleus; SCP, superior cerebellar peduncle; VTt, ventral trigeminothalamic tact.

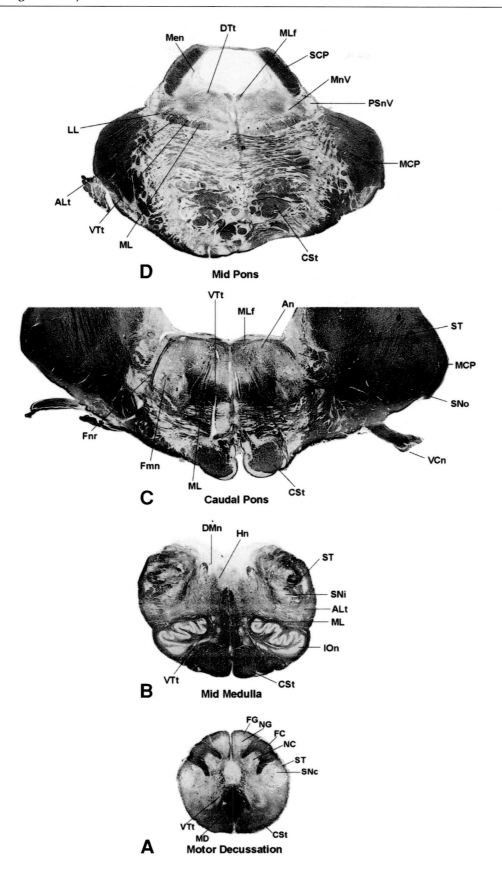

D Mid Pons

C Caudal Pons

B Mid Medulla

A Motor Decussation

general (crude) tactile sensations also terminate in the principal sensory nucleus. Anatomically, the principal sensory nucleus is continuous caudally, and overlaps to some extent, with the subnucleus oralis of the spinal trigeminal nucleus (Figs. 3,5C).

The separation of sensory modalities in the trigeminal system nuclei is not as sharp as once believed. Nevertheless, most neurons of the principal sensory trigeminal nucleus respond to mechanical stimuli in a manner that suggests perception of fine (discriminatory) tactile sensations. Moreover, at least some neurons in all sensory trigeminal nuclei respond when mechanical, thermal, or nociceptive stimuli are applied to their receptive fields. Nonetheless, certain nuclear subdivisions respond more prominently to a particular sensory modality. For example, tactile stimuli that correspond to light touch or deflection of hair on the skin activate neurons in the principal sensory trigeminal nucleus and in all subnuclei of the spinal trigeminal nucleus. Most neurons in the principal sensory nucleus and the spinal trigeminal subnucleus oralis are activated by stimuli applied to well-defined sensory fields and conveyed by large-diameter, well-myelinated primary sensory fibers associated with rapidly adapting mechanoreceptors and discriminatory tactile perception. Prominent internuncial connections between all trigeminal sensory nuclei have been revealed, indicating that complex integration of sensory modalities occurs in these structures.

The *trigeminal mesencephalic nucleus* extends from mid-pontine levels into the midbrain and lies just lateral to the periaqueductal gray (Figs. 3,5D; Chapter 11, Figs. 5B,C,6A). It consists of unipolar primary sensory neuron-cell bodies and is the only example of primary sensory neuron-cell bodies located in the central nervous system (CNS). The peripheral processes of these neurons are large-diameter, myelinated axons that form the *tract of the trigeminal mesencephalic nucleus* (Fig. 5D; Chapter 11, Figs. 5C, 6A) and terminate as pressure and stretch receptors from the orofacial musculature. The trigeminal mesencephalic nucleus provides bilateral proprioceptive input to the trigeminal motor nuclei, the surrounding RF and to other cranial-nerve motor nuclei for reflex functions. Other trigeminal mesencephalic neurons project proprioceptive information to the cerebellum by way of the superior cerebellar peduncle (Fig. 3; Chapter 2, Fig. 2). It should be noted that current evidence suggests that most proprioceptive stimuli originating from extra-ocular muscles are conveyed by primary sensory neurons with cell bodies in the trigeminal ganglion.

The *trigeminal motor nucleus* is a well-defined cluster of neurons located in the lateral tegmentum of the pons. It lies ventromedial to principal sensory trigeminal nucleus and extends from the level of the abducens nucleus caudally to the level of the superior colliculus rostrally (Figs. 3,5D). The trigeminal motor nucleus consists mostly of large and some small multipolar neurons. The larger neurons are the lower motor neurons for the skeletal muscles innervated by the trigeminal nerve, and participate in important reflexes and other responses. The smaller neurons are probably interneurons associated with trigeminal motor functions.

Cortical control (e.g., upper motor neurons) of skeletal muscles innervated by the trigeminal motor neurons (e.g., lower motor neurons) originates from the *face region of the precentral gyrus* (Chapter 2, Fig. 10) and other cortical motor areas. There are about equal ipsilateral and contralateral cortical projections (e.g., corticobulbar tracts) to the trigeminal motor nuclei and surrounding RF. Some corticobulbar-tract terminals directly innervate trigeminal motor neurons, yet most corticobulbar innervation is indirectly conducted through small internuncial neurons in the surrounding RF. Inputs to the motor trigeminal nuclei from the tri-geminal mesencephalic nuclei are direct and probably form the sensory limb of the *jaw-jerk reflex* (Fig. 3).

Diffuse connections from the hypothalamus and other limbic structures through the RF activate the trigeminal motor nuclei, along with other cranial-nerve motor nuclei, to produce facial expressions in response to emotion. Orofacial reflex activities, such as chewing, swallowing, and speaking, also involve the trigeminal system and other cranial nerves. The functions of these structures are integrated through the RF, and other integrating axons may follow the *medial longitudinal fasciculus* (Fig. 5C,D).

4. ASCENDING TRIGEMINAL-SYSTEM PATHWAYS

The *principal sensory trigeminal nucleus* neurons convey tactile and mechanical information via axons that join the contralateral medial lemniscus and ascend to the *ventral posteromedial nucleus* of the dorsal thalamus. Some axons form an ipsilateral ascending pathway located in the dorsal tegmentum. These bundles of axons are the *ventral* and *dorsal trigeminothalamic tracts*, respectively (Figs. 5,6). The related thalamocortical axons project, by way of the *posterior limb of the internal capsule*, to the *face region of the postcentral gyrus* (Chapter 2, Fig. 10) and other cortical areas. The cortical projections provide for the conscious appreciation of the character and precise location of tactile and proprioceptive sensations originating in the trigeminal sensory field.

Axons from the *spinal trigeminal nucleus*, especially the *subnucleus caudalis* (Figs. 3,5A) and surrounding RF, form the ventral trigeminothalamic tract, which transmits pain, thermal, and some general tactile (light touch) sensations to the contralateral thalamus. Thalamocortical projections subsequently relay these sensations to the *face region of the postcentral gyrus* (Fig. 6; Chapter 2, Fig. 10). These axons cross the midline through the upper cervical cord and tegmentum of the medulla, join the medial lemniscus and spinothalamic tracts in the pons, and terminate in the *ventral posteromedial thalamic nucleus* (Figs. 5D,6). It should be noted that all sensory modalities, including taste, are integrated first in the ventral posteriomedial nucleus of the thalamus before projection to the postcentral gyrus.

5. FUNCTIONS AND MALFUNCTIONS OF THE TRIGEMINAL SYSTEM

5.1. Nociception in the Trigeminal System Involves the Spinal Trigeminal Nucleus and the Surrounding Neurons of the RF

The spinal trigeminal nucleus, specifically the subnucleus caudalis, provides integration and relay of nociceptive stimuli from the face and oral structures to the cerebral cortex for conscious appreciation. Nociceptive stimuli are also relayed through the RF and the thalamus to limbic-system structures in the cerebral hemispheres (Chapter 12, Fig. 4). These connections are believed to evoke the disagreeable characteristics of pain. Other RF circuits activate neurons in the raphe nuclei (Chapter 11, Figs. 4C,D,5), which project serotonergic terminals to the enkephalinergic interneurons in the spinal trigeminal nucleus. This circuit modulates pain transmission from trigeminal sensory fields.

5.2. Trigeminal Peripheral Sensory and Motor Distributions Have Important Functional and Diagnostic Implications

Several aspects of the peripheral trigeminal sensory distribution deserve further emphasis. As illustrated in Fig. 2, branches of the ophthalmic division innervate the forehead, anterior scalp, upper eyelid, bridge of the nose, and cornea. Branches of the maxillary division innervate the upper lip, alar region of the nose, most of the cheek, and the lower eyelid. The mandibular divi-

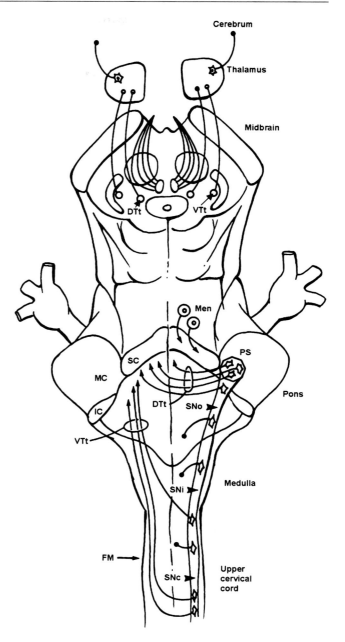

Fig. 6. Posterior view of the brainstem with the cerebellum removed, illustrating the major ascending pathways of the trigeminal system. DTT, dorsal trigeminothalamic tract; FM, level of the foramen magnum; IC, inferior cerebellar peduncle; MC, middle cerebellar peduncle; Men, mesencephalic nucleus; PS, principal sensory nucleus; SC, superior cerebellar peduncle; SNc, spinal nucleus—subnucleus caudalis; SNi, spinal nucleus—subnucleus interpolaris; SNo, spinal nucleus—subnucleus oralis; VTt, ventral trigeminothalamic tract.

sion innervates the lower lip chin and mandibular region. However, branches of spinal nerves C_2 and C_3 innervate the skin of the angle of the jaw, the posterior scalp, and the neck.

The boundaries of the sensory regions innervated by each division of the trigeminal nerve on the face and scalp are sharp, and display little overlap with one another or across the midline. In contrast, there is considerable overlap in the sensory regions (dermatome patterns) innervated by the spinal nerves on the body surface.

A discussion of the etiologies of headache is beyond the scope of this chapter, but it is important to remember that most of the meninges, falx and tentorium receive sensory innervation from the trigeminal system. In addition, trigeminal sensory nerves also innervate the major intracranial blood vessels. Intracranial lesions could evoke pain by exerting tension on or displacing these structures. However, the pain perceived by the patient is often not an accurate reflection of the anatomical location or size of the lesion.

Axons that form the root and main divisions of the trigeminal nerve follow a course partly in the posterior and middle cranial fossae and thus could be affected by lesions in either of these anatomical compartments (Fig. 1; Chapter 2, Fig. 4).

Corneal (blink) response is frequently used to test the integrity of the peripheral components of the trigeminal and facial nerves and their internuncial brainstem connections. The examiner touches the cornea with a wisp of cotton; the normal response is that both eyes blink. The *afferent limb of the corneal response* consists of the primary sensory axons in the ipsilateral ophthalmic division, which terminate on the sensory trigeminal nuclei that serve tactile sensations. Secondary axons arising from the sensory trigeminal nuclei project to both the ipsi- and contralateral facial motor nuclei in the caudal pons (Fig. 5C). Axons originating from the facial motor nuclei follow the facial nerves and innervate the respective orbicularis oculi muscles providing the *efferent limb of the corneal response*. As a result, touching one cornea normally evokes both direct (in the ipsilateral eye) and consensual or indirect (in the contralateral eye) responses.

Lesions that affect the ophthalmic division or the trigeminal root result in no (or diminished) direct and consensual responses if the ipsilateral cornea is touched. However, if the contralateral cornea is touched, both eyes blink because of the bilateral input to the facial motor nuclei.

The corneal responses are also altered in patients with facial-motor nucleus or facial-nerve lesions. Thus, touching the cornea evokes no direct blink response if the ipsilateral facial nucleus or nerve is lesioned, but the contralateral eye does respond. However, touching the contralateral cornea activates a direct but not a consensual response.

Other trigeminal sensory reflexes are activated by sensory trigeminal nuclei through the RF and other pathways. Through these circuits, brainstem and spinal nuclei that regulate emesis, lacrimation, swallowing, and other responses are influenced by the trigeminal system (Fig. 6).

The *masseter* or *jaw-jerk reflex* is activated by depressing the mandible or tapping the chin resulting in bilateral contraction of the masseter and temporalis muscles. The response is dependent on proprioceptive input to the trigeminal mesencephalic nuclei and direct activation of the trigeminal motor nuclei (Fig. 3).

5.3. Trigeminal-System Components Can Be Involved in a Number of Neurological Conditions

Skull fractures involving the petrous portion of the temporal bone may damage the trigeminal root as it passes from the posterior cranial fossa to the middle cranial fossae (Fig. 1; Chapter 2, Fig. 4). In this case, all sensory modalities, except taste, would be lost on the ipsilateral face. In addition, opening the mouth would result in deviation of the jaw toward the side of the lesion because of a lower motor-neuron paralysis of the ipsilateral muscles of mastication—specifically, the lateral pterygoid muscle. It is important to remember that axons originating from neurons in the facial (Chapter 11, Fig. 5A) and hypoglossal (Chapter 11, Fig. 4C) nuclei innervate muscles of facial expression and the tongue, respectively, and would not be affected.

A fracture traversing the foramen ovale on the floor of the middle cranial fossa (Chapter 2, Fig. 4) could damage the mandibular division and its motor component, but would spare ophthalmic- and maxillary-division functions. This could result in diminished cutaneous sensations of the ipsilateral lower lip, chin, and jaw region, as well as a lower motor-neuron paralysis of the ipsilateral muscles of mastication.

Space-occupying lesions (such as tumors and aneurysms) in the posterior or middle cranial fossae could exert pressure on the trigeminal-nerve root (Fig. 1; Chapter 2, Fig. 4) or its divisions, and alter functions on the ipsilateral face. Tumors in the posterior cranial fossa (e.g., acoustic neurinoma or cerebellopontine angle tumor) may exert pressure on the lateral aspect of the brainstem, and thus on the spinal trigeminal tract and nucleus (Chapter 11, Fig. 1). Pain and thermal sensations from the ipsilateral face could be altered (either diminished or exacerbated), but tactile sensations—most of which relay in the principal sensory trigeminal nucleus—would be spared (Fig. 3). The tumor could also influence the functions of the ipsilateral spinothalamic tracts, inferior cerebellar peduncle, facial, vestibulocochlear, glossopharyngeal, and/or vagus nerves (Chapter 11, Fig. 4C). Alternately, a tumor could exert pressure on the trigeminal root (Fig. 1; Chapter 11, Fig. 1). In fact, an early sign of this type of tumor is decreased sensitivity of the ipsilateral cornea resulting in an asymmetric corneal response.

Trigeminal neuralgia (tic douloureux) is characterized by sudden onset of excruciating pain, lasting for a period of seconds to minutes. It does not respond to common pharmacological methods of pain control. The pain is often triggered by tactile stimulation of a particular location, or trigger zone, on the face. The trigger zone is usually in the perioral region or oral cavity. Jaw movements or food in the mouth may evoke bursts of pain. The pain is restricted to the territory of one division of the trigeminal nerve—usually the maxillary, rarely the ophthalmic (Fig. 2). Episodes of pain usually become more frequent and present a progressively debilitating condition for the patient. Some pharmacological therapies are helpful, but surgical treatment is usually required for relief. Surgical treatment options include various methods for placing a small lesion in the portion of the trigeminal ganglion that contains the primary sensory neurons innervating the affected region of the face. The lesions are produced by injection of alcohol or coagulation. One approach for injection of the trigeminal ganglion is by way of the foramen ovale, obviating the need for a major neurosurgical procedure. Recently, focused gamma radiation ("gamma knife") has been used to "lesion" the root of the trigeminal nerve where it enters the pons. In some of these procedures the neurons that convey pain are more susceptible to the destructive treatment than the tactile neurons, therefore some tactile sensations on the affected portion of the face are spared. Transection of the spinal trigeminal tract in the caudal medulla is a neurosurgical procedure that is now rarely used to treat patients with trigeminal neuralgia.

Pseudobulbar palsy is caused by brainstem vascular lesions that interrupt the corticobulbar tracts (e.g., upper motor neurons) that innervate cranial nerve somatic motor nuclei, including the motor trigeminal

nucleus. The resulting weakness (paresis) of skeletal muscles innervated by cranial nerves interferes with ocular, facial, jaw and tongue movements.

Posterior inferior cerebellar artery (PICA) *syndrome* (lateral medullary syndrome, Wallenberg's syndrome) is a cerebrovascular accident involving the intrinsic vasculature supplying the lateral aspect of the medulla (Fig. 5B). It can result in the destruction of several neural structures in the lateral medulla, leading to the dysfunctions characteristic of this syndrome. Specific to the trigeminal system, the disruption of blood supply to the spinal trigeminal nucleus and tract results in an ipsilateral loss of pain and thermal sensations in the face, but tactile sensations and trigeminal motor function, which depend on the principal sensory trigeminal and trigeminal motor nuclei in the pons, are unaffected (Fig. 5).

ACKNOWLEDGMENTS

The invaluable assistance of Ms. Mary Gail Engle and Dr. Bruce Maley, University of Kentucky, in the preparation of illustrations for this chapter is greatly appreciated.

Dr. Marina Del Fiacco, University of Cagliari, Monserrato, Italy provided the illustrations of immunohistochemical preparations for SP and CGRP in the human trigeminal system (Fig. 6). Her generosity is greatly appreciated.

The Weigert-stained sections of human brainstem were photographed from the Yakovlev Collection, housed at the Armed Forces Institute of Pathology, Washington, DC.

SELECTED READINGS

Bowsher D. Trigeminal Neuralgia: An anatomically oriented review. Clinical Anatomy 1997; 10:409–419.

Edvinsson L, Cantera L, Jansen-Olesen I, Uddman R. Expression of CGRP receptor mRNA in human trigeminal ganglion and cerebral vessels. Neurosci Letters 1997; 229: 209–211.

Brodal A. Cranial Nerves—"The Trigeminal Nerve." In Neurological Anatomy in Relation to Clinical Medicine, 3rd ed. New York:Oxford University Press, 1981; 508–532.

Esser MJ, Pronych SP, Vallen G. Trigeminal-reticular connections: nociception-induced cardiovascular reflex responses in the rat. J Compar Neurol 1998; 391:526–544.

Gundmundsson K, Rhoton AL, Rushton JG. Detailed anatomy of the intracranial portion of the trigeminal nerve. J Neurosurg 1971; 35:592–600.

Hassanali J. Quantative and somatotopic mappings of neurones in trigeminal mesencephalic nucleus and ganglion innervating teeth in monkey and baboon. Arch Oral Biol 1997; 42: 673–682.

May A, Goadsby PJ. The trigeminovascular system in humans: Pathophysiologic implications for primary headache syndromes and the neural influences on cerebral circulation. J Cerebral Blood Flow Metabol 1999; 19:115–127.

Miles JB, Eldridge PR, Haggett CE, Bowsher D. Sensory effects of microvascular decompensation in trigeminal neuralgia. J Neurosurg 1997; 86:193–197.

Paxinos G, Törk I, Halliday G, Mehler WR. "Human homologs to brainstem nuclei identified in other animals as revealed by acetylcholinesterase activity". In Paxinos G (ed). The Human Nervous System. New York:Academic Press Inc. 1990; 149–202.

Quartu M, Diaz G, Floris A, Lai ML, Priestly JV, DelFiacco M. CGRP in the huma trigeminal sensory system at developmental and adult life stages: immunohistochemistry, neuronal morphometrics and coexistence with SP. J Chem Neuroanat 1992; 5:143–157.

Sessle B. "Physiology of the trigeminal system," In Fromm GH, Sessle BJ (eds). Trigeminal Neuralgia: Current Concepts Regarding Pathogenesis and Treatment, Boston: Butterworth-Heinemann, 1991; 71–104.

Sugimoto T., Yi-Fen HE, Funahashi M, Schikawa H. Induction of immediate-early genes c-fos and Zif268 in subnucleus oralis by noxious tooth pulp stimulation. Brain Res 1998; 794:353–358.

14 The Oculomotor System

Robert F. Spencer* and John D. Porter

1. INTRODUCTION

The oculomotor system has the dual tasks of maintaining stability of eye position and directing eye movements toward novel features of our environment. This system operates under very fine tolerances. The fovea, the region of highest visual acuity on the retina, "sees" only an area about the size of a quarter held at arm length. Thus, the eyes must be precisely directed toward an object of interest and held in that position for precise and clear vision. Drift of the eyes produces blurred vision, and misalignment of both eyes (strabismus) causes double vision, or diplopia.

The oculomotor system is known as the efferent limb for the visual system and vestibular system, but

*Deceased.

From: *Neuroscience in Medicine, 2nd ed.* (P. Michael Conn, ed.),
© 2003 Humana Press Inc., Totowa, NJ.

it is important to remember that eye movements are also directed by the senses of hearing or touch. The five distinct eye movement systems described in this chapter are responsible for maintaining stability of eye position and directing the eyes to new targets. The extra-ocular muscles mediate all movements of the eyes, and are characteristic to all of the eye-movement systems. These muscles are controlled by precise connections with several brainstem structures that are related to eye movements in the vertical and horizontal planes. Extra-ocular muscle-fiber types and their elegant organization in the extra-ocular muscles are unmatched by any of the skeletal muscles that are controlled by spinal cord motor systems. Because the premotor structures that control eye movements also have connections with motor neurons in the cervical spinal cord that innervate muscles of the neck, the motor behavior produced by these structures is known as gaze. Gaze is a combination of coordinated eye and head movements, and is the result of a complex interaction between the visual and vestibular systems that allows us to see clearly and precisely.

The mechanisms related to eye movements and gaze can best be appreciated by understanding the brainstem, cerebellar, and cortical connections of the pre-oculomotor structures. It is sometimes clinically possible to separate the various visual and vestibular components so that lesions in different portions of the cerebral cortex, the brainstem, and the cerebellum produce specific eye movements, or gaze deficits. This chapter will link the neuroanatomical pathways to the five types of eye-movements, and illustrate the consequences of lesions at various points in eye-movement control pathways.

2. TYPES OF EYE MOVEMENTS

Eye movements are classified into five categories: vestibular, optokinetic, smooth pursuit, saccadic, and vergence. Of these, the vestibular, optokinetic, smooth pursuit, and saccadic eye movements are *conjugate movements*, in which both eyes move in the same direction at the same time. Conjugate eye-movement types share some components of the brainstem neural circuitry. Vergence eye movements are *disjunctive movements*, in which the eyes move in opposite directions at the same time. This is achieved by using very different neural control mechanisms than those used for conjugate eye movements. Vergence and conjugate eye-movement systems overlap only in their sharing of the same motor neurons and extra-ocular muscles.

Movements of the head that activate the semicircular canals elicit *vestibular eye movements*. The *vestibulo–ocular reflex* (VOR) is a compensatory eye movement that replicates a head movement, but in the opposite direction. The function of the VOR is to maintain the stability of the visual field while the head moves. For example, rotation of the head to the right produces a compensatory conjugate eye movement to the left so that images in the visual field remain stationary on the retina. To understand the interaction of the VOR and vision, hold your thumb out in front and turn both head and arm while maintaining focus on your thumb. Note that your thumb stays in focus while the rest of the world is blurred as you *cancel* the VOR. If you did not have a VOR, any movement of the head would cause

blurring of vision in the same way that moving a camera blurs the image on the film. The VOR works best for brief or rapid movements of the head, as the semicircular canals are best at detecting these types of movements.

Optokinetic eye movements are tracking movements elicited by movement of the entire visual field, such as occurs while looking out of the window of a moving train. The *optokinetic reflex* is the smooth eye movement that tracks a moving stimulus. *Optokinetic nystagmus* (OKN) is characterized by a slow-phase eye movement in the direction of a moving stimulus and a quick-phase return eye movement in the opposite direction when the excursion limit of the oculomotor range has been reached. The optokinetic system works synergistically with the vestibular system to stabilize images in the visual field on the retina during movements of the head. The optokinetic reflex effectively compensates for those types of head movements that are not detected well by the vestibular apparatus—sustained or slow movements of the head.

Smooth-pursuit eye movements track images that move across the visual field. These movements maintain the focus of moving targets in the visual field on the fovea of the retina. Smooth-pursuit eye movements that are accompanied by movement of the head in the same direction require suppression or *cancellation* of the VOR.

Saccadic eye movements are typically rapid scanning movements that change foveal fixation from one point in the central visual field to another point in the periphery. Saccades are used as you skip from word to word in reading this book or in scanning a picture, but also replace or augment smooth pursuit when an image moves too rapidly across the visual field. Intentional saccades, such as those made to a remembered target, are differentiated from reflexive saccades, which are made in response to a novel object that appears in the peripheral visual field.

Vergence eye movements are associated with changing the point of foveal fixation from a distant object to a near object. Vergence movements are disjunctive, because they are produced by contraction of the medial rectus muscles in both eyes. Vergence eye movements also are associated with changes in the shape of the lens of the eye (e.g., accommodation) and constriction of the pupil (e.g., miosis) as a part of the process is known as the near triad or near response.

3. EXTRA-OCULAR MUSCLES

Regardless of the category of eye movement, all changes in eye position result from coordinated contraction and relaxation of extra-ocular muscles. There are six extra-ocular muscles responsible for eye movements: the superior rectus, lateral rectus, medial rectus, inferior rectus, superior oblique, and inferior oblique muscles. The superior and inferior recti are the primary elevators and depressors of the eye, respectively. The lateral rectus abducts and the medial rectus adducts the eye. Actions of the oblique muscles are more complex, but the superior oblique is the primary intorter (inward rotation of the eye) and the inferior rectus is the primary extorter (outward rotation). Damage to individual extra-ocular muscles, or to one of the three cranial nerves involved in eye movement, is easily detected by routine ophthalmic examination. Upward deviations of the eyes are known as hypertropias, and downward deviations—hypotropias, and lateral deviations—are known as exotropias. Medial deviations are known as esotropias. An additional extra-ocular muscle, the levator palpebrae superioris, elevates the upper eyelid. Damage to the levator muscle or its nerve results in drooping of the eyelid, or ptosis.

4. EXTRA-OCULAR MOTOR NUCLEI

Motor neurons in the extra-ocular motor nuclei (e.g., cranial nerves III, IV, and VI) are the final common pathway on which inputs converge from several brainstem premotor structures that are related to the control of different types of eye movements. The cranial nerves with which these motor neurons are associated provide *general somatic efferent* innervation of the extra-ocular muscles.

4.1. The Oculomotor Complex Contains Somatic and Visceral Motor Neurons

The somatic division of the oculomotor complex (e.g., cranial nerve III) contains motor neurons that innervate the ipsilateral medial rectus, inferior rectus, and inferior oblique muscles and innervate the superior rectus and levator palpebrae superioris muscles bilaterally with contralateral predominance. Axons of the superior rectus and levator palpebrae superioris decussate in the vicinity of the oculomotor nucleus before coursing ventral to exit the brainstem with the remainder of the third cra-

nial nerve. The oculomotor nerve then exits the brainstem from the ventral surface of the mesencephalon, through the interpeduncular fossa. At this location, the nerve passes between the superior cerebellar and posterior cerebral arteries, a clinically important anatomic configuration. Note the difference between oculomotor nucleus lesions, which would affect eye movements bilaterally, and oculomotor nerve lesions, which affect only the ipsilateral eye.

The motor neurons that innervate different muscles are arranged in a precise topographic organization within the oculomotor nucleus. The medial rectus and inferior rectus motor neurons are in close proximity to each other, and the superior rectus and levator palpebrae superioris motor neurons occupy adjacent subdivisions. Inferior oblique motor neurons are located in the vicinity of superior rectus motor neurons. This arrangement is largely a reflection of the synergistic actions of the muscles and the common inputs of the different populations of motor neurons. Levator palpebrae superioris motor neurons are considered to occupy the *caudal central nucleus* subdivision of the oculomotor complex.

In addition to motor neurons, the somatic oculomotor nucleus and the overlying supraoculomotor region contain *internuclear neurons* which have descending brainstem connections with abducens nucleus and facial nucleus. At least some of the internuclear neurons are contacted by motor neuron axon collaterals, and may be involved in the coordinated activity of extra-ocular and facial muscles, which can occur during blinking.

The *anteromedian, Edinger-Westphal nuclei* are a collection of midline *preganglionic parasympathetic neurons* that overlie the rostral portion of the somatic oculomotor nucleus and curve ventrally rostral to the somatic nucleus. An additional population of autonomic neurons lies along the midline, between the somatic portions of the oculomotor nucleus. The *general visceral efferent* axons of these neurons course via the third cranial nerve to synapse in the ciliary ganglion, with postganglionic fibers distributed primarily to the sphincter pupillae muscle of the iris and ciliary body. The postganglionic fibers that innervate the sphincter pupillary muscles are related to the *pupillary light reflex*, and those that innervate the ciliary body control lens accommodation. Both autonomic and somatic divisions of the oculomotor nucleus function together in the viewing of near objects—the *near triad*, consisting of convergence, accommodation, and pupillary constriction. Another population of coexistent neurons located in the same region projects to the upper thoracic spinal cord (the site of preganglionic sympathetic neurons for the head and neck), and may be involved in the coordination of parasympathetic-constriction and sympathetic-dilation control of pupillary function.

The combination of somatic and parasympathetic components in the third cranial nerve forms the basis for characteristic deficits that are associated with a third-nerve palsy. The loss of parasympathetic innervation is manifested by pupillary dilatation (e.g., mydriasis), with a complete loss of the direct and consensual light reflexes for the affected eye, and anisocoria. Damage to the somatic portion of the oculomotor nerve produces an abnormal deviation of the eye, or strabismus. In the resting position, the apparent motility deficits are manifested as exotropia (e.g., external strabismus caused by an unopposed lateral rectus) and ptosis (e.g., drooping eyelid). The loss of inervation to the vertical eye muscles becomes apparent only when the patient is asked to move the eyes upward or downward. Routine ophthalmic examinations test movements of the eyes in each direction, starting from different positions of gaze, and can precisely diagnose the site of brainstem or nerve lesions.

4.2. The Trochlear Nucleus Innervates the Contralateral Superior Oblique Muscle

The trochlear nucleus (e.g., cranial nerve IV) contains motor neurons that predominantly innervate the contralateral superior oblique muscle, but approx 10% of the motor neurons innervate the ipsilateral muscle. The axons exit the dorsomedial portion of the nucleus, course around the medial longitudinal fasciculus and periaqueductal gray, decussate in the anterior medullary velum, and exit the dorsal surface of the brainstem immediately caudal to the inferior colliculus. The trochlear nerve is the only one of the cranial nerves to exit from the dorsal surface of the brainstem. The small size of the fourth cranial nerve and its anatomic relationship to the tentorium cerbelli make it especially vulnerable clinically in trauma. Lesions of the fourth nerve (e.g., fourth-nerve palsy) are associated with an overacting inferior oblique muscle, which usually is manifested only if the lesion is bilateral (a

V-shaped pattern is seen—the eyes move together when looking down and apart when looking up).

4.3. The Abducens Nucleus Is the Center for Conjugate Horizontal Eye Movement

The abducens nucleus is composed of both motor neurons and interneurons that collectively participate in conjugate horizontal movements of the eyes (Fig. 1). Approximately 70% of the neurons of the abducens nucleus (e.g., cranial nerve VI) are abducens motor neurons that innervate the ipsilateral lateral rectus muscle. Their axons exit the ventral surface of the brainstem at the pontomedullary junction, just lateral to the pyramids as they emerge from the basilar pons. The sixth-cranial nerve has the longest intracranial course of any of the cranial nerves, and because of its size, it is clinically vulnerable (e.g., sixth-nerve palsy, which produces an exotropia), especially in the regions where it courses ventral to the basilar pons and where it traverses the petrous portion of the temporal bone.

The remaining 30% of neurons in the abducens nucleus are abducens internuclear neurons, whose axons cross the midline at the level of the abducens nucleus, ascend in the contralateral medial longitudinal fasciculus (MLF), and establish extensive excitatory synaptic connections with medial rectus motor neurons in the contralateral oculomotor nucleus. The abducens nucleus is known as the *center for conjugate horizontal eye movement*, because it controls the ipsilateral lateral rectus muscle directly and the contralateral medial rectus muscle indirectly. This arrangement allows the abducens nucleus to elicit co-contraction of the lateral rectus muscle on the ipsilateral side and the medial rectus on the contralateral side, resulting in movement of both eyes in the ipsilateral direction.

Lesions of the abducens nucleus and the abducens nerve produce markedly different deficits in ocular motility (Fig. 1). Because the abducens nucleus contains both motor neurons and internuclear neurons, a lesion involving the nucleus produces paralysis of conjugate horizontal eye movements toward the side of lesion (lesion 3 in Fig. 1). Lesions of the sixth nerve are manifested by esotropia (e.g., internal strabismus caused by unopposed medial rectus) at rest and a paralysis of ipsilateral attempted abduction (lesion 1 in Fig. 1). Lesions of the MLF cause the syndrome of *internuclear oph-*

Control of Conjugate Horizontal Gaze

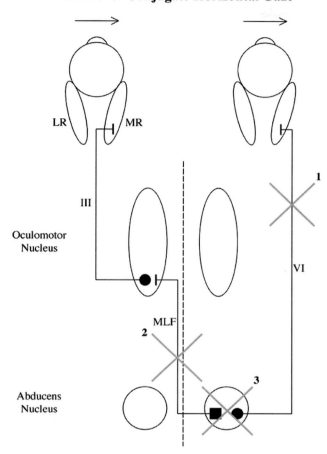

Fig. 1. The organization of conjugate horizontal eye movements. Medial and lateral rectus motor neurons (*filled circles*) are shown projecting through cranial nerves III and VI, respectively, to innervate the medial (MR) and lateral rectus (LR) muscles. Abducens internuclear neurons (*filled square*) send their axons across the midline and up the MLF to target contralateral medial rectus motor neurons. In this way, conjugate horizontal signals are sent equally to abducens motor neurons and abducens internuclear neurons, which then relay the signals faithfully to contralateral medial rectus motor neurons. Thus, activation of the ipsilateral abducens nucleus causes abduction of the ipsilateral eye and adduction of the contralateral eye. Because of the organization of horizontal gaze, there are differing consequences of abducens nerve (**1**), MLF (**2**), and abducens nucleus (**2**) lesions (*see* Section 4.3.).

thalmoplegia, resulting in loss of adduction (medial rectus activation) during conjugate movements of the eyes (lesion 2 in Fig. 1). Internuclear ophthalmoplegia is not a rare occurrence, frequently resulting from a stroke or multiple sclerosis. A more complete explanation of internuclear ophthalmoplegia appears in Section 5.1.

5. PRE-OCULOMOTOR NUCLEI

Four brainstem premotor areas are individually significant for the control of eye movement and gaze in the vertical and horizontal planes. These structures have direct, monosynaptic connections with motor neurons in the extra-ocular motor nuclei.

5.1. The Vestibular Nuclei Control the Vestibulo–Ocular Reflex

The VOR originates from the semicircular canals in the ear (*see* Chapter 25). In its simplest form, this reflex is mediated by, an arc of three neurons—primary vestibular neuron to secondary vestibular neuron to eye-movement motor neuron. The superior vestibular nucleus and rostral portions of the medial and inferior vestibular nuclei receive afferents from semicircular canal-related primary vestibular axons and centrally from the flocculus and fastigial nuclei of the cerebellum. Canal-specific efferent projections of the second-order vestibular neurons target motor neurons in the extra-ocular motor nuclei, thereby providing the basis for the VOR. Each semicircular canal is related to two pairs of muscles in each eye through reciprocal excitatory and inhibitory synaptic connections with the extra-ocular motor neurons. The basis of this interaction is explained by the relationship of the spatial orientation of the semicircular canals with the pulling actions of the extra-ocular muscles.

Axons from second-order anterior and posterior canal-related superior vestibular neurons ascend the ipsilateral MLF and are inhibitory to all vertical motor neurons in the oculomotor and trochlear—nuclei (Fig. 2). Axons from second-order anterior canal-related neurons in the superior vestibular nucleus and from posterior canal-related neurons in the medial and inferior vestibular nuclei ascend the contralateral MLF and are excitatory to all vertical motor neurons in the oculomotor and trochlear nuclei. Horizontal canal-related medial or inferior vestibular neurons are excitatory to contralateral abducens neurons (both motor neurons and internuclear neurons) and inhibitory to ipsilateral abducens neurons. Medial rectus motor neurons in the oculomotor nucleus receive the majority of their vestibular inputs via the MLF. However, the medial

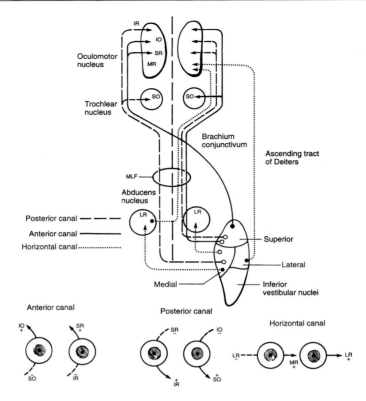

Fig. 2. The vestibulo–ocular pathways that relate each of the semicircular canals to the activation of specific pairs of extra-ocular muscles. Excitatory neurons are indicated by filled circles; inhibitory neurons are indicated by open circles. Excitatory fibers ascend contralateral to their cells of origin, and inhibitory fibers ascend ipsilateral to their cells of origin. The actions of extra-ocular muscles influenced by activation of the individual canals are indicated at the bottom of the drawing.

rectus motor neurons also receive a small direct ipsilateral excitatory input from neurons located in the ventral portion of the lateral vestibular nucleus, whose axons ascend via the ascending tract of Deiters, which is lateral to the MLF.

The basic three-neuron reflex arc (e.g., first-order vestibular ganglion neuron→second-order vestibular nucleus neuron→extra-ocular motor neuron) is necessary but insufficient for the normal functional operation of the VOR. When a compensatory eye movement is made in response to rotation of the head, the head velocity signals of vestibular neurons are incapable of maintaining gaze in the new position. The prepositus hypoglossi nucleus, which is located in the periventricular dorsal aspect of the medulla extending from the rostral pole of the hypoglossal nucleus to the abducens nucleus, plays a fundamentally important role in gaze holding (Fig. 3). The prepositus hypoglossi nucleus has extensive reciprocal connections with the vestibular nuclei, and is regarded as the *neural integrator* responsible for converting the head velocity signals of vestibular neurons to eye-position signals that

are carried by extra-ocular motor neurons. Damage to the prepositus hypoglossi nucleus interferes with integrator function, making it difficult to maintain gaze positions. Consistent with its function related primarily to horizontal eye movements, the excitatory and inhibitory connections of prepositus hypoglossi neurons are directed predominantly to the abducens nucleus. A similar neural integrator function has been postulated for the neurons in the interstitial nucleus of Cajal, in the rostral midbrain, which controls vertical gaze.

Lesions of the vestibular nerve or nuclei and of the MLF produce quite different deficits. Vestibular nerve or nucleus lesions are characterized by spontaneous nystagmus, an enhanced vertical nystagmus induced by caloric stimulation of the contralateral ear, and positional nystagmus. These deficits underscore the importance of balanced inputs from the semicircular canals and otolith organs on both sides. However, deficits associated with peripheral lesions are only transient because of compensation mediated by commissural connections between the vestibular nuclei on each side.

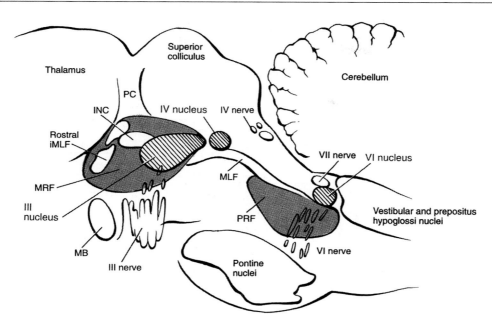

Fig. 3. A midsaggital view of the brainstem, indicating the locations of premotor neurons that are related to the control of gaze. The mesencephalic reticular formation (MRF) rostral to the oculomotor (III) nucleus contains the interstitial nucleus of Cajal (INC) and the rostral interstitial nucleus of the medial longitudinal fasciculus (rostral iMLF); both of these are related to the control of vertical upward and downward gaze. The paramedian pontine reticular formation (PRF) rostral and ventral to the abducens (VI) nucleus contains neurons that are related to the control of horizontal gaze. MB, mamillary body.

Lesions of the MLF in the pons and caudal midbrain, as noted previously, are responsible for the clinical syndrome of *internuclear ophthalmoplegia* (*see* Fig. 1). This syndrome is characterized by paralysis of ipsilateral adduction on attempted conjugate horizontal eye movements to the opposite side and nystagmus in the abducted eye, but the preservation of vergence eye movements. In this case, the motor nerve innervation of the medial rectus and lateral rectus muscles is intact and muscle function is normal, but the axons of abducens internuclear neurons have been disrupted, and signals related to conjugate horizontal eye movements are not relayed to the oculomotor nucleus. Vergence eye movements are unaffected, because the premotor neurons and motor neurons that are responsible for these movements are located in the midbrain, rostral to the lesion.

5.2. The Mesencephalic Reticular Formation Controls Vertical Gaze

The region of the mesencephalic reticular formation in the vicinity of the oculomotor complex contains two structures that are intimately related to the control of vertical upward and downward gaze (*see* Fig. 3). The *rostral interstitial nucleus of the medial longitudinal fasciculus* is located at the junction of the mesencephalon and diencephalon, lateral to the periventricular gray in the region of the subthalamus and the field H of Forel. Extending caudally from this location into the rostral midbrain, the *interstitial nucleus of Cajal* is lateral to the MLF at the level of the rostral portion of the somatic and visceral oculomotor nuclei. Neurons in both structures have afferent synaptic connections with the superior colliculus and the vestibular nuclei. Excitatory and inhibitory efferent connections are established bilaterally with vertical motor neurons in the oculomotor nucleus and trochlear nuclei (Fig. 4). Contralateral projections that are related specifically to vertical upward eye movements cross the midline through the *posterior commissure*. The rostral interstitial nucleus of the MLF contains burst neurons that discharge before the initiation of vertical saccadic eye movements. This region is physiologically differentiated from the tonic neurons in the interstitial nucleus of Cajal, whose activity is related to eye position. Many of the neurons in these structures also project to the spinal cord, forming the basis for their role in the control of vertical gaze.

Lesions of the rostral interstitial MLF at the mesodiencephalic junction produce paralysis of vertical upward or downward gaze (e.g., Parinaud's syndrome), and direction depends on the extent of

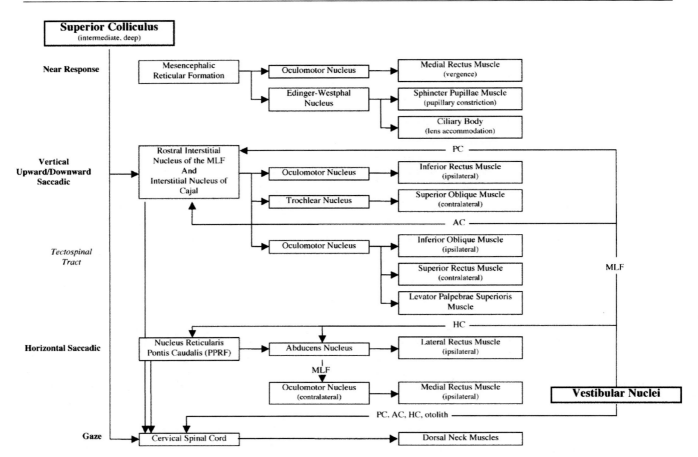

Fig. 4. Flow diagram of the major efferent connections of the superior colliculus and the vestibular nuclei that are related to the control of gaze. Connections related to accommodative vergence also are indicated. AC, anterior semicircular canal; HC, horizontal semicircular canal; MLF, medial longitudinal fasciculus; PC, posterior semicircular canal. Note how information from specific semicircular canals is distributed to the muscles that are appropriate for making the correct eye movements.

the lesion. Lesions of the posterior commissure have a selective effect on vertical upward saccadic eye movements and produce deficits in the pupillary light reflex as a result of the proximity to the pretectal area (e.g., pretectal syndrome).

5.3. The Pontine Reticular Formation Is the Center for Conjugate Horizontal Gaze

The paramedian zone of the pontine reticular formation in the vicinity of the abducens nucleus contains neurons that discharge with a burst of activity before the initiation of conjugate horizontal gaze. The *nucleus reticularis pontis caudalis* is rostral to the abducens nucleus and contains *excitatory burst neurons* that project to ipsilateral abducens neurons, and to the cervical spinal cord. *Inhibitory burst neurons* are located caudal to the abducens

nucleus and project to contralateral abducens neurons. Both populations of neurons receive inputs from the superior colliculus and vestibular nuclei (*see* Fig. 4). A third type of neuron, known as the *omnipause neuron*, is also located in the vicinity of the burst neurons. The tonic activity of omnipause neurons inhibits the burst neurons, except during saccades. Omnipause neurons then serve as a gating mechanism that prevents spurious saccades. This function is seen in lesions of the omnipause neurons, which produce constant saccadic oscillations of the eyes (oscillopsia). Collectively, the region of the paramedian pontine reticular formation is known as the *center for conjugate horizontal gaze.* Lesions of this area result in paralysis of ipsilateral conjugate horizontal gaze (eye plus head movements), in contrast to lesions of the abducens nucleus, which affect only conjugate horizontal eye movements.

6. ROLE OF THE CEREBRAL CORTEX AND CEREBELLUM IN EYE MOVEMENT

Although many of the functions of the oculomotor system appear to involve mainly brainstem structures, the cerebral cortex plays an important role in their proper operation. Despite the direct projections from the retina to the superior colliculus and pretectum, the binocularity and directional-selectivity features of the neuronal receptive fields in the superior colliculus and pretectum rely on descending connections from the primary and secondary visual areas of the cortex. Association areas of the cortex (e.g., frontal eye fields, occipitotemporal, and posterior parietal cortices) are largely responsible for the voluntary motor behaviors that are mediated by subcortical structures.

In contrast to the definitive role of the descending corticospinal and corticobulbar control from Brodmann's area 4 over spinal and other brainstem motor nuclei (e.g., trigeminal, facial, and hypoglossal), the cortical motor control of eye movement, which originates from area 8 of the prefrontal cortex (e.g., "frontal eye fields"), is less direct. This cortical region has afferent corticocortical connections with visual cortical areas, and is a major source of cortical input to the intermediate and deep layers of the superior colliculus. Lesions of this region produce only transient deficits in eye movements. The main deficit appears to be in eye movements that require attention to a particular stimulus in the visual field. Only combined lesions of the frontal eye field and the superior colliculus have a significant effect on voluntary eye movements, which is manifested by deficits in visually guided saccadic eye movements, particularly in the horizontal plane.

The *superior colliculus* is regarded as a site of sensorimotor transformation, and its function is related to orientation behavior. Inputs from any of the sensory systems can be converted into an eye movement that is directed toward the stimulus. The superficial layers of the superior colliculus are associated predominantly with visual inputs from the retina and the visual cortex. The deeper layers of the superior colliculus receive somatosensory, auditory, and visual inputs from a variety of cortical and subcortical areas (Fig. 5). The maps of the visual field, auditory space, and the body lie in register with one another, and are superimposed on the motor map. This arrangement allows for stimulation of different points in the superior colliculus to produce saccades that differ in amplitude and direction. Thus, saccades are precisely directed to a target, regardless of whether that target is visual, auditory, or another sensory modality.

The output neurons in the deeper layers of the superior colliculus project by way of the *tectospinal tract* to brainstem premotor areas in the mesencephalic and pontine reticular formation that control vertical and horizontal saccadic eye movements and to motor neurons in the cervical spinal cord that innervate the muscles of the neck (*see* Figs. 4 and 5). The activity of these deep-layer efferent neurons encodes information about the direction, velocity, and amplitude of saccades.

Cortical projections to the *pretectum*, (e.g., nucleus of the optic tract) and *accessory optic nuclei* are involved in the optokinetic reflex (*see* Fig. 6). In the basic reflex, visual projections through pretectum and accessory optic nuclei are relayed through the nucleus reticularis tegmenti pontis, the inferior olive, and the prepositus hypoglossi nucleus to the cerebellar flocculus. From there, movements generated by the optokinetic pathway converge upon the vestibular nucleus, where they share projections with the VOR, to motor neurons for the appropriate eye movements. Regions of the occipitotemporal and pareito-occipital cortex also appear to be important for the modulation of optokinetic responses, because lesions of the posterior parietal cortex can alter the bilateral, direction-specific response of this reflex.

The last class of smooth eye movements—smooth pursuit—lso converges upon second-order vestibular neurons to share the same pathways for sending eye-position signals to motor neurons. Pursuit signals originate with visual inputs to cortical area 19, pass through pontine nuclei (the *dorsolateral pontine nucleus*) that are distinct from those used by the optokinetic reflex, pass through the cerebellar flocculus, and then to the vestibular nuclei, which in turn carry the pursuit signal to motor neurons (Fig. 6).

The cerebellum appears to play a key role in integrating sensory inputs from a variety of sources and using these to direct and recalibrate eye movements. Total cerebellectomy produces persistent

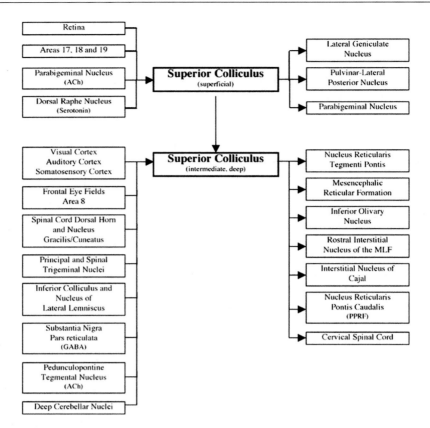

Fig. 5. Flow diagram of the major afferent and efferent connections of the superficial and deep layers of the superior colliculus. Ach, acetylcholine; GABA, ψ-aminobutyric acid; PPRF, paramedian pontine reticular formation.

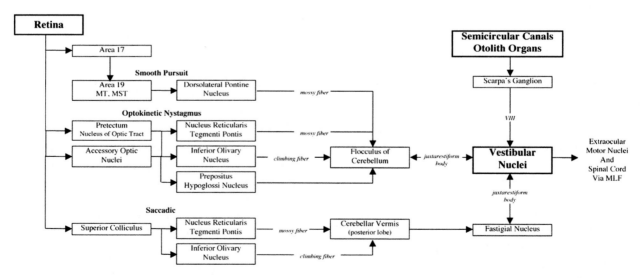

Fig. 6. Flow diagram of the structures and pathways related to the convergence of visual and vestibular information in the cerebellum and their role in smooth pursuit, optokinetic, and saccadic eye movements. The superior colliculus, pretectum, and accessory optic nuclei project to precerebellar relay nuclei in the basilar pons (nucleus reticularis tegmenti pontis, dorsolateral pontine nucleus) and medulla (inferior olivary nucleus). These regions project visual information to the same areas of the cerebellum that receive input from neurons in the vestibular ganglion and vestibular nuclei. The output of the cerebellum is directed to neurons in the vestibular nuclei that projects to the extra-ocular motor nuclei and the spinal cord through the MLF.

deficits in smooth pursuit, optokinetic nystagmus, and holding eccentric positions of gaze. Moreover, loss of total cerebellar function interferes with the ability to use visual information to re-calibrate eye movements after paresis of one or more extra-ocular muscles. The vestibulocerebellum, which includes the *flocculus*, nodulus, and uvual, specifically controls eye movements that stabilize images on the retina whether the head is still (e.g., smooth pursuit) or moving (e.g., cancellation of the VOR). The *flocculus* of the cerebellum is the site of convergence of primary vestibular fibers and axons from brainstem precerebellar nuclei (e.g., nucleus reticularis tegmenti pontis (via mossy fibers), dorsolateral pontine nucleus (via mossy fibers), and inferior olivary nucleus (via climbing fibers). Since both optokinetic reflex and smooth pursuit are smooth eye movements that result from visual stimuli, their convergence at the flocculus allows the conservation of neurons into a common pathway that serves similar purposes (Fig. 6). The *fastigial nucleus* of the cerebellum is primarily related to the visual portion of the vermis of the posterior lobe, which also has afferent connections from the same brainstem nuclei, but to those regions that are synaptically related to the superior colliculus (*see* Fig. 6). The dorsal cerebellar vermis and fastigial nuclei are important for the control of saccadic amplitude and accuracy. In summary, the cerebellum can be considered as the principal site of convergence of visual and vestibular information, which is transmitted to the oculomotor system by means of cerebellovestibular projections from the flocculus and fastigial nuclei to the vestibular nuclei.

7. ROLE OF THE BASAL GANGLIA IN EYE MOVEMENT

Diseases of the basal ganglia, including parkinsonism and Huntington's chorea, are characterized by deficits in saccadic eye movements. The gamma-aminobutyric acid-mediated inhibitory projection from the pars reticulata of the substantia nigra to the intermediate layer of the superior colliculus provides one pathway through which the basal ganglia may influence oculomotor control. This region of the substantia nigra receives input from the caudo-putamen (e.g., striatum) and the subthalamus, and forms part of an indirect corticotectal circuit by which sensory information from widespread regions of the cerebral cortex gain access to the superior colliculus. Neurons in the substantia nigra and the caudate nucleus discharge before intentional saccades.

Another link between the basal ganglia and the oculomotor system may be provided by an excitatory cholinergic projection to the superior colliculus, which arises from a collection of neurons in the caudal mesencephalic and rostral pontine tegmentum that partially corresponds to the pedunculopontine tegmentum nucleus or cholinergic-cell group Ch5. This region receives afferent connections from the pars reticulata of the substantia nigra, and has efferent connections with the pars compacta of the substantia nigra and the subthalamus. This region of the tegmentum has been the only location from which the resting tremor that is the hallmark of Parkinson's disease has been produced by experimental lesions.

8. CONTROL OF VERGENCE EYE MOVEMENTS

Vergence eye movements consist of the coordinated contraction of medial rectus muscles bilaterally for convergence and coordinated contraction of the lateral rectus muscles bilaterally for divergence. Although these movements are in the horizontal plane, they do not use the MLF pathway, since they are not conjugate eye movements. The neural control of vergence eye movements is perhaps the least understood of all eye-movement systems. However, there is a loosely organized population of neurons that cap the oculomotor nucleus that discharge tonically in relationship to vergence angle—the angle formed between the two eyes as they converge or diverge. The cerebellum appears to play a key role in vergence eye movements, particularly in combined conjugate-vergence movements. Neurons in parietal and visual association cortices discharge in relationship to vergence, but the precise anatomical pathways are not well-understood. Lesions of these cortical areas have been shown to compromise vergence.

SELECTED READINGS

Averbuch-Heller L. Supranuclear control of ocular motility. Ophthalmol Clin North Am 2001; 14:187.

Delgado-Garcia JM. Why move the eyes if we can move the head? Brain Res Bull 2000; 52:475.

Hanes DP, Wurtz RH. Interaction of the frontal eye field and superior colliculus for saccade generation. J Neurophysiol 2001; 85:804.

Leigh RJ, Zee DS. The neurology of eye movements, 3rd ed. New York: Oxford, 1999.

Mays LE, Gamlin PD. Neuronal circuitry controlling the near response. Curr Opin Neurobiol 1995; 5:763.

Sparks DL. Conceptual issues related to the role of the superior colliculus in the control of gaze. Curr Opin Neurobiol 1999; 9:698.

Straumann D, Haslwanter T. Ocular motor disorders. Curr Opin Neurol 2001; 14:5.

Disorders of Ocular Motility

Gregory Cooper and Robert L. Rodnitzky

Coordinated eye movements occur via saccades, smooth pursuit, the vestivular ocular reflex and convergence. These movements depend on intact supranuclear control mechanisms, brainstem gaze centers, certain cranial nerves, extra-ocular muscles, and neuromuscular transmission. Dysfunction of any of these components impairs ocular motility and produces a variety of distinct visual and neurologic signs and symptoms.

CAUSES OF EYE-MOVEMENT DISORDERS

Several Supranuclear Systems Guide Eye Movement

The saccadic system allows visual refixation on an object of interest seen in the periphery by moving the eyes rapidly until the image of the object is moved onto the fovea and into central vision. Saccades may be either intentional or reflexive. The pursuit system moves the eyes at the appropriate speed to hold the image of a slowly moving object on the fovea. The vergence system allows the eyes to move apart or toward one another so that images of objects at various distances can be kept on the fovea of both eyes simultaneously. The vestibular system moves the eyes to compensate for head movements so that images remain on the fovea during such activity.

Abnormalities of saccadic eye movement can result from lesions of the frontal eye fields, supplemental eye fields, parietal eye fields, pontine and mesencephalic reticular nuclei, the cerebellum, or the basal ganglia, which constitute some of the major structures of the system responsible for the generation of this form of ocular movement. Acute lesions of the eye fields in the frontal lobe result in the inability to voluntary initiate a saccade in the direction opposite the lesion. In a patient with a stroke involving the right frontal lobe, the eyes are deviated to the right and cannot voluntarily be moved to the left beyond the midline. However, by evoking reflex movements of the eyes, they can be moved to the left, indicating that the cranial nerve nuclei, cranial nerves, and extra-ocular muscles used for movement in this direction are still intact. This form of eye-movement disturbance in the face of intact cranial nerves and nuclei is known as a supranuclear gaze palsy. Another way in which saccadic movements can be abnormal is in relationship to their speed. In certain degenerative conditions of the cerebellum or basal ganglia, saccades become slowed. In Huntington's disease, for example, the appearance of slow saccades may be one of the earliest signs of neurologic dysfunction.

Like the saccadic system, the pursuit system incorporates several CNS structures, including the striate and extrastriate cortex, pontine nuclei, vestibular nuclei, and the cerebellum. Lesions in a variety of anatomic sites may interfere with pursuit movement. When pursuit fails, the speed of eye movement does not keep pace with a moving target. To compensate, corrective saccades are periodically generated, giving the otherwise smooth eye movements a jerky or ratchet-like character. These jerky movements are known as saccadic pursuit. A lesion of the parietotemporal cortex on one side can impair pursuit, resulting in saccadic pursuit when following objects moving toward the side of the lesion. The ipsilateral nature of this impairment has been attributed to a double decussation of the brainstem pathways. After cortical projections reach pontine nuclei, there are decussations between these pontine nuclei and the cerebellum and then between the vestibular nucleus, and the abducens nucleus.

ABNORMALITIES OF CONJUGATE GAZE IMPLY BRAINSTEM PATHOLOGY

When both eyes move in the same direction at the same speed, maintaining a constant alignment, gaze is said to be conjugate. The center controlling horizontal conjugate gaze is located in the pons in the vicinity of the abducens nucleus, and is known as the paramedian zone of the pontine reticular formation. A lesion involving the pontine parareticular formation on one side results in inability to move either eye beyond the midline toward that side. Unlike supranuclear gaze paralysis caused by frontal lobe lesions, this form of gaze paresis cannot be overcome by inducing involuntary reflex eye movements. The vertical conjugate gaze center is located in the midbrain. Lesions in this region, such as a tumor of the pineal gland compressing the dorsal midbrain, produce paralysis of conjugate vertical gaze, which in this case is an inability to gaze upward.

The cranial-nerve nuclei on both sides of the brainstem subserving conjugate eye movements are connected by the medial longitudinal fasciculus (MLF) fiber tract. An isolated lesion of this tract produces a specific abnormality of ocular motility. Because the cranial-nerve nuclei are left intact by a MLF lesion, eye movements in all directions are still possible, but because the nuclei are disconnected, the eyes do not move in a conjugate manner in the horizontal plane. When left lateral gaze is attempted by an individual with a right MLF lesion, the right eye, which must move inward, cannot cross the midline, although the outward-moving left eye responds normally. The same eye that could not move inward during attempted voluntary lateral gaze can do so when both eyes converge on a near target, proving the intactness of the third cranial nerve and medial rectus muscles underlying this movement. This pattern of deficient inward eye movement resulting from a MLF lesion is referred to as an *internuclear ophthalmoplegia*. This abnormality can be caused by any lesion interrupting the MLF, but multiple sclerosis is the most common cause, especially when the MLF is affected on both sides.

DISTINCT PATTERNS OF IMPAIRED OCULAR MOTILITY RESULT FROM LESIONS OF INDIVIDUAL CRANIAL NERVES

Abnormalities of the third (oculomotor), fourth (trochlear), or sixth (abducens) cranial nerves produce distinct patterns of impaired ocular motility. In an oculomotor-nerve palsy, the superior, inferior, and medial recti are paralyzed, as is the inferior oblique muscle. The affected eye deviates downward and laterally. This position results from the action of the two functioning ocular muscles, the lateral rectus and the inferior oblique, which are innervated by the abducens and trochlear nerve, respectively. In a complete oculomotor nerve palsy, the pupil is dilated and the eyelid droops. The patient complains of double vision (diplopia) in several directions of gaze because of the number of different muscles paralyzed. The oculomotor nerve can be damaged by ischemia in diabetes, be impinged on by an arterial aneurysm on the surface of the brain, or be compressed by brain tissue being forced downward by an expanding mass such as a tumor within the cranium. The latter turn of events often signals imminent death from compression of other vital brain structures if the causative mass effect is not corrected.

In an abducens nerve palsy, only the lateral rectus is weakened. The affected eye deviates medially, and the globe cannot be moved laterally beyond the midline. The patient complains of double vision that is worse during lateral gaze toward the side of the lesion. The abducens nerve pursues a long intracranial course and is angled over bony structures at the base of the skull. Because it pursues this path, the nerve is susceptible to stretch after any displacement of the brainstem to which it is attached. An abducens-nerve palsy may appear in patients with increased intracranial pressure of any cause if the pressure results in slight downward displacement of the brainstem or after blunt trauma to the skull, for the same reason.

In a trochlear-nerve palsy the superior oblique muscle is weak, resulting in inability to depress the globe, especially in the adducted (e.g., medial) position. In this syndrome, diplopia may occur, which is improved by tilting the head in the direction of the normal eye. The presence of head tilt, especially in a child, is often the first indication of the presence of a trochlear nerve-palsy.

DISORDERS OF MUSCLE OR NEUROMUSCULAR TRANSMISSION CAN AFFECT OCULAR MOTILITY

Ocular motility is involved in some disorders of muscle. This is especially true of the muscle disorder associated with thyroid disease and that seen in the mitochondrial disorders. In these two conditions, the degree of weakness of ocular muscles may be much greater than that seen in appendicular or truncal musculature.

Abnormalities of ocular motility are extremely common, and often the presenting sign in myasthenia gravis, a disorder of neuromuscular transmission. In this condition, any one or all of the ocular muscles can be involved. Most commonly, there is associated weakness and drooping of the eyelid. Myasthenia is characterized by abnormal fatigability, and unlike motility disturbances related to central nervous system disorders, the degree of motility impairment may vary from day to day and hour to hour, depending on the use of the eyes. For example, patients with myasthenia gravis often notice diplopia only after sustained gaze in the same direction, which may occur while watching TV or looking at an object in the sky. When impaired ocular motility and eyelid weakness appear in a myasthenic, a diagnosis of oculomotor-nerve palsy may be mistakenly made, but the absence of pupillary abnormality and the response to cholinesterase-inhibiting medications clearly establish myasthenia as the cause.

NYSTAGMUS IS AN ABNORMAL PATTERN OF REPETITIVE EYE MOVEMENTS

Nystagmus is a rhythmic to-and-fro oscillation of the eyes. It can occur in the vertical or horizontal plane, and sometimes can be rotatory. It is usually phasic; the oscillation in one direction is faster than in the other direction. In pathologic states, nystagmus may occur when the eyes are in the primary position or after they are moved to their limit in one direction. *Gaze-evoked nystagmus* is usually seen in patients receiving sedative drugs, and also occurs in cerebellar diseases. It occurs when gaze is directed away from the middle position in the vertical or the horizontal plane. *Downbeat nystagmus*, evident when the eyes are in the primary position, is most commonly caused by lesions in the vicinity of the craniocervical junction.

Vestibular nystagmus results from dysfunction of the vestibular apparatus or vestibular nerve. If the dysfunction is unilateral, the nystagmus has its fast phase directed away from the side of the lesion. There is often a rotatory component to the nystagmoid movement. Vertigo, a spontaneous hallucination of movement (often a sense of spinning), commonly accompanies vestibular nystagmus. Vestibular nystagmus can result from causes as diverse as a tumor of the eighth cranial nerve or viral labyrinthitis. Vestibular nystagmus can be readily provoked in normal persons by instilling ice water into the ear canal. This caloric stimulation sets up convection currents in the endolymph within the semicircular canals, resulting in nystagmus toward the side of stimulation and a profound sense of vertigo. This procedure can be used as a test of the intactness of the vestibular system.

Pendular nystagmus differs from most other types in that it is not phasic; the speed of the nystagmoid movement is equal in both directions. It is often congenital, in which case it may be associated with poor vision. If pendular nystagmus is acquired, it usually indicates brainstem pathology, usually related to multiple sclerosis or stroke. *Physiologic nystagmus* appears at the extremes of gaze in normal persons, especially when the eye muscles are fatigued or when the eyes are held at the extreme of lateral or vertical gaze for an extended period. Approximately 5% of the population is capable of producing *voluntary nystagmus*, consisting of a 10- to 25-s burst of extremely rapid back-and-forth horizontal movements.

SELECTED READINGS

Eggenberger ER, Kaufman DI. Ocular motility review for 1997-1998: Part I. J Neuro-Ophth 2000; 20:73–84.

Eggenberger ER, Kaufman DI. Ocular motility review for 1997-1998: Part II. J Neuro-Ophth 2000; 20:192–206.

Glaser JS (ed.). Neuro-opthalmology, 2nd ed. Philadelphia: JB Lippincott, 1990; 299, 361.

Pierrot-Deseilligny C, Gaymard B, Muri R, Rivaud S. Cerebral ocular motor signs. J Neurol 1997; 244:65–70.

15 The Hypothalamus

Marc E. Freeman and Thomas A. Houpt

1. INTRODUCTION

1.1. Functions of the Hypothalamus

The hypothalamus is part of the limbic portion of the brain in vertebrates, which regulates the *internal milieu* of the cells within narrow limits as it compensates for changing external conditions, such as variations in temperature, energy, or defensive requirements. The constancy of the internal environment resulting from these fine adjustments made by the hypothalamus is known as *homeostasis*. The hypothalamus maintains homeostasis by exerting control over the two regulatory systems of the organism: the *nervous system* and the *endocrine system*.

In regulating the nervous system, the hypothalamus controls *autonomic processes*, such as cardiovascular, thermoregulatory, and visceral function. In addition, *behavioral processes* that include ingestive, sexual, maternal, and emotional behaviors are also regulated by the hypothalamus. The role of the hypothalamus in the regulation of the nervous system is summarized in Table 1.

In its regulation of the function of the endocrine system, the hypothalamus exerts control of the two subdivisions of the *pituitary gland*. The *anterior pituitary* or *adenohypophysis* synthesizes hormones that regulate adrenal, thyroid, and gonadal function as well

as growth and lactation. The synthesis and secretion of anterior pituitary hormones, in turn, are regulated by peptides and amines. These are synthesized by and secreted from specific hypothalamic neurons, and are transported to the adenohypophysis through a microscopic vascular route, known as the *hypothalamo–hypophyseal portal system* (Fig. 1) to either stimulate or inhibit the synthesis and secretion of specific hormones of the adenohypophysis. These peptides and amines are known collectively as *releasing* or *release-inhibiting hormones* (Table 2).

The hormones of the *posterior pituitary* or *neurohypophysis* are synthesized by specific hypothalamic neurons and transported to the neurohypophysis axonally by the *hypothalamo–hypophyseal tract* (Fig. 1), released into sinusoids and ultimately into the peripheral circulation to directly regulate blood pressure, water balance, and milk ejection (Table 2).

The fact that certain neurons can subserve two functions—the receipt and transmission of electrical information as typical nerve cells and as endocrine cells that secrete their products into a minute blood supply to regulate the adenohypophysis, or into the neurohypophysis and ultimately into the peripheral circulation to regulate visceral processes—led to the concept of *neurosecretion* and ultimately to the birth of the science of *neuroendocrinology*.

It is important to note that hypothalamic control of any one process is not exerted in a manner that is exclusive of other processes. Thus, the hypothalamus

From: *Neuroscience in Medicine, 2nd ed.* (P. Michael Conn, ed.),
© 2003 Humana Press Inc., Totowa, NJ.

Table 1
Neural Processes Regulated by the Hypothalamus

Category	System or activity	Process
Autonomic Process	Cardiovascular	Blood flow ($\downarrow$ or $\uparrow$) vasodilation or vasoconstriction
	Thermoregulatory	Blood flow, shivering, panting
	Visceral	Digestive acid secretion ($\uparrow$)
Behavioral Process	Sexual	Sexual receptivity ("heat")
	Maternal	Nest building
	Emotional	Aggression ($\uparrow$)
	Ingestive	Eating and drinking ($\uparrow$ or $\downarrow$)

$\uparrow$ = increase; $\downarrow$ = decrease.

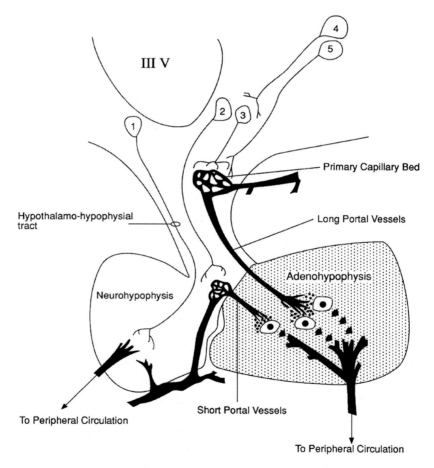

Fig. 1. Diagrammatic representation of the control of the neurohypophysis and adenohypophysis by the hypothalamus. *Neuron 1* is a peptidergic magnocellular neuron from the supraoptic or paraventricular nuclei of the hypothalamus that secretes oxytocin or vasopressin into sinusoids in the neurohypophysis. The axons of these two nuclei travel to the neurohypophysis in the hypothalamo–hypophyseal tract. *Neuron 2* could be a hypophysiotropic peptidergic or aminergic neuron terminating adjacent to the short portal vessels, which represent a potential route of communication between the neurohypophysis and adenohypophysis. The hypothalamic release or release-inhibiting peptidergic neurons are of this type. The tuberohypophysial dopaminergic neurons are also of this type. *Neuron 3* could also be a hypophysiotropic peptidergic or aminergic neuron. In this case, the neuron terminates on the primary capillary bed of the median eminence (ME). It also secretes release or release-inhibiting peptides into portal blood, which reach the adenohypophysis via the long portal vessels. The tuberoinfundibular dopaminergic neurons are also of this type.

Table 2
Neuroendocrine Regulators of Hypothalamic Origin

System regulated	Site of regulation	Action	Hypothalamic regulator
Thyroid gland	Adenohypophysis	Stimulation of thyrotrophin secretion	Thyrotrophin-releasing hormone
Adrenal cortex	Adenohypophysis	Stimulation of adrenocorticotrophin secretion	Corticotrophin-releasing hormone
Gonads	Adenohypophysis	Stimulation of luteinizing hormone and follicle-stimulating hormone secretion	Gonadotrophin-releasing hormone
Muscle, bone, liver	Adenohypophysis	Stimulation or inhibition of growth hormone secretion	Growth hormone-releasing hormone, somatostatin
Milk synthesis and secretion from the mammary gland	Adenohypophysis	Inhibition of prolactin secretion	Dopamine
Cardiovascular, Renal muscle, renal tubule	Vascular smooth water reabsorption	Vasoconstriction, (antidiuretic hormone)	Vasopressin
Mammary Gland, Uterus of mammary ducts and uterus	Smooth muscle pressure inducing milk ejection; increase uterine contraction in labor	Increase intramammary	Oxytocin

exerts *integrative function* over physiological processes. For example, thermoregulatory processes are governed by both the autonomic nervous system and the endocrine system. Exposure to extremes of temperature results in the adjustment of blood flow through autonomic processes and metabolic adjustments through regulation of thyroid hormone secretion. Both of these seemingly unrelated controls are under the influence of the hypothalamus.

1.2. Historical Perspective

Although there are indications that the ancients may have appreciated the vital role of higher centers in normal physiology, the role of the hypothalamus did not begin to crystallize until a series of clinical observations made from the late nineteenth to the early twentieth centuries. Most of the early studies focused on hypothalamic control of pituitary function because

pituitary pathologies were the most overt. A connection between the hypothalamus and pituitary gland was not appreciated at that time; thus, many of the early observations were often mistakenly attributed directly to "pituitary tumors." In 1901, Dr. Alfred Fröhlich, a Viennese physician, correctly reported a case of adiposogenital dystrophy in a 14-yr-old boy suffering from a pituitary tumor that compressed the optic tract and hypothalamus, which was subsequently relieved by surgery. Shortly thereafter, Erdheim described gonadal atrophy and obesity directly caused by hypothalamic damage without damage of the pituitary gland. Camus and Roussay (1913) later demonstrated polyuria in dogs bearing surgical lesions of the hypothalamus without damage to the pituitary gland. These were the first direct observations that the hypothalamus controls the pituitary gland. The development of a parapharyngeal procedure to surgically remove the

---

(*Fig. 1. continued*) Neurons with cell bodies that lie within the arcuate and periventricular nuclei and terminate on the primary capillary bed in the ME comprise the infundibular tract. The link between the rest of the brain and the pituitary gland is represented by *neurons 4 and 5*. These neurons secrete catecholamines (and in some cases peptides) that act as neurotransmitters or neuromodulators on the hypophysiotropic neurons. The termination of neuron 4 is axo-dendritic or axo-somatic, and that of neuron 5 is axo-axonic.

pituitary gland of rats (hypophysectomy) by Philip Smith (1926) led to a flurry of studies of the pituitary gland and brain. It was appreciated at that time that the pituitary gland must remain intact with the brain for coitus to induce ovulation in rabbits. The classical, yet, crude experiments of Marshall and Verney (1936) demonstrating ovulation-induction in rabbits by passage of an electrical current through the brain were soon followed by the experiments of Geoffrey Harris (1937), which showed that more localized stimulation of the hypothalamus also led to ovulation induction in rabbits. Subsequent studies revealed that coitus would not result in ovulation in the rabbit if the pituitary stalk was cut and a foil barrier was placed between the hypothalamus and pituitary with the (mistaken) intention of preventing the regrowth of severed "nerves" (Westman and Jacobsohn, 1937). A "fast forward toward the future" allows us to determine that coitus stimulated the release of the decapeptide gonadotropin-releasing hormone (GnRH) into portal blood, and its role was to stimulate the release of an ovulation-inducing amount of luteinizing hormone (LH) into the peripheral circulation.

Perhaps the most significant early contribution to the science of neuroendocrinology was the development of the concept of *neurosecretion* by the husband-and-wife team of Ernst and Berta Scharrer. Beginning in the early 1930s, they proposed that the cells of the hypothalamus must have a unique function distinct from other brain cells based on their multinucleated appearance, the abundance of protein-containing colloid-like vacuoles, and the unique proximity between these cells and the surrounding capillary network. The Scharrers proposed that these nerve cells must therefore have a glandular function. At about the same time, Popa and Fielding (1930) described the vascular connection between the hypothalamus and adenohypophysis in rabbits, although they mistakenly believed that the direction of blood flow was from the gland toward the hypothalamus. The first report of flow toward the pituitary was made in a study of toads by Houssay (1935). The developing concept of neurosecretion coupled with the description of the portal vasculature opened the door to an innovative series of experiments demonstrating that the hypothalamus controlled the adenohypophysis with messages transported over a vascular route. However, experiments involving transection of the stalk connecting the hypothalamus with the pituitary gland led to varying results, leading some to doubt the importance of a vascular connection until Green and Harris (1947) suggested

that the cut portal vessels could regenerate and Harris (1950) subsequently showed that reproductive function was restored to a degree proportional to portal vessel regeneration in stalk-sectioned rats. Finally, the elegant experiments of Harris and Jacobsohn (1952) convincingly demonstrated the primacy of the hypophyseal-portal vasculature in anterior pituitary function. In these experiments, rats were hypophysectomized, and adenohypophyses from their newborns were transplanted to either the temporal lobe of the brain or, by a transtemporal route, immediately beneath the median eminence (ME) of the hypothalamus. Only those animals with transplants beneath the ME that had been re-vascularized by the portal vasculature showed a resumption of reproductive function. In support of this, Nikitovich-Weiner and Everett (1958) autografted anterior pituitaries to the kidney capsule and demonstrated a loss of thyrod-stimulating hormone, or thyrotropin (TSH); adrenocorticotropic hormone (ACTH); follicle-stimulating hormone (FSH); and LH secretion, but an enhancement of prolactin secretion from the transplants. These transplants were subsequently removed and placed under the temporal lobe of the brain or beneath the ME. Only those rats bearing transplants to the ME showed a resumption of normal anterior pituitary function.

The dawning of the science of neuroendocrinology was completed with the focus on the chemical nature of the activities of the adenohypophysis and neurohypophysis. After the studies of Van Dyke and associates (1941) established the existence of separate oxytocic and pressor principals, du Vigneaud identified the structure of oxytocin (OT) (1950) and then vasopressin (1954). This was followed by a multitude of studies between the mid 1960s through the 1970s by Andrew Schally and Roger Guillemin's laboratories on the chemical nature of the hypothalamic neuropeptides, which control the secretion of TSH, LH/FSH, ACTH, and growth hormone from the anterior pituitary. The "arrival" of the science of neuroendocrinology was recognized by the Nobel Prizes awarded to these two investigators in 1977.

2. ANATOMY OF THE HYPOTHALAMUS

2.1. The Boundaries of the Hypothalamus are Distinctly Defined

The hypothalamus is situated in the lowermost portion of the *diencephalon* (Figs. 2 and 3). The human hypothalamus presents well-defined boundaries. The rostral border is limited by a vertical line drawn

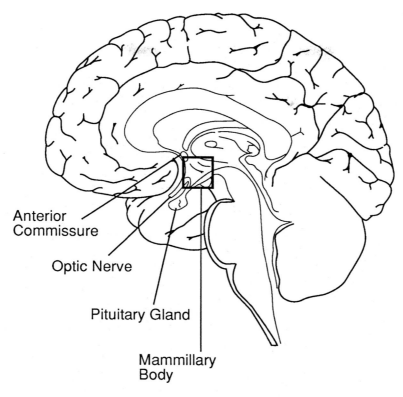

Anterior
Commissure

Optic Nerve

Pituitary Gland

Mammillary
Body

Fig. 2. The position of the hypothalamus and pituitary of the human relative to the rest of the brain. The hypothalamus is bounded by the *dark-bordered box*.

through the anterior border of the *anterior commissure*, *lamina terminalis*, and *optic chiasm*. The hypothalamus is bordered caudally by a vertical line drawn through the posterior border of the *mammillary body* as it bounds the *interpeduncular fossa*. The superior border of the hypothalamus is the *hypothalamic sulcus* as it borders the *thalamus*, and the inferior boundary is the bulging *tuber cinereum*, which tapers to form the *infundibulum*, the funnel-shaped functional connection between the hypothalamus and the pituitary gland. Laterally, the borders are poorly defined as a result of the blending of the hypothalamic gray matter with adjacent structures. However, by convention, the lateral borders are confined by the *internal capsule* and its caudal limits.

2.2. The Divisions of the Hypothalamus are Described as Functional Groupings

The hypothalamus is divided into clusters of perikarya embedded in gray matter. These are known as *nuclei* (singular: *nucleus*). Several problems are inherent in this designation. In most cases, the nuclei are not morphologically distinct structures with boundaries that are distinct in histological preparation. The dendrites and axons of these neurons may extend for distances beyond the limits of the nucleus. Moreover, chemically and functionally, the nuclei may be heterogeneous to varying degrees. Thus, only vague functional and anatomical boundaries can be drawn for hypothalamic nuclei.

The groupings of the nuclei may be described in a *rostro-caudal* direction as (i) *anterior* or *supraoptic* (Fig. 4), located between the lamina terminalis and the posterior edge of the optic chiasm; (ii) *medial* or *tuberal* (Fig. 5), located between the optic chiasm and the mammillary bodies; and (iii) *posterior* or *mammillary* (Fig 6), including the mammillary bodies and the structures just dorsal to them. The hypothalamus can also be described longitudinally in mediolateral zones (Figs. 4–6) known as *periventricular*, bordering the third ventricle; *medial*, comprising the major hypothalamic nuclei, which are sites of limbic-system projections; and *lateral*, which is separated from the medial zone by the *fornix*, a large C-shaped tract that interconnects limbic-system structures.

The most anterior hypothalamic areas are poorly defined. Rather than being grouped as diencephalic structures, the *medial preoptic* and *septal* areas are

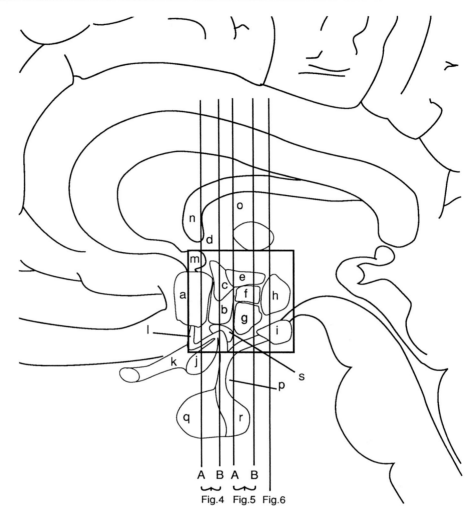

Fig. 3. The position of hypothalamic nuclei and adjacent structures in sagittal section. The vertical lines represent the planes of frontal Figs. 4A,B; 5A,B; and 6. The box outlines the corresponding area of Fig. 2. *a*, preoptic nucleus; *b*, anterior hypothalamic area; *c*, paraventricular nucleus; *d*, hypothalamic sulcus; *e*, dorsal hypothalamic area; *f*, dorsomedial nucleus; *g*, ventromedial nucleus; posterior hypothalamic area; *i*, mamillary body; *j*, optic chiasm; *k*, optic nerve; *l*, lamina terminalis; *m*, anterior commissure; *n*, fornix; *o*, thalamus; *p*, infundibulum; *q*, adenohypophysis; *r*, neurohypophysis; *s*, suprachiasmatic nucleus.

actually part of the telencephalon (Fig. 4A). However, modern embryology has shown that the preoptic area has the same embryonic origins as many diencephalic structures. Thus, the preoptic area is often considered to be part of the hypothalamus. The *medial preoptic area* (Fig. 4A, part *g*) has been shown to possess sexually dimorphic features. As described later, uniquely stained groups of neurons form in this area in organisms exposed to testosterone prenatally or neonatally. The *lateral preoptic area* (Fig. 4A, part *f*) is not morphologically distinct from the medial preoptic area, but subserves uniquely distinct physiological roles. More caudally, the *anterior* and *lateral hypothalamic areas* appear (Fig. 4B, parts *d,c*). The cells of these

areas are small, with few dendritic branches. The lateral hypothalamic area receives fibers from the medial forebrain bundle. Chemical lesion of this area leads to aphagia. As discussed later, this area plays a stimulatory role in feeding behavior. The *paraventricular nucleus* (Fig. 5A, part *f*) is wedge-shaped, and as its name implies, lies adjacent to the third ventricle. The deeply staining neurons are of two types: *magnocellular*, or neurons with large perikarya, and *parvicellular*, or neurons with small perikarya. The axons of the magnocellular neurons terminate in the neurohypophysis, and the axons of the parvicellular neurons terminate on the primary capillary bed of the hypophyseal portal vasculature in the ME. The *supraoptic*

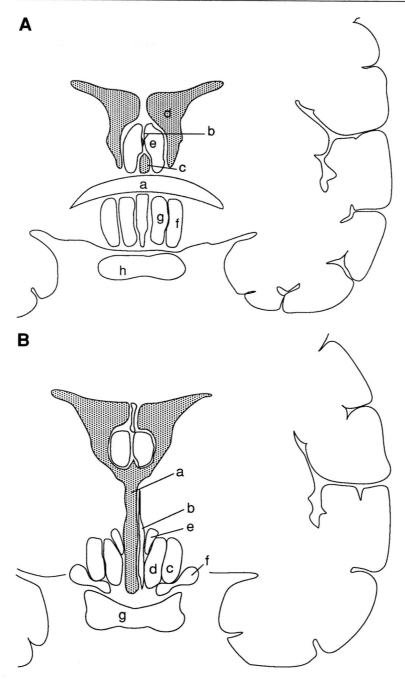

Fig. 4. The hypothalamic and adjacent structures of the anterior or supraoptic groupings. (**A**) *a*, anterior commissure; *b*, septal area; *c*, third ventricle; *d*, lateral ventricle; *e*, column of fornix; *f*, lateral preoptic area; *g*, medial preoptic area; *h*, optic chiasm. (**B**) *a*, third ventricle; *b*, periventricular nucleus; *c*, lateral hypothalamic area; *d*, anterior hypothalamic area; *e*, paraventricular nucleus; *f*, supraoptic nucleus; *g*, optic chiasm.

nucleus (Fig. 5A, part *j*; Fig. 5B, part *h*) is located directly above the beginning of the optic tracts, and consists of a large anterolateral subnucleus and a smaller posteromedial subnucleus connected by a thin strand of cells (Fig. 5A). As in the paraventricular nucleus, the neurons of the supraoptic nucleus stains darkly and consists of magnocellular perikarya with axons that terminate in the neurohypophysis. The axons of the supraoptic and paraventricular nuclei travel in a bundle, known as the *hypothalamo–hypo-*

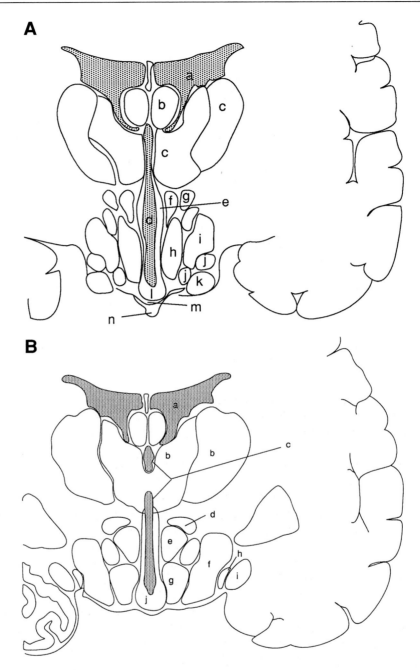

Fig. 5. The hypothalamic and adjacent structures of the medial or tuberal groupings. (**A**) *a*, lateral ventricle; *b*, body of fornix; *c*, thalamus; *d*, third ventricle; *e*, periventricular nucleus; *f*, paraventricular nucleus; *g*, dorsal hypothalamic area; *h*, anterior hypothalamic area; *i*, lateral hypothalamic area; *j*, supraoptic nucleus; *k*, optic tract; *l*, arcuate nucleus; *m*, median eminence; *n*, infundibulum. (**B**) *a*, lateral ventricle; *b*, thalamus; *c*, third ventricle; *d*, dorsal hypothalamic area; *e*, dorsomedial nucleus; *f*, lateral nucleus; *g*, ventromedial nucleus; *h*, supraoptic nucleus; *i*, optic tract; *j*, arcuate nucleus.

physeal tract, to the neurohypophysis (Fig. 1). The magnocellular and parvicellular cells of these regions produce vasopressin and OT. The *suprachiasmatic nuclei* (Fig. 3, part *s*) are distinctly staining paired structures (in rodents) overlying the *optic chiasm*

(Fig. 3, part *j*). In humans, the suprachiasmatic nuclei are not strikingly distinct morphologically. In all mammals, the cells of this area receive retinohypothalamic input, and are believed to be the "circadian clock" that controls the temperature cycle, sleep/wake cycle, and

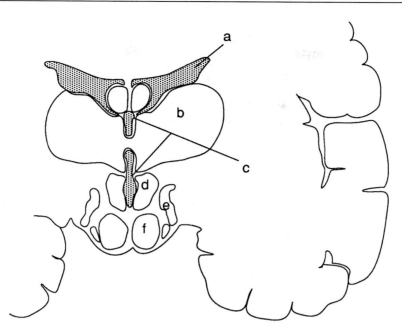

Fig. 6. The hypothalamic and adjacent structures of the posterior or mammillary groupings. *a*, lateral ventricle; *b*, thalamus; *c*, third ventricle; *d*, posterior hypothalamic area; *e*, lateral hypothalamic area; *f*, mammillary body.

the circadian changes in the timing of certain hormone systems such as those pituitary hormones that control the adrenal cortex (ACTH) and the reproductive system (LH and prolactin). The *periventricular nuclei* (Fig. 5A, part *e*) have small perikarya, which contain some of the release and release-inhibiting factors controlling the pituitary gland. Also associated with the anterior hypothalamic area are the morphologically indistinct telencephalic structures known as *circumventricular organs* (CVOs). One of these is the *organum vasculosum of the lamina terminalis (OVLT)*, and the other is the *subfornical organ (SFO)*. These are areas where the blood–brain barrier is absent, and thus can sense plasma osmolality. These areas play a role in the regulation of blood pressure and thirst because they contain angiotensin II (AII) receptors, and may even be able to synthesize their own AII. The OVLT has also been implicated in the control of LH secretion by GnRH. The other *"leaky"* CVOs are the *subcommissural organ (SCO)* and the *area postrema* (AP).

In the medial area the optic tracts separate, the lateral hypothalamus continues caudally, and the caudal termination of the supraoptic nucleus is located. Also in this area, the anterior hypothalamic area ends (Fig. 5A), and is replaced by two distinct nuclei, the *dorsomedial* and *ventromedial nuclei* (VMN) (Fig. 5B, parts *e,g*). The two can be separated by the small cells

of the dorsomedial nucleus and the dense grouping of the neurons in the VMN. Both of these nuclei play a role in food intake. Lesions of both nuclei cause hyperphagia. Thus, this area regulates food intake in an inhibitory manner. The VMN in particular contains glucose-sensitive cells, which are believed to be the site through which caloric intake is monitored. The cells of the VMN are also rich in receptors for the gonadal steroids estrogen and testosterone, and thus are believed to play a major role in reproductive behavior and regulation of hormone secretion from the adenohypophysis. Finally, the *arcuate nucleus* begins in this medial hypothalamic area (Fig. 5A, part *l*; Fig. 5B, part *j*). The parvicellular neurons in this area have short axons, and some of these terminate on the *primary capillary bed* of the hypothalamo-hypophyseal portal system. The primary capillary bed is located in the underlying *median eminence* (ME) (Fig. 5A, part *m*). The neurons of the arcuate nucleus have several functions. In some mammals—such as the guinea pig, human, most monkeys bats, ferrets, cows, and the horse, cat, dog, and rabbit—GnRH neurons are in the basal portion of the medial hypothalamus. However, in others such as the rat and sheep, this area is devoid of GnRH neurons, or small numbers of such neurons are found in a so-called *cell-poor zone*. In those species in which the arcuate nucleus contains GnRH neurons, the fibers continue to the ME and some continue through the infundibular stalk and into the neurohypo-physis (human). A second function is in the control of prolactin and growth-hormone secretion. This area is populated by cells that contain dopamine, the prolactin-inhibiting hormone and growth hormone-releasing hormone (GHRH), the peptidergic stimulator of growth-hormone secretion. Finally, the arcuate nucleus is abundant in cells that contain β-endorphin, the endogenous opioid that is a cleavage product of the larger peptide, pro-opiomelanocortin (POMC). These neurons project to various hypothalamic and forebrain sites, and are believed to play a role in emotional behavior as well as endocrine function.

The posterior hypothalamic area contains the continuation of the lateral hypothalamic area as well as the *posterior hypothalamic nuclei and mammillary bodies* (Fig. 6, parts *d,f*). The posterior hypothalamic nucleus contains both small and large cell bodies, which give rise to efferent fibers descending through the central gray matter as well as the reticular formation (RF) of the brainstem. These neurons are believed to play a role in temperature regulation because they respond to cooling with the induction of shivering as well as the burning of brown adipose tissue. The mammillary nucleus is actually a complex consisting of medial and lateral nuclei. The mammillary bodies are critical circuits that link the hypothalamus with the limbic forebrain and midbrain structures lying rostral and caudal, thus implying a role in hypothalamic activity.

2.3. The Afferent and Efferent Connections are the Information Pathways of the Hypothalamus

The afferent and efferent connections of the hypothalamus reveal that this part of the brain is a complex integration center for somatic, autonomic, and endocrine functions.

2.3.1. INTRINSIC TRACTS

There are two main intrinsic tracts in the hypothalamus (*see* Fig. 1). The *infundibular tract* arises from neurons in the arcuate nucleus and periventricular nucleus with terminals on capillaries within the ME. These tracts axonally transport substances such as dopamine to the portal vessels. The *hypothalamo–hypophyseal tract* arises in the supraoptic and paraventricular nuclei and terminates in the neurohypophysis. As noted earlier, these axons transport vasopressin and OT, respectively. Both of these transfer

information unidirectionally, from the hypothalamus to the pituitary gland.

2.3.2. EXTRINSIC TRACTS

The lateral hypothalamus is reciprocally connected with the *thalamus*, the *paramedian mesencephalic area (limbic midbrain area)*, and the *limbic system*. The medial hypothalamus also receives connections from the limbic system (Fig. 7). It is quite clear that higher cortical centers communicate with the hypothalamus through the limbic system. In addition to the hypothalamus, the limbic system includes the *hippocampus*, the *amygdala*, the *septal area*, the *nucleus acumbens* (part of the *striatum*), and the *orbitofrontal cortex*. Anatomically, the hypothalamus is intimately related to the amygdala, which sits in the temporal lobe just rostral to the hippocampus. Efferents from the amygdala enter the hypothalamus through the *ventral amygdalofugal pathway*. The rostral amygdalofugal fibers form the *diagonal band of Broca*. More caudally, these fibers fan out and enter the hypothalamus, and many of them terminate near the VMN. A second afferent to the hypothalamus arises from the *corticomedial amygdala*. This pathway, the *stria terminalis*, terminate near the VMN of the hypothalamus. The other major limbic afferent to the hypothalamus arises from the hippocampus. The body of the hippocampus gives rise to the columns of the *fornix*, which courses toward the *anterior commissure* and then splits into two portions. The *post-commissural fornix* terminates in the mammillary bodies at the caudal end of the hypothalamus. Arising from the mammillary bodies is the *mammillothalamic tract*, which extends to the anterior nuclei of the thalamus, and then projects to the cingulate gyrus and the parahippocampal gyrus before returning to the hippocampus. A second efferent projection from the mammillary bodies, the *mammillotegmental tract*, turns caudally to the ventral tegmentum. A reciprocal pathway from the ventral tegmentum to the mammillary bodies is the *mammillary-pudendal tract*. The *Dorsal-longitudinal fasciculus of Schütz* are efferents from the periventricular nuclei of the hypothalamus, which terminate in the mesencephalic central gray. Stimulation of this fiber bundle produces fear and adverse reactions. A subset of ganglion cells in the retina projects to the suprachiasmatic nucleus of the hypothalamus by way of the *retinohypothalamic tract*. This tract transmits lighting periodicity information to be transduced by the

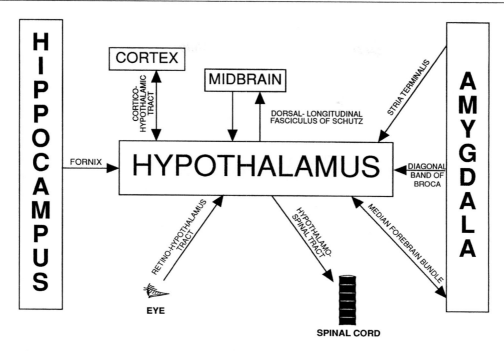

Fig. 7. A diagrammatic representation of some afferents and efferents of the hypothalamus.

suprachiasmatic nucleus. The *hypothalamospinal tract* originates in the supraoptic and paraventricular nuclei (parvicellular division), which projects down the spinal cord to the thoracic level and terminates in the intermediolateral column, and from there to the preganglionic sympathetic nerves. Based upon the anatomy, this pathway clearly must be important as the pathway over which the hypothalamus influences autonomic function. The other major hypothalamic fiber tract is the *median forebrain bundle*. This is a collection of tracts with ascending and descending fibers that run in the lateral hypothalamus between the midbrain RF and the basal forebrain. The descending fibers originate from structures in the basal forebrain, including the olfactory cortex, the preoptic area, the septal area, the accumbens, and the amygdala. The ascending portion comes from spinal cord and RF and visceral and taste nuclei in the brainstem as well as monoaminergic centers in the brainstem.

2.4. Blood Flow as a Means of Communicating Hypothalamic Information

The key neurohumoral link between the hypothalamus and the pituitary gland is the *hypothalamo–hypophyseal portal vasculature* (Fig. 8), which arises from a *primary capillary plexus* that extends from the ME

to the adenohypophysis. This plexus is supplied with blood from three sources: rostrally by the *superior hypophyseal artery*, caudally by the *inferior hypophyseal artery* and mediorostrally by the *anterior hypophyseal artery (or Trabecular artery)*. All three of these arise from the *internal carotid artery*. In some species (rat, rabbit, and cat) they unite to form a single artery that supplies the infundibular stem. These arteries encircle the ME. The inferior hypophyseal artery also supplies the neurohypophysis. The primary capillary plexus in the ME is drained by the fenestrated *long portal vessels*, which course to the adenohypophysis, where they branch to a *secondary capillary plexus*. The primary capillary plexus is the site at which axon terminals converge to release their quanta of hypophysiotropic peptides into portal blood. After transport through the long portal vessels, they are released from the secondary capillary plexus to the surrounding adenohypophyseal cells. A set of *short portal vessels* arise from the anterior hypophyseal artery. These connect the infundibular stem, the neurohypophysis, and the intermediate lobe of the pituitary gland to the adenohypophysis. The short portal vessels are the route through which neurohypophyseal and intermediate-lobe peptides travel to the anterior pituitary.

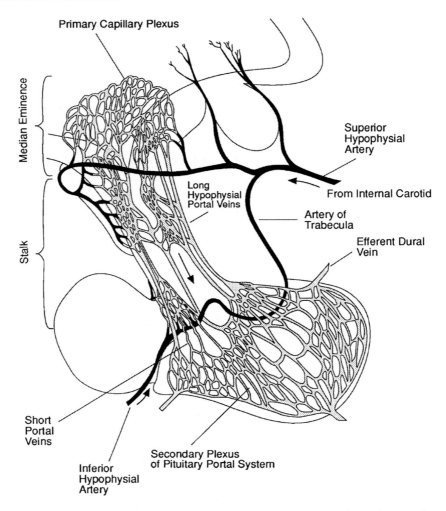

Fig. 8. A schematic representation of the hypothalamo–hypophyseal portal vasculature in man. *See* text for details.

2.5. The Chemiarchitecture Describes the Functions of the Hypothalamus

2.5.1. MONOAMINES

There are essentially three monoamines of importance to hypothalamic function, and their distributions have been described. These are dopamine, norepinephrine, and serotonin.

2.5.1.1. Dopamine. There are two major dopaminergic systems with long axons that originate from outside the hypothalamus (Fig. 9). The *nigrostriatal system*, has cell bodies in the substantia nigra with long axons that terminate in the caudate-putamen and globus pallidus. The *mesolimbic system*, has cell bodies in the ventral tegmentum that send projections through the hypothalamus and terminals in areas of the limbic system such as the nucleus acumbens, olfactory tubercle, cingulate cortex, and frontal cortex. Axons

of both of these areas travel through the medial forebrain bundle. The hypothalamus contains three intrinsic dopaminergic pathways with short axons. The cell bodies of the *incertohypothalamic neurons* are located in the caudal hypothalamus, zona incerta, and rostral periventricular nucleus, with axons terminating in the dorsal hypothalamus, preoptic area, and septum. The cell bodies of the *tuberoinfundibular neurons* are located in the arcuate and periventricular nuclei, with short axons that terminate in the ME. These converge upon the primary capillary bed of the hypophyseal portal system, and thus have been shown to play a direct role in the release of hormones from the adenohypophysis. The *tuberohypophyseal neurons* have cell bodies in the rostral arcuate and periventricular nuclei, with axons terminating in the intermediate and posterior lobes of the pituitary gland. In the neurohypophysis, these axons lie in close proximity to vascular

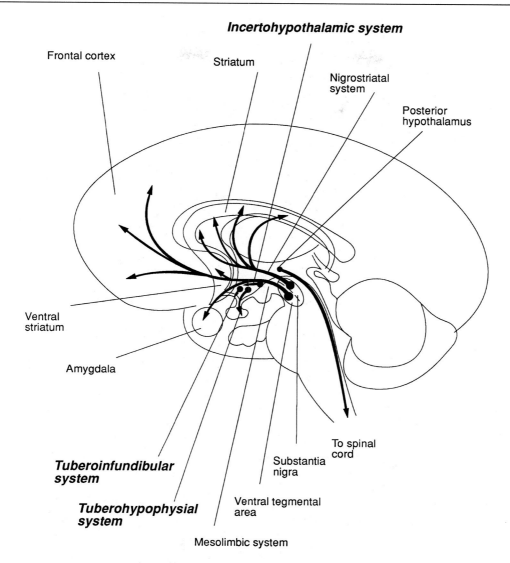

Fig. 9. Diagrammatic representation of the dopaminergic system. Two dopaminergic systems originate and terminate outside of the hypothalamus: the *nigrostriatal* and *mesolimbic*. The hypothalamus contains three intrinsic dopaminergic systems: (i) the *incertohypothalamic*, with cell bodies in the caudal hypothalamus, zona incerta and rostral periventricular nucleus with terminals in the rostral preoptic area and septum; (ii) the *tuberoinfundibular*, with cell bodies in the arcuate and periventricular nuclei and terminals in the external zone of the ME adjacent to the primary capillary bed; (iii) the *tuberohypophysial*, with cell bodies in the rostral arcuate and periventricular nuclei and terminals in the intermediate and posterior lobe of the pituitary gland. The tuberoinfundibular and tuberohypophysial dopaminergic systems are responsible for delivering dopamine to the adenohypophysis through the portal vasculature.

spaces, neurosecretory axons, and pituicytes (modified astroglial cells). Within the intermediate lobe, these axons terminate on secretory cells known as melanotropes. It is believed that a portion of the dopamine that acts within the adenohypophysis originates from the axon terminals in the intermediate and posterior lobes, and ultimately reaches the anterior pituitary through short portal vessels. Within the hypothalamus, the incertohypothalamic dopaminer-

gic neurons appear to play a neuromodulatory role, and the tuberoinfundibular and tuberohypophyseal neurons subserve a neuroendocrine role.

2.5.1.2. Norepinephrine. The noradrenergic cell bodies of greatest importance to the hypothalamus are the *locus coeruleus* (Fig. 10). The efferents course toward the hypothalamus as the large *dorsal noradrenergic* (or *tegmental*) *bundle* and the *rostral limb of the dorsal periventricular pathway*. The former path-

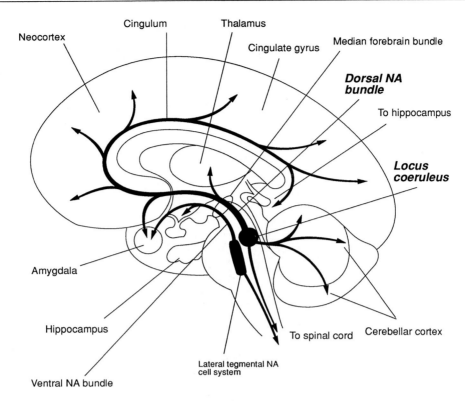

Fig. 10. Diagrammatic representation of the noradreneregic system. The cell bodies of greatest importance to the hypothalamus are located in the locus coeruleus, whose efferents course toward the hypothalamus as the dorsal noradrenergic bundle. These terminate in the paraventricular and arcuate nuclei of the hypothalamus as well as in the preoptic area.

way joins the ascending *ventral noradrenergic bundle* from the *lateral tegmental noradrenergic* cell groups. The dorsal and ventral noradrenergic pathways unite in the *median forebrain bundle* to enter the amygdala (dorsal) and hypothalamus (ventral).

2.5.1.3. Serotonin. Two groups of serotonergic cell bodies are found in the brain, in the *dorsal* and *medial raphe nuclei* (Fig. 11). Axons from the dorsal raphe nucleus form the *ventral ascending serotonergic pathway*, which sweep ventrally and then curve rostrally through the ventral tegmentum to join noradrenergic fibers of the median forebrain bundle in the lateral hypothalamic area. Two large fiber groups leave the ventral ascending pathway as it courses through the lateral hypothalamus—one directed laterally and the other ventromedially. The ventromedial fibers innervate many hypothalamic areas, including the lateral, medial preoptic, and anterior hypothalamic areas as well as the dorsomedial and VMN, the infundibulum, and the suprachiasmatic nuclei. In addition, the OVLT is rich in serotonin terminals.

2.5.2. Peptides

Time-honored steps must be taken to identify peptides as physiologically significant in the hypothalamus (Table 3). First, a quantitative bioassay must be established. A specific, dose-dependent relationship must be established between the amount of peptide and the biological response. Second, evidence must be provided that the biologically active material is peptidic in nature. This can be established by demonstrating that proteolytic enzymes diminish or destroy the biological activity. Third, a scheme for extraction and separation of maximal yields of the purified peptide must be devised. Fourth, chemical and physical characterization of the peptide must be performed. This would consist of mol-wt characterization as well as amino acid composition and sequencing. Fifth, once the sequence is known, the peptide must be synthesized and the synthetic product must be tested for biological activity in the bioassay. Sixth, antibodies to the peptide must be produced, and the purified antibodies must be characterized using synthetic analogs of the

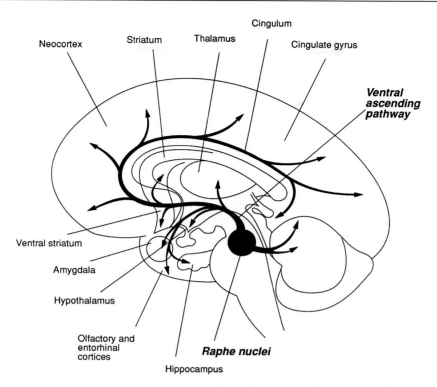

Fig. 11. Diagrammatic representation of the serotonergic system. The cell bodies of importance to hypothalamic function are found in the dorsal and medial raphe nuclei. Axons from the dorsal raphe form the ventral ascending serotonergic pathway, and enter the hypothalamus ventromedially to terminate in the anterior hypothalamus, dorsomedial and ventromedial nuclei, the suprachiasmatic nuclei, and the infundibulum. In addition, serotonergic terminals are found in the lateral and medial preoptic areas as well as the OVLT.

Table 3
Strategies in the Analysis of a Hypothalamic Neuropeptide

1. Development of quantitative bioassay.
2. Proof of peptidic nature.
3. Development of extraction scheme.
4. Chemical and physical characterization.
5. Synthesize peptide and determine its bioactivity.
6. Produce antibodies to the peptide.
7. Use antibodies for immunocytochemical localization and radioimmunoassay.
8. Isolate the cDNA encoding the precursor of the peptide.

peptide. Several immunologic approaches with the antibodies must be developed. This would consist of immunocytochemistry for visualization of peptides in neural tissue, as well as radioimmunoassay for quantitation of the concentration of the peptide in neural tissue and portal blood. Finally, the cDNA that encodes the precursor of the peptide must be isolated, and methods such as *in situ* hybridization histochemistry and Northern blotting must be developed for detecting the mRNA of the precursor. Most of these approaches have been taken to identify the peptides of importance to hypothalamic function.

Six arbitrary classes of peptides are involved in hypothalamic function (Table 4): *hypophysiotropic peptides* (Fig. 12), which affect the function of the adenohypophysis; the *neurohypophyseal peptides* (Fig. 13), which control blood pressure, water retention, milk ejection, and smooth-muscle contraction;

Table 4
Classes of Hypothalamic Peptides

Class	Function	Example
1. Hypophysiotropic peptides	Regulate adenohypophysis.	TRH, GnRH, GHRH, CRH, somatostatin
2. Neurohypophysial peptides	Regulate water retention, blood pressure, milk ejection, uterine contraction.	Vasopressin, oxytocin
3. Brain-gut peptides	Neuromodulatory, neuroendocrine.	VIP, CCK, substance P
4. POMC-derived peptides	Neuromodulatory, neuroendocrine.	Endorphins, ACTH
5. Dynorphin-derived peptides	Neuromodulatory, neuroendocrine.	Met-enkephalin, leu-enkephalin
6. "Other" peptides	Neuromodulatory, neuroendocrine.	Angiotensin II, NPY, galanin, endothelins

LHRH: p^1Glu-His-Trp-Ser-Tyr-Gly-Leu-Arg-Pro-Gly^{10}-NH$_2$

TRH: p^1Glu-His-Pro^3-NH$_2$

CRH: ^{1}Ser-Gln-Glu-Pro-Pro-Ile-Ser-Leu-Asp-Leu-Thr-Phe-His-Leu-Leu-Arg-Glu-Val-Leu-Glu-Met-
(ovine) Thr-Lys-Ala-Asp-Gln-Leu-Ala-Gln-Gln-Ala-His-Ser-Asn-Arg-Lys-Leu-Leu-Asp-Ile-Ala^{41}NH$_2$

GHRH: ^{1}Tyr-Ala-Asp-Ala-Ile-Phe-Thr-Asn-Ser-Tyr-Arg-Lys-Val-Leu-Gly-Gln-Leu-Ser-Ala-Arg-Lys-
Leu-Leu-Gln-Asp-Ile-Met-Ser-Arg-Gln-Gln-Gly-Glu-Ser-Asn-Gln-Glu-Arg-Gly-Ala-Arg-Ala-
Arg-Leu^{44}-NH$_2$

Somatostatin: ^{1}Ala-Gly-Cys-Lys-Asn-Phe-Phe-Trp-Lys-Thr-Phe-Thr-Ser-Cys^{14}

Fig. 12. Amino acid sequences of the *hypothalamic hypophysiotropic peptides*, so named because they all regulate pituitary function directly. The superscript "1" represents the amino terminus, and the carboxyl terminus is designated with the greater suprascript number. Note that the Glu at position 1 of LHRH and TRH is designated pyro (p) and that LHRH, TRH, CRH, and GHRH all are amidated at their carboxy termini.

Arginine Vasopressin: ^{1}Cys-Tyr-Phe-Glu-Asn-Cys-Pro-Arg-Gly^9-NH$_2$

Oxytocin: ^{1}Cys-Tyr-Ile-Glu-Asn-Cys-Pro-Leu-Gly^9-NH$_2$

Fig. 13. Amino acid sequences of the *neurohypophyseal peptide* hormones. Note that they share common features: both are nonapeptides, have an intramolecular disulphide bond and are amidated at the carboxyl terminal. The differences that account for their differing bioactivities are found at positions 3 and 8. In addition, a closely related *pressor peptide*, lysine vasopressin, differs from AVP by substituting lys for arg in position 8.

brain-gut peptides (Fig. 14), which serve a predominantly neuromodulatory function; the *POMC-derived peptides* (Fig.15), which also subserve a neuromodulatory role in hypothalamic function; the *enkepha-* *lins* (Fig. 16), which also serve as modulatory peptides that are found in the hypothalamus and those found outside of the hypothalamus that effect hypothalamic function. Other peptides, such as *angiotensin II*, neu-

Substance P: ^{1}Arg-Pro-Lys-Pro-Glu-Glu-Phe-Phe-Gly-Leu-Met^{11}-NH$_2$

VIP: ^{1}His-Ser-Asp-Ala-Val-Phe-Thr-Asp-Asn-Tyr-Thr-Arg-Leu-Arg-Lys-Glu-Met-Ala-Val-Lys-Lys-Tyr-Leu-Asn-Ser-Ile-Leu-Asn^2-NH$_2$

CCK (8): ^{1}Asp-Tyr-Met-Gly-Trp-Met-Asp-Phe^8-NH$_2$
                    |
                   SO$_3$

NT: p^{1}Glu-Leu-Tyr-Glu-Asn-Lys-Pro-Arg-Arg-Pro-Tyr-Ile-Leu^{13}

Fig. 14. Amino acid sequences of the hypothalamic *brain-gut peptides*, so named because they are localized and active in both the brain and gastrointestinal system.

ACTH: ^{1}Ser-Tyr-Ser-Met-Glu-His-Phe-Arg-Trp-Gly-Lys-Pro-Val-Gly-Lys-Lys-Arg-Arg-Pro-Val-Lys-Val-Tyr-Pro-Asn-Gly-Ala-Glu-Asp-Glu-Leu-Ala-Glu-Ala-Phe-Pro-Leu-Glu-Phe^{39}

β-LPH: ^{1}Glu-Leu-Thr-Gly-Gln-Arg-Leu-Arg-Glu-Gly-Asp-Gly-Pro-Asp-Gly-Pro-Ala-Asp-Asp-Gly-Ala-Gly-Ala-Gln-Ala-Asp-Leu-Glu-His-Ser-Leu-Leu-Val-Ala-Ala-Glu-Lys-Lys-Asp-Glu-Gly-Pro-Tyr-Arg-Met-Glu-His-Phe-Arg-Trp-Gly-Ser-Pro-Pro-Lys-Asp-Lys-Arg-Tyr-Gly-Gly-Phe-Met-Thr-Ser-Glu-Lys-Ser-Gln-Thr-Pro-Leu-Val-Thr-Leu-Phe-Lys-Asn-Ala-Ile-Ile-Lys-Asn-Ala-Tyr-Lys-Lys-Gly-Glu^{89}

α-MSH: Ac-^{1}Ser-Tyr-Ser-Met-Glu-His-Phe-Arg-Trp-Gly-Lys-Pro-Val^{13}-NH$_2$

γ-LPH: ^{1}Glu-Leu-Thr-Gly-Gln-Arg-Leu-Arg-Glu-Gly-Asp-Gly-Pro-Asp-Gly-Pro-Ala-Asp-Asp-Gly-Ala-Gly-Ala-Gln-Ala-Asp-Leu-Glu-His-Ser-Leu-Leu-Val-Ala-Ala-Glu-Lys-Lys-Asp-Glu-Gly-Pro-Tyr-Arg-Met-Glu-His-Phe-Arg-Trp-Gly-Ser-Pro-Pro-Lys-Asp^{56}

β-END: ^{1}Tyr-Gly-Gly-Phe-Met-Thr-Ser-Glu-Lys-Ser-Gln-Thr-Pro-Leu-Val-Thr-Leu-Phe-Lys-Asn-Ala-Ile-Ile-Lys-Asn-Ala-Tyr-Lys-Lys-Gly^{31}

β-MSH: ^{1}Asp-Glu-Gly-Pro-Tyr-Arg-Met-Glu-His-Phe-Arg-Trp-Gly-Ser-Pro-Pro-Lys-Asp^{18}

γ-MSH: ^{1}Tyr-Val-Met-Gly-His-Phe-Arg-Trp-Asp-Arg-Phe-Gly^{12}

Fig. 15. Amino acid sequences of the hypothalamic peptides derived from *proopiomelanocortin*.

Met-Enk: ^{1}Tyr-Gly-Gly-Phe-Met^5

Leu-Enk: ^{1}Tyr-Gly-Gly-Phe-Leu^5

Fig. 16. Amino acid sequences of the *enkephalins*. Note that the sole difference between them is in position 5.

ropeptide Y and the endothelins (Fig. 17) could stand as a class by themselves because they may play a variety of neuroendocrine, neuromodulatory, neurotransmitter, and hormonal roles.

2.5.2.1. Hypophysiotropic Peptides. Of all the neuropeptides that control the function of the adenohypophysis, the chemiarchitecture of *luteinizing hormone-releasing hormone (GnRH)* is perhaps the most

Table 5
Localization of the Hypophysiotropic Peptides

Peptide	Cell Bodies	Fibers	Terminals	Present in portal blood
GnRH	Medial septal nucleus, nucleus of the diagonal band of broca, bed nucleus region of stria terminalis, OVLT, medial preoptic nucleus, anterior hypothalamic area, arcuate nucleus, ME, olfactory tubercle.	Continuum from septal region to premammillary nucleus.	ME, neurohypophysis, suprachiasmatic nucleus, ependymal lining of ventricles, olfactory bulb, amygdala.	+
TRH	Periventricular area, paraventricular nucleus, dorsomedial/ventromedial nuclei, arcuate nucleus.	Paraventricular nucleus, periventricular hypothalamic area, dorsomedial nucleus perifornical region, nucleus accumbens, bed nucleus of stria terminalis, spinal cord.	ME	+
CRH	Paraventricular nucleus, supraoptic nuclei, arcuate nuclei dorsal raphe nucleus, hippocampus, OVLT, medial preoptic nucleus, bed nucleus of stria terminalis, locus coeruleus.	Septal nuclei, stria terminalis, median forebrain bundle.	ME	+
GHRH	Arcuate nucleus.		ME	+
SS	Preoptic/anterior hypothalamic area, paraventricular nucleus.		ME, suprachiasmatic nucleus.	+

+ = Yes, in concentrations greater than peripheral blood.
– = No, concentrations the same as or lower than peripheral blood.

widely studied. GnRH-positive cell-body fibers and terminals are not restricted to the hypothalamus. They are scattered over a continuum extending from the septal region from the septal region to the premammillary region (Table 5). These are found in the medial septal nucleus, the nucleus of the diagonal band of Broca, the bed nucleus of the stria terminalis, the OVLT, the medial preoptic nucleus, the anterior hypothalamic area, the supraoptic nucleus, and the arcuate nucleus. Cell bodies in the arcuate nucleus and the adjacent medial ME area give rise to short axons, which pass to the infundibulum and form a dense plexus around the primary capillary bed of the hypothalamo-hypophyseal portal system in the ME. These are the cells that control the secretion of LH from the adenohypophysis. In some mammals, these same cells have axons that terminate directly in the neurohypophysis. These axons are of unknown function, but their termini in the neurohypophysis adjacent to the adenohypophysis suggests that they may play a role in adenohypophyseal function. GnRH-positive cells in the medial preoptic nucleus send projections to the suprachiasmatic nucleus and the ME. Cells in the medial septal nucleus and the diagonal band of Broca also contribute to this projection. Other GnRH-positive cells from these areas terminate in the OVLT to form a dense plexus around the capillary network, suggesting another vascular route through which the peptide reaches the anterior pituitary. GnRH-positive cells originating in the medial preoptic nucleus, the bed nucleus of the stria terminalis, and the septum send fibers that terminate on the ependymal linings of the third and lateral ventricles. This suggests that the cerebrospinal fluid (CSF) may be an additional vehicle for transport of GnRH. In the medial septal nucleus, the diagonal band of Broca, and the olfactory tubercle, a few groups of GnRH-positive cells terminate upon blood vessels in this area. In addition, GnRH-positive cells in the medial preoptic nucleus, medial septal nucleus, and the diagonal band of

Angiotensin II: ^{1}Asp-Arg-Val-Tyr-Ile-His-Pro-Phe^8

Human NPY: ^{1}Tyr-Pro-Ser-Lys-Pro-Asp-Asn-Pro-Gly-Gln-Asp-Ala-Pro-Ala-Gln-Asp-Met-Ala-Arg-Tyr-Tyr-Ser-Ala-Leu-Arg-His-Tyr-Ile-Asn-Leu-Ile-Thr-Arg-Gln-Arg-Tyr^{36}-NH$_2$

Rat Galanin: ^{1}Gly-Trp-Thr-Leu-Asn-Ser-Ala-Gly-Tyr-Leu-Leu-Gly-Pro-His-Ala-Ile-Asp-Asn-His-Arg-Ser-Phe-Ser-Asp-Lys-His-Gly-Leu-Thr^{29}-NH$_2$

Endothelin 1: ^{1}Cys-Ser-Cys-Ser-Ser-Leu-Met-Asp-Lys-Glu-Cys-Val-Tyr-Phe-Cys-His-Leu-Asp-Ile-Ile-Trp^{21}

Endothelin 2: ^{1}Cys-Ser-Cys-Asp-Ser-Trp-Leu-Asp-Lys-Glu-Cys-Val-Tyr-Phe-Cys-His-Ile-Ile-Trp^{21}

Endothelin 3: ^{1}Cys-Thr-Cys-Phe-Thr-Tyr-Lys-Asp-Lys-Glu-Cys-Val-Tyr-Tyr-Cys-His-Leu-Asp-Ile-Ile-Trp^{21}

Fig. 17. Amino acid sequences of some of the *other peptides* localized in the hypothalamus and controlling hypothalamic function. Among the unusual features, note that the endothelins have two intramolecular disulphide bonds.

Broca terminate in the external plexiform and glomerular layers of the olfactory bulb. The medial preoptic nucleus also provides fibers to the amygdala through the stria terminalis. Although the GnRH neurons originating in the preoptic and arcuate nuclei that terminate in the ME have been shown to play a direct role in cyclic LH release, termini in other areas such as the olfactory system, the amygdala, the habenula, and the mesencephalic gray have not been assigned a firmly established functional role in reproductive processes. It is likely that these areas play a role in control of pituitary hormone secretion and the behaviors related to reproduction that are controlled by GnRH not as a neurohormone but as a neuromodulator. Finally, it is interesting to note that GnRH is not confined to the central nervous system (CNS). In the sympathetic ganglia of the bullfrog, a peptide that resembles GnRH and is co-localized with acetylcholine elicits prolonged excitatory postsynaptic potentials (EPSPs) with long latencies. This would categorize GnRH as a neurotransmitter.

The *Thyrotropin-Releasing Hormone (TRH)*, the physiological stimulator of TSH release from the adenohypophysis, is found widely throughout the nervous system of mammals (Table 5). In fact, only approximately one-third of the total amount of the peptide found in the brain is localized to the hypothalamus. Thus, TRH is believed to play both a neuromodulatory and neuroendocrine role. The highest concentration of TRH in the hypothalamus is found in the ME with significant levels in the dorsomedial,

ventromedial, and arcuate nuclei. Extrahypothalamic structures such as the preoptic and septal areas as well as the motor nuclei of some cranial nerves also contain significant levels of TRH. Within the hypothalamus, TRH-positive cell bodies are found in the periventricular area, the paraventricular nucleus, the dorsomedial and ventromedial nuclei, and the arcuate nucleus/ME area. TRH-positive nerve terminals are found in the greatest abundance in the external layer of the ME, with dense fiber networks in the parvicellular part of the paraventricular nucleus, the periventricular hypothalamic area, the dorsomedial nucleus, the perifornical region, the nucleus acumbens, and the bed nucleus of the stria terminalis. TRH-positive fibers are also found in the spinal cord.

Corticotropin-releasing hormone (CRH), the physiological stimulator for the release of ACTH from the adenohypophysis, has been localized in hypothalamic and extrahypothalamic sites (Table 5). CRH-positive cells are found in greatest abundance in the paraventricular nucleus of the hypothalamus. Although most of the cells are parvicellular, some are members of the magnocellular population of this nucleus. Axons from the CRH-positive cells of the paraventricular nucleus project to a so-called *neurohemal area* that encompasses the external zone of the ME. These cells provide the CRH to the portal vasculature, bathing the adenohypophysis and stimulating the release of ACTH and β-endorphin. CRH-positive cell bodies have also been identified in the supraoptic and arcuate nuclei in the hypothalamus, with additional groups of cell bodies in the dorsal raphe nucleus, the hippocampus, and the OVLT. Scattered CRH cell bodies are found throughout the lateral preoptic lateral hypothalamic continuum, and numerous cell bodies have been identified in the medial preoptic nucleus and the bed nucleus of the stria terminalis. In the midbrain, CRH-staining cells are found in the reticular formation (RF) and the periaqueductal gray. Moreover, CRH has been co-localized with the catecholamines in the locus coeruleus. CRH-immunoreactive fibers originating from the bed nucleus of the stria terminalis enter the lateral and medial septal nuclei. Numerous fibers found within the stria terminalis and the ventral amygdalofugal pathway connect the rostral hypothalamus and basal telencephalon with the amygdala. Fibers originating from the telencephalon/diencephalon course caudally through the median forebrain bundle and split into a dorsal pathway throughout the brainstem and a ventral pathway to the lateral part of the RF. Although a well founded physiological role has been ascribed to the hypothalamic paraventricular-ME pathway, a role for the other pathways has not been similarly characterized. Since ACTH-immunoreactive cell bodies and fibers of unknown function have been found throughout the brain localized closely with CRH, it is possible that this reflects the same regulatory relationship described for pituitary ACTH.

Growth hormone-releasing hormone (GHRH), the physiological stimulator of growth-hormone secretion from the adenohypophysis, has been found in hypothalamic, non-hypothalamic, and even non-neural sites (Table 5). The concentration of immunoreactive GHRH in the hypothalamus is highest in the arcuate nucleus/ME area, which is probably a reflection of its neuroendocrine role at the pituitary gland. Immunocytochemical localization studies have revealed GHRH-positive cell bodies in the arcuate nucleus, with short axons terminating in the arcuate nucleus and the ME. Some of these GHRH cell bodies also contain neurotensin, and others contain galanin. The physiological significance of this dual packaging is unknown. Interestingly, surgical isolation of the medial basal hypothalamus does not lead to a significant decline in the concentration of GHRH in the arcuate nucleus ME area. Thus, virtually all of the hypothalamic GHRH originates from cells in this area. Significant amounts of GHRH are also found in some nonneural sites. Specifically, both GHRH-messenger RNA and newly synthesized GHRH are found in somatotropes of the adenohypophysis. This has led to the belief that some degree of growth-hormone secretion is intrinsic

through an autocrine relationship. Other locations of GHRH cells lack a compelling physiological explanation. GHRH has been found in the ovary and the placenta—sites for which a role for GHRH has yet to be described.

Growth hormone release-inhibiting hormone or somatostatin (SS), as its name implies, inhibits the secretion of growth hormone or somatotropin from the adenohypophysis. However, the name does not fully represent the variety of roles played by this neurohormone. SS also inhibits the release of thyrotropin and prolactin from the adenohypophysis. In addition to its location in the hypothalamus, SS is widely distributed throughout the CNS (Table 5), suggesting that it may be a neurotransmitter or neuromodulator as well as a neurohormone. Of interest to control of growth-hormone secretion, SS-positive cell bodies are quite abundant in the preoptic-anterior hypothalamic area. Parvicellular SS-positive cells are also found in the paraventricular nucleus. These areas send axons as a group caudally to terminate in the suprachiasmatic nucleus, as well as the arcuate nucleus/ME area. Fibers pass from the preoptic area terminate in the primary capillary bed of the ME. This is the source of SS, which directly inhibits growth-hormone secretion from the adenohypophysis. Moreover, these same preoptic SS fibers synapse on GHRH cell bodies in the arcuate nucleus. This suggests two levels of inhibition of growth-hormone secretion by SS: directly at the somatotrope and secondarily at the GHRH neuron. Finally, SS can be found outside of the nervous system. Within the endocrine pancreas a specific cell type—the delta cell—synthesizes and secretes SS that is identical to that made by hypothalamic neurons. Pancreatic SS plays numerous roles in the gastrointestinal tract. In addition, SS directly affects pancreatic insulin and glucagon secretion.

2.5.2.2. Neurohypophyseal Hormones. *Arginine-vasopressin (AVP)*—which is also known as *antidiuretic hormone (ADH)*—and another neurohormone, *oxytocin (OT),* are produced in magnocellular (e.g., large) neurons whose cell bodies are located in the *supraoptic* (AVP) and *paraventricular* (OT) nuclei of the hypothalamus (Table 6). They are synthesized as *prohormones,* or precursor proteins, in the cell body (Fig. 18). These large molecules consist of packaging peptides and specific axonal transport peptides, *neurophysins (NP),* as well as the bioactive fragment AVP or OT, which is ultimately found in the peripheral circulation. There are actually two forms of the NPs. NP-I, or estrogen-linked neurophysin, is

Table 6
Localization of Neurohypophyseal Peptides

Peptide	Cell bodies	Fibers	Terminals	Presence in portal blood
OT	Paraventricular nucleus, supraoptic nucleus.	Hypothalamo–hypophysial tract.	Neurohypophysis, ME.	+
AVP	Supraoptic nucleus, paraventricular nucleus, suprachiasmatic nucleus, bed nucleus of stria terminalis, nucleus of diagonal band of broca, amygdala.	Hypothalamo–hypophysial tract, septum, thalamus, hippocampus.	Neurohypophysis, ME OVLT, dorsomedial nucleus.	+

+ = Yes, in concentrations greater than peripheral blood.
− = No, concentrations the same as or lower than peripheral blood.

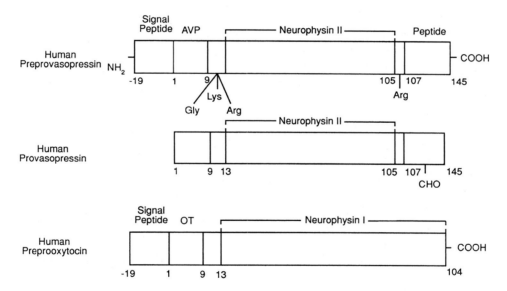

Fig. 18. The structure of human preprovasopressin, provasopressin, and preprooxytocin. Note that preprovasopressin is 21 K_d and consists of a signal peptide, the AVP sequence; a tripeptide spacer, neurophysin II (also called nicotine-linked neurophysin); a spacer glycosylation signal (Arg), and a 39-amino-acid carboxyl terminal. Provasopressin is a 19-K_d product of preprovasopressin from which the signal sequence has been deleted and carbohydrate (CHO) added to the C-terminal peptide posttranslationally. Preprooxytocin is smaller than preprovasopressin, with a different neurophysin, and the posttranslational modifications do not include glycosylation.

associated with OT and NP-II, or nicotine-linked neurophysin is associated with AVP. Both NPs are 9.5–10 K_d The translation product of the AVP gene is a 21-K_d protein known as *preprovasopressin* (Fig. 18), which in humans consists of a 19-aa signal peptide at the amino terminal, vasopressin (9 aa), a 3-aa spacer sequence, NP-II (93 aa), another spacer sequence (1 aa), and a 39-aa peptide at the carboxyl terminal. *Provasopressin* (19 K_d) is the peptide with the 19-aa

signal sequence cleaved and carbohydrate added posttranslationally to the C-terminal peptide. Oxytocin is synthesized in a similar fashion, with the exception that there is no glycopeptide at the carboxyl terminus and the prohormone is significantly smaller—15 K_d (Fig. 18). In both cases, the NP is required as a carrier protein to the axon terminal and presumably prolongs the half-life of the neuropeptide. The peptide-NP complex is exocytosed into fenestrated capillaries, where the respective NP is cleaved from either OT or AVP. Originally it was believed that the cell bodies of the supraoptic nucleus exclusively contained AVP, and the cell bodies of the paraventricular nucleus contained exclusively OT. We now know that both types of nuclei are found in each area. Axons from each of these nuclei form the *hypothalamo–hypophyseal tract*, which terminates upon sinusoids in the neurohypophysis. OT and AVP can also be transported from the neurohypophysis to the adenohypophysis through the short portal vessels connecting these two areas. The paraventricular nucleus also sends fibers to the ME, where they terminate upon the primary capillaries from which the long portal vessels project to bathe the adenohypophysis. This is the pathway by which AVP reaches the corticotrope and stimulates ACTH secretion. It is well-known that AVP is an *accessory* ACTH-releasing factor of hypothalamic origin. Also, the caudal portion of the paraventricular nucleus contains *parvicellular* or small neurons, which contain mostly OT and some AVP. These neurons also project to the ME as well as other parts of the brain and spinal cord. Therefore, significant quantities of OT are found in portal blood. The parvicellular part of the paraventricular nucleus also sends fibers to the locus coeruleus, the parabranchial nuclei, the dorsal motor vagal nucleus, the nucleus of the solitary tract, the midbrain central gray and the dorsal horn of the spinal cord. Localization of AVP and OT fibers in the lower brainstem and autonomic centers may reflect their roles in such peripheral processes as the regulation of blood pressure and lactation. Other parvicellular neurons are found in the suprachiasmatic nucleus. These almost exclusively contain AVP and project to the OVLT, the dorsomedial hypothalamic nucleus, and the thalamus. Also outside of the supraoptic and paraventricular nuclei, AVP cells have been found in the bed nucleus of the stria terminalis to the nucleus of the diagonal band of Broca and lateral septum, the anterior amygdala, the lateral habenular nucleus , the mesencephalic central gray, and the locus coeruleus. The location of AVP fibers in the septum is compatible with a role of the peptide in thermoregulation, and the presence of fibers in the mediodorsal thalamic nucleus, the hippocampus, and the neocortex is compatible with a role for this peptide in learning and memory.

2.5.2.3. Brain-Gut Peptides.

This group of peptides is so named because the activities have been characterized by immunocytochemistry within the gastrointestinal tract as well as the hypothalamus (Table 7). In addition to many of them being localized in the hypothalamus, a neuroendocrine role for some have been identified.

Substance P has been found in extracts of the brain and intestine. Its structure is known, and it has been implicated in pain perception, baroreception, and chemoreception. In the monkey, substance P cell bodies have been found in the most lateral portions of the arcuate nucleus. Fibers pass to the external zone of the ME and also to the neurohypophysis. In the rat, substance P-positive cells are found in the medial and lateral preoptic areas, the anterior hypothalamic area, and the dorsomedial and ventromedial nuclei. Substance P-containing afferent pathways project to the supraoptic and paraventricular nuclei as well as the arcuate nucleus. However, despite the location of substance P fibers in the neurohemal zone of the ME, the levels of substance P in portal blood is essentially equivalent to that of peripheral blood; thus eliminating it as a neurohormone. Substance P and its receptors are also found within the adenohypophysis. Alternatively, substance P may be found in the anterior lobe as a paracrine agent rather than as a neurohormone. Substance P plays a role in the secretion of all the important anterior pituitary hormones, either by acting directly on the specific cells of the gland or indirectly as a neuromodulator affecting the release of the releasing hormones of hypothalamic origin.

Vasoactive intestinal polypeptide (VIP) is present in large quantities throughout the gastrointestinal tract, where it plays multiple roles in digestive processes. For example, it is vasodilatory, glycogenolytic, and lipolytic. It enhances insulin secretion, inhibits gastric acid production, and stimulates secretion from the exocrine pancreas and small intestine. Since it exerts some of its effects through vascular pathways, it fits the description of a true hormone. Neuronal VIP is found in highest concentrations in the cerebral cortex, where it acts as an excitatory neurotransmitter or neuromodulator. Within the hypothalamus, the suprachiasmatic nuclei contain very dense concentrations of VIP-positive cell bodies. Efferents from these course dorsally and then split into a dense rostro-dorsal component and a less dense caudal component. The rostrodorsal fibers terminate on the paraventricular nucleus, and the caudal fibers terminate at the dorsomedial, ventromedial, and premammillary nuclei. Like substance P, VIP is found in high concentrations

Table 7
Localization of Brain-Gut Peptides

Peptide	Cell bodies	Terminals	Presence in portal blood
Substance P	Arcuate nucleus, preoptic area, anterior hypothalamic area, dorsomedial/ventromedial nuclei.	ME, neurohypophysis, supraoptic nucleus, paraventricular nucleus, arcuate nucleus.	+
VIP	Suprachiasmatic nucleus.	Paraventricular nucleus, dorsomedial/ventromedial nuclei.	+
CCK	Cortex, striatum, amygdala supraoptic nucleus, para-ventricular nucleus, neurohypophysis, preoptic area, dorsomedial nucleus.	ME.	−
NT	Preoptic area, anterior hypothalamic area, medial preoptic area, paraventricular nucleus, dorsomedial nucleus, arcuate nucleus.	ME, neurohypophysis.	+

+ = Yes, in concentrations greater than peripheral blood.
− = No, concentrations the same as or lower than peripheral blood.

in the adenohypophysis. However, unlike substance P, it is also found in high concentrations in portal blood. There is also evidence that it may be synthesized in the adenohypophysis. VIP has been shown to affect adenohypophyseal hormone secretion as a transmitter/neuromodulator, as a neurohormone, and as a local autocrine or paracrine agent.

Cholecystokinin (CCK) is synthesized in the duodenum, and stimulates the secretion of pancreatic enzymes and the ejection of bile from the gallbladder. Unfortunately, CCK occurs in multiple molecular forms, which complicates the description of its tissue distribution. Duodenal CCK is composed of 33 or 39 amino acids. The carboxy-terminal octapeptide of CCK (CCK8) which has full biological activity, shares a pentapeptide sequence with gastrin, another gastrointestinal hormone. However, for the most part, whereas CCK8 occurs throughout the CNS, gastrin-like peptides are found only in the pituitary gland and hypothalamus. The highest concentrations of immunoreactive CCK8 are found in the cortex, striatum, and amygdala, with lesser amounts in the hypothalamus. CCK-like immunoreactivity has been found in the

magnocellular systems of the supraoptic and paraventricular nuclei of the hypothalamus, as well as the neurohypophysis. In some neurons, OT and CCK are co-localized. Physiological perturbations that stimulate the release of AVP and OT lower neurohypophyseal CCK. Parvicellular CCK-positive cells project axons that terminate in the ME. In addition to these, CCK cells are found in the medial preoptic area as well as the dorsomedial and supramammillary nuclei. Functionally, CCK has been implicated as a neuromodulator in the control of pituitary hormone release. As such, it probably facilitates the release of the hypothalamic-releasing hormones as well as OT and AVP. It has also been shown that CCK may be copackaged with many of the hypothalamic peptides. There is no definitive direct evidence implicating CCK as a neurohormone.

Neurotensin (NT) is a peptide consisting of 13 amino acids, which was first isolated from the brain and later from the intestine. In general, NT is a peptide neurotransmitter is found in highest concentrations in the hypothalamus, and seems to play a role in the control of release of the adenohypophyseal hormones.

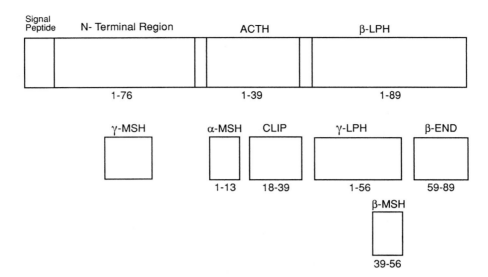

Fig. 19. Human POMC and its cleavage products. The numbers below each bar represent the number of amino acids of the parent peptides (*upper bar*) or the position in the parent peptides from which the products are cleaved (*middle* and *lower bars*).

NT-positive cell bodies are found in the preoptic and anterior hypothalamic areas, the medial preoptic nucleus, the magnocellular and parvicellular zones of the paraventricular nucleus, the arcuate nucleus, and the dorsomedial nucleus. In the arcuate nucleus, NT is colocalized in tuberoinfundibular dopaminergic neurons. The biological significance of this common packaging is not yet fully appreciated. However, it has been suggested that NT mediates the release of dopamine into the portal vasculature. NT-positive fibers are also localized to the external zone of the ME. In addition, NT is present in portal blood, and thus may assume the role of a classic neurohormone. When placed into the brain, NT can affect the secretion of prolactin, growth hormone, TSH, and LH, yet its placement directly into pituitary-cell cultures is only effective at supraphysiological doses. This suggests that NT acts within the hypothalamus as a neuromodulator/neurotransmitter, and perhaps not directly at the pituitary cell. In addition to NT fibers terminating at the external zone of the ME, some NT-positive axon terminals are found in the neurohypophysis. These probably originate in the paraventricular nucleus and play a role in the release of OT and AVP. Finally, the adenohypophysis contains cells that stain NT-positive. It seems unlikely that this material arises from neuronal sources, but it is probably synthesized directly in the pituitary, where it plays a paracrine or autocrine role in the secretion of one or more of the adenohypophyseal hormones.

2.5.2.4. POMC-Derived Peptides.

POMC is a large mol-wt precursor protein (265 aa), which in the human (with subtle differences between mammals) is post-translationally cleaved into moieties *ACTH (39 aa), β-lipotropin (β-LPH; 89 aa)* and a *16-K N-terminal fragment* of 76 aa (Fig. 19). Each of these is further cleaved enzymatically to yield: *α-melanophore-stimulating hormone (α-MSH=ACTH$_{1-13}$)*, and *corticotropin-like intermediate-lobe peptide (CLIP=ACTH$_{18-39}$)*. β-LPH is further cleaved into *γ-LPH (β-LPH$_{1-56}$)* and the endogenous opioid *β-endorphin (β-end=β-LPH$_{59-89}$)*. β-MSH is a cleavage product of LPH $_{(39-56)}$, and *γ-MSH* is a fragment of the 16k N-terminal peptide. These are widely distributed in the CNS (Table 8).

Aside from the adenohypophysis, ACTH is found in cells of the arcuate nucleus/ME area. The cells are diffusely distributed throughout this area, which extends rostrally to the retrochiasmatic area, caudally to the submammillary region, and dorsally to the area between the ventricular surface and the VMN of the hypothalamus. The fact that hypophysectomy does not influence the amount of ACTH in this area indicates that this activity is *not* a product of the corticotropes of the adenohypophysis. Thus, ACTH is actually formed in the brain. Since ACTH and other peptides are common products of POMC, it is not surprising that β-LPH, α-MSH, β-MSH, and β-END are colocalized with ACTH in these neurons. These neurons give rise to numerous ACTH-positive fibers, which are distributed widely throughout the brain. Within the hypothalamus, ACTH fibers terminate in the anterior, mediobasal, and periventricular areas of the hypothala-

Table 8
Localization of POMC-Derived Peptides

Peptide	Cell bodies	Terminals	Presence in portal blood
ACTH	Arcuate Nucleus, ME Area.	Anterior Hypothalamic Periventricular area dorsomedial nucleus, para-ventricular Nucleus, OVLT, ME, preoptic area.	+*
β-LPH	Same as ACTH		ND
γ-MSH	Same as ACTH		+*
β-END	Same as ACTH		+

+ = Yes, in concentrations greater than peripheral blood.
− = No, concentrations the same as or less than peripheral blood.
ND = Not determined.
* = Probably by retrograde blood flow from pituitary gland.

mus. In the periventricular area, the fibers actually penetrate the ependymal lining of the third ventricle. ACTH is measurable in the CSF. ACTH terminals are found in the dorsomedial nucleus, the magnocellular and parvicellular portions of the paraventricular nucleus, and the OVLT. In addition, ACTH terminals are found in the external zone of the ME close to the portal capillaries, as well as within the neurohypophysis. Terminals are also found in the medial preoptic area.

β-LPH cell bodies are also found in the arcuate nucleus/ME area, with fibers projecting to various areas of the brain. In general, ACTH-positive fibers and β-LPH fibers project to the same areas of the brain. β-LPH is also found in the corticotropes of the adenohypophysis. These common distribution patterns are reasonable, considering the common precursor of both.

α-MSH is secreted from the intermediate lobe of the pituitary gland in all vertebrates. Although it has a dramatic skin-coloring effect in poikilotherms, the role of α-MSH in homeotherms is uncertain. There is some suggestion that it may play a role in the secretion of hormones from the adenohypophysis. Within the hypothalamus, α-MSH-positive cell bodies and fibers are found in the same areas of the arcuate nucleus/ME that were described for ACTH. The fibers, for the most part, project to the same areas as the ACTH-positive groups. There is also a second group of α-MSH-positive cells, which are distinct from those in the medial basal hypothalamus. These cells are concentrated in the area between the dorsomedial nucleus and in the

fornix and in the lateral hypothalamic area. These cells do not colocalize α-MSH with any other of the POMC-derived peptides, suggesting that the biosynthetic route of α-MSH in these cells may be quite different than that of the mediobasal hypothalamus or the intermediate lobe of the pituitary gland. Fibers from this group project to the caudate-putamen complex, the neocortex and various parts of the hippocampus. As with the POMC-derived peptides, β-END-positive cell bodies are most numerous in the arcuate nucleus/ME area of the hypothalamus, and the course of their efferent projections is similar to ACTH, LPH, and MSH. Similarly, β-END is also found in the intermediate lobe of the pituitary gland. β-END is also found in significant concentrations in hypophyseal portal blood. Thus, β-END qualifies as a neurotransmitter/neuromodulator as well as a neurohormone. Since β-END binds to opiate receptors throughout the nervous system, it has been classified an endogenous opioid.

2.5.2.5 Enkephalins. The opioid peptides are derived from three different precursors. The derivation of β-END from POMC has been described. Smaller opioids known as the enkephalins (ENK) are pentapeptides derived from larger molecules known as *proenkephalins* (Fig. 20). One, proenkephalin A (50 K_d, 267 aa), contains four copies of *methionine-ENK (met-ENK)* and one copy of *leucine-ENK (leu-ENK)*, and one copy each of a met-ENK C-terminal heptapeptide and a met-ENK C-terminal octapeptide. The other, proenkephalin B (also known as prodynorphin) contains three copies of leu-ENK. The

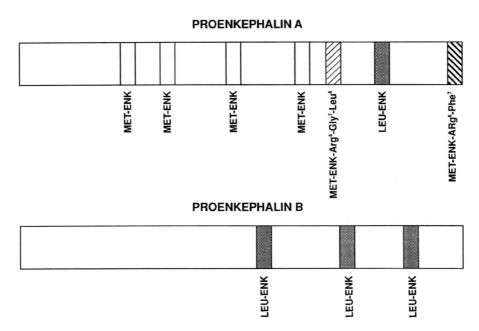

Fig. 20. The structure of proenkephalin A and proenkephalin B. Note the four repeating met-ENK sequences, the single leu-ENK, and each single met-ENK heptapeptide and octapeptide characteristic of proenkephalin A. Proenkephalin B is characterized by three intramolecular leu-ENK sequences.

Table 9
Localization of Enkephalins

Peptide	Cell bodies	Terminals	Presence in portal blood
Met-ENK	Supraoptic nucleus, paraventricular nucleus preoptic area, dorsomedial/ventromedial nuclei.	ME, neurohypophysis.	+
Leu-ENK	Same as Met-ENK.		+

+ = Yes, in concentrations greater than peripheral blood.
− = No, concentrations the same as or less than peripheral blood.

most widely distributed opioid peptides are the ENKs, with met- and leu-ENK found in the same areas. In general, met-ENK is found in higher concentrations than leu-ENK. With regard to the hypothalamus (Table 9), ENK-positive cell bodies are found in the supraoptic and paraventricular nuclei. ENK-positive efferents project from these areas and terminate in the external zone of the ME adjacent to the portal vessels and in the neurohypophysis. Met-ENK is reported to be present in portal blood. In addition, cells in the intermediate lobe of the pituitary gland contain the hepta- and octapeptide of met ENK, but not free met-ENK. In the adenohypophysis, gonadotropes contain all forms of met-ENK. These are not the same gonadotropes that colocalize β-END. Moreover, there is a population of gonadotropes that also contain prodynorphin. The medial preoptic nucleus as well as the dorsomedial and ventromedial hypothalamic nuclei also contain ENK-positive cell bodies. The ENKs appear to regulate pituitary hormone secretion by act-

Table 10
Localization of "Other" Hypothalamic Peptides

Peptide	Cell bodies	Terminals	Presence in portal blood
AII	Paraventricular nucleus, Supraoptic nucleus, adenohypophysis.	ME, neurophypophysis, dorsomedial nucleus.	–
NPY	Arcuate nucleus, ME, dorsomedial nucleus, locus coeruleus.	Medial preoptic area, anterior hypothalamic area, periventricular area, suprachiasmatic, supraoptic, paraventricular, arcuate, and ventromedial nuclei, ME.	+
Galanin	Supraoptic, paraventricular and arcuate nuclei.	ME, neurohypophysis.	+

+ = Yes, in concentrations greater than peripheral blood.
– = No, concentrations the same as or less than peripheral blood.

ing as neuromodulators/neurotransmitters. In the neurohypophysis, ENK inhibits the release of OT and AVP. In the adenohypophysis, ENK inhibits LH and stimulates prolactin, growth hormone, and ACTH secretion by acting within the hypothalamus as a neuromodulator/neurotransmitter. The colocalization of the ENKs with pituitary hormones suggests a paracrine or autocrine role of ENK, but the only direct effect has been shown in the neurohypophysis on the inhibition of OT and AVP.

2.5.2.6. Other Hypothalamic Peptides. Within the past few years, several neuropeptides have been described, on the basis of their neuroanatomical location and pharmacologic studies, as potentially significant regulators of hypothalamic function (Table 10). Although the evidence for their physiological significance is incomplete, they should be considered as potential physiological regulators of hypothalamic function.

One peptide, *angiotensin II (AII)*, plays a role in vasoconstriction, sodium retention, antidiuresis, and drinking behavior through direct actions on peripheral structures such as the adrenal cortex and kidney, an action on the CVOs such as the OVLT, the AP and the SFO, and a direct action on the hypothalamus. There is also physiological evidence that *AII* affects the secretion of LH and prolactin from the adenohypophysis through a neuromodulator/neurotransmitter, neurohumoral and even a paracrine or autocrine role. *AII* is formed by the action of a renal proteolytic

enzyme, *renin*, acting upon a peptide produced in the liver, *angiotensinogen*, to form a circulating decapeptide known as *angiotensin I (AI)*. AI, in turn, is cleaved by an *angiotensin-converting enzyme (ACE)* produced in the lungs to form the biologically active octapeptide *AII*. Peripherally, *AII* acts on smooth muscle in arterial walls to promote vasoconstriction and raise blood pressure. Application of AII directly to the CVO also evokes an increase in blood pressure, secretion of AVP and short-latency drinking behavior. The CVOs are outside of the blood–brain barrier, and possess a significant number of AII receptors. AII stimulates the adrenal cortex to secrete aldosterone, the hormone that promotes sodium retention by the nephron. Certain hypothalamic and extra-hypothalamic structures bear *AII* receptors and are sensitive to the application of *AII*. The preoptic area contains a large number of *AII* receptors, and its cells increase their firing rate when *AII* is applied microiontophoretically. These cells mediate the dipsogenic effects of *AII*. The paraventricular nucleus is also sensitive to *AII*. It is not clear how peripheral *AII* gains access to these centers. However, there is abundant evidence for the existence of *AII*-producing elements within the CNS. In fact, *AII*-producing cell bodies are found within the magnocellular cells of the paraventricular nucleus as well as within the supraoptic nucleus. The efferent projections of these cells terminate within the ME as well as within the neurohypophysis. *AII* terminals are also found concentrated in the dorsomedial nucleus of the hypothalamus and scattered throughout the medial basal hypothalamus. It has been reported that *AII* and AVP are copackaged, and that *AII*, renin, and OT are also copackaged. In the adenohypophysis *AII* has been reported to be packaged in gonadotropes. Taken together, these various locations of *AII*-positive cells and terminals would explain the neuromodulator/neurotransmitter roles (CVO), the neuroendocrine role (supraoptic, paraventricular nuclei; neurohypophysis), and the paracrine/autocrine role (gonadotrope of the adenohypophysis) subserved by *AII*.

Neuropeptide Y (NPY) is a highly conserved 36-aa peptide, which is widely distributed in the CNS in many mammals. Of particular importance to hypothalamic function are the extensive networks of NPY-positive fibers and terminals within the medial preoptic area, the periventricular and anterior hypothalamic areas, the suprachiasmatic, supraoptic and paraventricular nuclei, and the arcuate and ventromedial nuclei as well as the ME. Significant concentrations of NPY are found in hypophyseal portal blood. Within the hypothalamus, NPY-positive cells are distributed in the arcuate nucleus/ME area and in the dorsomedial nucleus. Interestingly, much of the hypothalamic NPY originates from noradrenergic cells outside of the hypothalamus. These cells are found in the lateral reticular medulla, the nucleus tractus solitarius region, the locus coeruleus, and the subcoeruleus. Transection of ascending noradrenergic fibers does not eliminate but substantially decreases NPY immunoreactivity in various hypothalamic areas. NPY has multiple actions within and outside the CNS. Most striking is its effect on the adenohypophysis and on some behaviors. Specifically, NPY plays a role in the regulation of gonadotropin secretion by acting within the hypothalamus—as a neuromodulator/neurotransmitter that affects GnRH secretion and as a neurohormone that affects LH secretion directly. NPY has also been implicated in the control of secretion of ACTH, growth hormone, and prolactin from the pituitary gland. It may act as a neurotransmitter, affecting the secretion of AVP from the neurohypophysis. Moreover, NPY is synthesized in a subpopulation of thyrotropes in the adenohypophysis, suggesting a paracrine/autocrine role. Finally, NPY controls eating behaviors through intrahypothalamic pathways.

Galanin is a highly conserved 29-amino-acid peptide that is widely distributed throughout the central and peripheral nervous systems. Within the hypothalamus, galanin-positive cell bodies are found in the supraoptic and paraventricular nuclei as well as the arcuate nucleus. Dense efferent fibers from these areas terminate in the external and internal layer of the ME as well as in the neurohypophysis. Galanin-like immunoactivity and its message are expressed in somatotropes, lactotropes, and thyrotropes within the adenohypophysis. Expression in thyrotropes and in lactotropes is positively regulated by thyroid hormones and estrogen, respectively. Galanin has been implicated as a neurotransmitter/neuromodulator in the control of growth hormone, ACTH, TSH, LH, and prolactin secretion. It has also been found to colocalize with CRH and GnRH in the hypothalamus. Galanin is secreted from cells of the adenohypophysis and is present in portal blood. Taken together, galanin affects pituitary hormone secretion as a neurotransmitter/neuromodulator, as a neurohormone and as a paracrine/autocrine factor.

Endothelins (ETs) are a family of regulatory peptides with vasoconstrictor activity, originally isolated from incubation media of vascular endothelial cells. One, designated ET-1, is a 21-residue peptide that contains two intramolecular disulphide bonds. Two related peptides, designated ET-2 and ET-3, differ by two and six amino acid residues, respectively. The localization of the ETs in the supraoptic and paraventricular nuclei of the hypothalamus, and the adenohypophysis and neurohypophysis—and the presence of ET-receptors in the hypothalamus as well as the adenohypophysis and neurohypophysis—has prompted active inquiry into the role of the ETs in pituitary hormone secretion. In general, the ETs act within the hypothalamus to enhance LH secretion via stimulation of GnRH. Within the pituitary, they are capable of directly stimulating LH, FSH, TSH, and ACTH secretion. In addition, they are potent inhibitors of prolactin secretion, but exert no action on growth-hormone secretion from the pituitary gland. It is not known whether the ETs are in the portal circulation. These data suggest that the ETs can act as neuromodulators/neurotransmitters, or even act in a paracrine/autocrine manner to affect pituitary hormone secretion.

3. TECHNIQUES FOR STUDYING HYPOTHALAMIC FUNCTION

Many techniques have been used to study hypothalamic function. Below is a partial description of some of the approaches available.

3.1. Sampling Methods

The response to stimuli suspected of involving the hypothalamus are studied at several levels. The end point or dependent variable may be the response itself.

Table 11
Sampling Methods for Studying Hypothalamic Function

Methods	Use
Micropunch	Determine amine or peptide content of various areas of the hypothalamus.
Push–pull perfusion	Measure amine or peptide dynamics in CSF.
Microdialysis	Measure amine or peptide dynamics in CSF.
Collection of hypophysial portal or peripheral plasma	Measure neurohormones in portal blood and peripheral plasma.

Thus, one might manipulate the hypothalamus and observe alterations of behaviors, temperature regulation, or pituitary hormone secretion. In addition, the alterations of the biogenic amines and neuropeptides accompanying natural or artificial stimuli may be measured directly. In making these measurements, the investigator is confronted with two problems: a method of collecting the sample that will not impact upon the quantitation of material and reliable measuring tools.

The content of neurotransmitters and neurohormones in hypothalamic tissue can be measured (Table 11). Although there are several *brain microdissection techniques* available, a particularly innovative and useful approach is the *micropunch technique*. This involves the punching from fresh or frozen sections of brain—areas as small as nuclei—for subsequent measurement of content of biogenic amine or neuropeptide. The area is "punched" with needles constructed from stainless steel tubing. The dimensions of the punched area are determined by the size of the needle. The pellet is blown out into a dish or tube for subsequent homogenization and extraction. Using this technique, large numbers of samples can be rapidly processed.

Although the micropunch technique represents a highly useful method for estimating the tissue content of neurotransmitters and neurohormones, its utility is limited by the fact that a single animal can only be sampled at a single point in time. This has been overcome by two related methodologies: *push–pull perfusion* and *microdialysis* (Table 11). Each method has the distinct advantage of multiple sampling over time. To use push–pull perfusion, concentric stainless steel cannulae are implanted so that the tip of the inner cannula is located at the desired site of study (Fig. 21). Artificial CSF lacking the biogenic amines and neuropeptides is "pushed" through the inner cannula and instantaneously "pulled" through the outer cannula into an appropriate receptacle. Assuming the push-pull rates are matched, the "pulled" CSF should be rich

in biogenic amines and neuropeptides. The related technique, microdialysis, has been likened to the implantation of an artificial blood vessel in tissue. A probe bearing a small piece of semipermeable dialysis membrane at the end is implanted into the hypothalamus. The end is localized in the area of interest for study. Artificial CSF or saline is pumped through the probe and recovered. Theoretically, amines or peptides will diffuse from the area of higher concentration in the brain to the area of lowest concentration on the probe side of the dialysis tubing. The size-exclusion selectivity of the membrane will determine the size of the molecule diffusing into the probe, and the length of the membrane will determine the amount of tissue sampled.

The concentration of biogenic amines and neuropeptides can even be measured in the microscopic vessels, the hypothalamo–hypophyseal portal vessels connecting the ME with the adenohypophysis (Table 11). Collection of the blood in these vessels free from dilution by peripheral blood involves a complex ventral surgical approach to expose the ME. Once exposed, the stalk is cut and placed inside a polyethylene cannula. Using this procedure, blood is collected from all of the cut portal vessels simultaneously. Although this procedure involves experimental manipulation and collection of portal blood under anesthesia in rats, surgical approaches have been developed to collect portal blood from unanesthetized sheep and monkeys.

3.2. Methods of Quantitating Hypothalamic Function

3.2.1. Assay Techniques

There are two modern assay techniques currently used to measure catecholamines and indolamines in tissue, media, CSF, and blood (Table 12). One technique, the *microradioenzymatic assay*, takes advantage of the fact that the catecholamines and indolamines are methylated in vivo. Dopamine, norepinephrine, and epinephrine are O-methylated in vivo to form metho-

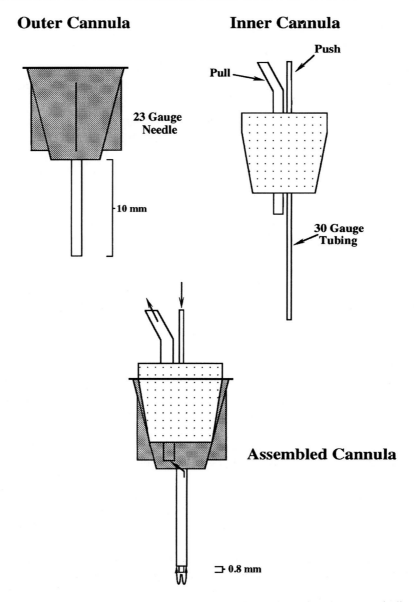

Fig. 21. The structure of the inner, outer, and assembled push–pull perfusion cannula. The arrows indicate the direction of flow through the assembled cannula.

Table 12
Methods of Quantitating Hypothalamic Function

Methods	Use
Microradioenzymatic assay	Measure catecholamines or indoleamines.
High-performance liquid chromatography/ electrochemical detection	Measure catecholamines or indoleamines.
In situ voltammetry	Measure catecholamines or indoleamines.
Radioimmunoassay	Measure neuropeptides or pituitary hormones.
Hybridization assay	Measure peptide message.

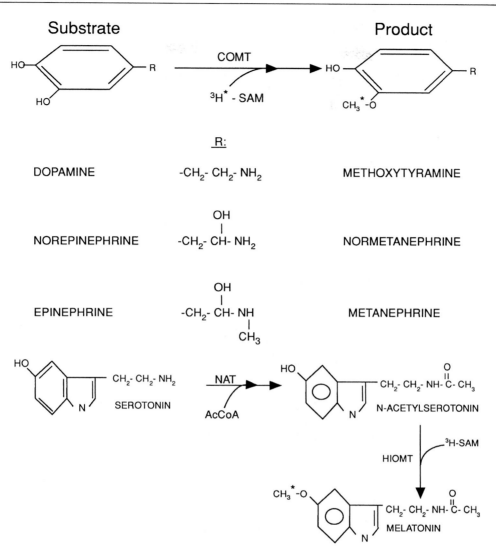

Fig. 22. The critical reactions in the microradioenzymatic assay for catecholamines (dopamine, norepinephrine, and epinephrine) and indoleamines (serotonin). COMT=catecholamine-o-methyl transferase; ^{3}H-SAM=tritiated S-adenosyl methionine; NAT= N-acetyl transferase; AcCoA=Acetyl CoA; HIOMT=hydroxyindole-O-methyl transferase. The amount of the tritiated methylated products (methoxytyramine, normetanephrine, metanephrine, and melatonin) is proportional to the amount of the respective starting substrate (dopamine, norepinephrine, epinephrine, or serotonin). *=position of ^{3}H donated by ^{3}H-SAM.

xytyramine, normetanephrine, and metanephrine, respectively, and serotonin is O-methylated and N-acetylated to form melatonin (Fig. 22). Radio-enzymatic assays exploits these metabolic fates by incorporating ^{3}H into the structure of the O-methylated derivatives. In the case of the catecholamines, this is accomplished by using the enzyme catechol O-methyl transferase and as methyl donor, ^{3}H-S-adenosyl methionine (^{3}H-SAM). Similarly, the serotonin assay is based upon the ability of hydroxyindole O-methyl transferase to catalyze the transfer of the ^{3}H-methyl group of SAM to N-acetyl serotonin and thus form

melatonin. Since the amount of radiolabeled product is proportional to unlabeled substrate, the isolation of these products by thin-layer chromatography represents a quantitative estimate of substrate. The other modern widespread approach to quantitating the catecholamines is through the use of *high-performance liquid chromatography* coupled with *electrochemical detection (HPLC-EC)* (Table 12). Using this technique, separation of catecholamines is achieved with an analytical column packed with C_{18} reverse-phase material. This material allows resolution of catecholamines, their precursors and metabolites as well as serotonin and its metabolites. Resolution of sample molecules takes place by their differential interactions with the mobile-phase solvent and the column packing material. Distinct bands of solute form during passage through the column. Resolution of the solutes are controlled by pH, ionic strength, and the nature and concentration of aqueous phase as well as the concentration of the organic components of the mobile organic phase. Quantitation is achieved by eluting the resolved solutes through the electrochemical detector. The potential applied to the detector's cell favors oxidation of the catecholamine. For a given set of operating conditions, the oxidative current is directly proportional to the concentration of electroactive species in solution. Related to the HPLC-EC procedure is a method for determining catecholamine flux in vivo in neural tissue. This procedure, known as *in situ voltammetry*, involves stereotaxic placement of a carbon-based microelectrode. As a potential is applied and increased, the catecholamines in a thin surface adjacent to the electrode are oxidized. The magnitude of the oxidizing current generated is a function of the concentration of electroactive species in solution. The potential at which the current appears is specific for particular catecholamines. Unfortunately, this technique cannot differentiate subtle differences in side-chain groups and thus dopamine, norepinephrine, and epinephrine cannot be adequately differentiated.

Neuropeptide content in various areas of the hypothalamus or concentration in portal blood is routinely measured by *radioimmunoassay (RIA)* (Table 12). Similarly, RIAs are used to measure the hormones of the anterior and posterior pituitary gland that the hypothalamus controls. RIAs are dependent upon the ability of relatively specific antibodies to recognize the unlabeled species of neuropeptide or hormone after it has been labeled with a radioactive tag such as [125]I. Since the binding sites on the antibody are the same and are specific, there is a competition between labeled and unlabeled species for that binding site. Thus, the amount of binding of labeled peptide is inversely proportional to the amount of unlabeled peptide with which it competes. The unlabeled peptide would either be varying known amounts of standard or unknown amounts extracted from tissue or blood.

With the advent of modern molecular biological techniques, it is possible to measure the amount of peptide in the hypothalamus, and even to measure the regulation of neuroendocrine peptide gene expression by quantitation of specific messenger RNA. In general, most of the methods for measuring neuroendocrine peptide message are some variant of a *hybridization assay* (Table 12). The basis for the assay is to manipulate the animal in vivo or the cells in vitro with a specific treatment and then to isolate cell nuclei. During the isolation, RNA polymerases remain bound to the genes being transcribed. The nuclei are then incubated in vitro with radiolabeled nucleotide triphosphates, and the polymerases will continue to transcribe the genes for several hundred nucleotides. Thus, the newly synthesized transcripts are being labeled. The critical requirement of this type of assay is the availability of specific cDNA probes for the neuropeptide under study. The specific RNA transcripts are now *hybridized* to the cDNA probes bound to an inert matrix such as nitrocellulose filter, which are subsequently washed and counted in a scintillation counter. The amount of radioactivity counted is proportional to the amount of *specific* mRNA.

3.2.2. ELECTROPHYSIOLOGY

Electrophysiological studies of the hypothalamus have provided a great deal of information on the firing patterns of hypothalamic neurons. However, this information is most valuable only when the firing patterns are correlated with a hypothalamic-dependent event such as pituitary hormone secretion, or behavioral responses. In general, hormone release from cells or neuropeptide release from axon terminals in the hypothalamus follows an influx of calcium through membrane depolarized during action-potential activity.

Extracellular recordings from hypothalamic nuclei in vivo can be used for topographical or functional identification (Table 13). For example, magnocellular neurons in the paraventricular nucleus can be excited antidromically and identified by electrically stimulating the neurohypophysis. The topographical origin of those neurons terminating in the neurohypophysis can be identified by this method. Similarly, these neurons can be recorded orthodromically after application of a suckling stimulus and correlated with the release of oxytocin into peripheral plasma. Such a relationship suggests, but does not prove, a functional role for the neurons recorded from in control of pituitary hormone secretion.

Several in vitro electrophysiological approaches can be used to study neurotransmitter effects on hypothalamic neurons or effects of hypophysiotropic substances of hypothalamic origin on target cells

Table 13
Electrophysiological Methods
for Studying Hypothalamic Function

Methods	Use
Extracellular recordings	Topography of neurons.
Hypothalamic slice recordings	Characterize neuronal excitation.
Voltage clamp or current clamp	Neurosecretory mechanisms.

Table 14
Neuroanatomical Methods for Studying Hypothalamic Function

Methods	Use
Immunocytochemistry	Visualize location of amines and peptides, activity of neurons.
Tract tracing	Visualize axons.
Autoradiography	Characterize transmitter binding sites, peptide message.

(Table 13). Slice preparations of whole hypothalami allow for introduction of drugs or other factors by superfusion close to the neuron being recorded. Excitable membrane properties of pituitary cells can be studied after application of suspected neurohormones of hypothalamic origin. *Voltage-clamp* or *current-clamp* approaches are used to study the effects of hypophysiotropic substances on the secretory function of pituitary cells (Table 13). These yield valuable information about the identity of ion channels involved in secretion.

3.2.3. Neuroanatomical Approaches

At the present time, *immunocytochemistry* is the favored approach for visualizing neuropeptides in neuronal cell bodies, dendrites, axons, and axon terminals (Table 14). The technique involves saturating histologically prepared sections of hypothalamus with antisera that are specific for the neuropeptide in question. The reaction complex is then treated with an anti-immunoglobulin that has been bonded with an enzyme that will cause a visible precipitate. Alternatively, the antibody can be conjugated with a fluorescent chromogen, which will produce a distinctive fluorescent color.

Localization of peptide in different parts of neurons requires different approaches and produces different information. For example, in order to study neuropeptides in cell bodies, axonal transport must be blocked with agents that disrupt microtubules such as colchicine. Cell-body density can then be estimated. Topographical three-dimensional localization of neuropeptide-containing neurons can be determined. Axons are most difficult to visualize by immunocytochemistry because neuropeptides are transported from the cell body to the nerve terminal by fast axoplasmic flow, and thus not enough material is available for immunostaining. Nerve terminals, however, can be visualized by immunocytochemistry under the light microscope.

Tract-tracing techniques can be employed either alone or in combination with immunocytochemical approaches to determine the path taken by axons of particular neurons (Table 14). Two approaches can be used. Tracts can be visualized from the neuronal-cell body to the axon terminal (anterograde) or from the nerve terminal to the cell body (retrograde). An enzyme—horseradish peroxidase, a glycoprotein capable of catalyzing the oxidation of some chromogens—can be used for both anterograde and retrograde tracings. Fluoro-gold is a fluorochrome that is used specifically for retrograde tracings.

Neurons can also be labeled for activity. The product of the protooncogene c-fos—Fos—can be detected in the nuclei of active neurons by immunocytochemistry (Table 14). Neuronal activity can also be quantitated autoradiographically with the 2-deoxyglucose technique. Active neurons preferentially utilize glucose for oxidative metabolism. 2-deoxy-{D-}^{14}C glucose

Table 15
Methods for Creating Deficits of Hypothalamic Function

Methods	Use
Hypophysectomy	Create deficits of neurohypophysial and adenohypophysial hormones and targets for adenohypophysial-releasing hormones.
Stalk transection	Create deficits of neurohypophysial hormones and releasing hormones at their targets.
Surgical lesions	Destroy groups of cells or fibers suspected of involvement in hypothalamic function.
Chemical lesions	Destroy groups of cells which synthesize and secrete specific neurotransmitters or neurohormones.

is injected intravenously, the hypothalami are prepared and sectioned by conventional histological techniques, and the concentration of grains in particular nuclei is evaluated microdensitometrically.

Autoradiography can be used to localize neurotransmitter-binding sites, trace axonal connections, locate sites of steroid receptors, and evaluate neuronal activity. The system to be studied is labeled, brain sections are prepared histologically, the slides are covered with a radiosensitive emulsion, and the emulsion is developed photographically.

Just as there are immunocytochemical techniques to study the localization of neuropeptides, enzymes for catecholamine biosynthesis and neurotransmitter or steroid receptors, there are also immunocytochemical techniques for studying the transcription of the message. The technique in widest use is *in situ hybridization* histochemistry. In this case, specific cDNA is used in place of specific antibody (Table 14). The hybridization of the specific cDNA occurs on the brain section, which is then developed by autoradiographic techniques similar to those previously described. Alternatively, nonradioactive probes are now available that allow visualization of a chromogenic reaction.

Finally, the great advantage of these approaches is that they can be used in combination. For example, one might wish to identify hypothalamic neurons that have steroid receptors. Under these circumstances, it is possible to combine immunocytochemistry with steroid autoradiography.

3.3. Creation of Deficits of Hypothalamic Function

3.3.1. SURGICAL MANIPULATIONS

In general, most surgical manipulations involving the hypothalamus and its targets such as the pituitary

gland are performed in order to create deficit symptoms (Table 15).

3.3.1.1. Hypophysectomy. This procedure for removal of the pituitary gland from the sella turcica by a parapharyngeal approach was first described in the rat by Philip Smith in 1927. Since the hypothalamus produces neurohormones that control the adenohypophysis and neurohormones that are released from the neurohypophysis, hypophysectomy creates many, but not all, of the deficits of hypothalamic hypofunction. Although hypophysectomy creates deficits of *all* of the adenohypophyseal and neurohypophyseal hormones, a hypofunctional hypothalamus creates deficits of all of the pituitary hormones *except* prolactin. Whereas prolactin levels in blood are virtually undistinguishable after hypophysectomy, circulating prolactin levels increase as a result of a hypofunctioning hypothalamus. This is caused by the removal of the pituitary lactotrope from the influence of dopamine, the physiological prolactin-inhibiting hormone. It is often difficult to verify completeness of hypophysectomy until postmortem inspection. A further problem associated with hypophysectomy is that it is difficult to prevent partial functional regeneration of the hypothalamo–hypophyseal tract, and thus permanently create deficits in OT and vasopressin secretion. In some cases, the aspirated gland can be *transplanted* to sites distant from the hypothalamus. Deficit symptoms of all the hormones except prolactin persist. When transplanted to the sella turcica to allow revascularization by the hypophyseal portal vessels, the deficit symptoms are reversed. These types of procedures allowed early anatomists to conclude that the critical link between the hypothalamus and adenohypophysis was *neurovascular*. Finally, the stalk ME connecting the hypothalamus with the pituitary gland can be *transected*. This procedure causes disruption of

Table 16
Methods for Stimulating Hypothalamic Function

Methods	Use
Natural stimuli	To study the relationship between physiological stimuli and hypothalamic function.
Chemical stimuli	To study the relationship between neurotransmitters and hypothalamic function.
Artificial stimuli	To excite groups of hypothalamic neurons and study the effect on a hypothalamically dependent end point.

the hypothalamo–hypophyseal portal vasculature as well as the hypothalamo–hypophyseal tract. This disruption is permanent if regrowth is prevented by placement of a foil barrier in the transected area. Under these circumstances, the deficit symptoms would be the same as hypophysectomy followed by transplantation to a site that is distant from the sella turcica.

3.3.1.2. Lesions. It order to destroy deep-seated nuclei of the brain in areas such as the hypothalamus, the nuclei must be located with accuracy. This is achieved by placing the head of the subject in a device known as a stereotaxic apparatus, which holds it in a predefined, rigid position. With the aid of a map of the brain (a stereotaxic atlas), as well as anatomical landmarks on the skull and the surface of the underlying brain, focal lesions that destroy discrete anatomical groupings of cell bodies can be placed by sending a current through an electrode. Similarly, fibers of passage may be destroyed by placement of a small knife, which can be manipulated to deafferentiate specific axons that control the hypothalamus.

3.3.2. Chemical Lesions

Selective lesions induced by neurotoxins have become a modern tool to study the role of the hypothalamus (Table 15). They can be either site-selective or transmitter-selective. *Monosodium glutamate* or its more potent analog, *kainic acid*, have site selectivity for neuronal cell bodies and dendrites, sparing fibers of passage and axon terminals in areas outside of the blood/brain barrier such as the arcuate nucleus/ME, the OVLT, and the pre-optic area. Thus, glutamate, kainate, or its less toxic analog, *ibotenic acid*, may be injected systemically and will lesion only those areas. Selectivity is further enhanced by local injections stereotaxically. *Gold thioglucose* will selectively lesion the VMN of the hypothalamus.

Neurotoxic lesions can be made in catecholamine or indolamine neurons. *6-hydroxydopamine* or *6-hydroxydopa* will deplete catecholamines in the

brain when injected in the third ventricle. They pass the blood-brain barrier, so their specificity may be restricted by stereotaxic injection in small volumes locally. The indolamine neurotoxins are *5,6-* or *5,7-dihydroxytryptamines*, which are injected intraventricularly or locally.

Cysteamine, 2-mercaptoethylamine, depletes SS in the CNS and the periphery. In the CNS, cysteamine depletes SS in both cell bodies and axons.

Certain plant lectins, such as *ricin*, are taken up and transported retrogradely along axons to cell bodies, and ultimately kill the cell. Specificity is conferred by coupling an antiserum to the peptide made by the cell so that when the antiserum binds to the peptide, specific cells are killed. Alternatively, the cytotoxic plant lectins can be conjugated to hypophysiotropic peptides in order to selectively kill target cells.

3.4. Stimulation of Hypothalamic Function

There are essentially three approaches to studying excitation of the hypothalamus and its consequences (Table 16). One can study hypothalamic function in response to *natural stimuli*. For example, one can record from specific areas of the hypothalamus or study the activities of specific neuropeptides or amine transmitters in the hypothalamus in response to exteroceptive stimuli such as suckling, mating, volume expansion (hypertonic saline), volume depletion (hemorrhage), or alterations in temperature. The activity of hypothalamic neurons can be studied in response to their natural *chemical stimulators* including neurotransmitters as well as neurotransmitter agonists and antagonists. Moreover, the effects of endogenous peripheral factors such as hormones can be described. Under these circumstances, for example, the activity of estrogen on excitation of hypothalamic neurons involved in sexual behavior can be studied. Hypothalamic neurons can be excited by *artificial means*, and the consequence of their activity can be studied. The usual approach is to stimulate electrically or electrochemically. In the former case, neurons are excited by electrical depolarization, and in the latter case, depolarization is caused by deposition of iron by the stimulating electrode. Using either of these approaches, one can stimulate an area of the hypothalamus and measure a visceral end point.

3.4.1. The Direct Application of Active Hypothalamic Peptides or Amines to Physiological Targets Reveals Their Physiologic Role

One can study the response of target cells to their physiological affecters. For example, cells of the anterior pituitary gland can be enzymatically dissociated and placed in short-term culture. Hypothalamic peptides can be applied to the cultures by perifusion or by static incubation in monolayer cultures. The release of pituitary hormones into the media can be monitored, and intracellular transduction events can be studied with this approach. Using similar approaches, the receptors for the neuropeptides can be studied.

4. PHYSIOLOGICAL PROCESSES CONTROLLED BY THE HYPOTHALAMUS

4.1. The Hypothalamus Regulates Pituitary Hormone Secretion

4.1.1. General Concepts

4.1.1.1. Characteristics of a Neuroendocrine System. As noted previously, the key feature of a neuroendocrine system is the existence of the neurohemal area; the external zone of the ME, at which neurosecretory axon terminals converge upon a capillary bed that ultimately leads to and affects the secretions of the adenohypophysis. Similarly, neurosecretory axons comprising the hypothalamo–hypophyseal tract terminate on sinusoids in the neurohypophysis, and ultimately secrete their products to the peripheral circulation to affect visceral processes. The axons that terminate in the external zone of the ME secrete release- and release-inhibiting *hormones* into the hypothalamo–hypophyseal portal plasma. In order to meet the definition of release- or release-inhibiting hormones, the substances in portal plasma must meet certain criteria (Table 17): (i) They must be *extractable* from hypothalamic or ME tissue; (ii) They must be present in hypophyseal portal blood in *greater amounts* than in the systemic circulation; (iii) Varying concentrations of a particular release- or release-inhibiting hormone in portal plasma must be *correlated with* varying secretion rates of one (or more) of the anterior pituitary hormones in a variety of experimen-

tal conditions; (iv) The suspected hormone should stimulate or inhibit one or more pituitary hormone(s) when administered in vivo or applied to pituitary cells or tissues in vitro; (v) *Inhibitors* that antagonize the actions of the release- or release-inhibiting hormones should block or stimulate anterior pituitary hormone secretion; and (vi) Target cells should have *receptors* for the release or release-inhibiting hormones.

4.1.1.2. Concept of Feedback. The hypothalamo-pituitary-target axes can be characterized as a set of links over which information flows. As information is transmitted from link-to-link, it stimulates or depresses a biological response in the next link, but it also influences the activity of an earlier link. Such an influence is referred to as a *feedback*. In general, there are two types of feedbacks. A *negative feedback* (Fig. 23) is one in which the activity of the downstream link inhibits the activity of one or more upstream links. Conceptually, regulation of room temperature by a thermostatically driven furnace fits this model. The furnace, in response to regulation by a thermostat, raises the temperature of the room to a point that is preset on the thermostat. Once that temperature is achieved, the thermostat senses that level and turns off the furnace. If the thermostat is inoperative, the furnace runs extensively, and the temperature in the room rises to the limits of the furnace. In neuroendocrinology, an example of a negative feedback is the ability of adrenal corticosterone to inhibit CRH secretion into portal blood. A *positive feedback* is one in which the downstream link enhances the activity of one or more upstream links. Conceptually, this is a more difficult mechanism to describe accurately. A voice-activated recording device is perhaps the best example of a positive feedback. The voice begins the recording device. When the voice ceases, the recording device stops. Unlike negative feedback, which is a long-term dampening process, positive feedback is relatively brief and inherently unstable. The feedback signal can be provided by a hormone itself or by a nonhumoral metabolite. The classical example of a positive feedback in neuroendocrinology is the ability of ovarian estradiol to stimulate GnRH secretion into portal blood.

Feedback loops can take several routes (Fig. 24). In the case of the hypothalamo-pituitary-target gland axis, a *long-loop feedback* would be blood-borne from the peripheral target gland to affect the hypothalamus or pituitary. A *short-loop feedback* might be exemplified by a pituitary hormone influencing the secretion of its hypothalamic release- or release-inhibiting fac-

Table 17
Required Characteristics of Neurohormones

1. Activity must be extractable from whole hypothalamus or ME tissue.
2. Concentration in hypophysial portal blood must be greater than systemic circulation.
3. Dynamics in portal plasma must be correlated with dynamics of adenohypophysial hormone secretion.
4. Extracted material must be active in vivo and in vitro.
5. Inhibitors of neurohormones should affect physiological end point.
6. Target cells should have receptors for neurohormones.

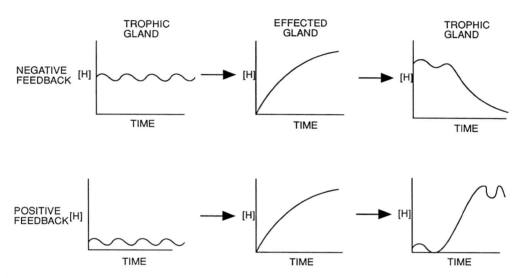

Fig. 23. Diagrammatic representation of a negative feedback (*upper sequence*) and positive feedback (*lower sequence*) in the endocrine system. In a negative-feedback system, the trophic gland (such as the adenohypophysis) secretes a signal (such as TSH), which stimulates the target gland (the thyroid) to secrete its product (thyroid hormone), which in turn feeds back to inhibit TSH secretion. In a positive-feedback system, the trophic gland (the adenohypophysis) secretes a signal at low rates (such as LH), which stimulates the target gland (the ovary) to secrete its product (estradiol), whose increasing secretion rate allows the trophic gland to secrete LH in larger amounts. [H]=hormone concentration in blood.

tor. Finally, an *ultra-short-loop* feedback is represented by a pituitary hormone effecting its own secretion through an autocrine mechanism.

4.1.2. Regulation of the Adenohypophysis by the Hypothalamus

4.1.2.1. Gonadotropes. Overwhelming evidence indicates that the hypothalamic decapeptide known as luteinizing hormone-releasing-hormone (LHRH or GnRH) is the peptide in hypophyseal portal blood that is the physiological humoral stimulator of LH and FSH secretion. Although FSH-releasing activities devoid of LH-releasing activity have been isolated from the hypothalamus, a distinctive FSH-RH has not yet been identified. GnRH regulates LH and FSH secretion

from the gonadotropes of the adenohypophysis in both basal and ovulation-inducing "surge" states in female mammals. In rodents, the "surge" center is the medial preoptic area and the basal center is in the medial basal hypothalamus. Males lack a functional "surge" center. The ovarian steroids, estrogen and progesterone, inhibit LH and FSH secretion by acting directly at the gonadotrope, and also at the medial basal hypothalamus to inhibit GnRH release into portal blood. The ovarian steroids also stimulate a preovulatory surge of LH and FSH secretion by acting at the medial preoptic area to stimulate a surge of GnRH into portal blood. This process is presumed to be the result of a noradrenergic mechanism. In rodents, surgical isolation of the medial preoptic area from the medial basal hypo-

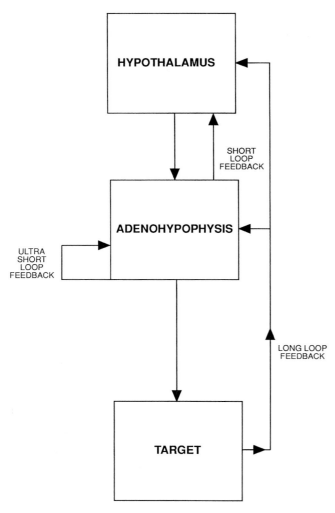

Fig. 24. Diagrammatic representation of feedback loops. In the hypothalamo-pituitary-target gland axis, a long-loop feedback would be blood-borne from the peripheral target gland to effect the hypothalamus or pituitary. A short-loop feedback could be exemplified by a pituitary hormone provoking the secretion of its hypothalamic release- or release-inhibiting hormone. An ultra-short-loop feedback is characterized by a pituitary hormone effecting its own secretion through an autocrine mechanism.

thalamus will prevent a steroid-induced surge of LH secretion. Ovarian and testicular steroids will not induce an LH surge in males. But the gonadal steroids will inhibit LH and FSH secretion, regardless of the sex of the recipient. In primates, there is evidence that the surge center may reside in the basal hypothalamus, and that the ovarian steroid merely sensitizes the gonadotropes to respond to unvarying pulses of GnRH. Monkeys bearing surgically isolated medial basal hypothalami and infused with pulsatile GnRH respond to estradiol with an LH surge. This has led to the con-

cept that the medial basal hypothalamus is a *pulse generator* for GnRH release into portal blood. There is a clear sexual dimorphism of the medial preoptic area: males have a more intensely stained medial preoptic nucleus within this area than females. Such differentiation occurs perinatally. In rodents, castration of males within the first few days of life prevents the appearance of this sexually dimorphic area in adults. Moreover, as adults, neonatally castrated males can respond to an estradiol challenge with a preovulatory-like LH surge. If testosterone is administered to phenotypic female rodents within the first few days of life, they develop the male-type sexual dimorphic nucleus and the male pattern of gonadotropin secretion. Since they lack a surge center, they are anovulatory. Although GnRH is the physiological regulator of LH and FSH secretion, other neuropeptides subserve a similar function, either as neurohormones, neurotransmitters, or neuromodulators. These are listed in Table 18.

4.1.2.2. Lactotrope. As noted earlier, the dominant hypothalamic control over pituitary prolactin secretion is inhibitory. Removal of hypothalamic influence over the adenohypophysis results in an enhanced secretion of prolactin. Thus, stalk transection, destruction of the medial basal hypothalamus or placement of pituitary fragments or cells in culture results in hypersecretion of prolactin. Moreover, in vivo treatment with dopamine antagonists results in hypersecretion of prolactin. Conversely, in vitro treatment with dopamine agonists depresses pituitary prolactin secretion. These data, coupled with the inverse relationship between dopamine levels in portal blood and peripheral blood levels of prolactin, suggest that dopamine is the prolactin release-inhibiting hormone. However, recent studies of the dynamics of prolactin release in response to lowered dopaminergic tone suggest that the lactotrope must also be under the influence of prolactin-*releasing* hormones (PRH) of hypothalamic origin. Although thyrotropin-releasing hormone (TRH) is one of the most widely studied candidates, others (listed in Table 18) have prolactin-releasing properties and may also play a role. Prolactin secretion in response to exteroceptive stimuli such as suckling may thus involve a reduction of dopamine levels in portal blood as well as an increase in the portal-blood concentration of a putative PRH.

4.1.2.3. Thyrotropes. There is little doubt that the tripeptide pyro glu-his-pro-NH$_2$ is the thyrotropin-releasing hormone (TRH; Table 18). TRH is the physiological stimulator of TSH secretion from the adenohypophysis. The cell bodies with axons that ter-

Table 18
Peptide and Amines that Act Directly
on Adenohypophyseal Cells

Cell Type	Peptide or amine	Other peptides or amines
Gonadotrope	GnRH	VIP
		CCK
		NPY
		Substance P
		Galanin
		Neurotensin
Lactotrope	Dopamine*	TRH
		OT
		VIP
		Angiotensin II
		Somatostatin
		GnRH
Thyrotrope	TRH	Somatostatin*
Corticotrope	CRH	AVP
Somatotrope	GHRH	TRH
	Somatostatin*	

* = inhibit function of cell.

minate upon the external zone of the ME are found primarily in the paraventricular nucleus. In turn, TSH, stimulates thyroid hormone (thyroxine and triiodothyronine) secretion from the thyroid gland. The thyroid hormones, in turn, diminish the release of TSH by lowering the response of the thyrotrope to TRH. This is a classical negative-feedback control system. Removal of the thyroid gland enhances the release of TSH into the peripheral circulation without affecting portal-blood levels of TRH. This further suggests that primary control of TSH secretion by thyroid hormones *does not* reside at the hypothalamus. The hypothalamus provides the drive (TRH), but the thyroid gland negatively regulates (by thyroid hormone) the response of the thyrotrope (TSH) to that drive.

4.1.2.4. Corticotrope. ACTH secretion from the corticotrope is controlled primarily by CRH released into portal blood. ACTH stimulates the release of the steroid hormones of the adrenal cortex, which in turn feed back negatively to inhibit ACTH release by acting at the hypothalamus as well as the adenohypophysis. It is now apparent that arginine vasopressin (AVP) is also a potent ACTH-releasing hormone. Portal blood levels of both AVP and CRH are positively correlated with ACTH-releasing stimuli such as stress. Thus, ACTH release is not caused by the action of a single peptide, but is the result of the actions of a hypothalamic *complex*.

4.1.2.5. Somatotrope. Though the somatotrope is predominantly under the stimulatory influence of hypothalamic GHRH, it is also under the opposing influence of a growth-hormone release-inhibiting hormone, SS. Each neurohumoral peptide affects growth-hormone secretion through distinct receptor sites on the somatotrope, but each plays a reciprocal neuromodulatory role on the other. The SS neurons also directly innervate GHRH neurons with the result of diminishing GHRH release into portal blood, and consequently reducing GH release into the peripheral circulation. Conversely, stimuli known to release growth hormone also suppress release of SS into portal plasma. Feedback control of growth-hormone secretion does not fit the models of classical negative or positive feedback by target endocrine organs. For example, hypoglycemia will stimulate growth-hormone secretion by stimulating the release of GHRH into portal blood. Conversely, hyperglycemia will inhibit growth-hormone secretion by increasing SS and decreasing GHRH levels in portal blood.

4.1.3. The Hypothalamus
and Neurohypophyseal Function

4.1.3.1. Mechanism of Secretion of Neurohypophyseal Hormones. The hormone-neurophysin complex (vasopressin-neurophysin II or oxytocin-neurophysin I) are synthesized in cell bodies of the supraoptic or paraventricular nuclei. The complexes, still undergoing posttranslational processing, are transported down the long axons that comprise the hypothalamo–hypophyseal tract to terminals adjacent to fenestrated capillaries in the neurohypophysis (Fig. 25). Adjacent to the fenestrated capillaries in the neurohypophysis are specialized glial-like cells known as *pituicytes* that regulate the microenvironment of the terminals. During this voyage they are packaged in neurosecretory granules. Once at the axon terminal, the granule membrane fuses with the membrane of the axon terminal and the hormone-neurophysin complex is exocytosed. The process coincides with the arrival of the action potential, which depolarizes the membrane and allows entry of sodium ions. These in turn permit the opening of calcium channels, which plays an unambiguous role in the exocytotic process. After exocytosis of the neurohormone, intracellular calcium is packaged into microvesicles and extruded, and the membrane potential is restored by a sodium-potassium pump. The membranes of the evacuated neurosecretory granules are reformed from the surface of the axon terminal, where they are either packaged into lysosomes and degraded or recycled, usually in areas of nonterminal swelling known as Herring bodies.

4.1.3.2. Stimuli for Secretion of Vasopressin.

The two main stimuli for vasopressin secretion are an increase in osmolality of the plasma and a decrease in plasma volume (Table 19). These can be either interrelated or independent stimuli. Water deprivation causes an increase in plasma osmolality and a diminution of intracellular water. A change in plasma osmolality of as little as 1% is detected by osmoreceptive neurons, which are distinct from the vasopressin magnocellular neurons in the hypothalamus. The osmoreceptive neurons stimulate vasopressin synthesis and release from the magnocellular neurons in the supraoptic area at a threshold of 280 mosM/kg. The osmoreceptor neurons can also stimulate thirst, but with a greater sensitivity of 290 mosM/kg. Vasopressin release is also stimulated by a 5–10% decrease in blood volume, blood pressure, or cardiac output. Hypovolemia is perceived by pressure receptors in the carotid and aortic arch, as well as stretch receptors in the walls of the left atrium, pulmonary veins, and the juxtaglomerular apparatus of the kidney. The afferent impulses of these sensors are carried via the ninth and tenth cranial nerves to the medulla, and then through the midbrain over noradrenergic synapses to the magnocellular vasopressinergic neurons of the supraoptic nucleus. In the absence of any change in pressure, the receptors tonically inhibit vasopressin secretion. With acute volume depletion such as that caused by hemorrhage, noradrenergic inhibitory tone from the medulla to the hypothalamus is decreased, resulting in an increase in the secretion of vasopressin. Volume depletion also stimulates central renin-dependent angiotensin release, which also stimulates vasopressin secretion and thirst.

4.1.3.3. Stimuli for Secretion of Oxytocin.

Suckling is the best-described stimulus for OT secretion (Table 19). As one might expect, the pathways are similar to that of vasopressin. The suckling stimulus is carried over afferent spinal pathways to the medulla and midbrain, and then through cholinergic synapses to the paraventricular nucleus. OT release is pulsatile. Nipple suction by the young leads to synchronized activation of action potentials for 2–4 s in the paraventricular nucleus. From a resting "spontaneous" background of 1–10 spikes/s, these neurons generate a synchronized series of 70–80 action potentials within 3–4 s of application of the stimulus, resulting in the secretion of 0.5–1.0 mI.U. of oxytocin. This is followed by milk ejection from the mammary gland, 12–15 s later. These pulses of neuronal activity occur uniformly every 4–8 min. This characteristic of periodic bursting of action potentials at high frequency appears to be important for OT secretion and consequent milk ejection. The stimuli for OT release during labor appear to be multiple. The activation of cervicovaginal stretch receptors by the growing conceptus is an important signal, and a hormonal background of diminishing placental progesterone and elevated fetal free cortisol act in concert to stimulate OT secretion sufficient to enhance contractions of the uterus. Interestingly, OT secretion has a significant sensory component. In the human female, merely playing with the infant or sensing the cries of a hungry infant will cause milk ejection. In contrast, emotional stress will inhibit the secretion of OT.

4.2. The Hypothalamus Regulates Autonomic Processes

4.2.1. Cardiovascular Function

Independent of the control of blood pressure through the neuroendocrine function of the hypothalamus, the cardiovascular system is influenced by the hypothalamus through the autonomic nervous system (Table 20). These effects are mediated primarily by the sympathetic system through the vagus nerve. Stimulation of the posterior and lateral hypothalamus increases arterial pressure and heart rate, whereas stimulation of the preoptic area decreases heart rate and arterial pres-

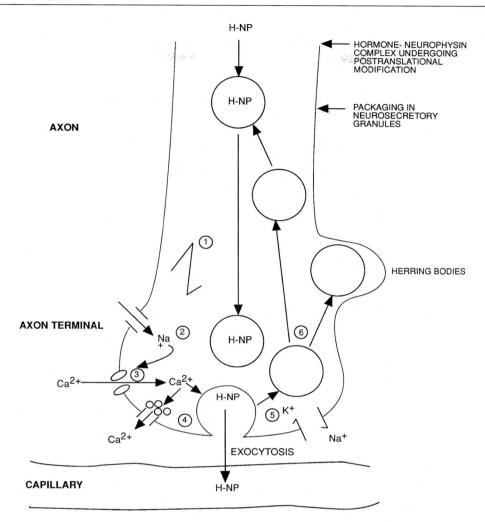

Fig. 25. The mechanism by which the neurohypophyseal peptide-neurophysin complex is axonally transported, processed, packaged, and secreted from the axon terminal. As the hormone neurophysin complex is transported down the axons in the hypothalamo–hypophyseal tract, further posttranslational processing is taking place. The mature complex is then packaged into neurosecretory granules, whose arrival at the axon terminal coincides with the arrival of the action potential (*1*). The membrane of the granule fuses with the axon-terminal membrane, and the product is exocytosed. The action potential is believed to play a role in the process by causing depolarization and entry of sodium (*2*), which in turn allows entry of calcium through specific channels (*3*). Calcium plays a partially understood role in the exocytotic process. The intracellular calcium is then packaged into microvesicles (*4*) and extruded, and the membrane potential is restored by a sodium–potassium pump (*5*). The membranes of the evacuated neurosecretory granules are reformed (*6*), and are either packaged into lysosomes and degraded or recycled in areas of nonterminal swelling known as Herring bodies.

sure. These effects are mediated by the cardiovascular centers in the medulla and pons. Cardiovascular regulation in response to alterations in environmental temperature or defense reactions is also mediated by the hypothalamus. In response to a hot environment, dilation of blood vessels of the skin and constriction of deep visceral vessels occur, and cold exposure induces the opposite responses. These are controlled by the preoptic/anterior hypothalamic areas. The defense reaction that is characterized by cutaneous vasoconstriction and muscular vasodilation is the result of discharge of sympathetic cholinergic vasodilators as well as sympathetic adrenergic excitation. These effects can be induced by selective stimulation of the anterior and posterior hypothalamus.

4.2.2. THERMOREGULATORY FUNCTION

The control of body temperature by the hypothalamus is a classical example of an *integrative* approach to alteration of the *internal milieu*. The hypothalamus oversees *autonomic compensations* such as alterations of blood flow and sweating, *endocrine compensations*

Table 19
Physiological Inputs for Stimulation
and Inhibition of Vasopressin and OT Secretion

Hormone	Stimulation	Inhibition
Vasopressin	↑ Plasma osmolality ↓ Plasma volume ↓ Blood pressure ↓ Cardiac output (α↑,β↓) noradrenergic tone	↓ Plasma osmolality ↑ Plasma volume ↑ Blood pressure ↑ Cardiac output
Oxytocin	Suckling ↑ Activation of cervico–vaginal stretch receptors ↓ Placental progesterone ↑ Fetal cholesterol ↑ Sensory stimulation	Stress

↑ = Increase.
↓ = Decrease.

Table 20
Control of Cardiovascular Function
by the Hypothalamus

Area	Response
Lateral and posterior hypothalamus	↑ arterial pressure ↑ heart rate
Preoptic area	↓ arterial pressure ↓ heart rate

↑ = increase.
↓ = decrease.

such as metabolism-regulating alterations of thyroid function, and *musculoskeletal compensations* such as shivering, panting and piloerection (Table 21). Temperature regulation by the hypothalamus is also a nonendocrine example of a feedback mechanism. The regulatory system actually collects temperature information from two sources: peripheral sources such as the skin, visceral structures, and spinal cord, and central sources such as thermosensors in the preoptic area/anterior hypothalamus, whose neurons are activated or inactivated by the temperature of the blood bathing them. The hypothalamus bears dual mechanisms for controlling heat dissipation and heat conservation. The heat dissipation centers lie in the preoptic area/anterior hypothalamus, and the heat conservation centers lie in the posterior hypothalamus. Electrical stimulation of the preoptic area/anterior hypothalamus favors dilation of cutaneous blood vessels, panting, and suppression of shivering. All these result in a drop in body temperature. Conversely, electrical stimulation of the posterior hypothalamus leads to cutaneous vasoconstriction, visceral vasodilation, shivering, and a suppression of panting. The metabolic response to temperature alteration also involves the hypothalamus. Exposure to cold enhances the animal's heat-generating metabolic rate by stimulating TRH-activated TSH secretion and subsequent thyroid-hormone secretion. It is clear from recordings of neurons in the preoptic area/anterior hypothalamus that thermosensitive neurons are of two separate types: warm-sensitive and cold-sensitive. Thus, warming of either the skin or hypothalamus results in enhanced firing of warm-sensitive neurons and decreased firing of cold-sensitive neurons. Conversely, cooling of the skin or hypothalamus leads to opposite effects. Thus, these neurons serve to integrate information from the periphery as well as the CNS.

Interestingly, the hypothalamus coordinates voluntary behavioral adjustments to extremes in environmental temperatures sensed at both the hypothalamus and the skin. For example, in both rats and monkeys trained to make behavioral adjustments to a hot environment, local warming of the hypothalamus in the face of normal ambient temperature results in the appropriate behavioral adjustment to warmth. The hypothalamus will also integrate a summation of the responses. Thus when both the hypothalamus and the environment are warmed, the behavioral response is greater than either alone. In a hot environment, cooling of the hypothalamus will completely suppress the behavioral adjustment to elevation of environmental

Table 21
Thermoregulatory Function of the Hypothalamus

Compensation	Area	Response
Autonomic	Preoptic area	Dilation of cutaneous blood vessels sweating
	Posterior hypothalamus	Vasoconstriction
Musculoskeletal	Preoptic area	Panting Suppression of shivering
	Posterior hypothalamus	Shivering Suppression of panting Piloerection
Endocrine	Preoptic area	Thyroid function

temperature. Thus, the hypothalamus assumes supremacy in the behavioral responses to alteration in temperature. Finally, the hypothalamus mediates the response to pyrogens in pathological states. Body temperature is regulated around a set-point. Substances that allow the temperature to deviate from that set-point—*pyrogens*—can be produced by macrophages in disease state. The preoptic area appears to respond to one such pyrogen, interleukin-1. It has been suggested that the prostaglandins mediate the response to certain pyrogens and act at the preoptic area. Antipyretics such as indomethacin may act by blocking the synthesis of prostaglandins. The brain also contains a nearby *antipyretic area* within the septal nuclei. This area may use the peptide vasopressin. Injection of vasopressin directly into this area counteracts the effects of many known pyrogens. Thus, antipyretics may also act by stimulating the release of vasopressin. Injection of a vasopressin antagonist prevents the antipyretic effects of indomethacin.

4.2.3. DEFENSIVE FUNCTION

The hypothalamus is also responsible for the preparation of the organism to respond to threatening or stressful situations. The so-called *flight-or-fight* response actually represents an integrated constellation of responses to prepare for stressful situations (Table 22). Many of these responses are directly controlled by the hypothalamus, and others are indirectly controlled by the hypothalamus through its control of the endocrine system. The hypothalamus stimulates a variety of cardiovascular compensations. In response to a perceived threat, blood pressure, heart rate, force of contraction, and rate of cardiac conduction velocity increase. The rate and depth of respiration increases. There is a shift of blood flow from the skin and splanchnic organs to the skeletal muscles, heart, and brain.

Metabolic adjustments are made in anticipation of increased energy requirements. These are enhanced glycogenolysis and lipolysis. In addition to the cardiovascular adjustments, there are other autonomic alterations. These would be: mydriasis, ocular accommodation for far vision, contraction of the spleen capsule leading to increased hematocrit, piloerection, inhibition of gastric motility and secretion, contraction of gastrointestinal sphincters, and sweating. Some of these are regulated by the autonomic nervous system directly, and others are controlled by hormones secreted in response to stressful stimuli. Classically, epinephrine is secreted from the adrenal medulla in response to acute stressors. This catecholamine controls many of the metabolic demands of the flight-or-fight response. Additionally, glucocorticoids are secreted from the adrenal cortex in response to stressful stimuli. Secretion of glucocorticoids are controlled by ACTH secreted from the pituitary gland under the influence of hypothalamic CRH and AVP. In long-term stressful situations, this leads to suppression of the immune system. Other hormones whose secretion is stimulated in response to stress (and their putative roles in stress responses) are: β-endorphin (pain perception), vasopressin (renal function), glucagon (carbohydrate mobilization), and prolactin (immune responses). Growth hormone and insulin are typically inhibited during stressful circumstances. Many of these autonomic and hormonal responses are controlled by the anterior and ventromedial hypothalamus.

4.3. Regulation of Behavioral Processes

4.3.1. INGESTIVE BEHAVIOR

4.3.1.1. Hypothalamic Control of Feeding Behavior. The role of the hypothalamus is to coordinate ingestion with parallel neuroendocrine responses and long-term regulation of metabolism and adipos-

Table 22
Components of the Flight-or-Fight Response

1. Increase in: blood pressure, heart rate, force of contraction, rate of conduction velocity.
2. Increase in: rate and depth of respiration.
3. Shift in: blood flow from skin and splanchnic organs to skeletal muscles, heart, and brain.
4. Metabolic adjustments: enhanced glycogenolysis and lipolysis.
5. "Other" autonomic adjustments: mydriasis, accomodation for far vision, contraction of spleen capsule, piloerection, inhibition of gastric motility and secretion, contraction of gastrointestinal sphincters, sweating.

ity. Ingestion during short-term meals is coordinated by brainstem sensory and motor circuits. The nucleus of the solitary tract (NST) relays gustatory and visceral information about ingested food during individual meals by direct and indirect pathways to the hypothalamus. To achieve long-term weight regulation, the appetitive systems of the hypothalamus must also monitor energy storage (in peripheral adiposity) and generate neural signals back to the brainstem to increase or decrease food intake. Body weight is regulated by the balance of energy expenditure (e.g., basal metabolism and locomotor activity) and food intake. Total food intake is the product of number of meals (meal frequency) and meal size. Therefore, body weight can be altered through changes in hunger or appetite (e.g., to change meal initiation and frequency) or sensitivity to satiety signals (e.g., to alter meal size). The regulation of body wt and food intake is achieved by a complex network in the hypothalamus involving multiple transmitter and neuropeptide systems (Fig. 26).

4.3.1.2. Leptin is a Negative-Feedback Adiposity Signal. In order to regulate body weight and long-term energy balance, the hypothalamus must monitor the amount of long-term energy storage in the fat. Although the hypothalamus is sensitive to several other adiposity signals such as insulin, the adipose hormone leptin serves as the primary negative-feedback signal to the brain to regulate fat mass. Leptin is a 127-amino-acid peptide secreted into the circulation from adipocytes; plasma leptin levels are proportional to total body adiposity. Weight loss and food deprivation, which rapidly decrease fat mass and the metabolic rate of adipocytes, lead to a rapid decrease in plasma leptin. Overfeeding, refeeding after fasting, or increased adipose tissue mass increases plasma leptin. Because leptin is a negative-feedback signal, increased

leptin secreted by increased fat will reduce food intake; decreased leptin during weight loss causes increased appetite to drive compensatory hyperphagia. Exogenous systemic or central administration of leptin in animals reverses many of the physiological and behavioral correlates of fasting. In normally feeding or obese animals, leptin administration decreases appetite and food intake, and increases metabolic rate, resulting in weight loss. The leptin system is functional in humans, because of a mutation in the leptin gene that blocks leptin synthesis, or a mutation in the leptin receptor that results in functional hypoleptinemia, causes profound obesity and other neuroendocrine deficits. In mutants without leptin signaling, the hypothalamus responds as if the body has no fat reserves of energy: in order to compensate for the apparent starvation state, profound hunger and overeating occurs.

Leptin enters the arcuate nucleus and is transported across the blood–brain barrier to act on hypothalamic neurons that express leptin receptors. The leptin receptor is a member of the cytokine-receptor superfamily, and leptin binding activates Janus Kinasey Signal Transducer and Activator of Transcripton (JAK-STAT) signaling pathways that have both acute effects on neuronal firing rate and long-term effects on gene transcription. Leptin receptors are particularly highly expressed in NPY neurons and POMC neurons of the arcuate nucleus, and to a lesser degree on other cell types of the paraventricular nucleus and lateral hypothalamus. The neurons of the arcuate nucleus comprise interconnected but distinct and opposing pathways regulating food intake: the NPY system and the melanocortin system.

4.3.1.3. NPY System. The NPY neurons of the arcuate nucleus form the major orexigenic or appetite-stimulating system of the hypothalamus. They contain

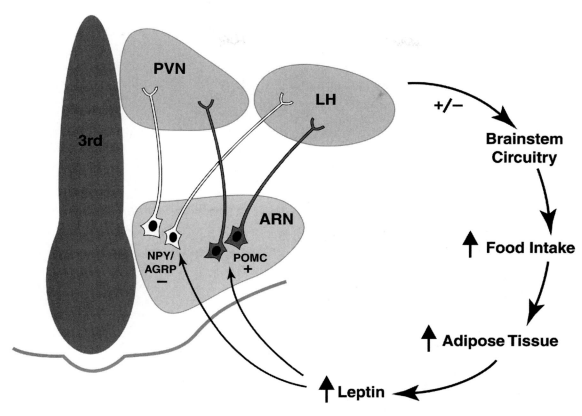

Fig. 26. Hypothalamic integration of ingestive behavior and adiposity. The acute behavior of food intake is largely regulated by neural networks of the pons and medulla. Increased food intake leads to increased fat mass and elevated leptin levels. Leptin provides negative feedback to the hypothalamus to decrease feeding, primarily by decreasing synthesis and release of NPY/AGRP (orexigenic peptides) and increasing synthesis of POMC and thus αMSH (an anorexic peptide) in neurons of the arcuate nucleus (ARN). The ARN neurons project to the paraventricular nucleus (PVN) and the lateral hypothalamus (LH), which in turn modulate brainstem circuitry to decrease food intake and maintain a stable level of adiposity. Food deprivation and reduced fat mass has the opposite effect (to increase food intake), reducing negative feedback by leptin.

the highest concentration of NPY within the brain; they are also unique in their co-expression of agouti-gene-related peptide (AGRP). The primary projection of the NPY neurons is from the arcuate nucleus to the hypothalamic paraventricular nucleus, but they also have long projections to midbrain, pons, and medulla, where they can interact directly with brainstem ingestive circuitry.

Exogenous NPY administered into the third ventricle or the paraventricular nucleus is the most potent orexigen known: nanogram quantities of NPY acting at Y1 and Y5 receptors cause rodents and primates to eat voraciously for hours. Consistent with the NPY system as a positive signal for food intake, food deprivation, and other hunger-inducing treatments cause an increase in NPY mRNA synthesis, peptide synthesis, and NPY release onto the paraventricular nucleus. Furthermore, negative feedback adiposity signals such

as leptin and insulin decrease NPY mRNA and peptide levels.

4.3.1.4. Melanocortin System. Intermingled with the NPY neurons of the arcuate nucleus are POMC neurons, which have projections to the paraventricular nucleus and LH that parallel the NPY projections. Although POMC serves as a precursor for several neuropeptides, α-melanocyte-stimulating hormone (αMSH) is the primary product found in the cells of ARN. Although NPY induces appetite, αMSH from POMC neurons acting on MC4 receptors has an opposing satiating effect. In many ways, POMC neurons respond to adiposity signals with a negative effect to balance NPY's positive effects on food intake. Thus, decreased plasma leptin after food deprivation or weight loss decreases POMC mRNA and peptide levels, and increased plasma leptin (e.g., after involuntary overfeeding) increases POMC expression in the arcuate nucleus in parallel with decreased eating. Injection of αMSH or other MC4 agonists into the hypothalamus reduces food intake; antagonism of the MC4 receptor causes increases in food intake. POMC neurons and MC4 receptors are also present in the brainstem, where they may contribute to local ingestive circuitry. The melanocortin system is critical to human physiology, as mutations in POMC or the MC4 receptor cause obesity in humans.

In an intriguing twist, NPY neurons of the ARN also produce AGRP, an endogenous peptide antagonist of the MC4 receptor. Like NPY, AGRP is a potent orexigen, but it acts by postsynaptically antagonizing αMSH signaling from the POMC neurons to reduce satiety and increase food intake. NPY neurons and POMC neurons have opposing responses to leptin and other adiposity signals, and opposing functional consequences at their target neurons, but the orexigenic NPY/AGRP neurons directly antagonize the satiating effects of the POMC neurons. Thus, the response of the hypothalamus to peripheral adiposity levels is an adjustment of the balance between NPY/AGRP orexigenic and POMC anorexic systems.

4.3.1.5. MCH and Other Peptide Systems. In
recent years, a large number of other peptides within the paraventricular nucleus and LH have been implicated in the control of feeding and body weight, including melanin-concentrating hormone (MCH), CRH, galanin, oxytocin, hypocretin/orexin, cocaine-and-amphetamine-regulated-transcript (CART) and TRH (Table 23). These other peptide systems are presumed to be secondary to the major modulatory role of leptin on NPY and POMC neurons of the arcuate nucleus, and can receive input from one or both types of ARN neurons. MCH is a particularly significant member of the secondary systems, because MCH injection into the brain potently induces food intake, and mice lacking MCH are lean, with reduced body fat mass.

4.3.1.6. Serotonin and Norepinephrine. The
hypothalamus receives dense innervation of serotonin fibers and norepinephrine fibers from the raphe nuclei and locus ceruleus, respectively, which can modulate the effects of the peptidergic systems. Stimulation of serotonin 5HT-2C receptors reduces food intake by decreasing meal size, and mice lacking 5HT2C receptors show mild obesity in adulthood. Similarly, norepinephrine release into the paraventricular nucleus

acting at beta-2 receptors decreases food intake and causes weight loss. Because the agonists of the monoamines are better characterized and are easier than peptidergic compounds to administer systemically, the serotonin and norepinephrine systems are more accessible targets for the pharmacological treatment of obesity than the peptide systems. Thus, the serotonin agonist fenfluramine and the mixed serotonin/norepinephrine reuptake inhibitor subitramine have been used to decrease food intake and induce weight loss in humans.

4.4. Obesity and Pharmacological Control of Appetite

Obesity (defined as a body mass index—weight divided by height squared—of 30 kg/m² or greater) is a growing problem in developed countries. Body-fat mass is rapidly increased by easy access to highly palatable, calorie-rich foods. Indeed, by engaging the dopaminergic reward pathways of the limbic system, palatability can override or reset the hypothalamic regulation of body weight. Because it contributes to many other illnesses (e.g., diabetes and cardiovascular disease), obesity is a major public health problem.

In many cases, there may be a genetic contribution to obesity. Mutations that cause obesity or leanness demonstrate the critical role of specific genes in normal behavior and physiology; however, mutations that are homologous to obese rodent mutations are exceedingly rare in humans. The genetic predisposition to obesity in some individuals is probably the result of more subtle interactions of polymorphisms in multiple appetite-regulating genes.

There are many potential points of body-weight regulation that might be targets for therapeutic manipulation. Because of its primary role as an adiposity signal, leptin signaling is an obvious candidate. However, human obesity is accompanied by leptin resistance because plasma levels of leptin are greatly elevated in obese individuals. As mentioned previously, serotonin and norepinephrine are the most accessible factors. Serotonin and norepinephrine receptors are widely distributed in the brain and periphery, and thus, monoamine treatments are usually accompanied by unwanted side-effects. Because the hypothalamus contains unique peptide systems that engage both endogenous appetitive and satiating mechanisms, future treatments may be able to mimic

Table 23
Peptides Involved in the Hypothalamic Regulation of Ingestion

Peptide	Source	Effect
Leptin	Adipocytes	Anorexic

Val[1]-Pro-Ile-Gln-Lys-Val-Gln-Asp-Asp-Thr-Lys-Thr-Leu-Ile-Lys-Thr-Ile-Val-Thr-Arg-Ile-Asn-Asp-Ile-
Ser-His-Thr-Gln-Ser-Val-Ser-Ser-Lys-Gln-Lys-Val-Thr-Gly-Leu-Asp-Phe-Ile-Pro-Gly-Leu-His-Pro-Ile-
Leu-Thr-Leu-Ser-Lys-Met-Asp-Gln-Thr-Leu-Ala-Val-Tyr-Gln-Gln-Ile-Leu-Thr-Ser-Met-Pro-Ser-Arg-
Asn-Val-Ile-Gln-Ile-Ser-Asn-Asp-Leu-Glu-Asn-Leu-Arg-Asp-Leu-Leu-His-Val-Leu-Ala-Phe-Ser-Lys-
Ser-Cys-His-Leu-Pro-Trp-Ala-Ser-Gly-Leu-Glu-Thr-Leu-Asp-Ser-Leu-Gly-Gly-Val-Leu-Glu-Ala-Ser-
Gly-Tyr-Ser-Thr-Glu-Val-Val-Ala-Leu-Ser[127]

AGRP	ARN	Orexigenic (αMSH antagonist)

Leu[1]-Ala-Pro-Met-Glu-Gly-Ile-Arg-Arg-Pro-Asp-Gln-Ala-Leu-Leu-Pro-Glu-Leu-Pro-Gly-Leu-Gly-Leu-
Arg-Ala-Pro-Leu-Lys-Lys-Thr-Thr-Ala-Glu-Gln-Ala-Glu-Glu-Asp-Leu-Leu-Gln-Glu-Ala-Gln-Ala-Leu-
Ala-Glu-Val-Leu-Asp-Leu-Gln-Asp-Arg-Glu-Pro-Arg-Ser-Ser-Arg-Arg-Cys-Val-Arg-Leu-His-Glu-Ser-
Cys-Leu-Gly-Gln-Gln-Val-Pro-Val-Val-Asp-Pro-Cys-Ala-Thr-Cys-Tyr-Cys-Arg-Phe-Phe-Asn-Ala-Phe-
Cys-Tyr-Cys-Arg-Lys-Leu-Gly-Thr-Ala-Met-Asn-Pro-Cys-Ser-Arg-Thr[108]

CART	ARN	Anorexic

Gln[1]-Glu-Asp-Ala-Glu-Leu-Gln-Pro-Arg-Ala-Leu-Asp-Ile-Tyr-Ser-Ala-Val-Asp-Asp-Ala-Ser-His-Glu-
Lys-Glu-Leu-Ile-Glu-Ala-Leu-Gln-Glu-Val-Leu-Lys-Lys-Leu-Lys-Ser-Lys-Arg-Val-Pro-Ile-Tyr-Glu-
Lys-Lys-Tyr-Gly-Gln-Val-Pro-Met-Cys-Asp-Ala-Gly-Glu-Gln-Cys-Ala-Val-Arg-Lys-Gly-Ala-Arg-Ile-
Gly-Lys-Leu-Cys-Asp-Cys-Pro-Arg-Gly-Thr-Ser-Cys-Asn-Ser-Phe-Leu-Leu-Lys-Cys-Leu[89]

MCH	LH	Orexigenic

Asp[1]-Phe-Asp-Met-Leu-Arg-Cys-Met-Leu-Gly-Arg-Val-Tyr-Arg-Pro-Cys-Trp-Gln-Val[19]

Hypocretin1/Orexin A	LH	Orexigenic/Wakefulness

Gln[1]-Pro-Leu-Pro-Leu-Cys-Cys-Arg-Gln-Lys-Thr-Cys-Ser-Cys-Arg-Lys-Tyr-Glu-Leu-Leu-His-Gly-Ala-
Gly-Asn-His-Ala-Ala-Gly-Ile-Leu-Thr-Leu-Gly[34]

Hypocretin2/Orexin B	LH	Orexigenic/Wakefulness

Arg-Ser-Gly-Pro-Pro-Gly-Leu-Pro-Gly-Arg-Leu-Pro-Arg-Leu-Leu-Pro-Ala-Ser-Gly-Asn-His-Ala-Ala-Gly-
Ile-Leu-Thr-Met-Gly[29]

See other tables for the sequences of the two major arcuate peptides, orexigenic NPY and anorexic αMSH. Neurons of the arcuate nucleus (ARN) containing NPY/AGRP or POMC/CART are the major targets of leptin; neurons containing MCH, hypocretin/orexin, and other peptides such as galanin, CRH, and TRH are targets of the arcuate neurons. There are two peptide products of the hypocretin/orexin gene; note that they may exert an orexigenic effect by regulating wakefulness and arousal rather than appetite.

or antagonize these endogenous systems specifically and efficaciously.

4.5. Hypothalamic Control of Drinking Behavior

Thirst is regulated by tissue osmolality and vascular volume. These are controlled, in turn, by AVP secreted from magnocellular neurons in the supraoptic nucleus and also by *AII* formed in the plasma as well as the brain. Although the drive for water ingestion is through enhanced tissue osmolality and/or decreased vascular volume sensed by osmoreceptors in the brain and baroreceptors in the brain and periph-ery, there appears to be a direct effect of hormones acting at the hypothalamus to mediate the behavioral response. The SFO lies near the third ventricle, and has fenestrated capillaries permitting entrance of blood-borne materials. The SFO responds to low levels of AII in the blood and conveys information to the hypothalamus. It is possible that the communication is by way of a neuronally derived *AII* that affects the preoptic area. In addition, the preoptic area receives information from peripheral baroreceptors. Thus, when water ingestion is required, the baroreceptors and *AII* stimulate the preoptic area, which in turn activates other areas of the brain to begin drinking.

The drive for termination of drinking is less understood. However, it is clear that cessation of drinking is not merely the absence of the baroreceptor and osmoreceptor-initiating signal.

4.6. Sexual Behavior

The circumscribed behaviors leading to pregnancy and propagation of the species depend on the interaction of the gonads and the hypothalamus. In subprimate mammals, these events are driven by a heightened period of female sexual receptivity known as *estrus*, which coincides with the availability of a potentially fertilizable egg in the oviduct. Since these female mammals have reproductive cycles characterized by a heightened receptivity, the cycles are referred to as *estrous cycles* (noun:estrus; adjective:estrous). A similar coincidence of gamete availability is not discretely defined in most primates. Since primate cycles are overtly characterized by a period of breakdown of the lining and blood vessels of the uterus known as *menses*, these are referred to as *menstrual cycles*. Obviously, sexual receptivity is best studied in mammals that overtly display the behavior at discrete periods. For this reason, the rat is the most widely studied model of hypothalamic control of sexual behavior.

4.6.1. HYPOTHALAMIC CONTROL OF SEXUAL BEHAVIOR IN FEMALES

Sexual receptivity can be quantitated in female rats by a *lordosis quotient*, or *LQ*. Lordosis is the process by which the female arches her back, deflects her tail, and stands rigid to allow mounting and intromission by the male. The LQ is the number of times this event takes place divided by the number of attempts at mounting by the male multiplied by 100. Although the effects of various hormones on sexual behavior are species-specific, the common hormone that regulates most sexual behaviors is the ovarian hormone *estrogen* (Table 24). Estrogen receptors are present in the areas of the hypothalamus known to control sexual receptivity. Estrogen secretion is highest when sexual receptivity is increased. Although estrogen, by itself, will enhance sexual receptivity, sexual receptivity is greatest when both estrogen and *progesterone* secretion is highest. Progesterone, by itself, exerts little effect on sexual receptivity. Only in an estrogen-primed animal will progesterone further enhance sexual receptivity. Estrogens act by stimulating progesterone receptors in areas of the hypothalamus known to control sexual receptivity. Prolonged exposure to progesterone (as in pregnancy) causes a downregulation of progesterone receptors in the hypothalamus, and subsequently a decrease in sexual receptivity. Four parts of the nervous system have been shown to play a role in the control of female sexual behavior: *the forebrain, the ventromedial hypothalamic nucleus (VMN), the midbrain central gray*, and *the lower brainstem and spinal cord*. Within the hypothalamus, lesions of the VMN depress sexual behavior in response to estrogen and progesterone. The VMN bears receptors for the ovarian steroids. This hypothalamic nucleus is believed to modulate the intensity or interpretation of sexually related sensory input. Estrogen receptors are also localized in the midbrain central grey. Neurons from both the VMN and spinal cord project to the midbrain central grey. The spinal projection transmits tactile information provided by the male's mounting required for the induction of lordosis. The neurotransmitter control of female sexual behavior is well-described, but cannot be reduced to participation by a single transmitter. Among the catecholamines, ascending noradrenergic fibers from the locus coeruleus regulate lordosis behavior by acting upon α_1-noradrenergic receptors in the medial preoptic area and VMN. Norepinephrine may act in these areas by modulating progesterone receptors. Dopamine, however, does not play a role in lordosis behavior, but appears to modulate proceptive behaviors such as ear wiggling, hopping, or darting. Acetylcholine plays a role in the facilitation of lordosis behavior through estrogen. This steroid not only increases the activity of choline acetyltransferase, and increases the activity of acetylcholine receptors in the VMN. Moreover, acetylcholine applied directly to the medial preoptic area or VMN increases lordosis behavior, and acetylcholine antagonists applied to these same areas abolish or attenuate lordotic behavior. Among the indolamines, serotonin appears to play an inhibitory role in sexual receptivity. Inhibition of serotonin synthesis excites lordosis behavior, and thus it has been suggested that serotonin is a *sexual satiety* neurotransmitter. A similar role has been proposed for gamma-aminobutyric acid (GABA). Some of the hypothalamic peptides that serve a neuroendocrine role in regulating the pituitary gland also serve a neurotransmitter role in regulating sexual behaviors in the female. The best example is GnRH. When GnRH is applied directly to the hypothalamus of ovariectomized female rats receiving an ineffective dose of estradiol, lordosis behavior is exhibited. This suggests that GnRH both stimulates LH secretion and consequent ovulation and subsequent sexual behavior in the female. In addition, not

Table 24
Hypothalamic Control of Sexual Behavior in Females

Chemical mediator	Site of action	Effect
Estrogen	Ventromedial nucleus Midbrain central gray	Increase LQ*
Progesterone	Ventromedial nucleus Preoptic area	Increase LQ response to estrogen
Norepinephrine	Ventromedial nucleus Preoptic area	Modulate progesterone receptors
Acetylcholine	Ventromedial nucleus Medial preoptic area	Modulate LQ response to steroids
Serotonin		Inhibit sexual behavior
GnRH	Midbrain central gray	Heighten response to estradiol
Prolactin	Midbrain central gray	Heighten response to estradiol

*LQ = lordosis quotient.

only do preoptic GnRH neurons project to the arcuate nucleus/ME area and subsequently release the peptide into portal blood to bathe the adenohypophysis, but they also project to the midbrain central grey, the site mediating sexual receptivity. GnRH applied to the midbrain cenral grey stimulates sexual receptivity, and GnRH antisera applied to this area depresses sexual receptivity. Aside from neuropeptides, pituitary hormones themselves may play a role in sexual receptivity. Indeed, prolactin applied directly to the MCG enhances sexual receptivity in rats receiving a low dose of estradiol. Conversely, pharmacologic depression of prolactin secretion at the time of anticipated onset of estrus depresses the magnitude of sexual receptivity. Finally, pituitary hormones are released in response to the mating stimulus. It is well-established that prolactin is released from the adenohypophysis of rodents in response to excitation at the uterine cervix by the act of mating, which is transmitted to the hypothalamus through spinal pathways. It has been shown that the mating stimulus acts at the hypothalamus by lowering tuberoinfundibular dopaminergic tone, which subsequently leads to the release of prolactin. Prolactin, in turn, activates the corpora lutea to maintain progesterone secretion, which maintains the subsequent pregnancy. The other pituitary hormone released in response to the mating stimulus is OT. Once again, the stimulus is transmitted over spinal pathways to enhance the activity of magnocellular neurons in the paraventricular nucleus. It has been suggested that once OT is released in response to the mating stimulus,

it acts to enhance uterine contractions and thus favor sperm transport from the site of deposition at the mouth of the cervix to the site of fertilization at the oviduct. The lone weakness in this theory is that rather than enhancing contractions of the uterus from the cervical toward the ovarian direction, the contractions are enhanced in the ovarian–cervical direction. This process would appear to retard sperm transport at best.

4.6.2. Hypothalamic Control of Sexual Behavior in Males

The sexual behavior of male rodents is characterized as having both *motivational* and *consummatory* components (Table 25). Motivational are those behaviors required to gain access to the female in heat. Consummatory behaviors are those required for copulation. These would include mounting, erection, intromission, and ejaculation. Stereotypical male sexual behaviors are provoked by testosterone secreted from the Leydig cells of the testis. Testosterone controls male sexual behavior through two mechanisms. In peripheral tissues, testosterone is converted to dihydrotestosterone (DHT). DHT is responsible for stimulating sensory receptors, and thus may play a role in penile erection. Testosterone acts on the preoptic area of the hypothalamus to integrate the various consummatory components of male sexual behavior. The amygdala controls the motivational components of male sexual behavior. This function of estrogen appears to have been aromatized from testosterone intraneuronally. Among the catecholamines, dopam-

Table 25
Hypothalamic Control of Sexual Behaviors in Males

Chemical mediator	Site of action	Effect
Testosterone	Preoptic area	Control consummatory behaviors.
Estradiol	Amygdala	Control motivational behaviors.
Mesolimbic dopamine	Amydala	Control motivational behaviors.
Incertohypothalamic	Preoptic area	Control consummatory behaviors.
GnRH	Preoptic area	Control consummatory behaviors.
Endorphins	Preoptic area	Inhibit consummatory behaviors.

ine from mesolimbic neurons appears to be the neurotransmitter that controls the motivational component of male sexual behavior. The incertohypothalamic dopaminergic system appears to be responsible for the consummatory component. Neuropeptides have been shown to modulate both motivational and consummatory behaviors. GnRH appears to act within the preoptic area to control consummatory behaviors. Endorphin neurons projecting from the amygdala to the preoptic area appear to have the opposite effects, they inhibit many consummatory behaviors. Other peptides that have been implicated in male sexual behaviors include substance P, NPY, α-melanophore-stimulating hormone and oxytocin. However, the physiological significance of their role has not been fully determined. As mentioned earlier, the preoptic area of the hypothalamus is sexually dimorphic, which is reflected in the pattern of LH secretion from the adenohypophysis. The dimorphic nature of the hypothalamus is also reflected in stereotypical male or female sexual behaviors. Just as males who are deprived of testosterone neonatally present a female cyclic pattern of LH secretion when challenged with estrogen as adult, so they will also present the typical female receptive lordotic pattern in response to estrogen and an aggressive male. Conversely, a female treated neonatally with testosterone will show the non-cyclic pattern of LH secretion as an adult and, if treated with testosterone as adult, will mount females in heat. Some of this sexual differentiation occurs in utero but in rodents most of it is determined neonatally. Thus, all hypothalami develop potentially as functionally female, and the differentiating event is the presence of androgen prenatally or neonatally.

4.7. Maternal Behavior

The hypothalamus is also intimately involved in mediating maternal behaviors stimulated by both ovarian and pituitary hormones (Table 26). Again, the rodent model is the most frequently studied. There are essentially four components of maternal behavior in the rat. *Nestbuilding* is the first behavioral sign. Late in pregnancy, the rat will gather bedding and any other materials available, and prepare a nest in which she can deliver, nurse, and care for the young. She designs this to be the center of all her activities while the young are present. After the pups are born, the dam spends a large amount of time *licking* the neonates for the purpose of cleaning. The typical behavior rodents share with all mammals is assumption of a *nursing* posture to allow the hungry young access to the mammary glands for retrieval of milk. Finally, as the nursing young mature, they tend to leave the convenience and safety of the mother's nest. The nursing mother then spends much time *retrieving* the young to the nest. The hormonal drive for the onset of maternal behavior actually occurs during the prepartum period (Table 26). By supplying foster pups late in pregnancy, the development of these behaviors can be characterized. The signal appears to be the gradual decline in progesterone secretion by the placenta, coupled with the increase in ovarian estrogen secretion as the time of parturition approaches. The prepartum period can therefore be envisioned as a period of *hormonal priming*. Maternal behaviors are not only the result of the combined actions of estradiol in the face of the withdrawal of progesterone, but they also influenced by adenohypophyseal (or perhaps even neural) prolactin. OT may also play a role. Estrogen exerts its effect on maternal behavior largely through an action at the medial preoptic area. Much of the action of estrogen at the medial preoptic area is through stimulation of estrogen receptors. In general, throughout pregnancy estrogen receptors are much greater in the preoptic area than in the entire hypothalamus. On the last day of pregnancy, estrogen receptors in the rest of the hypothalamus rise to levels equivalent to those of the preoptic area. In addition to stimulating parental

Table 26
Hypothalamic Control of Maternal Behavior

Chemical mediator	Site of action	Effect
Estrogen after decline of progesterone	Medial preoptic area	Stimulate maternal behaviors.
Prolactin	Preoptic area	Stimulate maternal behaviors in estrogen-primed rats.
OT	Ventromedial nucleus	Stimulate maternal behaviors in estrogen-primed rats.

behaviors directly, estrogens also stimulate prolactin secretion. Moreover, it is the withdrawal of progesterone at the end of pregnancy that allows prolactin to exert its actions on the mammary gland to initiate and maintain lactation. Prolactin, when secreted after parturition, has been implicated in the control of maternal behaviors. Indeed, hypophysectomy or treatment with the DA agonist bromocryptine, will prevent many of the components of maternal behavior. In contrast, the infusion of prolactin directly into the preoptic area or into the CSF through the third ventricle stimulates maternal behaviors in estrogen-primed female rats. Thus, prolactin can act upon cells in the preoptic area as well as the circumventricular organs. Since prolactin is a large polypeptide, it is unlikely that it can cross the blood-brain barrier to affect neural structures. There are essentially three possibilities from the route prolactin may take to affect neural structures and subsequently maternal behavior. One is that pituitary prolactin arrives at the hypothalamus by *retrograde blood flow* through the portal circulation. Alternatively, it has been shown that circulating prolactin has access to the CSF and brain through a receptor transport system located in the choroid plexes of the lateral, third, and fourth ventricles. Finally, the most recent evidence indicates that specific areas of the hypothalamus contain prolactin mRNA leading to the suggestion that prolactin is synthesized in these areas distinct from pituitary prolactin. Since estrogen can enhance brain and CSF levels of prolactin in *hypophysectomized rats*, it has been suggested that estrogen stimulates central prolactin synthesis and that centrally prolactin may enhance the sensitivity of estrogen-sensitive cells in the hypothalamus that regulate maternal behavior. Among the hypothalamic peptides, OT has been shown to promote maternal behavior when injected into the CSF of estrogen-treated rats. OT is ineffective when injected peripherally. Moreover, an OT antagonist is effective in delaying maternal behavior when

injected centrally. Destruction of the paraventricular nucleus, the source of OT, also modifies maternal behaviors. The effects of OT are correlated with the appearance of OT cell-membrane receptors in areas of the brain known to mediate maternal behavior. These include the VMN of the hypothalamus, the bed nucleus of the stria terminalis, the anterior olfactory nucleus, and the central nucleus of the amygdala.

4.8. Emotional Behaviors

It has long been appreciated that the hypothalamus participates in emotional responses. For example, electrical stimulation of the lateral hypothalamus of cats results in many of the somatic and autonomic characteristics of *anger* such as piloerection, pupillary constriction, arching of the back, raising of the tail, and increased blood pressure. Similar rage-like responses can be elicited by decortication or merely separating the hypothalamus from the cortex. The anger that is elicited is referred to as *sham rage*. Such animals respond to seemingly innocuous stimulation with a multitude of aggressive responses. The hypothalamus appears to act as an integrating center for these responses.

4.9. Regulation of Rhythmic Events

4.9.1. TYPES OF RHYTHMS

Rhythms (Fig. 27) are characterized by their *period* (the time needed to complete one cycle), *frequency* (number of cycles per unit time), *phase* (points of reference on a time scale), and *amplitude* (the magnitude of variation from the mean). Biological rhythms are endogenous and self-sustaining. The only external cues may be provided by *Zeitgebers* or time-givers such as lighting periodicity in some rhythms. Biological rhythms fall into one of four categories based on their period (Table 27): *circadian* (approximately one day and thus driven by zeitgeber), *ultradian* (less than one day and of much greater frequency such as heart

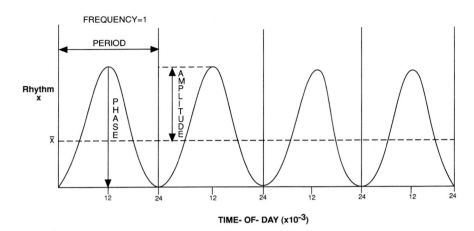

Fig. 27. Parameters of a *rhythm* (x) over four complete cycles of any *zeitgeiber*. For purposes of this example, imagine that the zeitgeber is the lighting periodicity of an artificial 24-h day with daylight lasting from 7 a.m. to 7 a.m. The *period* is the time to complete one cycle of the rhythm. In this example the period is 24 h. The *frequency* is the number of cycles per unit of time. Here the frequency of rhythm x is one (per day). The *phase* is the maximum of the rhythm in reference to a time scale such as that provided by the lighting periodicity or a clock. The *amplitude* is the deviation from the mean of the rhythm, x̄.

Table 27
Categories of Biological Rhythms

Rhythm	Approximate period	Example
Ultradian	Much less than 24 h	Respiration, heart rate
Circadian	Approx 24 h	Corticosterone rhythm
Infradian	Greater than 24 h but much less than 365 d	Menstrual cycles
Circannual	Seasonal, approx 365 d	Hibernation

beat or respiration), *circannual* (greater than one day and usually synchronized with seasonal events, such as seasonal fat deposition) and *infradian* (greater than one day but shorter than a year, such as menstrual or estrous cycles).

4.9.2. ROLE OF THE HYPOTHALAMUS IN BIOLOGICAL RHYTHMS

We have already described the role of hypothalamic neurohormones and neurotransmitters in infradian rhythms characterized by the menstrual and estrous cycles. Indeed, the cyclic release of luteinizing hormone every 28 d in the human female involves participation of parts of the hypothalamus, ranging from the most rostral to the most caudal boundaries. In rodents, it is particularly useful to appreciate the multifaceted roles of various areas of the hypothalamus regulating the various rhythms that comprise the estrous cycle. For example, it is well-known that

GnRH neurons in the preoptic area respond to estrogen secreted every 4–5 d by secreting the peptide into portal blood and consequently release a large bolus of LH into peripheral plasma. Thus the preoptic area controls an infradian rhythm. The preoptic area also controls a circadian rhythm. Again, in rodents, ovariectomy and estrogen replacement results in not just a single preovulatory-like surge of LH secretion, but a surge at the same time on each day for the next several days. Shifting the lighting phase will shift the time of the occurrence of each surge an equivalent amount. Thus, the lighting periodicity is the zeitgeber and the biological event is a true circadian rhythm. It is well-known that hypothalamic circadian rhythms require the participation of a timing device or *clock* within the hypothalamus. This role is served by the *suprachiasmatic nucleus* (SCN) of the hypothalamus. Destruction of the SCN will result in the inability of the rat to transduce the lighting periodicity. A circadian rhythm generalizable to virtually all mammals is the adrenal corticosterone rhythm. In response to entrainment by lighting periodicity (rodents) or activity rhythms (man), corticosterone levels in the blood begin to increase and reach peak magnitudes at the same time each day. This process has been shown to be driven by pituitary ACTH and hypothalamic CRH as described previously. In rodents, the stimulus is the onset of darkness, whereas in man it is the onset of activity or wakefulness cycles. It is quite clear that the secretion of most pituitary hormones is not merely biphasic (basal and surge pattern), but is actually pulsatile, and that blood levels of hormone at any time represent the summation of an ultradian pattern of hormone secretion from the cell. Such a rhythm is probably the result of the activity of a *pulse generator* within the hypothalamus, regulating neurohormone secretion into hypophyseal portal blood. A pulsatile ultradian rhythm of LH secretion is revealed in ovariectomized rats and monkeys. Measurement of multiple-unit activity in the medial basal hypothalamus of monkeys reveals that the pulsatile pattern of LH secretion coincides with spikes of multiple-unit activity in the medial basal hypothalamus. This implies that the pulse generator for GnRH and subsequent LH secretion (at least in monkeys) resides within the medial basal hypothalamus. Annual or circannual rhythms are not exclusively linked to the hypothalamus. Annual behavioral rhythms are of two types. Type I annual rhythms are dependent upon the environment, and type II are dependent upon an endogenous biological clock. Type I rhythms are generally photoperiodic driven because they require transduction of seasonal changes in day length. For example, as day length shortens during the late summer through early fall (short days) voles reduce their food intake and their gonads involute. Under long days of spring, food intake and gonadal weights return to normal. Type II annual rhythms are those that *free run*, (e.g., require no environmental input and thus persist under constant environmental conditions). European starlings store fat prior to their demanding spring migration. Under constant light, temperature, and food availability, the rhythm of fat deposition persists. Each animal free runs with a period of 1 yr, and eventually become desynchronized under constant environmental conditions. We have already mentioned that photoperiodic time measurement involves the SCN of the hypothalamus. Fibers from the retina of the eye terminate within the SCN. It is over this *retinohypothalamic tract* that the lighting periodicity is transduced.

Efferent fibers from the SCN terminate in the paraventricular nucleus, which in turn sends efferent fibers via the medial forebrain bundle to the spinal cord, which terminates upon the *intermediolateral cell column*. Processes from these cells synapse in the *superior cervical ganglion of the sympathetic chain*. Postganglionic noradrenergic fibers from this area then project to and innervate the *pineal gland*. Through this pathway, the SCN generates a circadian rhythm in the pineal hormone *melatonin*, which is synchronized to the light-dark cycle. Melatonin is produced in greatest amounts during dark phases of the cycle, and appears to be most important in mediating the effects of annual rhythms. The testes of male hamsters are most competent to produce sperm and normal levels of testosterone during the long days of summer. Pinealectomy prevents the loss of competency when animals are placed in the abbreviated illumination of short days. However, if pinealectomized hamsters receive long melatonin pulses (signaling short days or long nights) the testes regress independently of the environmental photoperiod. There appears to be a strain difference in the sensitivity to melatonin. In addition, not all mammals are dependent upon the pineal gland for generation of biological rhythms. For example, the rat, a photoperiodic mammal, has normally timed ovulation-inducing surges of LH release from the pituitary gland when pinealectomized. In those animals responsive to melatonin, the sites in the CNS and periphery where melatonin acts to regulate biological rhythms are unclear. Although there are marked species differences, the anterior hypothalamus, the SCN and the adenohypophysis apear to be candidate sites.

5. CONCLUSION

By now, the neuroscience student must appreciate a point made in the Introduction to this chapter. The hypothalamus does not exert control over one process exclusive of other processes. Thus, the hypothalamus plays an *integrative role* in adapting the organism to demands placed upon it by its environment. Because of its multifaceted role in allowing the organism to respond to the environment, the hypothalamus can be appropriately characterized as an organ that most uniquely ensures the perpetuation of the species.

SELECTED READING

Conn PM and Freeman ME. (eds) Neuroendocrinology in Physiology and Medicine. Totowa, NJ: Humana Press, 2000.

16 The Cerebral Cortex

Michael W. Miller and Brent A. Vogt

1. INTRODUCTION

As the name implies, the cerebral cortex forms a shell that covers the brain. In fact, the cortex forms most of the visible surface of the brain. Below its surface is a complex network of neurons and axons. The cerebral cortex is not uniform; rather, it is composed of many structurally and functionally unique subunits that perform a wide range of sensory, motor, and mnemonic processes associated with cognition. Cortex organizes affective behaviors, including responses to painful stimuli, maternal and sexual behaviors, and the expression of rage and other emotions. Like other parts of the CNS, the cerebral cortex does not function in isolation, but it is a part of an intricate plexus of overlapping circuits. This chapter describes the morphology of cortical neurons and the way in which these neurons are assembled into clusters, columns, and areas. In addition, this chapter describes the intrinsic and extrinsic circuitries that subserve the principal functions of the cerebral cortex.

2. SURFACE FEATURES OF THE CEREBRAL CORTEX

Magnetic resonance images of the cerebral cortex, like those in Fig. 1, show that the cortex has a corrugated appearance. The crest of each fold is known as a gyrus, and a depression between adjacent gyri is a sulcus. Very deep sulci are known as fissures. Two principal fissures are the space between the hemispheres, the interhemispheric fissure, and the lateral fissure (of Sylvius). The lateral surface of the cerebral cortex is composed of four lobes: the frontal, parietal, temporal, and occipital lobes. The medial surface contains extensions of each of these lobes and the limbic lobe.

The *frontal lobe* is the large anterior segment of the cerebral cortex. It extends from the rostral pole of each hemisphere to the central sulcus (of Rolando) and from the cingulate sulcus on the medial wall to the lateral

From: *Neuroscience in Medicine, 2nd ed.* (P. Michael Conn, ed.),
© 2003 Humana Press Inc., Totowa, NJ.

fissure on the lateral surface. The frontal lobe is composed of five major gyri. The precentral gyrus, which contains the motor cortex, runs parallel to the central sulcus and is bounded by the central and precentral sulci. Coursing perpendicular to the precentral gyrus on the lateral surface of the frontal lobe are the superior, middle, and inferior frontal gyri. The inferior frontal gyrus is further subdivided into the opercular, triangular, and orbital parts. An operculum is an extension of the cortex that overlies or overhangs another region. In this instance, the operculum overlies the cortex in the depths of the lateral fissure, the insular cortex (Fig. 1E,F). The opercular and triangular divisions of the inferior frontal gyrus contain Broca's speech area. The fronto-orbital gyri form the ventral part of the frontal lobe and rest on the orbital plate of the frontal bone.

The *parietal lobe* is bounded rostrally by the central sulcus, medially by the cingulate sulcus, posteromedially by the parieto-occipital sulcus, posterolaterally by an imaginary line between the parieto-occipital sulcus and the preoccipital notch, and ventrally by the lateral fissure. The parietal cortex includes the postcentral gyrus, a strip of cortex that is located posterior to the central sulcus and parallel to the precentral gyrus. The postcentral gyrus contains the somatosensory cortex. Caudal to the postcentral gyrus are the superior and inferior parietal lobules, which are divided by the intraparietal sulcus. The inferior parietal lobule is composed of two gyri, the supramarginal gyrus that caps the lateral fissure and the angular gyrus, which straddles the border with occipital cortex and forms the banks of the end of the superior temporal sulcus. Two regions form the medial surface of the parietal lobe. One is the paracentral lobule, which surrounds the medial tip of the central sulcus. This lobule also includes a segment of the frontal cortex. Caudal to the paracentral lobule is the precuneal cortex, which ventrally blends with the limbic lobe.

The *insula* is an island of cortex in the depths of the lateral fissure. It is covered by the opercular cortex of the frontal, parietal, and temporal lobes. The dorsal border of the lateral fissure is composed of the opercu-

lar part of the inferior frontal gyrus and the parietal operculum, whereas the ventral border is composed of the temporal operculum. The rostral insula is part of the limbic system, although its specific functions are not fully understood. The posterior part of the insula is mainly involved in processing somatosensory information.

The *temporal lobe* is ventral to the lateral fissure. This lobe includes the superior, middle, and inferior temporal gyri that run parallel to the lateral fissure. The dorsal surface of the superior temporal gyrus contains the transverse gyri (of Heschl), where the primary representation of audition is located. The ventral part of the temporal lobe includes the occipito-temporal gyrus. The *occipital lobe* includes the cortex caudal to an imaginary line through the parieto-occipital sulcus and notch, which demarcates it from the temporal lobe. The occipital lobe includes the calcarine fissure, and within and around this is the visual cortex.

In 1868, the comparative neurologist Paul Broca defined the *limbic lobe*. This lobe is composed of the cingulate gyrus and hippocampal and parahippocampal gyri. The limbic lobe contains areas that are a major part of the anatomical limbic system, as discussed in Chapter 17. This cortical region is involved in olfaction, memory, and visceral, skeletal, and endocrine functions associated with emotional behaviors.

3. CORTICAL CYTOLOGY

3.1. Projection Neurons

Most cortical neurons are projection neurons, and the most common cortical projection neuron is the pyramidal neuron. The general features of projection neurons are described in Table 1. A typical pyramidal neuron has a large pyramid-shaped cell body that gives rise to two sets of dendrites (Fig. 2). One set is a prominent dendrites that issues from the apex of the cell body. This apical dendrite often reaches layer I, where it arborizes in a tuft of dendrites. In addition, the apical dendrite gives rise to smaller caliber collateral processes that often branch at right angles. The second set of dendrites are processes that emanate from the base

---

Fig. 1. (*Opposite page*) Magnetic resonance imaging is used to examine the structure of the brain. (**A**) A lateral view of the cerebral cortex can be appreciated in a brain reconstructed from serial magnetic resonance images. This image is a compilation of a series of 1.5-mm thick sections. (**B**) The sulci and gyri are labeled. The labels for the sulci are placed around the brain, whereas the labels for the gyri are placed at the appropriate site on the brain. (**C,D**) A parasagittal section reveals a number of the features characteristic of the medial surface of the brain. The horizontal and vertical lines shown in **C** identify the planes of section used in the horizontal and coronal sections shown in **E** and **F**, respectively. cg, cingulate gyrus; co-collateral sulcus; cs, cingulate sulcus; hf, hippocampal formation; in, insula; lf, lateral fissure. (MRI images courtesy of Nancy Andreasen, University of Iowa, Iowa City, IA.)

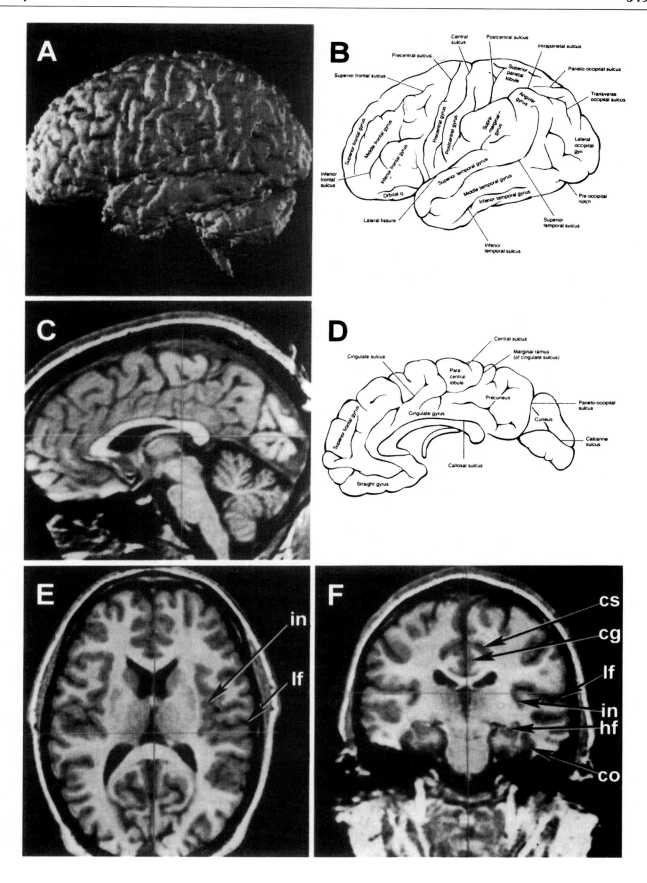

Table 1
Features of Types of Cortical Neurons

Feature	Projection neurons	Local circuit neurons
Dendrites	Spinous	Aspinous
Axons	Local arbors and distant projections	Local arbors only
Synapses formed by: Axo-somatic afferents	Symmetric	Symmetric and asymmetric
Efferents	Asymmetric	Symmetric
Neurotransmitter	Glutamate and aspartate	GABA and neuropeptides
Discharge properties	Regular spiking	Fast spiking

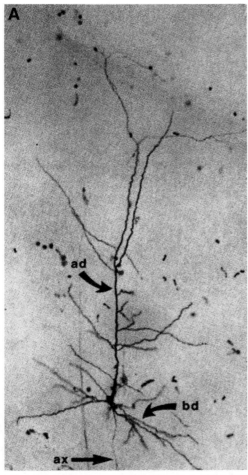

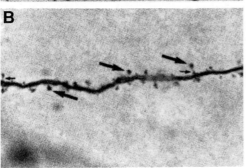

of the cell body. In contrast to the apical dendrite, the branches of the basal dendrites bifurcate at acute angles. All of the dendrites (with the exception of the dendritic segments proximal to the cell body) are densely covered with small protuberances known as spines. A spine typically has the appearance of a lollipop, with a large rounded head that is attached to the dendritic shaft by a slender neck.

Apical dendrites of pyramidal neurons are often aggregated together into clusters. Each cluster contains the apical dendrites of pyramidal neurons, whose cell bodies are distributed in superficial and the deep cortex. The apical dendrites of neurons whose cell bodies are in the deep cortex form the core of the cluster, whereas the apical dendrites of neurons whose cell bodies are in the superficial cortex are distributed at the periphery of the cluster. Such clusters may define a functional unit or module.

With few exceptions, the axons of pyramidal neurons arise from the base of the cell body. In addition to emitting a local plexus of collaterals, the axons of pyramidal neurons have one of two projection patterns. They either project from one region of cortex to another in the ipsilateral cortex (association projections) or contralateral hemisphere (callosal projections) or descend to subcortical structures. The axons of projection neurons usually release the excitatory

Fig. 2. (A) (*left*) This pyramidal neuron was intracellularly injected with the tracer, horseradish peroxidase, which was subsequently localized histochemically. This neuron has an apical dendrite (ad), which ascends from the apex of the pyramid-shaped cell body and reaches layer III. At this point, it branches to form an apical tuft that ramifies within layers I and II. The base of the cell body gives rise to a set of dendrites (bd) and an axon (ax) that descends toward the white matter. **(B)** Each dendrite is invested with a coat of spines. A spine has a bulbous head (*large arrows*), which is attached to the dendritic shaft by a long, thin neck (*small arrows*).

amino acids aspartate and/or glutamate as neurotransmitters.

Two subpopulations of projection neurons do not have apical dendrites. Notable among these are the spinous stellate neurons in the middle of sensory cortices and the large, nonoriented neurons in the superficial entorhinal cortex. Like the typical pyramidal neurons, these projection neurons have spinous dendrites, and they excite the postsynaptic neurons through the release of glutamate.

Most projection neurons respond to a stimulus with a series of spikes that are followed by prolonged after hyperpolarizations and after depolarizations (Fig. 3). These regular spiking neurons adapt to sustained stimuli.

3.2. Local Circuit Neurons

Based on their somatodendritic morphology, two groups of local circuit neurons can be discerned. One group is the stellate neuron. The stellate neurons have round cell bodies and an array of dendrites that radiate uniformly from their somata (Fig. 4). The second group of local circuit neurons has a polarized form. Their cell bodies are elongated, and may be oriented either radially or horizontally. Regardless of their orientation, the dendrites tend to arise from the attenuated poles of the cell body. The dendrites of all local circuit neurons are aspinous, or at most sparsely spinous.

The pattern of the axonal arbors of local circuit neurons is highly variable. The axon may arise from virtually any site on the cell body or from a proximal dendrite. The distribution of these axons are restricted to the sphere of the dendritic arbors or extend beyond the dendritic field. Local circuit neurons use γ-aminobutyric acid (GABA) as their neurotransmitter (Fig. 4A). Release of this neurotransmitter inhibits the activity of postsynaptic neurons. In addition, local circuit neurons can release other neuroactive substances from their axonal terminals (Fig. 4B,C). These peptides include cholecystokinin, neuropeptide Y (NPY), somatostatin (SS), substance P, and vasoactive intestinal polypeptide (VIP). It is not yet clear how these other neuroactive substances interact with GABA on postsynaptic neurons to modulate neurotransmission. On the other hand, it does appear that the release of the secondary substances is activity-dependent. Thus, at low levels of excitation, local circuit neurons release only GABA, whereas at high levels of excitation, they release both GABA and the other neuroactive compound (Table 1).

Intracellular recordings of local circuit neurons reveal that cortical local circuit neurons have mem-

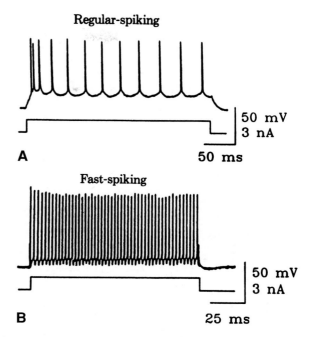

Fig. 3. Intracellular recordings show that projection and local circuit neurons exhibit different firing patterns. **(A)** Projection neurons have a phasic, regular spiking pattern. **(B)** Stimulation of a local circuit neuron results in a continuous, and maintained stream of fast spikes. (With permission of Barry Connors and Michael Gutnick, Trends Neurosci 1990;13:99–104.)

brane and spiking properties that differentiate them from projections neurons. Following a suprathreshold stimulation, local circuit neurons discharge fast spikes of less than 0.5-ms duration (Fig. 3). These neurons exhibit little or no adaptation during a prolonged stimulation, e.g., the spike frequency remains the same. Thus, the local circuit neurons transmit inhibitory information to postsynaptic targets with great fidelity.

3.3. Cortical Synaptology

Two structurally and functionally unique types of synapses are formed by cortical neurons. *Asymmetric synapses* are formed by axons that contain large vesicles and excitatory neurotransmitters, e.g., primarily glutamate. These synapses have postsynaptic densities that are composed of a protein kinase, and activation of these synapses leads to depolarizing potentials or excitatory responses in postsynaptic neurons. In contrast, *symmetric synapses* have presynaptic axons with small synaptic vesicles that contain the inhibitory transmitter GABA. The pre- and postsynaptic densities of these synapses are approximately of equal thickness. The activation of symmetric synapses evokes hyperpolarizing potentials or inhibitory responses in postsynaptic neurons.

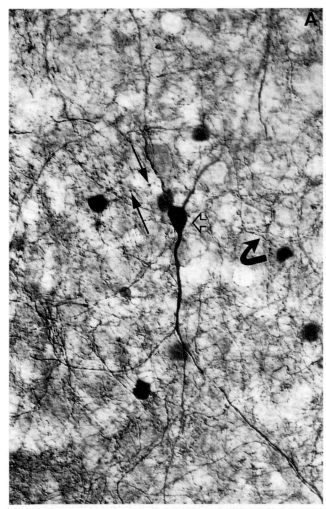

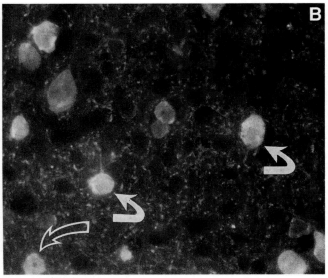

Fig. 4. (A) Cortical local circuit neurons use γ-aminobutyric acid (GABA) as a neurotransmitter. The open arrow indicates the cell body of an aspinous stellate neuron, that was labeled immunohistochemically with an antibody directed against glutamic acid decarboxylase (GAD). GAD is the enzyme that catalyzes the rate-limiting step in GABA synthesis. GAD-immunoreactivity is evident in the axonal processes (*curved solid arrow*) and in GABAergic axonal terminals (*straight solid arrows*). Many GABAergic neurons colocalize with a peptide neurotransmitter. Immunofluorescence techniques were used to identify GABA-immunoreactive neurons (indicated by *solid arrows* in **B**), which were double-labeled with an anti-substance P antibody (indicated by corresponding *solid arrows* in **C**). Note that not all of the GABAergic neurons colocalize substance P (*open arrows* in **B** and **C**). (Courtesy of Stewart Hendry, Johns Hopkins University, Baltimore MD.)

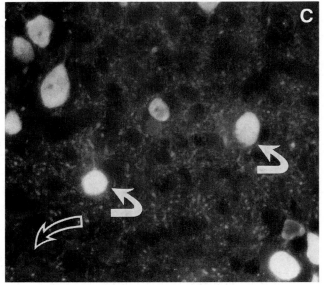

The distributions of asymmetric and symmetric synapses are among the many features that distinguish projection neurons from local circuit neurons. The two types of synapses are largely segregated on projection neurons. The most common target of axons that form asymmetric synapses is the heads of dendritic spines. In contrast, most symmetric synapses are formed in the perisomatic region. This region includes the soma, the smooth surfaces of proximal dendrites, the axon hillock, and the initial segment of the axon. The result of this organization is that excitatory responses can be evoked over a large area of the pyramidal-cell dendritic tree. The summed excitatory input is gated by inhibitory activity in the perisomatic region. Since the action-potential initiation zone is in the initial segment of the axon, the symmetric synapses are strategically placed to modulate the discharge frequency of cortical pyramidal neurons. In contrast, asymmetric and symmetric synapses are intermingled along the smooth dendrites of local circuit neurons. The dispersion of inhibitory synapses in relationship to excitatory ones results in a less pronounced gating of excitatory activity by local circuit neurons.

The efferents of the two classes of cortical neurons have different patterns of connectivity. The local arbors and projections of pyramidal neurons form excitatory, asymmetric synapses with postsynaptic targets. The axons of local-circuit neurons form inhibitory, symmetric synapses. Thus, the two neuronal populations effect their targets in opposite ways.

The functional and connectional differences of the two populations of cortical neurons are evident during an epileptic seizure. In the absence of local circuit neuron-mediated inhibition, the activity of the projection neurons is unchecked. Projection neurons discharge without inhibitory modulation, and produce depolarizing shifts that are composed of very large excitatory postsynaptic potentials. A common treatment for seizure activity is administration of compounds that have actions similar to GABA, such as valproic acid.

4. STRUCTURE AND DISTRIBUTION OF CORTICAL AREAS

The size and packing densities of neurons are not uniform in the cerebral cortex. *Cytoarchitecture* refers to the unique distributions of neurons in different parts of the cortex. The underlying tenet of this approach to neuroscience is that structural differences in the cerebral cortex are associated with functional unique areas. Figure 5 has Nissl-stained sections through soma-

tosensory and motor cortices—e.g., areas caudal and rostral to the central sulcus, respectively. One of the striking features of cortical architecture is the horizontal alignment of its neurons into layers. It is generally accepted that neocortex or *isocortex* contains six layers.

The differentiation of cortical layers is largely based upon the distinctive population of projection neurons in a layer. (NB, A neuron is described as being in a layer by the position of its cell body. Thus, a pyramidal neuron with a cell body in layer V may be referred to as a layer V neuron, or a layer may be described as having pyramidal neurons.) The most superficial cortical layer—the layer which abuts the pia mater—is layer I. Layer I is also referred to as the plexiform or molecular layer. Layer I is composed mainly of the apical tuft dendrites of pyramidal neurons and afferent axons. This layer is virtually devoid of neuronal cell bodies; it has only a few local circuit neurons, and projection neurons are absent from layer I. Layer II has a granular appearance and is densely populated by the cell bodies of small pyramidal neurons. Layer III is composed of medium and large pyramidal neurons. The size of their cell bodies increases with the depth so that the largest layer III neurons are deep, near the border with layer IV. Layer IV has a granular appearance. It is composed of the small, round cell bodies of stellate projection neurons and pyramidal neurons that do not have orienting apical dendrites. Often, the cell-packing density in layer IV is the greatest of all the cortical layers. Layer V contains the largest pyramidal neurons. The cell-packing density in this layer is the lowest of all cortical laminae. Layer VI has multiform projection neurons; thus, the cell bodies of layer VI neurons have many different shapes. Local circuit neurons are distributed in all cortical layers; however, their distribution does not facilitate the cytoarchitectonic differentiation of cortical layers and areas.

A comparison of somatosensory and motor cortices (Fig. 5) provides an example of how cortical areas can be differentiated on the basis of their cytoarchitecture. The superficial layers I–IV of the somatosensory cortex contain many small neurons that endow it with a granular appearance. This granularity is particularly evident in layers II and IV. The somatosensory cortex also is characterized by relatively small layer V pyramidal neurons. In contrast, motor cortex has almost no layer IV, and relatively few small neurons in layers II and III. Instead, there are many large pyramidal neurons, particularly in layer V. The largest layer V pyramidal neurons are known as Betz cells, named after the nineteenth-century scientist who first described them. The Betz cells and other layer V projection neurons

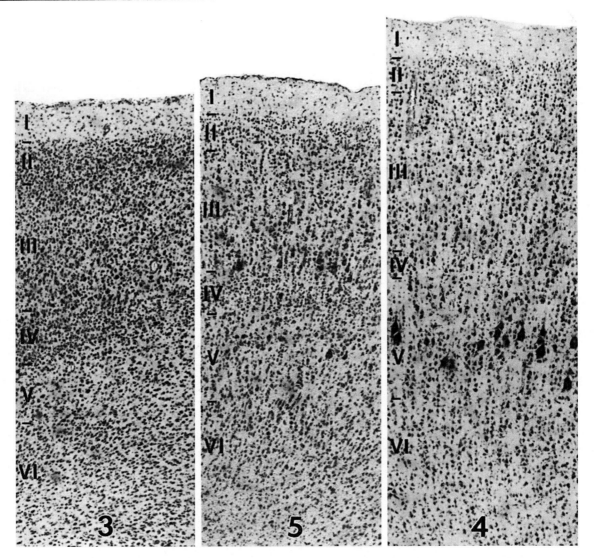

Fig. 5. Photomicrographs of Nissl-stained sections through three sensorimotor areas to show differences in cytoarchitectural organization: primary somatosensory cortex, *area 3*; first somatosensory association cortex, *area 5*; motor cortex, *area 4*. Notice the highly granular layers II and IV in area 3 and large pyramidal neurons in the deep part of layer III in area 5 and in layer V of area 4.

project axons to the spinal cord via the corticospinal tract. Although the pyramidal neurons in layer V of the somatosensory cortex are smaller, some of them also contribute axons to the corticospinal tract.

Early in the twentieth century, Karl Brodmann produced one of the most thorough and enduring cytoarchitectural studies of the human cerebral cortex. Figure 6 is a copy of the classic cytoarchitectural map that summarizes his conclusions about the distributions of cortical areas. Each cytoarchitectural area is designated with an Arabic numeral in the order in which he studied them. Accordingly, the somatosensory cortex is area 3 (as described here), as well as

adjacent areas 1 and 2. These areas are in the postcentral gyrus of the parietal lobe. The motor cortex is area 4 (as described here), and is in the precentral gyrus of the frontal lobe. The auditory cortex, areas 41 and 42, is located in the transverse gyri on the dorsal aspect of the superior temporal gyrus. The visual cortex, area 17, is found in the banks of the calcarine sulcus and the lateral wall of the occipital lobe. Other numbers used in this text refer to cortical areas designated by Brodmann.

Although most of the cytoarchitectonic areas on the lateral surface of the cerebral cortex are isocortical, many on the medial surface do not have six layers. For

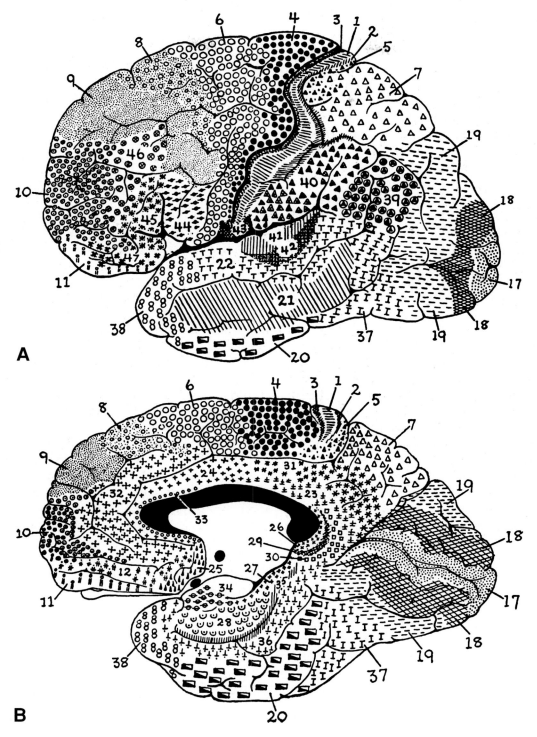

Fig. 6. Brodmann's maps of the distribution of cortical areas on the lateral (*top*) and medial (*bottom*) surfaces of the cerebral cortex.

example, the hippocampus has a pyramidal-cell layer sandwiched between two plexiform layers. Cortical areas with fewer than six layers are referred to as *allocortex*. The allocortex is part of the "anatomical limbic system."

The allocortex is very heterogeneous, and is subdivided into three parts or moieties: (i) The archicortex includes the hippocampal formation—e.g., the hippocampus, dentate gyrus, and subiculum. (ii) The paleocortex includes the olfactory piriform area and the rostral insula. (iii) The periarchicortex includes many transitional or mesocortical areas, such as the entorhinal, posterior parahippocampal, and cingulate cortices. An example of the cytoarchitecture of some allocortical moieties are represented by drawings of neuronal perikarya in Fig. 7. The allocortical subiculum has a single pyramidal layer; the junction of this layer with the neuron-sparse molecular layer is indicated with an open arrow in this figure. The entorhinal cortex or Brodmann's area 28 is an example of the periarchicortex, and forms a major part of the parahippocampal gyrus. One of its prominent features are the islands of large star neurons in layer II; these neurons are surrounded by a dashed line in Fig. 7 to emphasize this "insular" arrangement. These neurons project into the hippocampal formation via the perforant pathway. Finally, neocortical area 20 forms much of the inferior temporal gyrus. This area has six layers, including large-layer III pyramidal neurons and granular layers II and IV.

One simple conceptualization of the cortical mantle is to view it as a sheet of layer V pyramidal neurons that is continuous from the hippocampus to the isocortex. To this basic layer of neurons is added the superficial layer of pyramidal neurons, which is differentiated in the periarchicortical and isocortical areas to form the many cytoarchitectural variations that compose the cerebral cortex.

The various components of the cerebral cortex are affected differently in some neurological and psychiatric diseases. This is exemplified by Alzheimer's disease. Figure 8 has examples of neurons from three regions of the brain of a person afflicted with Alzheimer's disease. The tissue is stained for neurofibrillary tangles with the fluorescent dye thioflavin S. Observe the flame-shaped neurofibrillary tangles that fill the perikarya of projection neurons. The structure of neurofibrillary tangle-laden projection neurons is shown for the hippocampal formation, layer II of the entorhinal cortex, and layer III in the isocortex. Neurofibrillary tangles also accumulate in layer V neurons of the entorhinal and isocortical areas. The presence of this pathology in large-projection neurons is indicative of ongoing degenerative processes. In many instances, the somata completely disappear, and only "ghost" neurofibrillary tangles remain. Since many of these large neurons are corticocortical projection neurons, there is a disruption of major efferent projection systems of the cerebral cortex in this disease. Therefore, degeneration of these neurons contributes to the cognitive and emotional impairments in Alzheimer's disease.

5. FUCTIONAL SUBDIVISIONS OF THE CEREBRAL CORTEX

Combined structural and functional studies led to systematic classification schemes of the principal functions of individual cortical areas. The main tools for functionally defining cortical areas are neuronal recording, electrical microstimulation, positron emission tomography (PET) techniques, and functional magnetic resonance imaging.

5.1. Sensory Areas

Cortices involved in different aspects of sensation are subdivided into primary, first sensory association, second sensory association, and multimodal cortices. *Primary sensory cortices* contain neurons with spatially restricted receptive fields and properties that are dominated by thalamic afferents. For example, the lateral geniculate thalamic nucleus has neurons with receptive fields that are round and subtend as little as 1° of the visual field. Layer IV of primary visual area 17 (the lamina in which thalamic afferents principally arborize) has neurons with rectangular receptive fields, and their size and orientation are the product of multiple thalamic inputs that terminate on individual neurons.

Sensory spaces can have *multiple representations* in the primary sensory cortices. In the primary somatosensory cortex (SI), for example, there are four separate body representations. These separate sensory representations are contained within unique cytoarchitectural areas. Thus, the primary somatosensory cortex is composed of areas 3a, 3b, 1, and 2 and each area has its own representation of the body surface. These body representations are known as homunculi. Each area is involved in the high-resolution localization and discrimination of somatic stimuli. Body regions with the highest density of receptors, such as the face and hands, also have the largest area of representation in the cortex, thus improving localization and discrimination of sensory stimuli in these areas. Likewise, in the visual cortex, a relatively large area of cortex is devoted to the central visual fields—the cortex that responds to stimuli focused on the fovea. Each of the primary sensory areas are indicated with vertical lines in Fig. 9.

Parasensory association cortices receive their inputs mainly from the primary areas. Neuronal responses in these areas are more complex, and involve the integration of a number of cortical inputs as well as those from the thalamus. As shown in Fig. 9, each primary sensory area has a first parasensory associa-

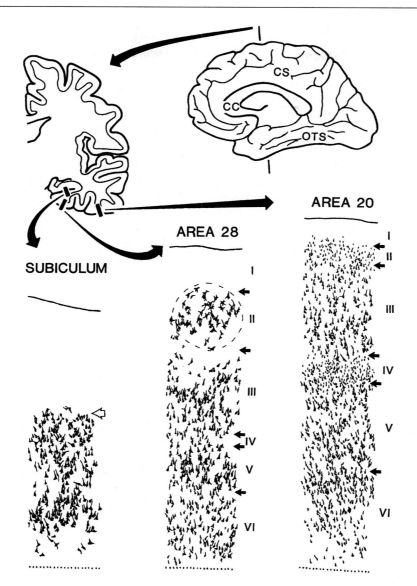

Fig. 7. The cerebral cortex is not cytoarchitecturally uniform, and has a progressive elaboration in its architecture in the medial to lateral direction. This is true for both dorsal and ventral surfaces, although it is illustrated here with areas from the ventral part of the cortex. The medial view of the brain shows the corpus callosum (CC), cingulate sulcus (CS), and occipito–temporal sulcus (OTS), as well as the plane of section through which a coronal section was taken for Nissl staining. The *top arrow* indicates this section. The transverse section has three black rectangles through the subiculum—area 28 and area 20, respectively, in the medial-to-lateral direction. The three strips of cortex below are perikaryal drawings to show the distribution of neurons in each of these areas. The junction between the molecular and pyramidal-cell layers of the subiculum is demarcated with an *open arrow*. In area 28, an island of layer II star pyramidal neurons is presented, with a *dashed line* around it in order to emphasize that this is not a continuous layer of neurons as in most other cortical areas. Notice that each area in the medial-to-lateral direction has a progressively more differentiated laminar architecture.

tion area: the first visual association area (VA1) for the primary visual cortex includes areas 18 and 19, the first auditory association area (AA1) for the primary auditory cortex includes part of area 22, and the first somatosensory association area (SA1) for the primary somatosensory cortex includes area 5 and rostral area 40. In the left hemisphere, there is a specialization of the first auditory association area known as Wernicke's area. Wernicke's area is a posterior part of AA1, and is involved in recognition of spoken language. It is important to note that layer III pyramidal neurons are the main source and target of corticocortical projections. Therefore, layer III neurons are particularly well developed in sensory association

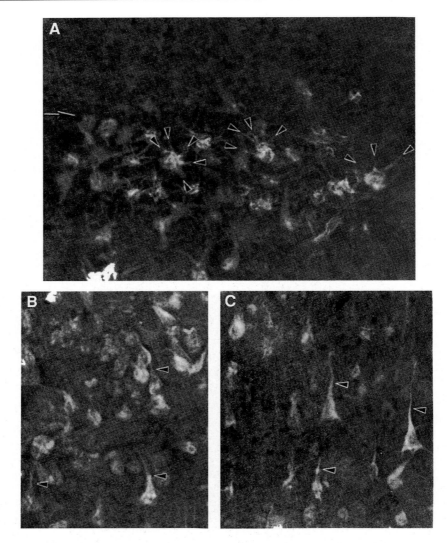

Fig. 8. Micrographs of thioflavin S-stained neurofibrillary tangles in layer II of area 28 (**A**), the subiculum (**B**), and layer III of area 20 (**C**) of a case of Alzheimer's disease. Note in **B** and **C** that the apical dendrites of pyramidal neurons (*arrowheads*) are filled with these tangles, as are the somata. The border of layers I and II of the entorhinal cortex are marked with an arrow in **A**. In this island of layer II neurons, there are almost no primary, or orienting, apical dendrites. Rather, neurons in this layer have dendrites that radiate from around the soma (*arrowheads*), and thus these neurons are known as star cells.

areas. Figure 5 shows the architecture of area 5 with its large layer III pyramidal neurons.

Secondary sensory-association cortices are characterized by their corticocortical connections. The second sensory association areas receive inputs from the first sensory association cortices and project to multimodal areas. There is a second sensory association cortex adjacent to each of the first association areas; VA2 for visual cortex, AA2 for auditory cortex, and SA2 for somatosensory cortex (Fig. 9).

Multimodal association areas receive inputs from more than one sensory modality, and thus provide for intermodal associations among stimuli arriving in two

or more second sensory-association cortices. Thalamic nuclei that project to multimodal areas include the pulvinar, lateral posterior, and mediodorsal nuclei. These thalamic nuclei do not have a singular sensory function and are themselves probable sites for multimodal interactions. Multimodal areas can be classified into bimodal and trimodal cortices. Although there are many bimodal areas, Fig. 9 presents only one as an example of these areas. This one is on the angular gyrus dorsal to the tip of the superior temporal sulcus, and it receives inputs from the second association areas for the visual and somatosensory modalities. There are three major trimodal association areas (two are shown

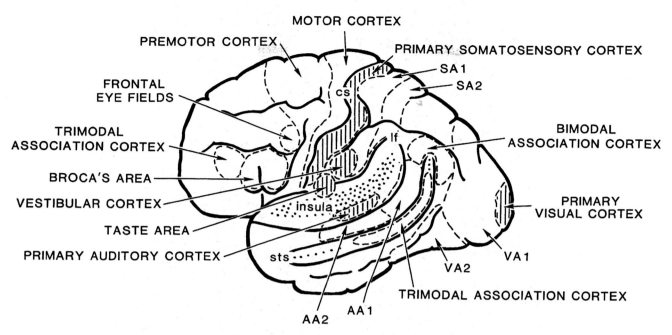

Fig. 9. Topographical distribution of functional areas in the cerebral cortex. These regions were determined from a wide range of physiological and anatomical studies in human and nonhuman primate brains, and thus are highly schematic. They were plotted onto the same hemisphere as that used by Brodmann in the top of Fig. 6, so that functional regions can be compared with their associated cytoarchitectural areas. Primary sensory cortices are indicated with vertical hatching. A few sulci are labeled for orientation purposes, and include the central sulcus (cs), lateral fissure (lf), and superior temporal sulcus (sts). Furthermore, the lateral fissure and superior temporal sulcus were "opened" so that the depths of these sulci can be visualized. By lifting the frontal, parietal, and temporal opercula, the underlying insula can be seen. The taste area extends onto the upper bank of the parietal operculum, whereas the primary auditory cortex is on Heschl's gyri on the superior-temporal plane—e.g., the planum-temporale. The superior-temporal sulcus was "opened" in order to expose one of the trimodal, association cortices.

in Fig. 9). One is in the ventral part of area 46 in the prefrontal cortex, one is in the depths of the superior temporal sulcus, and a third is in the posterior parahippocampal cortex on the ventral surface of the cerebral cortex.

Each multimodal association area has projections to cingulate and rostral parahippocampal cortices. These limbic areas are believed to be involved in monitoring the sensory environment because they have neurons that respond to large sensory stimuli, and lesions in the cingulate cortex disrupt attention to sensory stimuli. Furthermore, ablations in parahippocampal, hippocampal, and cingulate cortices disrupt memory formation and spatial orientation. Thus, these cortices likely form an "end stage" in cortical processing of sensory inputs, and provide mechanisms for memory that apply to complex patterns of sensory stimuli.

5.2. Motor Cortex

Activity in the various sensory spaces leads to environmentally adapted behaviors. The relationships

between sensory and motor cortices and the mechanisms by which particular motor sequences are generated are leading issues in clinical neuroscience. Motor cortices have direct projections to the spinal cord and/ or brainstem motor nuclei, and are classified according to their contributions to movement based on responses to electrical microstimulation and the length of time by which neuronal firing precedes movement. *Primary motor cortex* (MI), Brodmann's area 4 in the precentral gyrus, has the lowest threshold for electrically evoked movements. Thus, activation of neurons in the motor cortex engages a limited number of muscle groups such as the lumbrical muscles for each finger. Neuronal activity in MI occurs just prior to movement. Thus, the finest control of motor activity is mediated by MI.

A dramatic example of the topographic representation of the musculature in the motor cortex, the homunculus, occurs when seizure activity spreads through the motor cortex in what is termed the "Jacksonian march." When seizure activity is initiated in one part of the homunculus, it induces convulsions in the associated part of the body. As the seizure activity spreads through the network of local axon collaterals of projection neurons, the large depolarizing shifts in projection neurons induces hyperexcitability in adjacent cortical areas. The result is convulsions that progressively include adjacent parts of the body. This seizure activity can spread across the entire motor cortex as well as though connections from the corpus callosum to the contralateral hemisphere. Thus, convulsions that originally start in one focus can spread across the body surface and involve both sides of the body.

Classical accounts of the motor cortex defined a secondary or supplementary motor area (SMA) on the superior frontal gyrus medial to the MI. SMA is one of a number of separate *premotor areas*. Neurons in premotor areas have direct projections to the MI and to the spinal cord and/or brainstem motor nuclei. Electrical microstimulation in these areas can activate larger groups of muscles; the movements elicited have a longer latency than those resulting from stimulation of units the in primary motor cortex. One of the premotor areas directs eye movements and is shown in Fig. 5 as the frontal eye fields. Another area controls movements of the mouth during speech and is termed "Broca's area." Broca's area is directly connected to Wernicke's area, which is part of the first auditory association cortex in the left hemisphere. Thus, language comprehension in Wernicke's area can control speech via Broca's area.

The classic studies of epileptic patients by the neurosurgeons Wilder Penfield and Herbert Jasper had a profound impact on our understanding of the functional organization of the cerebral cortex. They surgically exposed the cerebral cortex under general anesthesia, and then allowed the patient to regain consciousness so that the patient's sensations could be reported following electrical stimulation or during seizure activity. In addition to observing sensory and motor phenomena following electrical stimulation of sensory and motor cortices, respectively, Penfield and Jasper observed that stimulation of limbic cortical areas evoked visceral and emotional sensations and memories. Case NC, for example, had seizure activity that began with a "far-off" feeling. She smacked her lips, swallowed, and complained of nausea. Borborygmi could be heard from her abdomen during the seizure, and these attacks were often associated with a feeling of panic. Electrical stimulation of the anterior temporal lobe and rostral insula evoked similar feelings and intestinal activity, and ablation of these cortices alleviated the seizure activity and associated emotions and autonomic activity. Thus, the limbic cortex contributes to visceromotor activity and emotion as well as operating as an end stage in sensory processing, as noted previously. These limbic areas include orbital, insular, temporal pole, and anterior cingulate cortices.

6. CORTICAL CONNECTIVITY

6.1. Thalamocortical Relationships and the Cortical Column

One of the principles of neuroscience is that the activity of sensory thalamic afferents defines the primary functions of a sensory cortical area. Thus, as noted here, the receptive field characteristics of neurons in the lateral geniculate nucleus determine the visual properties of neurons in area 17. The thalamic projections terminate chiefly in layer IV, with minor projections to layers I and VI. As a result, the thalamic afferents synapse with any element (cell body or dendrite) that compose these layers (regardless of where the cell body is located). Projections from the ventrolateral and ventroanterior thalamic nuclei contribute to the motor functions of motor and premotor areas, respectively. The pivotal role of the thalamic input is confirmed by transplantation studies. After transplanting the fetal somatosensory cortex to visual cortex, the neurons from the somatosensory cortex respond to visual stimuli.

The termination of thalamic afferent axons in the cerebral cortex determines functional cortical modules or columns. Vernon Mountcastle and his colleagues first showed that neurons in a vertical column of the somatosensory cortex shared similar response properties. Thus, one column contains neurons with preferential responses to stimulation of joints and deep tissues, whereas an adjacent column may contain neurons with preferential responses to a light touch of the skin. The columns in the visual cortex represent ocular dominance and orientation specificity (Fig. 10). In sensory cortices, these columns measure 500–1000 μm in diameter and reflect the distribution of thalamic axon terminals in the cortex.

Aggregates of neurons form columns in the motor cortex. Unlike the columns in sensory cortices, the columns of functionally similar neurons are evaluated in terms of the output of the motor cortex, by microstimulation techniques rather than receptive field mapping. The output columns in the motor cortex are larger than in sensory cortices—up to 2 mm in diameter. These large sizes are the result of the size of dendritic fields of particularly large pyramidal neurons in the motor cortex, and are specified according to the

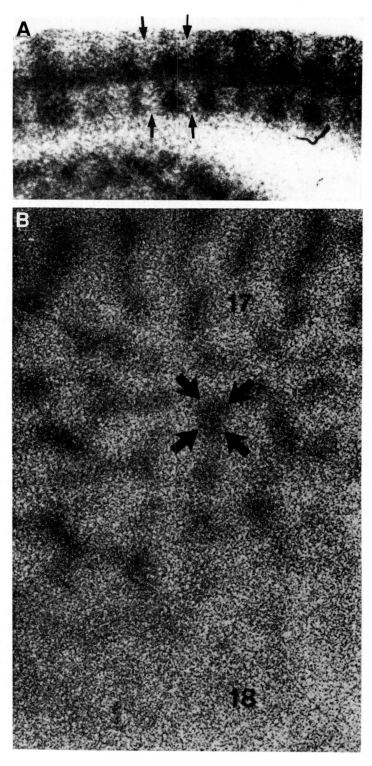

Fig. 10. (A) Presentation of a bar of light with a particular orientation results in partial stimulation of visual cortex. The responsive neurons in area 17 are organized in vertical, or radial columns (*arrows*). These columns were visualized autoradiographically using 2-[14C]deoxyglucose, radioactive tracer for glucose. This tracer was taken up and trapped in metabolically active neurons. The highest activity occurred in layer IV, the termination site of the thalamic afferents. (With permission of Hubel, Weisel, and Stryker, J Comp Neurol 1978; 177:361–380.) **(B)** An autoradiograph of a tangential section through the superficial cortex reveals a complex patchwork of activity. Note that the orientation specific columns (*arrows*) are present only in area 17, but not in visual association cortex, area 18. (With permission of Charles Gilbert and Torsten Weisel, J Neurosci 1989; 9:2432–2442.)

amount of cortex that must be electrically stimulated to evoke contraction in a small group of muscles.

Thalamocortical connections are reciprocal. That is, a column of neurons defined by a particular thalamic input to layer IV contains pyramidal neurons in layer VI that project to the thalamus. These return projections are organized in a point-to-point fashion so that, for example, cortical points representing the central visual fields project to similar places in the lateral geniculate nucleus. These reciprocal connections are believed to be involved in modulating the receptives field properties of thalamic neurons.

6.2. Monoaminergic Afferents and Sleep

The cerebral cortex is innervated by two ascending monoaminergic afferent systems. The noradrenergic and serotonergic systems arise from brainstem nuclei and project throughout the ipsilateral hemisphere. These projections are widely distributed and cross cytoarchitectonic borders.

Noradrenergic afferents project from neurons in pontine and mesencephalic nuclei. The most notable of these nuclei is the locus coeruleus, so named because it appears as a blue site in the fresh brain. This is a small, pigmented nucleus near the floor of the fourth ventricle. The noradrenergic afferents terminate in all layers of the cortex, but predominantly in layers I–IV. The cortical terminals of the noradrenergic afferents contain dense core vesicles. These vesicles package the norepinephrine prior to its exocytotic release into the synaptic cleft, where the norepinephrine binds with α- and β-adrenoceptors. The laminar distribution of these receptors differs. α_1-adrenoceptors are distributed in layers I–IV, whereas α_2-adrenoceptors are most common in layers I and IV. β-adrenoceptors are most densely distributed in layers I–III. The interaction of norephinephrine with these receptors produces different responses. For example, activation of α_2-adrenoceptors (which presumably are on the presynaptic membrane) opens potassium channels, inhibiting further release of norepinephrine. In contrast, binding of norepinephrine with the α_1- and β-adrenoceptors closes potassium channels in postsynaptic neurons that are excited.

The serotonergic afferents arise from the dorsal and median raphe nuclei. These are small clusters of neurons that are located along the midline of the pons and caudal midbrain. Interestingly, raphe neurons also co-localize neuroactive peptides such as substance P, Leu-enkephalin, and thyrotropin-releasing hormone. Serotonergic afferents innervate layers I, III, and IV. Likewise, the cortical serotonin receptors are largely confined to layers III and IV. The release of serotonin results in changes in the permeability of potassium channels, which in turn lead to complex modulation of the activity of postsynaptic neurons.

The monoaminergic afferents to the cortex are believed to be involved in the regulation of sleep and arousal. Serotonergic neurons in the dorsal raphe exhibit a slow, rhythmic activity. The pacemaker activity is modulated by the activity of noradrenergic afferents. This pacemaker activity is accelerated by the closing of potassium channels by norepinephrine. The activity of the pacemaker neurons changes with the state of arousal—highest when the person is awake, lower during periods of "slow-wave" sleep, and lowest during periods of dream (or rapid eye movement, REM) sleep. The activity of noradrenergic raphe neurons rises during slow-wave sleep and falls during periods of REM. The phasic activity of a population of cholinergic neurons in the reticular formation, or RF (the gigantocellular tegmental field) rises during REM sleep. Interestingly, these neurons are innervated by descending cortical projections that serve in a feedback capacity. Thus, it appears that an interaction of a number of neurotransmitter systems regulates the states of consciousness.

6.3. Cortical Cholinergic Connections and Memory

Memory formation is a process that involves short- and long-term events, as well as many cortical areas and a number of cortical afferents. It is beyond the scope of this chapter to detail what is known about the mechanisms of memory. A thumbnail sketch, however, should note the following observations. The hippocampus is critical for short-term memory, whereas long-term memories are likely stored in many of the multimodal association and limbic cortices. Since acetylcholine-receptor antagonists interfere with memory formation, it is believed that cholinergic afferents are important for the operation of cortical circuits involved in memory formation. For example, it is possible that cholinergic connections operate as an "enabling switch" that allows particular memories to be transferred from short- to long-term storage.

There are two sources of acetylcholine in the cerebral cortex. About 70% originates in neurons with cell bodies in the magnocellular basal forebrain nuclei, and 30% arises from a subpopulation of cortical local-circuit neurons. The basal forebrain nuclei include the medial septum, the basal nucleus of Meynert, the diagonal band of Broca, and the substantia innominata. Medial septal neurons project to the hippocampus.

Projections from neurons in the basal nucleus of Meynert and medial segments of the diagonal band of Broca terminate in medial cortical areas, including the entorhinal, medial prefrontal, and cingulate cortices. Neurons in the substantia innominata and lateral segments of the diagonal band of Broca project to many neocortical areas including temporal, parietal, and occipital neocortical areas. Projections to the cerebral cortex generally terminate in layers V and VI, although there are projections to the superficial layers.

Disruption of cholinergic connections may contribute to memory loss and spatial disorientation observed in patients with Alzheimer's disease. Neurofibrillary tangles and neuronal degeneration occur in the basal forebrain nuclei and are considered to be pathological hallmarks of Alzheimer's disease. Memory deficits in Alzheimer's patients are associated with damage—to the hippocampus that is engaged during short-term memory formation, to multimodal and periarchicortical limbic areas involved in long-term memory storage, and to the cholinergic system that may be involved in enabling these structures to convert short- to long-term memories.

6.4. Neurotrophin Systems

Cholinergic projections from the basal forebrain to cortex are supported by growth factors, neurotrophins, that are elaborated by cortical neurons. The family of neurotrophins includes nerve growth factor (NGF), brain-derived growth factor (BDNF), and neurotrophin 3 (NT-3). Neurons throughout the depth of cortex express the neurotropohins, indeed, many co-express multiple neurotrophins. Alterations of cortical neurotrophins lead to deficits in neural plasticity and in learning and memory. For example, the brains of people with Alzheimer's Disease or of people who have chronically abused alcohol are characterized by deficits in neurotrophins.

Neurotrophins binds to specific receptors. One set of recptors binds neurotrophins with high affinity. An active part of the intracellular portion of these receptors is a tyrosine kinase, hence they are known as trk's. Three trk's have been identified: trkA, trkB, and trkC. They differ in their extracellular domains and have high preference for NGF, BDNF, and NT-3, respectively. Another receptor, p75, binds neurtrophins with lower affinity. All of the neurotrophin receptors are highly expressed by cortical neurons, especially by layer V pyramidal neurons.

A neurotrophin is realeased by cortical neurons at synaptic sites, takes up by cholinergic axons expressing trk, and retrogradely transported back to the basal forebrain. Using such a retrograde system, cortical neurons are considered to be invaluable for supporting basal forebrain cholinergic projections, which in turn are important in gating cortical processing (*see* above). Interestingly, neurotrophin receptors are most commonly exhibited at dendritic and somatic synaptic sites. Only few axons express neurotrophin receptors. Thus, it appears that neurotrophins can act through systems that parallel neurotransmission systems, i.e., autocrine and paracrine mechanisms as well as anteograde systems. This implies that the role of neurotrophins in learing and memory primarily is a product of intracortical processing.

6.5. Interhemispheric Connections and the Unification of Cognitive Activity

Each hemisphere contains the representation of the contralateral sensory field. Although there is slight overlap at the midline, such as in the region of central vision and the somatotopic representation of the trunk, the separation of the two perceptual spaces is rather clean. Despite this division, each person perceives a seamless representation of the world. The coordination of the processing that goes on in each hemisphere depends upon axons that cross the *corpus callosum.*

Many cortical areas on one side of the brain are connected with areas in the contralateral hemisphere via callosal connections. Although the details about the callosal system vary among discrete cytoarchitectonic areas, some general patterns can be described. The axons of the callosal pathway arise from pyramidal neurons in layer III, and to a lesser extent from layer V projection neurons. These axons descend into the white matter and pass across the corpus callosum. After entering the contralateral hemisphere, the axons follow a mirror-image course and terminate in layers I, III, and IV of the homotopic, or corresponding site in the contralateral hemisphere.

The function of callosal connections can be determined from studies by Roger Sperry and colleagues, who examined people whose corpora callosa and anterior commissures were transected. Overtly, such people with "split" brains operate perfectly well, but when challenged with certain tasks, it is clear that each hemisphere is not capable of executing all tasks. In one experiment, a split-brain subject was presented with an apple in his/her right or left visual fields. Following presentation to the right visual field, a subject was able to verbally describe the object. In contrast, when the apple was placed in the left visual field, the person was unable to come up with the word "apple," but s/he was able to point to an image of the apple when offered a choice of images. This experiment shows that both hemispheres receive sensory information, but differ in their communicative capabilities. The functional separation of abilities characterizes some of the hemispheric asymmetries. Although it is difficult to make generalizations about the functions of each hemisphere, each hemisphere is best able to mediate either verbal or nonverbal communication. At the risk of oversimplifying the situation, it appears that the left hemisphere is expressive and best at analytical, rational thought, whereas the right hemisphere is perceptive and capable of emotional, intuitive thought.

The lateralization of function is expressed in normal, intact people as cerebral dominance in language and handedness. Virtually all right-handed people have dominant left hemispheres. As might be expected, a significant percentage (15%) of left- or mixed-handed people express right hemispheric dominance, but interestingly, the dominant hemisphere for language in most of these people (70%) is the left hemisphere. Thus, regardless of the outward expression of handedness, the left hemisphere is usually the dominant hemisphere for language.

6.6. Projections to Nonthalamic Subcortical Systems

In addition to the corticospinal (pyramidal) pathway (mentioned above), the axons of layer V neurons project to extrapyramidal targets as summarized in Fig. 11. These targets are sensory, motor, and integrative centers. Cortical afferents innervate *sensory* cranial-nerve nuclei such as the trigeminal brainstem nuclear complex and the solitary nucleus. These projections serve as feedback controls, modulating the output from second-order sensory nuclei. Other descending axons project to motor centers. These targets include *motor* cranial-nerve nuclei that have direct projections to skeletal muscle. Specifically, these nuclei are the trigeminal motor, facial, supraspinal, and hypoglossal nuclei. These corticobulbar projections serve as upper motor neurons that are analogous to the corticospinal projections. In addition, the cerebral cortex projects to three structures that in turn project to the spinal cord. (i) Projections from frontal, parietal, occipital, and temporal lobes project to the superior colliculus. These afferents carry somatosensory, visual, and auditory information that enables the superior colliculus to execute its role in coordinating complex behaviors such as tracking and attending to moving stimuli. (ii) Cortical afferents, primarily from

the precentral gyrus, synapse with neurons throughout the red nuclei. (iii) Two nuclei in the RF receive cortical input, the gigantocellular region of the medullary RF, and the oral area of the pontine RF. Extrapyramidal projections from layer V neurons also terminate in nuclei that are *integrative* centers. These targets include the caudate nucleus, the periaqueductal gray, and the pontine nuclei.

The cortical projections that innervate brainstem structures follow a pathway that is common with the corticospinal tract. That is, the cortical projections pass through the subcortical white matter, the internal capsules, the crus cerebri, the base of the pons, and the pyramidal tracts. The only difference is that the axons exit from the common pathway at the level of the structure being innervated. For example, corticobulbar fibers that innervate the hypoglossal nuclei descend with the corticospinal neurons, but perpendicular arbors leave the pyramidal tract in the caudal medulla. Thus, the size of the descending common pathway decreases as the axons exit.

The cortex also is interconnected with the *claustrum*. The claustrum is a small sheet of neurons embedded in the subcortical white matter. The corticoclaustral interconnections largely parallel the corticothalamic interconnections. The claustrum sends cortical afferents to layer IV, and to a lesser extent to layer VI. The cortex in turn projects to claustrum; these projections originate in layer VI neurons in many cortical areas including the primary auditory, somatosensory, and visual cortices. The function of the claustrocortical relationship largely remains a mystery; however, they may play a role in the modulation of sensory receptive field properties. For example, claustral afferents to the visual cortex contribute to the property of end-inhibition, whereby the sizes of certain receptive fields are limited by antagonistic effects. The corticoclaustral connections, like the corticothalamic projections, probably feedback on the claustrum to modulate the activity of the claustral neurons. These reciprocal projections may also provide a system for the integration of the three sensory spaces within the claustrum.

7. SUMMARY OF THE ORGANIZATION OF THE CEREBRAL CORTEX

The organization of the cerebral cortex, from the perspectives of intrinsic circuitry and afferent and efferent connections, is summarized in Fig. 11. It is built around a small group of layer III and V neurons

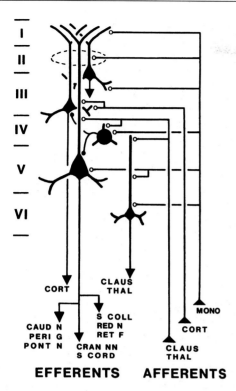

I
II
III
IV
V
VI

CORT
CLAUS
THAL
MONO

CAUD N
PERI G
PONT N
S COLL
RED N
RET F
CRAN NN
S CORD
CORT
CLAUS
THAL

EFFERENTS   AFFERENTS

Fig. 11. A summary diagram of the intrinsic organization and connections of a "generic" neocortical area. Three pyramidal neurons forming a cluster (within the *dashed lines*) are shown. Excitatory connections are indicated with open axon terminals, whereas inhibitory ones are shown with black axon terminals. Abbreviations for these connections are as follows: caud n, caudate nucleus; claus, claustrum; cort, corticocortical connections for both ipsilateral and contralateral hemispheres; cran nn, sensory and motor cranial-nerve nuclei; mono, monoamines including norepinepherine and serotonin; peri g, peri-aqueductal gray; pont n, pontine nuclei; red n, red nucleus; ret f, reticular formation; s coll, superior colliculus; s cord, spinal cord; thal, thalamus.

whose apical dendrites are aggregated into a cluster. Afferent connections are shown to the right, and include excitatory thalamic afferents to layer IV, excitatory cortical connections from ipsilateral and contralateral cortices to layer III, and a diffuse distribution of serotonergic and noradrenergic projections that innervate elements in all cortical laminae. A single local circuit neuron is shown in layer IV with its inhibitory connections with pyramidal neurons; however, it should be remembered that these neurons are diffusely distributed throughout all layers of the cortex.

Cortical neurons project to a number of extrinsic sites. The actual density of any one of these projections depends upon the specific cortical area under consideration. All cortical areas have ipsilateral cortical projections that originate in layer III, and projections to the thalamus, pontine, and caudate nuclei that originate from layer V neurons. Fig. 11 does not intend to imply that each layer V pyramidal neuron makes all of these projections. It is likely that a single pyramidal neuron in layer V has axon collaterals that project to one to three subcortical sites. Specialization in projection systems for each cortical area occurs in terms of inputs to the superior colliculus, RF, sensory and motor cranial-nerve nuclei, and the red nucleus. Many of these connections are unique to parts of particular motor and premotor areas.

Sensory and motor information interact in the cortex; visual, auditory, and somatosensory information can be integrated, stored, and recalled so that the appropriate motor system(s) can be activated. All of these processes are essential for mnemonic mechanisms and cognition. In fact, the cortex is pivotal for all of the processing that underlies the complex thought and communication that are considered to be uniquely human. Nevertheless, it cannot be emphasized enough that the cerebral cortex does not act in isolation. The cortex can function only because of the diverse interconnections with other CNS structures.

SELECTED READINGS

Connors BW, Gutnick MJ. Intrinsic firing patterns of diverse neocortical neurons. Trends in Neuroscience 1990; 13:99–104.

Elston GN, DeFelipe J. Spine distribution in cortical pyramidal cells: a common organizational principle across species. Progress in Brain Research 2002; 136:109–133.

Goldman-Rakic PS. Working memory and the mind. Scientific America 1992; 267:110–117.

Kalaska JF, Crammond DJ. Cerebral cortical mechanisms of reaching movements. Science 1992; 255:1517–1523.

Maunsell JH. The brain's visual world: representation of visual targets in cerebral cortex. Science 1995; 270:764–769.

Marin Padilla M. The evolution of the structure of the neocortex in mammals: a new theory of cytoarchitecture. Revista de Neurologia 2001; 33:843–853.

Martin KA; Microcircuits in visual cortex. Current Opinion in Neurobiology 2002; 12:418–425.

Miller MW. Expression of nerve growth factor and its receptors in the somatosensory or motor cortex of the *Macaca nemestrina*. Journal of Neurocytology 2000; 29:453–469.

Okhotin VE, Kalinichenko SG. The histophysiology of neocortical basket cell. Neuroscience and Behavorial Physiology 2002; 32:455–470.

Passingham RE, Stephan KE, Kotter R. The anatomical basis of functional localization in the cortex. Nature Reviews 2002; 3:606–616.

Roland PE. Dynamic depolarization fields in the cerebral cortex. Trends in Neurosciences 2002; 25:183–190.

Sejnowski TJ, Destexhe A. Why do we sleep? Brain Research 2002; 886:208–223.

Squire LR, Zola-Morgan S. The medial temporal lobe memory system. Science 1991; 253:1380–1386.

Super H, Uylings HB. The early differentiation of the neocortex: a hypothesis on neocortical evolultion. Cerebral Cortex 2001; 11:1101–1109.

Thoenen H. Neurotrophins and activity-dependent plasticity. Progress in Brain Research 2000; 128:183–191.

Willis WD Jr, Westlund KN. Pain System. In; Paxinos G, Mai JK (eds) Human Nervous System. Academic Press, San Diego, CA, 2003.

Vogt BA, Hof PR, Vogt LJ. Cingulate Cyrus. In: Paxinos G, Mai JK (eds) Human Nervous System. Academic Press, San Diego, CA.

Dementia and Abnormalities of Cognition

Gregory Cooper and Robert L. Rodnitzky

Dementia is a state of cognitive impairment resulting from the progressive loss of previously acquired mental abilities. There may be a mild decline in cognitive function that occurs with normal aging, but it seldom results in serious functional disability. In dementia, cognitive dysfunction is sufficient to prevent the normal accomplishment of standard activities of daily living such as dressing, cooking a meal, or balancing a checkbook.

REGIONAL BRAIN PATHOLOGY

The individual signs and symptoms of dementia reflect the underlying regional pathology. For example, the clinical characteristics of dementia occurring in diseases affecting primarily the cerebral cortex differ from those of subcortical dementia. In cortical disorders such as Alzheimer's disease, symptoms specific to cortical dysfunction include aphasia, suggesting involvement of perisylvian cortices, apraxia (e.g., inability to organize and perform a motor task despite normal strength and coordination), and agnosia (e.g., inability to recognize), suggesting temporal and parietal cortical involvement. Visuospatial difficulties indicate the involvement of parietal cortices and impairments in visual processing suggest involvement of visual-association cortices. In other conditions affecting frontal cortices, marked alterations in personality and behavior may be seen. In dementias primarily related to subcortical pathology, such as that occurring in Parkinson's disease, these features are usually absent. In both forms, memory loss occurs, but it is typically less severe in subcortical dementia. The memory loss associated with subcortical dementia is frequently amenable to cuing, and usually a hint will bring the forgotten thought to mind. It has been said that those with cortical dementias forget, and those with subcortical dementia, who can recall after being cued, forget to remember. In other words, memory loss in cortical dementia reflects an impairment in learning and in subcortical dementia and impairment of recall. Subcortical dementia is also marked by a general cognitive slowing.

ALZHEIMER'S DISEASE

Alzheimer's Disease Is the Most Common Cause of Severe Dementia

Although more than 70 causes of dementia have been identified, Alzheimer's disease is responsible for up to 60% of cases of dementia in persons older than 65 yr of age. This condition is characterized histologically by the presence in the brain of abnormal aggregations of cytoskeletal filaments known as *neurofibrillary tangles* and by abnormal structures referred to as *senile plaques*. Both of these microscopic abnormalities are predominantly found in the neocortical areas and the hippocampus. The major componenet of senile plaques is the β-amyloid protein (Aβ), which is derived from the larger amyloid precursor protein (APP). Aβ is formed when the APP is cleaved by β- and γ-secretase. The the exact function of the APP has not been resolved. However, it has been suggested that Aβ, possibly through direct neuronal toxicity, is responsible for the cascade of events leading to the signs of symptoms of Alzheimer's disease. Support for the amyloid hypothesis comes from findings in cases of familial Alzheimer's disease. Mutations in the APP-encoding gene on chromosome 21 and in the presenilin genes on chromosomes 1 and 14 all lead to increased production of Ab. In addition, the ε4 allele of the APOE gene has been identified as a risk factor for Alzheimer's disease in a dose-dependent fashion. It has been proposed that this risk is mediated through alterations in Ab metabolism, and it has been shown that subjects with one or more ε4 alleles have higher amyloid plaque burdens. These findings have led to considerable interest in developing agents that will alter APP metabolism or promote clearance of Ab.

Memory Loss Is the Most Constant Feature of Alzheimer's Disease

The clinical hallmark of Alzheimer's disease is memory loss. Recent memory is affected initially, reflecting an impairment in learning new facts. This may manifest as repetitive questioning, missed appointments, or misplaced objects. In contrast, memory of more remote events is often relatively preserved in the early stages. The onset of memory loss is insidious, and impairment is slowly progressive. In Alzheimer's disease, memory loss may in part be related to neuronal loss in the hippocampus, and a reduction in the number of cholinergic neurons projecting from the basal nucleus of Meynert in the forebrain. Attempts to augment or restore cholinergic transmission through the use of cholinesterase inhibitors have proven to be modestly effective in improving memory and cognition in Alzheimer's disease.

SUDDEN ABNORMALITIES OF MEMORY AND COGNITION

Sudden abnormalities of memory and cognition are more likely caused by brain tumors or stroke than degenerative conditions. Symptoms similar to those seen in Alzheimer's disease can occur as a result of localized damage to specific regions of the brain from a brain tumor or cerebral ischemia. *Transient global amnesia* is the sudden but temporary inability to encode new memories. This syndrome is usually caused by temporary dysfunction of both hippocampi resulting from causes such as epileptic discharges or ischemia. Affected patients remain alert, but repeatedly ask the same orienting questions, because they cannot retain the information provided in previous answers. Within minutes to hours, the episode passes, but there is little or no recall of the total event.

Brain tumors or stroke involving the right parietal lobe often result in agnosia, an inability to recognize. Autotopagnosia refers to the inability to recognize a part of one's own body. After a right parietal stroke, a person with autotopagnosia may identify his or her own left hand as belonging to the examiner instead. Prosopagnosia is a specific agnosia that can result from highly localized cortical damage. It is characterized by the inability to recognize and identify familiar faces. This condition occurs in persons who have suffered damage to the visual-association cortices in both hemispheres.

Apraxia is the inability to perform skilled motor movements despite normal coordination and preserved motor, sensory, and cognitive function. The apractic patient may properly grasp and lift a spoon, but he cannot demonstrate how it is used. Apraxia most commonly occurs after damage to the inferior parietal region of the dominant hemisphere. Certain forms of apraxia are more related to impaired perception of spatial relations, and are caused by lesions of the nondominant hemisphere. Dressing apraxia is an example of this phenomenon. The affected person cannot correctly perform acts such as putting an arm into the sleeve of a coat, buttoning buttons, or placing a garment on the correct part of the body.

SELECTED READINGS

Chan YM, Jan YN. Presenilins, processing β-amyloid precursor protein, and notch signaling. 1999; 23:201–204.

Mayeux R, Sano M. Treatment of Alzheimer's disease. N Engl J Med 1999; 341:1670–1679.

Selkoe DJ. Translating cell biology into therapeutic advances in Alzheimer's disease. Nature 1999; 399(6738 Suppl):A23–A31.

St. George-Hyslop PH. Molecular genetics of Alzheimer's disease. Semin Neurol 1999; 19:371–383.

17 The Limbic System

J. Michael Wyss, Thomas van Groen, and Kevin J. Canning

CONTENTS

1. NEUROANATOMY OF THE LIMBIC SYSTEM

Willis (1664) was the first to refer to the cortical regions that form the medial edge of the telencephalon as *limbus* (i.e., Latin meaning border), but Broca (1878) was the first to popularize the designation of this cortex as "le grand lobe limbique," or limbic lobe. Broca envisioned the limbic lobe as comprising the entire gray mantle, namely the telencephalic cingulate and parahippocampal gyri that lay as a transition between the neocortex and the diencephalon and formed a circle around the interventricular foramen (Fig. 1). The limbic lobe is rostrally connected to the olfactory bulb and olfactory cortex, and is smaller in microsmatic animals and larger in macrosmatic animals. These facts led Broca to suggest that the function of the limbic lobe was related to olfaction, and several researchers expanded on this view, even to the point of suggesting that the limbic lobe was a "smell brain," or rhinencephalon. By 1940, several lines of evidence suggested that these regions of the cortex also received other types of sensory information and were involved in other functions, especially emotion.

In 1937, Papez hypothesized that there was an anatomical basis for the emotional disturbances of some

From: *Neuroscience in Medicine, 2nd ed.* (P. Michael Conn, ed.),
© 2003 Humana Press Inc., Totowa, NJ.

of his psychiatric patients. Papez proposed a circuit to explain these disturbances, now known as the *Papez circuit* (Fig. 2), which involved connections between limbic cortical areas and the diencephalon. Papez's original hypothesis was that the hippocampal formation received major input from sensory areas of the cerebral cortex, and that the hippocampal formation processed this information and projected this to the mammillary bodies from which the appropriate emotional response could be coordinated (Fig. 2). This circuitry has been elucidated in more detail, and it is clear that the afferent and efferent connections of the hippocampal formation are far more varied and complex than Papez's original model. Two years after Papez proposed this hypothesis, Klüver and Bucy demonstrated that extensive lesions to the temporal lobe that primarily damage two parts of the limbic system—especially the amygdala and hippocampal formation—profoundly influenced the affective behavior of subhuman primates.

On the basis of the studies of Klüver, Bucy, and others, MacLean (1949, 1952) suggested that the term *limbic system* (Fig. 1) should be applied to the limbic areas. MacLean emphasized that the limbic-system elements were at the interface between somatic and visceral areas of the brain, and thus could relate these systems to each other and to the ongoing behavior of the organism. Nauta later expanded on the definition of the limbic system by showing that areas of the

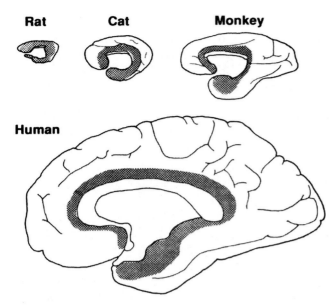

Fig. 1. In comparison to other animals, the limbic cortex, which encircles the upper brainstem, reaches its largest proportions in the human. These drawings of the medial surface of a hemisected brain, with brainstem and cerebellum removed, illustrate the size and position of the limbic cortex (*stippled region*) in the three animals in which it has often been studied experimentally, and in the human. Broca originally used the concept of the unity of "le grand lobe limbique" in the otter (Broca, 1878). Broca, like many neurologists of his day, often used macrosmatic (those with a highly developed sense of smell) animals such as the otter for anatomical studies. In these macrosmatic animals, the continuity of the limbic cortex with the olfactory bulb is very prominent, but in the primate, this attachment is less striking.

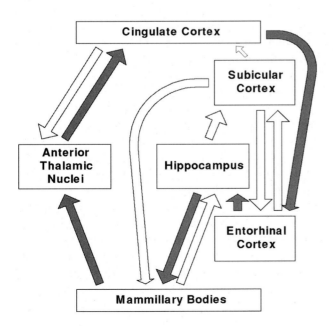

limbic cortex (but not neocortex) were connected directly to many areas of the hypothalamus and brainstem.

Thus, the limbic system is a concept that has undergone considerable redefinition since its introduction. The primary areas that are currently included under the umbrella of limbic system include the hippocampal formation, subicular cortices, entorhinal cortex, cingulate cortex, septal nuclei, and amygdala. All these regions are telencephalic, but they are structurally more primitive than the cerebral neocortex, and they are strongly interconnected by direct connections between the limbic regions and by indirect projections through diencephalic regions, including the mammillary bodies and the anterior thalamic nuclei. Together, these interrelated areas of the telencephalon and diencephalon form the limbic system. Although the individual limbic areas are functionally diverse—serving emotional responses and drive-related behavior on the one hand, and learning and memory on the other— the high degree of interconnection suggests that these areas have an underlying unity.

In contrast to the neocortex that can be divided into six layers (i.e., five neuronal-cell layers and one superficial molecular layer), the limbic cortical areas tend to be structurally simpler, and they arise earlier in mammalian phylogeny. These areas have often been called ancient (i.e., archicortex), old (i.e., paleocortex), and middle (i.e., mesocortex) cortices on the basis of the development of each individual area. Despite their phylogenetically early, immature appearances, many limbic areas of the cortex reach their greatest development in humans. The limbic cortex expands more rapidly in size from lower primates to humans relative to the primary sensory and motor cortex (Fig. 1). However, these areas are not antiquated remnants of earlier evolution, but are brain regions that have continued to develop both structurally and functionally throughout phylogeny.

Researchers may still differ as to the exact areas that comprise the limbic system; however, most agree that it includes the *hippocampal formation, subicular cortex, entorhinal cortex, cingulate (midline) cortex,*

Fig. 2. (*Left*) Papez's circuit as originally proposed (*gray arrows*) with additional connections now commonly considered important components of the limbic system (*open arrows*). In Papez's original work, the hippocampal formation was viewed as a single area.

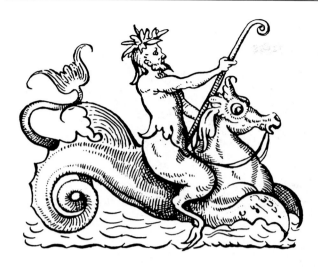

Fig. 3. The sixteenth-century Italian physician Aranzi displayed his vivid imagination when he named the hippocampus for its resemblance to the mythical seahorse (shown here being ridden by Triton in a seventeenth-century drawing).

septal nuclei, amygdala, mammillary bodies, and anterior thalamic nuclei.

1.1. The Hippocampal Formation Is a Major Landmark in the Temporal Cortex

1.1.1. OVERALL STRUCTURE

The hippocampal formation, or hippocampus, lies in the temporal lobe of the cerebral cortex, just medial to the inferior horn of the lateral ventricle. Some early anatomists believed its gross appearance looked like a seahorse and gave it the name hippocampus, which originates from the Greek word for seahorse, *hippokampos* (Fig. 3). Although the hippocampus stretches from the amygdala to the splenium of the corpus callosum, the intrinsic structure of the hippocampus proper is best appreciated in its mid portion (septotemporal). In this region, the cortical sheet of hippocampal tissue is folded over itself in the characteristic S-shape (Fig. 4). In more rostral regions of the hippocampus, the entire S-shaped hippocampal cortex bends back on itself, and the CA fields become much more difficult to differentiate with precision (Fig. 5C). Similarly, at caudal levels, the simple S-shape is obscured as the formation bends near the splenium of the corpus callosum. The hippocampus continues as a small band of neurons (i.e., the indusium griseum) above the entire length of the corpus callosum that extends around the genu of the corpus callosum and descends into the septal area, where it is known as the taenia tecta.

The hippocampus is one of the most easily discriminated regions within the cerebral cortex. Most of the hippocampus has a single compact layer of neuronal-cell bodies, and thus contrasts sharply with the five neuronal-cell layers present in most areas of the neocortex. This relative simplicity has led many researchers to use the hippocampus as a model system to illuminate the structure and function of the more complex neocortex.

Although some differences in nomenclature continue to confuse the hippocampal literature, the following terms are most widely used and are best-defined. The *hippocampal formation* consists of two facing and overlapping horseshoe-shaped cell layers, the *dentate gyrus* and the *hippocampus proper* (Ammon's horn or cornu Ammonis [CA]; Fig. 4). However, in most common usage, and in this chapter, the term "hippocampus" is used instead of hippocampal formation. The most common nomenclature divides the hippocampus proper into CA regions: CA_1, CA_2, and CA_3 (adapted from Lorente de Nó; Fig. 4). Rose divided the hippocampus proper into five fields, designated h1 through h5, and his terminology remains popular among some neuropathologists. The *subiculum*, which is a natural extension of the CA region, may also considered to be a part of the hippocampal formation, but it is usually considered as a separate entity.

1.1.2. REGIONS OF THE HIPPOCAMPUS

The *dentate gyrus* is a trilaminar structure that caps the distal tip of the CA fields (Fig. 4). The main cell layer is composed of tightly packed granule-cell neurons that have apical dendrites that project primarily toward the pial surface, but the granule-cell neurons also give rise to less conspicuous basal dendrites that extend toward the hilus. These granule cells are generated rather late in embryonic development, and some of these neurons continue to divide into adulthood, although at an extremely slow rate. Although proliferation was known to occur in the dentate gyrus, more recent work demonstrates that neurons can proliferate in many places in the mature brain.

Superficial to the granule-cell layer lies the molecular layer, which contains most of the dendrites of the granule cells, and deep to the granule-cell layer lies the polymorphic layer or hilus. Axons of the polymorphic neurons in this region project to the molecular layer of the dentate gyrus, but they do not project to the hippocampus proper.

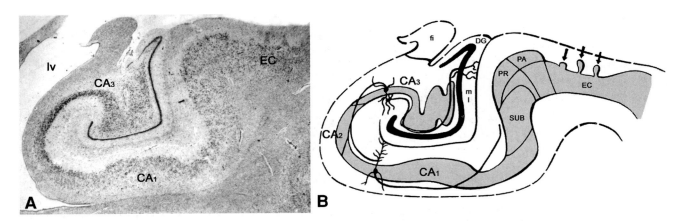

Fig. 4. (A) A Nissl-stained, coronal section of a human hippocampal formation taken from the mid-anterior-posterior level. **(B)** A line drawing that illustrates the divisions of the hippocampal formation and the relative appearance of the granule cells and pyramidal neurons in the dentate gyrus and CA fields, respectively. CA, the fields of the hippocampus proper; DG, dentate gyrus granule-cell layer; EC, entorhinal cortex; fi, fimbria: lv, lateral ventricle; ml, dentate gyrus molecular layer; PA, parasubiculum; PR, presubiculum; SUB, subiculum.

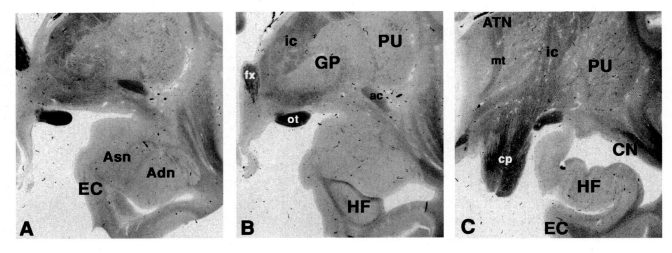

Fig. 5. Three photomicrographs of Weil-stained coronal sections through the human amygdala and rostral hippocampal formation. Ac, anterior commissure; Adn, deep nuclei of the amygdala; Asn, superficial nuclei of the amygdala; ATN, anterior thalamic nuclei; CN, caudate nucleus; cp, cerebral peduncle; EC, entorhinal cortex; fx, fornix; GP, globus pallidus; HF, hippocampal formation; ic, internal capsule; mt, mammillothalamic tract; ot, optic tract; PU, putamen.

The hippocampus proper is made up of one pyramidal-cell layer that is a few neurons thick. On the basis of cellular morphology, the hippocampus proper has been divided into three areas. Area CA_3 lies proximal to the dentate gyrus. Area CA_1 lies distal to the dentate gyrus and contains neurons that are slightly smaller in size and more widely scattered than CA_3. Area CA_2 consists of a short, mixed-cell region that lies between CA_3 and CA_1 (Fig. 4). Of the seven million neurons in the CA fields, approx 67% reside in CA_1, 30% lie in CA_3 and 3% are in CA_2.

Area CA_3 has a relatively compact pyramidal-cell layer. Within the dentate hilar area, CA_3 bends toward one blade of the dentate gyrus and then bends back toward the opposite blade (Fig. 4). In addition to the relatively large size of the CA_3 pyramidal neurons, the structure of the apical dendrites differentiates these neurons from those in CA_2 and CA_1. The apical dendrites of the CA_3 pyramidal neurons bifurcate close to their soma, but the apical dendrites of the CA_1 and CA_2 pyramidal neurons, apical dendrites have smaller branches along most of their length (Fig. 4B). The granule-cell neurons of the dentate gyrus send their axons, the *mossy fibers* (so named because of the large terminals that stud these axons) to the CA_3 neurons, and these axons terminate massively on the proximal shaft of the apical dendrites in a layer that is named *stratum lucidum*. In this layer, the postsynaptic specializations on the CA_3 dendrites resemble large thorns, a characteristic not seen on the CA_1 and CA_2 apical dendrites. The apical CA_3 dendrites extend from stratum lucidum into *stratum radiatum* and *stratum lacunosum-moleculare*; each of these layers contains distinct afferent inputs to the pyramidal neurons. Above the molecular layer of the CA fields is the obliterated *hippocampal fissure*. The CA_3 basal dendrites extend into the layer known as *stratum oriens*, where scattered basket and polymorphic neurons are also located. Between stratum oriens and the lateral ventricle lies the *alveus*, a major fiber bundle that carries information to and from the hippocampus. Many axons in the alveus course through the *fimbria*, a large fiber bundle that lies medial and dorsal to the CA fields (Fig. 4), and *fornix* en route to subcortical and diencephalic sites.

The borders of area CA_2 are not easily discriminated in Nissl-stained material because some neurons of CA_3 tend to lie deep to the CA_2 pyramidal cells. Other features differentiate the CA_2 area. For example, CA_2 contains many large pyramidal neurons that are similar in size to those in CA_3, but CA_2 has a more compact pyramidal-cell layer. In contrast, CA_1 has slightly smaller and more widespread pyramidal neurons (Fig. 4A). Further, the mossy fibers do not extend to the CA_2 neurons, and the CA_2 neurons can be selectively labeled for some neurotransmitters. Because the mossy fibers do not extend to area CA_2 or CA_1, these regions lack a stratum lucidum, and therefore the stratum radiatum is adjacent to the pyramidal-cell layer.

1.1.3. THE SUBICULAR CORTICES ARE THE PRIMARY AREAS RESPONSIBLE FOR THE EXTRINSIC CONNECTIONS OF THE HIPPOCAMPAL FORMATION

Researchers have identified up to six subregions in this area, but it is useful to consider three major divisions in the human subicular cortices (i.e., subiculum, parasubiculum, and presubiculum; Fig. 4). The *subiculum proper* has a much wider pyramidal-cell layer than CA_1 and can be subdivided into a superficial (large cell) and deep (small cell) sublayer. Several researchers suggest that there is a prosubicular division between CA_1 and subiculum proper, but the dif-

ferences between this area and the subiculum are not easily distinguished. The border of subiculum with *presubiculum* (area 27 of Brodmann) is marked by the appearance of a tightly packed layer of small pyramidal neurons (i.e., lamina principalis externa) that caps the inner layer (i.e., lamina principalis interna), which appears in the same position as the subiculum's pyramidal-cell layer. As in all areas of the hippocampal formation, adjacent areas tend to slide over or under each other in transition regions (Fig. 4). The *parasubiculum* (i.e., area 48 of Brodmann) lies between the presubiculum and the entorhinal cortex. Similar to the presubiculum, the parasubiculum has two major neuronal-cell layers, but the neurons in the lamina principalis externa are larger than those in the corresponding layer of the presubiculum.

1.1.4. THE ENTORHINAL CORTEX IS THE PRIMARY AREA RESPONSIBLE FOR CONNECTING THE HIPPOCAMPUS AND SUBICULAR CORTEX TO THE REMAINDER OF THE TEMPORAL CORTEX

The human entorhinal cortex (area 28 of Brodmann) lies ventral to the rostral half of the hippocampal formation and the entire amygdaloid complex (Figs. 4,5). The entorhinal cortex has been divided into as many as 23 separate areas, but all these areas are generally similar in morphology, and the cortical area is not subdivided in this chapter. The differentiating elements of the entorhinal cortex are present in layers II and IV. The neuronal-cell bodies in layer II form large prominent cell islands, especially at the rostral levels of the entorhinal cortex. In contrast, layer IV consists of a dense fiber plexus (i.e., the lamina dissecans) that clearly separates the small pyramidal neurons in layer III from the larger pyramidal neurons in layer V. The entorhinal cortex is bordered by area 35 (i.e., part of the perirhinal cortex). Although the entorhinal cortex was named for its proximity to the rhinal sulcus in subprimates and monkeys, the entorhinal cortex is caudal to the rhinal sulcus. Over most of the rostral-caudal extent of the human hippocampal formation, the perirhinal cortex is the border between the entorhinal cortex and the temporal neocortex, and it is primarily aligned with the collateral sulcus.

1.2. The Septal Nuclei Are a Major Subcortical Target of the Hippocampus

The *septal region* is a subcortical telencephalic region that is highly interconnected with the hippocampus through the fornix, and it lies near the genu of the corpus callosum and medial to the lateral ventricles

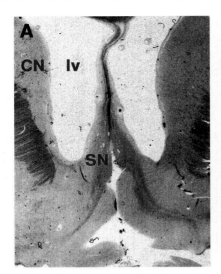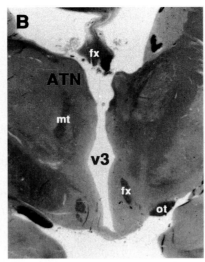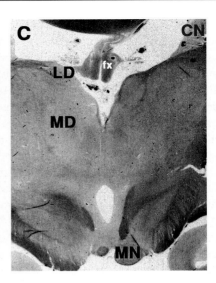

Fig. 6. Three photomicrographs of the Weil-stained (for myelinated axons) coronal sections through successively more caudal areas of the human brain. (**A**) Illustrates the septal nuclei; (**B**) the rostral anterior thalamic nuclei and mid-hypothalamus, and (**C**) the posterio and anterior thalamic nuclei, the lateral dorsal nucleus and the mammillary complex. Note that each of the the sections are cut asymmetrically—i.e., the left side of the brain is further caudal than the right side. ATN, anterior thalamic nuclei; CN, caudate nucleus; fx, fornix; ic, internal capsule; LD, lateral dorsal nucleus of the thalamus; lv, lateral ventricle; MD, medial dorsal nucleus of the thalamus; MN, mammillary nuclei; mt, mammillothalamic tract; ot, optic tract; SN, septal nuclei; VA, ventral anterior thalamic nucleus; v3, third ventricle.

(Fig. 6A). Few or no neuronal-cell bodies are within the septum pellucidum, which is the thin sheet of tissue that is dorsal and caudal to the anterior commissure and separates the lateral ventricles. Conversely, most septal neurons lie ventral to the septum pellucidum and rostral to the anterior commissure. The septal nuclei are separated into two major divisions, the *medial* and *lateral septal nuclei*. The lateral septal nucleus has relatively small neuronal-cell bodies, whereas the medial septal nucleus has larger neuronal-cell bodies and is the major origin of the hippocampal projections of the septal nuclei. In addition to the medial and lateral nuclei, the septal complex also includes the *septohippocampal, septofimbrial,* and *triangular septal nuclei,* the *bed nucleus of the stria terminalis,* and the *diagonal band of Broca.*

1.3. The Mammillary Complex Is a Major Limbic Hypothalamic Area

Although several areas of the hypothalamus are interconnected with limbic cortical regions, the mammillary bodies have the most prominent connections to this cortex. In humans, the *medial mammillary nuclei* bulge out from the base of the hypothalamus, thus giving rise to their suggestive name (Fig. 6C). The mammillary complex is typically divided into four

nuclei, and each of these regions has a distinct cytoarchitecture and connections. The largest nucleus is the *medial mammillary nucleus,* lateral to which is the *lateral mammillary nucleus,* and further lateral lies the *tuberomammillary nucleus.* The neurons in the latter two nuclei are much larger than those in the medial mammillary nucleus. Finally, above the medial mammillary nucleus is the *supramammillary nucleus.* The main input to the mammillary bodies is through the postcommissural fornix, and derives from the subicular cortices. The major projection arising from the mammillary bodies is through the *mammillothalamic tract,* which terminates in the anterior thalamic nuclei.

1.4. The Anterior Thalamus Is the Primary Limbic Thalamic Area

The anterior nuclei of the thalamus are situated dorsomedial to the internal medullary lamina, and classically are divided into three nuclei: the *anterior dorsal, anterior medial* and *anterior ventral thalamic nuclei* (Fig. 6B). In lower primate and subprimate species, the three nuclei are quite distinct, but in the human brain, the anterior medial nucleus is difficult to discriminate from the anterior ventral nucleus, and the two have often been grouped together and called the nucleus anterior principalis, but the connections of these areas are very different. The anterior dorsal nucleus is by far the smallest of the three anterior thalamic nuclei, and its relative volume does not increase substantially in humans compared to lower primates. In all species, the cytoarchitecture of the anterior dorsal nucleus is distinct from that of the anterior ventral and the anterior medial nuclei, because its neurons are more tightly packed and stain darker than the other nuclei.

The *lateral dorsal nucleus* lies on the dorsal surface of the thalamus and is surrounded by a fiber capsule, thus giving an appearance very similar to the anterior nuclei that it borders (Fig. 6C). Although its Nissl-stained appearance and location are distinct from those of the anterior nuclei proper, in fiber stains, the lateral dorsal nucleus appears to be a caudal continuation of the anterior group, and many of its connections are similar. Thus, it is often considered as part of the anterior thalamic group.

Several other thalamic nuclei have major projections to the limbic cortex. These include the *medial dorsal nucleus*, the *midline nuclei* (especially the parataenial, the paraventricular, and the reuniens nuclei), the *intralaminar nuclei*, and the *lateral thalamic nuclei* (i.e., lateral posterior and medial pulvinar nuclei). Modern tract tracing studies show that only distinct regions of these nuclei are limbic, and that other regions are primarily related to nonlimbic areas of the neocortex.

1.5. The Cingulate Cortex Comprises the Limbic Midline Cortex

The major projection of the anterior thalamic nuclei is to the cingulate cortex, an area that forms a major component of the circuit of Papez. This cortical region lies below the cingulate sulcus and surrounds the corpus callosum from its rostrum to its splenium. This cortex typically is designated according to the numbering system of Brodmann (1909) or the names suggested by Rose (1928). Both schemes recognize that a major division of the cingulate cortex lies immediately behind the splenium of the corpus callosum, deep within the sulcus of the corpus callosum. This part of cingulate cortex includes areas 26, 29, and 30 of Brodmann, and is the retrosplenial cortex of Rose. The part of the cingulate cortex that is rostral to the splenium of the corpus callosum includes areas 23, 24, 25, 32, and 33 of Brodmann. In humans, the Brodmann numbering system of the rostral cingulate cortex is preferred to Rose's six divisions of *infraradiata cortex*.

1.6. The Amygdala is Divided Into Two Major Regions

The amygdala, whose name reflects its almond-like appearance, is a mass of gray matter that is situated within the temporal lobe, immediately rostral to the inferior horn of the lateral ventricle (Fig. 5). In Weigert-stained sections, the amygdala looks similar to the striatum, and it appears continuous with the lentiform nucleus dorsally and the tail of the caudate nucleus caudally. Together with the fact that both the amygdala and the striatum develop from the embryonic striatal ridge, this suggested to early anatomists that the amygdala was part of the basal ganglia, but later connectional and immunohistochemical studies demonstrated that it is connected with and functions as part of the limbic system. Today, many researchers see the amygdala as the core of the extended amygdala system.

The amygdala is usually divided into two major regions: the *corticomedial* (or superficial) and the *basolateral* (or deep) nuclei. The deep nuclei, which take up a greater volume in the amygdala, contain four nuclei: the lateral, the basal lateral, and the basal medial nuclei and the amygdaloclaustral area. The superficial group of nuclei includes the anterior, the medial, and the cortical amygdaloid nuclei, the periamygdaloid cortex, and the nucleus of the lateral olfactory tract, a nucleus that is poorly developed in the human brain. On the basis of its structure and connections, the central nucleus is considered to be a separate region from the two large nuclear groups of the amygdala. At its caudal end, the superficial group is continuous with the amygdalohippocampal area, a transition zone between the amygdala to the hippocampal formation.

2. MAJOR CONNECTIONS OF THE LIMBIC SYSTEM

2.1. The Entorhinal and Subicular Cortices Are the Primary Gateways to the Hippocampus

2.1.1. AFFERENT CONNECTIONS

The majority of extrinsic inputs to the hippocampus initially terminate in either the *entorhinal* or *subicular cortices* (Fig. 7). The entorhinal cortex receives inputs from several areas of the temporal, frontal, and midline cortices. The perirhinal cortex and the temporal polar cortex project to the lateral portion of the

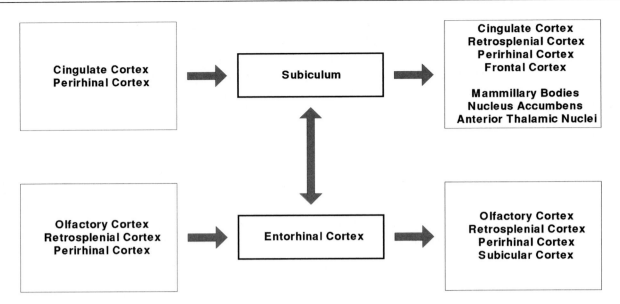

Fig. 7. The hippocampal formation is heavily connected to the subiculum and entorhinal cortex. The primary extrinsic connections the subiculum and entorhinal cortex are illustrated.

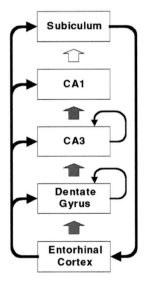

Fig. 8. The *gray thick arrows* show the trisynaptic pathway, and the feedback and feedforward collaterals are shown by the *black arrows*.

entorhinal cortex. The dorsal temporal, insular, orbitofrontal, infralimbic, prelimbic, cingulate, and retrosplenial cortices have significant projections to the entorhinal cortex. Several subcortical areas also have significant direct projections to the entorhinal cortex. The lateral nucleus of the amygdala has a dense projection to the lateral entorhinal cortex, and other areas of the amygdala have less prominent projections to the entorhinal cortex. The claustrum also projects to the entorhinal cortex, as do the paraventricular and reuniens nuclei of the thalamus.

The subicular cortices also receive many extrahippocampal projections. Temporal, frontal, dorsolateral parietal, and midline cortices project rather densely to distinct divisions of the subicular cortices. Areas of the visual cortex also project directly to the subicular cortices. Several subcortical areas also have significant direct projections to the subicular cortices—i.e., most of the thalamic input to the hippocampal formation terminates in the subicular cortices. Each of the anterior nuclei of the thalamus projects to selective areas of the presubicular and parasubicular cortex, and each nucleus has a distinctive terminal pattern in these cortical areas. The midline thalamic nuclei (i.e., parataenial and reuniens nuclei) also have prominent projections to the subicular cortices.

The inputs to the entorhinal cortex, including those from the subicular cortices, probably provide most of the sensory and motor information to the dentate gyrus and hippocampus, but a few other extrinsic inputs directly project onto the dentate granule cells and the fields of the hippocampus proper (CA) pyramidal neurons. The most prominent of these projections originates in the medial septal nucleus and nucleus of the diagonal band of Broca, and reaches the hippocampus through the fornix. Axons from the septal nuclei terminate throughout the hippocampal formation, but the major terminal field is in the molecular layer of the dentate gyrus and in area CA_3 (Fig. 4). Approximately 50% of the septal axons in this projection use acetylcholine as a neurotransmitter. A second direct projection to the dentate gyrus and CA fields originates in the supramammillary nucleus and terminates prominently on the proximal dendrites of the dentate gyrus granule cells and in the CA fields. The nucleus reuniens of the thalamus has a prominent projection to the distal part of the CA_1 apical dendrites and a weaker projection to other areas of the hippocampal formation.

Several brainstem nuclei that project to most of the telencephalon also project to the hippocampal formation. These include a noradrenergic projection from the *locus coeruleus*, a serotonergic projection from the *raphe nuclei* (i.e., dorsal raphe and central superior nuclei) and a smaller, dopaminergic projection from the *ventral tegmental area of Tsai*. The *periaqueductal gray*, the lateral and dorsal tegmental nuclei, and the reticular nuclei of the brainstem also project to the hippocampal formation.

2.1.2. INTRINSIC CONNECTIONS

The intrinsic connections of the hippocampal formation form a serial pathway with several collateral and feedback projections added onto the serial path. The serial connections of the hippocampal formation, traditionally called the *trisynaptic pathway*, i.e., the sequential projections from the entorhinal cortex to the dentate gyrus to CA_3 to CA_1 (Fig. 8). The entorhinal cortex projects to the dentate gyrus granule cells

and has collaterals to the CA fields as well as the subiculum. The largest input to the dentate granule neurons originates in *layer II neurons of the entorhinal cortex*; the axons terminate in the molecular layer of the dentate gyrus on the outer two-thirds of the granule cell dendrites. In contrast, the input to the CA fields originates in layer III neurons of the entorhinal cortex; the axons terminate in stratum lacunosum moleculare. The position of the cells of origin within the entorhinal cortex dictates the position of the terminals along the septotemporal axis of the hippocampus. In the monkey, axons from neurons in lateral parts of the entorhinal cortex terminate in the septal (dorsal) part of the hippocampus, whereas axons originating in medial parts of the entorhinal cortex terminate in the temporal part of the hippocampus. The polymorphic neurons of the dentate hilus project to the inner one-third (i.e., proximal portion) of the dentate molecular layer.

The granule cells of the dentate gyrus project to the pyramidal neurons in area CA_3 through their mossy fibers (Fig. 4B). The CA_3 pyramidal neurons, in turn, send out a projection, known as the *Schaffer collaterals*, to the apical and basal dendrites of CA_2 and CA_1. CA_1 has a massive projection to the subiculum, which in turn projects back to the entorhinal cortex (Fig. 8). The presubiculum and the parasubiculum do not receive direct input from the hippocampus, but they give rise to dense projections to the entorhinal cortex, with presubicular axons terminating in layers I and III and parasubicular axons terminating in layer II of the entorhinal cortex. All three areas of the subicular cortex have connections with the retrosplenial cortex.

Several feedback loops and local projections of interneurons (inhibitory) modify the information flow in the hippocampal formation. The dentate hilar, polymorphic neurons project back to the proximal dendrites and cell bodies of the granule cells and strongly influence information flow through the granule cells. Similarly, the interneurons in the CA fields provide local feedback to the CA pyramidal neurons. The primary cell layer of all CA fields and of the dentate gyrus contains basket-cell neurons that project to and potently inhibit neurons in the layer in which they reside. In distinction to all other hippocampal areas, the CA_3 neurons have extensive feedback excitatory intrinsic connections.

2.1.3. EXTRINSIC CONNECTIONS

Although CA_1 and CA_3 neurons give rise to significant projections to the septal nuclei, most of the major outputs of the hippocampal formation are routed through the subicular and entorhinal cortices (Fig. 7). The *postcommissural fornix* originates in the subicular cortices. These subicular axons innervate the anterior and lateral dorsal thalamic nuclei, the ventromedial hypothalamic nucleus (VHN) and the mammillary complex. The mammillary complex receives the densest of these diencephalic projections. Each component of the subicular cortices projects in a distinct pattern. For example, only the subiculum innervates the medial mammillary nucleus, but both presubiculum and parasubiculum densely innervate the lateral mammillary nucleus, and the subiculum has a much less dense projection to this nucleus.

The subicular and entorhinal cortices are also the origin of projections to other cerebral cortical areas. The subicular cortices project to the cingulate, retrosplenial, and medial orbital cortices and to the parahippocampal gyrus, including the perirhinal cortex. The entorhinal cortex provides a dense projection to the cerebral cortex, where its axons terminate prominently in perirhinal, caudal parahippocampal, retrosplenial, and temporal polar cortices, and it probably sends reciprocal projections to all other areas that project to it. The cortical areas to which subicular and entorhinal cortices project have widespread connections with almost all associational cortices. The hippocampal formation also projects directly and indirectly to the amygdala. The entorhinal cortex has a small projection to the lateral and basal nuclei of the amygdala, but most of the entorhinal axons in these nuclei are destined for the more rostral substantia innominata. The prosubiculum has a substantial amygdaloid projection that terminates in the basal nucleus as well as in the periamygdaloid nucleus. The subicular and entorhinal cortices are interconnected through direct reciprocal projections.

The constellation of these connections suggest that information flow in the hippocampal formation may be primarily serial, but as shown in Fig. 7, there are many feedback loops in this circuit.

2.2. Axons to and from the Septal Nuclei Course in the Fornix and the Medial Forebrain Bundle

The septal nuclei have dense reciprocal connections with the hippocampus. Most of the axons that connect these two regions course through the fornix. The septal nuclei receive projections from the amygdala, the hypothalamus, and the medial midbrain reticular region through the medial forebrain bundle. The septal nuclei are also innervated by the olfactory regions. Efferent axons of the septal nuclei course through the *stria medullaris* and the *medial forebrain bundle* to terminate in the habenula and hypothalamus, respectively. Some medial forebrain bundle axons arising from the septal nuclei extend to midbrain tegmentum and other brainstem nuclei.

2.3. The Mammillary Bodies Relay Hippocampal Information to the Anterior Thalamic Nuclei

The mammillary complex connections of the limbic system were important to Papez's hypothesized circuit of emotion. The *fornix* splits into two segments at the anterior commissure—the postcommissural fornix and the precommissural fornix. The postcommissural fornix originates in the subicular cortices, traverses through the hypothalamus, and terminates in both the hypothalamus and the mammillary complex. The dorsal and ventral tegmental nuclei and the anterior hypothalamus also innervate the mammillary complex.

The majority of efferent axons leave the mammillary nuclei by way of the *mammillothalamic tract* (ascending) and the *mammillotegmental tract* (descending). Through the mammillothalamic tract, the medial mammillary nucleus projects to the anterior ventral and anterior medial thalamic nuclei, and the lateral mammillary nucleus projects primarily to the anterior dorsal nucleus. The lateral dorsal thalamic nucleus also receives a small projection from the mammillary complex. The mammillotegmental tract carries axons to dorsal and ventral tegmental nuclei in the midbrain. The supramammillary nuclei have a significant direct projection to the dentate gyrus.

2.4. The Anterior Thalamic Nuclei Project Primarily to the Posterior Cingulate Cortex and the Hippocampal Formation

Three major pathways innervate the anterior thalamic nuclei. The mammillothalamic tract and the fornix from the subicular cortex supply approximately equal numbers of axons to all three nuclei. Corticothalamic fibers from the cingulate and the retrosplenial cortices provide the third major afferent. One other notable input is a small projection from the visual system. A direct projection from the retina to the anterior nuclei has been reported to exist in several species. The visual cortex projects to the anterior nuclei, although most of these projections terminate in

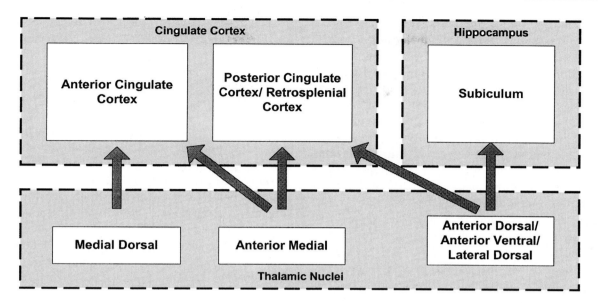

Fig. 9. Each of the thalamic nuclei that project to the cingulate cortex and hippocampus has a distinct terminal field (*arrows*).

the lateral dorsal nucleus. This nucleus also receives prominent inputs from retrosplenial and subicular cortices, and a small input from the mammillary complex.

The thalamocortical projections from the anterior thalamic nuclei supply the entire cingulate, retrosplenial, and subicular cortices with a thalamic innervation, but each of the thalamic nuclei ends in distinct regional and laminar patterns (Fig. 9). Data from subprimates indicate that unlike most thalamic projections, which terminate primarily in layer IV of the cortex, the projections from the anterior and lateral dorsal nuclei primarily terminate in layers I and IV of the cortex. The anterior dorsal and anterior ventral projections to the retrosplenial (i.e., area 29) and subicular cortices largely overlap in their regional spread, but are distinct in their laminar terminal patterns, with the anterior ventral nucleus projection largely confined to the outer third of layer I of the cortex and the anterior dorsal nucleus projection terminals spread throughout layer I. The anterior medial thalamic nucleus projects to the posterior cingulate cortex (i.e., area 23), but also provides a sparse projection to anterior cingulate cortex (i.e., area 24), an area that is densely innervated by the parataenial, paraventricular, and intralaminar nuclei. The anterior medial nucleus also projects to the prefrontal and orbitofrontal region of the cortex. Studies in the rat suggest that the projections to the posterior limbic cortex from the anterior ventral thalamic nucleus form a precise map in which

individual thalamic neurons project to restricted groups of cortical neurons.

The lateral and medial thalamic nuclear groups also project to the limbic cortex. The projection from the lateral dorsal nucleus largely overlaps the projections of anterior dorsal and anterior ventral thalamic nuclei to the posterior limbic cortex, and extends into the medial parietal cortex. The medial pulvinar thalamic nucleus projects to the posterior cingulate and retrosplenial cortex in primates. Two different parts of the medial dorsal nucleus—pars densicellularis and pars parvicellularis—project to the rostral cingulate cortex, including areas 25 and 32. The medial subnucleus of the ventral anterior thalamic nucleus projects to the cingulate cortex. Although these latter thalamic areas are not usually considered part of the limbic system, some data demonstrate that the portions of these nuclei that project to the limbic cortex do not project widely to other cortical targets, and these can be considered as limbic subnuclei.

2.5. In Contrast to the Anterior Cingulate Cortex, the Posterior Cingulate Cortex Is Connected Primarily to the Hippocampal Formation

2.5.1. Afferent Connections

The thalamic projections to the cingulate cortex are extensive, but the cortical connections are equally important. The entire cingulate cortex, including the retrosplenial cortex, is interconnected by extensive commissural and associational projections, and the latter interconnects up the posterior and anterior segments. Much of the caudal cingulate cortex also receives extensive projection from the subicular cortex. Several neocortical areas, including somatosensory, prefrontal, and association cortices (i.e., visual, parietal, and auditory) project to the cingulate cortex.

As in other parts of the cortex, the cingulate cortex is innervated by cholinergic (i.e., from the diagonal band of Broca), noradrenergic (i.e., from the locus coeruleus) and serotonergic (i.e., from the dorsal raphe and central superior nuclei) axons. The ventral tegmental area of Tsai sends a dense dopaminergic projection to the anterior cingulate cortex but only a limited dopaminergic projection to the posterior cingulate and the retrosplenial cortices. Each of these transmitter-specific systems terminates in a distinct laminar pattern.

2.5.2. EFFERENT CONNECTIONS

The projections of the cingulate and retrosplenial cortices to the subicular and entorhinal cortices, which course through the cingulum bundle, close the hypothesized circuit of Papez (Fig. 2). This projection is relatively dense and arises from many regions of the cingulate cortex, but it originates primarily in the retrosplenial cortex. The cingulate cortex is reciprocally connected with areas of associational neocortex. All areas of the cingulate cortex project to the medial striatum, and all areas are connected to the anterior and midline thalamic nuclei.

The anterior cingulate cortex also has substantial projections to the hypothalamus and brainstem, especially to areas related to visceral regulation. The cingulohypothalamic projection arises primarily from areas 23, 24, 25, and 32, and terminates primarily in the lateral hypothalamic area. Midbrain projections from the cingulate cortex arise primarily in areas 24 and 25, and these terminate in the periaqueductal gray matter, the raphe nuclei, and the deep layers of the superior colliculus. Areas 23, 24, 25, 29, and 32 project to the ventral pontine nuclei in a topographic manner. Sparse, medullary projections arise primarily from area 25 and end in the nucleus of the solitary tract (NST). A few axons from the cingulate cortex, primarily from dorsal areas 23 and 24 near the motor cortices, pass into the spinal cord, although their precise termination is unclear.

2.6. The Amygdala Is Connected to Both the Cerebral Cortex and the Hypothalamus

2.6.1. AFFERENT CONNECTIONS

The major afferent connections of the amygdala differentiate the two components of the complex. The *olfactory bulb* projects directly to the superficial amygdaloid nuclei through the lateral olfactory tract, but few or no olfactory bulb axons directly innervate the deep group of nuclei. Within the superficial nuclear group, dense-olfactory bulb and anterior-olfactory nucleus projections terminate in the anterior cortical nucleus, the nucleus of the olfactory tract, and the periamygdaloid cortex. Most areas of the deep nuclear group receive an olfactory-related input, but this originates in the piriform cortex and from intrinsic amygdaloid projections from the superficial nuclear group. The only major area of the amygdala that appears to lack either an olfactory bulb or a direct olfactory cortex input is the *central nucleus*. The olfactory bulb projections to the amygdala are reciprocated from the superficial amygdala (Fig. 10).

The amygdala, especially the lateral nucleus, is innervated directly by several other unimodal sensory areas of the cerebral cortex, but it receives no significant projections from primary sensory cortices except for the olfactory input. In addition to these single-modality sensory inputs, most other parts of the temporal lobe supply polysensory inputs to the amygdala, most of these projections are directed at the lateral and basal nuclei.

Somatosensory information reaches the amygdala through projections from the *insular* and *orbital cortices*. The most direct pathway for this information is from the secondary somatosensory cortex to the posterior insular cortex, which projects heavily to the lateral nucleus of the amygdala. The caudal orbital cortex projects to the basal nucleus, and this region may also project to the central nucleus. The anterior cingulate cortex (e.g., areas 24, 25, and 32) projects primarily to the basal nucleus.

Several *thalamic nuclei* project to the amygdala. Auditory input is directed to the lateral and central nuclei through projections from the medial geniculate nucleus. Gustatory projections reach the lateral nucleus from the ventral posterior medial nucleus (i.e., pars medialis). Other thalamic projections to the amygdala originate in the midline, intralaminar, and the medial pulvinar nuclei.

Chapter 17 / The Limbic System

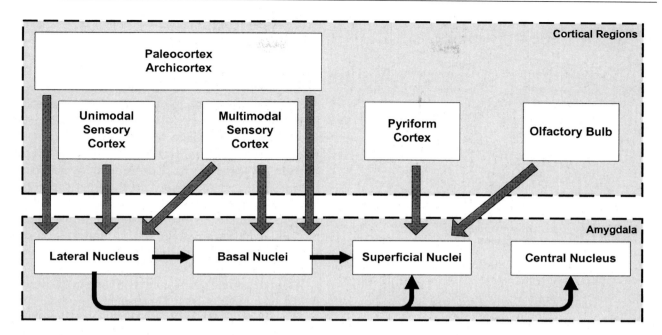

Fig. 10. The primary cortical inputs to the amygdala are shown by *thick gray arrows*, and the main intrinsic connections of the amygdala are shown by *black arrows*.

The *hypothalamus* sends a moderately dense projection to the amygdala, which reciprocates the amygdalohypothalamic projections. The most prominent projections originate in the ventromedial and lateral hypothalamic nuclei and terminate in the deep nuclei of the amygdala.

A significant cholinergic projection to the amygdala originates from the magnocellular neurons of the basal forebrain. Specifically, the nucleus basalis of Meynert and the horizontal and vertical limbs of the diagonal band of Broca project to the deep and superficial nuclei, and the substantia innominata projects to the central amygdaloid nucleus. Brainstem projections to the amygdala arise in the parabrachial nucleus (to the central nucleus), the pedunculopontine nucleus, the ventral tegmental area of Tsai (i.e., dopaminergic), the subcoeruleus (i.e., noradrenergic), the locus coeruleus (i.e., noradrenergic).

2.6.2. Intrinsic Connections

The intrinsic connections of the amygdala have been difficult to resolve with precision because of the small, irregular size of many amygdaloid nuclei and the fact that many axons pass through nuclei in which they do not terminate. Tracers placed in a nucleus could inadvertently label these axons. With the advent of several modern techniques that minimize these problems, the intrinsic circuitry of the amygdala has finally begun grudgingly to give way. The lateral nucleus, which receives the most direct sensory inputs, projects to all subdivisions of the amygdala. A connection that is of particular interest is the projection from the lateral nucleus to the basal nuclei, which are the main sources of the reciprocal projections to the sensory cortices. The basal nuclei project to all other amygdaloid nuclei except the lateral amygdaloid nucleus. The central and superficial nuclei have many intraamygdaloid connections, but few of these projections are to the deep nuclei. These connections suggest that processing through the amygdala occurs primarily in series (Fig. 10).

2.6.3. Efferent Projections

The amygdala projects directly to many cortical areas. Both the entorhinal cortex and the subicular cortex receive a substantial projection from the amygdala. Evidence suggests that some of these efferents may terminate on the distal dendrites of the hippocampus proper. The basal amygdaloid nuclei project densely to several areas of the unimodal sen-

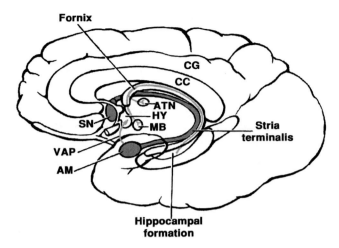

Fig. 11. This figure depicts the three major fiber bundles related to the limbic system. The first two carry the primary output axons from the amygdala (AMY) and include the stria terminalis and the ventral amygdalofugal pathway (VAP). The other major fiber bundle, the fornix, connects the hippocampal formation to subcortical and diencephalic sites. ATN, anterior thalamic nuclei; CC, corpus callosum; CG, cingulate gyrus, HY, hypothalamus; MB, mammillary bodies; NBF, basal forebrain including nuclei accumbens, diagonal band of Broca, and nucleus basalis; SN, septal nuclei.

sory cortex that project primarily to the lateral nucleus of the amygdala (Fig. 10). The amygdala projects to many polysensory regions of the cortex, and many of these projections arise from the lateral nucleus. Within the temporal lobe, the rostral one-third of the temporal cortex receives the most dense amygdaloid projections, but most of the temporal lobe and much of the occipital lobe are innervated to some extent. The amygdala also projects densely to the anterior cingulate cortex (e.g., areas 23–25, and 32) and the frontal and insular cortices.

Two major fiber tracts connect the amygdala with the diencephalon and brainstem (Fig. 11). The *stria terminalis* is the more obvious of the two, since it arches along medial to the entire extent of the body and tail of the caudate nucleus and descends lateral to the fornix at the level of the anterior commissure. Most axons in the stria terminalis terminate in the bed nucleus of the stria terminalis, which is located dorsal to the anterior commissure. This nucleus, which is considered by some to be a rostral extension of the amygdala, has dense projections to the hypothalamus and brainstem. Axons in the postcommissural stria terminalis project to the anterior hypothalamus, and some of these axons likely course further caudally to the brainstem through the medial forebrain bundle.

Other fibers terminate in the preoptic region, in the cell-poor region surrounding the VMN (i.e., these axons derive from the amygdalohippocampal area) and the core of the ventromedial hypothalamic nucleus (i.e., from the medial nucleus of the amygdala).

The *ventral amygdalofugal tract* provides a second pathway for amygdaloid axons that are destined for subcortical, diencephalic, and brainstem areas. This projection passes rostrally from the amygdala, courses beneath the lenticular nucleus through the substantia innominata, and terminates in the lateral preoptic nucleus and the lateral hypothalamic area. Caudal to the hypothalamus, axons from the central nucleus of the amygdala terminate in several brainstem nuclei (Fig. 12). A few axons appear to continue into the cervical spinal cord.

Amygdalofugal fibers also terminate in the medial dorsal thalamic nucleus. These axons originate from most areas of the amygdala (the medial and the central nuclei appear to be exceptions), but especially from the deep nuclei and the periamygdaloid cortex. There is also a reciprocal connection to the midline thalamic nuclei, primarily from the central and medial amygdaloid nuclei. The central and basal amygdaloid nuclei have a reciprocal connection with the basal forebrain. One of the most dense amygdalofugal projections is that from the basal nuclei to the striatum, although much of this terminates in the "limbic" striatum (i.e., the nucleus accumbens) there is a substantial projection to the ventromedial caudate and putamen.

3. FUNCTIONAL CONSIDERATIONS

3.1. The Limbic System Is Involved in Affective Behavior

A major insight into the neurological mechanisms controlling affective state (i.e., personality, emotion and social behavior) was Papez's 1937 paper in which he proposed that the "limbic lobe" of the cortex formed an anatomic circuit that coordinates emotion. Although this paper was very speculative and lacked rigorous experimental support, it quickly gained considerable acceptance, partially because of the dominant trend in psychology and psychiatry at that time. Freudian psychoanalytic theory readily welcomed the idea that the old and ancient parts of the brain were responsible for emotional and instinctive behavior, and that phylogenetically newer areas of the brain, such as the neocortex, were primarily attentive to conscious tasks and controlled behavior.

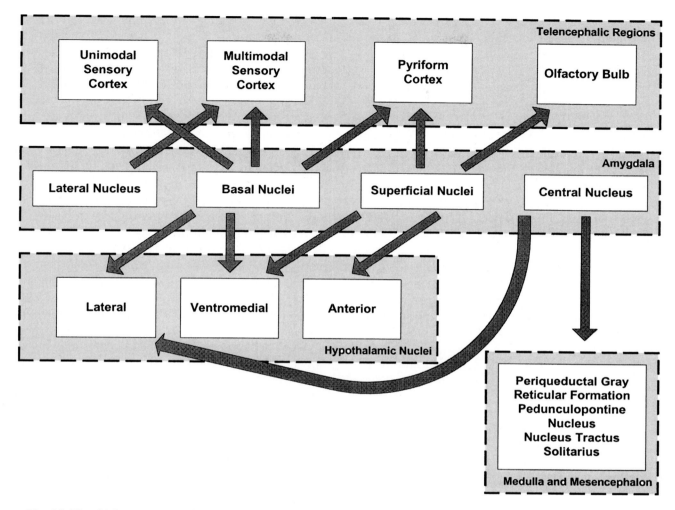

Fig. 12. The *thick gray arrows* show the major telencephalic, hypothalamic, and brainstem connections of the amygdala.

In a study published in 1939, Klüver and Bucy reported that bilateral temporal lobectomy in monkeys produced dramatic behavioral changes, most of which could be defined as affective disorders. The Klüver-Bucy syndrome was characterized by a markedly increased sexual activity that was often inappropriate (i.e., monkeys mounting other species or chairs), a loss of fear and a resulting flattening of emotions, an enormous increase in oral behavior (i.e., the animals that would put almost anything in their mouth), and indiscriminate dietary behavior. Subsequent studies have demonstrated that damage to the amygdala causes the sexual, appetitive, and affective dysfunctions in these animals. The visual and memory losses that Klüver and Bucy reported in their original primate experiments appear to be the result of collateral damage to other areas of the temporal cortex. The Klüver-Bucy

syndrome has been shown to occur in humans who have selective damage to the amygdala.

At around the time that Klüver and Bucy demonstrated the effects of amygdalectomy on emotional behavior, Jacobson reported on his neurosurgical studies in chimpanzees. In his presentation, he parenthetically alluded to the calming effect of a prefrontal lesion on the behavior of one particularly neurotic female chimp. This led Egas Moniz, the young Portuguese neuropsychiatrist, to return home immediately and begin treating severe mental disorders using prefrontal lobotomy. Moniz launched modern psychosurgery, for which he was awarded the 1949 Nobel Prize in Physiology and Medicine.

From the 1940s to the 1970s, many clinicians carried out psychosurgery on various limbic regions, especially the amygdala, the cingulate, and the prefrontal cortices. For a time, these lesion techniques became the method of choice to relieve severe emotional disorders. However, except for the study of Klüver and Bucy and the work of a few other behaviorists, the method lacked an empiric basis until the late 1960s, when critical animal experiments on the connections and functions of these areas were undertaken.

Whereas the questionable effectiveness of psychosurgery as a treatment for psychiatric diseases has considerably dampened enthusiasm for the treatment, studies of patients who received these surgical interventions and the experimental literature in this field have demonstrated that the circuit of Papez is not a major contributor to emotional control. The areas not included by Papez in his circuit (i.e., the amygdala, medial dorsal thalamic nucleus, and anterior hypothalamus) or that he believed were peripheral contributors to the circuit (i.e., the prefrontal cortex and rostral cingulate cortex) appear to play a major role in emotional control and the conscious perception of emotional experience.

Disorders in the limbic cortex have been linked to several psychiatric diseases, (i.e., *autism* and *schizophrenia*). Autistic children display abnormalities in temporal-lobe electroencephalographic patterns, and an enlargement of the temporal horn of the lateral ventricles along with some Klüver-Bucy-type affective disorders. In monkeys, lesions of the temporal lobe can mimic the behavioral signs of autism, but this only occurs if the lesions are made very early in the monkey's life. The linkage between schizophrenia and limbic-system dysfunction is suggested by several clinical and pathologic studies. The frontal and temporal cortices appear to be somewhat smaller in schizophrenic patients, and pyramidal neurons in the CA fields of the hippocampus are often abnormally oriented in these patients. In schizophrenic patients, there appear to be several imbalances in neurotransmitters that are selective for the limbic system. Most prominent among these is the dopamine system, which has a particularly dense projection to anterior limbic-system regions. Many effective therapies for schizophrenia target the dopamine system. In schizophrenics, the areas of the limbic system that receive a dense dopamine projection display selective imbalances, including decreased glucose uptake. Lesions of the cingulate cortex can result in akinetic mutism.

3.2. The Limbic System Contributes to Normal Learning and Memory

Although the relationship between emotional dysfunction and the limbic system appears to primarily involve the amygdala and anterior cingulate cortex, learning and memory deficits that accompany affective disorders seem to be the product of damage to more caudal limbic regions, especially the hippocampal formation and the posterior cingulate and retrosplenial cortices.

Before discussing the relationship between the limbic system and learning and memory, it is useful to clarify certain terms that define memory. Memory can be divided into *short-term memory*, which endures for a very brief time, and *long-term memory*, which is retained long after the conscious perception and consideration of an event. Long-term memories are further divided into *declarative memory*, which refers to the memory of facts that can be recalled to consciousness, and *procedural memory*, which refers to patterns of behavior that are learned (i.e., motor skills and procedural skills). The limbic system appears to be primarily involved in the transfer of declarative memory from short-term to long-term.

Much of our early understanding of the relationship between learning and memory and the limbic system came from studies of patients with damage to the brain. At the turn of the 19th century, Bekhterev suggested that damage to the temporal lobe was related to severe memory impairments in one of his patients, but it was not until the late 1950s that the relationship was widely accepted. In 1953, William Scoville operated on a patient who presented with intractable, severe, and generalized epileptic seizures. The bilateral temporal-lobe resection was a successful treatment for the epilepsy, but it left the patient with a severe anterograde memory deficit (i.e., he was unable to convert short-term to long-term memory). The patient displayed very little retrograde memory deficit (i.e., he was able to recall events that occurred prior to his operation). During the subsequent half century, this patient (designated HM) has been studied intensively. An example of HM's dysfunctional state comes from the detailed 1968 report of Milner and colleagues, in which HM failed to recall almost any event that occurred after his surgery, even very traumatic events such as the death of his father. Only those events that were continuously repeated were remembered and these were remembered only vaguely. For instance, when riding home with Dr. Milner in 1966, HM was asked to provide directions to his new home, in which he had lived for over 8 yr. Instead, he led Dr. Milner to the house he lived in before his surgery. He recognized this was not the correct location, but he could not provide any directions to the new home. In contrast to his obvious deficit in declarative memory, HM is quite accomplished in tasks requiring procedural learning skills, such as the mirror-draw task in which he displays normal memory. The case of HM (and similar cases) demonstrates the importance of the temporal lobe in declarative memory, and they show that there is a dissociation between the areas of the brain that subserve declarative compared to procedural memory.

Deficits in many other patients have confirmed the role of the posterior limbic cortex in mnemonic tasks, but patient RB provides the clearest clinical picture of the relationship because rigorous testing of this patient has been followed by clear histological findings. While undergoing coronary bypass surgery, RB had a transient ischemic episode, after which he displayed severe anterograde amnesia but no significant retrograde amnesia. His memory of past events appeared somewhat improved compared to normal subjects. Postmortem examination five years after the ischemic episode revealed a very selective bilateral lesion of the CA_1 fields of the hippocampus, and no apparent damage to any other limbic region of the brain (Zola-Morgan et al., 1986). Remarkably, the severe deterioration of declarative memory ability in RB was not accompanied by any apparent alteration in emotion or cognitive function.

Animal studies have supported the role of the hippocampus and posterior limbic cortex in mnemonic tasks. In monkeys, damage to the hippocampal formation impairs memory but has little effect on emotional behavior. In contrast, selective damage to the amygdala causes affective alterations but few or no alterations in learning and memory.

Several other areas of the limbic cortex also appear to contribute to learning and memory. As would be expected from the connections, damage to the subicular and entorhinal cortices affects learning and memory. The retrosplenial cortex, with which the hippocampal formation is highly interconnected, has been shown to participate in learning and memory. Animal studies suggest that the retrosplenial cortex contains areas that are involved in mapping out spatial relations, and lesion of this region in rat cause a significant decline in learning. Valenstein reported a case in which severe anterograde memory impairment was present in a patient with very selective neurologic damage that was confined to the retrosplenial cortex. Animal studies suggest that the cingulate cortex, like the retrosplenial cortex, may play a role in learning and memory. Damage to the cingulate cortex causes a decrease in learning ability in monkeys, but these deficits may relate more closely to an inability of the animal to correctly weight the importance of events.

Two subcortical limbic regions should be mentioned in relation to learning and memory. Some patients with relatively selective vascular lesions of the basal forebrain and patients with *Alzheimer's disease* display dementia and loss of the cholinergic projection to the limbic cortex. Animal studies suggest that selective lesions of the basal forebrain projection to the limbic cortex reduce learning and memory abilities, and reestablishing this pathway by means of transplantation of embryonic basal forebrain tissue ameliorates the lesion-induced deficits. These data suggest that the basal forebrain projection to the limbic system is a contributor to learning and memory.

The diencephalon appears to play a role in learning and memory. In 1887, Korsakoff characterized a syndrome in which a severe loss of memory was present in chronic alcoholics. Patients with *Korsakoff's syndrome* display anterograde amnesia, especially for paired-association tasks, extensive retrograde amnesia for events that occurred throughout their adult life, confabulation (i.e., making up stories that are relatively plausible, to attempt to cover up their memory impairments), reduced frequency of speech, little perception of their memory loss, and generalized apathy. The cause of Korsakoff's syndrome in many patients appears to be a lack of dietary thiamine (i.e., vitamin B_1) which is caused by the malnutrition that accompanies the long drinking bouts characteristic of chronic alcoholics. The syndrome consists of variable damage, primarily to the medial dorsal nucleus of the thalamus, the frontal cerebral cortex, and the mammillary bodies, and their connecting fiber tracts. The pivotal position of the mammillary bodies in the posterior limbic circuitry suggests that this damage is critical to Korsakoff's syndrome, but the anatomical mechanisms underlying the disease remain unresolved. The severe retrograde amnesia and affective disorders in Korsakoff's syndrome are not observed in amnesic patients with primary temporal-lobe dysfunction. Although amnesia and Korsakoff's syndrome involve memory deficits that are related to limbic-cortex dysfunction, the two diseases have different neuropathologic and functional attributes.

3.3. The Hippocampal Formation Plays a Role in Epilepsy

The hypothesized relationship between hippocampal formation damage and epileptic seizures dates to the early nineteenth century, and by 1880 Sommer had clearly identified an area of the hippocampus proper (*Sommer's sector* or area CA_1) which was consistently damaged in the epileptic patients he studied. Several

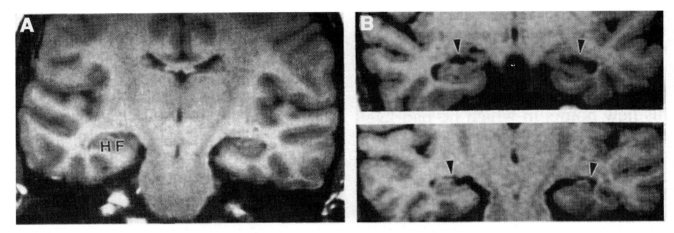

Fig. 13. A magnetic resonance imaging (MRI) coronal section through the temporal lobes of a normal adult (**A**) and an adult with severe, long-standing epilepsy (**B**). Note the marked bilateral atrophy of the hippocampus (*arrowheads*) in the epileptic patient (**B**).

subsequent reports have supported the idea that, in patients with temporal-lobe epilepsy, the epileptogenic focus is often in the hippocampus proper, and that limited resection of the hippocampal focus can eliminate subsequent seizure activity. In many patients, analysis of the degree of hippocampal sclerosis (Fig. 13) compared to the frequency and severity of epileptic activity suggests that the damage to the hippocampus was present before the initial epileptic activity.

The pyramidal neurons (especially in field CA_3) in the hippocampus are contributors to the initiation of epileptic seizure activity, and are damaged by recurring seizures. This pattern occurs in children and adults, and could create enlarged sclerotic foci that would increase the probability and or intensity of additional seizure activity.

3.4. Limbic-System Abnormalities Are Present in Alzheimer's Disease

In the normal course of aging, some neurons in the limbic cortex degenerate, potentially compromising limbic memory circuits. In contrast, persons with Alzheimer's disease display extensive neuronal damage (i.e., neurofibrillary tangles and β-amyloid plaques) and cell loss, especially in limbic and olfactory cortical regions. The entorhinal cortices are among the first and most severely affected cortical areas. Within the hippocampal formation, area CA_1 and the subicular cortices are the most severely affected. Damage to neurons in the subiculum would significantly affect the major outputs of the hippocampal formation, i.e., the fornix projection to septal and

diencephalic nuclei, and the innervation of entorhinal cortex. The prominent damage to the layer II pyramidal neurons of the entorhinal cortex compromises the entorhinal cortex input to the hippocampus. Together, these lesions isolate the hippocampal formation, and thus presumably produce the short-term memory impairments that are characteristic of Alzheimer's disease.

Damage to other limbic areas probably contributes to many of the affective changes in Alzheimer's patients. The olfactory regions of telencephalon, the amygdala, the cingulate cortex, and the hypothalamus are consistently compromised in Alzheimer's patients, and each of these areas plays an important role in the regulation of emotional stability. The cholinergic neurons in the diagonal band of Broca and nucleus basalis of Meynert are damaged (shrunken) in Alzheimer's disease, thereby significantly reducing the cholinergic input to the (limbic) cortex.

The pathogenesis of Alzheimer's disease is discussed in detail in Chapter 16.

3.5. The Hippocampus as a Model System Has Provided Important Insights into the Function of the Cerebral Cortex

The relative simplicity of the limbic cortex, and especially the hippocampus, has made it a useful model system for investigating several types of neuronal plasticity. Many studies have investigated the ability of axons to reinnervate areas of the hippocampus that have been denervated. Together these studies have shown that the hippocampus displays a high degree of active reorganization, an attribute that may account for its central role in learning and memory and its contribution to epilepsy.

At the synaptic and molecular level, the hippocampal system has been the major model in which *long-term potentiation* (LTP) has been studied. LTP is a long-term (i.e., 15 min to several days) increase in the efficiency of synaptic transmission that can be induced by a short-term high-frequency stimulation. This phenomenon was first identified in the projection from the entorhinal cortex to dentate gyrus granule cells, and was subsequently demonstrated in many other areas of the nervous system. Many researchers believe that LTP-like phenomena may underlie memory consolidation and storage in the brain.

4. LIMBIC-SYSTEM OVERVIEW

The limbic system is a highly interconnected group of regions that receive diverse multimodal sensory information. The anterior portions of the system (i.e., the amygdala and the anterior cingulate cortex) primarily regulate affective behavior and visceromotor function, and the posterior portions (i.e., the hippocampal formation and retrosplenial cortex) are predominantly involved in the temporary storage of information, including the encoding of spatial relations. In contrast to this diversity, the limbic cortical areas are highly interconnected, and have prominent connections with limbic subcortical, diencephalic, and brainstem nuclei, suggesting that these areas are functionally interrelated. Emotional states can significantly influence learning and memory, and the inverse is also true (i.e., elements of learning and memory such as habituation and orientation can significantly alter emotional states and arousal). Riding the wave of the rapidly progressing neurobiological techniques, future studies should quickly begin to illuminate the unity and diversity of the limbic system.

SELECTED READINGS

Aggleton JP. The Amygdala: Neurobiological Aspects of Emotion, Memory, and Mental Dysfunction. New York: Wiley-Liss, 1992.

Broca P. Anatomie comparée des circonvolutions cérébrales. Le grand lobe limbique et la scissure limbique dans la série des mammifères. Rev Anthrop 1978; 2:285–498.

Chan-Palay V, Köhler C. The Hippocampus. Neurology and Neurobiology, vol. 52, New York: Alan R. Liss, 1989.

Isaacson RL. The Limbic System, 2nd ed. New York: Plenum Press, 1982.

Klüver H, Bucy PC. Preliminary analysis of function of the temporal lobes in monkeys. Arch Neurol Psychiatry 1939; 42:979–1000.

Kolb B, Whishaw IO. Fundamentals of Human Neuropsychology, 4th ed. New York: W.H. Freeman and Company, 1996; 110–140.

Lopes Da Silva F, Witter MP, Boeijinga PH, Lohman A. Anatomical organization and physiology of the limbic cortex. Physiol Rev 1990; 70:453–511.

MacLean PD. Psychosomatic disease and the "visceral brain": Recent developments bearing on the Papez theory of emotion. Psychsom Med 1949; 11:338–353.

MacLean PD. Some psychiatric implications of physiological studies on the frontotemporal portion of the limbic system (visceral brain). Electroencephalogr Clin Neurophysiol 1952; 4:407–418.

Papez JW. A proposed mechanism of emotion. Arch Neurol Psychiatry 1937; 38:724–744.

Scoville WB, Milner B. Loss of recent memory after bilateral hippocampal lesions. J Neurol Neurosurg Psych 1957; 20:11–21.

Valenstein ES, Bowers D, Verfaellie M, Heilman KM, Day A, Watson RT. Retrosplenial Amnesia. Brain 1987; 110: 1631–1646.

Valenstein ES. Brain Control: A critical examination of brain stimulation and psychosurgery. New York: John Wiley & Sons, 1973.

Van Hoesen G, Rosene DL. The hippocampal formation of the primate brain: A review of some comparative aspects of cytoarchitecture and connections. Cereb Cortex 1987; 6: 345–456.

Vogt BA, Gabriel M. The neurobiology of cingulate cortex and limbic thalamus. New York: Springer-Verlag, 1992.

Zola-Morgan S, Squire LR, Amaral DG. Human amnesia and the medial temporal region: Enduring memory impairment following a bilateral lesion limited to field CA1 of the hippocampus. J Neurosci 1986; 6:2950–2967.

18 The Basal Ganglia

Marie-Francoise Chesselet

CONTENTS

1. INTRODUCTION

1.1. Definition

The basal ganglia comprise subcortical regions of the brain that are involved in both motor and cognitive functions. The definition of the basal ganglia has evolved over the years as functional relationships between regions that were previously believed to be unrelated began to emerge. Classically, the "basal ganglia" included the caudate-putamen, the pallidum, and the amygdala. In the human brain, the caudate nucleus and putamen are separated by the internal capsule and have a characteristic "striated" appearance caused by the presence of bundles of myelinated fibers (pencils of Willis), hence the name "striatum." More modern definitions of the basal ganglia include the substantia nigra and subthalamic nucleus, which have close functional relationships with the striatum and the pallidum. The amygdala is now considered to be a separate functional entity, although it has anatomical connections with some regions of the basal ganglia.

From: *Neuroscience in Medicine, 2nd ed.* (P. Michael Conn, ed.),
© 2003 Humana Press Inc., Totowa, NJ.

1.2. Clinical Relevance

The existence of numerous motor disorders associated with loss of neurons in the basal ganglia has focused attention on the role of these regions in motor control. However, more recent work has emphasized the role of these regions in certain forms of memory and reward. Dysfunction of specific aspects of cognition is indeed often present in diseases of the basal ganglia. From the motor point of view, symptoms vary with the site of lesion, although a range of overlapping symptoms can be seen in different disorders that affect these regions. A common characteristic of movement disorders originating in the basal ganglia is the absence of muscle paralysis, a feature that differentiates them from defects resulting from cortical or spinal lesions. This has led to the concept of "extrapyramidal systems," comprised of the basal ganglia on the one hand and the cerebellum on the other. This concept is still used in the clinical setting, however modern physiology emphasizes the close relationships that exist between "pyramidal" and "extrapyramidal systems," and no longer considers them to be separate entities.

The best-characterized an most frequent disorder that is primarily the result of dysfunction in the basal ganglia is Parkinson's disease. Parkinson's disease is caused by the loss of pigmented neurons in the substantia nigra pars compacta that contain the neurotransmitter dopamine. Its cardinal signs include difficulty to initiate movements (akinesia), muscle rigidity, and tremor. Dystonia (a movement disorder caused by the co-contraction of opposing muscles) is often present in these patients. Dyskinesia, or abnormal involuntary movements, can appear as a result of the most common treatment for Parkinson's disease—the chronic administration of L-dopa, a dopamine precursor. Abnormal movements are a major symptom of Huntington's disease, hereditary disease caused by an expanded CAG repeat in the gene that encodes a protein called huntingtin. Through a mechanism that is still largely unknown, this mutation causes a progressive loss of neurons in the caudate nucleus and the putamen. Patients present dance-like abnormal movements (chorea), often evolving toward dystonia and akinetic states.

1.3. General Organization

Modern anatomical methods have led to the concept of a high degree of organization both within each region of the basal ganglia and within these regions. Current models of basal ganglia organization are centered around the striatum (caudate nucleus and putamen), which is considered the "receiving" region of the basal ganglia. Indeed, it receives massive, topographically organized inputs from the entire cerebral cortex as well as other inputs. The striatum in turn projects to two distinct regions that together form the pallidum: the external pallidum and the internal pallidum. These are anatomically and functionally very different: in contrast to the internal pallidum, the external pallidum projects mainly within the basal ganglia, specifically to the subthalamic nucleus and to both the internal pallidum and substantia nigra pars reticulata. These latter two regions are considered the "output structures" of the system because they mainly project outside the basal ganglia. Thus internal pallidum and substantia nigra are responsible for relying information processed by the striatum and the internal circuits of the basal ganglia to other brain regions, primarily the thalamus and the brainstem. Although this description overemphasizes some connections to the detriment of others and is an obvious simplification, it has had an enormous heuristic value for the design of working models of basal ganglia functions that integrate anatomical, cellular, molecular, and clinical data.

2. THE STRIATUM

The striatum is the largest component of the basal ganglia, and is considered a main processing station for information originating from outside the basal ganglia, particularly the cerebral cortex, the thalamus, and the brainstem. Anatomically, the striatum is divided into the caudate nucleus and the putamen, and also includes the nucleus accumbens. This ventral portion of the striatum is considered a component of the limbic system, and is not discussed here. The largest region of the striatum is the putamen. The caudate nucleus is medial to the putamen, and is separated from it by the internal capsule. It can be divided into three parts: the largest, the head, borders the lateral ventricle; the body is dorsal to the thalamus, and the tail is the narrower portion located posterior to the thalamus before proceeding ventrally in a caudo-rostral direction (Fig. 1). It is of interest to note that a distinct anatomical region is interposed between the head of the caudate nucleus and the lateral ventricle: the subventricular zone or, more accurately, the subependymal layer in adults. This region is distinguished by the presence of continuously dividing cells, even in adults. In rodents, it is well-established that these dividing cells migrate toward the olfactory bulb, where they differentiate into neurons. Their existence in primates, including humans, has recently been confirmed.

2.1. The Internal Organization of the Striatum

With classical histological methods, such as Nissl or hematoxylin-eosin (H&E) stains, the striatum appears to be a remarkably homogenous structure comprised of very similar neurons. This appearance is deceptive, as more refined techniques have revealed a high level of molecular diversity and a fine anatomical organization within the striatum. First, studies have revealed a macroscopic organization of the striatum in two compartments, the striosomes and the extrastriosomal matrix. These compartments are characterized by the presence of neurons with distinct birth dates, molecular properties and anatomical connections. This organization is reminiscent of the functional subdivisions of the cerebral and cerebellar cortices; however, the implications of these differences for the overall function of the basal ganglia remains largely unknown.

The anatomical relationships of the basal ganglia with other regions of the brain ("extrinsic connections") is described before the connections between

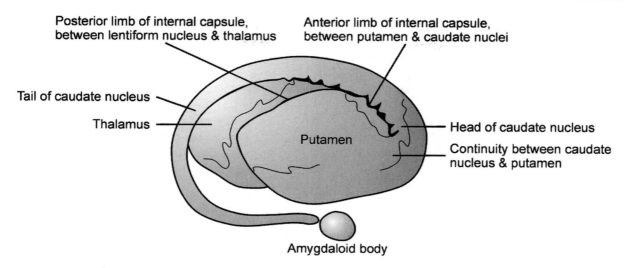

Fig. 1. Drawing of the putamen and caudate nucleus (striatum) indicating their close relationship with the thalamus, after removal of the internal capsule, which normally courses where indicated.

regions of the basal ganglia ("intrinsic connections"). This emphasizes the position of the basal ganglia in relation to other brain regions before addressing the anatomical substrate for information processing within the basal ganglia, which is likely to determine its functional role.

2.2. Extrinsic Inputs to the Striatum

As indicated in the introduction, this chapter focuses on inputs to the caudate-putamen, or its equivalent in rats, the dorsal part of the striatum. These regions are involved primarily in the control of movement.

2.2.1. THE CORTICOSTRIATAL INPUT

The cerebral cortex provides the major input to the striatum. This projection is excitatory, originating from all cortical regions except the primary auditory and visual cortices (Fig. 2). Importantly, this is a unidirectional projection: the striatum does not project back to the cortex directly. Therefore, cortical information received by the striatum must be processed by the striatum, as well as its projection areas, the pallidum and substantia nigra, before reaching back to the cortex by way of the thalamus. The fine organization of the corticostriatal projection has been examined in great detail over the years in many different species. Indeed, since the striatum is positioned between the cerebral cortex and the remainder of the basal ganglia, it is likely that the structural organization of this pathway provides insight into the type of computation performed by the striatum, and can help in the understanding of its function.

Two different types of organization of basal ganglia circuits have emerged from mapping studies. The maintenance of a clear topographical organization of inputs and outputs throughout the basal ganglia suggests that information originating from different regions of the cerebral cortex—for example, from limbic vs motor cortical regions—is processed in parallel. However, a comparison of the large number of corticostriatal vs the much smaller number of striatal and pallidal output neuron indicates that convergence must also exist within this system. Thus, it is likely that these two forms of organization are superimposed throughout the basal ganglia. Indeed, corticostriatal neuron projections follow a mediolateral organization so that the more medial cingulate cortex projects to the caudate nucleus, whereas the more lateral motor cortex projects primarily to the putamen. However, corticostriatal neurons form each cortical region do not project uniformly onto striatal neurons. Projections from any given cortical area form synapses with distributed clusters of striatal neurons. In turn, clusters of striatal neurons receive multiple projections form various cortical areas. In some cases, these converging inputs originate from either anatomically connected or functionally related cortical areas—for example, motor and sensory regions linked to the same part of the body. The organization of the corticostriatal pathway also follows the distinction between striosomes and matrix outlined earlier in a highly organized manner, too complex to be described here in detail. Most corticostriatal inputs originate from neurons located in the deep part of layer III and the superficial part of

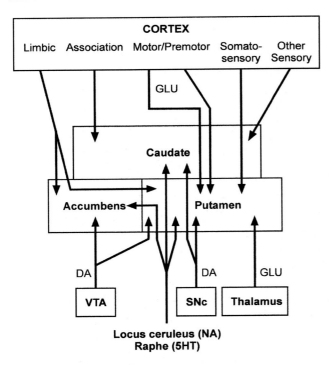

Fig. 2. Schematic representation of the main inputs to the striatum, indicating the topographical relationship between inputs to the striatum and the nucleus accumbens. 5-HT, serotonin; DA, dopamine; Glu, glutamate; NA, noradrenaline; SNc, substantia nigra pars compacta; VTA, ventral tegmental area.

layer V. A small portion of the corticostriatal pathway projects to the contralateral striatum, but the majority is ipsilateral.

The corticostriatal input uses the excitatory amino acid glutamate as a neurotransmitter, and projects onto all classes of striatal neurons. Medium-sized neurons with highly spinous dendrites (the medium-sized spiny neuron) form the largest majority (95%) of striatal neurons (Fig. 3). These neurons have axons that project outside the striatum (efferent neurons). They receive the bulk of cortical inputs, and these inputs form synapses on their dendritic spines. The striatum also contains much less numerous but functionally critical interneurons. These are either large (cholinergic) or medium-sized (GABAergic) cells with smooth dendrites (aspiny neurons). The large cholinergic interneurons are likely to correspond to the "tonically active neurons" or TAN that have been shown to play a critical role in motor learning in the striatum. GABAergic interneurons can be further divided into several classes based on their level of expression of GABA. Neurons with low GABA levels contain the neuropeptides somatostatin (SS) and neuropeptide Y (NPY),

and their role is poorly understood. In contrast, interneurons that express very high levels of GABA—and of its synthetic enzyme, glutamic acid decarboxylase—have been shown to play a critical role in the corticostriatal circuitry. Indeed, these neurons have a high rate of firing—they are driven by cortical inputs to their soma, and synapse onto the medium-sized spiny projection neurons that they inhibit. Therefore, they mediate the feed-forward inhibition of striatal projection neurons by the cortex.

2.2.2. THALAMOSTRIATAL INPUTS

The second largest input to the striatum, also glutamatergic, originates in the thalamus. The bulk of this projection originates from the diffusely projecting thalamic nuclei, a property that distinguishes them from the "specific" motor and sensory relays. The most massive projections originate from the centromedian nucleus, which projects preferentially to the putamen and from the parafascicular nucleus, which projects to the caudate nucleus. The striatum also receives moderate inputs from thalamic motor nuclei. Some of the thalamic regions that project to the striatum also receive inputs from the substantia nigra, suggesting that they represent a site of convergence of projections to and from the basal ganglia.

Like corticostriatal inputs, thalamic projections innervate medium-sized spiny neurons, and their organization respects the compartmental boundaries between striosomes and matrix, with projections from intralaminar nuclei (centromedian and parafascicular nuclei) preferentially innervating the matrix, and neurons from midline nuclei preferentially innervating the striosomes.

2.2.3. OTHER STRIATAL INPUTS

In addition to glutamatergic inputs from the cortex and the thalamus, the striatum receives an important projection from the substantia nigra pars compacta. These nigrostriatal neurons are dopaminergic, and have been the focus of extensive studies because it was discovered in the early 1960s that their loss was a hallmark of Parkinson's disease. More minor projections to the striatum originate in the amygdala—specifically, the basolateral nucleus, the dorsal raphe, which sends a dense serotonergic innervation particularly to the ventral part of the striatum, the external pallidum (GABAergic), and the subthalamic nucleus (glutamatergic). Interestingly, the GABAergic projection from the external pallidum, long neglected, seems to project specifically to the rapidly-firing

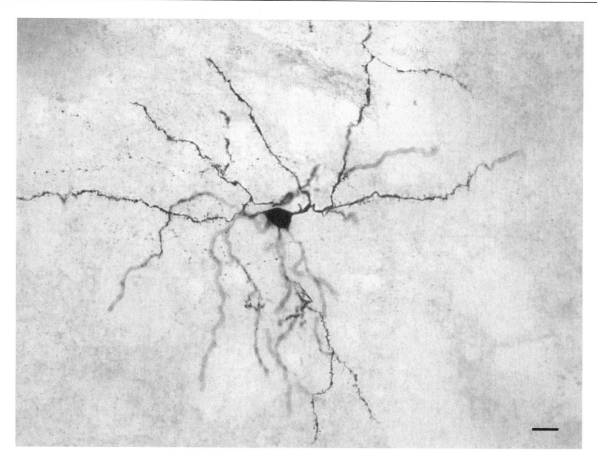

Fig. 3. Photomicrograph of a biocytin-filled medium-sized spiny neuron in the striatum. This type of neuron represents the majority of striatal neurons, and projects outside the striatum. It receives cortical and thalamic excitatory inputs on the head of its dendritic spines. Scale bar: 10 μm. (Courtesy of Dr Michael Levine, UCLA.)

GABAergic interneurons of the striatum. In contrast to glutamatergic inputs, GABAergic and dopaminergic inputs terminate preferentially on the neck of spines and dendritic shafts, suggesting that these inputs can interfere with the effect of cortical and thalamic excitatory inputs at the level of individual neurons.

3. OTHER BASAL GANGLIA NUCLEI

3.1. Extrinsic Inputs to the Globus Pallidus, Substantia Nigra, and Subthalamic Nucleus

Whereas it is conceptually useful to center a study of the basal ganglia around the striatum as the main receiving area of the basal ganglia, connections to other regions should not be overlooked. Most importantly, the subthalamic nucleus and substantia nigra, and to a lesser extent the external pallidum, receive inputs from the cerebral cortex. All basal ganglia regions also receive inputs from the tegmentopedun-culopontine nucleus, a region of the reticular formation (RF) that has emerged as a critical player in several movement disorders of the basal ganglia, including Parkinson's disease. Finally, they receive a diffuse serotonergic projection from the dorsal raphe, which is particularly abundant in the external pallidum.

Inputs to the substantia nigra pars compacta should be considered separately because of the critical role of this pathway in basal ganglia function, as indicated by the profound effect of its loss in Parkinson's disease. Inputs from regions outside the basal ganglia to the substantia nigra pars compacta originate in the cerebral cortex, the central nucleus of the amygdala, the tegmentopedunculopontine nucleus, the dorsal raphe, and importantly, the nucleus accumbens. This region is often considered part of the striatum, but differs from the dorsal striatum by its connections with limbic structures, such as the cingulate cortex, the hippocampus, and the ventral tegmental area. The projection

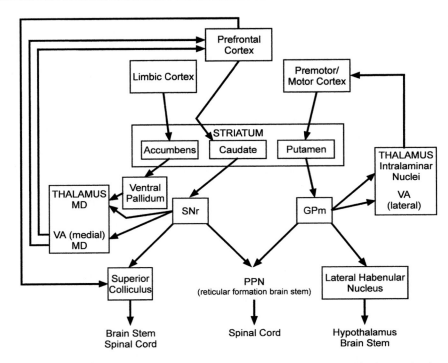

Fig. 4. General organization of output pathways from the striatum, showing the topographical organization of outputs from the striatum and nucleus accumbens. MD, mediodorsal nucleus; GPm, globus pallidus, medial (or internal) segment; PPN, pedunculopontine nucleus; SNr, substantia nigra pars reticulata; VA, ventroanterior nucleus.

from the nucleus accumbens to the substantia nigra pars compacta may represent an important functional link between the limbic system, which is primarily involved in emotional behaviors, and the motor system.

3.2. Outputs from the Pallidum and Substantia Nigra Pars Reticulata

The internal segment of the pallidum (entopeduncular nucleus in rats) and the substantia nigra pars reticulata are the only regions of the basal ganglia to send prominent projections outside the basal ganglia. Their main targets are the motor nuclei of the thalamus, which in turn project to the cerebral cortex. The major output of the internal pallidum forms distinct fiber bundles: a compact fiber bundle that travels around the internal capsule, the ansa lenticularis, and small facsicles that cross the internal capsule to form the lenticular facsiculus above the subthalamic nucleus. Both facsicles combine rostrally before entering the lateral aspect of the ventroanterior nucleus of the thalamus. Pallidal efferents are primarily involved in the control of limb movements. Nigral-output neurons reach the thalamus through diffuse fibers. They project more medially that the pallidum into the ventrolateral

nucleus, and also innervate the mediodorsal nucleus. Nigral ouputs are primarily involved in the control of orofacial, eye, head, and neck movements.

Parallel circuits are maintained in the pallidothalamic and thalamocortical pathways. The substantia nigra pars reticulata projects to regions of the thalamic motor nuclei, adjacent to but distinct from those innervated by the internal pallidum (Fig. 4). In addition, it projects to the paralamellar part of the mediodorsal nucleus, an area that projects to regions of the frontal cortex that are involved in the control of eye movements. Another common projection is the tegmentopedunculopontine region of the RF. Although similar in many respects, the external pallidum and substantia nigra differ in the detail of their inputs and output pathways. Most notably, the substantia nigra pars reticulata also projects to the deep layers of the superior colliculus, a region of the brainstem involved in the control of eye movements. This explains the high frequency of alteration in eye movements in disorders of the basal ganglia. All output neurons of the basal ganglia are GABA-ergic.

Recent studies have shown that, at least in rats, individual nigral neurons project to several of these targets, and their combination depends on the position of the neurons within the substantia nigra. Finally, the substantia nigra pars reticulata, but not the internal pallidum, projects to the reticular nucleus of the thalamus, a group of GABAergic neurons that surround the body of the thalamus, control corticothalamic and thalamocortical connections, and play a role in attention and sleep. Dysfunction of this pathway may contribute to the cognitive deficits and sleep disorders that are frequently observed in patients with basal ganglia lesions. Although generally considered an internal component of basal ganglia circuitry, the external pallidum also projects to the reticular nucleus of the thalamus (Fig. 5).

4. INTRINSIC CONNECTIONS WITHIN THE BASAL GANGLIA

4.1. The Nigrostriatal Pathway

The substantia nigra pars compacta is not homogenous. Neurons in its dorsal tier contain the calcium-binding protein calbindin, which is absent from neurons in its venral tier. These neurochemical distinctions may be related to the greater vulnerability of ventral dopaminergic neurons in Parkinson's disease and provide some clues to the pathophysiology of Parkinson's disease. Like other pathways in the basal ganglia, the nigrostriatal dopaminergic pathway is organized topographically, with the medial and lateral substantia nigra projecting to the medial and lateral striatum, respectively.

Nigrostriatal dopaminergic terminals can be visualized in vivo with positron emission tomography (PET) with labeled fluoro-dopa, a precursor of dopamine. This method allows the researcher to follow the loss of dopaminergic terminals in patients with Parkinson's disease. In addition to the striatum, where dopaminergic nerve terminals normally form a dense network, the nigrostriatal dopaminergic pathway also projects—probably through collaterals—to the pallidum and subthalamic nucleus. Furthermore, dendrites of the nigrostriatal pathway release dopamine within the substantia nigra pars reticulata. All these regions contain dopaminergic receptors, suggesting that the direct effects of dopamine in the basal ganglia are not limited to the striatum.

Connections among regions of the basal ganglia are numerous, which has led to the consideration of and have led to a series of reverberating "loops." A more modern view, is to consider how the flow of information travels from the striatum to the output regions of

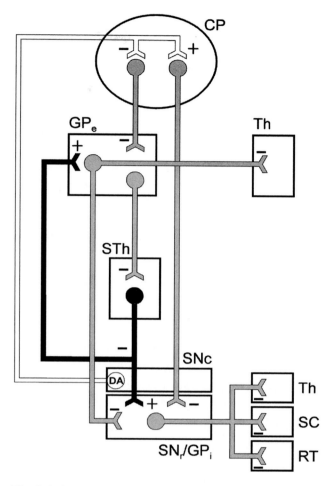

Fig. 5. Schematic representation of the basic intrinsic organization of basal ganglia circuits and their main projections. Gray pathways are GABAergic (inhibitory); dark pathways are glutamtergic (excitatory); white pathway is dopaminergic. CP, caudate-putamen; DA, dopaminergic neurons; Gpe, globus pallidus, external segment; Gpi, globus pallidus, internal segment; RT, reticular formation; SC, superior colliculus; SNc, substantia nigra pars compacta; SNr, substantia nigra pars reticulata; STh, subthalamic nucleus; Th, thalamus.

the basal ganglia, the internal pallidum, and the substantia nigra pars reticulata.

4.2. Striatal Efferent Pathways

A fundamental principle of this organization is that striatal outputs are largely segregated into two main pathways. A direct pathway that connects the striatum to the internal pallidum and substantia nigra pars reticulata and an indirect pathway that does this by way of two relays: the first in the external pallidum and the second in the subthalamic nucleus (Fig. 5). Accordingly, each output region of the basal ganglia receives a direct GABAergic input form the striatum and a glutamatergic input from the subthalamic nucleus. The external pallidum also projects directly to the internal pallidum and the substantia nigra, thus bypassing the subthalamic nucleus. This GABAergic projection exerts a powerful inhibitory effect on neurons of the internal pallidum and substantia nigra pars reticulata because it terminates on the proximal region of their dendrites.

As described previously, information processed through the indirect pathway is under the control of multiple afferents to the external pallidum and the subthalamic nucleus, and the latter includes a significant projection from the motor cortex. In addition, the flow of information is not unidirectional in this pathway. Indeed, the subthalamic nucleus sends a reciprocal glutamatergic projection to the external pallidum. Finally, the two systems (direct and indirect) are not independent. Indeed they are connected within the striatum, in particular by cholinergic neurons, and by collaterals from the direct striatal efferent neurons to the external pallidum.

4.3. Functional Organization of Intrinsic Connections in the Basal Ganglia

Based on anatomical studies, both parallel and convergent processing can occur in the basal ganglia. Experimental evidence in primates indicates that very few neurons have coordinate firing in the external pallidum; however, the proportion of coordinated units markedly increases in animals with a lesion of the nigrostriatal dopaminergic pathway. This suggests that parallel processing is necessary for normal movement, and is partially maintained by the neurotransmitter dopamine. Recent research has emphasized the relationship between neuronal activity in the basal ganglia and complex behavior, including rewards and memory.

In the normal brain, the GABAergic output structures of the basal ganglia (internal pallidum and substantia nigra pars reticulata) have a high level of activity, resulting in a tonic inhibition of their target neurons. The striatum normally has a low level of spontaneous activity. Activation of the striatum by cortical inputs leads to both a direct and an indirect (by way of the external pallidum and subthalamic nucleus) inhibition of the internal pallidum and substantia nigra pars reticulata, thus releasing their target cells from inhibition. This effect is transient because activation of the corticostriatal pathway also activates

GABAergic interneurons, which project onto striatal output neurons, thus inducing a secondary inhibition of striatal outputs.

Although the function of each nucleus in the basal ganglia is far from clear, a better understanding of the organization of striatal output pathways has led to a useful model of basal ganglia function that predicts how the loss of the nigrostriatal dopaminergic pathway leads to akinesia (e.g., difficulty to initiate movements) and bradykinesia (e.g., slowness of movements) in Parkinson's disease. This model is based on the observation that dopamine exerts opposite effects on the direct and indirect output pathways of the striatum (Fig. 5). Since the early 1980s, imaging studies in rats have shown that dopamine stimulates the direct and inhibits the indirect pathway. This was confirmed by studies of the distinct neuropeptides present in these neurons (subtsance P in the direct and enkephalin in the indirect pathway) (Fig. 6). By considering the fact that all intrinsic basal ganglia pathways except that originating from the subthalamic nucleus are GABAergic, it can be predicted that loss of dopamine will result in increased GABAergic output from the basal ganglia, leading to increased inhibition of thalamocortical pathways. Imaging studies in human patients have supported this theory. Furthermore, lesions of the internal pallidum or silencing of the subthalamic nucleus improve akinesia and bradykinesia in patients with Parkinson's disease.

Hyperkinetic movement disorders have proven more difficult to understand. One form of hyperkinesia is the chorea or dance-like movements characteristic of Huntington's disease. Huntington's disease is a hereditary disease caused by the expansion of a stretch of CAG repeats that encode glutamine in the protein huntingtin. Although the pathophysiology of the disease is not fully understood, current theories favor a toxic effect of the accumulation of the abnormal protein in the nucleus and/or cytoplasm, where it could bind essential molecules such as transcription factors. This leads to neuronal dysfunction and a progressive loss of neurons in the striatum and the cortex. However, the basis for this regional selectivity is not yet understood. Striatal neurons of the indirect pathway are affected first, leading to an imbalance between the direct and the indirect pathways, decreased activity in basal ganglia outputs, and chorea. Other hyperkinetic movement disorders include dystonia (co-contraction of opposing muscles), and various dyskinesia (involuntary movements) that can be

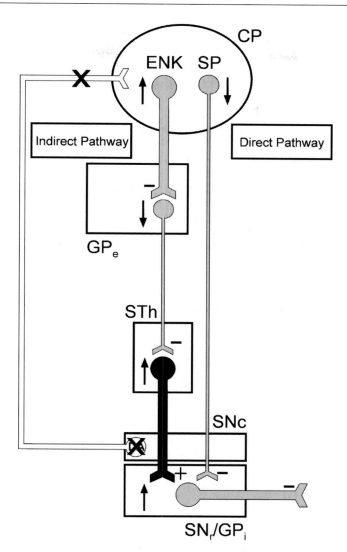

Fig. 6. Parkinson's disease: Schematic representation of the main changes in neuronal activity in intrinsic pathways and outputs of the basal ganglia. *See* Fig. 5 for color coding. Because dopamine exerts opposite effects on the two output pathways of the striatum (*see* Fig. 5), after the loss of the nigrostriatal dopaminergic neurons (*X*), firing increases in the direct output pathway from the striatum and decreases in the indirect pathway. Increased activity in the enkephalinergic-GABAergic pathway from the striatum to the GPe (*direct pathway*) increases inhibition of the Gpe-STh pathway, resulting in a decreased inhibition of the STh. Increased excitatory output from the STh, together with decreased activity in the inhibitory, substantce P-GABAergic direct pathway, result in an increased activity in the output neurons originating in the SNr and the Gpi. CP, caudate-putamen; ENK, enkephalinergic neurons; Gpe, globus pallidus, external segment; Gpi, globus pallidus, internal segment; SNc, substantia nigra pars compacta; SNr, substantia nigra pars reticulata; SP, substance P-containing neurons; STh, subthalamic nucleus.

the side effects of longterm L-dopa therapy for Parkinson's disease or of antipsychotic treatments. The pathophysiology of these disorders is poorly understood.

4.4. Therapeutic Implications

The overactivity of the subthalamic nucleus plays a critical role in the symptoms of Parkinson's disease.

Indeed, lesions of the subthalamic nucleus improve akinesia in primates that have a lesion of the nigrostriatal pathway. Simulation of the subthalamic nucleus at high frequency (deep brain stimulation) in patients with Parkinson's disease leads to a remarkable improvement in symptoms. By analogy with the effects of lesions, this effect is believed to result from an inhibition of hyperactivity of the subthalamic nucleus through depolarization block. This mechanism, however, remains controversial. In contrast to their beneficial effects shown in Parkinson's disease, lesions of the subthalamic nucleus in primates—including humans—with an intact dopaminergic system lead to large amplitude abnormal movements known as hemiballismus.

An alternative surgical approach to subthalamic stimulation is to lesion the internal pallidum, which, as a main target of the subthalamic nucleus, is also hyperactive in Parkinson's disease. Unexpectedly, both high-frequency stimulation of the subthalamic nucleus and lesions of the intrernal pallidum (commonly referred to as "pallidotomy") improve akinesia as well as dyskinesia, a frequent side effect of treatment with the dopamine precursor L-dopa, the most common treatment for Parkinson's disease. This effect highlights to the importance of abnormal firing patterns in the pathophysiology of movement disorders of the basal ganglia.

SELECTED READINGS

Chesselet M-F. Mapping the basal ganglia. In Toga AW, Mazziotta JC (eds). Brain Mapping: the Systems. Academic Press, 2000; 177–206.

DeLong MR. Primate models of movement disorders of basal ganglia origin. Trends Neurosci 1990; 13:281.

Graybiel AM. The basal ganglia and cognitive pattern generators. Schizophr Bull 1997; 23:459.

Middelton FA, Strick PL. Basal ganglia output and cognition: Evidence from anatomical , behavioral and clinical studies. Brain Cognition 2000; 42:183.

Olanow CW, Brin MF, Obeso JA. The role of deep brain stimulation as a surgical treatment for Parkinson's Disease. Neurology 2000; 55:S60.

Smith Y, Bevan MD, Shink E, Bolam JP. Micorcircuitry of the direct and indirect pathways of the basal ganglia. Neuroscience 1998; 86:353.

Disorders of the Basal Ganglia

Gregory Cooper and Robert L. Rodnitzky

The classic clinical syndromes that result from abnormalities of the basal ganglia are disorders of movement. These may take the form of excessive involuntary movements (i.e., hyperkinesia) or decreased movement (e.g., hypokinesia). Hypokinesias such as bradykinesia (e.g., slow movement) or akinesia (e.g., absence or difficult initiation of movement) are often seen in Parkinson's disease and a few conditions that mimic this disorder. There are several forms of hyperkinesias, and many different disease states that cause these symptoms. Among the most common forms of hyperkinesia are chorea, dystonia, tremor, and tics. The complex anatomic connections and physiologic associations of the basal ganglia often make it difficult to determine the anatomic locus of disease responsible for these abnormal patterns of movement. Similarly, with the exception of Parkinson's disease, the neurotransmitter aberrations responsible for many movement disorders are unknown, and are often defined only by the mode of action of the drugs used to treat them.

CHOREA

Chorea is an involuntary movement with a variety of causes. It is characterized by arrhythmic, rapid, involuntary movement that flows from one part of the body to another in nonstereotypic fashion. When chorea is severe, of high amplitude, and prominent in proximal parts of an extremity, it is referred to as ballism. There are many causes of chorea, including rheumatic fever, metabolic imbalance (e.g., hyperthyroidism), and the use of certain drugs (e.g., amphetamines, levodopa). The form associated with rheumatic fever is known as *Sydenbam's* chorea. One of the most common non-drug-related causes of chorea is

Huntington's disease, an autosomal dominant condition that invariably progresses to severe disability and death.

It has long been known that examination of the brains of patients with Huntington's disease at autopsy reveals remarkable gross atrophy of the head of caudate nucleus. Modern neuroimaging techniques such as computerized tomography or magnetic resonance imaging can demonstrate this finding during the patient's life. At the cellular level, the chorea of Huntington's disease has been related to a loss of striatal GABA-enkephalin neurons that are the origin of the indirect inhibitory pathway to the external segment of the globus pallidus (GPe). It is theorized that reduced inhibition of these pallidal cells leads to increased inhibition of the subthalamic nucleus (STN) by the GPe, in turn reducing the excitatory drive on neurons in the internal segment of the globus pallidus (GPi) from the STN. Decreased inhibitory output from the GPi to the thalamus results in increased cortical activation and chorea.

This explanation of the origin of chorea in Huntington's disease is consistent with the fact that the most severe and acute form of chorea, ballism, is usually associated with a direct lesion of the STN. The most common of these direct lesions is an infarction of the subthalamic nucleus, resulting in contralateral ballism or *hemiballism*.

In the chorea of Huntington's disease and the ballism of STN infarction, dopamine-blocking (e.g., haloperidol) or dopamine-depleting (e.g., reserpine) drugs are effective in reducing the abnormal movements, and dopaminergic drugs worsen them. Although dopaminergic cells are not the focus of pathology in either of these conditions, dopamine blockade is effective in reversing the chorea associated with them.

These drugs, by reducing the inhibitory effect of dopamine on striatal GABA-enkephalin neurons, enhance the inhibiting influence of these cells, resulting in less inhibition of the subthalamic nucleus. The often remarkable effect of antidopamine drugs on chorea is a prime example of the fact that the researcher cannot always infer from a salutary pharmacologic response which cell group or neurotransmitter is primarily affected by the disease process in basal ganglia disorders. One obvious exception to this observation is *Parkinson's disease*, for which replenishment of a deficient neurotransmitter, dopamine, does reflect the primary neurochemical abnormality.

DYSTONIA

Dystonia—an abnormal hyperkinetic movement that is distinct from chorea—is an involuntary movement that is twisting, somewhat sustained, and often repetitive. With time, the body part affected by this abnormal movement may develop a fixed, abnormal posture.

Dystonia can be described according to its distribution within the body as focal, segmental, or generalized. Focal dystonia implies involvement of a single part of the body such as the hand, and segmental dystonia involves two or more adjacent areas of the body, such as the neck and arm. Generalized dystonia is defined as involvement of the lower extremities plus any other body part. Examples of focal dystonia are writer's cramp, an involuntary contraction of hand or finger muscles that occurs while writing, and torticollis, an involuntary turning or tilting of the head. Torticollis plus facial or eyelid dystonia constitute segmental dystonia.

Idiopathic torsion dystonia is the most common condition that causes generalized dystonia. It is an autosomal dominant disorder with variable penetrance that typically begins in childhood or adolescence. The gene for this condition, torsine A, is on the long arm of chromosome 9 at the DYT1 locus. The function of the resultant protein is currently unknown. In this disorder, like most spontaneously occurring dystonic disorders, no apparent structural abnormalities of the basal ganglia and no abnormalities of neurotransmitter function have been consistently demonstrated. However, neurotransmitter manipulation sometimes results in marked reduction of dystonia. The most effective results are obtained with anticholinergic agents. A smaller subset of patients respond remarkably to the dopamine precursor l-dopa. This dopa-responsive

dystonia is inherited in an autosomal dominant fashion, resulting from a mutation to the gene encoding GTP cyclohydrolase, which is involved in dopamine synthesis.

Although there is no obvious structural pathology of the basal ganglia in the idiopathic dystonias, discrete structural lesions of these structures caused by tumor, trauma, or stroke can result in an identical movement disorder. In these cases, the brain abnormality leading to dystonia is most likely to be located in the putamen, but it can also be found in areas related to the basal ganglia through efferent or afferent pathways, such as the thalamus or cerebral cortex. Typically, dystonia caused by unilateral structural abnormalities of the basal ganglia or their connections is confined to the extremities on the contralateral side of the body, and is referred to as *hemidystonia*.

Pending the development of better pharmacologic therapies for dystonia based on a fuller understanding of its etiopathogenesis, the use of botulinum toxin has emerged as one of the most effective treatments for this condition. Partial weakening of the muscles responsible for the dystonic movement can be accomplished by directly injecting them with small amounts of botulinum toxin. This substance works by inhibiting release of acetylcholine from nerve terminals, effectively producing chemical denervation of muscle with resultant weakness and atrophy.

TICS

Tics are sudden, brief, stereotyped movements. The movement is involuntary and complex, such as blinking of the eye or shrugging of the shoulder. Movements such as these are known as *motor tics*. When the vocal apparatus is involved, a tic may consist of a nonspecific vocalization, such as a grunt or a distinct verbalization, including recognizable words or phrases. *Tourette's syndrome* is a condition in which motor and vocal tics occur. Tourette's syndrome, believed to be a hereditary disorder, begins in childhood and is more common in boys. It is often associated with certain behavioral abnormalities such as attention deficit disorder, or a variety of compulsions or ritualistic behaviors. Interestingly, first-degree relatives are at a substantially higher risk for Tourette's syndrome, simple motor tics and obsessive-compulsive disorder (OCD). Like idiopathic torsion dystonia, its anatomic and neurochemical basis are not fully understood. However, the results of structural and functional imaging studies have suggested impaired function of the basal ganglia. A failure to inhibit subsets of the cortico-striato-thalamocortical circuits has been hypothesized to result in the symptoms of both Tourette's syndrome and obsessive-compulsive disorder. Tics, like chorea, are effectively suppressed by dopamine-blocking drugs, but no definite abnormalities of dopaminergic cells or pathways have been demonstrated in the brains of affected persons.

BASAL GANGLIA DISORDERS CAUSING MULTIPLE FORMS OF ABNORMAL MOVEMENT

Some basal ganglia disorders can result in several different forms of abnormal movement. Several distinct diseases of the basal ganglia can result in several or all of the previously described abnormal movements. *Hallervorden-Spatz syndrome*, a condition associated with neuronal loss and increased iron storage primarily in the substantia nigra pars reticulata (SNr) and internal globus pallidus (GPi) can result in chorea, bradykinesia, or dystonia in any combination. This same spectrum of disordered movements plus tremor can occur in *Wilson's disease*, a condition characterized by neuronal loss and excessive copper storage in the brain, especially the putamen. In this condition, symptoms can be reversed by decoppering the central nervous system (CNS) with medications.

Tardive dyskinesia is a syndrome in which abnormal movements occur after prolonged administration of dopamine-blocking drugs such as chlorpromazine or metoclopramide. In this condition, the abnormal movement is usually chorea, but occasionally is dystonia. The abnormal movements of tardive dyskinesia can affect any part of the body, but they are most often focused on the mouth and tongue. A common but unproven explanation for the pathogenesis of this condition is that dopamine receptors develop compensatory supersensitivity as a result of being subject to chronic pharmacologic blockade.

The class of dopamine receptor that is blocked seems to be important in the pathogenesis of this syndrome, because dopamine-blocking drugs that preferentially block the D3 rather than the D2 dopamine receptor are much less likely to cause tardive dyskinesia.

19 The Thalamus

Yoland Smith and Mamadou Sidibe

CONTENTS

1. INTRODUCTION

The thalamus is the largest structure of the mammalian diencephalon. It comprises many nuclear groups, each concerned with transmitting characteristic afferent signals to specific areas of the cerebral cortex. The thalamus is often described as the gateway to the cerebral cortex. The term "thalamus" is a Greek word meaning inner chamber. Its origin dates back to the 2nd Century AD, when Galen traced the optic-nerve fibers to an oval mass closely associated with the ventricles. This part of the brain known as the optic thalamus was later defined as a large mass of gray matter, involved with visual stimuli, and in the processing of all sensory modalities, except olfaction. The size of the thalamus is relatively small compared to that of the neocortex, but the functions of each major neocortical areas largely depend on the interactions with a well-defined thalamic-cell group. For this reason, an increase in size of any neocortical areas is correlated with a corresponding increase in the related thalamic nuclei. The nomenclature of the different nuclear sub-divisions of the primate thalamus is more complex than in rodents. Although the thalamic cytoarchitecture in monkeys and humans is relatively similar, the nomenclature used to define thalamic nuclei in simians and humans has diverged so much over the years that non-specialist readers surely believe that the thalami of humans and monkeys are fundamentally different (Table 2). The main difference between human and nonhuman primate thalami is the relative growth of specific thalamic nuclei relative to other nuclear subdivisions; the pulvinar is the most representative example of a thalamic nucleus that has overgrown in the human brain.

This chapter provides an overview of the main features that characterize the anatomy and functional organization of the primate thalamus. For additional information, the reader is referred to recent reviews and compendiums (Steriade and Deschenes, 1984; Jones, 1985, 1998; McCormick, 1990; Steriade and McCarley, 1990; Deschenes et al., 1998; Sherman and Koch, 1998; Kultas-Ilinsky and Ilinsky, 2001; Sherman and Guillery, 2001).

From: *Neuroscience in Medicine, 2nd ed.* (P. Michael Conn, ed.),
© 2003 Humana Press Inc., Totowa, NJ.

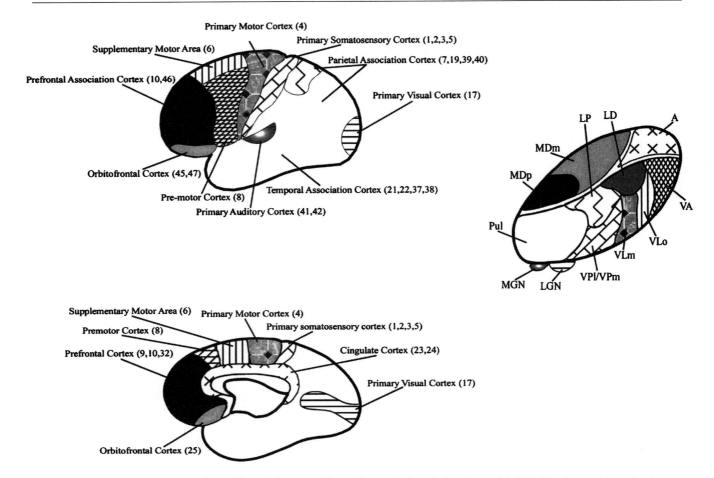

Fig. 1. Thalamocortical connections of modality-specific and association thalamic nuclei. The Brodmann's cortical areas are indicated in parentheses. A, anterior thalamic nuclei; LD, lateral dorsal nucleus; LGN, lateral geniculate nucleus; LP, lateral posterior nucleus; MDm, mediodorsal nucleus, magnocellular part; MDp, mediodorsal nucleus, parvocellular part; MGN, medial geniculate nucleus; Pul, pulvinar; VA, ventral anterior nuclei, VLm, ventrolateral nucleus, pars medialis; Vlo, ventrolateral nucleus, pars oralis; VPl, ventroposterolateral nucleus; VPm, ventroposteromedial nucleus.

2. NUCLEAR SUBDIVISIONS OF THE THALAMUS

The dorsal portion of the diencephalon comprises three major parts: the epithalamus, the dorsal thalamus, and the ventral thalamus. The *epithalamus* consists of the pineal body, the habenular nuclei, the stria medullaris, and the associated paraventricular nuclei. This part of the diencephalon is a major component of the limbic system, and is not discussed further in this chapter. The *dorsal thalamus* is divided into anterior, medial, ventrolateral, and posterior nuclear groups by a band of myelinated fibers, the internal medullary lamina of the thalamus (Fig. 1). The *anterior nuclear group* forms a rostral swelling that protrudes from the dorsal surface of the rostral thalamus. It is separated from other thalamic nuclei by a myelinated capsule. The *lateral nuclear group* comprises two main nuclear

masses, and the ventral nuclear mass, which extends throughout the entire rostrocaudal extent of the thalamus, is divisible into separate nuclei: (i) the ventral posterior nucleus, medial geniculate nucleus, and dorsal lateral geniculate nucleus caudally, (ii) the ventral lateral nucleus at intermediate levels, and (iii) the ventral anterior nucleus rostrally. These are the ventral-tier thalamic nuclei. The lateral nuclear mass, located dorsal to the ventral nuclear mass, also comprises three major nuclei: (i) the pulvinar, which occupies a large part of the caudal thalamus; (ii) the lateral posterior nucleus, located at an intermediate level; and (iii) the lateral dorsal nucleus, the most rostral component of this nuclear mass. These are known as the dorsal-tier thalamic nuclei. The *medial nuclear group*, located medial to the internal medullary lamina, is largely made up of the mediodorsal nucleus, a major relay center for cognitive information to the prefrontal cortex. A fourth thalamic nuclear group, confined within the boundaries of the internal medullary lamina, is the *intralaminar nuclei*. These nuclei, which are often considered as nonspecific or diffusely projecting nuclei, are divided into two main groups: the anterior group, which contains the paracentral and centrolateral nuclei, and the posterior group represented by the centromedian and parafascicular nuclei. The so-called *midline thalamic nuclei* are more or less distinct cell clusters along the medial portion of the thalamus. These nuclei are smaller and more difficult to delimit in humans and monkeys than in rodents. The main cell groups are the paraventricular, rhomboid, median central, and reuniens nuclei. These nuclei are directly connected with cortical and subcortical limbic-related brain regions. Along the lateral border of the thalamus, near the internal capsule, lies the external medullary lamina, which separates the *reticular nucleus* from the remainder of the thalamus. The reticular nucleus forms a thin outer envelope that tightly surrounds the entire extent of the dorsal thalamus. In contrast to all other thalamic nuclei that project to the cerebral cortex, the reticular nucleus does not provide cortical inputs, but instead innervates other thalamic nuclei and the brainstem. The *ventral thalamus* comprises the ventral lateral geniculate nucleus, the zona incerta, and the fields of Forel.

In general, most thalamic nuclei can be classified either as modality-specific nuclei, multimodal-association nuclei, and nonspecific, diffusely projecting nuclei (Fig. 1). The modality-specific nuclei are reciprocally connected with well-defined cortical areas that are related to specific motor or sensory functions. However, the multimodal-association nuclei have widespread cortical connections, with association areas in the frontal, parietal and temporal lobes. Unlike modality-specific nuclei, they do not receive inputs from one dominant subcortical structure, but are rather innervated by many different afferent inputs that have equal weight. Consistent with such a pattern of innervation, the functions of association nuclei are not precise and modality-specific, but are related to higher functions such as language and learning. Finally, the nonspecific or diffusely projecting nuclei comprise the intralaminar and midline thalamic nuclei that provide widespread cortical projections and innervate the striatum more massively than the cerebral cortex.

3. CELL TYPES OF THE THALAMUS

The mammalian thalamus comprises three major cell types; (i) the relay cells, which project their axons to the cerebral cortex or the striatum, (ii) the interneurons, which are not present in all nuclei in nonprimates, and have their axons and synaptic connections confined within the nuclei in which they lie, and (iii) the reticular neurons, which have their perikarya confined within the limits of the reticular nucleus and sends their axons to the dorsal thalamus (Fig. 2). Relay neurons are glutamatergic, whereas both interneurons and reticular neurons use GABA as a neurotransmitter. The morphology of these three cell types is strikingly different. In most thalamic nuclei, relay cells have a bushy appearance, containing a relatively symmetrical dendritic field with occasional dendritic appendages or protrusions, but with no apparent morphological characteristics that correspond to their physiological properties. In the lateral geniculate nucleus (LGN), relay cells in the parvocellular laminae have smaller somata and bitufted dendrites confined to the lamina in which they lie, whereas magnocellular neurons have larger somata and more radial dendritic fields that cross laminar boundaries. Overall, relay cells have a larger somata than those of interneurons, but they exhibit a broad range of sizes. For instance, the perikarya of relay cells in the ventral posterior and ventral lateral nuclei of monkeys range from 70 μm^2 to more than 400 μm^2. In the LGN of monkeys, magnocellular neurons have somata that range from 25 to 40 μm in size, whereas cells in the parvocellular laminae range from 16–25 μm in diameter. However, cells in the S and interlaminar zones have 8–10 μm soma (Fig. 2).

The GABAergic interneurons, which are found in all thalamic nuclei in primates, are much smaller than relay cells. In general, their somata is less than 10 μm in diameter, with a few short dendrites that give off numerous lengthy processes that end in terminal boutons and form dendro-dendritic synapses. Interneurons form approx 30% of the total neuronal population in all thalamic nuclei, except in intralaminar nuclei, where they are slightly less abundant and account for about 15–20% of neurons (Fig. 2).

The cells of the reticular nucleus are relatively large, with somal diameters ranging from 25–50 μm in monkeys and humans. The cells are flattened so that the dendritic field is commonly discoidal, and they densely overlap at all levels of the nucleus. The axons of reticular neurons have short intranuclear collaterals, and in some species, the dendritic branches form dendro-dendritic synapses. All reticular cells are GABAergic and project to all dorsal thalamic nuclei, except the anterior nuclei in rats and cats, although some reticular projections to these nuclei have been found in primates. Other chemicals found in reticular

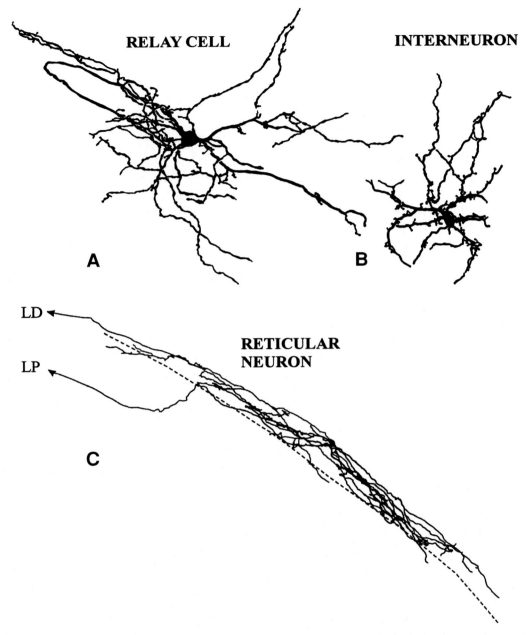

Fig. 2. The three major cell types of the mammalian thalamus drawn from Golgi preparation (**A,B**) (From Jones E. The Thalamus. New York, Plenium Press, 1985, with permission) or intracellular filling (**C**).

neurons include parvalbumin and somatostatin. Both corticothalamic and thalamocortical neurons give off axon collaterals to very specific sectors of the reticular nucleus. The topographical arrangement of these projections makes different sectors of the reticular nucleus specifically dedicated to a particular dorsal thalamic relay nucleus. Projections to and from intralaminar and midline nuclei are more diffuse and less topographic. The large dendritic field of reticular neurons

allow a high degree of functional convergence in the somatosensory sector of the nucleus (Fig. 2C). In line with this, reticular neurons are not modality-specific, and have larger receptive fields than cells in the somatosensory cortex and the ventroposterolateral thalamic nucleus. The reticular nucleus also receives dense brainstem inputs from cholinergic, noradrenergic, and serotonergic cell groups. These modulatory afferents control the firing rate and pattern of reticular neurons

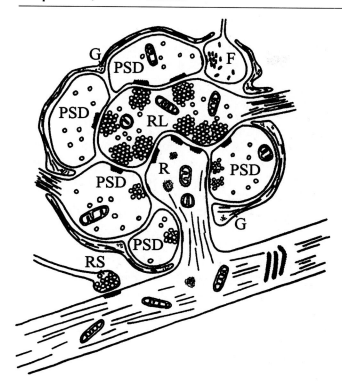

Fig. 3. Complex glomerular synaptic arrangement of major synaptic inputs to thalamic relay neurons in the thalamus. G, glial processes; R, relay neuron. *See* text for other abbreviations.

in different states of vigilance, and influence all thalamocortical activity. Basal forebrain cholinergic and GABAergic inputs from the basal nucleus of Meynert, substantia innominata, and globus pallidus have also been reported.

4. BASIC SYNAPTIC ORGANIZATION OF THE DORSAL THALAMUS

In most relay and intralaminar thalamic nuclei, four types of synaptic terminals are found and named according to their size and the shape of vesicles they contain. They are termed: (i) RL, round vesicles and large size; (ii) RS, round vesicles and small size; (iii) F, flat vesicles; and (iv) PSD, presynaptic dendrites. The RL terminals are relatively abundant, are packed with small synaptic vesicles, usually contain many mitochondria, and form asymmetric synapses. They (Fig. 3) arise mainly from the main extrinsic afferents to relay nuclei, which include the medial lemniscus, cerebellum, optic tract, mammillothalamic tract, and inferior colliculus. The RS terminals, which are much more numerous than RL terminals, also contain small, round vesicles and form asymmetric synapses mostly

with distal dendrites of thalamocortical neurons. They largely originate from layer VI of the cerebral cortex. The F terminals are GABAergic, contain flattened synaptic vesicles, and form symmetric synapses. The reticular nucleus and axons of interneurons, when present, are the main sources of these terminals. The PSD terminals contain aggregates of pleomorphic synaptic vesicles, significant quantities of rough endoplasmic reticulum (ER), and clusters of free ribosomes. They arise from dendrites of GABAergic interneurons. In general, the RL and PSD terminals form synapses with the proximal part of relay neurons, whereas RS boutons mostly terminate on distal dendrites of relay neurons, although a substantial proportion also innervates dendrites of interneurons. F-terminals end on the proximal part of relay neurons and interneurons as well as on the PSD of interneurons (Fig. 3). Detailed quantitative measurements of the relative abundance of these different types of terminals on specific neuronal populations in cats and monkeys have been performed. Overall, the pattern of distribution of afferent terminals on thalamic neurons is relatively similar across primates and non-primates—e.g., subcortical afferents are concentrated on the proximal dendrites and cell bodies, corticothalamic terminals converge on distal dendrites, and inhibitory terminals are evenly distributed across the somatodendritic domain. The degree of convergence of cortical and subcortical afferents from various sources onto individual thalamocortical neurons varies between thalamic nuclei. For instance, in the LGN, each relay neuron is innervated by a single type of retinal ganglion-cell axon, whereas in the ventroposterior nucleus, indirect evidence suggests that spinothalamic and medial lemniscus afferents partly converge on the same neurons. It is very likely that RS terminals that end onto individual thalamocortical neurons arise from cortical layer VI neurons. There is also evidence that a subpopulation of corticothalamic terminals arise from layer V neurons. These terminals display the ultrastructural features of RL boutons and form asymmetric synapses with dendrites of relay neurons and PSD of interneurons. The F terminals that arise from the reticular nucleus innervate the full length of relay-cell dendrites, whereas F terminals from the basal ganglia output structures, the substantia nigra pars reticulata (SNr), and the internal globus pallidus (GPi) which are largely confined to the proximal part of relay neurons in the ventral anterior and ventral lateral nuclei. In general, interneurons receive a much less dense innervation from RL and RS terminals than relay cells. For instance, less than 10% of cerebellar RL terminals end on PSD in the monkey ventrolateral nucleus. Axons from single cerebellar neurons form 3–4 times more synapses with dendrites of relay neurons than interneurons. Despite this relatively light innervation, electrophysiological data clearly demonstrate that stimulation of either the cerebral cortex or subcortical glutamatergic afferents induces disynaptic inhibitory postsynaptic potentials (IPSPs) in relay neurons, indicating the effectiveness and strength of these connections. Similarly, IPSPs were recorded in relay neurons of the anterior nuclei following stimulation of the mammilothalamic tract in cats. The fact that anterior nuclei do not receive GABAergic inputs from the reticular nucleus in this species indicates that these IPSPs were generated by PSDs and the axon terminals of interneurons.

5. SYNAPTIC CONNECTIVITY OF THE RETICULAR NUCLEUS

As mentioned previously, the reticular nucleus does not project to the cerebral cortex, but rather provides GABAergic inputs to most thalamic relay nuclei and the brainstem. In turn, reticular neurons receive glutamatergic inputs from axon collaterals of corticothalamic and thalamocortical neurons as well as modulatory cholinergic and monoaminergic inputs from the tegmental pedunculopontine nucleus, nucleus raphe, and locus coeruleus. In addition, neurons in the basal forebrain and globus pallidus as well as axon collaterals and/or PSD of reticular neurons provide substantial GABAergic inputs to reticular neurons. There is considerable evidence that the ascending brainstem inputs, acting both on the reticular nucleus and other thalamic nuclei, control the functional state of the thalamus as well as the transition from wakefulness to sleep. Reticular neurons have complex firing patterns that depend on the subject's state of vigilance. During deep sleep, thalamic neurons fire in rhythmic bursts that increase hyperpolarization of thalamocortical neurons, thereby inhibiting transfer of sensorimotor information to the cortex. In an awake state or during paradoxical sleep (REM sleep), the ascending brainstem projections suppress reticular neuron activity and activate other thalamic nuclei, thereby facilitating the relay of information through the thalamocortical system. Under these conditions, thalamocortical neurons function in a relay-type mode, actively process arriving subcortical information, and transmit it to the cortex.

The role of corticothalamic inputs and intrinsic GABAergic connections has been the subject of intensive research. Corticothalamic projections facilitate synchonized activity in thalamo-cortico-thalamic circuits, and thereby initiate and maintain thalamic rhythms that underlie changes in the electroencephalogram that accompany changes in conscious states. Stimulation of cortical neurons induces fast monosynaptic excitatory postsynaptic potentials (EPSPs) followed by fast GABA-A-mediated and slow GABA-B-mediated IPSPs in cat reticular neurons. Although the exact functions of these IPSPs has not yet been determined, there is strong evidence that they may play an important role in controlling burst discharges in reticular neurons, thereby influencing oscillations in the thalamic network. Projections from the reticular nucleus to the dorsal thalamus are topographically organized—e.g., sectors of the reticular nucleus that project to a particular thalamic nucleus receive projections back from this nucleus.

6. NEUROTRANSMITTERS AND RECEPTORS IN THE THALAMUS

6.1. Glutamate

As discussed previously, glutamate and GABA are the two transmitters released at most synapses in the dorsal thalamus. The corticothalamic and major spinal, tegmental, and cerebellar afferents to modality-specific thalamic nuclei use glutamate as neurotransmitter. Overall, the thalamus is enriched in all types of glutamate receptors. Both ionotropic, AMPA, NMDA, and kainate-receptor subunits, as well as various subtypes of metabotropic glutamate receptors, are expressed to varying degrees in relay neurons and thalamic interneurons in primates and nonprimates. For instance, in the monkey thalamus, there are low levels of gene expression for the AMPA/kainate subunits GluR1, GluR2, GluR5, and GluR7, whereas GluR3, GluR4, and GluR6 subunits are expressed at a moderate level. The five genes (NMDAR1 and NMDAR2A–D) that encode subunits of the NMDA receptors are all found to some extent in the dorsal thalamus. In general, the NMDAR1 and NMDAR2B subunits are expressed at higher levels than the other NMDAR2 subunits. The mRNAs for the three main groups of metabotropic glutamate receptors (Group I: mGluR1,5; Group II: mGluR2–3; Group III: mGluR4–8) have been identified in the rodent and primate thalamus. The mRNAs for mGluR1, mGluR4 and mGluR7 are highly expressed throughout the dorsal thalamus, whereas mGluR3 mRNAs are particularly abundant in the reticular nucleus. Very low levels of mGluR2 mRNAs are found throughout the thalamus.

6.2. GABA

In most thalamic nuclei, GABA is derived from both reticular neurons and local interneurons. In the ventral and posterior intralaminar nuclear group, basal ganglia afferents from GPi and SNr also provide strong GABAergic influences. Both GABA-A and GABA-B receptors mediate inhibitory transmission throughout the thalamus. At least 10 of the 15 GABA-A-receptor subunits have been identified in thalamic nuclei. GABAA-receptor densities, identified by autoradiographic ligand-binding studies, are high throughout the thalamus, except in the reticular nucleus. In fact, the reticular nucleus displays a pattern of GABA-A-receptor subunits that differs from dorsal thalamic nuclei. Many subunit mRNAs expressed at very high levels in dorsal thalamic nuclei and throughout the brain ($\alpha1$, $\alpha2$, $\beta2$ subunits) are either undetectable or expressed at low levels in the reticular nucleus. GABA-B-receptor binding is very dense in both the rat and primate thalamus, which is consistent with electrophysiological studies showing that GABA-A and GABA-B-mediated fast and slow IPSPs can be induced in thalamic relay neurons following stimulation of extrinsic inputs or reticular afferents. Similarly, connections between reticular thalamic neurons elicit their effects through both GABA-A and GABA-B receptors.

6.3. Monoaminergic and Cholinergic Systems

In addition to glutamate and GABA, modulatory inputs from brainstem monoaminergic and cholinergic cell groups are needed to modulate the activity of ensembles of thalamocortical neurons, thereby setting the state of brain activity. The serotoninergic, noradrenergic, and cholinergic terminals and receptors are found, to some extent, in all thalamic nuclei. A small histaminergic projection from the tuberomammilary region to the paraventricular, as well as the lateroposterior, lateral and medial geniculate nuclei have been described. Both muscarinic and nicotinic cholinergic receptors mediate slow-inhibitory and fast-excitatory effects of acetylcholine in thalamic neurons, respectively. For instance, reticular neurons are slowly inhibited by acetylcholine application, probably through activation of M2 muscarinic receptors, whereas nicotinic receptors mediate fast cholinergic excitation of relay neurons. Of the five muscarinic-receptor subunit mRNAs, M2 and M3 are very abundant throughout the dorsal thalamus and reticular nucleus, whereas M1 and M4 are practically absent. Similar degree of heterogeneity is also found for nicotinic-receptor subunits.

6.4. Calcium-Binding Proteins and Neuropeptides

Thalamic neurons show differential expression of calcium-binding proteins, parvalbumin, calbindin D 28k, and calretinin. In the primate thalamus, relay neurons stain for either parvalbumin and calbindin, but almost never for both. Calretinin is found in a subpopulation of calbindin neurons. Virtually no GABAergic interneurons express calcium-binding proteins, which is drastically different from other regions of the CNS where inhibitory GABAergic interneurons are enriched in these proteins. In the primate thalamus, calbindin and parvalbumin show a marked reciprocity of distribution—e.g., the thalamic nuclei strongly labeled for calbindin (anterior intralaminar nuclei, anterior pulvinar, laterodorsal nucleus, and medial geniculate nucleus) are usually devoid of parvalbumin immunoreactivity and vice versa. GABA cells in the reticular nucleus display strong parvalbumin immunoreactivity.

Many neuropeptides are found in cells and afferent fibers to various thalamic nuclei. Among the most abundant neuropeptides identified thus far are: tachykinin, cholecystokinin, somatostatin (SS), neuropeptide Y (NPY), neurotensin (NT), galanin, bombesin, angiotensin II (AII), enkephalin, and vasoactive intestinal peptide (VIP).

7. SPECIFIC CONNECTIONS OF THALAMIC NUCLEAR GROUPS

This section describes the organization of the main cortical and subcortical connections of thalamic nuclei. For simplification , thalamic nuclei are pooled into three major groups based on their cortical projections: (i) the modality-specific nuclei, (ii) multimodal or association nuclei, and (iii) nonspecific or diffusely projecting nuclei (Fig. 1).

7.1. The Modality-Specific Nuclei

This group includes six major thalamic nuclei: the anterior, ventral anterior, ventral lateral, ventroposterior, medial geniculate and lateral geniculate nuclei.

7.1.1. THE ANTERIOR NUCLEI

In most animal species, the anterior nuclei comprise two distinct subdivisions, the anteromedial and anteroventral nuclei. In humans, the principal anterior nucleus is the major component of this nuclear group.

Table 1
Nomenclature of Various Subdivisions
of the VA/VL Nuclear Complex in New World and Old World Monkeys

Olszewski	Vlo	VPLo	Area X	Vlc (and VLps)	VLm	VApc	Vamc
Jones	VLa	VLp			VMp	VA	
Illinsky and Kultas-Ilinsky	VAdc	VL	VLd	VM	VApc	Vamc	
Paxinos et al.	VAL (Vo)	VLL	VLM	VAL	VAM	VAL(Vo)	VAM
Stepniewska et al.	VLa	VLp	VLx	VLd	VM	VApc	Vamc

VA, ventral anterior nucleus; VAdc, ventral anterior nucleus, densocellular part; VAL, ventral anterior nucleus, lateral part; VAM, ventral anterior nucleus, medial part; VAmc, ventral anterior nucleus, magnocellular part; VApc, ventral anterior nucleus, parvocellular part; VL, ventral lateral nucleus; VLa, ventral lateral nucleus, anterior division; VLc, ventral lateral nucleus, pars caudalis; VLd, ventral lateral nucleus, dorsal division; VLL, ventral lateral nucleus, lateral part; VLM, ventral lateral nucleus, medial part; VLo, ventral lateral nucleus, pars oralis; VLp, ventral lateral nucleus, principal division; VLps, ventral lateral nucleus, pars postrema; VLx, ventral lateral nucleus, Area X; VM, ventral medial nucleus; VMp, ventral medial nucleus, principal division; Vo, ventralis oralis nucleus; VPLo, ventral posterior lateral nucleus, pars oralis.

The laterodorsal nucleus shares many anatomical similarites with the anterior group. The anterior nuclei are part of the limbic system and play important roles in controlling emotions, behavior, learning, and memory. All nuclei of this group have reciprocal connections with the cingulate cortex. They also project to suprasplenial and retrosplenial areas, extending as far as the parasubiculum. Afferents to the limbic thalamus arise from many sources, and the most important of these is the mammilary bodies that give rise to the mammilothalamic tract that ascends and terminates in various subdivisions of the anterior nuclei. Cells located in the medial part of the mammilary bodies project to the ipsilateral principal anterior nucleus, whereas fibers from the lateral mammilary body terminate in the anterodorsal nucleus bilaterally. Another main afferent to the limbic thalamus derives from the subiculum and presubiculum region of the hippocampal formation.

7.1.2. THE VENTRAL ANTERIOR AND VENTRAL LATERAL NUCLEI

The ventral anterior and ventral lateral nuclei are the main targets of basal ganglia and cerebellar inputs to the thalamus. These two nuclear groups are divided into various subnuclei that are based on cytological criteria. The nomenclature of these nuclei is extremely confusing, which makes understanding of papers published in this field difficult for nonspecialists (Tables 1 and 2). Here, we use the nomenclature of Jones (1985)

to describe projections of these nuclei. According to this nomenclature, the ventral anterior (VA) nucleus is the main recipient of GABAergic inputs from the SNr, the anterior ventrolateral nucleus (VLa) receives inputs from the Gpi, whereas the posterior ventrolateral nucleus (VLp) is the main target of ascending cerebellar afferents. There is little or no overlap between these three projection systems in the primate thalamus (Fig. 4). On the other hand, a higher degree of convergence of cerebellar and basal ganglia inputs is found in rats and cats. Both SNr and GPi projections are largely ipsilateral, use GABA as neurotransmitter, and terminate on the proximal part of thalamocortical neurons and PSDs in VA and VLa, whereas cerebellar inputs are glutamatergic and arise from the contralateral dentate nucleus. Because of these close relationships with motor-related subcortical regions, the VA/VL nuclei are often termed motor thalamic nuclei. In contrast to the long-held belief that basal ganglia outflow was conveyed exclusively to premotor (PM) and supplementary motor (SMA) cortical areas, it is now established that a substantial contingent of information from the basal ganglia is sent to the primary motor cortex (MI). Conversely, the cerebellar outflow, which was believed to be directed exclusively to MI, also reaches PM and SMA cortical regions. Both cerebellar and basal ganglia thalamic projections, terminate in motor thalamic territories, and reach major associative and limbic regions of the primate thalamus, which in turn innervate various cortical areas in the frontal,

Table 2
Correlation Between Nomenclature of Ventral Thalamic Nuclei
in Humans and Two Commonly Used Nomenclatures in Macaque Monkeys

Human/monkey	Jones	Olszewski
N. ventro-caudalis anterior internus (V.c.a.i)	VPM	VPM
N. ventro-caudalis portae (V.c.por)	Pla	Plo
N. ventro-caudalis parvocellularis internus (V.c.pc.i)	VMb + Sm	VPMpc
N. ventro-caudalis parvocellularis externus (V.c.pc.e)	VPI	VPI
N. zentrolateralis caudalis (Z.c.)	VPLa (Posterodorsal)	VPL (part)
N. Ventr-intermedius (V.im)	VLp (ventral part)	VPLo
N. dorso-intermedius (D.im)	VLp (dorsal part)	VLc
N. zentro-intermedius (Z.im)	VLp/VPLa (parts)	VLc/VPLc (parts)
N. ventro-oralis anterior (V.o.a)	VLa	———
N. ventro-oralis posterior (V.o.p)	VLa/part VLp	Vlo
N. ventro-oralis medialis (V.o.m)	VM	VLm
N. ventro-oralis internus (V.o.i)	VLp (anteromedial)	Area X
N. zentrolateralis oralis (Z.o)	VLa (parts)	Vlo (parts)
N. dorso-oralis (D.o)	VA (parts)	———
N. lateropolaris (L.po)	VA	VA
N. lateropolaris magnocellularis (L.po.mc)	VAmc	VAmc

parietal, and temporal lobes involved in cognitive functions (Fig. 4). These projections provide a substrate by which basal ganglia and cerebellar functions extend beyond motor control and involve complex cognitive and learning processes. The ventral anterior and mediodorsal thalamic nuclei are the main targets of nigrothalamic projections. In monkeys, inputs from the medial part of the SNr terminate mostly in the medial magnocellular division of the VA (VAmc) and the mediodorsal nucleus (MDmc), which in turn innervate anterior regions of the frontal lobe, including the principal sulcus (Walker's area 46) and the orbital cortex (Walker's area 11). Neurons in the lateral SNr project preferentially to the lateral posterior region of the VAmc and to different parts of MD that are mostly related to posterior regions of the frontal lobe, including the frontal eye field and areas of the premotor cortex. Nigral outputs to the thalamus flow along separate channels that target various cortical areas involved in cognitive, sensory, and oculomotor functions (Fig. 4).

7.1.3. THE VENTROPOSTERIOR NUCLEI

The ventroposterior nucleus is the main recipient of ascending somatosensory information. Two major subnuclei are recognized based on topographic and cytoarchitectonic organization—the ventroposterolateral (VPl) and ventroposteromedial (VPm) nuclei. In both nuclei, cells are arranged in clusters involved with the same modality and receptive fields. The main sources of inputs to the VPl are the medial lemniscus and spinal lemniscus, which carry sensory information related to the extremities and the trunk. Terminations of the medial lemniscus and spinothalamic tracts end on different targets in VPl. Medial lemniscal afferents contact projection neurons and interneurons and represent major components of complex synaptic arrangements, whereas spinothalamic fibers almost exclusively innervate projection neurons and avoid complex synaptic arrangements. The main input to the VPm arises from the trigeminal lemniscus that carries all somatic sensory modalities of the face. The gustatory sense is also represented in the VPm. Both VPm and VPl contain precise somatotopic maps of corresponding body parts. Lemniscal axons terminate in a rod-like fashion that encompasses clusters of thalamic neurons. Terminals within each rod carry a specific somatosensory modality that is transferred to specific columns of the primary somatosensory cortex. These precise connections provide the basis for preserving the somatotopic organization within the somatosensory system. The main cortical projection sites of VPl and VPm is the primary somatosensory cortex that comprises Brodmann's areas 1, 2, 3a, and 3b in the postcentral gyrus. In turn, these cortical regions provide inputs to the ventroposterior nucleus. Additional inputs from VPl and VPm to non-somatosensory cortical regions of the parietal lobe have also been shown.

Pallidal Output Channels

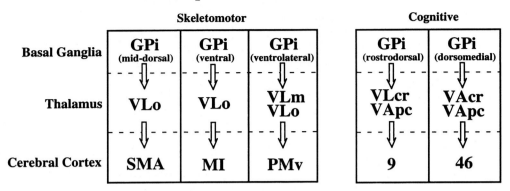

Nigral Output Channels

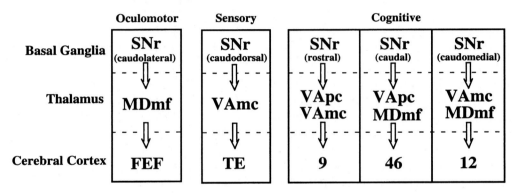

Cerebellar Output Channels

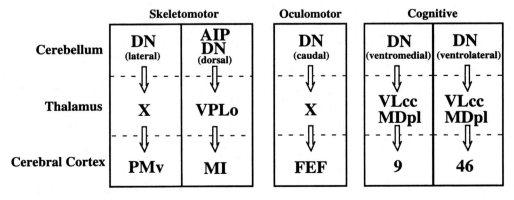

Fig. 4. Segregated basal ganglia and cerebellar motor and nonmotor thalamocortical output channels in monkeys. The GPi, SNr, and deep cerebellar nuclei project to different subdivisions of VA/VL and MD nuclei, which in turn reach functionally segregated cortical areas involved in motor, cognitive, and sensory functions. The nomenclature of thalamic nuclei used in this diagram is that of Olszewski (*see* Table 1 for abbreviations). AIP, interpositus nucleus; FEF, frontal eye field; MDmf, mediodorsal nucleu, pars multiformis; MD pl, Mediodorsal nucleus, pars lateralis; TE, area of inferotemporal cortex. (Reproduced from Middleton and Strick. Basel ganglia and cerebellar loops-motor and cognitive circuits. Brain Res Rev 2000, with permission from Elsevier Science.)

7.1.4. THE MEDIAL GENICULATE NUCLEUS

The medial geniculate nucleus is cytoarchitectonically subdivided into three main parts in primates. These regions are termed ventral, dorsal, and magnocellular. The ventral nucleus is the primary auditory relay to the primary auditory cortex located in Brodmann's areas 41 and 42 in Heschl's gyri. There is a point-to-point representation, called a tonotopic map, of the cochlea in this region. Neurons show high-frequency tuning and respond preferentially to inputs from the contralateral ear, although inputs from the ipsilateral ear also influence these neurons. Inputs to this subnucleus arise from the contralateral cochlea, with only one synaptic relay in the central nucleus of the inferior colliculus, which then sends fibers through the brachium of the inferior colliculus. The dorsal and magnocellular nuclei receive less direct auditory inputs than the ventral nucleus; neuronal responses in these regions are less frequency-specific and the tonotopic maps are not as well-defined, or even absent. The dorsal subnucleus receives auditory inputs from various brainstem nuclei and projects outside, but around, the primary auditory cortex. On the other hand, the magnocellular region receives auditory, somatosensory, and vestibular afferents by collaterals of the spinothalamic, medial lemniscal, and brachium of the superior colliculus tracts, and provides more widespread projections to non-auditory cortical areas than the two other subnuclei.

7.1.5. THE LATERAL GENICULATE NUCLEUS

The LGN is the main thalamic center for processing visual information. It is one of the most distinctive nuclei of the thalamus by its lamination into six distinct layers that receive completely segregated inputs from the two eyes. The ventralmost two layers (1 and 2) are composed of large cells and are called "magnocellular layers," whereas the dorsal layers (3–6) comprise small cells, thereby called "parvicellular layers." The major afferent inputs to the lateral geniculate nucleus arise from the retina. The axons of retinal ganglion cells travel through the optic tract and terminate in an orderly fashion into specific layers of the LGN, preserving a point-to-point map of the visual space. Layers 2, 3, and 5 receive inputs from the ipsilateral eye, whereas layers 1, 4, and 6 are the main targets of the contralateral eye. The information is then conveyed to primary and secondary visual areas (Brodmann's areas 17–19) in the occipital lobe. The terminations of fibers that arise from the LGN laminae

and are innervated by the ipsilateral and contralateral eyes do not overlap in the primary visual cortex. Instead, they terminate in a series of alternating left- and right-eye domains of 400–500-μm wide—known as ocular dominance columns—primarily in cortical layer IV. A main feature of LGN neurons is their center-surround receptive field, first described in the primary visual cortex by Hubel and Wiesel in the 1960s. In brief, a center-surround receptive field means that cells have a central zone in which a flash of light elicits excitation (on-center) or inhibition (off-center) of the cell, and a concentric surround in which flashed-light stimuli inhibit an on-center cell or excite an off-center cell. The LGN GABAergic interneurons play a major role in defining the extent of these receptor fields. Most retinal ganglion cells can be divided into two main categories based on the functional organization of their center-surround receptive fields: The M or P-α cells (parasol ganglion cells), which account for about 10% of the total ganglion-cell population, are not color-coded, display a broad-band spectral sensitivity, and have large concentric receptive fields. They respond to changes in brightness and have fast-conducting axons. The P or P-β cells (midget cells) have much smaller receptive fields, are color-coded, and are thereby excited by certain wavelengths and inhibited by others. Overall, the axons of M and P cells are segregated among laminae of the LGN; the M cells exclusively innervate the magnocellular layers 1 and 2, whereas the P cells terminate preferentially in the parvocellular layers. Another way to categorize retinal ganglion cells is by their pattern of innervation and neuronal targets in the LGN. The so-called X-type retinal axons are involved in complex synaptic associations, known as glomeruli, with relay neurons and interneurons, whereas the Y-type axons terminate directly on relay neurons and are usually not part of synaptic glomeruli. Additional afferents to the LGN come from primary and secondary visual cortical areas, the superior colliculus, the pretectal nucleus, brainstem oculomotor regions, and tegmental monoaminergic and cholinergic cell groups.

7.2. The Multimodal Association Nuclei

As mentioned previously, these nuclei differentiate themselves from the modality-specific nuclei by their diversity in sources of innervation and widespread cortical projections to association cortices. The major association nuclei of the primate thalamus are the mediodorsal and lateral posterior-pulvinar nuclei.

7.2.1. THE MEDIODORSAL NUCLEUS

The mediodorsal nucleus is a large nuclear mass located dorsomedial to the internal medullary lamina. It is tightly connected with the prefrontal agranular cortex, and plays major roles in high-order cognitive functions. In primates, the MD is cytoarchitectonically divided into three subnuclei: a medial, magnocellular nucleus, a parvocellular nucleus, which encircles the magnocellular compartment, and a lateral, multiform nucleus. Olfactory inputs from the prepiriform cortex and olfactory tubercle as well as the amygdala are considered to be the main sources of afferents to the magnocellular region of the nucleus. GABAergic inputs from basal ganglia nuclei—such as the ventral pallidum and SNr—terminate in all subdivisions of the nucleus, whereas the parvocellular and multiform subnuclei receive additional inputs from the superior colliculus, midbrain tegmentum, and brainstem mono-aminergic and cholinergic neurons. Each subnucleus has a preferential termination site in the prefrontal cortex—the magnocellular nucleus projects mainly to orbital areas (Brodmann's areas 10, 11, 12, 13), and projections from the parvocellular nucleus are more widespread and include lateral and medial areas of the frontal lobes (Brodmanns' areas 9, 24, 32, 45, 46, etc...). Finally, the multiform nucleus innervates preferentially more caudal regions of the frontal lobe, particularly the frontal-eye field. In line with these anatomical connections, neurons in the magnocellular MD and the orbital prefrontal cortex are activated following electrical stimulation of the olfactory cortex or olfactory bulb, and respond to odors. The MD's tight connections with the prefrontal cortex explain why it is involved in various cognitive brain diseases such as schizophrenia and Korsakoff's syndrome, which are characterized by changes in emotional behavior and loss of memory.

7.2.2. THE LATERAL POSTERIOR/PULVINAR NUCLEI

The lateral posterior/pulvinar complex is much larger and more highly differentiated in primates than in any other animal species. In monkeys and humans, one lateral posterior nucleus and four pulvinar subdivisions (anterior, lateral, medial, and inferior) have been identified. The main afferent inputs to this nuclear group arise from visuomotor regions of the midbrain, especially the superficial and deep layers of the superior colliculus and pretectum. There is also a direct retinal input to the inferior pulvinar nucleus. The superficial layers of the superior colliculus provide an indirect route through which retinal inputs reach these nuclei. Deep layers of the superior colliculus are likely to provide motor-related inputs from the basal ganglia, cerebellum, and brainstem centers that process various sensory modalities. Cortical projections arise from widespread regions of the parieto-temporo-occipital cortices. The inferior and lateral pulvinar nuclei contain one or more representations of the contralateral visual fields, probably as a result of their topographically organized projection from the superior colliculus. Based on these connections, the lateral posterior nucleus-pulvinar complex is often considered to be an integrative center for sensory and motor information related primarily to vision.

7.3. The Nonspecific or Diffusely Projecting Nuclei

This nuclear group includes two major sets of thalamic nuclei named for their location in the thalamus. The intralaminar nuclei are found within the internal medullary lamina, whereas the midline nuclei lie along the medial wall of the thalamus, just along the third ventricle. The main feature of these nuclei is that they provide rather diffuse projections to the cerebral cortex and project mainly to the striatum and other subcortical regions.

7.3.1. THE INTRALAMINAR NUCLEI

The intralaminar nuclei comprise two major groups, namely the anterior and posterior intralaminar nuclei. Two main nuclei are recognized in the anterior group—the paracentral and the centrolateral—whereas the posterior group comprises the centromedian and parafascicular nuclei. The main projection site of the intralaminar nuclei is the striatum. In primates, the centromedian (CM) and parafascicular nuclei (Pf) are the main sources of the thalamostriatal projection (Fig. 5). The CM projects preferentially to the post-commissural putamen—the sensorimotor striatal territory—whereas the Pf innervates preferentially the pre-commissural putamen, the caudate nucleus, and nucleus accumbens—the associative and limbic striatal territories, respectively (Fig. 5). The anterior intralaminar nuclei project mainly to the nucleus accumbens. The thalamostriatal projection is glutamatergic, and terminates preferentially in the matrix compartment of the striatum. At the electron microscopic level, thalamic boutons form asymmetric synapses with dendrites, and less frequently with spines, of medium-sized-projection neurons and subpopulations of interneurons. The pattern of innervation of striatal projection neurons by CM/Pf is different from

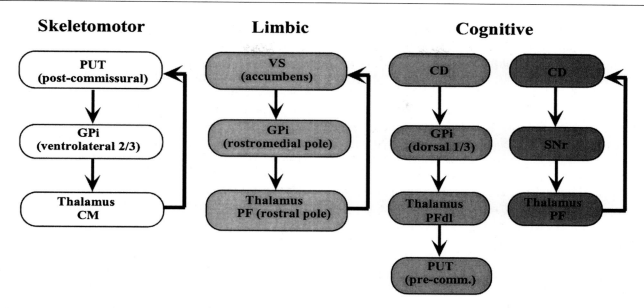

Fig. 5. Basal ganglia-thalamostriatal loops through the caudal intralaminar thalamic nuclei, CM and Pf, in monkeys. CD, caudate nucleus; PFdl, dorsolateral part of Pf; PUT, putamen; VS, ventral striatum. *See* text for other abbreviations.

that of cortical afferents, the other major glutamatergic afferent to the striatum. Most cortical boutons form synapses on the head of dendritic spines, yet thalamic inputs from CM/Pf preferentially end on dendritic shafts. Another main difference between thalamic and cortical inputs to the striatum is synaptic interactions with dopaminergic afferents. Whereas cortical and dopamine terminals often converge on the same postsynaptic targets, thalamic boutons from CM and dopamine terminals are never found in close proximity to each other in the monkey striatum. This suggests that the dopaminergic inputs are located to subserve a more specific control of corticostriatal than thalamostriatal influences in primates. Furthermore, it appears that thalamic inputs from CM selectively target a subpopulation of striatal projection neurons that innervate preferentially the internal globus pallidus (GPi), so-called "direct striatofugal neurons." This represents the first evidence that an extrinsic input to the striatum selectively targets a subpopulation of striatofugal neurons. In turn, the CM and Pf are the main targets of basal ganglia outputs from GPi and SNr. Recent anatomical studies show that these projections are massive, and display a high level of functional specificity. For instance, the sensorimotor, associative, and limbic territories of GPi innervate segregated regions of CM/Pf; the sensorimotor inputs are confined to the CM, and the associative and limbic GPi project mainly to Pf. This specific pattern of functional organization of basal ganglia-thalamostriatal

connections indicates that information flows through these circuits in segregated parallel channels, a common feature for processing of information in the basal ganglia (Fig. 5).

Other subcortical targets of intralaminar nuclei include the amygdala, substantia innominata, globus pallidus, subthalamic nucleus, and claustrum. Although less massive than thalamic inputs to the striatum, intralaminar nuclei also project to various cortical regions. Cortical projections from the anterior intralaminar nuclei are partly collaterals of the thalamostriatal pathways, whereas cortical and striatal afferents from CM/Pf largely arise from segregated neuronal populations. Although considered to be diffuse and primarily confined to layer I of the cortex, it appears that clusters of cells in intralaminar nuclei project to relatively restricted cortical areas, and that layer VI also receives some intralaminar projections. Based on data largely obtained in nonprimates, the cortical projections of intralaminar nuclei are organized as follows: anterior intralaminar nuclei project mainly to various functional areas in the prefrontal, cingulate, parietal, temporal, prepiriform, and entorhinal cortices as well the hippocampus; the CM is reciprocally connected with motor and somatosensory cortical regions, and the Pf projects to prefrontal, premotor, and cingulate cortices.

The anterior intralaminar nuclei receive subcortical inputs from various brainstem, cerebellar, and spinal cord nuclei. Additional inputs from the amygdala, substantia nigra, superior colliculus, and pretectal nuclei have also been found. As discussed previously, the CM/Pf are the main targets of basal ganglia projections from GPi and SNr, which largely arise from collaterals of the basal ganglia outputs to the VA/VL. Brainstem cholinergic and monoaminergic inputs from the pedunculopontine nucleus, raphe nuclei, and locus coeruleus have also been established. Notably, projections from the pedunculopontine nucleus are mainly directed toward Pf and display a high degree of chemical heterogeneity using acetylcholine, GABA, and glutamate as co-existing neurotransmitters. The reticular formation (RF) also provides massive inputs to anterior and posterior intralaminar nuclei. By virtue of these strong associations with the RF, the intralaminar nuclei are traditionally seen as part of the "reticular activating system" that regulates the mechanisms of cortical arousal and attention. Other functions of intralaminar nuclei include the regulation of tolerance to pain, and motor control mediated by spinothalamic and basal ganglia afferents, respectively.

7.3.2. The Midline Nuclei

The midline nuclei comprise three main cell groups that are much better defined in nonprimates than in monkeys and humans. The most prominent nuclei are the paraventricular, rhomboid, and reunions nuclei. The bulk of efferents from these regions are directed toward limbic-related cortical and subcortical areas. Similarly, they receive inputs from various limbic structures such as the amygdala and hypothalamus, as well as several midbrain and medullary regions including the nucleus of solitary tract (NST), the periacqueductal gray, the parabrachial region, the raphe nucleus, and the locus coeruleus. Collaterals of the spinothalamic tract also reach these nuclei. By virtue of their pattern of connectivity, midline thalamic nuclei are likely to be involved in emotional and motivational behaviors and autonomic functions.

8. SYMPTOMS FOLLOWING THALAMIC LESIONS

As discussed previously, the thalamus is the main relay center for sensory information to the cerebral cortex. Because of the high degree of functional specificity, lesions of specific thalamic nuclei would be expected to result in an impairment or loss of specific sensations in the opposite half of the body. However,

since thalamic nuclei are relatively small and very close to each other, lesions that affect only one of them are very rare. Furthermore, the fact that large ascending and descending fiber bundles travel through the thalamus, often makes thalamic lesions multi-symptomatic and difficult to interpret. Tumors and especially vascular lesions related to the middle and posterior cerebral artery may involve the thalamus and induce various kinds of behavioral changes. In cases where the entire thalamic area receiving somatosensory modalities is destroyed, deep sensibility and discriminating senses are severely impaired, whereas the sense of touch, temperature and pain perception are less affected. A distinguishing feature of thalamic lesions is the appearance of spontaneous "burning" pains, often refered to as thalamic pain syndrome. The thalamic pains are usually very intense, frequently irradiate to the entire half of the body, and are usually intractable to analgesics. They are often present together with a sensory loss, although they may occur without this loss, and usually then as an initial symptom. No universally accepted explanation for these pains has been given. Some believe that they are the result of vasomotor disturbances in the thalamus, and others assume that disappearance of cortical inhibition or lack of intrathalamic association may be the cause. These pains usually occur with small vascular lesions, and can be partly abolished by stereotactic thalamotomy. The thalamus, particularly the caudal intralaminar nuclei, is also the target of some neurodegenerative diseases such as Parkinson's disease. Some persons with multinutritional deficiencies resulting from starvation or alcoholism suffer from Wernicke-Korsakoff's syndrome, characterized by various motor and short-term memory problems. Autopsy often reveals neuronal degeneration of the mediodorsal thalamic nucleus in these patients.

The thalamus is the main target for neurosurgical therapies of various movement disorders. Thalamotomy has been used in the management of Parkinson's disease for more than 40 yr. Investigators largely agree that lesions or deep brain stimulations of the ventral intermediate nucleus markedly reduce tremor, but have little effect on other parkinsonian symptoms such as rigidity or bradykinesia. Two major pathways are interrupted by thalamic lesion—the pallidofugal projection from GPi and the cerebellar outflow from the contralateral deep cerebellar nuclei. The mechanisms of action of thalamotomy are unknown, but may be the result of destruction of autonomous neural activity, that is, neurons that fire at tremor frequency. The mortality rate for thalamotomy in parkinsonians is less than 0.3%.

9. CONCLUDING REMARKS

This chapter briefly reviews the main anatomical features of the thalamus and explores some of the basic functional characteristics of specific thalamic nuclei. The basic circuitry of the thalamus relies upon three major sets of neurons—the glutamatergic relay neurons that project to the cerebral cortex and two classes of GABAergic intrinsic neurons arising from the reticular nucleus and local interneurons. The afferents to the thalamus come from a variety of cortical and subcortical sources that provide modality-specific information to different sets of thalamic nuclei, which in turn convey this information to the cerebral cortex through parallel segregated channels. These parallel pathways are particularly evident for modality-specific nuclei. The reticular nucleus, in concert with the corticothalamic projections and brainstem modulatory afferents from cholinergic and aminergic cell groups, play a major role in inducing oscillations in large ensembles of thalamic neurons that underlie changes in the conscious state. It is clear that the thalamus is not a passive relay of information to the cerebral cortex. Instead, it actively filters the flow of information according to patterns that may vary with the state of consciousness and attention. The thalamus is connected with the cerebral cortex, and also provides major inputs to various subcortical structures related to limbic and motor functions. The thalamostriatal projection from intralaminar nuclei is particularly important in that regard. Although specific lesions of the thalamus are not common because of the size and close proximity of modality-specific subnuclei, loss of somatic sensibility, cognitive deficits, memory impairment, and motor problems have been described following thalamic lesions. Furthermore, the loss of neurons in caudal intralaminar nuclei of parkinsonians

supports the involvement of the caudal intralaminar nuclear group in basal ganglia functions and motor control. Neurosurgical therapies directed at lesioning specific thalamic subnuclei are often used for thalamic pains and tremor.

SELECTED READINGS

Deschenes M, Veinante P, Zhang Z-W. The organization of corticothalamic projections: reciprocity versus parity. Brain Res Rev 1998; 28:286–308.

Hassler R. Anatomy of the thalamus. In Schaltenbrand G, Bailey P, (eds). Introduction to stereotaxis with an atlas of the human brain New York: Thieme, 1959; 230–290.

Ilinsky IA, Kultas-Ilinsky K. Sagittal cytoarchitectonic maps of the Macaca mulatta thalamus with a revised nomenclature of motor-related nuclei by observations on their connectivity. J Comp Neurol 1987; 262:331–364.

Jones E. The Thalamus. New York: Plenum Press, 1985.

Jones E. The Thalamus of Primates. In Bloom FE, Bjorklund A, and Hokfelt T, (eds). Handbook of Chemical Neuroanatomy. Vol. 14: The Primate Nervous System, Part III. Amsterdam: Elsevier, 1998; 1–268.

Kultas-Ilinsky K, Ilinsky IA. Basal Ganglia and Thalamus in Health and Movement Disorders. New York: Kluwer Academic/Plenum, 2001.

McCormick DA. Cellular mechanisms of cholinergic control of neocortical and thalamic neuronal excitability. In Steriade M, Biesold B (eds). Brain Cholinergic Systems Oxford: Oxford Univiversity Press, 1990; 236–259.

Middleton FA, Strick PL. Basal ganglia and cerebellar loops: motor and cognitive circuits. Brain Res Rev 2000; 31:236–250.

Olszewski J. The thalamus of the Macaca mulatta. An atlas for use with stereotaxic instrument. Basel: Karger, 1952.

Paxinos G, Huang X-F, Toga AW. The rhesus monkey brain in stereotaxic coordinates. San Diego: Academic Press, 2000.

Sherman SM, Koch C. Thalamus. In Shepherd GM, (ed). The Synaptic Organization of the Brain, 4th ed. New York: Oxford University Press, 1998; 289–328.

Sherman S, Guillery RW. Exploring the Thalamus. San Diego: Academic Press, 2001.

Stepniewska I, Preuss TM, Kaas JH. Architectonic subdivisions of the motor thalamus of owl monkeys: Nissl, acetylcholinesterase, and cytochrome oxidase patterns. J Comp Neurol 1994; 349:536–556.

Steriade M, Deschenes M. The thalamus as a neuronal oscillator. Brain Res Rev 1984; 8:1–63.

Steriade M, McCarley RW. Brainstem control of wakefulness and sleep. New York: Plenum Press, 1990.

20

Spinal Mechanisms for Control of Muscle Length and Force

C. J. Heckman and W. Zev Rymer

CONTENTS

A BRIEF REVIEW OF MUSCLE FUNCTION
MECHANICAL PROPERTIES OF WHOLE MUSCLE
MUSCLE RECEPTORS
AFFERENT PATHWAYS TO THE SPINAL CORD
MOTONEURONS AND THE MOTONEURON POOL
REFLEX REGULATION OF MOVEMENT
SELECTED READINGS

1. A BRIEF REVIEW OF MUSCLE FUNCTION

1.1. Introduction: Muscle as a Mechanical System

All motor commands from the central nervous system (CNS) are expressed through changes in the magnitude of neural excitation of skeletal muscle. These changes in muscle excitation give rise to force generation and to motion, whose magnitude depends on the properties of muscle, and the mechanical loads experienced by the muscle. It is therefore necessary to begin a description of the neural regulation of movement with a short description of the relevant mechanical properties of muscle, with particular emphasis on the dual roles of skeletal muscle as a force generator, and as a mechanical impedance with both elastic (e.g., spring-like) and viscous (frictional) properties.

1.2. Muscle as a Force Generator

Skeletal muscle acts as a machine that transforms chemical energy, stored in the form of high-energy phosphate bonds in the molecule adenosine 5' triphosphate (ATP) into mechanical energy, that is to force,

or to motion. The means by which this transduction of energy takes place is relatively well-understood, yet space does not permit a full exposition here. Nonetheless, a short description of the cellular basis for the mechanical actions of muscle is important to our understanding of movement regulation, because many of the characteristics of neural activity are related to the special stimulus requirements of muscle.

As shown in Fig. 1A, muscle is made up of muscle fibers, which are, in effect, the cells of the tissue. These muscle fibers contain slender fibrils, known as myofibrils, which bear a striated pattern. (The fact that the striations are in register on different fibrils within the muscle fibers gives rise to the striated appearance of the skeletal muscle fiber under the light microscope). The force generating element of the myofibril is the sarcomere, (*see* Fig. 1B), which is defined as the segment of the myofibril between two adjacent thin dark vertical lines, called the Z lines. It is this recurring structure which gives rise to the striated pattern of the fibril, and ultimately, to the striated pattern of the whole fiber. The sarcomere contains thick and thin filaments, which bear the chemical moieties responsible for force generation.

The *thick filament* is made up primarily of myosin, which is a long-tailed molecule with a globular head

From: *Neuroscience in Medicine, 2nd ed.* (P. Michael Conn, ed.),
© 2003 Humana Press Inc., Totowa, NJ.

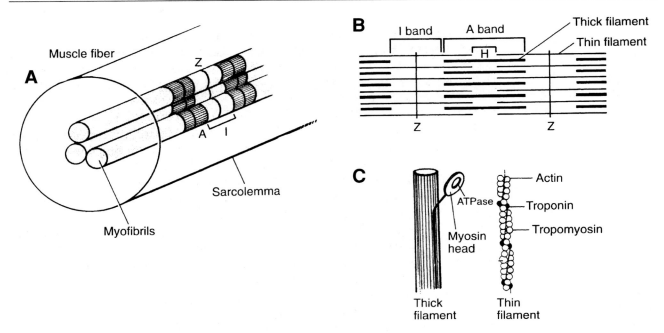

Fig. 1. (A) The constituent elements of the muscles include the muscle fiber, the membrane or sarcolemma, and the myofibrils, which appear striated because of the A and I bands, which have different optical properties. The myofibrils are the bundles of filaments that comprise the sarcomeres, which are the segments between adjacent Z lines. **(B)** Components of the sarcomere: Each sarcomere contains thick and thin filaments. Thick filaments reside in the center of the sarcomere, and the thin filaments traverse the area from one sarcomere to another through the boundary, known as the Z line. The thick filaments carry the myosin crossbridges, which interact with the thin filaments. The thin-filament actin carries a receptor that binds the myosin crossbridge. **(C)** Molecular constituents of the sarcomere: The thick filament is composed primarily of myosin, which has a long tail and a protruding head forming the crossbridge. The head incorporates an ATPase-binding location, which is needed for establishing the high-energy mechanical state of the crossbridge. The thin filament is made up of actin monomers, which are organized in a helical chain, forming F-actin. Regulatory proteins lie in the grooves of the F-actin strands. These are tropomyosin, an elongated molecule that lies in each of the two grooves of the actin helix, and troponin, a peptide that occurs at periodic locations along the thin filament.

and a flexible neck. The myosin molecule is made up of two heavy chains, which form the body of the molecule, and four light chains, which are sequestered in the head of the myosin molecule. Different types of muscle tissue (skeletal, cardiac, smooth), muscle at different stages of development (e.g., embryonic and neonatal), and muscles from various animal species show differences in the myosin heavy-chain isoforms. The myosin molecules are laid out in the thick filament so that their tails are packed in parallel, oriented along the long axis of the filament, and the heads protrude at regular spatial intervals around the circumference of the thick filament (*see* Fig. 1C).

As shown in Fig. 1C, the myosin head is a key locus at which the chemical to mechanical transduction takes place. This transduction requires binding of the myosin head to receptor sites on the thin filament, and there are subsequent conformational changes in the crossbridge, which are instrumental in producing muscle contraction. The myosin head is also the locus for an important ATPase, which facilitates the process of muscle contraction.

The *thin filament* has a more complex structure, because it is composed of several different proteins. The major protein, actin, is a globular monomer that is packed in the form of a twisted chain, known as F actin (*see* Fig. 1C). The thin filament also contains so called "regulatory" proteins, including *tropomyosin,* an elongated, rod-shaped molecule lying along the actin molecular helix, and *troponin,* which appears as a globular molecule, placed at periodic intervals along the thin filament. The troponin consists of various subunits, including Tn-C, which binds calcium, $4\,Ca^{2+}$, on each subunit, TnI, which is a major inhibitory subunit, and TnT, which binds to Troponin. These two proteins regulate contraction by controlling access of the myosin head to the actin-receptor sites on the thin filament. The process of force generation takes place when myosin heads bind to exposed actin-receptor sites on the thin filament.

1.2.1. Sliding Filament Theory

In 1954, A. F. Huxley (with Neidergeke) proposed that force generation in sarcomeres of skeletal muscle takes place when myosin crossbridges on the thick filament bind to actin-receptor sites on the thin filament, and induce sliding movement of thin filaments between thick filaments, toward the center of the sarcomere (*see* Fig. 1B). This was called the "sliding filament" theory, because force was generated by filament motion, rather than by length or force changes within one or another type of filament. This theory is now widely accepted as the most plausible mechanism for muscle-force generation. We also know that in the process of binding crossbridges to actin-receptor sites, there is a degradation of chemical energy, and an associated conformational change in the crossbridge, driving the thin filament toward the center of the sarcomere. This sequence usually results in a reduction of sarcomere length.

The process of crossbridge binding and detachment can occur repeatedly within a given contraction cycle, so that a given crossbridge may bind, undergo conformational change, detach, and then rebind to a different actin-receptor site. This process can continue as long as the level of free calcium ion (Ca^{2+}) in the sarcoplasm remains high, and as long as ATP synthesis keeps pace with the need for high-energy phosphate.

1.3. How Is Muscle Contraction Initiated?

1.3.1. The Role of Free Intracellular Calcium Ions in Excitation–Contraction Coupling

Calcium ions (Ca^{2+}) are widely believed to regulate many cellular processes, including cell motility, secretion, and synaptic transmission. Calcium also appears to be important for muscle contraction in at least two ways. Initially, increases in the concentration of calcium ions (Ca^{2+}) appear to control the sequence of events of contraction directly, by regulating myosin interaction with actin. Subsequently, calcium ion reductions act to terminate contraction.

The processes of excitation-contraction coupling rely on specialized structures known as the T tubule, and the sarcoplasmic reticulum (SR) (*see* Fig. 2A,B). The T tubule, or transverse tubule, is a tube that communicates with the muscle-fiber membrane surface, and extends into the cell interior. It is apparently capable of supporting action-potential propagation, well into the cell interior. The SR is a closed set of tubules and cisterns, which does not communicate with the cell surface, but which approaches the T tubule,

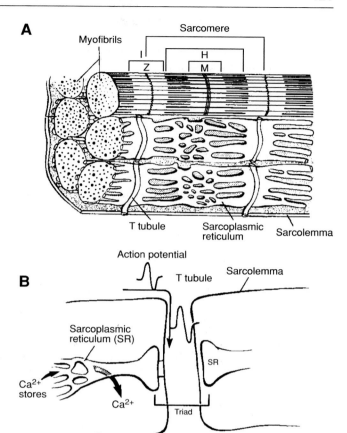

Fig. 2. (A) Components responsible for excitation–contraction coupling within the muscle. The muscle contraction is initiated by CA^{2+} release from stores within the sarcoplasmic reticulum (SR). An action potential, initiated in the end-plate region, traverses the sarcolemma and is propagated inward toward the fiber center by conduction of the action potential into the T tubule. (B) The structures responsible for excitation-contraction coupling are seen in more detail. The terminal cisternae of the SR are arranged symmetrically around the sarcolemma of the T tubule, forming a triad. Depolarization of the plasma membrane of the muscle cell induces calcium release from the adjacent SR by chemical or voltage signals.

forming specialized structures known as triads. These regions of apposition form the locus for chemical—or perhaps voltage—signaling between electrical and chemical intracellular events. These various tubes are utilized to regulate signal transmission from the cell surface to the interior, and to control calcium flux within the cell. We now believe that calcium ions are released from storage sites in the SR in response to electrical and perhaps chemical cues, which are emitted following depolarization of the surface membrane (the sarcolemma) and the transverse "T" tubule.

Under normal resting conditions, the concentration of free calcium ions (Ca^{2+}) in the sarcoplasm is held at barely detectable levels ($<10^{-12}$ M). In response to neurally initiated depolarization of the sarcolemma, calcium release occurs very swiftly, reaching concentrations of 10^{-7} M or higher in some types of muscle cells. The effect of these calcium-ion increases is to change the conformation of the regulatory proteins on the thin filament, allowing nearby myosin crossbridges to access and to bind to exposed actin-receptors sites.

Our present understanding is that the binding of crossbridges to actin and the subsequent conformational change represent an energy-releasing process, which does not require initial ATP degradation. (This helps to explain the phenomenon of muscle *rigor*, in which muscle becomes quite stiff after death. Loss of ATP production gives rise to calcium accumulation in sarcoplasm, exposing actin-receptor sites to myosin crossbridge interaction. Crossbridges then bind, giving rise to increased muscle stiffness, or rigor). Subsequently, energy absorption is required to detach the myosin from the actin-receptor site, and to allow the crossbridge to be reconfigured to its original high-energy state. This detachment is necessary in to order for crossbridge cycling and for force generation or muscle shortening to continue.

1.4. How Does Muscle Contraction End?

Since an increase in calcium-ion concentration is the primary event that initiates contraction, it is reasonable to suppose that calcium-ion reduction act to terminate contraction, and this does appear to be the case. When calcium release is terminated, governed by the recovery of the muscle-fiber membrane potential to normal levels, calcium is reabsorbed swiftly by active transport from the sarcoplasm into the SR. This reabsorption process is energy-dependent, because the calcium must be reabsorbed against a substantial concentration gradient. One molecule of ATP is degraded for two molecules of calcium absorbed.

1.5. Energetics of Muscle Contraction: Specialization of Muscle Fibers

ATP is used to promote crossbridge detachment and conformational change in crossbridges, and also to support active transport of calcium into the SR. Therefore, ATP plays a pivotal role in many processes that are responsible for muscle contraction. ATP is generated as a result of several biochemical processes in the muscle fiber, including degradation of free fatty (FFA) acids (that are absorbed from the bloodstream) and/or degradation of glucose. This glucose may also originate directly from capillary absorption, or it may be generated by the degradation of intracellular glycogen stores. The breakdown of glucose or FFA can then proceed using the machinery of either oxidative metabolism, or of glycolytic metabolism when oxygen-dependent mechanisms are less readily available.

1.5.1. Relevance of Metabolic Specialization to Specialization of Muscle Fibers

Fibers in different skeletal muscle, and even fibers in the same muscle, often exhibit differences in metabolic properties, to allow functional specialization of mechanical muscle performance. These specializations include the speed of muscle contraction and the degree of muscle fatigability.

Some muscle fibers contain very high glycogen concentrations, and these appear to rely primarily on glycolytic pathways to generate the ATP needed for contraction. Glucose is released from stored glycogen by a phosphorylase enzyme, then is degraded to lactate, generating a few molecules of ATP per molecule of glucose degraded. ATP may also be generated on a short-term basis by transfer of high-energy phosphate ($\sim$P), from a storage location on creatine. Other muscle fibers rely on oxidative metabolism, which is a far more efficient means to generate the high-energy phosphate of ATP. These fibers typically utilize absorbed glucose or FFA and oxygen, and have a highly specialized metabolic apparatus for oxidative phosphorylation, including large numbers of mitochondria, substantial intracellular myoglobin (which is a binding compound, rather like hemoglobin, which facilitates oxygen storage), and relatively modest or absent glycogen stores. These latter (oxidative type) fibers are usually surrounded by a dense capillary network, presumably to facilitate oxygen and FFA delivery to fibers.

These topics are also covered in the section that describes the use of functional groups of muscle fibers, known as the *motor units*, in the regulation of muscle-force generation.

2. MECHANICAL PROPERTIES OF WHOLE MUSCLE

Neurally activated muscle has several important mechanical properties, which are instrumental in the performance of movement.

2.1. Muscle Behaves Like a Spring

When an active muscle is stretched, muscle-force output increases progressively with increasing muscle length. This proportional relationship between force and length is the defining property of a spring. As shown in Fig. 3A, for a given level of neural excitation, the force increases with increasing muscle extension, until maximum physiological length is reached. When maximum length is exceeded, muscle force begins to decline, although this length is not normally achieved in intact limbs. The form of the length-tension relationship also varies somewhat with the rate of neural excitation—the length at which the force begins to increase steeply depends upon stimulus rate, and the peak tension occurs at different lengths. The reasons for these length-dependent changes in force are not entirely clear, but changes in the available population of bound crossbridges, and length-related increases in calcium release from the SR are both potentially significant factors.

This spring-like description of muscle mechanics is broadly accurate for *isometric*-length conditions (in which the length of the muscle is clamped at each measurement point), but it becomes even more precise for slow stretches, which generate a near-linear force-length relationship, resembling a simple spring even more closely. The significance of these spring-like responses will become more clear after we describe the added effects of reflex action; however, one clear benefit of these spring-like properties is that muscle forms a compliant interface with the external world, and thus acts somewhat like a shock absorber.

2.1.1. Deviations from Spring-Like Behavior

If active muscle without reflex control is stretched rapidly from an initial isometric state, then the spring-like behavior is disrupted, and muscle stiffness can be seen to change sharply with increasing stretch. As shown in Fig. 3B, once the stretch exceeds a fraction of 1 mm (typically 300–400 μm), the initial steep rise in force is interrupted, and muscle force declines sharply, sometimes even falling below the initial pre-stretch level. The initial high-stiffness region is known as the *short-range stiffness*, and the subsequent sharp decline in force the muscle *yield*. Although this short-range stiffness and yield are most apparent in slow-twitch muscles (such as the soleus), there is a routine change in stiffness during stretch even in fast-twitch muscle, once the length change exceeds a fraction of a millimeter. The initial high stiffness is attributable to

the stiffness of a population of attached myosin crossbridges, and the steep decline in force (and in stiffness) is a result of stretch induced crossbridge rupture.

2.1.2. Asymmetry of Muscle Mechanical Response to Stretch and Release

There is also a profound asymmetry of the force response to symmetrical stretch and release, which represents a substantial deviation from classic spring-like behavior. Although the force changes after a few hundred microns stretch or release is usually symmetrical, the two responses then depart substantially from this pattern. Specifically, muscle remains quite stiff during release, but as described previously, it often shows a substantial decline in overall stiffness during stretch.

These mechanical characteristics represent a significant departure from spring-like behavior of muscle, and they pose substantial difficulties for any neural control mechanism, because the force changes develop so quickly, and because they are so profound.

2.1.2.1. Force-Velocity Relations. Although muscle shows spring-like behavior for both slow extensions and slow shortening, the magnitude of the force generated during shortening of muscle is determined primarily by the speed with which the shortening occurs. Conversely, there is a well-defined relationship between the speed with which a muscle can shorten and the load which it can carry. For example, when a muscle is activated electrically and allowed to shorten against a load, a characteristic sequence of length and force changes has been observed, in which the shortening speed declines with increasing load magnitude.

A typical shortening experiment is diagrammed in Fig. 3C,D. Initially, as the muscle force develops, it may not be sufficient to overcome the opposing load, and no motion takes place. (This is the *isometric* phase, in which force is increasing without an accompanying reduction in muscle length). Once the force generated exceeds the magnitude of the opposing load, the muscle begins to shorten progressively at a constant velocity. The shortening velocity is very rapid when loads are small, and the shortening velocity declines when the applied load is increased. Ultimately, shortening velocities become very slow when loads are very large, when measured with respect to the maximum force-generating capacity of the muscle.

The relationship between shortening velocity and applied load has been studied extensively, and is well-

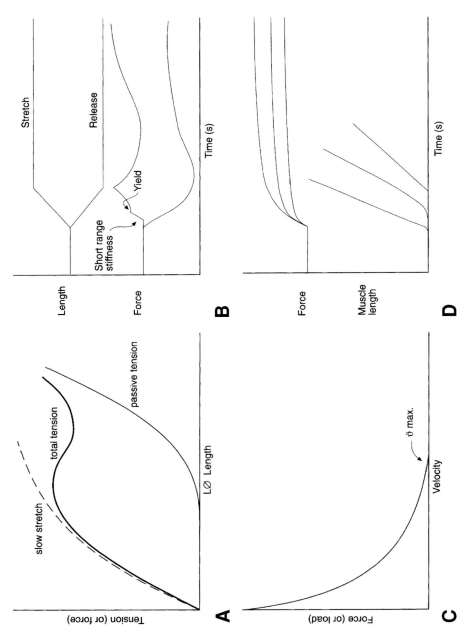

Fig. 3. Mechanical properties of skeletal muscle: (**A**) Length of tension properties: The isometric length-tension relationship is derived by stimulating the muscle nerve at a constant intensity and frequency while holding the muscle rigidly at a designated length. If this length is progressively increased, muscle force increases progressively until it reaches a maximal value at extreme lengths. If extension is continued beyond this maximum, the muscle force begins to fall, before ultimately increasing again at extreme lengths. This decline and subsequent increase in force at longer isometric lengths is attributable to the contribution of passive tissues surrounding the fibers. (**B**) Mechanical properties of active muscle subjected to symmetric stretch and release: When electrically stimulated muscle or deafferented active muscle is subjected to symmetric stretch and release of comparable velocity and amplitude, the force responses are grossly asymmetric. During stretch, the muscle initially has a region of elevated stiffness known as the short-range stiffness, which is followed by an abrupt decline in stiffness, called the yield. At the end of the stretch, there is a secondary decline in force, which gradually recovers, with the muscle reaching a steady state only after several hundred milliseconds. During shortening, there is a relatively smooth decline in force, which settles to an isometric value. (**C**) Force-velocity relationship: When muscle is allowed to shorten against a constant load, the magnitude of the shortening velocity, when measured at a constant length, is related to the load magnitude as a hyperbolic function. (**D**) Correlations between load and shortening velocity: If muscle force is generated with the muscle attached to the load, no shortening can occur until muscle force exceeds the load magnitude. When the load is minimal, this level is reached quickly, and muscle shortening begins relatively early and takes place at a relatively high velocity. When the load is maximal, the shortening begins after a longer period, and takes place at a relatively slow velocity.

424

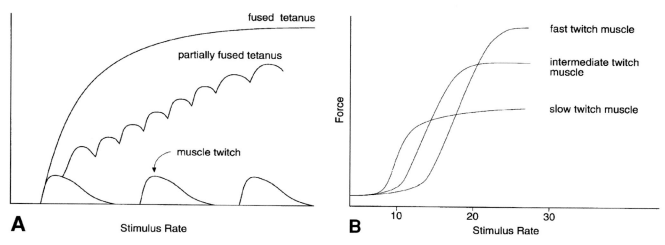

Fig. 4. Relationship between stimulus rate and muscle force. (**A**) Affect of stimulus frequency on muscle-force output. When muscle is stimulated with a single, short stimulus to the muscle nerve, the resulting force change is described as a muscle twitch in which the force rises quickly to a maximum and then decays slowly. If stimuli are applied at low rates, there is no net force accumulation. If the stimulus rate is increased so that the mean force-level accumulates, the force rises progressively, and it is described as a tetanus. If the individual twitch transients are still visible, the tetanus is known as an unfused tetanus, and if the force trace is entirely smooth, the tetanus is described as a fused tetanus. (**B**) Force-rate relations for different muscles: When a slowly contracting muscle such as the soleus is stimulated at different rates, the force begins to rise at relatively low rates, and the plot is a sigmoidal curve, demonstrating a maximal force arising at 20–30 pulses/s. For a fast-twitch muscle, the steep portion of the sigmoidal curve is moved significantly to the right of the plot, and may not be reached until rates of more than 10 pulses/s are applied. Maximal force values may not be reached until rates exceed 50 or 60 pulses/s.

characterized. Fig. 3C illustrates a typical force-velocity relationship drawn from mammalian skeletal muscle, showing that the decline in force (relative to the isometric state) is very steep, even at modest shortening velocities, indicating that the effect of movement on muscle-force generation is quite profound.

The form of the force–velocity relationship is given by the classic Hill equation, which shows that

$$(P + a)(V + b) = c \qquad (1)$$

where P is the load (in newtons), V is the shortening velocity (in mm/sec), and a, b, and c are constants.

Although the classical force-velocity relationships were described using muscle shortening against controlled loads, the converse relationship also applies, in that the maximum force generated falls steeply when muscle *velocity* is regulated by the experimenter. Although these force–velocity relationships may seem somewhat arcane, they are very important in regulating the speed of human movement, and they are ultimately limiting to motor performance.

2.2. Neural Excitation of Muscle

In the beginning of this chapter, we described the sequence of events lying between the neural excitation of muscle and the resulting force generation. We will now describe the relationship between the frequency of neural excitation and the resulting muscle force.

2.2.1. FORCE–FREQUENCY RELATIONS

When the motor axon is electrically activated by a single short pulse, or naturally by synaptic excitation of the motoneuron, a single action potential is transmitted from nerve to muscle, producing a transient increase in muscle force, described as the *muscle twitch*. There is a substantial delay between the arrival of the excitatory potential in the muscle, and the beginning of muscle-force generation. This delay is described as the *excitation contraction delay*, and it may reach 3–5 ms or more, depending on the type of muscle being examined. In all mammalian skeletal muscles, however, the twitch has a characteristic form, in which there is a relatively rapid rise from onset to peak force, and then a more gradual decay. This time to peak force—and time to half-peak force during the declining phase—vary greatly in different types of muscles, but the twitch is routinely asymmetric, with a more prolonged declining phase.

As shown in Fig. 4A, when muscle is activated repeatedly by a train of action potentials, the mean force level generated varies greatly with the rate of neural activation. When the excitation rate is sufficiently low, so that the force generated by the twitch has returned to baseline between each twitch, there is no net force increase, and the maximum force reached is simply that generated at the peak of each individual twitch. However, as the rate of stimulation is increased, the new nerve impulse arrives before the force generated by the previous twitch has completely dissipated. There is then force summation, and successive twitches generate a progressively increasing force level. This force level increases over the first few impulses, then reaches a plateau level that remains relatively constant for several seconds. When the individual twitches are still discernible, this plateau in force is described as a *partially fused tetanus*. When no individual twitch transients are evident, and the force trace is smooth, the response is described as a *fused tetanus*.

The practical implications of this force-frequency relationship are twofold. First, as shown in Fig. 4B, there is a nonlinear relationship between the stimulus rate at which motor axons are activated, and the resulting mean muscle force, although the effects of such rate increases vary in different kinds of muscle. The plot of this relationship is sigmoidal in shape. The example illustrated in Fig. 4 shows that at very low rates (usually between 3–6 impulses/s) significant relative increases in rate produce very little increase in mean force. However, after rates of 8–10 impulses/s are reached, increases in rate produce substantial increases in mean force, and this high sensitivity to increasing rate continues until relatively high rates are achieved. For one of the muscles illustrated in the figure, the rates may ultimately reach 30 or 40 pulses/s, but this rate varies widely in different kinds of muscles.

This nonlinear relationship between rate and force is extremely important, because it requires that the motor units must be activated at particular rates in order for muscle to be an optimally effective force generator. In most instances, the nervous system generates motoneuron discharge rates, which do indeed lie within the steeply rising portion of the sigmoidal relationship for each motor unit. However, although the form of the rate–force relationship is routinely sigmoidal, the exact magnitude and shape of the sigmoidal curve varies greatly for different types of muscle fibers. Slowly contracting muscle fibers reach the steep portion of their sigmoidal curve at relatively low discharge rates, whereas rapidly contracting fibers need more frequent neural activation to achieve a full tetanus. As a result, in rapidly contracting muscles, the sigmoidal relationship is moved to the right. In addition, the form of the force–rate relationship will change

for a muscle fibers as they become fatigued, or as they are activated repeatedly, and achieve a state known as *potentiation*, in which twitch size increases during repetitive activation.

The means by which the motoneuron rate is tuned to match the contractile properties of the associated muscle fibers is not entirely clear, although this "matching" must also be achieved acutely to accommodate the changing contractile properties of muscle fibers during repetitive activation. For example, in fatigue, the muscle-fiber contraction time and relaxation times slow substantially, meaning that lower motoneuron discharge rates are required to achieve maximal force. However, when other fibers are activated repeatedly, twitch size may increase, and contraction times may change as a result of potentiation.

3. MUSCLE RECEPTORS

3.1. Muscle Receptors: What is Transduced?

3.1.1. INTRODUCTION

Skeletal muscle contains several types of specialized receptors, and their properties, structure and functional contributions to movement regulation are now relatively well-understood. Fig. 5 illustrates the three main classes of muscle receptors in muscle—namely, muscle-spindle receptors, Golgi tendon organs, and free nerve endings.

3.1.2. MUSCLE-SPINDLE RECEPTORS

As shown in Fig. 5A, the *muscle spindle* consists of a cluster of slender muscle fibers, called *intrafusal fibers*, contained within a fluid-filled capsule. The muscle spindle lies adjacent to other regular muscle fibers and traverses the length of the muscle (or a substantial fraction of it), from the tendon of origin to the tendon of insertion. Because of this arrangement, the muscle spindle is said to lie "in parallel" with regular skeletal-muscle fibers. Under isometric conditions, active muscle-force increases, such as those mediated by neural excitation of muscle fibers, will elongate series elastic elements, including the tendon, and reduce tension on the spindle and on the spindle receptors, causing a *reduction in afferent discharge rate*. This force induced reduction of discharge is known as *unloading*, and it is often used as a test to distinguish muscle-spindle receptors from the in-series receptors, the tendon organ, which increases its discharge during active muscle-force increase.

The muscle spindle carries two kinds of specialized sensory terminals, and a dense and highly specialized

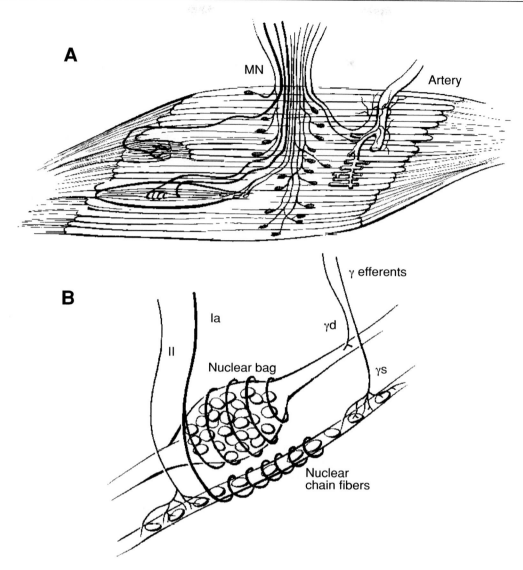

Fig. 5. Organization of muscle receptors: (**A**) Extrafusal muscle, with fibers reaching from the tendon at one end to the tendon of the other end. The motor innervation terminates as a motor point in which end-plates are distributed across the muscle. Two of the key encapsulated muscle-receptor organs are the muscle spindle and the tendon organ. The muscle spindle consists of an encapsulated structure in which small fibers, the intrafusal fibers, reach from tendon on one end to tendon on the other. Around the central portion of the spindle, there is a receptor terminal with an annulospiral structure known as the primary ending. In the polar regions of the spindle, there is a separate spindle innervation, known as the fusimotor innervation. (**B**) Expanded view of the intrafusal fibers and receptor terminals of the muscle spindle. The spindle contains large nuclear-bag fibers, which are characterized by a cluster of nuclei in the central or equatorial region. Other intrafusal fibers, called nuclear-chain fibers, have the nuclei arranged serially. The primary ending usually has an annulospiral appearance, in which the receptor is coiled around all of the intrafusal fibers. The secondary ending has a branched or coiled structure and is located more peripherally. Gamma efferent innervation (γ) is illustrated with gamma plates on the bag fiber and branching terminals on the chain.

efferent innervation. The structure of these receptor terminals is shown in Fig. 5B. There is a large, typically annulospiral-shaped ending, wrapped around the central portion of all intrafusal fibers in the spindle, and a smaller, often branching sensory terminal, which is located more peripherally, toward the polar regions of the spindle. Based on their differing responses to muscle-length increase, the first is known as the *primary ending*, and the other is the *secondary ending*.

Intrafusal fibers display specialized anatomical features, which separate them into two broad categories. A small fraction of the intrafusal fibers (usually only

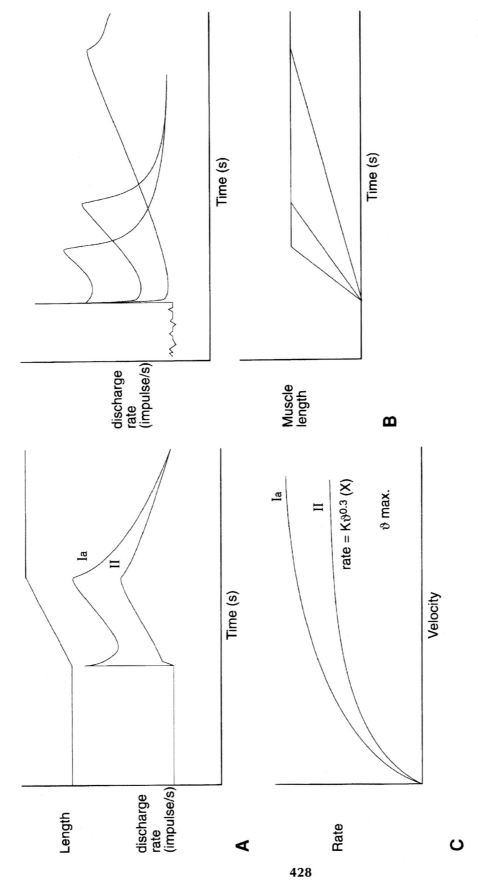

Fig. 6. (A) Responses of primary and secondary endings to constant-velocity stretch of a given amplitude: The primary ending shows a very steep, step-like increment in the discharge rate at the beginning of the stretch, terminating in a brief cluster of action potentials, emitted at a very high frequency. This is known as the initial burst. The rate increases progressively with increasing length, and then falls steeply at the end of the ramp of the plotted curve, returning to a substantially lower level. The secondary ending has a much smaller incremental increase at the beginning of the ramp of the curve, and may have a limited dynamic overshoot. **(B)** Velocity dependence of the primary ending discharge-rate: Three velocities are illustrated, but the discharge-rate increment changes modestly. **(C)** The rate increment changes modestly with increasing velocity. A 100-fold increase in stretch velocity produces a twofold to threefold increase in the discharge rate. The form of this correlation is that of a power function, with the velocity exponent ranging between 0.2 and 0.3. The graph also demonstrates that primary and secondary endings are scaled versions of each other.

428

1–2 in each spindle) show clusters of nuclei in the central or *equatorial* region of the fiber, and are known as *nuclear-bag fibers*. The majority of the intrafusal fibers are slender and elongated, with nuclei arraigned in chains. These are labeled as *nuclear-chain intrafusal fibers*. We now know that there are further subspecializations of these intrafusal fibers (e.g., bag_1 bag_2, long- and short-chain), but these distinctions are not essential to our understanding of spindle-receptor function at the present time.

The behavior of the muscle-spindle receptor appears to be governed primarily by the mechanical properties of the supporting intrafusal muscle fiber, although the intrinsic biophysical properties of the primary- and secondary-receptor terminal areas may also be somewhat different. Nuclear-bag fibers have little or no contractile material present in the equatorial regions where the nuclei are located. Instead, the contractile regions are confined to the intrafusal fiber poles. This has two consequences. First, if intrafusal fibers are stretched, the mechanical resistance exerted by the pole is likely to be different from that of the equatorial region, even at rest. Since the poles are more viscous in character, more rapid stretches would extend the equatorial regions disproportionately, because the poles would be more resistant to stretch under these conditions. Because the primary ending terminals are located mainly around the equatorial regions, more rapid muscle stretches will impact the receptor terminals to a greater extent.

A second way in which intrafusal structure impacts spindle-receptor behavior is that efferent spindle innervation, which activates the polar regions of the muscle spindle, will produce increased force and shortening of the polar regions, at the expense of the more elastic equatorial zone. This is especially likely in the bag fibers, which appear to have the greatest difference between the mechanical properties of poles and equator. Although the nuclear-chain fiber shows less structural inhomogeneity, mechanical observations indicate that the polar regions may also be somewhat less stiff than the equatorial zones in these fibers. These differences in the structural and mechanical properties of the polar region may help to explain the different responses of primary and secondary endings to muscle stretch.

Figure 6 illustrates the different responses of primary and secondary spindle-receptor afferent fibers to constant velocity stretches of the receptor-bearing muscle, beginning at a relatively short length. The primary spindle afferent shows a substantial increase of discharge during the dynamic phase of stretch, and this discharge rate drops to a much lower level when a new constant length is achieved. This appearance is broadly comparable to that of a velocity sensor, which would be expected to increase its output substantially during the dynamic phase of stretch, where the velocity reaches a constant level, and to drop the output substantially when the velocity falls to zero. In contrast, the secondary-spindle afferent is much less influenced by the speed of the stretch, and appears to follow the length changes more closely, displaying relatively little dynamic overshoot during the ramp stretch.

When characterized in this fashion, it is possible to attribute predominant *velocity* sensitivity to muscle-spindle primary receptors, and predominant *length* sensitivity to the secondary endings. In fact, a more extensive comparison of the impact of different stretch velocities on various receptor types as shown in Fig. 6B,C indicates that primary or secondary endings are not especially sensitive to stretch velocity, since a hundredfold increase in stretch velocity induces only a two- to threefold increase in discharge rate in either type of receptor. Furthermore, the relative increase in discharge with increasing velocity is quite comparable between the two classes of receptors, presumably reflecting the similarities in mechanical properties of intrafusal fibers that support both receptor types.

3.1.3. DEPENDENCE OF SPINDLE-RECEPTOR AFFERENT DISCHARGE ON STRETCH AMPLITUDE

The response of the spindle receptor is also strongly influenced by the amplitude of stretch. Indeed, stretches of 100–200-μm amplitude produce disproportionately large increases in discharge rate, which would be unsustainable if continued over many millimeters of length change. This high-sensitivity region is frequently called the *small signal* region, and is responsible for the so-called *initial burst*, which is visible at the very beginning of a large-amplitude, constant velocity stretch (*see* Fig. 6A). This high-sensitivity "small signal" response is also visible during other kinds of length stimuli, such as sinusoidal or square wavelength change, and it is noteworthy in that the behavior of spindles in this region is essentially linear, which means that spindle afferent discharge-rate scales with increasing stretch amplitude and velocity.

3.1.4. EFFERENT INNERVATION OF THE MUSCLE SPINDLE

As outlined earlier, and illustrated in Fig. 7, all muscle spindles receive several types of efferent, or motor, innervation. This efferent innervation, which is

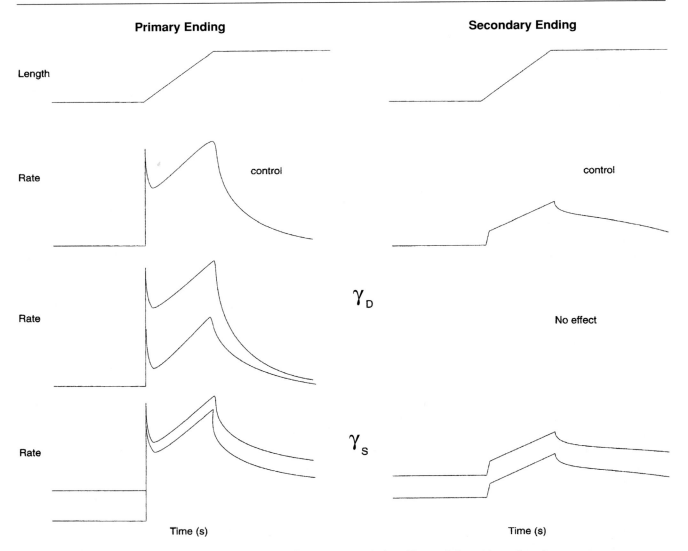

Fig. 7. Fusimotor effects on spindle afferents. This figure compares the effects of dynamic and static gamma motor neuron stimulation on primary and secondary muscle-spindle afferents exposed to similar stretches. The second panel (*from the top*) on each side illustrates the control responses of primary and secondary endings, without added fusimotor input. Stimulation by gamma efferents of bag fibers produces a substantial increase in the dynamic response without a significant change in the initial and final firing rates. The dynamic motor neurons are known as gamma$_d$ fibers. The efferent innervation of the chain fibers enhances the length sensitivity and discharge rate of both the primary and secondary endings. Because both initial and final or plateau rates are increased by gamma neuron stimulation, with little or no effect during the dynamic phase, this static efferent innervation is known as gamma$_s$.

broadly described as *fusimotor* innervation, arises from small motoneurons in the ventral horn, via small-diameter, slowly conducting myelinated fibers, known as γ fibers. Alternatively, the efferent innervation may come from branches of regular, large-diameter skeletomotor fibers, displaying more rapid-fiber conduction velocity. These larger fusimotor fibers are referred to as β, or *skeletofusimotor* fibers because they originate from branches of regular motoneuron efferents.

The actions of these two types of innervation (e.g., γ and β) on the muscle spindle are known to be broadly comparable, and are not discussed further here. Yet the relative use of these pathways is undoubtedly quite different, given their differing cellular origins, and the likely difference in recruitment and rate behavior of the originating spinal neurons.

The effect of the fusimotor innervation on spindle afferent discharge depends essentially on the particular intrafusal fiber that is innervated. Those fusimotor efferents that innervate bag fibers enhance the dynamic responsiveness of the primary endings, because these endings are present on the bag fiber; thus, they are described as γ_d (or β_d) dynamic fibers. However, fusimotor fibers that innervate nuclear-chain fibers enhance both the length, sensitivit, and static background discharge rate of *both* primary and secondary endings. For this reason, they are described as static fusimotor (again, γ_s or β_s fibers).

Figure 7 illustrates the different responses elicited by activating one or another class of fusimotor efferent fibers individually. (Of course, this situation is unlikely to take place in life, because both types of efferents are normally activated together). Nonetheless, activation of individual fusimotor γ_d fibers shows that primarily spindle-ending responses increase substantially, and γ_s activation produces changes mainly during the constant length, or isometric phase, of muscle extension.

3.1.5. Muscle Afferent Recordings in Intact Subjects

In recent years, several methods that allow recording of afferent discharge in essentially intact, unanesthetized animal and human subjects have been developed. These include recordings from dorsal-root afferents in the cat using fine wire electrodes, dorsal-root ganglion recordings in the cat and monkey using sharp pin-like electrodes, and intraneural (or microneurographic) recordings in human subjects with insulated tungsten electrodes. The dorsal-root and dorsal-ganglion recordings in the cat have revealed the patterns of afferent discharge in a range of motor behaviors, including stance and locomotion, and the human studies have allowed accurate quantification of spindle afferent discharge during changing voluntary force, and during voluntary movements of controlled velocity.

In many of these studies, a consistent pattern of spindle afferent excitation has been shown, in which motoneurons are activated broadly in concert with spindle afferent rate increases, suggesting that fusimotor activity increases with increasing skeletomotor activity. In many experiments in which α and γ discharge is recorded simultaneously, γ neurons appear to be largely activated before skeletomotor (e.g., α)activity begins, so that by the time extrafusal muscle-fiber activation takes place, large-scale activation of γ fibers has already occurred, giving rise to "α-γ coactivation." At the present time, the rules governing the activation of fusimotor neurons are not entirely clear, although it

has been demonstrated that fusimotor (e.g., γ) neurons may sometimes be activated without concurrent activation of α motoneurons. Whether the capacity to independently control fusimotor and skeletomotor activation exists (e.g., spinal motoneurons) has not yet been determined.

Studies from intact human subjects have revealed important details on afferent discharge during voluntary muscle contraction in either isometric contractions, or during slow movements. Such studies, which have been performed in muscles of both the upper and lower limbs of human subjects, have the capacity to define the relationship between fusimotor and skeletomotor activation more thoroughly than is possible in animal models, because of the voluntary cooperation provided by the human subjects. These human studies have shown that there is substantial variation in the level of fusimotor input during most naturally occurring movements, and that this fusimotor input is quite powerful in its effects on spindle afferent discharge.

As shown in Fig. 8, during voluntary isometric contraction, the discharge rate of muscle-spindle afferents increases substantially, reaching a level much greater than that recorded at rest. In most of these studies, the impact of γ-efferent innervation to the spindle is difficult to determined, because increasing force will induce elongation of tendon and other series of elastic components, allowing internal spindle shortening to occur. This elongation offsets fusimotor action, at least in some degree. However, the finding (illustrated in Fig. 8A) that the afferent discharge rate increases during force increase indicates that fusimotor input is more than able to offset the change in length series elastic elements. In addition, when muscle activation produces voluntary shortening, muscle-spindle discharge rates may fall very little, provided that the rate of muscle shortening is modest; (*see* Fig. 8C).

As a whole, these studies have shown that primary muscle-spindle afferents are strongly activated during voluntary contraction, that this activation is very strong at the lowest force levels, and that it may then increase relatively little with increasing force. This fusimotor activation can compensate for muscle-fiber shortening to a large degree, except when muscle shortening is rapid.

Finally, with respect to the type of fusimotor input activated in various movements, studies of both human and animal models also suggest that γ-dynamic and γ-static fusimotor activation takes place together,

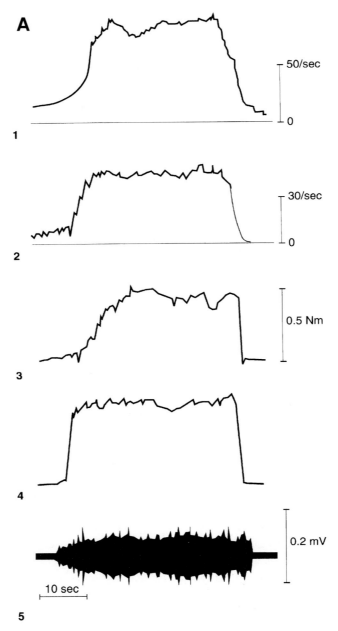

Fig. 8. (*Above and opposite page*) Response of human muscle-spindle afferents during voluntary contraction: (**A**) Response of a primary ending in a finger flexor during isometric contraction. *Panel 1* shows the afferent firing rate; *Panels 2 through 4* show the torque increase; and *Panel 5* shows the associated electromyographic (EMG) response. The afferent rate increases steeply, even before there has been a significant increase in torque or EMG activity. The fact that the afferent rate increases sharply and is sustained even with progressive force increase indicates that a substantial increase in fusimotor activity must have taken place to offset tendon elongation and the associated internal shortening of the spindle. (**B**) Torque rate relations: The responses of one primary and two secondary endings illustrate that the discharge rate increases modestly but significantly with increasing isometric torque. (**C**) Response of muscle-spindle afferent (nerve) from a finger flexor during a slow voluntary shortening. The visual target for movement is the command trace. The next series of traces (joint angle) depicts the sequence of actual movements. The plots labeled nerve are raster plots, in which the occurrence of an action potential appears as a dot. The lowest panel is a histogram, summarizing mean firing of the afferent during each phase of movement. Under conditions of slow voluntary motion, the fusimotor input to a muscle spindle may be sufficient to offset the muscle-length change. In this sequence of voluntary movements, the recording of muscle-spindle primary afferent responses is shown as a raster diagram. The response during the shortening and plateau phases is somewhat higher than that during the initial static or hold phase. However, the rate changes are modest, indicating the efferent innervation is able to compensate almost exactly for the change in muscle length.

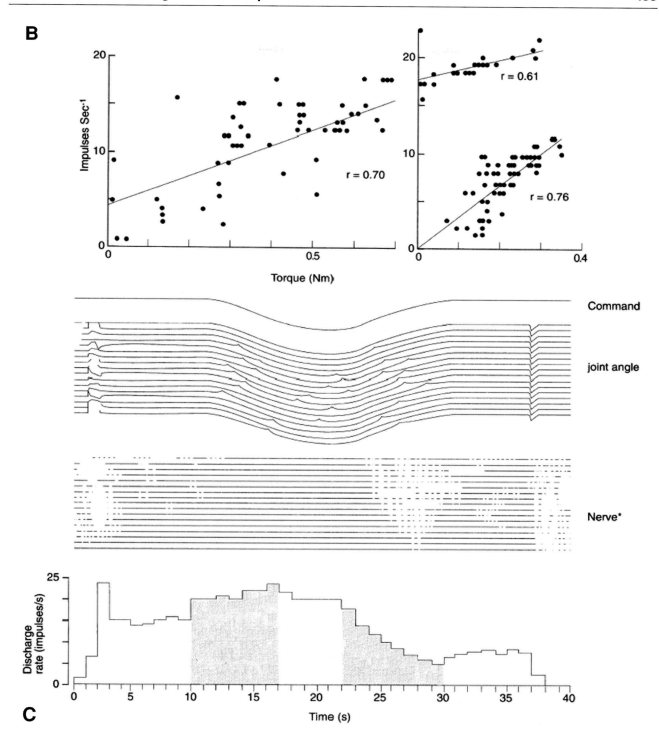

although the possibility that there may be independent activation of γ_d-dynamic and γ_s-static fibers under some naturally occurring conditions may exist.

3.1.6. SUMMARY

The mode of operation of fusimotor input to muscle spindles and its functional role are a matter of continu-ing debate; however, it is likely that at least some of the following functions are fulfilled.

1. γ_s activation takes up the slack in muscle spindles, allowing both primary and secondary endings to respond sensitively to added small length changes. This raises the possibility that with the help of

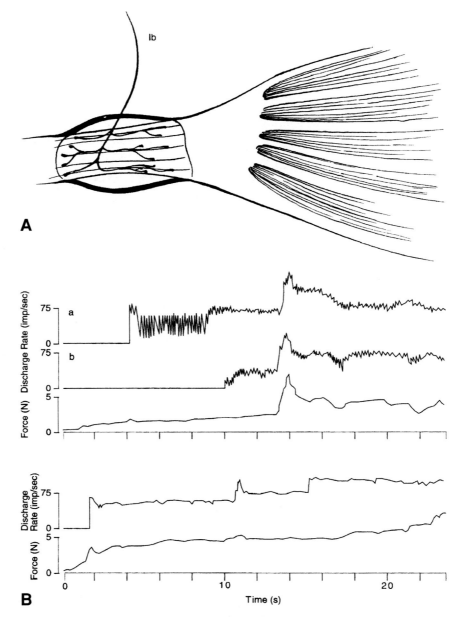

Fig. 9. (*Above and opposite page*) (**A**) Expanded view of a Golgi tendon organ, showing the encapsulated receptor area around the tendon fascicles and the limited number of muscle fibers attached to those collagen fascicles. (**B**) The sequence of activation of the two tendon organs was recorded from the same soleus muscle in a decerebrated cat preparation. Although the thresholds of the two receptors are somewhat different and the initial discharge rates are variable, the rates become quite smooth and follow accurately the minor fluctuations in force after a significant force level is achieved. (**C**) There is a straight-line relationship between reflexively generated static isometric force and the discharge rate. The relationship is not strictly linear, because there is a non-zero intercept on the ordinate. (**D**) The graph summarizes the relationship of a population of tendon organ afferents; the data was drawn from the soleus muscle in different preparations.

fusimotor input, spindle receptors are able to maintain a broad dynamic range, yet are still able to respond sensitively to small length perturbations.

2. Fusimotor innervation (either γ and/or β in type) may serve to match muscle spindles to the chang-

ing mechanical properties of muscle. For example, muscle becomes stiffer and more viscous as its level of activation increases. It is conceivable that efferent innervation to the spindle adjusts the mechanical properties of the intrafusal fibers to

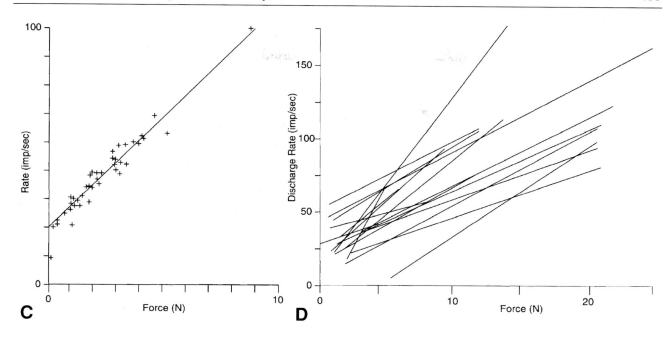

optimize the pattern of spindle response to compensate for these altered mechanical muscle properties.

3. γ_d input induces a substantial increase in the dynamic spindle response during muscle stretch, but has much less effect during muscle shortening. These effects may be important in providing appropriate asymmetry of reflex action in the stretch and release of muscle.

3.2. Golgi Tendon Organs as Force Transducers

3.2.1. STRUCTURE–FUNCTION RELATIONSHIP OF THE TENDON ORGAN

As illustrated in Fig. 9A, the tendon organ is an encapsulated receptor, which consists of a branching nerve terminal, interwoven with collagen and elastic fibers lying between a group of muscle fibers and the tendon proper. The tendon organ lies "in-series" with this small cluster of muscle fibers, and it is therefore subjected to mechanical strain when these muscle fibers are active.

3.2.2. ENCODER MECHANISMS

We do not yet precisely know the means by which muscle force is transduced by the tendon-organ receptor, but it is likely to be mediated by regional strain on nerve terminals, as they are compressed among the tendinous fascicles. It is also important to note that the tendon organ is not located within the body of the tendon itself, but within the muscle, at the muscle fiber-tendon boundary. Furthermore, tendon organs may be scattered through many muscles in regions quite distant from the tendon, although their locations are often near collagenous tissue planes.

3.2.3. TENDON ORGAN RESPONSES TO MUSCLE-FORCE CHANGE

Tendon organs are excited most readily by active force increases, such as those produced by neural activation of muscle, rather than by passive muscle force increases, such as those induced by muscle stretch. Typically, under conditions of physiological activation, tendon-organ discharge increases more or less proportionately with increasing force, and the tendon-organ will follow changes in force quite closely.

Fig. 9B shows a typical sequence of excitation of two different tendon organs, showing that each begins to discharge at a particular threshold force, and their rate increases irregularly at low forces, depending upon the recruitment of particular muscle fibers belonging to the subset of fibers attached to the tendon-organ receptor. Once many muscle fibers are active, the impact of added muscle-fiber activity on tendon-organ discharge is diminished, and the discharge rate of the tendon organs follows the changing force quite accurately.

Although recordings of tendon-organ afferents in intact conscious animal or human models are relatively rare, a number of studies have shown that tendon-organ activity in physiologically activated muscle closely reflects instantaneous muscle force recorded at the

Table 1
Muscle Afferent Nerve Fiber Diameters and Conduction Velocities

Type of afferent	Mean nerve fiber diameter (μm)	Mean nerve fiber conduction velocity (m/s)	Functional roles of afferents
Group I	15	90	Primary muscle spindle endings (Ia)
Group II	8	48	Golgi tendon organs (Ib) Secondary spindle endings
Group III	4	24	Free nerve endings, myelinated
Group IV	<1	1	Free nerve endings; unmyelinated

tendon, with relatively little sensitivity to the rate of change of muscle force. This pattern of response is summarized in Fig. 9C, which shows that rate of tendon-organ discharge increases linearly with increasing force over much of the force range, although the force-rate relationship often displays an upward convexity at higher forces. This relative linearity and sensitivity of the tendon-organ response is unexpected, because the numbers of muscle fibers sampled by any tendon organ are relatively small; typically 12–16 muscle fibers/tendon organs in large limb muscles of the cat (*see* Fig. 9A). Despite this rather limited sample, the response patterns of individual tendon organ are surprisingly close to the force variations of the whole muscle, as registered at the tendon (*see* Fig. 9B), except at very low forces, when only one or two of the muscle fibers attached to the tendon organ may have been activated.

3.3. Other Muscle Mechanoreceptors

The major muscle-spindle and tendon-organ afferents usually constitute less than 50% of the total sensory innervation from a typical muscle, as estimated from the total number of afferent fibers in the muscle nerve. There is also a substantial population of unmyelinated fibers in the nerve, and their receptor terminals have the appearance of free nerve endings, which are distributed throughout the muscle, including the muscle and tendon surfaces. These afferent fibers show differing conduction velocities, including a few belonging to the most rapidly conducting afferent fiber group (group I). However, in most cases these free-nerve-ending afferents exhibit conduction velocities of small myelinated (group III) and group IV fibers (which are largely unmyelinated). Although some of these afferent fibers arise from specialized nerve ter-

minals such as Pacinian corpuscles, most of them originate in free nerve endings, which have no discernible specialized terminal structure on light microscopy.

Although the nerve terminals of free nerve endings are not visibly specialized structurally on light microscopy, they do exhibit a range of functional specialization. Some terminals are responsive to nociceptive input, and others respond primarily to mechanical stimuli, such as pressure or tension, although with much less sensitivity than the encapsulated receptors (spindle and tendon organs) described previously. Some other small afferents arise from receptors that respond to thermal and metabolic changes in the muscle, which may indicate that they play a role in cardiovascular and neuromuscular responses to exercise, as well as in neuromuscular compensation for fatigue.

4. AFFERENT PATHWAYS TO THE SPINAL CORD

4.1. Afferent Classification

As summarized in Table 1, muscle afferents display a range of diameters and conduction velocities. The most rapidly conducting fibers, which are also those with largest diameter (group I) typically conduct at velocities of up to 100 *M*/s or more. In the cat, in which such fibers are most extensively studied, conduction velocities and diameters are well-established and primary endings afferent conduction velocities may reach 120 *M*/s. Secondary spindle afferents conduct at velocities ranging from 24–72 *M*/s and small myelinated and unmyelinated fibers from skin and muscle (group III and IV) from less than 1 *M*/s to 24 *M*/s. Conduction boundaries for the various fiber populations are not as well-defined in man, and in particular, there is no clearly defined conduction velocity boundary between primary and secondary spindle afferents.

4.2. Central Connections and Central Projections of Afferent Pathways

Sensory fibers enter the spinal cord primarily through the spinal dorsal roots, although a small number of unmyelinated nerve fibers, are recognized, and even a few myelinated fibers that enter through the ventral roots. The anatomical distribution of the major afferent pathways within the spinal cord is well-known, and is described in more detail in an earlier Chapter 9.

As shown in Fig. 10, large myelinated muscle afferents (groups I and II) entering through the dorsal roots tend to segregate medially as they enter the spinal cord, and then travel ventrally through medial portions of the dorsal spinal gray matter before diverging to make synaptic connections with neurons in the intermediate spinal gray matter and ventral horn. Some fibers terminate by making synaptic connections on regional interneurons, and others continue on to make synaptic connections directly with motoneurons in the ventral horn.

Small myelinated (A δ and unmyelinated (C) fibers make synaptic connections with neurons in dorsal gray matter, including the most superficial regions of spinal gray, known as lamina I, which is largely involved with the processing of pain-related or "nociceptive" information (*see* Fig. 10A). Other mechanoreceptor group III and IV afferents project to deeper regions of the dorsal gray (lamina IV, V) before they are propagated to other spinal and supraspinal sensory systems.

4.3. Spinal Circuitry

Muscle afferent information is relayed to interneurons in the dorsal horn or intermediate gray, or to motoneurons in ventral gray matter, with either monosynaptic or oligosynaptic connections in each location. The majority of the interneuronal elements of the spinal cord have not been fully identified in mammalian preparations. Only a small number of different interneuron types have been characterized, primarily because of the availability of specific and practical diagnostic electrophysiological tests.

4.3.1. GENERAL FEATURES OF SPINAL INFORMATION PROCESSING

Cutaneous and muscle afferent information follows several routes in the nervous system. Large myelinated afferents enter the spinal cord via the dorsal roots, and then may follow one of two distinct paths.

Large myelinated afferents from the skin, muscles, or joints may branch to send the fibers into dorsal column and dorsolateral column white matter, where they may travel rostrally for many centimeters. (Some of these large afferents may re-enter dorsal gray matter in proximal segments, where they may synapse with regional neurons, with new postsynaptic fibers re-entering dorsal and dorsolateral columns). A small number of fibers may traverse dorsal white matter without relay all the way to dorsal-column nuclei (gracile and cuneate). Muscle afferents in particular may circumvent gracile and cuneate relays and may make a separate relay in the brainstem, (although this relay has not yet been shown to be important in primates). The fibers from gracile, cuneate, and the brainstem muscle afferent relay nuclei then pass to higher centers, including the thalamus, cerebellum, and eventually, the cortex. The alternative afferent destination is directly to interneuronal and motoneuronal circuits, as described previously.

Muscle Ia afferents make extensive monosynaptic connections with virtually all motoneurons that innervate the muscle from which the spindle afferents originate (e.g., the homonymous motoneuron pool), and with many motoneurons from nearby synergists. The result is extensive divergence of afferents to many motoneurons, and extensive convergence of Ia afferents onto individual motoneurons.

4.3.2. SPINAL INTERNEURONAL SYSTEMS

Spinal interneurons are defined largely on anatomical grounds. Interneurons are simply neurons whose axons extend relatively short distances within the cord, usually no more than a few spinal segments. The cell bodies of these neurons are usually of small diameter, less than 50 μm, and many neurons are even smaller. Although muscle afferents from muscle spindles (primary and secondary spindle afferents) make some direct, or *monosynaptic* connections with spinal motoneurons in the ventral horn, almost all afferents—including those from primary and secondary endings—make their first synaptic connections with neurons in dorsal or intermediate spinal gray matter.

4.3.3. INTERNEURONAL INFORMATION PROCESSING

Interneurons are an important component of spinal information processing, because they perform several important computational operations. Fig. 10B illustrates the most common types of operation performed by interneurons. The most common computational operation is a *sign change* (e.g., inhibition) in which, for example, an afferent originating from muscle or skin produces synaptic excitation at the first synaptic

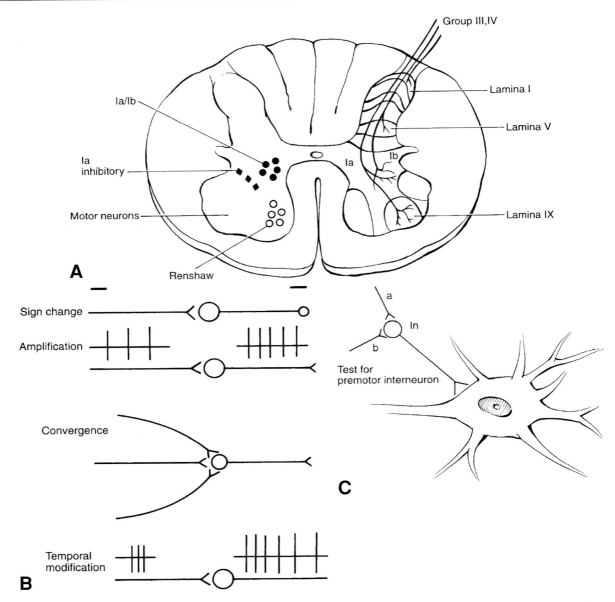

Fig. 10. (A) Interneuronal circuitry and afferent connections of the spinal cord: The spinal cord gray matter is composed of a variety of neurons that have specialized features demonstrated on light microscopy. These features have been used to classify the regions of the gray matter into the twelve laminae, with lamina I located more superficially in the dorsal gray matter. These laminae are useful for describing the preferred destination for particular classes of muscle afferent fibers. Large-diameter muscle afferents (e.g., Ia and Ib) travel medially through dorsal gray matter. Ib fibers terminate in the intermediate gray matter in laminae V through VII. Group Ia fibers may emit collaterals before proceeding into the ventral horn toward laminae IX, the location of spinal motor neurons. The cross-sectional drawing shows the major neuronal elements of the spinal cord, including spinal motor neurons, Renshaw interneurons located medial to the motor neuron core, Ia inhibitory interneurons, and Ia and Ib inhibitory interneuronal groups located dorsal or medial to the to the motor neuron pool. **(B)** Types of computational operations performed by spinal interneurons: The most common operation is a sign change, in which an excitatory input, such as an afferent, activates an inhibitory interneuron, which induces inhibition at its postsynaptic sites. Interneurons can amplify their input by transforming a low-frequency input train to a high-frequency output. Interneurons may also integrate spatially by means of a convergence of afferent inflow from different sources onto a particular interneuron. They may also induce changes in the temporal pattern, such as changing a transient input consisting of a few impulses into long-lasting discharge. **(C)** Key factors underlying a commonly used test for a premotor interneuron. Activation of afferent a or b individually may not be sufficient to cause the interneuron to reach the threshold, and the subsequent synapse at the neuron reveals no synaptic potential. However, if a and b are activated simultaneously, the interneuron is recruited, and postsynaptic potentials are manifested in the spinal motor neuron.

relay, then activates an inhibitory interneuron, producing inhibition at subsequent postsynaptic sites.

Excitatory interneurons may also act to *amplify information* received from the periphery, or they may change the *spatial distribution* of this information by virtue of the pattern of divergence of their nerve terminals. Interneurons may also change the time-course and the frequency content of incoming signals, by *filtering* out high frequencies or by providing *integrator* types of operations. Interneurons may provide other signal processing, such as *reshaping* or changing the transmitted signal from a step to a more transient or pulse-like response.

Because the input from a single afferent is sometimes modest, it may be necessary to combine the input from several sources to reach the interneuron threshold. A single afferent fiber input may not elicit a interneuron response by itself, but may reach neuron threshold when two or more afferent inputs are excited simultaneously. Furthermore, if these afferent sources are widely dispersed, the interneuron may serve to integrate spatial information as well.

As shown in Fig. 10C, the subliminal effect of single afferents on interneurons is useful as a diagnostic test for the existence of an interneuron in a projection pathway from afferent to motoneuron. For example, an interneuron is believed to be present when activation of an individual afferent pathway (such as a peripheral nerve) gives rise *no* synaptic potential in a motoneuron, yet simultaneous activation of two afferent inputs does induce a visible synaptic potential [which could be either an excitatory postsynaptic potential (EPSP) or inhibitory postsynaptic potential (IPSP)].

Alternatively, some interneurons are specialized for spinal relay; these are known as *propriospinal neurons*. Finally, others may promote *rhythm generation*, especially in the more proximal lumbar spinal segments, where they may contribute to the cyclical motoneuron excitation that takes place as part of locomotion.

In summary, the primary role of interneurons appears to be as summing or integrating elements, in which convergent input from a variety of sources, sometimes including differing sensory modalities, is integrated and passed onto the next step of information processing.

4.3.4. Transmitter Systems

Most interneurons are inhibitory in their postsynaptic effects, and release inhibitory transmitters such as glycine or GABA from their presynaptic terminals.

Others are excitatory, presumably releasing glutamate, aspartate, or other excitatory amino acids from their presynaptic terminals. The effects of these various transmitters are described in more detail elsewhere in this volume.

4.3.5. Actions of Identified Interneurons

Most of the interneuronal systems of the mammalian spinal cord are not fully identified, and those interneurons that are named are not necessarily the most important. This is because interneuron naming is often arbitrary, and frequently depends on some distinctive electrophysiological feature (such as the neuron response to synchronous antidromic ventral-root stimulation), which may have little relationship to the interneuron's functional roles.

Some of the named spinal interneurons are:
1. Ia inhibitory.
2. Renshaw.
3. Ia/Ib inhibitory.
4. II Excitatory.
5. Presynaptic inhibitory.

4.3.5.1. Renshaw Neurons (Figs. 10A,11A).
Identification of interneurons has been based upon a variety of circumstantial electrophysiological findings, which may either be unrelated or only obliquely related to the functional role of these interneuronal systems. For example, Renshaw interneurons, which are small interneurons located in the ventral horn medial to the spinal motor nuclei, display a unique, high-frequency bursting discharge following antidromic excitation of spinal motor axons in the ventral root. These interneurons receive excitatory input from motor axon collaterals, and make synapses on regional spinal motoneurons.

The transmitter released at the motoneuron axon collaterals to Renshaw neurons is acetylcholine, which is to be expected, because this transmitter is also released at the other terminal branches of the motor axon at the neuromuscular junction. The cholinergic postsynaptic receptors on the Renshaw neuron are *muscarinic* and *nicotinic* in type. Antidromic excitation of the Renshaw neuron is only partly impaired by separate administration of nicotinic or muscarinic acetylcholine antagonists, but essentially eliminated by the simultaneous administration of both cholinergic blockers. For example, combinations of cholinergic nicotinic antagonists (such as mecamylamine, and dihydro β erythroidine) and muscarinic antagonists (such as atropine) produce a severe reduction of anti-

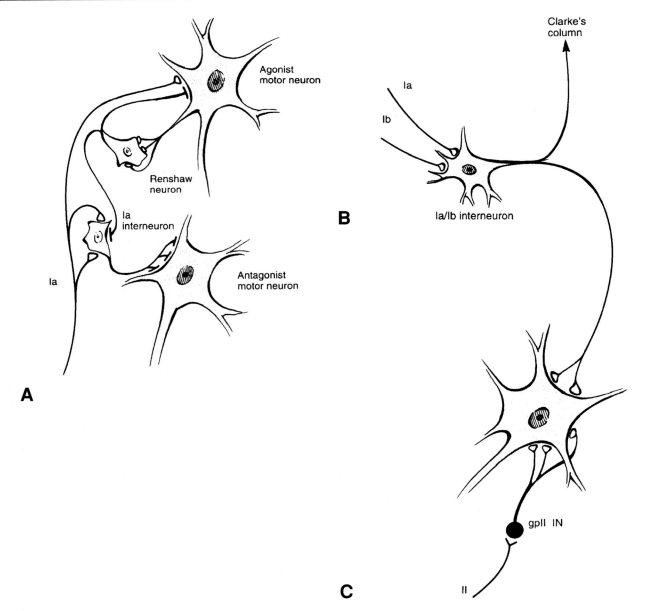

Fig. 11. Types of spinal interneurons. (**A**) This important circuit involves linkages among motor neurons and flexor and extensor muscle groups associated in interneuron pools. Flexor motor neurons produce collaterals that innervate and excite Renshaw interneurons. Renshaw axons may inhibit the originating motor neuron, the flexor, and the Ia inhibitory interneuron. The Ia inhibitory interneuron receives Ia afferent input from a flexor, which induces excitation of that flexor motor neuron. Activation of the Ia inhibitory interneuron inhibits the antagonist extensor motor neuron. Excitatory synaptic terminals are drawn as enclosed circles, and the inhibitory terminals are presented as bars. (**B**) The convergence of Ia and Ib afferents on an inhibitory interneuron inhibits the activity of a typical extensor motor neuron. The Ia and Ib interneurons also project to Clarke's column, which is the nucleus of origin of the dorsal spinocerebellar tract. (**C**) Group II afferents excite an interneuron, located in the proximal lumbar segments of the cord, which induces excitation of motor neurons in the lower lumbosacral segments.

dromically elicited Renshaw activity, confirming the diversity of postsynaptic cholinergic receptor types on the Renshaw neuron.

Axons of Renshaw neurons make synaptic connections with regional motoneurons as well as other inter-neurons, including Renshaw neurons of other motor neuron pools and regional Ia inhibitory interneurons. The transmitter released by Renshaw axon terminals is believed to be glycine, a naturally occurring amino acid. There has been some suggestion that GABA may also be released at Renshaw terminals, but this has not been independently verified.

4.3.5.2. Ia Inhibitory Interneuron (Figs. 10,11).

Another well-described interneuron is the *Ia inhibitory interneuron*. This interneuron is identified by the findings that it receives monosynaptic excitatory input from Ia afferents in one muscle, and then makes inhibitory synaptic connections to motoneurons of opposing, or antagonist, muscles. By virtue of these connections, the Ia interneuron is believed to promote *reciprocal innervation*, in which agonists and antagonists acting about a joint are prevented from being active simultaneously.

Although the functional role and utility of Ia inhibitory interneurons is relatively easy to comprehend, the identification of these interneurons is circumstantial, and depends upon the fact that they are inhibited by antidromic ventral-root excitation, apparently through Renshaw neurons. In other words, an interneuron activated by Ia afferents of a particular muscle but silenced by ventral-root stimulation, meets the necessary defining criteria.

The transmitter released at Ia interneuron axon terminals is believed to be *glycine*, for which no highly specific antagonists currently exist. Nonspecific antagonist effects are mediated by the agent strychnine, but the strychnine effects are not localized, and in fact may impact many synaptic locations within the CNS.

4.3.5.3. Ia/Ib Interneurons (Figs. 10,11).

Golgi tendon-organ afferents (identified as Ib afferents) are known to make synaptic relays in intermediate gray matter of the spinal cord, producing autogenetic inhibition of homonymous or synergist motoneurons. It is now apparent that these interneurons, which were originally called Ib, also receive muscle afferent input from Ia spindle-receptor afferents, making their integrative function more complex than originally perceived. Nonetheless, the major driving input is still primarily from Golgi tendon organs, which raises the possibility of a *force regulatory action* of this interneuronal system.

These interneurons also project to Clark's column neurons, which lie in proximal lumbar segments and give rise to axons that traverse the dorsal spinocerebellar tract. The existence of an inhibitory connection from muscle Ib afferents, via the Ib inhibitory interneuron to homonymous and other synergist motoneurons, raises the possibility of a closed-loop force regulator, in which force increases sensed by tendon organs give rise to inhibition of homonymous moto-

neurons. This force regulation has been difficult to demonstrate as a practical entity, because those animal preparations that allow study of intact-reflex spinal pathways, such as the decerebrate cat model, show substantial suppression of many segmental inhibitory interneuronal systems, including the Ia/Ib inhibitory pathway.

Several studies performed in man have provided indirect evidence for the operation of a force regulator. These studies have utilized fatigue as the test probe to evaluate force-feedback compensation, relying on the fact that fatigue induces a substantial short-term loss of muscle contractile force. However, although fatigue is the most common source of a loss of force-generating capacity, there are also likely to be substantial changes in afferent inflow from several types of muscle receptors, which may exaggerate the degree of responsiveness of the Ib pathway, as compared with the normal. Specifically, muscle fatigue induces changes in muscle temperature, pH, and metabolic state, all of which may change the spontaneous discharge patterns, and the mechanical responsiveness of group III and IV muscle afferents. Since free-nerve-ending afferents, and Ia and Ib afferents may all converge on the same set of Ib interneurons, alterations in the baseline discharge of group III and IV afferents might well alter the responsiveness of the Ib pathway.

4.3.5.4. Group II Excitatory Interneurons (Figs. 10,11).

Recently, an extended series of studies has demonstrated that interneurons exist that receive selective input from secondary-spindle afferents, which make excitatory synaptic connections to lumbosacral spinal motoneurons, and which are located in proximal lumbar spinal cord segments of the cat. The functional role of this interneuronal system is not yet understood, although interneuronal structural and electrophysiological properties and connections appear to be clearly defined.

4.3.5.5. Flexion Reflex Pathways.

There is (as yet) no uniquely identified set of interneurons involved in flexion reflexes. It is apparent that many of the interneurons located in the intermediate gray matter of the spinal cord and in deeper laminae are involved in processing information from cutaneous, subcutaneous sensory endings, and from high-threshold muscle afferents, especially those of smaller diameter (groups II, III, and IV). Excitation of any of these afferents often results in a coordinated pattern of flexor-muscle activation. Although the range of afferent input eliciting flexion reflexes is diverse, the ultimate effect is relatively stereotyped, in that activation of many of these afferent systems induces consistent excitation of flexors and inhibition of extensor muscles, primarily via the Ia inhibitory interneuronal system.

The individual neuronal elements of the flexion withdrawal reflex system are not clearly separable, and there appears to be an extensive polysynaptic chain involving multiple relay sites. The transmitters of such systems are also not clearly identified, although the excitatory synaptic connections are likely to be mediated by excitatory amino acids (glutamate and aspartate), and it is likely that GABA plays an important role in mediating inhibition.

4.3.5.6. Presynaptic Inhibitory Interneurons.
There are also known to be interneurons located in dorsal gray matter of the cord, which terminate on presynaptic terminals of afferents and of other interneurons. These interneurons release GABA, which depolarizes presynaptic terminals and reduces the amount of transmitter released by each incoming action potential. This reduction of transmitter release is mediated by reducing the amount of calcium that enters the terminal with the arrival of each action potential.

5. MOTONEURONS AND THE MOTONEURON POOL

5.1. Introduction

The physiology of CNS neurons began with the study of spinal motoneurons, primarily by John Eccles and colleagues in Canberra, Australia in the 1950s and 1960s. For many years, the motoneuron was the prototype for the study of central neurons, and it still remains one of the most extensively studied neurons in the mammalian nervous system.

5.2. Definitions

A spinal motoneuron (*see* Fig. 12) is the neuron that directly innervates skeletal muscle, primarily via axons traversing the ventral roots. All of the motoneurons innervating a given muscle are together termed the *motoneuron pool* (*see* Fig. 11). Each motor axon innervates a group of muscle fibers in the muscle. The motoneuron, together with the innervated muscle

fibers, is called the *motor unit*. The group of muscle fibers innervated by one motor axon is known as the *muscle unit*.

5.2.1. Intrinsic Properties of Motoneurons

Spinal motoneurons are of two general types. The first, characterized by a relatively large cell body (or cell soma), innervates muscle fibers in skeletal muscle. This type of motoneuron is referred to as α or *skeletomotor* neurons. A group of smaller motoneurons, known as γ or *fusimotor* neurons innervates muscle spindles (*see* earlier discussion of muscle-spindle efferent innervation). α and γ motoneurons are interspersed throughout the ventrolateral portion of spinal gray matter. An additional class of neurons known as β or skeletofusimotor motoneurons, is also present in many vertebrate systems, but these neurons have no features that distinguish them structurally or physiologically from α motoneurons, at least as far as we know. β motoneurons are characterized solely by the fact that they jointly innervate skeletal muscle and intrafusal fibers of muscle spindles in the same muscle.

Although the soma of spinal motoneurons may be quite large, approaching 100 μm or more, the dendritic arbor is even larger, and may extend for several millimeters radially from the cell soma out into white matter and far up into the dorsal gray.

Spinal motoneurons are characterized by a range of specific chemically or voltage-activated conductances.

5.2.1.1. Chemical Conductances.
Activation of excitatory synaptic projections to spinal motoneurons, such as those originating from Ia afferents, produces an EPSP. As shown in Fig. 12, the synaptic potential begins very quickly after the arrival of the action potential in the presynaptic nerve terminal. (This small delay is important because it indicates that the effects are not mediated by direct electrical transmission). After an interval of about less than 1 ms, there is a rapidly depolarizing voltage change, which may reach a peak in 3–5 ms and then decay gradually over the ensuing 15 or 20 ms.

From a variety of biophysical studies of motoneurons, it is now evident that the time-course of the synaptic potential is dependent jointly upon the magnitude and time-course of synaptic current injection (which may last only 100–300 μs), and on the electrical prop-

Fig. 12. (*Opposite page*) (**A**) Diagram of a motor neuron, showing the cell soma and dendrites (SD segment), the initial segment (IS) or axon hillock, and the first node of Ranvier (*see arrows*). The changes in action potential formation result as a motor neuron is stimulated antidromically. At –87 mV, only a small potential, called the M potential, is visible, as the potential reaches –80 mV, a partial action potential, called the A spike is visible, indicating invasion of the initial segment of the motor neuron. As the motor

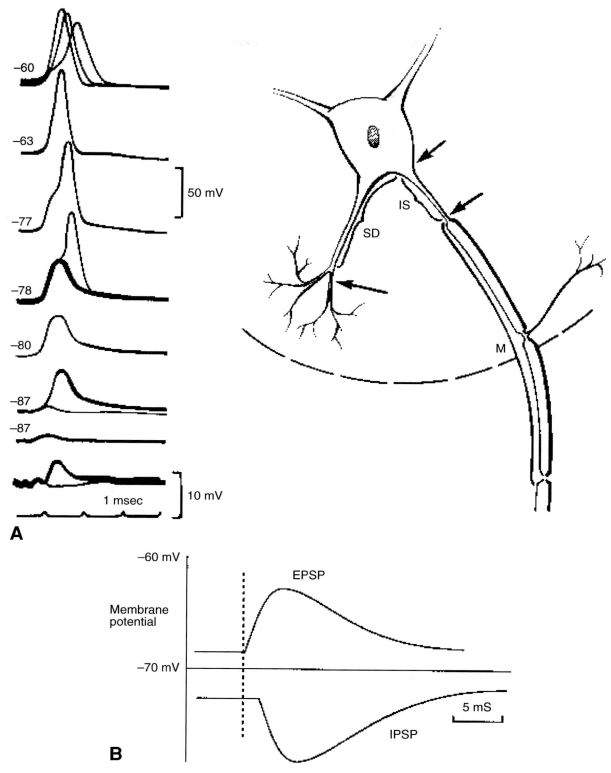

A

B

(*Fig. 12 continued*) neuron potential is further depolarized to –78 mV, a full action potential is visible, with a clear inflection still evident at the transition between A and B spikes. (**B**) The diagram plots the time course of an EPSP and IPSP. Both have a relatively similar rise time, reaching a peak in 3–5 ms, and a prolonged decay. The inhibitory postsynaptic potential begins a few milliseconds after the excitatory potential because of the intervening inhibitory interneuron.

erties of the cell membrane. The latter is referred to as the resistance-capacitance or "RC" properties of the membrane. The excitatory synaptic potential follows its particular time-course, primarily because of charge storage and distribution on the membrane "capacitor." This membrane charge is then slowly dissipated over the subsequent 10–20 ms, with a time-course that depends on the electrical properties of the membrane, and on the physical location of the synaptic terminals on the cell surface.

Specifically, the effective current flow seen at the axon hillock, the preferred site of action-potential initiation of the motoneuron, is strongly influenced by membrane properties, and by the cell geometry, especially the pattern of dendritic branching. In particular, excitatory synaptic potentials that originate on distal dendrites are greatly attenuated and are filtered by the electrical properties of the cell.

When some inhibitory inputs are activated, such as those from Ia inhibitory interneurons or from Renshaw cells, the IPSPs will begin 1–2 ms later, because of the time needed to activate one or more intervening interneurons, but the synaptic potentials have a broadly comparable time-course, although with hyperpolarizing voltage changes. A typical sequence and time-course of these synaptic potentials is diagrammed in Fig. 12.

5.2.1.2. Voltage-Gated Conductances. In addition to the chemically activated conductances described here, there are a number of voltage-gated conductances. As in all neurons, these conductances are differentially distributed over the initial segment, soma, and dendrites of the motoneuron. The rapid-activating Na^+ and K^+ conductances that generate the action potential are highly concentrated in the first node of Ranvier, and on the regional membrane close to the axon (the axon hillock), but they are relatively less concentrated over the cell soma and the dendrites. This means that when current is injected into a cell, the first point at which action-potential generation is initiated is at the axon hillock and first node, and this is then followed by the retrograde invasion of the action potential into the soma and dendrites, (as well as the standard orthodromic invasion of the motor axon). This discontinuity in activation sequence is visible during standard intracellular recordings as a minor

inflection on the rising edge of the voltage recording of the action potential.

High-threshold calcium (Ca^{2+}) channels allow for a significant rise in intracellular Ca^{2+} levels during the action potential, activating a Ca^{2+}-sensitive potassium (K^+) channel that generates a medium duration after hyperpolarization (AHP) after each spike. This medium AHP (50–200 ms) is much longer than the fast AHP (2–4 ms) generated by the K^+ channel that repolarizes the action potential. In addition, motoneuron dendrites now appear to contain both inward and outward voltage-sensitive channels. These channels are subject to regulation by neuromodulatory inputs, especially those that release the monoamines serotonin and norepinephrine.

5.2.1.3. Monoaminergic Control of Motoneuron Electrical Behaviors. The monoamines serotonin and norepinephrine originate in nuclei in the brainstem, which contains cells that project to many parts of the nervous system. The monoaminergic projection to the spinal cord is especially strong. In motoneurons, both serotonin and norepinephrine act to enhance activity of a long lasting Ca^{2+} current and to decrease K^+ currents . Most of these effects appear to be on the dendritic portions of the cell. As a result, a brief input to the cell can evoke a sustained output (Fig. 13). If the sodium (Na^+) conductances that generate the action potential are blocked, this output is revealed as a sustained depolarization known as a plateau potential. In normal conditions without blockade of Na^+ channels, the brief input evokes a long-lasting train of action potentials, giving self-sustained firing without input. Because both plateau potentials and the self-sustaining firing are turned off by a brief inhibitory input, the cell is said to behave in a *bistable* manner, with sustained firing being switched on and off by brief excitatory and inhibitory inputs (*see* Fig. 13). Equally or more important is the effect of the dendritic Ca^{2+} current on input while it is still being applied. Recent studies show that this voltage-sensitive dendritic conductance can amplify excitatory input by a factor of 2 to 5 times, depending on the level of monoaminergic drive. As the brainstem cells that release the monoamines are tonically active in the waking state, it is highly likely that amplification and bistable behavior play a major role in defining motorneuron output during normal motor behavior.

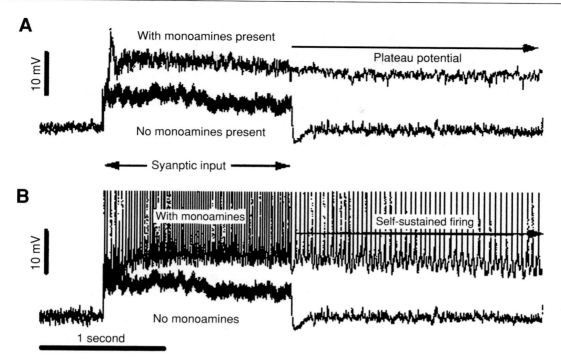

Fig. 13. Transformation of motoneuron electrical properties by the monoamines. (**A**) In the absence of the monoamines serotonin and norepinephrine, a 1-s period of synaptic input generates a sustained EPSP with a sharp onset and offset (*lower trace*). When monoamines are present, the same input generates a stronger depolarization and thus amplifies the input (action potentials are blocked in this cell). In addition, the depolarization continues on after the input ends, yielding a plateau potential. (**B**) When the cell is allowed to fire action potentials normally, the presence of monoamines allows generation of strong firing during the input and continued self-sustained firing after the input ends. Both the plateau potential and the self-sustained firing behave in a bistable manner, in that a subsequent inhibitory input returns the cell to the resting state.

5.3. Reflex Activation of Motoneurons

5.3.1. How Does the Spinal Cord Regulate Muscle Force?

There are two broadly different ways in which activation of the motoneuron pool occurs by afferent inflow, by segmental interneuronal input, or by descending spinal pathways. These are summarized in Fig. 14.

The first mode is *recruitment* of motoneurons, which is simply the transition from a passive state, in which the motoneuron is quiescent, to an excited state, in which the motoneuron is emitting action potentials. The second mode of force regulation is achieved by *increasing the rate of discharge of individual motoneurons*. This is known as *rate modulation*. In effect, the first option progressively activates more and more motoneurons (and muscle fibers), progressively filling in all the elements in the pool until the pool is completely recruited. The second option, *rate modulation*, alters the individual force output of single motor units by virtue of their capacity to produce a partially fused tetanus, in which the mean force output becomes progressively greater with increasing rate of motoneuron discharge.

In life, these two regulatory mechanisms are closely interwoven, with recruitment as the dominant source of force increase at low levels of motoneuron pool excitation, and rate modulation generating a progressively greater and greater impact on muscle-force output as more and more motoneurons are activated.

5.3.1.1. Characteristics of Motoneuron Recruitment.
When a motoneuron from a particular motoneuron pool is subjected to increasing excitatory synaptic input, such as from muscle-spindle Ia afferent fibers, the resulting progression of excitation and recruitment in different motoneurons is very orderly and virtually

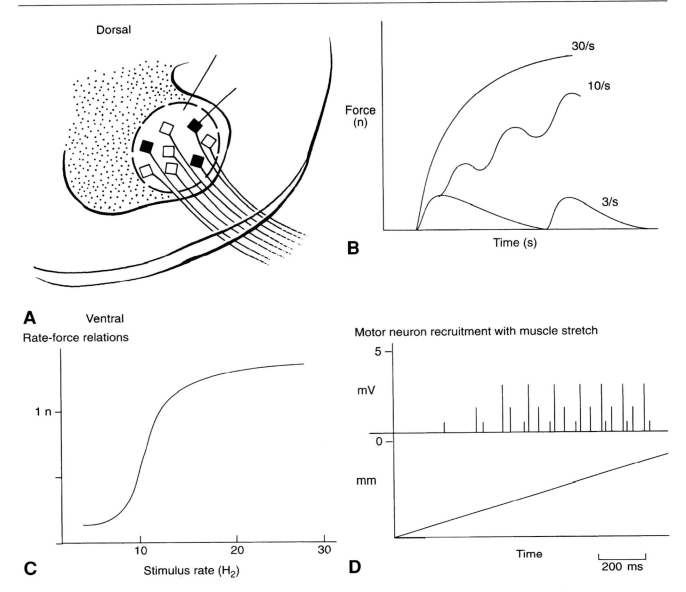

Fig. 14. Regulation of muscle force: (**A**) Recruitment of motor neurons is manifested as activation of the elements in the motor neuron pool. Recruitment can augment muscle force only if motor neurons are completely activated. (**B**) Rate modulation is available at all levels of recruitment. The discharge rate of the motor neuron strongly influences the net force output of the motor unit. At very low discharge rates, individual twitches generated by motor neuron excitation do not summate significantly, but at rates exceeding 6–8 pulses/s, a partially fused tetanus develops. Under normal conditions, motor units operate in a response region in which their tension output is partially fused. (**C**) The characteristic force and stimulus-rate relationship for an individual motor unit, demonstrating the sigmoidal curve describing the operating region in which small changes in the impulse rate (10–20 pulses/s) induce substantial changes in force. (**D**) Typical outcome of an experiment in which motor units are recruited progressively during slow muscle stretch. The first motor units to be activated have small action potentials, and as the excitation is increased, progressively larger action potentials are introduced, reflecting the recruitment of larger and larger motor neurons.

Fig. 15. (*Opposite page*) Relation between recruitment and rate modulation for different motor units recruited at different motor forces. (**A**) Three motor units were recruited during progressively increasing isometric force (*abscissa*). Unit 1 is recruited at a low force at a rate of 8 pulses/s, and subsequent units are recruited at slightly higher rates. The slope of the relationship between firing rate and force is somewhat steeper for the later units, indicating an increasingly important contribution from rate modulation. (**B**) The range of rate modulation and recruitment forces was recorded from motor units in the human extensor digitorum communis muscle. Voluntary force is depicted on the abscissa in a logarithmic scale, and the unit firing rate is shown on the ordinate. There are units recruited across a broad range of force, with units recruited at the lowest forces activated routinely at 8 pulses/s, but these

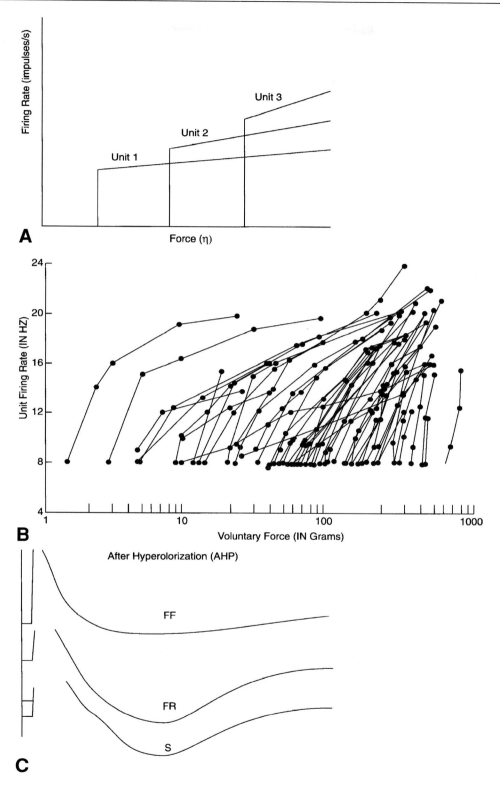

(*Fig. 15 continued*) lower-threshold units often increase their rate over a limited range and then saturate. Units recruited at higher forces showed a steeper force-rate relation. (**C**) Relationship between after-hyperpolarization (AHP) and motor neuron type. S-type motor neurons show the largest and most long-lasting AHP, and FF-type motor neurons show the smallest and the shortest AHP. FR motor neurons show intermediate AHP depth and duration. The magnitude of the AHP is closely correlated with the maximal firing rates of these different units.

stereotypic, obeying a principle known as the *size principle*. This principle, elucidated first by Henneman and colleagues in 1965, states that motoneurons are recruited in a defined rank order, in which small-sized motoneurons are recruited first, and these are followed progressively by larger and larger motoneurons. Conversely, if motoneurons in a pool are already active, the application of an increasing inhibitory input, such as from antagonist muscle Ia afferents, causes a derecruitment of motoneurons, in which the largest motoneurons are the first to drop out. With increasing inhibition, derecruitment continues progressively, and the smallest motoneurons are the last to be silenced.

5.3.1.2. What is Meant by Size of Motoneurons?
The original description by Henneman of the relationship between recruitment rank order and size was derived from studies using ventral-root recordings of motor axons, in which the size of the extracellular action potential recorded from the ventral root was used as an indication of the size of the motor axon, and by inference, as an indication of the size of the associated motoneuron. A typical pattern of activation is illustrated in Fig. 14C, which shows that increasing muscle extension gives rise to recruitment of ventral-root action potentials of progressively greater and greater amplitude. This correlation between action-potential size and motoneuron somatic size is broadly applicable to the bulk of motoneuron axons recorded in the ventral root, but it may not hold in fine detail. This is partly because unrelated technical factors may influence the size of the recorded action potential, but mostly because motoneuron size itself may not be the primary factor governing motoneuron recruitment order.

For example, when motoneuron recruitment order is plotted against tetanic tension of the associated motor unit, the relationship with size becomes much clearer (and is more linear than is the relationship between recruitment rank order and axon action potential size). Recruitment "reversals," in which the larger motoneuron appears to be the first activated, are much less common. Although tetanic-motor unit force has no obvious causal relationship to neuronal factors governing recruitment, it presumably provides a more sensitive marker of net motor-unit properties than is available by relying simply on action potential size.

5.3.1.3. Physiological Mechanisms of the Size Principle.
The physiological factors responsible for the orderly recruitment of motoneurons by size are not yet fully understood, despite intensive and continuing investigation. Originally, Henneman proposed that

motoneuron size itself could be the governing factor. The idea was that for a particular synaptic current, applied to all motoneurons in the pool, the magnitude of the resulting excitatory synaptic potentials in motoneurons would be determined by the effective electrical "input resistance" of the motoneuron, which is inversely related to the surface area of the cell. All other things being equal, a small neuron would present a higher input resistance than a large neuron because of the reduced membrane area available to transmit the current, and the resulting excitatory potentials in smaller motoneurons would be expected to be larger. Since the neuron voltage threshold is essentially constant in different motoneurons, the differences in EPSP size would then dictate the order of recruitment. The changes in motoneuron electrical properties mediated by the monoamines are also correlated with cell size, because the dendritic Ca current that generates amplification of synaptic input and bistable behavior has a substantially lower voltage threshold in smaller motor neurons.

Many synaptic inputs are distributed among motoneurons in a non-uniform fashion, with some inputs systems that tend to generate larger synaptic currents in larger motoneurons (e.g., descending input from the rubrospinal nucleus and some cutaneous inputs). This inputs do not seem to be capable of reversing the normal order of recruitment. Therefore, it seem that the large differences in the intrinsic electrical properties of motoneurons maintain the size principle, no matter what the organization of synaptic input.

5.3.1.4. Factors Governing Motoneuron Discharge Rate.
There is some tendency for the firing rate of motoneurons at their recruitment threshold to vary systematically with recruitment rank order. This is very clear with injected current during intracellular recording, but may be obscured by synaptic noise during normal motor behavior in humans. In Fig. 15, for example, no systematic differences in the initial rate are evident. Perhaps the most striking feature of motoneuron rate modulation in humans is the phenomenon of *rate limiting*, in which low-threshold units undergo a dramatic reduction in firing rate as higher-threshold units are recruited. The mechanism of this effect is unclear, but the initial steep increase may reflect a surge in firing caused by activation of the dendritic plateau potential. Rate limiting aids in energy efficiency, as the slow-twitch fibers innervated by early recruited motoneurons are already driven effectively by the low rates achieved before rate limiting commences.

5.4. Motor Units: The Functional UNITS of Motor Control

When a motor axon is excited directly (for example, by electrical stimulation of a small ventral-root fascicle), or the related motoneuron is activated electrically by intracellular current injection, the muscle fibers innervated by this motor axon are excited, and show a twitch, whose mechanical features are related to the number and mechanical properties of the innervated muscle fibers. There has been extensive study of these motor-unit properties, and of the relationship between the mechanical behavior of the muscle fibers and the electrophysiological properties of the innervating motoneuron. Some of these findings are summarized in Fig. 16.

Motor units vary in the size and time-course of the twitch elicited by a single stimulus, and in the resistance to fatigue manifested during repetitive activation. The magnitude of the motor-unit twitch varies greatly between different mammalian muscles, and for different motor units in the same muscle; however, much of our current knowledge is drawn from the hindlimb muscles of the cat, especially the medial gastrocnemius (MG). These studies have shown that many muscles, such as the MG, are quite heterogeneous, possessing units with a spectrum of mechanical and biochemical properties.

5.4.1. TWITCH SIZE (FIG. 16)

When the twitch responses of different units in a given muscle are compared, the twitch tension, or force amplitude varies from several grams of weight, to only a few milligrams. The reasons for these differences are complex, but a number of factors contribute to the differences in twitch tension.

First, large motor units may have more muscle fibers innervated by a motor axon. In other words, the number of muscle fibers innervated by a single motor axon, which is called the *innervation ratio*, could be larger in those units that generate larger tensions. In the case of the MG muscle, the innervation ratio for large-twitch units is indeed greater than for small units, but the difference is not enough to explain the difference in twitch force. For example, the innervation ratio may vary from 250–700 muscle fibers/axon, a threefold range, but the differences in force may vary by 50- or even 100-fold.

A second factor contributing to the generation of muscle force is *the cross-sectional diameter of the muscle fiber*. The cross-sectional diameter is important, because it reflects the number of myofibrils that

can contribute to force generation, since these myofibrils are arranged in parallel, and can add to net fiber force independently. The average cross-sectional area of individual muscle fibers in large-twitch motor units is substantially greater than that of small-twitch units, although the difference in area is not quite enough to explain the differences in twitch and tetanic force.

The third and final factor is the specific force-generating capacity of each fiber type, or the *specific tension*. It is possible that fibers belonging to different types of motor units are capable of generating different forces, even when the effects of innervation ratio and of cross-sectional area are eliminated. In other words, the *force/unit area*, which is the measure of specific tension, is potentially greater in fast-twitch than in slow-twitch fibers. Attempts to calculate the specific tension of different muscle fibers have been made, and they show at most a threefold difference between fast- and slow-twitch units. However, the accuracy of such estimates is open to question, and the contributions of specific tension are likely to be even more modest than the previously mentioned twofold difference.

Taken overall, it is likely that differences in innervation ratio and cross-sectional area are the more important sources of difference in twitch tension for different motor-unit types, although specific tension differences may also contribute.

5.4.2. TWITCH TIME-COURSE (FIG. 16)

Different motor units vary greatly in the speed of their contraction, which is measured from the onset of the twitch transient to the peak of the twitch. This speed of contraction is an important marker of unit specialization, and an excellent correlate and predictor of the fatigability of the unit during repetitive activation.

For the case of the cat medial gastrocnemius, units are broadly divisible into *fast* and *slow twitch*, with a boundary value of 55 ms. Units with twitch contraction times longer than 55 ms are known as slow twitch, or S -type. These units are able to generate only small twitches, and modest levels of tetanic force during repetitive activation. The *fast-twitch* units, or F-type units, have contraction speeds less than 55 ms, and are usually able to generate much larger twitches and correspondingly greater tetanic forces. However, they are unable to sustain this tetanic force without change during prolonged repetitive activation.

The physiological basis of the differences in twitch contraction times is not fully established; however, the use of an array of histochemical techniques has revealed a systematic difference in the staining of

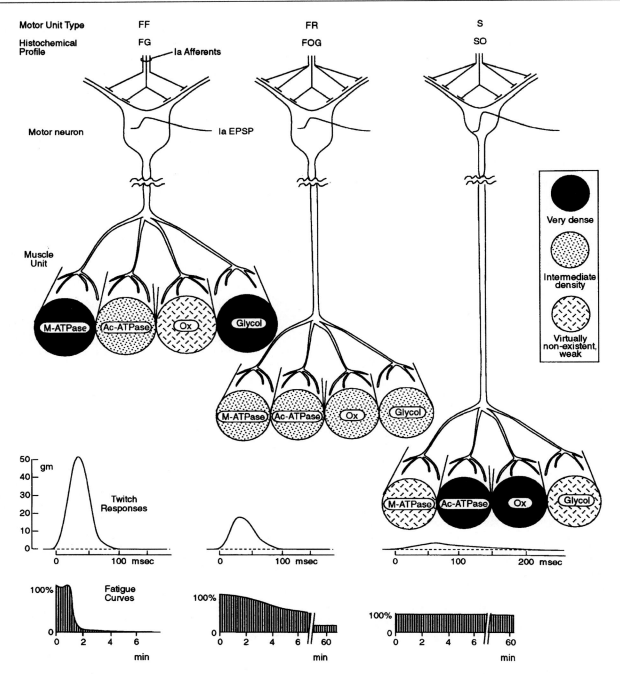

Fig. 16. Relationship between motor neurons and the muscle fibers they innervate. Three different-sized motor neurons innervate muscle fibers of varying diameters (*upper section*). The twitch induced by transient motor neuron, and has the lowest peak force and slowest rise time for the smallest motor neuron. Repetitive activation of the large neuron (*left*) results in a force tetanus which declines very rapidly, decaying almost completely within 2 min, whereas the smaller neuron (*right*) generates a smaller tetanus, which does not decline over many minutes; the intermediate unit shows a partial decline in tetanic force. These differing degrees of fatigue sensitivity are used in conjunction with differences in twitch contraction time to classify motor units (*see upper table and text*). Metabolic correlates of the physiological differences are also shown (*central portion*). S-type units show dense concentrations of oxidative (Ox) and mitochondrial (Ac-ATPase) enzymes. FF units stain strongly for glycolytic enzymes. These staining differences support an alternative histochemical classification scheme (*top*); fast glycolytic (FG), fast oxidative glycolytic (FOG), and slow oxidative (SO). The largest neurons receive the most extensive Ia afferent input, but with low terminal density; and the smallest motor neurons receive the highest density of Ia afferent input.

muscle fibers for a particular myosin ATPase. This ATPase is located on the myosin head, and may regulate the speed of crossbridge recycling during muscle-fiber excitation. Current evidence does not support the view that this ATPase is entirely responsible for regulating the speed of twitch contraction, but it may be implicated as one component of the regulatory process.

5.4.3. Fatigability of Motor Units (Fig. 16)

When a motor unit is subjected to repetitive activation at high frequency (such as 30 pulses/s for 300-ms bursts), the unit generates a sustained tetanus, with a force magnitude that may be several times greater than that of the twitch. This force response to prolonged repetitive activation has proven to be a helpful classification tool. For example, when an S-type motor unit is activated repetitively, the force response reaches a sustained tetanus, and remains at the same level for prolonged periods of time, often up to several hours. When measured at 2 min, the time chosen arbitrarily for evaluation, the force will have dropped by less than 25%.

When these motor-unit fibers are examined with histochemical stains, these S-type fibers contain many mitochondria, and stain heavily for mitochondrial enzymes (such as succinic dehydrogenase, and mitochondrial ATPases). These S-type fibers also contain substantial concentrations of myoglobin, and are surrounded by a dense capillary network. There is usually relatively little intracellular glycogen stored. The enzymatic profile indicates that these fibers are specialized for oxidative phosphorylation, and depend on transported blood glucose or FFA to generate the necessary ATP. Since oxidative phosphorylation is an efficient means of generating ATP production, muscle contraction can continue without decrement for prolonged periods of time, provided that blood flow is sufficient to deliver the needed metabolic substrates.

In contrast, *fast-twitch units* show a broad range of mechanical behaviors during repetitive activation, and a correspondingly broad range of metabolic/enzymatic features on histochemical analysis. During repetitive excitation, some motor units fail to sustain the tetanic force for even 2 min, falling to less than 25% of the initial level. These are classified as *FF*, or *fast-twitch, fatigable* units. Other fast-twitch units are able to sustain their tetanic force more readily, falling to between 25% and 75% of the initial tetanic force, at the 2-min mark. These are called *fast-twitch, fatigue-resistant*, or *FR* units.

Histochemical analyses of these fast-twitch units shows an array of histochemical profiles. The most fatigable units (FF) show high concentrations of myosin ATPase, few mitochondria, little or no myoglobin, a meager capillary network, and substantial glycogen stores. These units appear to rely on glycolysis to generate the necessary ATP to sustain contraction, and are therefore called *FG* units, in current metabolic classification schemes.

The units showing *intermediate degrees of fatigability* reveal some residual oxidative machinery on histochemical analysis, including mitochondria and associated mitochondrial enzymatic staining. Because the histochemical profile is mixed, these units are classified as FOG in metabolically based schemes.

It appears that the degree of fatigue, estimated from the loss of force, is related to the capacity to sustain high levels of ATP production. In FF (FG) fibers, ATP synthesis declines when glycogen is lost and muscle contraction declines, whereas in FR (FOG) fibers, the residual oxidative contributions delays the onset of fatigue.

6. REFLEX REGULATION OF MOVEMENT

6.1. Introduction

Thus far, this chapter has described the spinal elements that are implicated in the control of muscle force, including the neurons of the spinal cord, the muscle receptors, and the muscle itself. The sections that follow address the functional contribution of these various elements to the control of movement.

Broadly speaking, the spinal cord is engaged in three aspects of movement regulation.

6.1.1. Information Transmission

The spinal cord *relays afferent information* to higher centers in the spinal cord, brainstem, and beyond, and *transmits efferent commands* from higher centers to the motor nuclei of the spinal cord.

6.1.2. Reflex Action

Spinal cord neurons and their connections form the substrates for a variety of *sensory-motor reflexes*.

6.1.3. Pattern Generators

Spinal and brainstem interneurons form the basis for *oscillatory neuronal discharge*, which underlies rhythmical behaviors such as *locomotion*, *respiration* and *mastication*.

6.2. Definition of Reflexes

A reflex is defined as a *stereotypic motor response to a particular sensory input*. Reflexes vary broadly in the complexity of their motor response, and in the number and diversity of neural elements that are utilized. Reflexes may be relatively simple, involving sensory afferents such as Ia afferents from one muscle, and inducing activation of motoneurons innervating the same muscle. Such reflexes, which include the *tendon jerk* and the *tonic stretch reflex*, are often referred to as *autogenetic*, or *homonymous* in type. Reflexes elicited by muscle afferents of one muscle acting on motoneurons of a neighboring muscle are often described as *heteronymous* in type. When such reflexes result in coordinated responses between two or more muscles with similar mechanical actions, the muscles are said to be acting as *synergists*.

At a somewhat higher level of reflex organization, there is the *"reciprocal"* pattern of activation, in which inhibition is exerted by Ia afferents of one muscle on motoneurons of the antagonist muscle via the *Ia inhibitory* interneuron (*see* Section 4.3.5.2.).

At the next level, there is a more complex array of reflexes in which the response to a sensory input may be relatively complex and even repetitive, or rhythmical in character. These reflexes include such responses as *the flexion withdrawal* reflex, in which a noxious or sometimes even non-noxious stimulus to skin or other deep tissues evokes a broad-scale coordinated withdrawal of a limb, by systematic activation of flexor muscles at several joints.

Beyond the flexion withdrawal reflex, there is an array of complex goal-directed reflexes such as *wipe and scratch reflexes*, in which local excitation of skin surface gives rise to a coordinated and often repetitive motion by the animal to remove the irritant focus from the skin. In mammalian quadrupeds, this is usually known as the *scratch reflex*, and in amphibians it may be referred to as the *wipe reflex*. The fact that the action attempting to eradicate the irritant focus is repetitive and rhythmical in character suggests that the response may also involve an *oscillator* or *pattern generator*, which gives rise to rhythmical excitation of spinal circuits.

6.2.1. STRETCH REFLEX: SPRING-LIKE PROPERTIES OF THE STRETCH REFLEX

Since the work of Sherrington, it has been well-known that stretch of muscle in a physiologically active animal, such as an unanesthetized decerebrate preparation, gives rise to a substantial increase in motor output, which is reflected as an increase in muscle force. (This increase in force is induced by orderly recruitment and rate modulation of motoneurons, in a pattern characterized in earlier sections of this chapter). This increase in motor output results in a systematic increase in muscle force, in which the force rises smoothly and approximately in proportion to the degree of muscle extension. Conversely, when the muscle is allowed to shorten, the reduction in force is essentially proportional to the reduction in muscle length.

These features of the stretch reflex response can be characterized as being "spring-like" in character, in that a change of length is accompanied by a proportional change of force, the defining feature of a simple spring. Furthermore, when the muscle stretch is maintained, the increase in force is also maintained, verifying the spring-like property, since a spring continues to resist when extended. However, when muscle is stretched at a constant velocity, it also shows a force overshoot at the end of the stretch, suggesting that there is some degree of dynamic, or velocity sensitivity.

A detailed comparison of the forces generated over a broad range of velocity indicates that the effect of increasing velocity is relatively modest. Specifically, a 100-fold increase in stretch velocity induces less than twofold change in muscle force. When the force increment induced by stretch—measured at a constant length increment—is plotted against stretch velocity, the relationship is seen to be nonlinear, and is well-described by a power-function relationship, in which force increases with velocity raised to the power of 0.2. (e.g., $F = K v^{0.2}$). In these cases, it appears then that muscle is a relatively weak viscous element, because the increase in force is much less than proportional to the increase in velocity. Notably, the force generated increases relatively steeply at very low velocities, so that muscle would emulate a frictional device, resisting motion most powerfully at the onset of motion, where velocities are small.

6.2.2. COMPARISON OF REFLEX AND AREFLEXIVE BEHAVIOR OF MUSCLE

To review briefly, (*see* Section 2.1.2.), when active muscle is removed from reflex control, such as by dorsal-root section, muscle displays an asymmetric response to stretch, because stiffness is modest during stretch, yet is quite large in shortening. When reflex

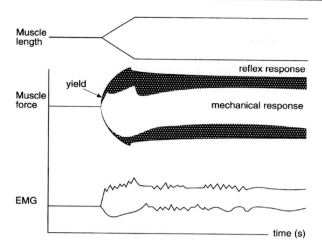

Fig. 17. Comparison of mechanical and reflex responses of reflexively active soleus muscle of the cat: Muscle is exposed to symmetric stretch and release of constant velocity. In the central part of the figure, the mechanical response is replicated, showing the short-range stiffness, yield, and asymmetric force characteristics. The overall reflex response (*top*) is much more spring-like, because stretch and release produce a smooth and progressive change in the force, which is essentially symmetric. Force changes are sustained even during the plateau phase of the length change. The EMG responses are also asymmetric, reflecting the different reflex actions during stretch and release. During stretch, there is a modest EMG reduction that is relatively smaller in magnitude, although with a sustained component during the hold phase.

mechanisms are intact, these asymmetrical mechanical properties of muscle are fully compensated, preventing muscle yield from being manifested.

As shown in Fig. 17, if the mechanical (or areflexive) response to stretch and release is superimposed upon the reflex response (matched for the same initial force), it is evident that the early phase of the force response to muscle stretch in both cases is virtually identical, indicating that the response to stretch is initially governed by the intrinsic mechanical properties of active muscle. However, at the point that yielding should have taken place, the reflex response continues smoothly without discontinuity, indicating that effective compensatory mechanisms must have been operating.

In contrast, the response to muscle shortening is much more similar for reflex and mechanical (e.g., areflexive) responses, indicating that there is less requirement for neurally mediated compensation during the shortening phase of motion. These differences in the mechanical behavior are also mirrored in the electromyographic (EMG) responses, which show

substantial EMG increases during stretch, and relatively modest EMG reductions during shortening.

The finding that the more complex mechanical properties of muscle—such as the muscle yield—are obscured in the presence of reflex action indicates that the *reflexes serve to linearize and to smooth the mechanical behavior of muscle*. It is also clear that in the absence of reflex action, the onset of muscle yield occurs very early in relationship to stretch onset, so that muscle mechanical properties would normally be expected to change abruptly, approximately within 20–50 ms of stretch onset. This rapid change is likely to impose severe time constraints on compensatory responses, which may take an additional 25–50 ms to elicit an appropriate mechanical response. A second issue is that the mechanical response to muscle is highly asymmetric, requiring substantial reflex compensatory responses in stretch, but relatively modest responses in shortening. This substantial asymmetry of reflex action needs an explanation.

These dual *constraints of timing and asymmetry* indicate that straightforward feedback-control mechanisms are unlikely to be responsible for compensating both muscle yield and asymmetric muscle mechanical behavior, because the time constraints are too severe to allow errors to be detected and transmitted to the cord, and the corrective neural command relayed and implemented in the muscle. The debate about the nature and consequences of reflex action is still ongoing; however, we now believe that much of the compensatory response for muscle yield is built into the response characteristics of the muscle-spindle receptors.

This is an unexpected solution to the problem of controlling muscle force, since muscle-spindle receptors are usually designated as primary length sensors, rather than as sensors regulating muscle force. Furthermore, in most published experiments, muscle length is controlled by the stretcher, so that muscle-spindle responses would be expected to be essentially invariant, and independent of muscle force levels. Nonetheless, this receptor is the only candidate with a short onset time for activation, and it also has the requisite pattern of asymmetric response to stretch and release. It appears that the neural mechanisms that mediate stretch-reflex action act predictively, at least initially, in that the muscle-spindle receptor issues a response that is appropriate for correcting impending changes in muscle properties, such as muscle yielding and asymmetric muscle stiffness.

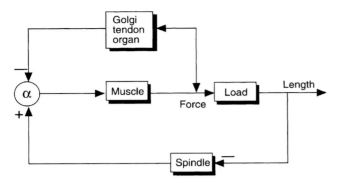

Fig. 18. Servocontrol of the spinal cord and the regulation of muscle length and force. The diagram documents the classic associations among the segmental motor apparatus and muscle sensors and the central connections in regulating force. The alpha motoneuron serves as a summing junction for the afferent inflow. Alpha motoneurons innervate muscle, which exerts force against the load of the limb or against additional superimposed loads. After muscle has acted on the load, there may be a resulting change in muscle length, which alters the spindle afferent discharge. Muscle-tendon organs are also activating by increasing force. Muscle-spindle receptors project directly to the spinal neurons. Increasing muscle length induces a force that opposes the length change in this negative-feedback loop. Muscle-force sensors, such as tendon organs, also inhibit homonymous motoneurons, closing a force-regulating loop. In combination, simultaneous force and length regulation achieves net regulation of muscle stiffness.

Although tendon-organ responses could contribute to and promote the improvement of muscle mechanical properties, the speed of tendon-organ-mediated feedback is too slow to prevent the manifestation of rapid-onset mechanical changes, such as muscle yielding. Furthermore, appropriate compensatory muscle mechanical responses occurs even when Ib interneuron responses are very modest or even absent.

6.3. Role of Force Feedback

6.3.1. An Assessment of the Hypothesis of "Stiffness Regulation"

As shown in Fig. 18, the dual and competing actions of muscle-length feedback (which would promote increased stiffness of muscle) and force feedback (which would induce reduced muscle stiffness) are simultaneously present and active under many conditions, suggesting that regulation of stiffness to some predetermined level could be a possible function of stretch reflex mechanisms. This view was advanced by Nichols and Houk (1976), who showed that the

stiffness of muscle was more constant in the presence of reflex action, although the actual magnitude was not held closely to any specific value.

We now believe that the evidence in support of a primary role of the stretch reflex as a stiffness regulator is limited, because muscle stiffness does not remain constant, or even approximately constant, under most operating conditions. However, it is clear that the presence of force and length sensors, together with their reflex connections, gives rise to a much more spring-like behavior of muscle, and it is this characteristic of muscle that is likely to be important in the control of movement.

For example, the presence of predictive reflex compensation means that the sharp extension of ankle extensors—such as the soleus extension, which takes place during the stance phase of locomotion—would induce a smooth force increase, and enhance effective damping of the contact point.

6.3.2. Pattern Generators

Virtually all nervous systems contain groups of neurons with the capacity to generate rhythmical bursting behavior, even when isolated from other neuronal systems. These neurons may show spontaneous bursting, or they may need a "gating" signal, such as that provided by monoaminergic agents including norepinephrine, but the pattern of discharge is not dependent on any incoming afferent or descending signals; thus the term *"pattern generator."*

On the basis of extensive studies from acute and chronic spinally transected preparations (including the cat and turtle), it is evident that such neuronal clusters can induce repetitive discharge sufficient to drive locomotion. In spinal cords removed from rodents and sustained in an artificial environment, stable locomotor patterns can be evoked from interneuronal circuits by appropriate tonic pharmacological drive (a combination of serotonin and the glutamate agonist NMDA work best). Thus, locomotion-like patterns of motoneuronal discharge are not dependent on either descending, ascending, or peripheral afferent inputs. These results support the view that locomotion emerges from the activities of a discrete oscillator, located primarily within the interneurons of the spinal cord. Normally, the spinal-pattern generator appears to be activated by descending inputs from locomotion-control regions in the mesencephalon and other areas of the brainstem.

The discharge of the spinal-pattern generators is subject to peripheral modulation because it can be modified in important ways by appropriate segmental afferent inflow. Specifically, cutaneous stimulation of a foot in a quadruped during the swing phase of locomotion gives rise to avoidance behavior in which the leg is caused to circumvent the obstruction, whereas when the leg is still weight-bearing, similar cutaneous stimulation is ineffectual, indicating that there is a substantial phase-dependent modulation of the effects of sensory input.

SELECTED READINGS

Binder MD, Heckman CJ, Powers RK. The physiological control of motorneuron activity. In Rowel L and Shepherd J (eds). Handbook of Physiology, sect. 12, New York, Oxford University Press), 1996; 3.

Burke RE, Levin DN, Tsairis P, Zajac FE. Physiological types and histochemical profiles in motor units of the cat gastrocnemius. J Physiol (Lond) 1973; 234:723.

Burke RE. Motor unit types of cat triceps surae muscles. J Physiol (Lond) 1967; 194:141.

Burke RE. Motor units: anatomy physiology and functional organization. In Brooks V(ed). Handbook of Physiology, sect I. Washington, DC: American Physiological Society, 1981; 345.

Crago PE, Houk JC, Rymer WZ. Sampling of total muscle force by tendon organs. J Neurophysiol 1982; 47:1069.

Henneman E, Mendell LM. Functional organization of the motoneuron pool and its inputs. In Brooks V (ed). Handbook of Physiology, sect. I. Washington, DC: American Physiological Society, 1981; 423.

Houk JC, Rymer WZ. Neural control of muscle length and tension. In Brooks V (ed). Handbook of Physiology, sect I. Washington, DC: American Physiological Society, 1981; 257.

Huxley AF, Niedergerke R. Structural changes in muscle during contraction. Nature 1954; 173:971.

Huxley HE, Hanson EJ. Changes in the cross-striation of muscle during contraction and stretch, and their structural interpretation. Nature 1954; 173:971.

Matthews PBC. Muscle spindles, their messages and their fusimotor supply. In Brooks V (ed). Handbook of Physiology, sect I. Washington, DC: American Physiological Society, 1981; 257.

Nichols TR, Houk JC. Improvement in linearity and regulation of stiffness that results from actions of the stretch reflex. J Neurophysiol 1976; 39:119.

Stein RB. What muscle variable does the nervous system control in limb movements? Behav Brain Sci 1992; 5:535.

Vallbo AB. Discharge patterns in human muscle spindle afferents during isometric voluntary contractions. Acta Physiol Scand 1970; 80:552.

21 Chemical Messenger Systems

Robert D. Grubbs and David K. Sundberg*

CONTENTS

1. NEUROTRANSMITTERS, NEUROHORMONES, AND NEUROMODULATORS

Neurotransmitters, neurohormones, and neuromodulators are the chemical messengers that allow one cell to communicate with another cell or with itself.

*Deceased.

From: *Neuroscience in Medicine, 2nd ed.* (P. Michael Conn, ed.), © 2003 Humana Press Inc., Totowa, NJ.

The concept of chemical messenger systems has come from studies of the peripheral nervous system, which started in the late 1800s and focused mainly on the somatic (e.g., neuromuscular junction) and autonomic (e.g., sympathetic and parasympathetic) nervous systems. These areas provided an accessible, discrete, and less complex model of interactions between neurons and target cells. Much of our current understanding of brain function derives from studies, which

Table 1
Steps to Identify a Substance as a Neurotransmitter

1. *Anatomical*: The substance must be present in appropriate amounts in the presynaptic process.
2. *Biochemical*: The enzymes that synthesize the substance must be present and active in the terminal, and enzymes that degrade it must be present in the synapse.
3. *Physiological*: Stimulation of the presynaptic axon should cause the release of the substance, and application of the specific substance should mimic stimulation of the nerve.
4. *Pharmacological*: Drugs that affect specific enzymatic or receptor-mediated effects of the proposed transmitter substance should alter nerve stimulation through changes in synthesis, storage, release, uptake, or stimulation or blockade of the receptor.

began in earnest in the middle 1800s, devoted to grinding up specific organs in an effort to extract their "vital essence."

2. NEUROTRANSMITTERS ARE SMALL ORGANIC MOLECULES THAT CARRY A CHEMICAL MESSAGE FROM A NEURONAL AXON OR DENDRITE TO ANOTHER CELL OR NERVE

Even in ancient times, remarkably accurate concepts suggested that the large nerves of the body, which could be easily visualized during dissection, carried a substance or substances that coordinated and activated the body. The Greeks and Romans called this substance *psychic pneuma*, a product of vital and animal pneuma from the lungs and heart. Early Hindus suggested that the spinal cord and the sympathetic-chain ganglia were channels, which they called *chakra*. These chakra carried a substance, called *pram*, the flow of which could be augmented by the practice of yoga. As early as 3000 BC, the Chinese taught about the flow of *chi*, an energy that flowed through the body in channels, which could be helped by the medical practice of acupuncture and by an exercise called *tai chi chuan*.

We now know that neurotransmitters are small molecules that are synthesized and stored in secretory granules or vesicles in the axons of nerves. These transmitters can be grouped chemically into families, including the biogenic amines (e.g., the catecholamines, norepinephrine, and dopamine and the indolamines, serotonin, and histamine), acetylcholine, amino acids (e.g., γ-aminobutyric acid [GABA], glutamate, glycine), and small proteins (peptides, such as substance P, vasopressin, and oxytocin [OT]). The peptide transmitters are generally synthesized in the cell body and carried to the axon terminal by axoplasmic transport, and the nonpeptide transmitters are generally synthesized in the axon terminal. By com-

bining with postsynaptic receptors, these transmitters either inhibit or stimulate a biological response in the target cell.

The process known as *nerve transmission* refers to the passage of biochemical information by means of a chemical messenger from a nerve across a specific junction to another cell. This should not be confused with *nerve conduction*, which is the passage of an electrochemical current down a nerve axon. Table 1 lists some proposed criteria for classifying a substance as a neurotransmitter.

3. NEUROHORMONES ARE CHEMICAL MESSENGERS THAT ARE SECRETED BY THE BRAIN INTO THE CIRCULATORY SYSTEM, AND ALTER CELLULAR FUNCTION AT A DISTANCE

The word *hormone* was originally coined by EH Starling in 1905 in reference to a "chemical messenger which, speeding from cell to cell . . . coordinates the activities and growth of different parts of the body." Thus, a neurotransmitter such as epinephrine, which is synthesized and released from the adrenal medulla, can also be a neurohormone. In the brain, certain hypothalamic neurons make small proteins, the *peptide neurohormones*. These are secreted from axons directly into a portal vasculature system, in which they are carried to the anterior pituitary to influence endocrine function. The early Greeks and the Romans ascribed a similar function to this part of the brain. Galen and later Vesalius suggested that the hypothalamus produced *pituita* (Latin for phlegm), which was distilled from the ventricular system and secreted through the hypothalamus into the pituitary, and then to the nose.

Just as a nonpeptide neurotransmitter can sometimes function as a neurohormone, peptide neurohormones appear to function as neurotransmitters in

Table 2
Coexistence of Neurotransmitters and Modulators

Neurotransmitter	Co-transmitter
Catecholamines	
Dopamine	Cholecystokinin, enkephalin
Norepinephrine	Neuropeptide Y, neurotensin, enkephalin
Epinephrine	Neuropeptide Y, enkephalin
Serotonin	CCK, enkaphalin, substance P
Acetylcholine	VIP, enkaphalin, enkephalin, CGRP
GABA	Enkephalin, neuropeptide Y, CCK
Glutamate	Substance P
Glycine	Neurotensin

CCK, cholecystokinin; CGRP, calcitonin gene-related peptide; GABA, γ-aminobutryic acid; VIP, vasoactive intestinal peptide.

some cells. Many of the neurohormone-producing cells have axons that project into other areas of the brain, the brainstem, and spinal cord to influence other somatic and behavioral functions. A full discussion of this subject is found in Chapter 9.

4. NEUROMODULATORS ARE TRANSMITTERS OR NEUROPEPTIDES THAT ALTER THE ENDOGENOUS ACTIVITY OF THE TARGET CELL

Excitable cells are unique because they have a specific complement of ion channels that dictate how these cells behave. The spontaneous behavior of cells is often referred to as *endogenous activity*. This activity is best observed when the cell or nerve is removed from its normal environment and studied in vitro. One of the best examples is the rhythmic activity of the heart, which is modulated by the autonomic nervous system. When removed from a frog, the heart continues to beat if it is incubated in an isotonic buffer containing calcium. The rate of contraction of the heart depends on the rhythmic activation of ion pumps that maintain a gradient of sodium and potassium across a relatively leaky membrane. Sympathetic nerves alter the strength and rate of contraction of the heart through cardiac β receptors that modulate the production of intracellular messengers and the activity of membrane ion channels.

Some neurons in the brain also have ionic pumps that rhythmically maintain an endogenous activity, or "firing pattern." Thus, neuromodulation allows a neuron to adapt its endogenous activity to changes that occur in its environment.

Although earlier investigators assumed that each neuron contained only one transmitter, more recent studies have shown that some neurons produce and release several transmitters. Studies have shown that the main transmitter and the cotransmitter can be specifically released from the same axon terminal at different frequencies of nerve activity because of the distribution of calcium channels within the terminal. As neuromodulators, cotransmitters serve a feedback role and are referred to as *autocoids*. By combining with the autoreceptors on its own presynaptic membrane, a transmitter can augment or inhibit further nerve activity. In some nerves, such as the peripheral sympathetic nerves, a substance can have both transmitter and modulator functions. For example, norepinephrine can activate a postsynaptic receptor and influence target tissue function (e.g., heart rate) or stimulate a presynaptic receptor (e.g., α_2) to inhibit further norepinephrine release.

An experimental technique known as *immunocytochemistry* can be used to visualize a transmitter or the specific enzymes needed to make a neurotransmitter within a nerve cell or axon. By using primary antibodies that are specific to the transmitter or enzyme and fluorescent secondary antibodies that bind to the primary antibodies, an investigator can visualize the transmitter and the cotransmitter within the same axon or nerve-cell body. In many cases, a typical small neurotransmitter and a neuropeptide coexist in nerves as the pair of cotransmitters. Either of the two substances may serve the neuromodulator function. For example, although norepinephrine functions as the transmitter and neuropeptide Y (NPY) as the modulator in sympathetic nerve endings, their roles may be reversed in specific neurons within the brain. A list of transmitters with documented co-transmitters is given in Table 2.

The classic small neurotransmitters are stored in synaptic vesicles (30 nm in diameter), which are manufactured and packaged within the axon terminal itself. The larger peptide cotransmitters are stored in large synaptic vesicles that are synthesized and assembled in the neuron-cell body (e.g., soma) and reach the terminal by axonal transport, a process that can take hours or days.

The small transmitter vesicles are concentrated in an active zone of the terminal, associated with an electron-dense area of membrane that contains many calcium channels. Low-frequency nerve stimulation causes a localized increase in calcium in the active zone that stimulates the release of the small transmitter by fusion of the anchored vesicle with the membrane. The intracellular calcium is rapidly sequestered by binding to neuronal proteins and being pumped out of the axon. In this way, calcium levels only reach a threshold value in the active zone during low-frequency stimulation. For the peptide cotransmitters, the larger vesicles are found in other parts of the axon terminal, distant from the active zone. Higher-frequency nerve stimulation results in increased calcium concentrations in these areas of the terminal with cotransmitter release. Low-frequency nerve stimulation can specifically release the small transmitter in the active zone, and higher frequencies effect cotransmitter release. These interactions are shown in Fig. 1.

5. THE RESPONSE TO TRANSMITTERS CAN BE EITHER FAST OR SLOW

Synaptic transmission can be rapid or slow, depending on the nature of the stimulus and the receptors involved. For example, certain amino acids (glutamate and γ-aminobutyric acid [GABA]) and acetylcholine at the nicotinic receptor cause a rapid alteration in postsynaptic function that can be measured in milliseconds. The molecular mechanism is mediated through the opening or closing of ionic channels. These acetylcholine and glutamate receptors are composed of five protein subunits that form a channel in the membrane for sodium or calcium (*see* Chapter 7). Activation of these receptors induces a rapid change in the ionic movement across the membrane. Whether this action persists for milliseconds, seconds, minutes, hours, or days is a function of the intensity of the stimulus, the specific transmitter, and the type of receptor mediating the postsynaptic response.

Other transmitter-receptor interactions induce slower cellular responses. Acetylcholine acting on

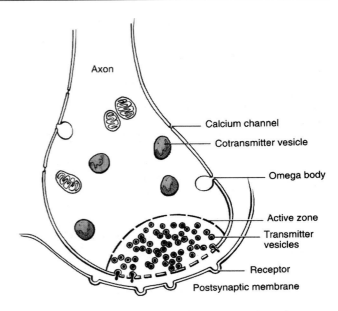

Fig. 1. The diagram of an axon terminal shows the active zone with many transmitter vesicles and calcium ion (Ca^{2+}) channels. Co-transmitters are localized in larger granules in the periphery of the terminal, where there are fewer Ca^{2+} channels. To achieve the necessary Ca^{2+} concentrations for co-transmitter release, a higher frequency of nerve stimulation is necessary.

muscarinic receptors and the catecholamines produce slow changes in the target cell that can take several seconds to minutes to manifest. These changes may include phosphorylation of proteins, activation of enzymes and second messengers, or even activation of genetic transcription and production of new proteins. The receptors that mediate these responses are single-subunit, 7 transmembrane (7-TM) domain proteins that activate a G protein to initiate a biochemical response within the cell. Thus, acetylcholine, catecholamines, and other transmitters acting on G-protein coupled receptors (GPCRs)—including neuropeptides and amino acids—can produce effects that extend over a period of hours or days.

The site of synthesis, the need for axonal transport of transmitters, and the location of enzymes needed for their metabolism, are important regulatory factors for synaptic transmission. Axonal transport occurs at a rate of 1–400 mm/d. The peptide transmitters, which are synthesized in the cell body and require transport to the axon terminal before release, could be easily depleted by persistent high-frequency nerve stimulation. In contrast, the nonpeptide transmitters are synthesized enzymatically and stored in the axon terminal. Conservation of the nonpeptide transmitters is achieved by re-uptake and storage into the nerve axon terminal. Thus, although transmitters usually produce an immediate response by changing the distribution of ions across a membrane and altering electrical potentials, the duration of this response depends on many factors that modify the biochemical changes within the cell.

6. NERVE ACTIVITY CAN BE MEASURED BY DETERMINING THE FIRING RATE OR RATE OF NEUROTRANSMITTER RELEASE OR TURNOVER

One of the most important issues in neurobiology is determining the activity of a specific nerve or type of nerve under various physiological or behavioral states. This challenge has been addressed primarily by electrophysiological or neurochemical methods.

6.1. Nerve Activity Estimated by Electrical Behavior

Nerve activity is usually characterized by measuring the electrical behavior of the cell under resting or basal conditions and following the application of some stimulus. This can be done by inserting an electrode into the brain and measuring electrical activity under these different conditions. However, it is extremely difficult to make these measurements in an awake, freely moving animal, in which movement of the electrode by as much as a few microns can confound results. Refinement of electrophysiological methods has progressed from extracellular recordings of nerve bundles to measurements of single neurons, and most recently to the technique of *patch clamping*. In this technique, a small patch of membrane from an individual neuron is sucked onto the end of a micropipet, and the electrical properties of this patch are studied. This technique is used to determine the types of ionic channels present on a small, isolated piece of membrane.

6.2. Nerve Activity Determined by the Rate of Transmitter Release or Turnover

Various techniques have been developed to measure the rate of release of a transmitter. These include monitoring the release from isolated neurons in tissue culture (in vitro), placing a small cannula (e.g., push-pull cannula) within a brain area of an anesthetized or awake animal and perfusing that area of the brain with physiological media, or implanting a similar perfusion cannula attached to a dialysis membrane (e.g., microdialysis) that restricts the recovery of brain ele-

ments to only specific molecular weights. Transmitter release can then be determined in the media, perfusate, or dialysate.

Several turnover techniques have been used to measure neuronal activity. The rate of transmitter use can be estimated by measuring its disappearance after chemically inhibiting its synthesis. An example of this technique is the use of α-methyl *p*-tyrosine to inhibit tyrosine hydroxylase, the rate-limiting enzyme in the synthetic pathway for norepinephrine and dopamine, and then measuring the rate of disappearance of norepinephrine or dopamine. Turnover can also be estimated by measuring the rate of accumulation of the transmitter after chemically inhibiting its metabolic breakdown or by measuring the rate of disappearance of its metabolite. An example is the measurement of the appearance of serotonin or the disappearance of its primary metabolite, 5-hydroxyindoleacetic acid, after inhibiting the enzyme monoamine oxidase (MAO) with the drug pargyline or iproniazid.

All of these techniques have provided valuable information about the activity of specific neurotransmitter pathways under different physiological conditions and behavioral states. They have led to the development of many behavioral models, such as the concept that the transmitter dopamine is involved in feelings of reward and reinforcement.

6.3. Small-Molecular-Weight Transmitters

The small-mol-wt transmitters are made locally within the nerve-cell axon or dendrite. The well-established small-mol-wt transmitters and modulators include three amino acids, five biogenic amines (essentially decarboxylate derivatives of amino acids), and acetylcholine. All of these molecules are synthesized and stored in the axon terminal, from which they are released after the arrival of an action potential. The response produced by these transmitters can be fast or slow, depending on the specific type of postsynaptic receptor present. If their synthesis required axoplasmic transport from the cell body, they would soon be depleted. The enzymes responsible for making these compounds are synthesized in the cell body and transported to the axon, where the actual transmitter synthesis takes place.

The discussion of these transmitters focuses on the history of the discovery of the transmitter, the mechanism of their biosynthesis, secretion and catabolism (e.g., degradation), their anatomic distribution, and their functions and physiologic actions. The function of many of these chemical messenger systems is still poorly understood. Our knowledge of these functions has often come from studying cases of behavioral or physiological alterations caused by disease states, specific lesions, or the effects of pharmacological intervention.

7. ACETYLCHOLINE IS THE PROTOTYPICAL NEUROTRANSMITTER

The first neurotransmitter to be isolated and identified was the small ester of the lipid choline, *acetylcholine*. The entire concept of neurotransmission developed from its discovery. In 1921 in Germany, Otto Loewi showed that a chemical substance, released on stimulation of the vagus nerve of an isolated frog's heart, would slow the beating of another frog's heart that was bathed in the same media. He called this substance *vagus-stuff* because it was released by stimulation of the vagus nerve. Nerve systems that use acetylcholine as a transmitter are called *cholinergic nerves*.

7.1. Anatomy and Function of Cholinergic Neurons

Cholinergic neurons are found in both the central and peripheral nervous system. Peripheral nerves that use acetylcholine include several important pathways, including the motor neurons that begin in the ventral root of the spinal cord and innervate striated skeletal muscle; the preganglionic sympathetic and parasympathetic nerves that begin in the intermediolateral column of the spinal cord or brainstem and activate all the autonomic ganglia; the postganglionic parasympathetic nerves that innervate the viscera (e.g., heart, pulmonary bronchi, gastrointestinal tract, bladder, eye, and exocrine glands); and the postganglionic sympathetic cholinergic nerves to the major sweat glands of the skin. Because of their simplicity and the relative ease of studying them, much has been learned about nerve transmission from these peripheral cholinergic nerves.

Although all of these pathways utilize the same neurotransmitter—acetylcholine—the postsynaptic receptors that trigger the cellular response are fundamentally different. The receptors located at the neuromuscular junction and the autonomic ganglia are known as *nicotinic* because they are activated specifically by the drug nicotine. In contrast, the receptors of the viscera (e.g., the gut, heart, and lungs) that are innervated by the parasympathetic nerves and the sweat glands are called *muscarinic* because they are activated by the compound muscarine, and do not

respond to nicotine. These different cholinergic receptors are also found in the brain, where the muscarinic types outnumber the nicotinic receptors by 10-fold to 100-fold.

Release of acetylcholine from spinal nerves is the initial signal from the central nervous system (CNS) in most peripheral response pathways. Acetylcholine release from somatic nerves triggers the contraction of skeletal muscle. In the autonomic ganglia, acetylcholine stimulates the postganglionic neurons that form both the sympathetic and parasympathetic nerves. Acetylcholine released from parasympathetic nerves slows down the heart rate; constricts the smooth muscle of the bronchi, stomach, intestines, bladder, and eye, and stimulates secretion of various enzymes, hydrochloric acid, and mucus from exocrine glands. A cholinergic receptor on the endothelium of the vasculature induces a biochemical event that produces nitric oxide from the amino acid arginine, which causes smooth-muscle relaxation. Recent studies have shown that nitric oxide synthetase is present all over the brain and may represent a very important transmitter or second-messenger system.

In the CNS, cholinergic pathways are present throughout the brain. Many of these pathways are diagrammed in Fig. 2. In the ventral forebrain, cholinergic cell bodies from the septum, diagonal band of Broca, and basal nucleus send axons to innervate the hippocampus, interpeduncular nuclei, and neocortex, respectively. Cholinergic cell bodies from the tegmentum of the brainstem innervate the hypothalamus and thalamus. There are also short cholinergic interneurons within the striatum.

The central cholinergic pathways in the striatum play an important role in the central motor control of muscles. This is evidenced by the fact that atropine, a drug that blocks muscarinic acetylcholine receptors, can alleviate the tremors associated with Parkinson's disease. Acetylcholine also seems to be important in memory consolidation, because cholinergic changes are found in the cortex of patients with Alzheimer's disease. Pharmacological evidence suggests that blockade of the central muscarinic cholinergic synapses (such as scopolamine) results in sedation and amnesia, and activation of nicotinic synapses increases alertness and is rewarding, as evidenced by cigarette smoking.

7.2. Neurochemistry of Cholinergic Neurons

The cholinergic axon has the capacity to synthesize, store, and secrete acetylcholine in a manner that

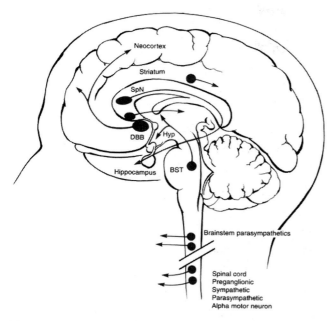

Fig. 2. Cholinergic pathways in the brain, brainstem, and spinal cord. In the brain, cholinergic cell groups are found in the septal nuclei (SpN), diagonal band of Broca (DBB), basal nucleus (BN), brainstem tegmentum (BST), and small interneurons in the striatum. Autonomic and somatic motor nuclear groups are also found in the brainstem and spinal cord. Major projection areas are found in the frontal and parietal neocortex, hippocampus, hypothalamus (Hyp), and thalamus.

is relatively independent from the nerve-cell body. The uptake of choline appears to be the rate-limiting step in acetylcholine synthesis.

Acetylcholine is synthesized from choline and acetylcoenzyme A in the nerve terminal by the enzyme choline acetyltransferase (Fig. 3). This enzyme, which has a mol wt of about approx 67,000 is synthesized in the cell body and transported to the axon. The enzyme is a cytoplasmic enzyme, but because it is positively charged, it is often associated with intracellular, mitochondrial or vesicular membranes. Choline is a component of the complex lipids of all cell membranes occurring as phosphatidylcholine and sphingomyelin, and all cells have a choline uptake mechanism. However, uptake pumps in noncholinergic cells are of low affinity (K_m of 40–100 μM). Acetylcoenzyme A is produced within the nerve terminal itself, using normal energy sources. Acetylcholine is synthesized in the cytoplasm and subsequently sequestered in small electron-opaque granules that are most prevalent in the active zone of the nerve terminal. Acetylcholine is stored within these granules with adenosine 5' triphosphate (ATP) at a concentration of about 1 M and with a charged anion protein known as vesiculin.

Acetylcholine Synthesis and Degradation

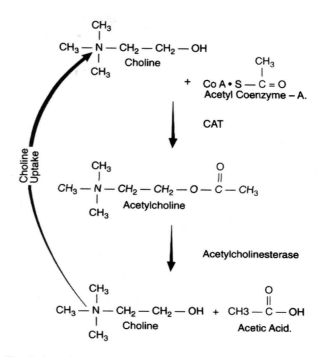

Fig. 3. Acetylcholine synthesis is catalyzed in the cytoplasm of cholinergic cells by the enzyme choline acetyltransferase (CAT). The transmitter is degraded outside of the cell by the enzyme, acetylcholinesterase, into choline and acetic acid. Choline is taken back up in the nerve by a high-affinity pump for reuse.

When acetylcholine is released, it is rapidly degraded by the enzyme acetylcholinesterase, which is found in high concentrations within the synaptic cleft and in other areas. True acetylcholinesterase is found in the synapse and is associated with the neuromuscular junction and cholinergic areas of the brain. This enzyme degrades acetylcholine to choline and acetic acid and is one of the fastest enzymes known. The maximal velocity of acetylcholine degradation has been measured at 75 g of substrate per hour using 1 mg of purified enzyme. It has been calculated that one molecule of cholinesterase can hydrolyze as many as 5000 molecules of acetylcholine per second. These biochemical events are diagrammed in Fig. 3. Acetylcholine can also be metabolized by pseudo- or butrylcholinesterase, which is found primarily in plasma.

The importance of acetylcholinesterase for the termination of cholinergic transmission can be demonstrated if this process is pharmacologically inhibited. Many drugs, insecticides, and even chemical warfare agents, such as sarin and soman, inhibit acetylcholinesterase in a slowly reversible or irreversible fashion. The pharmacological actions of these compounds produce overstimulation of the cholinergic receptor, which can lead to tetanic paralysis and death.

The choline that is formed from the degradation of acetylcholine is actively pumped back into the nerve terminal and reused to synthesize more acetylcholine. To accomplish this reuptake, the cholinergic neuron has developed a high-affinity choline pump (K_m of 0.4–4.0 μM) that rapidly sequesters any choline from the synaptic cleft. This process for supplying choline for transmitter synthesis appears to be the *rate-limiting step* for the production of this transmitter. Drugs that inhibit the uptake of choline, (such as hemicholinium), produce rapid paralysis of muscular activity. The muscles that are used most are those that become paralyzed first, indicating that the rate of cholinergic-nerve activity in these muscles leads to exhaustion and depletion of acetylcholine.

8. BIOGENIC AMINE TRANSMITTERS ARE DECARBOXYLATED AMINO ACIDS

The aminergic transmitter systems have been given several names, which can cause confusion. The biogenic amines that are synthesized from tyrosine are known as *catecholamines*, because their structure contains a catechol moiety (e.g., a phenol ring with two hydroxyls). They are also referred to as adrenergic after the English term, adrenalin. Serotonin or 5-hydroxytryptamine (5-HT) is also called a biogenic amine. Structurally, however, it is an indolamine because its ring structure arises from tryptophan. Histamine is a biogenic amine that is present in the brain and the enteric nervous system of the gastrointestinal tract. Chemically, it is the decarboxylated amino acid histidine, and it is present in high concentrations in mast cells and in some neuronal pathways.

8.1. Catecholamine Transmitters

The catecholamine transmitters norepinephrine, epinephrine, and dopamine serve a variety of functions in the peripheral and central nervous system. Around the turn of the century, when acetylcholine was being established as a neurotransmitter, the sympathetic nerves and the adrenal medulla were being extracted for substances that raised the blood pressure and accelerated the heart rate. Otto Loewi, one of the discoverers of acetylcholine, also worked with the sympathetic transmitter, and called it *acceleranse-stuff* because it increased the heart rate. The adrenal medulla is an autonomic ganglia where the

postganglionic neurons (designated chromaffin cells) do not possess long axons. They have the capacity, as do a variety of neurons in the brain, to synthesize the catecholamine transmitter and neurohormone, known as epinephrine.

When exposed to light or alkaline pH, catecholamines oxidize to colored substances known as quinones. This helped to establish the chemical identity of these amines and helped identify some of their pathways in the brain. The substantia nigra of the midbrain, for example, is the Latin term for black substance. This area of the brain, which contains dopamine, turns dark when exposed to light or air. In patients with Parkinson's disease, the dopamine producing neurons of the substantia nigra that send axons to the striatum die off, leading to the clinical manifestations of this disease.

The catecholamines serve as sympathetic-nervous-system transmitters and help to control most visceral activity. The major amine neurotransmitter is norepinephrine, and epinephrine and norepinephrine are secreted in a ratio of 4:1 from the adrenal medulla. Dopamine may also be an unrealized sympathetic neurotransmitter, particularly because specific dopamine receptors have potent actions on kidney blood flow.

The peripheral actions of the catecholamines are well-understood, because this is such an isolated system. The actions include constriction or dilation of the arteries that control blood pressure, the increase of heart rate and strength, dilation of the bronchioles of the lungs, a decrease in gastrointestinal activity, dilation of the iris of the eye, and a variety of metabolic effects, including glycogenolysis, lipolysis, and the release of renin.

The central actions of catecholamines can best be described as arousal. Because of the complexity of the brain, their functions are not fully elucidated, but they can be partially understood from experiments using specific lesions of catecholamine pathways or the actions of selective drugs.

8.1.1. Tyrosine Precursor

The amino acid tyrosine is the common precursor for all three catecholamine transmitters—dopamine, norepinephrine, and epinephrine. The biosynthesis of the catecholamine neurotransmitters occurs primarily in the nerve terminal, as for other small-mol-wt transmitters. The enzymes that catalyze this synthesis are made and packaged in the nerve-cell body, where they are synthesized by ribosomes before transport down the axon to the terminal.

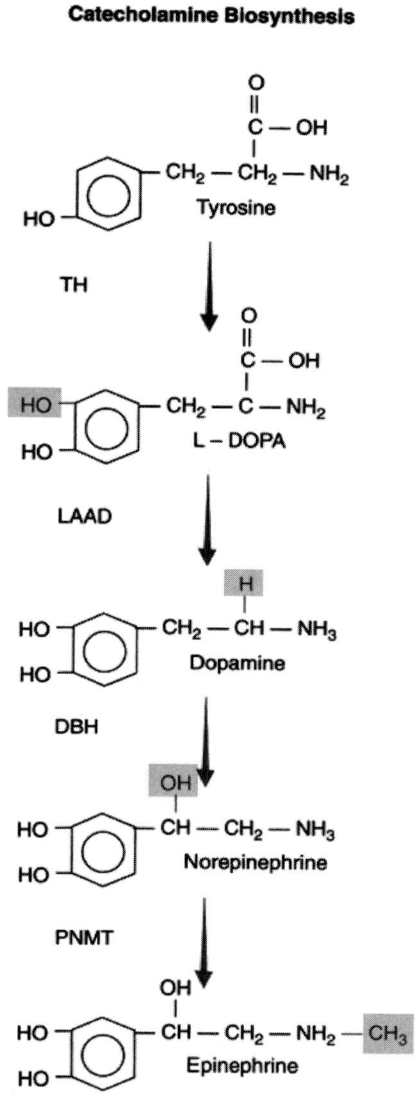

Catecholamine Biosynthesis

Fig. 4. The biosynthesis of the catecholamines, norepineph-rine, epinephrine, and dopamine from the common precursor, tyrosine. The enzymes involved are tyrosine hydroxylase (TH), L-amino acid decarboxylase (LAAD), dopamine-β-hydroxy-lase (DBH), and phenylethanolamine-*N*-methyltransferase (PNMT). The structural changes at each step are shaded.

Within the terminal, specific membrane pumps supply tyrosine or phenylalanine as the precursors for amine biosynthesis. The details of this pathway are shown in Fig. 4. Some of the biochemical parameters of the enzymes that synthesize the transmitters are also shown in Table 3. Tyrosine hydroxylase, the first and rate-limiting enzyme for the synthesis of all three catecholamines, is found in the cytoplasm. This enzyme requires molecular oxygen, iron, and a cofac-tor known as tetrahydrobiopterin. This cofactor helps

to maintain tyrosine hydroxylase in a reduced, active state. When catecholamines, such as dopamine or norepinephrine, build up in the cytoplasm, they inhibit the ability of the pteridine to activate tyrosine hydroxy-lase. This end-product inhibition provides one of the major regulatory steps in catecholamine synthesis. Other important regulatory steps include the phospho-rylation of tyrosine hydroxylase, which increases its affinity for the pteridine cofactor. This allosteric activation appears to be mediated by a variety of presynaptic receptors that use cyclic 3',5'-AMP or intracellular calcium concentration as second messen-gers. Thus, catecholamine synthesis is controlled by the rate-limiting enzyme tyrosine hydroxylase, which can be regulated by end-product feedback inhibition or by allosteric activation through second-messenger systems.

Hydroxylation of tyrosine by tyrosine hydroxylase yields the amino acid L-DOPA (L-3,4-dihydroxy-phenylalanine). This intermediate never reaches high concentrations in the cytoplasm because it is immedi-ately decarboxylated by the enzyme, L-amino acid decarboxylase. L-amino acid decarboxylase and dopamine-β-hydroxylase have activities that are 10 to 1000 times higher than tyrosine hydroxylase. The activity of these enzymes is not directly proportional to the affinity (K_m), but depends on the amount of enzyme present and on cofactor regulation (*see* Table 3). L-amino acid decarboxylase is very fast, uses the cofactor pyridoxal phosphate (e.g., Vitamin B_6), and yields dopamine, the first of the biogenic amine transmitters. Although dopamine was originally be-lieved to be only an intermediate in norepinephrine synthesis, it is the major catecholamine transmitter in the mammalian brain, is found in the autonomic ganglia and is a neurohormone in the hypothalamus, controlling pituitary prolactin secretion. In dopamin-ergic nerves, the transmitter is stored within secretory granules.

In noradrenergic nerves, dopamine is sequestered into secretory granules that contain the enzyme dopamine β-hydroxylase. This enzyme hydroxylates dopamine on the β-carbon atom by using the cofactors ascorbate (e.g., Vitamin C), molecular oxygen (O_2), and copper, producing norepinephrine. The inside of these granules are relatively acidic, which is ideal for the pH maximum of this enzyme. Many of the peptidergic transmitters are amidated on their car-boxyl-terminal ends by another vesicular enzyme that has identical pH and cofactor requirements. Noradr-energic nerves release the contents of these vesicles on

Table 3
Biochemical Properties of Emzymes

Enzyme	Mol wt	Cofactors	Affinity (K_m)
Tyrosine hydroxylase	60,000	Tetrahydrobiopterin, molecular O_2, Fe, NADPH	$0.4\text{-}2 \times 10^{-4}\,M$
L-amino acid decarboxylase	85,000–90,000	Pyridoxal phosphate (Vitamin B_6)	$4 \times 10^{-4}\,M$ (L-dopa)
Dopamine-β-hydroxylase	75,000	Ascorbate (Vitamin C), molecular O_2, Cu^{2+}	$5 \times 10^{-3}\,M$ (dopamine)
Phenylethanolamine-N-methyl transferase		S-adenosylmethionine	
Tryptophan Hydroxylase	60,000	Tetrahydrobiopterin, molecular O_2	$5 \times 10^{-5}\,M$ (tryptophan)
Choline Acetyltransferase	67,000	Acetylcoenzyme A	$7.5 \times 10^{-4}\,M$ (choline) $1 \times 10^{-5}\,M$ (coA)
Glutamic acid Decarboxylase	85,000	Pyridoxal phosphate (Vitamin B_6)	$7 \times 10^{-4}\,M$ (glut) $5 \times 10^{-5}\,M$ (Vitamin B_6)

stimulation. This type of nerve makes up the majority of sympathetic nerves in the periphery and many pathways in the brain. It is estimated that 10,000–15,000 transmitter molecules are stored in a single granule as a salt with calcium, ATP, and a protein known as chromogranin.

In adrenergic neurons in the brain or in the adrenal medulla, norepinephrine diffuses out of the secretory granules into the cytosol, where it is methylated by the last synthetic enzyme, called phenylethanolamine-N-methyltransferase (PNMT). This enzyme uses S-adenosylmethionine as a cofactor to add a methyl group to the amino side of norepinephrine. The product, epinephrine (called adrenaline by the British) is repackaged into secretory granules that contain ATP, the protein chromogranin, and dopamine-β-hydroxylase. The epinephrine-to-ATP ratio in these granules is about 4:1 in the adrenal medulla.

The activity of PNMT can be upregulated by the adrenal steroid known as cortisone. A specific portal vascular system between the adrenal cortex and medulla facilitates this activation. A diurnal early-morning increase in cortisol secretion activates PNMT to facilitate epinephrine synthesis. The resulting increase in epinephrine secretion stimulates liver glycogenolysis, gluconeogenesis, and prepares mammals for the upcoming daily activity.

8.1.2. TERMINATION OF CATECHOLAMINERGIC TRANSMISSION

Termination of catecholaminergic transmission is accomplished by active uptake of the released amines into the axon terminal, which are recycled or degraded enzymatically. Although the termination of cholinergic neurotransmission is accomplished exclusively by the enzymatic degradation of acetylcholine, termination of catecholaminergic transmission occurs primarily by active reuptake of the amines into the axon terminal.

Most cells, including platelets, appear to have some ability to pump catecholamines across their membranes. Catecholaminergic neurons have a very active high-affinity pump that sequesters the amines back into the axon before they can diffuse away from the synapse. This uptake, like that of choline, is sodium-dependent and has a K_m of 1–5 μM. The importance of this system for terminating aminergic transmission is demonstrated by the action of the stimulant drug cocaine, which inhibits uptake of the amines and increases their availability for the postsynaptic receptors. The norepinephrine-transporter protein has been cloned, and found to be a sodium-dependent membrane pump that is similar to the GABA transporter. It has 617 amino acids, and contains 12 hydrophobic (or lipophilic) amino acids sequences that span the lipid membrane.

The two enzymes that degrade the catecholamines are catechol-O-methyltransferase (COMT) and MAO. The biochemical action of these enzymes on the amine structure is shown in Fig. 5. Although COMT attaches a methyl group to the ring, MAO oxidizes the amine part of the molecule. The catecholamines can be acted on by both enzymes, forming compounds that are methylated and oxidized. These metabolites are often

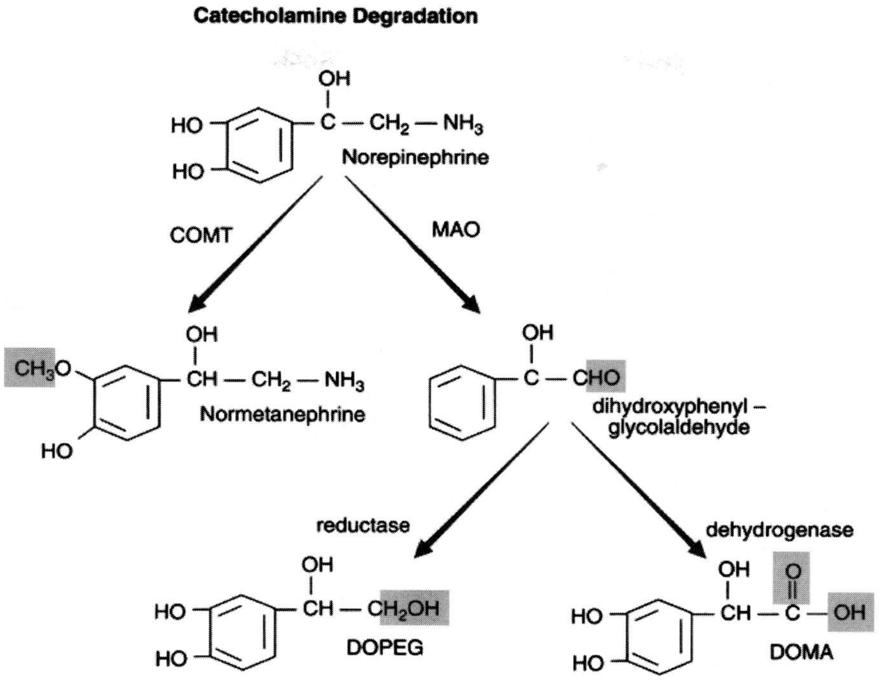

Catecholamine Degradation

Fig. 5. Changes induced by the degradative enzymes catechol-O-methyl transferase (COMT) and monoamine oxidase (MAO) on catecholamine structure. The intermediate product of MAO is an aldehyde that can be further metabolized by aldehyde reductase to 3,4-dihydroxyphenyl-ethyl-gylcol (DOPEG) or by aldehyde dehydrogenase to 3,4-dihydro-mandelic acid (DOMA). The structural changes at each step are shaded.

measured in the urine to evaluate sympathetic activity or the presence of an adrenal tumor known as a pheochromocytoma.

MAO is an intracellular enzyme found in the mitochondrial membranes of neurons and glial cells of the brain and in the liver, kidney, glandular tissues, and intestines. Its wide distribution suggests its importance in metabolizing other compounds. For example, when MAO is pharmacologically inhibited for treating depressive illnesses, tyramine—a normally innocuous substance found in aged cheeses and wines—becomes a potentially lethal toxicant. When tyramine, which is normally oxidized by MAO, is absorbed intact from the gastrointestinal tract, it can cause the release of sympathetic transmitter, leading to hypertensive crisis and death.

Monoamine oxidase has a mol wt of about 102,000 Daltons and occurs in two forms, MAO-A and MAO-B, based on substrate specificity and pharmacological inhibition. Nonselective MAO inhibitors are useful in the treatment of depressive illness, apparently because of their ability to make more biogenic amines available in the brain areas responsible for controlling mood. A selective inhibitor of MAO-B, known as

selegiline is used in treating Parkinson's disease, since dopamine is primarily metabolized by MAO-B.

MAO oxidizes the amines to their corresponding aldehydes. As shown in Figs. 6 and 7, the aldehyde product of norepinephrine and epinephrine can then be acted on by aldehyde dehydrogenase or aldehyde reductase to produce dihydroxyphenylethylglycol (DOPEG) or dihydroxymandelic acid, respectively. These can then be acted on by COMT to produce the 3-methoxy derivatives, 3-methoxy-4-hydroxy-phenylethylglycol (MHPG) and vanillylmandelic acid (VMA), respectively. The urinary excretion of these metabolic products, particularly VMA, is often used in the diagnosis of autonomic nervous system disorders. Since the aldehyde reductase pathway is believed to be more active in the CNS, MHPG or DOPEG would be the products of increased central noradrenergic and adrenergic activity.

The primary MAO metabolite of central dopamine is dihydroxyphenylacetic acid (*see* Fig. 7), which can be further metabolized by COMT to produce homovanillic acid. These metabolites are often used in research as a measure of noradrenergic or dopaminergic activity in the brain, and they may soon become clinically important.

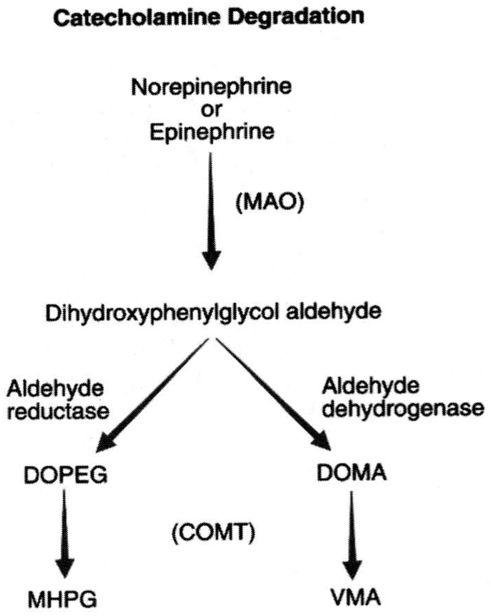

Catecholamine Degradation

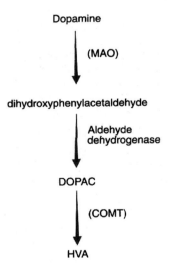

Fig. 6. MAO, aldehyde reductase, aldehyde dehydrogenase, and COMT catalyze the degradation of norepinephrine and epinephrine. The products include 3,4-dihydroxyphenylethylglycol (DOPEG), DOMA, 3-methoxy-4-hydroxyphenytethylglycol (MHPG), and vanillylmandelic acid (VMA).

Catecholamine Degradation

Dopamine

(MAO)

dihydroxyphenylacetaldehyde

Aldehyde
dehydrogenase

DOPAC

(COMT)

HVA

Fig. 7. The enzymatic degradation of dopamine is catalyzed by MAO and COMT. The major products are 3,4-dihydroxyphenyl acetic acid (DOPAC) and homovanillic acid (HVA).

COMT is a cytoplasmic enzyme that is distributed even more widely than MAO. It is found in high concentrations in the kidney and liver. The enzyme has a mol wt of about 24,000 Daltons and requires S-adenosylmethionine and the divalent cation, Mg^{2+}.

The enzyme transfers a methyl group from S-adenosyl-methionine to the 3-hydroxy group of the catecholamine. It can also methylate catechol-based drugs such as isoproterenol, a β-adrenergic-receptor-stimulating drug that is useful in treating asthma. Epinephrine, norepinephrine, and dopamine are methylated by COMT to produce metanephrine, normetanephrine, and 3-methoxytyramine, respectively. Measuring the amounts of these compounds excreted in the urine is useful in the diagnosis of the adrenal tumor, pheochromocytoma.

8.1.3. CATECHOLAMINE PATHWAYS

Specific catecholamine pathways have been mapped throughout the brain and appear to function in a variety of behavioral, cognitive, and physiologic processes. The three catecholaminergic pathways can be visualized by techniques known as fluorescent microscopy and immunocytochemistry.

Fluorescent histochemistry uses the property of the catechol molecules to fluoresce when exposed to chemicals such as formaldehyde. This method was initially used to map the catecholamine and indolamine (e.g., serotonin) pathways within the CNS. The drawback of this technique is that it is difficult to differentiate various catecholaminergic or indolaminergic pathways because of the similar wavelengths of emitted light.

Immunocytochemistry is a method that uses specific antibodies that are generated against the purified enzymes involved in catecholamine biosynthesis. The antibodies bind to the enzymes (or specific transmitters) that are fixed on histologic sections of the brain. This technique can be used to label the cell bodies, axons, and terminals of a specific neuronal pathway. The bound antibodies are detected by using chemical reactions that produce a color change or electron-opaque product in the neurons containing the antigen. In practice, if a pathway contains the enzyme PNMT, which methylates norepinephrine to epinephrine, it can be assumed that this pathway is adrenergic, although it would also contain dopamine-β-hydroxylase and tyrosine hydroxylase. If the pathway only contains dopamine-β-hydroxylase and tyrosine hydroxylase, it would probably be *noradrenergic*, but one that contains only tyrosine hydroxylase would be *dopaminergic*.

Dopamine is the major catecholamine neurotransmitter in the mammalian CNS. Dopamine was originally believed to be only a precursor in the synthesis of norepinephrine and epinephrine, but it was discovered that dopamine comprised as much as 50% of the

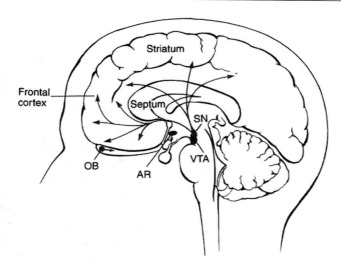

Fig. 8. The major dopaminergic pathways in the CNS. Dopaminergic cell groups from the substantia nigra (SN) project to the caudate and putamen. Cell bodies near the substantia nigra in the ventral tegmental area (VTA) project axons to the septum, limbic cortex (including the frontal and cingulate cortex), amygdala, nucleus accumbens (NA), and olfactory tubercle (OB). Other discrete dopaminergic systems exist in the hypothalamic arcuate (AR) and periventricular nuclei, in the olfactory bulb, and in the retina.

total catecholamines in the brain of mammals. Moreover, the localization of dopamine and norepinephrine within the brain did not always coincide. The dopaminergic neuronal systems are heterogeneous, and have been classified by the Swedish investigators who developed the fluorescent technique into several specific nuclear groups designated A8–A17.

Dopamine is found in interneurons in the peripheral autonomic ganglia. Similar dopaminergic interneurons with very short axons are also found in the retina and in the olfactory bulb, where they appear to modify sensory input through inhibition of their target neurons. In the retina, this is called lateral inhibition, which is important for processing visual information.

Dopaminergic neurons with intermediate-length axons include the tuberoinfundibular and hypophysial, incertohypothalamic cells, and the medullary periventricular group. The tuberoinfundibular neurons have a neurohumoral function; they secrete dopamine into a portal vascular system that supplies the anterior pituitary. This dopamine is responsible for inhibiting secretion of the anterior pituitary hormone, prolactin. Many of the dopaminergic pathways in the brain are diagrammed in Fig. 8.

The final subdivision of dopaminergic neurons includes the midbrain groups from the substantia nigra and the ventral tegmental area. These systems have long axons that innervate the basal ganglia, parts of the limbic system, and the frontal cortex. The neostriatal

system, which has cell bodies in the substantia nigra, innervates the caudate and putamen. This suggests that dopamine released from neostriatal areas has motor functions. The motor problems associated with Parkinson's disease are caused by a decrease in dopamine in these areas. Administration of the dopamine precursor L-DOPA bypasses tyrosine hydroxylase and alleviates some of the motor disturbances of Parkinson's disease.

The specificity and complexity of the dopaminergic systems is further demonstrated by the mesolimbic system. These neurons originate in the ventral tegmental area of the midbrain, next to the substantia nigra. Long axons from these neurons project to many parts of the limbic system, including the nucleus accumbens, olfactory tubercle, septum, amygdala, and limbic cortex (e.g., frontal and cingulate cortex). These areas are associated with mood alterations and cognitive function, indicating another important role of central dopamine. The nucleus accumbens is involved with reward, and the release of dopamine in this area generates positive feelings of reinforcement. It is in this area that the stimulant properties of cocaine and amphetamine (which releases axonal dopamine) are believed to act. The actions of many antidepressant drugs may also be associated with these brain areas. These agents, which inhibit MAO or the amine uptake pump, increase the amount of dopamine available for the dopamine receptor in these areas. The noradrenergic and serotonergic systems may also be involved in mood disorders.

The role of dopamine in cognition can be demonstrated by the action of a group of drugs used in treating schizophrenia. These agents, known as neuroleptics, block dopamine receptors and alleviate many of the hallucinations and ideations associated with this disease. However, prolonged therapy with some dopamine-blocking drugs can adversely affect the nigrostriatal system and produce a variety of adverse effects, including a Parkinson-like syndrome and an abnormal involuntary-movement syndrome called tardive dyskinesia.

The *noradrenergic pathways* of the brainstem are highly diffuse, project all over the brain, and are probably involved in activation of cognitive function and mood. The noradrenergic system in the brain comprises far fewer cells and is less specific than the dopaminergic system. Although there are 30,000–40,000 dopamine cells in the midbrain system alone, there are only about 10,000 noradrenergic neurons in the enire brain, which are localized in the brainstem. Specifically, noradrenergic cell bodies are found in the locus coeruleus and lateral tegmental nuclei of the brainstem (Fig. 9). Coeruleus means blue and refers to the pigment associated with this area. Although there are very few cells in these nuclei, the axons are highly branched and project to all parts of the CNS. Noradrenergic axons can be found throughout the cortex, limbic system, hypothalamus, olfactory bulb, cerebellum, medulla, and spinal cord.

Instead of forming discrete synapses at the ends of axonal branches, noradrenergic neurons elaborate varicosities all along their axons that contain norepinephrine filled vesicles. These are known as *diffuse synapses*, and resemble a string of beads or pearls when viewed by fluorescent microscopy. Presumably, the transmitter released at this type of synapse bathes the postsynaptic target area to initiate a response. These CNS noradrenergic neurons closely resemble the noradrenergic neurons found in the sympathetic nervous system. In contrast to the noradrenergic diffuse synapses, *contact synapses*, in which specific synaptic processes are formed at the end of the axons, are typical of most other transmitter systems, as exemplified by the neuromuscular junction.

Noradrenergic neurons, such as dopaminergic neurons, can inhibit or excite the postsynaptic cells, depending on which receptor subtype is present. Within the CNS, many neurons have been found to

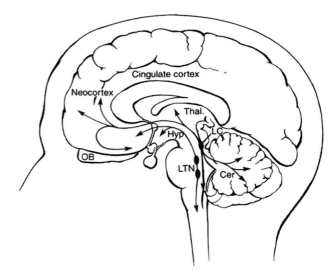

Fig. 9. The noradrenergic pathways in the CNS are restricted to several cell groups in the brainstem. The limited number of noradrenergic cell bodies in the locus ceruleus (LC) and the lateral tegmental nuclei (LTN) send highly branched axons to all areas of the brain, including the neocortex, cingulate cortex, thalamus (Thal), hypothalamus (Hyp), olfactory bulb (OB), and cerebellum (Cer).

express β-adrenergic receptors, which use cyclic AMP as a second messenger. Within the locus coeruleus, pharmacological studies have shown that α_2-adrenergic receptors influence firing rates. Noradrenergic activity inhibits spontaneous firing of large portions of the CNS and may enhance signal-to-noise levels in the brain.

The noradrenergic system appears to be important in arousal or motivation. Stimulant drugs, such as cocaine and amphetamine, and some tricyclic antidepressants (TCAs) and monoamine oxidase inhibitors (MAOIs) increase the amount of norepinephrine available for binding to adrenergic receptors, potentiating the noradrenergic system. Most studies suggest that increased noradrenergic activity is associated with heightened vigilance and behavioral awareness, and that decreased noradrenergic activity results in more vegetative processes. Central norepinephrine has also been implicated in pain pathways, memory, and the control of autonomic and endocrine function. The distribution of the noradrenergic neurons in the brain is diagrammed in Fig. 9.

Epinephrine-containing neurons in the brain are restricted to the brainstem, and may be important in regulating autonomic and endocrine function. Adrenergic neurons in the brainstem have been visualized by

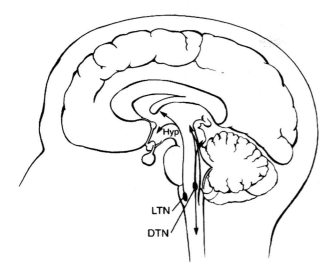

Fig. 10. The adrenergic pathways in the brain originate from a few cell groups in the lateral (LTN) and dorsal tegmental nuclei (DTN). These cell bodies send axons to the hypothalamus (HYP), locus coeruleus (LC), and to the intermediolateral-cell columns of the spinal cord.

staining for their unique enzyme, PNMT. Figure 10 shows the distribution of known adrenergic neurons in the brain. These cells are restricted to nuclei in the lateral and dorsal tegmentum (designated Cl-3 by the Swedish group that initially described them). They ascend to innervate the hypothalamus and descend the spinal cord to innervate the intermediolateral-cell column that gives rise to the preganglionic nerve cell bodies of the sympathetic nervous system.

Little is known about the function of epinephrine in the brain, although it does inhibit firing of neurons in the locus coeruleus. Based on epinephrine's anatomic distribution, it seems to be important in the regulation of autonomic and neuroendocrine hypothalamic function. Many studies attest to this supposition.

8.2. Serotonin

8.2.1. DISTRIBUTION

Serotonin is an indolamine present in neural pathways that parallel the distribution of norepinephrine in the brain. Serotonin is found in many cells of the body, such as blood platelets, mast cells, and the enterochromaffin cells of the gastrointestinal tract, and in brain cells. It was originally discovered in blood, where it has a vasoconstrictor effect on the arteries. For this reason, it was believed to be the cause of high blood pressure. So much serotonin exists in peripheral platelets, mast cells, and the gastrointestinal tract that the

amount in the brain only represents 1–2% of the total amount found in the body. Serotonin is also found in the pineal body of the brain, where it functions as the precursor for melatonin, an indolamine that is considered important in circadian cycles and reproductive function.

Serotonin is synthesized from the essential amino acid tryptophan, which crosses the blood-brain barrier by a mechanism that also supplies the brain with aromatic and branched-chain amino acids. The concentration of serotonin in the brain is sensitive to the availability of tryptophan in the diet, so that brain serotonin levels can be modified by competition for uptake by other amino acids. In the serotonergic neuron, tryptophan is hydroxylated to 5-hydroxytryptophan (5-HTP) by an enzyme known as tryptophan hydroxylase (Fig. 11). This enzyme is similar to tyrosine hydroxylase because both use molecular oxygen and a tetrahydropteridine cofactor. Like tyrosine hydroxylase, it is also regulated by phosphorylation, calcium, phospholipids, and partial proteolysis.

The genes for many hydroxylase enzymes have now been cloned and characterized, making it possible to compare their amino acid sequences. These studies show that tyrosine, tryptophan, and phenylalanine hydroxylases probably originated or evolved from a common ancestral gene. The catalytic and regulatory elements of all three enzymes show marked similarity, but there are also differences.

Unlike tyrosine hydroxylase, tryptophan hydroxylase is not regulated by end-product inhibition. Although dopamine or norepinephrine can feed back to inhibit their own synthesis, increased cytoplasmic serotonin does not inhibit tryptophan hydroxylase. For example, if an inhibitor of MAO (an enzyme that degrades catecholamines and serotonin) is administered, the concentration of serotonin in the brain increases by 300%. This is not the case with the catecholamines.

The second enzymatic step in the formation of serotonin is the decarboxylation of 5-HTP. This is accomplished by the aromatic amino acid decarboxylase, an enzyme that also decarboxylates L-DOPA to produce dopamine. Since this enzyme has a very high activity, it is not rate-limiting in the synthesis of serotonin, and therefore little 5-HTP is expected to be present in these neurons.

What regulates serotonin turnover? Several factors are probably involved. Presynaptic neuromodulation can regulate tryptophan hydroxylase activity by activation of second-messenger systems that phosphorylate and activate the enzyme. The K_m for tryptophan hydroxylase (*see* Table 3) is higher than the amount of tryptophan in the blood. This means that the enzyme is not saturated, and that the availability of substrate may also regulate activity. This suggests that in some circumstances, nutrition and diet can alter brain activity and mood.

As in the case of the catecholamines, serotonin is actively taken up and stored in a specific set of secretory granules. The pumping mechanism responsible for the uptake of serotonin (and the catecholamines) into these granules is inhibited by the drug reserpine. If the storage of the amines is inhibited by this drug, all four of the biogenic amines are depleted. Because of this action, this plant alkaloid has been used for centuries as a sedative, in psychosis, and for hypertension.

Once serotonin is released into the synaptic cleft, the serotonergic response is terminated by reuptake into the presynaptic axon terminal. An important class of antidepressant drugs, known as selective serotonin reuptake inhibitors (SSRIs), blocks the reuptake of serotonin from the synaptic cleft, thus prolonging and strengthening the postsynaptic response. Fluoxetine (Prozac), sertraline (Zoloft), and paroxetine (Paxil) are examples of SSRIs.

In the pineal gland, serotonin undergoes two additional biochemical steps to produce the pineal "hormone" melatonin. First serotonin is N-acetylated to make N-acetyl serotonin followed by methylation of the hydroxy group to melatonin by the enzyme 5-hydroxyindole-O-methyltransferase. The first enzyme in this pathway, N-acetyltransferase, is subject to regulation by the sympathetic nervous system-mediated β-adrenergic receptor, which alters cyclic AMP formation during the day-night cycle.

8.2.2. SEROTONIN CATABOLISM

The major pathways for the degradation of serotonin are reuptake into the nerve and degradation by MAO. There are many similarities between the catecholaminergic and indolaminergic metabolic pathways. Unlike the catecholamines, indolamines can not be degraded by methylation by COMT because of the difference in the ring structure and the presence of only one hydroxyl on the phenolic ring. The pathway for serotonin degradation is shown on Fig. 12. MAO oxidizes serotonin to 5-hydroxyindoleacetic acid through an indoleacetaldehyde intermediate or 5-hydroxytryptophol through an aldehyde reductase, depending on the $NAD^+/NADH$ ratio in the brain.

Serotonin Biosynthesis

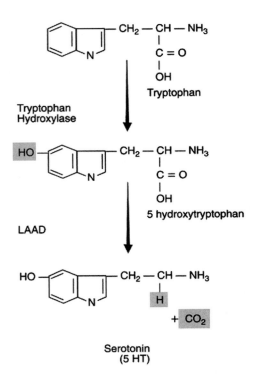

Fig. 11. Serotonin biosynthesis begins with the hydroxylation of tryptophan to 5-hydroxytryptophan (5-HTP) by tryptophan hydroxylase. This amino acid is decarboxylated by L-amino acid decarboxylase (LAAD) to serotonin (5-HT). The shaded groups represent enzymatic additions or deletions.

The similarities between the uptake and degradation processes are such that many of the same drugs that inhibit catecholamine uptake and MAO degradation do the same for serotonin. For example, many of the tricyclic antidepressants also inhibit neuronal serotonin uptake, and all of the MAO inhibitors inhibit serotonin degradation. Together with the SSRIs, these drugs are useful in the treatment of affective disorders such as anxiety and depression, a topic that is further discussed in the section on the aminergic theory of the affective disorders.

The *serotonergic pathways* originate in the raphe nucleus, area postrema (AP), and caudal locus coeruleus and generally parallel the noradrenergic pathways. Although the mapping of the serotonergic systems of the brain was initially hindered by some of the limitations of the histofluorescent microscopy, these systems are now well-delineated anatomically. The cell bodies of the serotonergic nerves in the brain arise from several groups of cells in a midline area of the pons and upper brainstem called the *raphe nuclei* (Fig. 13). They have been classified as the B1–B9 serotonergic nerve groups. The more rostral of the nuclei innervate the cortex, thalamus, and limbic systems, and the posterior nuclei (e.g., B1, B2, and B3) innervate the medulla and spinal cord. Unlike the organized nuclear distribution of the dopaminergic system, the serotonergic nuclei innervate much of the telencephalon and diencephalon in an overlapping manner.

The major functions of the serotonergic system remain relatively ill-defined. More than 90% of the brain serotonin can be depleted with p-chlorophenylalanine, a drug that inhibits tryptophan hydroxylase, with few gross effects on animal behavior. The serotonergic cells of the raphe possess a pacemaker-like activity that is modified by 5-HT autoreceptors and noradrenergic receptors. The rate of activity of these cells is high during wakefulness, low during sleep, and absent during *rapid eye movement* (REM) sleep. The raphe nucleus displays pacemaker-type activity similar to the sinoatrial node of the heart, which regulates the rate of the heart. Perhaps the raphe serotonergic neurons regulate the "rate of the brain function," in a manner analogous to altering the clock speed of a computer CPU. Although the serotonergic system has been linked to and modulates such phenomena as sleep, vigilance, arousal, sensory perception, and emotion, it does not appear to generate these phenomena.

Pharmacological observations have implicated the serotonergic system in higher cognitive function, schizophrenia, and hallucinations. Many of the hallucinogenic drugs resemble serotonin and interact with the 5-HT receptors. Dimethyltryptamine (DMT) and diethyltryptamine are hallucinogenic drugs of abuse, differing from serotonin by the addition of two methyl or ethyl groups on the amine terminal. The hallucinogenic drug lysergic acid diethylamide (LSD) also is chemically similar to serotonin, and has been shown to interfere with autoreceptor function at the raphe nucleus and increase serotonergic firing rates. Schizophrenia was once believed to be caused by the pathologic production of an abnormal serotonin, such as DMT.

8.2.3. AMINERGIC THEORY OF AFFECTIVE DISORDERS

The *affective disorders* are a group of psychiatric diseases that include mania, unipolar, and bipolar depression. Bipolar depression is characterized by exaggerated swings in mood that may cycle over a period of months or years. It is a serious, debilitating

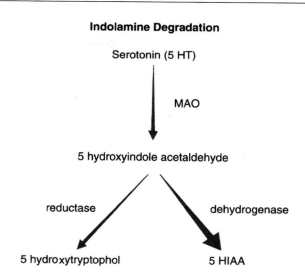

Fig. 12. Serotonin degradation is enzymatically catalyzed in a manner similar to that for the catecholamines. Serotonin or 5-hydroxytryptamine (5-HT) is acted on by MAO to yield 5-hydroxyindole acetaldehyde. This intermediate is metabolized by an aldehyde reductase or dehydrogenase to yield 5-hydroxytryptophol or 5-hydroxyindole acetic acid (5-HIAA).

disorder that can lead to suicide. About 80% of these patients respond to medication.

Although the medications fall into different groups, they all tend to make more biogenic amines available for receptor stimulation. The two major groups are the *tricyclic antidepressants*, which inhibit the uptake of the biogenic amines, and the MAO inhibitors, which inhibit their degradation. This information has prompted the *amine theory of affective disorders*.

There are still many unanswered questions regarding this theory. The specific amine that is responsible for the depressed mood is unknown. The tricyclic agents inhibit the uptake of norepinephrine, epinephrine, dopamine, and serotonin, while MAO is responsible for degrading all of the amine transmitters. There are selective uptake inhibitors for serotonin and norepinephrine, which are both effective in treating depression. The SSRIs are widely prescribed drugs, and have been shown to be effective. All of the antidepressants take several weeks to alleviate depression, although they are immediately effective in inhibiting amine uptake or MAO (in vivo and in vitro). One explanation for the delay is that they lead to slow changes in receptor populations that result in stabilization of mood. Depression is still an ill-defined disease that may result from several biochemical imbalances.

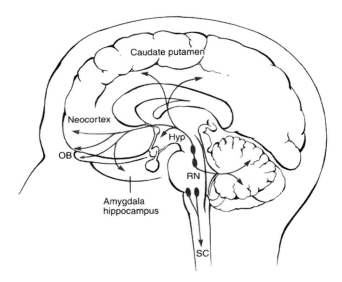

Fig. 13. The major serotonergic pathways in the brain originate in the midline pontine and upper brainstem area known as the raphe nuclei (RN). The posterior cell groups project to the spinal cord (SC), and the anterior serotonergic axons parallel the noradrenergic nerves to innervate diffusely the cortex, striatum, hypothalamus (HYP), olfactory bulb (OB), amygdala, hippocampus, and cerebellum.

8.3. Histamine

Histamine is found in mast cells and central neurons. This imidazole-containing substance has been studied since the early 1900s, when Henry Dale described its many actions. It was isolated and purified around 1930, and it has often been considered as a neurotransmitter candidate. Acceptance of this role for histamine, however, has been hampered by several factors. It is found in high concentrations in mast cells (also present in the brain), where it is important for immune responses. The histochemical techniques to visualize histamine-containing neurons were difficult to develop, and are only now being applied. Because the enzyme responsible for synthesizing this compound, histidine decarboxylase, is very much like the amino acid decarboxylase that produces catecholamines and serotonin, the specificity of its localization is questionable.

Histamine is produced by the decarboxylation of the essential amino acid histidine, as shown in Fig. 14. The enzyme that catalyzes this reaction resembles L-amino acid decarboxylase, although it has been difficult to isolate from adult mammalian tissue. A fetal liver histidine decarboxylase has been purified and is believed to be similar to the enzyme in central neurons. Like the other decarboxylases, it requires vita-

min B, (e.g., pyridoxal phosphate) and can be inhibited by drugs that interact with the same step in catecholamine and indolamine transmission. Similar to tryptophan hydroxylase, the affinity (K_m) for histidine decarboxylase is higher than the amount of substrate (e.g., histidine) available for decarboxylation. Since the enzyme is not usually saturated, dietary intake of this essential amino acid may affect the activity of this system. Histidine loading increases the amount of histamine in the brain.

The major catabolic pathway for the elimination of histamine in the mammal is through N-methylation to methylhistamine (*see* Fig. 14) by the enzyme histamine methyltransferase. This enzyme uses S-adenosylmethionine as the methyl donor. Methylhistamine can be further catabolized by MAO.

The concentration of histamine in the brain is about 50 ng/g, some of which is undoubtedly in mast cells. Administration of mast cell-degranulating agents (e.g., histamine-depleting agents) produces a 50% reduction of brain concentrations of histamine. During postnatal development, when the blood–brain barrier matures, the elevated histamine levels and the number of mast cells concurrently decrease.

Using antibodies against histidine decarboxylase and histamine itself, nerve pathways have been observed that originate in posterior basal hypothalamus and premammillary areas. These histaminergic neurons appear to ascend through the medial forebrain bundle to innervate the forebrain, including cortical, thalamic, and limbic structures. Lesioning of the medial forebrain bundle causes a complete depletion of the norepinephrine and serotonin, which has a timecourse similar to the degeneration of axons after lesioning. Studies have shown that similar lesions also cause a 70% decrease in histidine decarboxylase levels in the forebrain.

Many studies have indicated that central histamine pathways may be involved in the central control of autonomic and endocrine activity, food and water intake, and temperature regulation. Because blockers of the H_1 histamine receptor causes sedation, a role in arousal—like those of catecholamines and serotonin—is also suggested. This is easily demonstrated in the allergic patient, in whom antihistamines have the side effects of sleepiness and increased appetite.

This chapter does not cover all of the substances currently considered to be neurotransmitters, but focuses on those that are best-known, understood, and studied. Among the other potential candidates are taurine, octopamine, and ATP. The field offers a

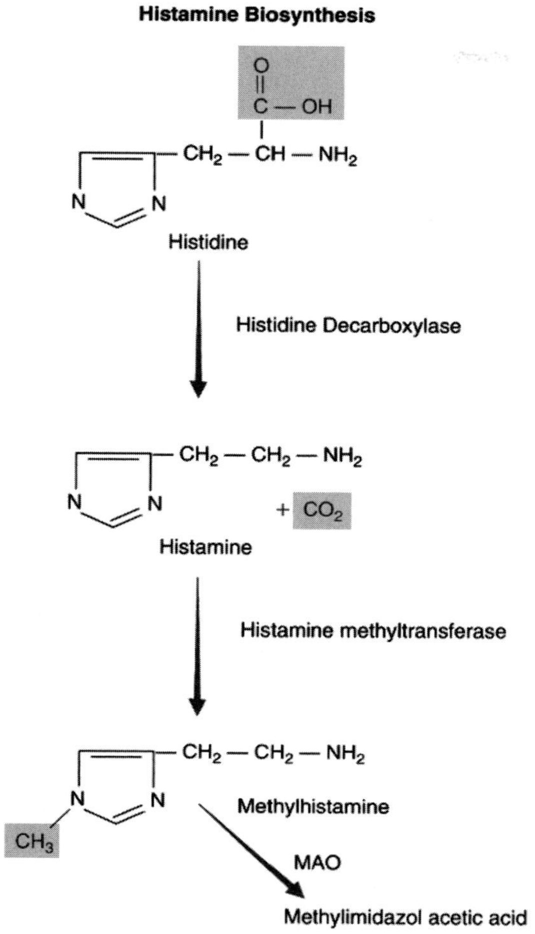

Histamine Biosynthesis

Histidine

Histidine Decarboxylase

Histamine

+ CO_2

Histamine methyltransferase

Methylhistamine

MAO

Methylimidazol acetic acid

Fig. 14. Histamine biosynthesis and degradation. The amino acid histidine is decarboxylated by histidine decarboxylase to produce the neurotransmitter histamine and CO_2. Histamine is degraded by methylation initially to methylhistamine before being oxidized by MAO to methylimidazol acetic acid. The shaded groups indicate enzymatic additions or deletions.

tremendous potential for further investigation of these candidates.

9. γ-GABA, GLUTAMATE, AND GLYCINE ARE MAJOR TRANSMITTER SYSTEMS IN THE MAMMALIAN BRAIN

Although the amino acid tyrosine is the common precursor for all three of the catecholamine neurotransmitters, glutamate is equally crucial for production of the amino acid transmitters in the CNS. Glutamate is a transmitter in the excitatory amino acid (EAA) pathway and is the precursor for the major inhibitory amino acid transmitter, GABA. The concentrations of these substances are almost 1000 times higher than the con-

ventional amine transmitters in the brain, which may reflect their relative importance.

The EAAs, glutamate and aspartate, depolarize their postsynaptic target neurons and can be compared with the accelerator pedal of an automobile. GABA in the brain and glycine in the spinal chord hyperpolarize their target neurons, and can similarly be compared with the brake pedal of the automobile. The inhibitory importance of GABA and glycine can be easily demonstrated if their receptors are blocked by drugs such as picrotoxin or strychnine, which block the GABA and glycine receptors, respectively. Administration of these drugs immediately induces life-threatening seizures and death.

Why were such important transmitter systems overlooked for so many years? The reason lies in the fact that amino acids are a common constituent of all cells. Although norepinephrine or serotonin could be specifically localized to certain neurons and brain areas, glutamate and glycine are universally present. New neurochemical, molecular, and immunochemical techniques have greatly expanded our understanding of the distribution and functioning of these transmitters.

9.1. γ-GABA

9.1.1. FUNCTION AND DISTRIBUTION

GABA serves as the principal transmitter involved in internal circuits within specific brain areas. GABA is found in the brain, spinal cord, and retina, with only trace quantities observed in other types of tissues or peripheral nerves. Quantitatively, the amount of the biogenic amine norepinephrine is in the range of nmoles/g, but GABA can be measured within the brain in units of μ moles/g. If the concentration of a transmitter is 1000-fold more, is it proportionally that much more important? The answer to this question is being sought in many laboratories.

The decarboxylation of glutamate to GABA is not very different from the decarboxylation of L-DOPA or tryptophan to dopamine and serotonin. The enzyme that does this is called glutamic acid decarboxylase (GAD), and it removes the α-carboxyl group to produce a γ-carboxyl amino acid. The biosynthesis and catabolism of GABA is shown in Fig. 15. Like the three other decarboxylases discussed in this chapter, GAD requires the cofactor pyridoxal phosphate (vitamin B_6). The saturation of GAD with its cofactor may be one of the rate-limiting steps in GABA synthesis, controlled by steric inhibition with ATP. This could explain why the concentration of GABA in the brain increases rapidly from 30–45% after death when ATP levels drop. The distribution of GAD does appear to be selective to endogenous GABA neurons, which generally have short axons. GAD is not present in glia or other types of neurons.

The GABA shunt, which is studied in conjunction with the Krebs cycle in biochemistry, is a unique feature of the brain and a viable form of energy production. The key aspects of this pathway are emphasized in Fig. 15. GABA is produced from α-oxoglutarate, through glutamate, degraded by two enzymes present throughout the brain, and reenters the Krebs cycle as succinic acid.

What is the significance of this energy-producing shunt? First, it generates ATP (three), although a little less efficiently (by one GTP) than the Krebs cycle. Estimates have indicated that the GABA shunt contributes to 10–40% of brain metabolism. Second, glial cells, which have high-affinity GABA pumps, are able to scavenge GABA and use it for energy. Third, glutamate is regenerated through the degradation of GABA in GABAergic nerves. Enzyme localization studies have shown that GAD is high in GABA-containing areas (e.g., GABA neurons), but the GABA-degrading enzymes, GABA transaminase (GABA-T) and succinic semialdhyde dehydrogenase (SSADH), are localized throughout the brain.

9.1.2. GABA Catabolism

GABAergic transmission is terminated by uptake into neurons and glia, where it is metabolized by enzymes that can regenerate glutamate and produce more ATP. The GABA-uptake transporter has been characterized and cloned. It is a large protein that appears to have 12 membrane-spanning domains containing hydrophobic amino acids that can insert through the lipid bilayer of the membrane. Like the catecholamine transporter, it is Na^+-dependent and has been shown to transport two Na^+ ions out of the cell in exchange for one GABA and one Cl^- ion. Because of the ionic redistribution, GABA uptake is electrogenic (e.g., changes the membrane potential) and can sequester GABA against a gradient of 10,000 to 1.

GABA is catabolized by several enzymes that are localized throughout the brain. GABA transaminase requires pyridoxal phosphate, and may under certain circumstances compete with GAD for the cofactor. The K_m of GABA-T for vitamin B_6 is much lower than that of GAD. The overall effect of vitamin B_6 deficiency is an increased susceptibility to seizures related to decreased GABA synthesis. These seizures are rap-

idly reversed after pyridoxine is administered. Transamination of GABA to succinic semialdehyde by GABA-T results in the regeneration of glutamate for decarboxylation to GABA. GABA-T catalyzes the formation of succinic semialdehyde, which is metabolized by SSADH to succinate. The K_m of SSADH is so low (10^{-6} M) that very little of its substrate, succinic semialdehyde, ever accumulates in the brain. An alternate pathway results in the formation of the metabolite γ-hydroxybutyrate.

Localization studies have hinged on the immunocytochemical distribution of GAD. Many of these pathways are outlined in the brain map in Fig. 16. Mapping studies have shown that GABAergic pathways make up the major endogenous circuits within specific brain areas. Most of these have short axonal pathways that interact locally. The best-understood systems are those in the Purkinje cells of the cerebellar cortex that inhibit the deep nuclei and the GABAergic system in the striatum that projects to the substantia nigra and globus pallidus (GPe). Other systems that are believed to be GABAergic are the granule cells of the olfactory bulb, some of the amacrine cells of the retina, basket cells of the hippocampus, and a long ascending projection from the hypothalamus to the cerebral cortex.

The major function of the GABA system is inhibition of the target pathways. This is accomplished by the opening of chloride channels and the resultant hyperpolarization. Several drugs that interact with the GABA system illustrate the inhibitory function of these nerves. GABA-blocking drugs such as picrotoxin, or drugs that decrease the availability of GABA lead to convulsions similar to epileptic seizures. This transmitter system is believed to be important in the cause of epilepsy. Drugs that increase the amount of GABA or potentiate the action of GABA result in central inhibition, and can lead to coma and death. Many drugs potentiate the GABA system, including the barbiturates, benzodiazepines (e.g., Valium and Librium), anesthetic steroids, and alcohol. The antianxiety and sedative characteristics of these agents provide a good idea of some of the actions and functions of central GABA systems. It is possible to speculate that death is not such an unpleasant experience because of the massive disinhibition and increase in GABA activity found postmortem.

This is an interesting, seemingly well-designed, inhibitory transmitter system that generates metabolic energy when it is active, regenerates its own substrate, and limits the rate of its own activity through produc-

Synthesis and Degradation

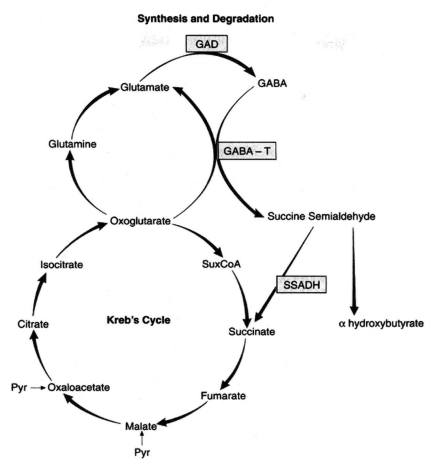

Fig. 15. GABA and glutamate synthesis and degradation are shown in relation to the Kreb's cycle and GABA shunt. The important enzymes in the pathway are shown in the *shaded boxes*. GABA is synthesized by the enzyme GAD from glutamate. GABA can be degraded by GABA transaminase (GABA-T) to succinic semialdehyde in a reaction that regenerates glutamate from oxoglutarate. Succinic semialdehyde can reenter the Kreb's cycle by the action of succinic semi-aldehyde dehydrogenase (SSADH), or can be degraded to α-hydroxybutyrate. The entire system is fueled by glucose, which enters the cycle after being converted to pyruvate (pyr) as indicated.

tion of ATP. It is well-suited to be the major inhibitory transmitter system in the brain.

9.2. Glycine

Glycine is an inhibitory transmitter that is principally localized in the brainstem and spinal cord. The transmitter role of glycine, like glutamate, was disputed for years based on the fact that it is an amino acid found in all cells as an important constituent of proteins, peptides, and precursor for porphyrins and nucleic acids. The concentration of glycine is very high in the spinal cord, as is glutamate and glutamine. Glycine is the simplest amino acid in the body, and is not considered to be essential for the diet.

Although glycine could originate from many metabolic sources, it appears to be predominantly gener-

ated from serine. This has been determined by following the incorporation of the radioactive carbon into glycine after administering various radiolabeled precursors. Similarly, although there are many possible degradation pathways, active uptake seems to be the preferred route of removal of this inhibitory amino acid from the synapse. Like the GABA and biogenic amine transporters, the glycine uptake mechanism is Na^+-dependent. Radiolabeled glycine preloaded into neurons can be released from spinal cord slices by depolarization in a Ca^{2+}-dependent manner. Glycinergic neurons are believed to mediate motor and sensory functions in the spinal cord, brainstem, and the retina.

Like GABA, glycine has important anticonvulsant properties. However, the anti-anxiety and sedative actions of glycine have not been demonstrated phar-

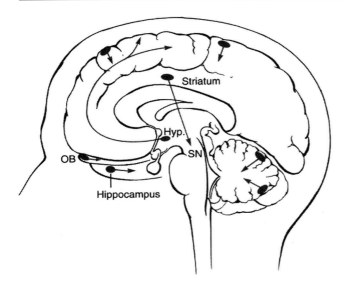

Fig. 16. The GABA-producing neurons in the brain consist mostly of interneurons with short axons that remain within the brain area from which the cells originate. GABA concentrations are about 100-fold higher than the catecholamines in most brain structures, including the cortex, limbic system, and cerebellum. In contrast, a group of GABA neurons in the striatum with long axons projects to the substantia nigra (SN), and another tract in the hypothalamus (Hyp) is believed to project to the forebrain. Tracts in the olfactory bulb (OB) and hippocampus are also depicted.

macologically. The Renshaw cell of the ventral root is an interneuron that has been characterized in terms of its ability to alter alpha motor neuron activity. This glycinergic interneuron receives its input from a collateral axon of the alpha motor neuron, and is stimulated by the release of acetylcholine when the motor neuron fires. The stimulated Renshaw cell then releases glycine onto dendrites or the cell body of the motor neuron to inhibit further motor activity. When this classic feedback mechanism is blocked by strychnine, the motor neuron fires without control, and convulsions result. Strychnine is a specific glycine-receptor blocker. It is a complex plant alkaloid found in the herb *Nux vomica*. It has been used as a rat poison, and is an ingredient in herbal, homeopathic, and proprietary drugs, although there is no generally accepted rationale for its use. Sensory actions of glycine in the spinal cord are also suggested by the use of small amounts of an extract of *Nux vomica* to increase tactile sensations.

Glycine also appears to be an important component of glutamatergic transmission. One of the glutamate receptors (e.g., NMDA receptor) has a glycine-binding site that, when occupied, increases the frequency

of Ca^{2+}-channel opening. This neuromodulatory response to glycine is not blocked by strychnine.

9.3. Glutamate

Glutamate is the major excitatory transmitter in the brain. Amino acids such as glutamate and aspartate stimulate (e.g., depolarize) many different types of neurons. For years, this action was considered to be nonspecific, which seemed to disqualify glutamate as a transmitter candidate. Glutamate and its precursor glutamine are found in very high concentrations in the brain and spinal cord. These high levels are apparently achieved without uptake from the periphery, since the influx of glutamate into the brain from the blood seems to be slower than its efflux from the brain to the periphery. The massive amounts of glutamate and glutamine in the brain arise from the metabolism of glucose by means of the Krebs cycle. Like glycine, these amino acids occur in all brain cells, including glia, which made it difficult for many years to map precise glutamate and aspartate pathways throughout the CNS. Now that several glutamate receptors have been identified and cloned, receptor subtype-specific antibodies have been generated and used to characterize the distribution of these receptors throughout the CNS.

Two possible pathways for the synthesis of glutamate in the CNS were discussed in the previous section on GABA and are diagrammed in Fig. 15. Synthesis can proceed from glucose via α-oxoglutarate (α-ketoglutarate) by the actions of GABA-oxoglutarate transaminase (GABA-T) or from glutamine by means of glutaminase. The synaptic activity of glutamate is terminated through the activation of high-affinity, Na^+-dependent glutamate transporters that sequester glutamate inside neurons and glia. In some brain areas, the glial uptake pathway is particularly important. Glia convert glutamate to glutamine via the enzyme glutamine synthetase, and then export it for surrounding neurons to take up via a low-affinity uptake system. In the dentate gyrus, for example, the active uptake of glutamine by neurons is required for continued availability of glutamate for signal transmission. The system has many similarities to the acetylcholine system, in which uptake of a precursor is a rate-limiting consideration in transmission.

EAA nerves serve the function of the major projection neurons between brain areas. Essentially every outgoing (e.g., efferent) system of the cortex appears to use glutamate, including the corticostriatal, thalamic, bulbar, and pontine pathways. The mossy fiber afferents of the cerebellum and pathways in the olfactory lobe may also use glutamate. Some of the glutamatergic pathways in the CNS are diagrammed in Fig. 17.

As can be seen from the distribution of fibers, the glutamatergic pathways appear to be the major stimulatory or driving pathway within the CNS. Pharmacologically, the effects of underactivity of this system are unknown, although many of the antagonists such as ketamine and phencyclidine (both hallucinogenic) have anesthetic properties. Overactivity of the glutamate system and the action of some highly potent agonists such as quisqualic acid, ibotenic acid, and kainic acid lead to overstimulation and neurotoxicity.

GABA and glutamate appear to be the major inhibitory and excitatory transmitter systems in the CNS and provide braking and acceleration systems, respectively, for neural activity. It is fascinating that these major systems use substances that are so intimately involved in brain metabolism. Through these systems, central energy metabolism, transmission, and nerve activity are inseparably linked.

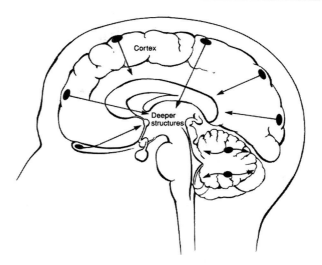

Fig. 17. Central EAA or glutamate pathways are the major efferent pathways from one brain area to another. These neurons possess long axons that project from the cortical and cerebellar areas to almost all brain areas. Concentrations of this transmitter are 1000-fold higher than the catecholamines. The glutamate neuronal pathways are denoted by black ovals and arrows.

10. NITRIC OXIDE

In the late 1970s, several groups demonstrated that nitroso and related nitro compounds, believed to decompose or be converted into nitric oxide (NO), were capable of activating the cytosolic form of guanylate cyclase to stimulate cyclic GMP production in mammalian tissues. These observations led others to consider that the well-known vasodilating effects of nitro compounds, such as *nitroprusside* and *nitroglycerin*, might be caused by the conversion of these compounds to NO by smooth muscle. Subsequent studies did show that NO is a potent smooth-muscle relaxant and that the resulting vasodilation is produced by the actions of cyclic GMP. Together, these observations suggested that smooth muscle and possibly other tissues possessed the capacity of generating NO from an unknown donor compound. The mystery was finally solved with the demonstration that L-arginine is converted to L-citrulline and NO by NO synthase in an NADPH-dependent manner.

Although most of the early NO research efforts were focused on vascular smooth muscle and platelets, the activation of guanylate cyclase from neuronal cells by L-arginine was demonstrated well before the NO synthetic pathway had been worked out. Eventually, the existence of the NO synthetic pathway in brain tissue was demonstrated, and the enzyme itself was purified from rat cerebellum. As other isoforms were discovered and characterized, the brain-derived isoform was designated neuronal NO synthase (nNOS). It is constitutively expressed in many different types of neurons, and is particularly abundant in the molecular layer of the cerebellum and the pediculopontine tegmental nucleus of the brainstem. Although a specific function for NO in the CNS has not been determined, nNOS has been shown to co-localize with NMDA receptors, and glutamate activation of these receptors is associated with increased production of NO. Since NMDA-receptor activation has been implicated in long-term potentiation (LTP) in the hippocampus and with neurotoxicity, NO production may also be involved in mediating these phenomena.

In the peripheral nervous system, both vascular and nonvascular smooth-muscle relaxation appear to be mediated by NO functioning as a neurotransmitter. The myenteric plexus of the gastrointestinal tract contains neurons that express nNOS and inhibit peristalsis when stimulated. NO functions as a neurotransmitter in the erectile tissue of the penis, where it mediates penile erection by inducing relaxation of both vascular and nonvascular smooth muscle. Recognition of this response pathway led to the development of the drug sildenafil (Viagra™), for the treatment of male impotence. This drug inhibits selectively the isoform of phosphodiesterase (PDE5) expressed in this tissue that metabolizes the cyclic GMP produced in response to NO.

11. NEUROACTIVE PEPTIDES

A variety of neuroactive peptides found in the brain are synthesized in the neuronal-cell body and transported axonally to the nerve terminal. Peptidergic transmission in the CNS is different from that of the small-mol-wt transmitters. More than 50 peptide transmitters have been described in the CNS and more are being discovered every year. This may not be so surprising, considering the fact that the human brain contains approx 10^{12} neurons.

The history of neuropeptides can be broken down into two periods: a 40-yr period from about 1930 to 1970, when only a few peptides were chemically characterized, and the 30-yr period from 1970 to the present, during which many neurally active peptides have been discovered and sequenced, mostly because of newer techniques and advances in molecular biology.

The first peptide transmitter to be identified, *substance P*, was discovered serendipitously around 1930, when U.S. Von Euler and John Gaddum were screening various tissues for concentrations of acetylcholine. A substance was found in the gut and in the brain that lowered blood pressure and increased gastrointestinal activity. The substance was not acetylcholine, and was called substance P because it was a powder that resembled a protein in several ways. The neurohypophyseal peptides, *oxytocin (OT)* and *vasopressin*, were isolated and characterized in the 1950s, partially because of the immense concentrations that were stored in the neural lobe of the pituitary. In a common laboratory animal, the white rat, almost half of a μg of each of these peptides is stored and released into peripheral blood to effect physiologic functions such as water retention and lactation. Because of the very small size of the neural lobe and the amount of peptide present, it was relatively easy to extract and characterize these peptides, each of which is nine amino acids long. The structure of substance P was determined by amino acid sequencing around 1970, when this new method became available. At that time, myriad new brain peptides were isolated and characterized.

11.1. Neuropeptides Are Synthesized in the Cell Body and Processed from Larger Precursors in the Endoplasmic Reticulum, Golgi, and Secretory Granules

The brain peptides are present in the axon in large secretory granules that are synthesized in the cell body and are moved to the nerve terminal by axoplasmic transport. The actions of these peptides on their target cells take some time to occur because their receptors are of the G-protein-coupled variety. Their rate of synthesis is also slow when compared to that of the catecholaminergic and amino acid transmitters. The process of *peptide synthesis* begins with the nuclear translation of specific messenger RNAs and their binding to ribosomes. When the mRNA is translated into protein, a 20- to 30-amino acid sequence known as the signal peptide is first formed. This hydrophobic sequence inserts itself into the endoplasmic reticulum (ER) and is followed by the gradually elongating protein chain. Some peptide processing occurs in the ER. The protein is glycosylated with a mannose-rich sugar that is attached to asparagine residues (flanked by other specific amino acids). These specific sequences of amino acids are called *consensus sequences*. In the ER the protein is folded, and disulfide bonds are formed. The disulfide isomerase that accomplishes this is not entirely characterized, but these bonds are important for maintaining the folded structure of the neuropeptide.

The mature propeptide is transported to the Golgi apparatus, where it can be further processed, sorted, and packaged into secretory granules. Much of the processing of the precursor to the active neuropeptide occurs within the secretory granule. These granules have a membrane-bound proton pump that maintains an acidic pH. An example of neuropeptide processing, using oxytocin, is shown in Fig. 18. Peptides are represented (by convention) with the amino-terminal on the left and carboxyl-terminal on the right.

Enzymes belonging to the subtilysin family of serine proteases are responsible for cleaving prohormones at paired basic amino acid residues (lysine and arginine). These enzymes have the characteristic active-site "catalytic triad" (D,H,S) and are active at an acidic pH (4.0–5.0) that allows them to work within the secretory granule. In the case of OT, this produces two products: an extended OT containing Gly-Lys-Arg on the carboxyl-terminal end and a 93-amino acid protein called neurophysin. Some proneuropeptides have more than a single neuropeptide sequence within their precursor. For example, proenkephalin-A has seven enkephalin sequences in the single precursor, and hypothalamic thyrotropin-releasing hormone (TRH) has five of these tripeptide sequences. The proteases that process the prohormone may differ in specificity between various tissues. For example, in the anterior pituitary, the hormone precursor, pro-opiomelanocortin (POMC), is converted into corticotropin (ACTH) and the opiate peptide β-endorphin. In the

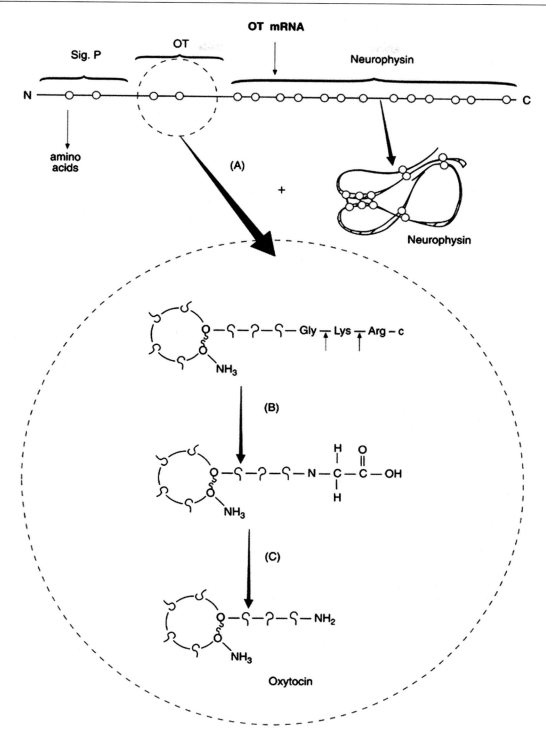

Fig. 18. Peptide biosynthesis in the CNS. Neuropeptides in the CNS are synthesized on ribosomes in the cell bodies of peptidergic neurons. This diagram describes the synthesis of oxytocin in the hypothalamus. The pro-neuropeptide contains the natural neuropeptide (OT) flanked by a signal peptide (Sig. P) and a binding protein known as neurophysin. The shaded dots on the propeptide represent the 18 cysteine residues (drawn relatively to scale). In the ER and Golgi apparatus, disulfide bonds are formed and the peptide is packaged in secretory granules. Within the secretory granule, the propeptide is cleaved by a serine protease (**A**) at a pair of basic amino acids. The extended OT is then acted on by a carboxypeptidase (**B**) to remove the extended basic amino acids and peptidyl glycine α-amidating monooxygenase (**C**) to produce the biologically active neuropeptide. The activity of these three enzymatic steps occurs in the synaptic vesicle while it is being transported to the axon terminal.

intermediate lobe, this same precursor POMC is cleaved to melanocyte-stimulating hormone (MSH), a peptide called corticotropin-like intermediate-lobe (CLIP), and β-endorphin.

The next enzymatic step eliminates the basic amino acids from the carboxyl-terminal of the neuropeptide. This enzyme is carboxypeptidase E/H, which has an acidic pH maximum and (in the case of OT) yields the nonapeptide with an additional glycine. Amidation is the next step in peptide synthesis, accomplished by an enzyme known as peptidylglycine α-amidating monooxygenase (PAM). Many peptides are amidated on the carboxyl-terminal end, including TRH, gonadotropin-releasing hormone, OT, vasopressin, angiotensin II (AII), substance P, and vasoactive intestinal peptide (VIP). The enzyme cleaves the additional glycine (of extended oxytocin or TRH) at the α-carbon atom, leaving the amide attached to the carboxyl residue (*see* Fig. 18). In terms of cofactor requirements, this enzyme is similar to dopamine-β-hydroxylase. As is the case for norepinephrine biosynthesis, copper and reduced ascorbic acid are required for the amidation of peptides to occur within the vesicles.

Much of this peptide processing occurs as the secretory granule is being transported down the axon to the nerve terminal. An investigator can follow the maturation of some peptides from the cell body down the length of the axon to the nerve terminal. Peptide-containing granules are usually larger than fast transmitter-containing granules. When they exist as co-transmitters, they can be differentially released, depending on the frequency of nerve action potentials and distribution of Ca^{2+} channels. This has been most completely worked out in the parasympathetic innervation of the salivary gland, where low-frequency stimulation releases acetylcholine, and high-frequency stimulation causes the secretion of VIP.

Termination of neuropeptide responses is achieved principally through enzymatic degradation. Uptake and reuse of peptides are not options, as there are no known peptide transporters. The enzymes that degrade peptides are called peptidases, and are classified by the amino acids or metals that are involved in their catalytic site (e.g., serine and metalloproteases) or by the location of the cleavage site of the peptide. Endopeptidases cleave internal peptide bonds at specific sequences. An example is the enzyme that degrades the opiate peptides, sometimes called enkephalinase. Exopeptidases remove one or two amino acids from the carboxyl or amino terminus of the peptide. The carboxypeptidases that remove the

basic amino acids from peptide precursors have already been discussed. Angiotensin II-converting enzyme (ACE), which removes a carboxyl-terminal dipeptide from its substrate, is the target for an important class of drugs used to lower blood pressure. Aminopeptidase A selectively removes acidic amino acids from the amino-terminal end of the peptide. A variety of peptidases are found in extracellular fluid or circulate in the blood. Aminopeptidase A and M, cathepsin D, and ACE all are found circulating in the blood.

Some of the characteristics of neuropeptides partially protect them from degradation by the peptidases. For example, the disulfide bonds and carboxyl-terminal amidation of OT and vasopressin are essential for biologic activity and protect these peptides from immediate destruction by circulating peptidases.

11.2. The Families of Neuroactive Peptides Mediate Endocrine, Neural, and Behavioral Functions

The peptides can be subdivided into several families of neurotransmitters. Because much of this information is discussed elsewhere in the text, only their major groupings, distribution, and some aspects of their function are discussed here.

11.3. Neurohypophysial Peptides

Hypothalamic neurons that secrete neurohypophysial peptides project to the posterior pituitary and higher brain centers. OT and vasopressin are synthesized in specific nuclei of the anterior hypothalamus and are transported by axons through the internal layer of the median eminence (ME) to the posterior pituitary (e.g., neural lobe). This small bundle of axon terminals and pituicytes store large amounts of both peptides, which contributed to their being among the first neuropeptides to be isolated and characterized.

Vasopressin is secreted into the blood, where its hormonal functions include constriction of vessels, as its name implies, and inhibition of water loss by the kidney (hence the name antidiuretic hormone). OT is usually associated with reproductive function, and is released to induce contraction of the uterus during parturition and the letdown of milk during suckling and lactation.

The axons of the neurons that produce these peptides project to other areas of the brain, brainstem, and spinal cord. Vasopressin has been associated with memory consolidation in the limbic system, and OT has been implicated in memory, maternal, social, and sexual behavior, and autonomic activity.

12. HYPOTHALAMIC NEUROHORMONES

The hypothalamus of the midbrain regulates autonomic functions, behavioral processes, and the endocrine system. Several small peptides reach the anterior pituitary through a portal blood system and regulate most humoral function. *Thyrotropin-releasing hormone* is a tripeptide that causes the release of thyroid-stimulating hormone (TSH) from the pituitary. *Gonadotropin-releasing hormone* is a decapeptide that releases pituitary luteinizing hormone (LH) and follicle-stimulating hormone (FSH) peripherally, and it has been implicated in some sexual behaviors such as lordosis, in the rodent.

Somatostatin (SS) occurs as both a tetradecapeptide (14 amino acids) that inhibits the release of growth hormone from the pituitary, and as a 28-amino-acid form found primarily in the gut where it inhibits the secretion of acid and gastrin. It has also been found in many higher brain areas, including the cortex and limbic system. Present in peripheral nerves, SS also plays a role in sensory function.

Corticotropin-releasing hormone (CRH) is found in many higher brain areas. It is responsible for regulating the secretion of ACTH and modulating the immune system. CRH activates a G-protein coupled receptor (GPCR) that stimulates adenylate cyclase, increasing cAMP levels and activating protein kinase A.

13. OPIATE PEPTIDES

In the mid-1970s, a peptide-like substance was isolated from the brain that displaced morphine from a membrane-bound receptor present in many areas of the mammalian brain. Morphine, which is an opium derivative from the dried resin of the oriental poppy plant, has been used for centuries to alleviate pain and as a drug of abuse. The discovery of this brain peptide answered a question that had been troubling pharmacologists and neurobiologists for some time—what is the endogenous substance that these plant alkaloids mimic so well?

Opiate peptides are found in almost all areas of the brain. Three major precursors give rise to the main opiate peptide groups: β-endorphin, the enkephalins, and the dynorphins. POMC, which was previously discussed, is the common precursor for ACTH and β-endorphin. It is present in the anterior and intermediate lobe of the pituitary, and in an ascending group of neurons in the hypothalamus.

Opiate peptides have similar pentapeptide sequences. Proenkephalin-A gives rise to several pentapeptides

(e.g., five methionine-enkephalins [Met-ENKs] and one leu-enkephalin [Leu-ENK]) that have potent opiate-like effects. Proenkephalin-B is the precursor for several leu-enkephalin pentapeptides, and the dynorphins. The common feature of all of these opiate peptides is the pentapeptide sequence Tyr-Gly-Gly-Phe-Met (or Leu), which seems to be important for binding to the opiate receptors that have been described. This family of neuropeptides is important in analgesia as well as a variety of other important inhibitory functions. The enkephalins and dynorphins are present throughout the CNS, particularly in the striatum, the limbic system, the raphe nuclei, and the hypothalamus.

14. BRAIN–GUT PEPTIDES

Since the discovery in 1930 of substance P, several peptides that are found in high concentrations in the gastrointestinal tract have been isolated and mapped in the brain. It has been proposed that the gastrointestinal tract has its own endogenous brain, known as the *enteric nervous system*, which is separate from the autonomic nervous system. The gut peptides that are also found in the brain include VIP, cholecystokinin (CCK), gastrin, secretin, neurotensin (NT), pancreatic polypeptide Y, neuropeptide Y (NPY), and many others. These peptides have been implicated in several physiologic processes, including pain, temperature regulation, satiety and hunger, and nausea and function as major cotransmitters in the autonomic nervous system (e.g., VIP and NPY).

15. OTHER PEPTIDES

The list of peptides that have been isolated and characterized in the brain and periphery is growing every day. Several others should be mentioned. *Angiotensin II (AngII)* and *bradykinin* are vasoactive peptides that have been localized within the brain. *AngII* has potent effects on water and fluid intake when injected directly into the hypothalamus. Various peptides, collectively called *sleep peptides*, are potent inducers of sleep. *Calcitonin gene-related peptide* (CGRP) was accidentally discovered when the gene for calcitonin in the thyroid was sequenced and translated into protein. Antibodies against a peptide coded for by the gene reacted strongly with peptidergic pathways in the trigeminal nerve and hypothalamus. Although it is a vasodilator, its central function is still unknown. *Galanin* is another peptide that is present in the brainstem, and it appears to regulate neuroendocrine activity.

16. CONCLUSION

In this chapter, about 100 neurotransmitters that are distributed among 1–10 billion neurons have been directly or indirectly discussed. If there were no other transmitters in the brain, each transmitter should occupy 10–100 million neurons, but this is not the case. For example, the noradrenergic nerves in the brain only occupy about 10,000 nerve cells, and the dopaminergic neurons in the midbrain number only 30,000–40,000. These calculations are obviously misleading, because the 100 transmitters are not evenly distributed, and there are probably more transmitters that are currently unknown. Our knowledge of "how the brain works" is undoubtedly very primitive. In the future, many new transmitter substances will be discovered, and new concepts will be offered to explain the complex neural interactions involved in thought, memory, mood, sensation, and maintenance of somatic and visceral function.

SELECTED READINGS

Bjorklund A, Hokfelt T. GABA and neuropeptides in the CNS, Part I. In Bjorklund A, Hokfelt T, Tohyama M (eds). Handbook of chemical neuroanatomy, (Vol 4). Amsterdam: Elsevier, 1985; 436–593.

Bjorklund A, Hokfelt T. Classical transmitters and receptors in the CNS, Parts I and II. In Bjorklund A, Hokfelt T, Kuhar MJ (eds). Handbook of Chemical Neuroanatomy, (Vols 2 and 3). Amsterdam: Elsevier, 1984; 1–156,1–403.

Bjorklund A, Hokfelt T, Tohyama M. Ontogeny of transmitters and peptides in the CNS. In Bjorklund A, Hokfelt T, Tohyama M (eds). Handbook of Chemical Neuroanatomy, (Vol 10). Amsterdam: Elsevier, 1992; 33–128.

Cooper JR, Bloom FE, Roth RH. The Biochemical Basis of Neurochemistry, 7th ed. New York: Oxford University Press, 1996.

Norman AW, Litwack G. Hormones, 2nd ed. San Diego: Academic Press, 1997.

Steinbusch HWM, De Vente J, Vincent, SR. Functional Neuroanatomy of the Nitric Oxide System. In Bjorklund A, Hokfelt T (eds). Handbook of chemical neuroanatomy, (Vol 17). Amsterdam: Elsevier, 2000; 1–39, 355–406.

Parkinson's Disease

Gregory Cooper and Robert L. Rodnitzky

In 1817, the English physician James Parkinson published a monograph entitled *An Essay on the Shaking Palsy*. He described six persons afflicted by a condition characterized by a flexed posture, slowness of movement, a tendency to walk rapidly with small steps, and an associated tremor of one or more extremities. Not all of the six cases were Parkinson's personal patients. Some were observed on the streets of London. To Parkinson's description of tremor and slowness of movement, the modern neurologist would add rigidity and loss of postural reflexes to complete the typical symptom complex of Parkinson's disease.

PARKINSON'S DISEASE SYMPTOMS
Parkinson's Tremor Is Most Prominent at Rest

Tremor is prominent in a variety of neurologic conditions, many of which are confused with Parkinson's disease. However, unlike most tremors, the *parkinsonian* tremor is most prominent at rest and is typically suppressed, at least temporarily, during action. In essential tremor, the condition most commonly con-fused with Parkinson's disease, tremor is typically absent at rest and only appears when the affected body part assumes a sustained, active posture. For instance, in essential tremor involving the hands, the tremor may only appear while holding the outstretched hands in front of the body or when attempting to bring a coffee cup to the mouth. The distribution also helps to identify Parkinson's tremor. In Parkinson's disease, the tremor usually affects the extremities, especially the hands. It occasionally affects the mandible, but unlike essential tremor, it almost never affects the head.

The term *pill-rolling* tremor is often used in Parkinson's disease. It refers to the tendency of the thumb and index finger to approximate one another while trembling as though an object were being rolled between the two fingers. This term is a reference to the turn-of-the-century technique used by pharmacists to fashion a pill by rolling a soft substance between the thumb and index finger. Like many of the symptoms of Parkinson's disease, tremor is often asymmetric, and in the early stages of the illness, it may be exclusively on one side. The typical frequency of the parkinsonian tremor is 4–6 cycles/s. The exact mechanism by which tremor arises in this condition is not clear, but most evidence strongly favors a central rather than a peripheral origin.

Parkinsonian Rigidity Differs from the Rigidity of Upper Motor Neuron Lesions or Other Basal Ganglia Disorders

In Parkinson's disease, limb rigidity can be demonstrated throughout the entire range of a large-amplitude passive movement. In contrast, the stiffness associated with an upper motor neuron lesions such as a cerebral infarction is referred to as clasp-knife rigidity, because there is considerable resistance at the beginning of the examiner's passive movement, which suddenly gives away as the passive movement is continued. When the examiner attempts to demonstrate parkinsonian rigidity, a rachet-like sensation known as cogwheeling can often be felt as the limb is moved. In Parkinson's disease, rigidity involves the extremities more than the axial musculature. In other degenerative conditions that mimick Parkinson's disease, such as progressive supranuclear palsy, axial rigidity predominates.

Bradykinesia Is One of the Most Disabling Symptoms of Parkinsons Disease

Bradykinesia is slowness of movement or inability to initiate movement. As a result of this dysfunction, automatic movements such as swinging the arms while walking become diminished or are totally lost. Similarly, eye blinking is decreased, and the normal range of facial expression is lost, resulting in a typical fixed stare. When severe slowness of movement evolves into a lack of movement, it is referred to as *akinesia*.

Patients with severe bradykinesia or akinesia find it difficult to perform motor tasks that require repetitive motions, such as finger tapping or combing the hair, and tasks that require manipulation of small objects, such as placing a button through a buttonhole. Difficulty in initiating movement results in the inability to arise from a chair, exit a car, or roll over in bed. Of the four cardinal clinical features of Parkinson's disease-tremor, rigidity, bradykinesia, and loss of postural reflexes, bradykinesia is the most severely disabling.

Another common clinical manifestation of bradykinesia is inability to properly manipulate a pen or pencil while writing. The resultant handwriting, referred to as *micrographia*, classically becomes progressively smaller as the affected person writes, reflecting an inability to carry out sustained repetitive movements in a normal fashion.

Like many of the clinical signs of Parkinson's disease, the exact physiologic basis of bradykinesia is not understood. The phenomenon of *kinesia paradoxia*, wherein an ordinarily bradykinetic patient demonstrates an unexpectedly rapid motor response to a sudden stimulus such as a thrown ball, suggests that alternate motor pathways may exist in individuals who can support movements of normal range and speed.

Impairment of Postural Reflexes Is Typically a Late Development in Parkinson's Disease

Postural reflexes are tested by applying a backward-directed perturbation to both shoulders in an attempt to pull a person off his base. The normal person takes one step at most to compensate for the perturbation. The Parkinson's patient with impaired postural reflexes cannot right himself, and continues to move backwards with a series of small and uncontrollable steps until stopped by the examiner. This inability to stop oneself from propelling backwards is referred to as retropulsion. The tendency to take uncontrollable steps in increasingly rapid fashion in the forward direction is referred to as a *festination* or propulsion. Patients with moderate to severe impairment of postural reflexes are at great risk for falls, because they cannot recover from the slightest naturally occurring perturbation, such as tripping over the edge of a rug.

The Cardinal Symptoms of Parkinson's Disease Can Appear in Different Combinations

Not all patients have all four of the cardinal symptoms of Parkinson's disease. Isolated resting tremor is a common presenting symptom of Parkinson's disease, and in some patients, it remains the predominant symptom for the entire course of the patient's illness. In a small percentage of patients, tremor never develops, and the parkinsonian syndrome consists solely of rigidity and bradykinesia with or without loss of postural reflexes. The absence of resting tremor makes establishing a diagnosis of Parkinson's disease slightly more difficult. If bradykinesia appears in isolation, it is commonly manifested as a change in handwriting or difficulty in performing fine motor tasks.

AGE-RELATED INCIDENCE OF PARKINSON'S DISEASE

In the United States, the estimated prevalence of Parkinson's disease is approx 187 per 100,000 persons in the general population, with an annual incidence of 20 per 100,000. Although occasionally beginning in persons as young as 30 yr of age, it classically presents in the sixth and seventh decades. Epidemiologic surveys suggest that the prevalence per 100,000 is between 30 and 50 in the fifth decade and between 300 and 700 in the seventh decade. The increasing occurrence with age has led to the speculation that normal age-related abiotrophy of dopaminergic cells is a contributory factor in the etiopathogenesis of the illness.

The role of genetic factors in Parkinson's disease has not been fully clarified. There are rare instances of a family with an apparent autosomal dominant pattern of inheritance, but for most patients, no familial pattern is apparent. Supporting the relatively minor role of heredity is the fact that twin studies have not consistently suggested a contribution of genetic factors in young-onset Parkinson's disease. It has been proposed that the inconsistent results from genetic studies may result from a complex interaction between genetic and environmental factors. In other words, an individual may inherit a genetic risk or predisposition for Parkinson's disease, but only develop this condition after a particular environmental exposure.

ETIOLOGY AND TREATMENT

A Toxin Can Cause a Syndrome Similar to Parkinson's Disease

Parkinsonism developed in a group of narcotic addicts who mistakenly injected themselves with the compound MPTP (1-methyl-4-phenyl-1,2,3,6-tetrahydropyridine). MPTP is metabolized by brain MAO to MPP+. MPP+ is conveyed into dopamine nerve terminals by the dopamine transporter, which normally acts to terminate dopaminergic neurotransmission by reaccumulating dopamine into presynaptic nerve terminals. The transporter also accumulates neurotoxins such as MPP+ that share structural features with dopamine.

Once inside dopaminergic cells, MPP+ accumulates within mitochondria, where it inhibits complex I of the mitochondrial respiratory chain, resulting in cell death. Decreased complex I activity has also been reported in naturally occurring Parkinson's disease, suggesting that the underlying mechanism of cell death may be similar to that documented in MPTP parkinsonism. Based on these processes, it can be appreciated why this toxin preferentially affects dopaminergic cells and why it causes a syndrome almost identical to that of ordinary Parkinson's disease.

In the laboratory, injection of MPTP into primates reliably produces parkinsonism. The remarkable resemblance of MPTP parkinsonism to naturally occurring Parkinson's disease raises the possibility that Parkinson's disease itself may be caused by a similar environmental toxin. Although MPTP itself has not been found in the environment, other potential toxins have been implicated. Epidemiologic studies have suggested that Parkinson's disease may be related to rural living, raising the possibility that agrichemicals may play a role in its causation.

Monoamine Oxidase Inhibition May Benefit Patients with Parkinson's Disease

Drugs that inhibit the enzyme MAO block MPTP from inducing experimental parkinsonism by preventing the conversion of this protoxin to its active toxic form, MPP+. The fact that MAO inhibitors prevent the development of MPTP-induced parkinsonism is one factor that has suggested their use to prevent or retard the development of naturally occurring Parkinson's disease, especially if that condition is caused by a neurotoxin biochemically related to MPTP.

There is another mechanism through which MAO inhibitors may benefit the Parkinson patient. MAO is normally involved in the catabolism of dopamine. MAO-inhibiting drugs slow this process, reducing the associated generation of potentially toxic free radicals, which may produce further nigral damage. Whether this effect of MAO-inhibiting drugs actually retards dopaminergic cell death and slows the progression of Parkinson's disease is not firmly established.

THE LEWY BODY IS THE PATHOLOGIC HALLMARK OF PARKINSON'S DISEASE

In Parkinson's disease there is severe neuronal loss in the pars compacta of the *substantia nigra*. Many of the remaining neurons contain a *Lewy body*, an eosinophilic cytoplasmic inclusion surrounded by a lighter halo. Lewy bodies can also be found, although in lesser numbers, in some other CNS degenerative conditions and occasionally in the brains of nonparkinsonian elderly persons. In Parkinson's disease, Lewy bodies are most prominent in the substantia nigra, but they are also found in the locus ceruleus, nucleus basalis of Meynert, raphe nuclei, thalamus, and cerebral cortex. To the extent the cerebral cortex and the nucleus basalis of Meynert contain Lewy bodies or other forms of pathology, dementia may appear in some Parkinson's patients.

Dopaminergic Preparations Are the Most Effective Therapy for Parkinson's Disease

In the 1950s, it was discovered that dopamine is profoundly depleted in the striatum of patients with Parkinson's disease. This led to initial attempts to treat parkinsonian patients with small, orally administered dosages of levodopa, a dopamine precursor that, unlike dopamine itself, can cross the blood-brain barrier. Once inside the brain, it was reasoned, levodopa could be transformed to dopamine by the enzyme dopa-decarboxylase. These initial attempts were unsuccessful because the small dosages of levodopa employed were almost entirely metabolized to dopamine peripherally by dopa-decarboxylase in the liver and gut and therefore lost to the brain. Subsequent attempts in the late 1960s using much larger dosages were successful in allowing some levodopa to escape peripheral decarboxylation and enter the brain. It was soon apparent that this strategy was remarkably effective in reversing the symptoms of Parkinson's disease. Levodopa remains the mainstay of therapy for Parkinson's disease. It is now administered with a peripheral dopa-decarboxylase inhibitor, and almost no conversion to dopamine occurs outside the brain, allowing smaller amounts of levodopa to be administered.

Recently, a new class of medications termed catechol-O-methyl-transferase (COMT) inhibitors have been developed. These medications inhibit the conversion of levodopa to 3-O-methyl-dopa by COMT, thereby promoting its conversion to dopamine by aromatic amino acid decarboxylase within the CNS. These agents therefore increase or prolong the action of levodopa when co-administered.

Similar but less reliable improvement of parkinsonian symptoms can be achieved by the administration of dopamine agonists, such as pergolide or bromocriptine, and more recently, pramipexole and ropinirole. These substances readily pass the blood-brain barrier and directly stimulate dopamine receptors, simulating the effect of dopamine. Because of concern regarding the potential complications associated with long-term levodopa use, dopamine agonists are being increasingly utilized in the early treatment of Parkinson's disease.

Severe Complications Can Occur After Years of Levodopa Therapy

After 5 yr of levodopa therapy, approx 50% of Parkinson's disease patients develop complications consisting of involuntary writhing, twisting movements of the extremities, trunk, and face, or episodes of sudden, transient, near-total loss of dopamine effect on their symptoms. The sudden loss of antiparkinson effect has been referred to as the *on-off effect*. Patients who experience this complication find that they may suddenly revert to total immobility as though someone had flipped a switch, followed by an equally sudden return to normal mobility. The unpredictability of these fluctuations in mobility can be extremely disabling. Both the on-off effect and the involuntary writhing movements, termed *dyskinesias*, that occur in patients with advanced Parkinson's disease are postulated to be related to the development of altered dopamine-receptor sensitivity. Whether these putative receptor changes are a function of the duration of the underlying disease or result from long-term nonphysiologic-receptor stimulation by dopaminergic drugs is unknown.

Tissue Transplantation May Improve the Symptoms of Parkinson's Disease

In the 1980s, there was considerable interest in transplantation of tissue into the CNS as a means of treating Parkinson's disease. Initial reports suggested improvement after transplantation of cells derived from the patients' own adrenal glands into the caudate nucleus. Cells from the adrenal medulla are metabolically capable of synthesizing dopamine, and it was reasoned that they could survive in the brain and elaborate this neurotransmitter. Although there were initial reports of improvement in patients who underwent this procedure, subsequent patients did not fare as well. The postmortem studies suggested that most transplanted cells did not survive.

A second wave of enthusiasm for cell grafting in treating Parkinson's disease has been generated by the early experience with the transplantation of tissue derived from human fetal mesencephalon and implanted into the caudate or putamen of patients. Careful study has shown that these cells do survive in the recipient's brain and effectively increase dopamine production, as demonstrated by positron emission tomography (PET). Clinically, the procedure results in a moderate reduction in neurologic symptoms and a reduced requirement for levodopa therapy, largely in patients under the age of 60.

Future therapies using cell or tissue grafting may depend on cells other than fetal tissue that have been genetically modified to produce dopamine.

Surgical Therapies Can Improve Parkinson's Disease

Microelectrode recordings in Parkinson's disease patients have demonstrated abnormal activity in basal ganglia structures, most notably overactivity in the subthalamic nucleus (STN). Accordingly various forms of ablative therapy of the STN or its efferent target, the internal segment of the globus pallidus, have been successfully employed to treat Parkinson's disease. Although thermocoagulation of cells in these structures is possible, the preferred mode of cellular suppression is administration of an electrical stimulation to the targeted nucleus (deep brain stimulation).

SELECTED READING

Freed CR, Greene PE, Breeze RE, et al. Transplantation of embryonic dopamine neurons for severe Parkinson's disease. New Engl J Med 2001; 344:710.

22 Pain

Mary M. Heinricher

Contents

1. PAIN IS A COMPLEX SENSORY EVENT

Pain is a useful warning signal, an alarm that prevents us from damaging our bodies irreparably as we go about daily life. However, pain arising late in the course of disease, or produced by dysfunction of the nervous system, has no survival value. Indeed, there is accumulating evidence that pain *per se* can have adverse health effects. For example, pain has been shown in animal studies to inhibit immune function, and to enhance tumor growth. In humans, appropriate

From: *Neuroscience in Medicine, 2nd ed.* (P. Michael Conn, ed.),
© 2003 Humana Press Inc., Totowa, NJ.

pain management can be shown to enhance healing. Pain is an thus important clinical issue in its own right.

Although pain is part of everyday life, a clinically and scientifically useful definition of pain is not straightforward, particularly when considering some of the types of pain with significant clinical impact. The International Association for the Study of Pain (IASP) has therefore developed a consensus definition of pain that is now widely accepted. According to the IASP, pain is an unpleasant bodily sensory experience commonly produced by processes that damage, or are capable of damaging, bodily tissue. Thus, the stimulus is generally tissue damage produced by some sort of injury or disease. (Processes that are harmful or at least potentially harmful to the body are known as *noxious*.) This definition also emphasizes that pain is a sensory experience, and leads to a distinction between pain and *nociception*, which refers to the neural mechanisms involved in detecting tissue damage. The primary reason for the distinction between pain and nociception is that the link between tissue damage and pain sensation can be rather loose. A given noxious stimulus may or may not give rise to a pain sensation, and it is possible to have significant tissue damage with little pain. Conversely, there are some situations in which very intense and very real pain occurs without any damage to tissue, or after healing is apparently complete. Finally, the definition recognizes that pain is multidimensional. It has an important emotional or *motivational* component, as well as the discriminative component related to judgments about intensity, quality, and location. Even mild pain is unpleasant, and both people and animals are highly motivated to escape from or avoid pain. Although this motivational aspect—suffering—is the most troubling aspect of pain for most individuals, it is valuable because it alerts the organism that something is wrong, and provides the motivation needed to escape from the damaging event and for subsequent recuperative behaviors. This aspect of pain also prompts us to avoid similar stimuli in the future.

2. SOMATOSENSORY PRIMARY AFFERENTS TRANSDUCE STIMULUS ENERGY AND TRANSMIT INFORMATION FROM THE PERIPHERAL TISSUES INTO THE CENTRAL NERVOUS SYSTEM

2.1. Somatosensory Receptors Are Specific in Their Response Properties

Somatosensory afferents are pseudo-unipolar neurons with cell bodies located in the dorsal-root gan-

glion at each spinal segment. Each *primary afferent neuron* has two branches: one travels out to the peripheral tissues, and a second shorter central branch enters the spinal cord (Fig. 1). (Note that the cell bodies of afferents that innervate the face reside in the trigeminal ganglion and project into the trigeminal system in the pons and medulla. Similar general principles apply to trigeminal as to spinal afferents; however, the subsequent discussion focuses on spinal systems.) The task of the primary afferents is to transduce stimulus energy into a form that can be used by the nervous system (e.g., action potentials), and to transmit that information into the central nervous system (CNS). The somatosensory system is unlike vision or audition because the sensory afferent itself is the primary sensory transducer, without a separate specialized receptor cell. Various primary afferents are specialized to respond to different forms of stimulus energy. Thus, *low-threshold mechanoreceptors* are activated by mechanical stimuli and not at all by heating or cooling, and *thermoreceptors* respond to innocu-ous warming or to cooling but not to mechanical stimuli. *Nociceptors* are more diverse, but are activated by various stimuli that have in common the ability to damage tissue. Adequate stimuli for a nociceptor may include intense mechanical, thermal, and/or chemical insults. The difference between a thermoreceptor that is responsive to innocuous warming, and a nociceptor responsive to intense heat is illustrated in Fig. 2. The thermoreceptor shows a gradual increase in activity as skin temperature is increased from a normal skin temperature around 30°C to about 42°C, the point at which the stimulus would be perceived as painful by humans and at which a prolonged stimulus can produce damage. Firing of the thermoreceptor is then depressed. In contrast, the threshold for a thermal nociceptor is around 42°C. The increased firing of the afferent as skin temperature increases parallels human ratings of the pain elicited by the thermal stimulus.

Primary afferents vary in the sizes of their axons and whether or not they are myelinated (Table 1). Axons that travel to skin are divided into Aβ, Aδ, and C classes. The largest fall into the Aβ group, and because of their large size and myelination, they conduct action potentials rapidly. The smaller myelinated axons are known as Aδ fibers, and these conduct more slowly than the Aβ fibers. Unmyelinated afferents are of extremely fine caliber, and thus conduct very slowly (<2 m/s). When activating the different classes using electrical stimulation, the amount of stimulation current required to activate the different classes varies inversely with diameter. Thus, the largest fibers have

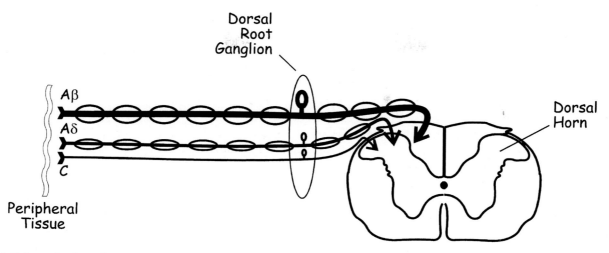

Fig. 1. Schematic view of somatic primary afferent axons in a cutaneous nerve. Pseudo-unipolar cells with cell bodies in the dorsal-root ganglion send a peripheral branch to the skin and a central branch into the dorsal horn of the spinal cord via the dorsal root. Afferents can be divided into Aβ fibers, which have large myelinated axons, Aδ fibers, which have smaller myelinated axons, and C fibers, which have small, unmyelinated axons.

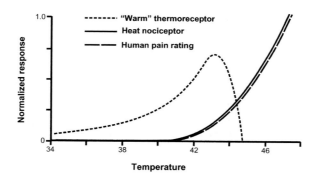

Fig. 2. Coding of innocuous and noxious heat by thermoreceptors and thermal nociceptors, respectively. Thermoreceptors exhibit a temperature-related activation as the skin is warmed above a holding temperature of about 30–34°C to about 42°C, the threshold for heat pain in humans. Activity then drops dramatically as temperature is increased into the noxious range. In contrast, heat nociceptors are not activated by innocuous warming, but show a temperature-related increase in activity that parallels human pain rating when the temperature is above 42°C. (Adapted with permission from the American Physiological Society for Kenshalo et al., J. Neurophysiol, 2000; 84:719–729.)

Table 1
Classification of Somatic Primary Afferents by Size and Myelination

	Cutaneous	Muscle	Viscera	Fiber diameter	Conduction velocity	Functional correlates
Myelinated		Ia, Ib		12–20 μm	80–120 m/s	Muscle-spindle afferents, GTO
	Aβ	II		6–12 μm	35–75 m/s	Low-threshold mechanoreceptors
	Aδ	III	Aδ	1–5 μm	2–30 m/s	Nociceptors, innocuous cooling, mechanoreceptors
Unmyelinated	C	IV	C	0.2–1.5 μm	0.5–2 m/s	Nociceptors, innocuous warming, mechanoreceptors

a low electrical threshold, and are relatively easily activated with electrical stimulation. A much higher current is required to activate C fibers. The various conduction velocities are reflected in the *compound action potential*, which is the summed activity that can be recorded from a peripheral nerve when it is stimulated electrically. The earliest peak recorded in the compound action potential represents discharges of the Aβ afferents, which travel rapidly down the axons to the recording site. The second peak is caused by activity in the Aδ fibers, and the final, much later, and more dispersed peak represents discharge of the C fibers.

Table 1 also outlines a parallel classification scheme using roman numerals, which is widely employed for afferents that innervate joints and muscle. Muscle afferents include a class of very large-diameter axons (Ia axons that innervate muscle spindles and Ib axons that innervate the Golgi tendon organs). Axons of this size are not found in cutaneous nerves. Visceral afferents are classified using the same system as cutaneous afferents, but lack the Aβ group.

At a gross level, the function of the different cutaneous afferents can be correlated with morphology and conduction velocity. The best-studied low-threshold mechanoreceptors are large myelinated afferents conducting in the Aβ range. These afferents have encapsulated endings, and are specialized for rapidly or slowly adapting responses to innocuous mechanical stimuli. Additional low-threshold mechanoreceptors, such as hair afferents, are found within the Aδ and C classes, as are thermoreceptors. The thermoreceptors that respond to innocuous cooling generally fall into the Aδ group, and those activated by warming into the C group. Like thermoreceptors, nociceptors are found among the small-diameter primary afferents with slower conduction velocities, the Aδ and C-fiber groups. Many nociceptors are *polymodal*, that is, they respond to both intense heat and intense mechanical stimuli, and in some cases to chemical irritants. Others are more selective, responding only to mechanical or chemical stimuli. In addition, there are large numbers of nociceptors that have extremely high thresholds for activation in healthy tissues. However, these unresponsive axons become highly sensitized following inflammation, and are thus sometimes referred to as *silent* or *sleeping* nociceptors, because they "awaken" following injury or inflammation.

2.2. Specific Response Properties of Somatosensory Primary Afferents Lead to Specificity of Function

The importance of small-diameter fibers for pain sensation was originally inferred from experiments using electrical stimulation of whole nerves. These experiments demonstrated that high-stimulus currents, sufficient to activate the smaller-diameter fibers, was required to produce painful sensations. Conversely, selective ischemic block of the activity in the largest afferents interfered with tactile sensibility, but not pain or thermal sensation. The functional specificity of individual primary afferents has since been confirmed in elegant experiments that use microneurography and intraneural microstimulation in conscious human subjects. In these experiments, the discharges of an individual sensory afferent are identified by recording with a microelectrode (*microneurography*). The response properties of the axon are then defined using natural stimulation of its receptive field on the skin (such as brushing, pinching, cooling or warming, or intense heating). The same electrode is then used to stimulate that same axon (*intraneural microstimulation*). Investigators who take this approach have shown that electrical stimulation of a *single* Aβ low-threshold mechanoreceptor causes the subject to report a sensation of tapping, vibration, or sustained pressure (depending on the type of mechanoreceptor stimulated and the stimulus frequency). These sensations are perceived as arising from the afferent's *receptive field*, the area of skin from which tactile stimulation activates the fiber. Stimulation of a large Aβ afferent does not evoke pain sensations under normal conditions, even when stimulus frequency is increased to drive the fiber at a high rate. In contrast, direct electrical stimulation of a single Aδ nociceptor produces a sensation of pain, usually sharp or pricking in character. Although stimulation of individual C-fiber nociceptors has not been possible because of their small size, stimulation of a small bundle of these fibers produces a dull, burning pain or itch. These findings demonstrate that activity in the low-threshold mechanoreceptors does not contribute to pain (again, at least under normal conditions), whereas activity in a single Aδ nociceptor is sufficient to produce pain. Activity in C fibers produces pain or itch, although we cannot say whether activity in one or many C fibers is required to produce a sensation.

Table 2
Chemical Mediators of Nociception and Inflammation Following Damage to Tissues

Leak from damaged cells or stimulated release:
- Ach: Released from damaged cells, causes pain.
- Protons: Inmigrating leukocytes secrete lactic acid, key aspect of inflammatory "soup" is low pH.
- 5HT: Released from platelets, intradermal application produces pain, activates nociceptors.
- ATP: Application produces pain, activates nociceptors.
- Histamine: Released by mast cells, produces itch not pain, but along with 5HT, BK, stimulates synthesis of prostaglandins.

Synthesized locally by enzymes from substrates released by damage or that enter area as part of inflammatory process (e.g., leukocyte migration):
- Bradykinin: Synthesized from protein precursor in plasma (kininogen), activates nociceptors to produce pain, sensitizes nociceptors to other inputs (including heat), triggers other elements of inflammatory process (including synthesis of prostaglandins and release of cytokines).
- Prostaglandins: Synthesized from arachidonic acid following injury. Contributes to inflammation by inducing vasodilation and plasma extravasation, attracts immune cells. Sensitizes nociceptors.

Released by activated nociceptors themselves:
- Substance P: Acts on other afferent fiber terminals to activate and/or sensitize, contributes to inflammation by causing vasodilation, plasma extravasation. Stimulates mast cells to release histamine.
- CGRP: Contributes to inflammation, dilates arterioles, synergizes with substance P in producing plasma extravasation.

2.3. Chemical Mediators of Nociception

Our understanding of how damage to tissue results in activation of the primary afferent nociceptors has been the focus of a great deal of research, but it is still incomplete. However, there are a number of chemicals that are released or synthesized when tissue is damaged. Some of the constituents of this "chemical soup" are listed in Table 2. Many of these substances are known to activate nociceptors and induce pain when applied to human volunteers. Others do not by themselves activate the nociceptors, but *sensitize* them, causing them to be more responsive to other inputs. As will be discussed in more detail here, the resulting sensitization of the primary afferent nociceptors is a major factor in enhanced pain following injury or inflammation.

2.4. Small Diameter Afferents, Including Nociceptors, Are Rich in Neuropeptides

With the physiological identification of nociceptive primary afferents came the hope that they would release a unique neurotransmitter. Interest in this idea was high, because a transmitter specific to nociceptors would provide an accessible and selective target for

potential pain treatments. Unfortunately, this was not the case.

The major fast excitatory transmitter in the small afferents is glutamate, an excitatory amino acid (EAA) neurotransmitter that is also expressed by large mechanoreceptor afferents. However, the small-diameter afferents (both nociceptors and thermoreceptors) are remarkable in also expressing an array of neuropeptides, among them substance P, calcitonin gene-related peptide (CGRP), vasoactive intestinal peptide (VIP) and somatostatin (SS). Indeed, many of these afferents co-localize several peptides in addition to glutamate. These peptides are released along with glutamate.

The best-studied of the many neuropeptides localized in small-diameter afferents is substance P, an 11-amino-acid neuropeptide that originally received considerable attention from investigators attempting to identify the "pain transmitter" in the spinal cord. However, blocking the action of substance P released from primary afferent nociceptors does not produce a potent analgesia. This indicates that although substance P may play a role in nociception, it is not the sole contributor. It is now recognized that the co-release of glutamate and various peptides plays an important role in the signaling of nociceptive information.

2.5. Primary Afferents Play an Active Role in Promoting Inflammation at a Site of Injury

Notably, *most* of the peptide manufactured by the primary afferent neurons is actually transported out to the periphery, rather than centrally into the dorsal horn. For example, approx 80% of the substance P produced by cells in the dorsal-root ganglion is transported out to the tissues. These peripherally released peptides have been shown to promote inflammation, and contribute to sensitization and activation of the primary afferent terminals (Table 2). Thus, the primary afferent neurons are not mere passive sensors for damage. Rather, they participate actively in dynamic alterations of peripheral sensory sensitivity and contribute to inflammation as part of the repair process.

3. NOCICEPTIVE SENSORY NEURONS PROJECT TO THE DORSAL HORN

3.1. The Pattern of Projection and Termination of Somatosensory Afferents Within the Spinal Cord is Highly Ordered

Somatosensory primary afferents travel through the dorsal root to enter the spinal cord (or in the case of the head and neck, the trigeminal nucleus, which can be considered the medullary homolog of the spinal somatosensory processing circuitry). The pattern of branching and termination within the dorsal horn shows a high level of anatomical ordering that can be related to function (Fig. 3). Upon entering the cord, the small fibers may travel within the white matter adjacent to the entry zone for several segments, but then terminate within the dorsal horn in two regions: the superficial layers (I and II) and lamina V. In contrast, the low-threshold mechanoreceptors course around the medial edge of the dorsal horn, and send branches rostrally towards the medulla in the dorsal columns and into the middle layers of the dorsal horn (laminae III and IV).

3.2. Nociceptive Dorsal Horn Neurons Include Some that Are Nociceptive-Specific, and Others that Respond to Both Innocuous and Noxious Stimulation

Considering the ordered distribution of primary afferents, it should not be surprising that dorsal horn neurons activated by tissue damage are found in the superficial layers and more deeply in lamina V. Dorsal-horn nociceptive neurons can be divided into two broad

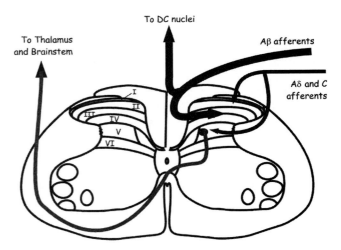

Fig. 3. Organization of somatosensory afferent terminations in the dorsal horn. As axons approach the spinal cord in the dorsal root, axons segregate by size, so that the Aβ afferents move dorsally and medially, and the Aδ and C afferents shift laterally. Large mechanoreceptive afferents then project through the dorsal columns to the medulla, and may send a branch into the middle layers of the dorsal horn (laminae III and IV). The smaller afferents terminate superficially (laminae I and II) and in the neck of the dorsal horn (lamina V).

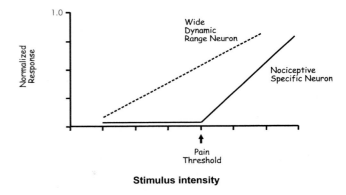

Fig. 4. Dorsal-horn nociceptive neurons include nociceptive-specific (NS) cells, which respond only to stimuli with intensity in the noxious range, and wide-dynamic range (WDR) cells, which are activated by both innocuous and noxious stimuli, with a graded increase in activity.

classes: nociceptive-specific (NS) and wide-dynamic range (WDR, Fig. 4). NS neurons are excited only by nociceptive primary afferents. They do not respond to brush or even moderate pressure. They generally have small receptive fields (e.g., only a toe and part of the foot), which suggests that they could be very important in coding the location of a noxious stimulus. WDR neurons receive input from low-threshold as well as nociceptive primary afferents, and show a graded increase in firing rate related to stimulus intensity.

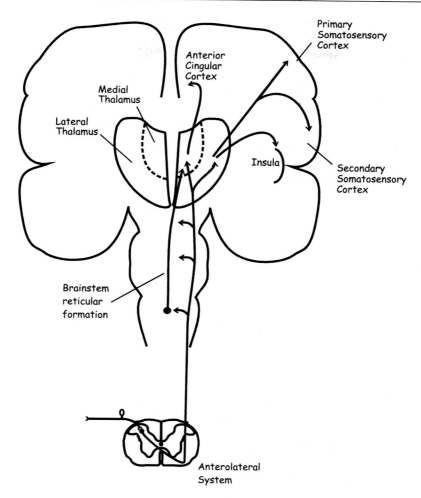

Fig. 5. Organization of the anterolateral system. Spinothalamic projections to lateral and medial thalamus and spinoreticular projections to brainstem reticular formation are shown.

Thus, unlike primary afferents, they respond to stimuli over a wide range of intensities, both innocuous and noxious. The receptive fields of WDR neurons are usually larger than those of NS neurons, suggesting that cells of this class do not contribute substantially to location coding. However, the firing rate of WDR cells is generally well-correlated with both stimulus intensity and subjective pain intensity in humans, so they are believed to code stimulus intensity.

4. PARALLEL ASCENDING PATHWAYS UNDERLIE DISTRIBUTED PROCESSING OF NOCICEPTIVE INFORMATION

4.1. Nociceptive Dorsal Horn Neurons Contribute to the Anterolateral System

Some of these nociceptive dorsal-horn neurons (NS and WDR) are interneurons (e.g., involved in processing either within the same segment or at other levels within the spinal cord), but many are projection neurons, that send their axons up to the brain. The axons cross to the contralateral side and ascend along with axons from thermoreceptive dorsal-horn neurons in the white matter of the anterolateral quadrant as part of the *anterolateral system* (Fig. 5). This stands in contrast with projections of large-diameter afferents, which are via the dorsal column ipsilateral to the site of entry (*see* Fig. 3). Hemisections of the spinal cord thus result, at least in the short term, in a loss of fine touch *ipsilaterally* and pain and temperature *contralaterally*. It should be noted that there is a small contingent of anterolateral system fibers that ascend ipsilaterally. This ipsilateral projection seems to make only a small contribution to sensation under normal conditions, but may contribute to intractable pain that sometimes develops after section of the contralateral anterolateral quadrant.

4.2. Parallel Pathways Within the Anterolateral System Form the Basis for Nociception

The anterolateral system has a number of targets in the brain. Among the most important is a direct spinothalamic projection to the lateral and medial thalamus (Fig. 5). Lateral spinothalamic targets (ventral posterolateral nucleus as well as more posterior and inferior regions that have not been as well-studied) in turn project to the primary and secondary somatosensory cortex and to the insula. These projections are believed to convey information needed for discriminative analysis of painful stimuli, and play an important role in monitoring of the "state of the body." At least as a first approximation, information related to the motivational component of pain is believed to involve projections to the medial thalamus, both direct and relayed through the brainstem reticular formation (RF). Some medial thalamic nuclei project to anterior cingulate cortex, a region believed to be closely linked to limbic processing of sensory information and decision-making. Recent functional imaging studies in humans confirm activation of the insula, anterior cingulate, and somatosensory cortex during painful stimulation. Spinoreticular projections that terminate in brainstem RF are believed to contribute to arousal, and as already noted, can also access medial thalamic structures indirectly (Fig. 5). The anterolateral system also includes spinal projections that extend directly to limbic and striatal forebrain structures, including the amygdala and hypothalamus. These are believed to play some role in sensory processing and/or neuroendocrine and autonomic adjustments needed to deal effectively with damage to the body.

Our understanding of the central neural mechanisms of pain sensation has increased substantially in recent years. A broad framework in which a crossed anterolateral system served as the pathway for sensations of pain can be traced by clinical and experimental observations made over a century ago. Indeed, as early as 1911, Head and Holmes suggested that discriminative and affective components of pain sensation were mediated by the lateral and medial thalamus, respectively. A role for cortical structures in pain sensation was generally discounted, because cortical lesions rarely altered pain sensation in patients. The recognition that the spinoreticular and spinothalamic projections can access and activate multiple cortical structures, as well as recent evidence that the antero-lateral system has direct projections to forebrain structures, demand a more complex view. Parallel ascending pathways target different areas in the brainstem, thalamus, and forebrain. These projections are likely to process different aspects of the noxious stimulus, and interact in a dynamic fashion to give rise to sensation. This fact, more than any other, probably accounts for our inability to produce durable analgesia through ablative central lesions. Whatever tract is cut or brain region is destroyed, there are always other circuits, redundant and plastic, that can reconstitute the nociceptive process.

5. VISCERAL NOCICEPTION

5.1. Stimuli that Give Rise to Pain Sensation Depend on the Tissue Stimulated

Although most clinically significant pains arise from deep somatic structures or viscera, the discussion thus far has been focused upon neural mechanisms of pain arising from the skin. That is at least partially because the skin is relatively easy to study, and as a result we know much more about it. However, the skin is a specialized tissue, important both as a sensory organ and as part of our defense against the outside world. Pain from deep structures, particularly the viscera, thus differs in a number of ways from the pain that arises from skin.

The effective stimuli are different, and extreme damage to a visceral organ does not necessarily give rise to pain. Indeed, surgeons have long known that it was possible to cut or burn visceral tissue without producing pain. This astonishing observation led to the idea that there was no such thing as pain from visceral structures, and pain that seemed to be derived from viscera actually arose because somatic structures were somehow involved. However, it later became clear that appropriate stimuli, which include the distention of hollow organs, ischemia (e.g., the heart), and inflammation, are important sources of visceral pain.

Another difference is that spatial summation seems to be important in visceral pain, although this is not the case with pain from skin. We all recognize that a pinprick is painful, although the area stimulated is quite small. With visceral structures, it is necessary to stimulate over a larger area, which may explain why visceral inflammation is painful, and more localized cutting or pinching is not.

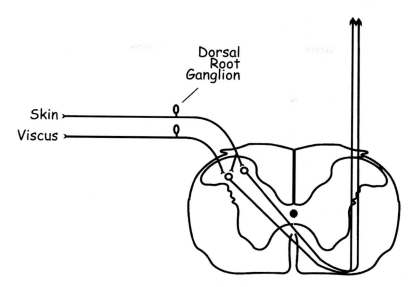

Fig. 6. Convergence-projection theory explains referral of visceral pain to skin. Dorsal-horn neurons with input from visceral structures also receive input from cutaneous afferents.

5.2. Visceral Pain is Poorly Localized

One of the real peculiarities of pain from visceral organs is that it is poorly localized, and is often perceived as arising in a body region remote from the actual pathology. The most commonly cited example is angina pectoris, in which a significant number of patients report pain in the left chest and shoulder or upper arm. This remote pain is known as *referred pain*, and it can be perceived either in other deep structures or skin. The pattern of referral is sometimes characteristic for a particular structure, and can be a helpful diagnostic aid.

5.3. Convergence of Somatic and Visceral Information in the Dorsal Horn Explains Referred Pain from Visceral Structures

Mechanisms of referred pain have been intensely debated. It should be recognized that the primary afferents innervating viscera are small in diameter (Aδ and C fibers) and project primarily to the superficial dorsal horn and deep dorsal horn, skipping laminae III and IV. Thus, they resemble cutaneous nociceptors in axon diameter and central projection. However, the innervation of the viscera is generally much less dense than that of the skin, and the projections within the dorsal horn are more diffuse. Visceral afferents show extensive spread along the rostro-caudal axis, and may even project to the contralateral dorsal horn. In addition, visceral afferents target dorsal-horn neu-

rons that also receive input from the skin or from musculoskeletal tissues. Thus, there are no specific "visceral" neurons in the dorsal horn. This suggests that referred pain is caused by convergence of inputs in the dorsal horn ("convergence-projection theory"). When the brain receives a signal from a dorsal-horn neuron, it has no way to determine the true source, and mistakenly "projects" the sensation to the skin or another somatic structure (Fig. 6). The projection of visceral input to skin rather than vice versa is likely a result of the fact that there are many neurons with strictly cutaneous input that bias supraspinal processing when active.

6. PAIN PROCESSES IN INJURED OR INFLAMED TISSUE

Thus far, we have discussed mainly the brief stimuli delivered to normal tissue that do not produce significant damage or inflammation. The pain that results in this situation is sometimes referred to as "normal" pain, and mildly painful stimuli are certainly encountered frequently as part of everyday life. In contrast, pain experiences that provide serious distress usually involve more serious destructive processes. In these situations, there is often a lingering tenderness and hypersensitivity. This increase in pain is loosely referred to as "hyperalgesia," and can involve a decrease in threshold (so that normally innocuous stimuli such as a light touch or gentle warmth are now

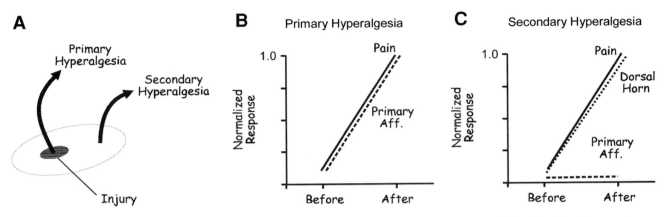

Fig. 7. Mechanisms of primary and secondary hyperalgesia. (**A**) Hyperalgesia within an area of injury is referred to as primary hyperalgesia, that in surrounding tissue is called secondary hyperalgesia. (**B**) Pain rating and activity in primary afferents before and after injury to the tissue. Sensitized primary afferents explain increased pain in the injured region. (**C**) Pain rating and activity in primary afferents and dorsal horn neurons with receptive fields in the area of secondary hyperalgesia. Primary afferents innervating the area of secondary hyperalgesia are not sensitized, whereas dorsal-horn neurons responding to stimulation of that area show increased responsiveness ("central sensitization").

perceived as painful, a state referred to as "allodynia") and increased sensation evoked by stimuli that normally would cause pain.

When considering the mechanisms underlying hyperalgesia following injury, it is important to distinguish between *primary hyperalgesia*, which is exaggerated sensitivity in the injured tissue, and *secondary hyperalgesia*, which refers to the increased sensitivity in the surrounding area (Fig. 7A). This distinction between primary and secondary hyperalgesia is significant because the underlying mechanisms are different.

6.1. Primary Hyperalgesia Involves Increased Sensitivity and Responsiveness in the Primary Afferent Nociceptors

Primary hyperalgesia is explained by increases in the sensitivity of the primary afferent nociceptors (Fig. 7B). Both Aδ and C fibers are sensitized by injury. Thresholds for activation are lowered, and the afferents display an increased response to suprathreshold stimuli. Primary afferents can also develop spontaneous activity, and show a prolonged afterdischarge so that activity in the nociceptor outlasts the stimulus. As previously noted, many nociceptors are silent under normal conditions, but become quite responsive to mechanical and thermal stimuli when the tissue is inflamed.

Mechanisms for peripheral sensitization involve the chemical "soup" that develops in injured tissues (Table 2). As already noted, a number of these com-

pounds do not excite the nociceptor directly, but will cause it to become sensitized. One effect of substance P released from the peripheral nerve terminals is to sensitize the terminals, making them more responsive to other components of the inflammatory soup. Bradykinin, formed from a plasma precursor, and prostaglandins, formed from membrane lipids by the actions of phospholipase A2 and cyclo-oxygenase (Fig. 8), also sensitize primary afferent terminals. Indeed, thermal sensitivity in inflamed tissue may be increased to the point that normal body temperature is now sufficient to activate nociceptive afferents and produce pain!

6.2. Central Sensitization Explains Secondary Hyperalgesia

Secondary hyperalgesia does not seem to be explained by primary afferent sensitization, because the properties of afferents with receptive fields in the area of secondary hyperalgesia are essentially unchanged. The significant alteration underlying hyperalgesia in tissue surrounding the injury instead seems to be in the dorsal horn (Fig. 7C). Thus, secondary hyperalgesia is explained not by sensitization of the primary afferents, but by *central sensitization*. Studies of dorsal-horn neurons with receptive fields in an area of secondary hyperalgesia show lowered thresholds and increased responses to frankly noxious stimuli. Many of these neurons also develop spontaneous activity. Changes are most pronounced in the WDR neurons, and the circuitry in the spinal cord is sensitized to the extent that inputs conveyed by large-

Tissue Injury

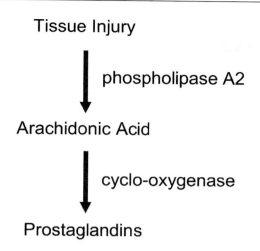

$\downarrow$ phospholipase A2

Arachidonic Acid

$\downarrow$ cyclo-oxygenase

Prostaglandins

Fig. 8. Prostaglandins are produced from membrane lipids following tissue injury. Aspirin and related analgesic drugs produce their effect by inhibition of cyclo-oxygenase.

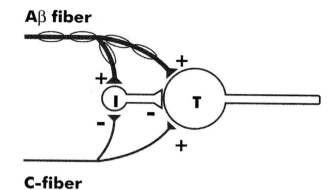

Aβ fiber

C-fiber

Fig. 9. Elements of the gate-control theory of Melzack and Wall. Activity in myelinated afferents closes the "gate," and activity in unmyelinated afferents opens it, leading to increased activity in the dorsal-horn transmission cell responsible for the sensation of pain. T, transmission cell; I, inhibitory interneuron that form the "gate."

diameter low-threshold mechanoreceptor afferents are now sufficient to elicit pain (although this is not the case under normal conditions).

7. REGULATORY MECHANISMS: GATE CONTROL AND DESCENDING MODULATION

Nociceptive information is not imposed on a passive nervous system. It is subject to a number of control mechanisms. These can be divided into segmental mechanisms (e.g., within the spinal cord), and descending controls, which are exerted on the dorsal horn from the brain.

7.1. Segmental Control Mechanisms Include That Described by "Gate-Control" Theory

The best-known example of segmental-control mechanisms is the "gate control" proposed by Melzack and Wall in 1965. Their theory was based on the observation that when conduction in large-diameter fibers is blocked (e.g., by pressure which interferes with conduction in myelinated fibers without affecting unmyelinated axons) most stimuli, ranging from a light touch to pinch gives rise to a very unpleasant, tingling, and burning pain. The implication of this finding is that activity in large-diameter fibers has a net inhibitory effect on nociceptive processes. Melzack and Wall thus proposed a model based on this idea. Their model had four elements (Fig. 9): unmyelinated afferents; myelinated mechanoreceptor afferents; a dorsal-horn transmission cell, activity in which gives rise to

pain; and an inhibitory interneuron, which is presumed to inhibit the transmission cell. The inhibitory interneuron is excited by myelinated input, but inhibited by unmyelinated activity. The ability of activity in the unmyelinated afferents to drive the transmission cell thus depends on whether the gate is "shut" as a result of myelinated input driving the inhibitory interneuron, or "open" because the myelinated fibers are not active. If the gate is "open," there will be a high level of activity in the transmission cell, and this will be sufficient to produce a sensation of pain.

Although the *specific* details of the gate-control theory as outlined here have not stood the test of time, the general idea that input conveyed over large-diameter, low-threshold afferents can interact with processing of nociceptive information does have some validity. A circuit similar to that proposed by Melzack and Wall is probably the basis for some treatments used clinically, such as TENS (trans-cutaneous electrical stimulation). TENS involves electrical stimulation of the skin at an intensity that activates large-diameter fibers (which have a lower threshold for electrical activation than smaller fibers). Use of TENS is particularly widespread in treatment of musculoskeletal pain states.

7.2. Brainstem Control of Spinal Nociceptive Processing

It has long been known that the relationship between stimulus intensity and pain sensation is not simple or constant. The magnitude of the response to a given noxious stimulus depends upon the individual and an array of situational and behavioral factors. Perhaps the

earliest systematic analysis of this variability was provided by Sir Henry Beecher, who found that soldiers
wounded in World War II experienced much less pain
than would have been expected from their injuries.
Subsequent psychophysical studies clearly demonstrated that the pain experience in humans can be
influenced by arousal, attention, learning, fear, and
stress.

The recognition that this variation in pain sensation
has an understandable neural basis, and that it is at
least in part caused by a central modulating circuit
specific for pain, is much more recent. This idea of
central modulation is usually traced back to the observation that electrical stimulation in the midbrain
periaqueductal gray of rats inhibited responses to
stimuli that would have been expected to produce pain
behaviors in normal animals. The significance of this
observation, which appeared in Science in 1969, was
in pointing to pain modulation as a specific function of
the CNS. Although a number of brain systems are now
known to regulate spinal nociceptive processing, the
best-studied and probably functionally most significant pain modulating network has links in the midbrain periaqueductal gray and rostral ventromedial
medulla (Fig. 10). Activation of the periaqueductal
gray in turn activates neurons in the rostral medulla
that project to the dorsal horn at all levels of the cord
and influence nociceptive processing at that level. The
periaqueductal gray has dense reciprocal connections
with limbic forebrain structures such as the amygdala
and hypothalamus. These connections link higher neural processes with pain regulation.

This descending modulatory system is also an
important substrate for opioid analgesia. Local administration of opioids in either the periaqueductal gray or
the rostral ventromedial medulla produces analgesia,
and studies at the single-cell level demonstrate that
this is a result of the ability of opioid analgesics to
activate pain-inhibiting neurons within the rostral
medulla. This system is also responsible for the inhibition of pain by various stressors. Interestingly, this
descending control system has now been shown to
contribute to *enhanced* nociceptive processing under
some conditions—for example, during illness or
inflammation. The neural basis for bi-directional control of nociception is two classes of neurons in the
rostral medulla: *off-cells*, which are activated by opioids and inhibit nociceptive processing, and *on-cells*,
which are inhibited by opioids and facilitate nociceptive processing.

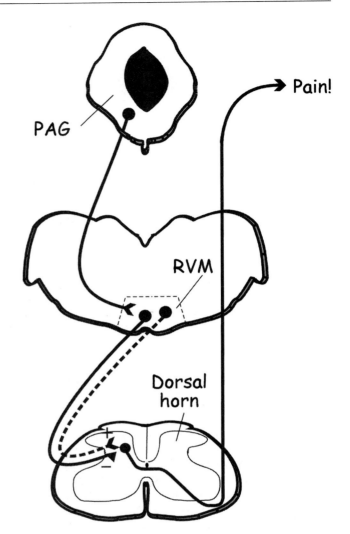

Fig. 10. Brainstem pain-modulating network has links in the
midbrain periaqueductal gray (PAG) and rostral ventromedial medulla (RVM). The RVM, which includes the nucleus
raphe magnus and adjacent reticular formation, receives a large
input from the PAG. The RVM in turns projects to the dorsal
horn, primarily to the superficial layers and lamina I, where it
can influence processing of nociceptive information. The RVM
includes two populations of cells, *off-cells*, which inhibit
nociception, and *on-cells*, which facilitate nociception at the
level of the dorsal horn

8. PAIN CAUSED BY INJURY TO PERIPHERAL OR CENTRAL NERVOUS SYSTEM

We have thus far been considering "nociceptive
pain,"—pain produced or at least triggered by tissue injury. However, there are situations in which the
source of pain is not in the tissue (where it is "perceived" to be), but in the nervous system itself. Vari-

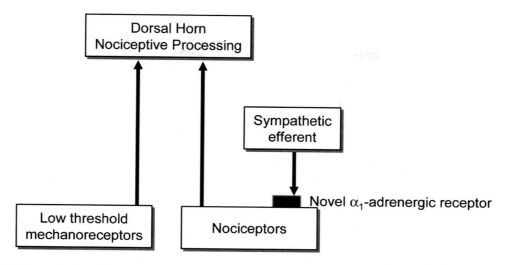

Fig. 11. Sympathetic mechanism of neuropathic pain. Initial injury causes nociceptors to develop a novel adrenoreceptor. Activity in sympathetic efferents thus evoke a continuing low level of activity in nociceptors, which in turn sensitizes dorsal-horn processing circuits. Because of this central sensitization, input from low-threshold mechanoreceptors now produces pain.

ous terms have been used to refer to pain of this type. The most general is "neuropathic," as it denotes pain arising from injury to the peripheral or CNS itself. Another frequently used term is "deafferentation pain," although this is falling out of favor, since only a subset of neuropathic pains involve deafferentation.

8.1. Features of Neuropathic Pain Distinguish It from Pain Produced by Tissue Injury

There are many neuropathic pain syndromes (examples include post-herpetic neuralgia, diabetic neuropathy, complex regional pain syndromes, phantom limb pain, and thalamic syndrome), and the character of pain in these syndromes is quite distinct from pain produced by injury to non-neural tissues. Neuropathic pain is persistent, generally burning or with a "shooting" or 'electric' quality. There is often extreme sensitivity to mechanical or thermal stimuli, so that everyday events such as the brush of clothing on the skin can be painful. In addition, the pain is often perceived as arising from a region of sensory deficit.

The mechanisms underlying these painful dysfunctions of the nervous system remain poorly understood, and in most neuropathic syndromes, there are probably multiple pathological processes at work. Nevertheless, we can consider mechanisms involving primary afferents, those caused by changes in central processing, and efferent mechanisms involving the sympathetic nervous system.

8.2. Damaged Primary Afferents Display Abnormal Activity

Normally, action potentials arise only at the peripheral terminals of primary afferents. However, when an axon is cut, new processes grow out toward the original target tissue. These sprouts often end up forming a tangle called a "neuroma." The axon sprouts within the neuroma are abnormally thin, and without the usual Schwann-cell sheath. These morphological abnormalities are associated with altered physiology, so that there is spontaneous activity and sensitivity to mechanical stimulation. Tapping the neuroma thus produces a sensation. Abnormal activity in these damaged afferents is called "ectopic," because it originates at an abnormal site—not at the terminal region, as is usually the case. Ectopic activity following injury may also arise from the region around the cell body in the dorsal-root ganglion. But wherever it arises, ectopic activity will be interpreted by central circuits as reflecting peripheral events, and it may contribute to a form of central sensitization, analogous to that underlying secondary hyperalgesia.

8.3. Central Factors in Neuropathic Pain Include Denervation Hypersensitivity and Central Sensitization

One mechanism that has been identified in the CNS is known as "denervation hypersensitivity," which refers to a hyperactivity that many central neurons exhibit when they lose their normal afferent input. When this hypersensitivity arises in pathways that would normally contribute to pain sensation, the result is likely to be neuropathic pain perceived as arising from the denervated region. This pain is thus particularly paradoxical because the region where the person "feels" the pain is at least partially anesthetic. Thus, for example, a pinprick in the painful region would not be perceived.

Central sensitization, as a factor in secondary hyperalgesia, is another mechanism believed to contribute to neuropathic pain. Thus, an intense nociceptive barrage or even just a low level of ongoing activity—possibly ectopic—in nociceptive primary afferents may trigger central sensitization. This would certainly explain the prominence of allodyia in many neuropathic pain states.

8.4. Sympathetic Efferent Mechanisms

It has been known since the last Twentieth Century that pain can be dependent on sympathetic activity in the painful area. This pain has been referred to as "reflex sympathetic dystrophy" or "causalgia," but is now termed "complex regional pain syndrome" (type I or II). Whatever you choose to call it, this syndrome of intense burning pain and allodynia usually develops after a traumatic lesion to peripheral nerve or deep tissue (muscle or bone). There are usually autonomic disturbances at some point in the course of the syndrome, and an important distinguishing feature is that pain can often be relieved by block of the sympathetic innervation to the painful area.

Because pain in complex regional pain syndromes is generally eliminated when activity in large-diameter afferents is blocked, it is believed that primary afferent nociceptors somehow become abnormally sensitive to norepinephrine released from sympathetic efferents. This promotes a continuous low level of activity in these neurons, which in turn produces a state of central sensitization. Because central circuits are sensitized, input from large-diameter mechanoreceptive afferents is now sufficient to induce pain (Fig. 11).

SELECTED READINGS

Casey KL. Forebrain mechanisms of nociception and pain: analysis through imaging. Proc Natl Acad Sci USA 1999; 96: 7668–7674.

Cervero F. Sensory innervation of the viscera: peripheral basis of visceral pain. Physiol Rev 1994; 74:95–138.

Fields HL. Pain. New York:McGraw Hill, 1987.

Fields HL, Heinricher MM. Anatomy and physiology of a nociceptive modulatory system. Philos Trans R Soc Lond B, 1985; 308:361–374.

Torebjörk HE, Lundberg LE, LaMotte RH. Central changes in processing of mechanoreceptive input in capsaicin-induced secondary hyperalgesia in humans. J Physiol (Lond) 1992; 448:765–780.

Wall PD, Melzack R (eds). Textbook of Pain. Edinburgh,: Churchill Livginstone, 1999.

Willis WD (ed). Hyperalgesia and allodynia. New York:Raven Press, 1992.

Willis WD, Coggleshall RE. Sensory mechanisms of the spinal cord. New York: Plenum Press, 1991.

Physical Trauma to Nerves

Gregory Cooper and Robert L. Rodnitzky

Nerve injury can occur as a result of major acute trauma, such as a gunshot wound, or develop more slowly as a result of milder but continuous trauma. The degree of neurologic deficit and the prospect for recovery depend on several factors. Typically, acute injuries resulting in anatomic disruption of the nerve cause more severe and lasting disability than slowly developing injuries that leave the nerve in anatomic continuity.

NERVE SEVERANCE RESULTS IN A PREDICTABLE SEQUENCE OF CHANGES IN THE NERVE AND MUSCLE

If nerve continuity is disrupted as a result of trauma, the nerve segment distal to the injury undergoes *wallerian degeneration*. This process involves disintegration of axoplasm and axolemma and ultimately results in the breakdown and phagocytosis of myelin, and the process takes several weeks to complete. Severe degeneration of the nerve implies that any recovery of function will require regeneration of nerve fibers from the intact nerve stump to the appropriate muscle or sensory organ.

After about 2 wk, significant changes appear in the denervated muscle. Acetylcholine receptors begin to proliferate at locations on the muscle fibers outside the endplate region, where they are usually concentrated. At the same time, spontaneous contractions of muscle fibers, known as *fibrillations*, appear. Fibrillations can be detected using electromyography, a common clinical electrodiagnostic technique in which the electrical potentials generated by muscle fibers can he measured through a small intramuscular needle electrode. Detection of fibrillation potentials suggests that the muscle is denervated. This finding can be considered indirect evidence that the nerve fiber innervating the muscle has undergone axonal disruption.

Fibrillations, which can only be detected by electromyographic techniques, should not be confused with *fasciculations*, which are gross muscle twitchings under the skin that are clearly visible to the naked eye. Unlike fibrillations, which strongly suggest muscle denervations, fasciculations can be seen in normal and denervated muscles.

NERVE-CONDUCTION TESTING IS USEFUL IN DETERMINING THE EXTENT AND LOCATION OF NERVE DAMAGE

Stimulation of a motor nerve segment distal to the point of injury can help determine whether the injury has disrupted the nerve's anatomic continuity. Within 8 d after severance of a nerve, stimulation of the distal segment no longer produces a response in the muscle it innervates. However, if the damage to the nerve has only resulted in a physiologic block of impulse conduction (e.g., *neuropraxia*) but not anatomic discontinuity, a muscle response occurs, implying intact conduction in the nerve segment beyond the point of injury.

Nerve stimulation can also help to determine whether an injury to a sensory nerve is preganglionic or postganglionic. In preganglionic injury, the distal nerve fibers are still in continuity with ganglion cells. Stimulation of the nerve produces propagated impulses that can be recorded over a distant portion of the nerve, proving its viability. In a postganglionic lesion, the distal segment of the nerve, after being disconnected from the nerve-cell body, degenerates and loses its ability to be stimulated.

CHRONIC COMPRESSION AND ENTRAPMENT ARE AMONG THE MOST COMMON FORMS OF NERVE INJURY

Compression, constriction, or stretching of nerves is common at certain anatomic sites that are vulnerable to these mechanical forces. A nerve may be susceptible to compression because of its superficial location. An example is the peroneal nerve below the knee, where it crosses over the lateral border of the top of the fibula just under the skin. Because of this superficial location, there is no protective layer of muscle or fat. The nerve is often damaged when one leg is crossed over the other and the fibular head comes to rest on the opposite knee. The ensuing peroneal-nerve palsy results in a pattern of muscle weakness, causing footdrop.

Nerve compression resulting from passage through a confining space is exemplified by carpal tunnel syndrome. At the wrist, the median nerve passes under a thick, fibrous ligament and can be chronically compressed, especially during repetitive flexion of the wrist. This syndrome, unlike peroneal-nerve palsy, typically develops over a period of months as a result of less severe but more prolonged trauma. In severe forms of carpal tunnel syndrome, neurologic symptoms develop, including weakness of the muscles controlling the thumb and tingling of the thumb and the next two digits.

Stretching is a form of trauma that often affects the ulnar nerve. This nerve courses over the elbow and can be stretched when the elbow is flexed. With repeated stretching, an ulnar-nerve palsy develops, producing symptoms that include weakness of the intrinsic hand muscles and numbness of the fourth and fifth digits of the hand. The susceptibility of the ulnar nerve to com-

pression at the elbow is known to anyone who has struck his or her "funny bone."

RECOVERY AFTER NERVE TRAUMA MAY DEPEND ON NERVE REGENERATION

After wallerian degeneration, nerve regeneration may occur, especially if the surrounding connective tissue elements of the nerve sheath are intact and guide the regenerating fibers in the proper direction. Even under these favorable circumstances, recovery may be delayed, because nerve regeneration proceeds at the rate of approx 1 mm per day. The forward progress of the regenerating nerve tip can be monitored by using Tinel's sign. Because the advancing edge of a regenerating nerve fiber is unmyelinated, it is unusually sensitive to minimal mechanical stimuli. By lightly tapping through the skin along the course of a regenerating nerve, the physician can identify the location of the advancing nerve tip. The tap produces a tingling sensation in the part of the body toward which the regenerating sensory nerve is growing.

One of the pitfalls of peripheral-nerve regeneration is that fibers, especially those with motor and autonomic functions, may become misdirected to a different muscle or gland than was originally innervated. This is known as *aberrant regeneration*. This misdirected growth often occurs in the face when regenerating facial-nerve fibers intended for eyelid muscles grow instead to perioral muscles. An attempted eye blink then produces a simultaneous twitch of the side of the mouth. This dual action, caused by aberrant regeneration, is called *synkinetic movement*.

SELECTED READING

Robinson LR. Traumatic injury to peripheral nerves. Muscle and Nerve 2000; 23:863–873.

Peripheral Neuropathy

Gregory Cooper and Robert L. Rodnitzky

The peripheral nerves are susceptible to toxic, metabolic, traumatic, and neoplastic damage. Regardless of the cause, the damage is known as *neuropathy*.

Circumstances can alter the nature of the damage to the nerve. In some neuropathies, the axon is the primary focus of involvement. In some, the myelin sheath is largely involved, and in others, the axon and sheath are equally affected. The anatomic distribution of nerve involvement also varies. In some neuropathies, the most proximal portion of the nerve is involved, but in others, the most distal segment is primarily affected. Involvement of a single nerve is referred to as *mononeuropathy*, and the term *polyneuropathy* is used when nerves throughout the body are diffusely affected.

There are too many causes of peripheral neuropathy to list here, but among the most common are diabetes, kidney failure, chronic alcohol use and its associated nutritional deficiencies, autoimmune diseases, and trauma.

AXONAL DEGENERATION CAN TAKE SEVERAL FORMS

Several processes can result in axonal degeneration. *Wallerian degeneration* is common after severe nerve trauma. After any insult that interrupts the axon, the segment distal to the lesion undergoes progressive degeneration over the next several days. The myelin components of the distal-nerve segment degenerate, and fragments of the axon and myelin sheath are ultimately cleared by macrophages.

Many neuropathies that primarily affect the axon, especially those of toxic origin, are characterized by degeneration of the distal portion of the axon through a process known as the *dying-back phenomenon*. This process usually involves the longest nerves in the body and is typically manifested first in the nerves innervating the feet and hands. This explains why sensory symptoms in many axonal neuropathies initially appear in the toes and feet or in the fingertips and hands. The dying back phenomenon is probably related to the failure of axonal transport to support sufficiently the portions of the nerve that are most distant from the cell body.

Neuronopathy refers to a destructive process primarily involving the nerve-cell body, producing degeneration and loss of neurofilaments within the axon, which reduces the caliber of the axon. The autoimmune sensory neuropathy associated with lung cancer is a neuronopathy of sensory neurons in the dorsal-root ganglia.

DEMYELINATION OF PERIPHERAL NERVES MAY BE PRIMARY OR SECONDARY

Segmental demyelination refers to the breakdown of the myelin sheath in the nerve segment between two nodes of Ranvier. These abnormal segments may be scattered along the length of the nerve. Because of the importance of the myelin sheath in facilitating rapid impulse conduction, segmental demyelination markedly slows nerve conduction and, in extreme forms, produces total conduction block. These conduction abnormalities can be easily demonstrated in the clinical electrophysiology laboratory using the technique of nerve-conduction velocity testing. The term *secondary demyelination* is used to describe the myelin breakdown that occurs as the result of an antecedent primary axonal insult.

THE TYPICAL SYMPTOMS OF PERIPHERAL NEUROPATHY INCLUDE POSITIVE AND NEGATIVE PHENOMENA

The most common negative signs of peripheral-nerve dysfunction are the loss of strength and sensation. In axonal neuropathies, these signs begin in the feet and progress proximally, correlating with the predominance of pathology in the distal portion of long peripheral nerves. Even in demyelinating neuropathies, a similar distal pattern of sensory and motor loss is often observed, because longer nerve fibers are more likely than shorter ones to contain randomly distributed demyelinated foci. In addition to muscle weakness, involved muscles may demonstrate atrophy and fasciculations, which are signs of denervation.

Any sensory modality can be lost in peripheral neuropathy. In conditions that primarily affect small fibers, pain and temperature sensation are preferentially lost, and in neuropathies involving large, myelinated fibers, there may a greater loss of vibratory and proprioceptive senses.

One of the most prominent negative signs of peripheral-nerve disease is the loss of muscle-stretch reflexes. Reduction or loss of stretch reflexes is one of the most sensitive signs of peripheral nerve disease. There are several mechanisms by which these reflexes can be affected. In neuropathies involving large, rapidly conducting fibers, Ia afferent fibers from the muscle spindle may be directly involved, interrupting the afferent arc of the reflex. In neuropathies involving smaller fibers, the gamma efferent fibers to the spindle may be the locus at which the reflex is affected. Although large- and small-fiber neuropathies can produce areflexia, it is more common in cases of large-fiber involvement.

Involvement of autonomic fibers can produce symptoms such as a loss of sweating, abnormal heart rhythms, or impaired control of blood pressure. In most neuropathies, autonomic dysfunction is not prominent, but there can be significant autonomic symptoms in conditions resulting in acute demyelination or those primarily affecting small myelinated and unmyelinated fibers. An example of the former is Guillain-Barre syndrome, and an example of the latter is the neuropathy of diabetes.

Sensory ataxia is another negative feature of peripheral neuropathy. It results from the severe loss of position sense in the feet. Involvement of large, myelinated fibers conveying proprioceptive sense prevents the patient from appreciating the exact position of the feet, resulting in an unsteady gait.

The most prominent positive symptoms of neuropathies are in the sensory realm. The term *paresthesia* is used to describe uncomfortable sensory perceptions occurring spontaneously without an apparent stimulus. These sensations are variously described as burning, tightness, tingling, or pins and needles. The term *dysesthesia* refers to an unusual or distorted sensation evoked by a stimulus such as a simple touch. *Hyperalgesia* is exaggerated pain perception that occurs in response to a stimulus that would ordinarily be painless. Spontaneously painful sensations are slightly more common in neuropathies involving small-diameter fibers.

Positive phenomena related to motor-nerve involvement include fasciculations and muscle cramps. A fasciculation is the spontaneous contraction of a denervated motor unit, which is a group of muscle fibers previously innervated by a single motor-nerve fiber. Fasciculations appear as flickering movements of muscles that can be seen through the skin. Normal muscles may occasionally exhibit fasciculations under conditions such as extreme fatigue.

NERVE-CONDUCTION TESTING IS USEFUL IN ANALYZING PERIPHERAL NEUROPATHIES

Nerve conduction velocity can be calculated by stimulating a nerve trunk at one point along its course and determining the time of arrival of the impulse at a measured distance along the nerve. This is a relatively painless procedure that requires a small electrical stimulus to be applied to the nerve through the skin. The technique can differentiate axonal from demyelinating neuropathies. Because an intact myelin sheath is critical to rapid nerve conduction, nerve-conduction velocity is markedly diminished in demyelinating neuropathies. Conduction block, another electrophysiologic feature typical of demyelinating neuropathies, can be demonstrated by this technique. In axonal neuropathies, conduction velocity is only minimally slowed, but the the amplitude of the evoked response in the nerve or in a muscle innervated by the nerve is clearly diminished.

In demyelinating neuropathies, recovery can occur through remyelination. However, even after recovery, nerve-conduction velocity may remain slow, because the nodes of Ranvier in remyelinated segments may be closer together, resulting in less efficient saltatory conduction.

PERIPHERAL NEUROPATHY MAY DEVELOP ACUTELY OR CHRONICALLY

Most neuropathies caused by metabolic, degenerative, or heritable abnormalities develop over a period of several months or years. Chronic evolution is seen in the neuropathies associated with diabetes, kidney failure, or lead exposure, and this pattern is typical of most familial neuropathies. A smaller subset of neuropathies develop more rapidly

The Guillain-Barre syndrome is an example of a neuropathy with a subacute onset. In this condition, autoimmune inflammatory demyelination of peripheral nerves occurs over a period of several days to 2 wk. Within this period, the affected person may revert from total normality to a profound state of weakness, immobility, and respiratory insufficiency.

The onset of traumatic nerve disorders can be acute or chronic. An example of acute traumatic neuropathy is the sudden development of footdrop caused by acute compression of the peroneal nerve as it crosses the outside of the knee. This condition is often caused by crossing one leg over the other. A more slowly developing traumatic nerve disorder is carpal tunnel syndrome. It is caused by chronic or repetitive compression of the median nerve as it courses under a tight ligament at the wrist. Dysfunction of the nerve results in sensory loss and paresthesias involving the first three or four digits of the hand and weakness of the muscles controlling the thumb. Footdrop caused by peroneal-nerve compression often recovers spontaneously if further trauma is avoided, but in carpal tunnel syndrome, trauma frequently continues, and the condition often requires treatment consisting of surgical release of the compressing ligament.

THERAPY FOR NEUROPATHIES CAN BE DIRECTED AT THE SYMPTOMS AND THE CAUSE

For most metabolic or toxic neuropathies, medical treatment is focused on correcting the underlying metabolic abnormality or reducing the amount of the toxic substance within the body. For example, in patients with kidney failure, renal dialysis is an extremely effective means of improving the associated neuropathy. In a toxic neuropathy such as that caused by lead intoxication, chelating agents, which promote the excretion of lead, are useful. Neuropathies that have an autoimmune basis are treated with immunosuppressive therapies. For patients with Guillain-Barre syndrome, plasma exchange and intravenous immunoglobulin (IVIg), both immunomodulatory treatments, have proven to be beneficial.

The treatment of the symptoms, as opposed to the cause of neuropathy, is largely confined to attempts at reducing pain and uncomfortable paresthesias. Anticonvulsant medications and tricyclic antidepressant drugs have been successfully used to reduce neuropathic pain. In neuropathies in which pain is localized to a discrete area such as the foot, capsaicin can be applied to the skin. This agent works by locally depleting substance P, a neuropeptide involved in the transmission of pain impulses.

23 Vision

J. Fielding Hejtmancik and Rafael C. Caruso

CONTENTS

1. INTRODUCTION

Components of the visual system include the optical components of the eye (cornea, aqueous humor, lens, and vitreous body), retina, optic nerves, optic tracts, optic radiations, visual cortex, and a variety of nuclei. Each of these structures plays an important role in receiving and interpreting visual signals.

The optical components of the eye focus light on the retina, which transduces the light signal into neural signals. It also performs some initial processing before passing the neural signals through the optic nerves and tracts to central structures that perform more elaborate processing, and integrate their information with that of the other senses. This chapter considers the visual process and the anatomic components that carry it out, as well as the critical periods during which intercellular communication by synaptic transmission alters the fate of connections in the primary visual pathway from the retina to the visual cortex. In keeping with the philosophy of this volume, general principles are emphasized instead of experimental results. Students who wish to learn more about the experimental bases

of these principles are directed to the Selected Readings provided at the end of this chapter.

2. REFRACTION

Initially, light passes through the cornea, aqueous humor, lens, and vitreous body (Fig. 1). Light travels through each of these relatively dense materials with a velocity that is inversely proportional to its density.

The *refractive index* of the material is defined as the ratio of the velocity of light in a vacuum to the velocity in that substance. When a light wave strikes the curved surface of the cornea at an angle, the waveform that enters the cornea first is slowed relative to that which travels a longer distance through the air. In this process, the path of a light ray is bent, a phenomenon known as *refraction*. If the components of the anterior segment of the eye—especially the cornea and lens—are shaped correctly, the light rays that emanate from a single point are focused onto a single point on the retina. The image of an object is projected onto the retina in an inverted fashion. Thus, the inferior part of the visual field is projected onto the superior part of the retina, the nasal visual fields are projected onto the temporal part of the retina, and the temporal visual fields are projected onto the nasal retina. Because

From: *Neuroscience in Medicine, 2nd ed.* (P. Michael Conn, ed.), © 2003 Humana Press Inc., Totowa, NJ.

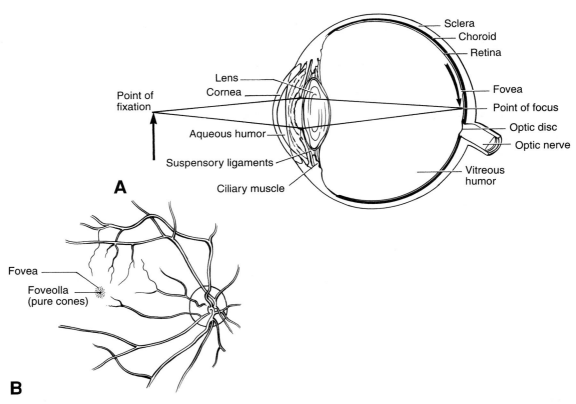

Fig. 1. (A) Overview of the eye and refraction. The refraction of light rays from the fixation point at the tip of the arrow to the focal point on the retina represents the summed effects of the anterior and posterior surfaces of the cornea and lens. The image of the arrow is projected in an inverted orientation on the retina. **(B)** View of the central retina, including the macular region.

human eyes are situated frontally, a significant fraction of each visual hemifield is viewed by both retinas, and is known as the binocular visual field.

The refractive power of the eye resides primarily in four surfaces, the anterior and posterior surfaces of the cornea and the anterior and posterior surfaces of the lens. Because the amount of refraction depends on the change in the refractive index between two substances, most refraction occurs at the anterior surface of the cornea, which is adjacent to air. When the eye is focused on a distant object, approximately one-third of the refractive power of the eye results from the lens. The degree of lens curvature depends on the contraction of the circular ciliary muscle. Contraction of the ciliary muscle decreases its diameter, allowing the lens to assume a more spherical shape. This change in the shape of the lens allows the eye to shift its focus from a distant point to a *near point*, and is called *accommodation.*

A variety of refractive errors can occur. Hyperopia (e.g., farsightedness) is usually caused by a globe that is shortened anteroposteriorly or a lens system that is too weak and focuses light on a point behind the retina. Myopia (e.g., nearsightedness) usually results from an elongated anteroposterior diameter, which causes light to be focused anteriorly to the retina, e.g., on a point in the vitreous body.

Astigmatism, a more complex refractive error, results from irregular curvature of the lens, or more commonly, of the cornea. This creates an optical element with stronger curvature in one meridian than another, which focuses a point source of light into a line rather than a point. These refractive errors can usually be corrected with appropriate lenses or, more recently, with surgery. Lens opacities (cataracts) may occur and, if they are sufficiently severe, may require surgery for correction.

After light has been focused on the retina, this structure effects the transformation from a light signal into a neural signal. The retina and the higher neuronal centers interpret the information transduced by the retina. Despite intensive research, the molecular events underlying the transformation of light energy into neural information are still being elucidated.

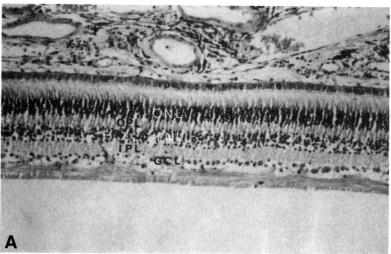

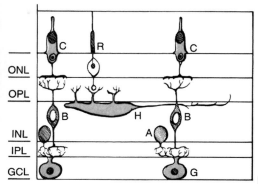

Fig. 2. The vertebrate retina. (**A**) Light microscopy section of a mouse retina. (**B**) Schematic of the cells in the retina. ONL, outer nuclear layer; OPL, outer plexiform layer; INL, inner nuclear layer; IPL, inner plexiform layer; GCL, ganglion-cell layer; R, rod cell; C, cone cell; B, bipolar cell; H, horizontal cell; A, amacrine cell; G, ganglion cell; RPE, retinal pigmented epithelium. (Photograph of hematoxylin & eosin [H&E] stain; mouse retina at original magnification ×200; courtesy of Dr. Chi Chao Chan, National Institute of Healthk, Bethesda, MD.)

3. THE RETINA

3.1. The Retina Consists of the Retinal Pigment Epithelium and the Neural Retina Containing Photoreceptors and Neuronal Processing Cells

The retina and its component cells have been described in great detail for vertebrate and invertebrate species. This discussion focuses on vertebrate vision, although much of the progress in understanding visual processes has come from studies of invertebrate models, which continue to be a valuable resource.

The structure of the vertebrate retina is shown schematically in Fig. 2. Many cell types contribute to the adult structure. The basic processes underlying retinal development are beginning to be understood, but are outside the range of this discussion. It is sufficient for our purposes to mention that the retina consists of two structural and functional components: the *retinal pigment epithelium* (RPE, the nonneural component) and the closely associated but physically distinct neural (e.g. sensory component) retina.

Cells of the retinal pigment epithelium contain melanin granules, which prevent light that is passed through the retina from being reflected by the sclera and degrading vision—a problem in disorders such as in albinism. The RPE cells also assist the photoreceptors with resynthesis of visual pigments and phagocytosis of shed outer-segment tips. Because this requires the outer segments containing these pigments to be closely approximated to the retinal-pigment epithelial layer, the neural processing networks of the retina are the anterior-most structures, and light must pass through them before stimulating the photoreceptor cells. The neural retina can be further divided into three nuclear layers separated by two plexiform (synaptic) layers. These layers are composed of six neuronal-cell types and the nonneuronal glial (Müller) cell. The interactions of these cell types are described later in this chapter

Phototransduction, the biochemical process of transforming light to electrical energy, occurs in the *photoreceptor cells*. The highly specialized photoreceptor cells can be divided into *rods* or *cones*, depending on their morphology and function. The most notable feature of these cells is the outer segment, which consists of a series of stacked membranous discs, from which the cells derive their names. Rhodopsin, which absorbs light energy and initiates the transduction cascade, is located in the discs of the rod cells (Fig. 3). Rod cells are found at greater density in the near periphery of the retina, and contain rhodopsin. Rods are able to detect light under dim illumination, are therefore important in night vision. The central retina, known as the macula, is densely populated with cone cells that mediate vision under strong (e.g. daylight)

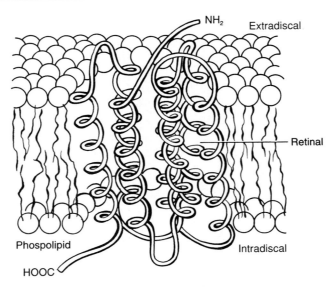

Fig. 3. The structure of human rhodopsin and its putative position in the membrane. A lysine in the seventh transmembrane (7-TM) domain is the site of the chromophore attachment (retinal).

illumination. Each cone contains one of three different opsins that vary in their peak wavelength absorption. Color vision relies on the comparison of the different degrees of stimulation of the three cone types by a colored stimulus. Another unique feature of the central portion of the macula—the fovea—that improves central vision is the absence of retinal elements other than photoreceptors. Axons from more peripheral retinal areas arc around the macula to minimize absorption and scattering of light in this critical part of the retina.

The photoreceptor cells, whose cell bodies make up the *outer nuclear layer*, synapse in the *outer plexiform layer* of the retina with horizontal cells and bipolar cells. The bipolar cells synapse in the inner plexiform layer with amacrine and ganglion cells. The cell bodies of the amacrine, bipolar, horizontal, and interplexiform cells comprise the inner nuclear layer, and the cell bodies of the ganglion cells constitute the ganglion-cell layer. The ganglion-cell axons traverse the nerve fiber layer of the retina and collect in the optic nerve, which leads to the brain. What is known of the specific nature of these neural interactions is considered in the following sections.

4. PHOTOTRANSDUCTION

4.1. Continuously Graded Signals are Generated in the Photoreceptors by Activation of Opsin–Chromophore Complexes

In the neural retina, the information contained in light absorbed by the photoreceptors is converted by

them into neural signals in a process called phototransduction. Phototransduction is a model for understanding more general signal-transduction processes. For example, opsins show homology to a family of hormone receptors, including adrenergic receptors that activate adenylyl cyclase through G-protein-coupled receptors (GPCRs). Figure 3 depicts the structure of the rhodopsin molecule in the disc membrane. Figure 4 shows a representation of the overall process of phototransduction. A photon of light is absorbed by the opsin–chromophore complex (e.g., rhodopsin in rods, cone opsins in cones) in the outer segment of the cone cell or rod cell, changing the chromophore retinal from the 11-*cis* to the all-trans conformation. This conformational change results in the activation of transducin (e.g., photoreceptor-specific G protein) by the exchange of a bound GDP for GTP. The activated transducin stimulates a cGMP phosphodiesterase (PDE), which then cleaves cyclic guanosine monophosphate (cGMP). Reduction of cGMP levels closes the cGMP-gated ion channels, causing intracellular hyperpolarization. This in turn results in closure of calcium channels and a subsequent decrease in glutamate release in the synaptic terminal of the photoreceptor (e.g., signal generation).

Rod cells have a low threshold of excitation, and react readily to the low intensities of light required for vision at twilight and at nighttime. The cones require a much higher intensity of stimulatory light, and are important for fine vision and color discrimination. This is especially true in the posterior pole, where the high

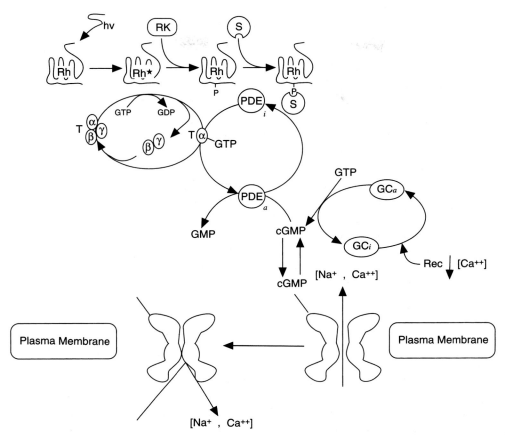

Fig. 4. Phototransduction. The light activation of rhodopsin (Rh → Rh*) activates transducin (T), the photoreceptor-specific G protein, by the exchange of GTP for GDP. The Tα subunit activates the cGMP phosphodiesterase (PDE), cleaving cGMP and closing the ion channels, resulting in hyperpolarization and subsequent propagation of the electrical impulse. Two pathways involved in modulating the photoresponse are also shown. The first involves phosphorylation of rhodopsin by rhodopsin kinase (RK), with subsequent binding by S-antigen, also known as arrestin or the 48-kDa protein (S). The second pathway involves the regeneration of cGMP through stimulation of guanylate cyclase by recoverin (rec) under a reduced calcium level. Recoverin is also known as the 26-kDa protein.

concentration of cones in the macula and fovea centralis are responsible for central vision. Because the eye must provide sensitivity over a range of light intensities and wavelengths, the basic transduction process is modulated by several mechanisms. For example, it is known that phosphorylation of rhodopsin by rhodopsin kinase after light stimulation is required for effective quenching of the signal through the interaction of phospho-rhodopsin and arrestin (also known as S antigen). The phosphorylation or dephosphorylation of a PDE subunit is also important in modulating the light-induced response. Other mechanisms involved directly or indirectly in the *transduction cascade* include modulation by Ca^{2+} levels, which are implicated in dark and light adaptation, regulation of cGMP concentration, and the dissociation and reassociation of the opsin protein moiety with its chromophore after

light activation. Phosphorylation and dephosphorylation of several different components of the cascade probably also play a regulatory role.

Other biochemical cascades appear to be initiated by photoactivation of rhodopsin. For example, activation of retinal phospholipase C, which cleaves phosphatidylinositol bisphosphate to diacylglycerol and inositol triphosphate and phospholipase A2, which releases arachidonic acid, have been shown to be light-dependent. The role of these pathways and probably others in the normal physiology of the retina is unclear. It is likely that they are involved in some type of second-order modulation of the photo response or possibly they are involved in housekeeping-type functions, such as signaling the turnover (e.g. shedding) of discs. The identification of molecules involved in these processes is important for understanding the molecular basis of vision and for identifying the possible causes of retinal lesions.

4.2. Neural Transmission and Processing in the Retina

Photoreceptor cells transduce visual stimuli to other cells of the neural retina as continuously graded changes in membrane potential. The efferent retinal neurons (ganglion cells) send this information through the optic pathways as a series of all-or-none signals (e.g., action potentials) with enhanced color, motion, and contrast detection. The interaction of the neural cells of the retina was described previously and is shown in Fig. 2. The importance of retinal processing is seen in the response of an individual ganglion cell within its receptive field. The *receptive field* of a cell is the part of the retina in which stimulation of photoreceptors with light causes activation of that cell, as demonstrated by an increase (for "ON" ganglion cells) or decrease (for "OFF" ganglion cells) in its firing rate. For ganglion cells, the receptive field is a roughly circular area of retina that corresponds to less than 1° of visual field at the fovea, which is the retinal area with tightly packed cones providing the finest visual discrimination, to 3°–5° at the retinal periphery. For "ON" ganglion cells, light that strikes the center of the receptive field is stimulatory, and light striking the periphery, known as the surround, is inhibitory. Conversely, for "OFF" ganglion cells light that strikes the center is inhibitory. Both types of ganglion cells are maximally stimulated by large contrasts in the intensity of light striking the center and periphery of their receptive fields, rather than an evenly spread illumination. It is a general principle that the visual system responds primarily to changes in the time, location, or intensity of visual input.

The importance of the concept of a receptive field is seen when retinal circuitry is examined in more detail. The photoreceptor cells send their input to the bipolar and horizontal cells. The horizontal cells appear to function as inhibitory neurons, using gamma-aminobutyric acid (GABA) as a neurotransmitter to perform negative-feedback control in the distal retina. They receive input from photoreceptors in the surround of a receptive field and pass an inhibitory signal on to the photoreceptors (negative feedback) and bipolar cells. This enhances contrast, emphasizing sharp edges and compensating for the blurring of the image caused by scattering of light by the various optical media of the eye.

Some bipolar cells are stimulatory (e.g., on), using glutamate to synapse to ganglion cells with their dendrites in the inner portions of the inner plexiform layer. Some are inhibitory (e.g., off), synapsing to ganglion cells with dendrites in the outer portion of the inner plexiform layer. The ganglion cells convert the graded light signal they have received from the bipolar cells into all-or-none signals (action potentials), typical of information-handling in the brain. They amplify visual signals and have on-center or off-center receptive fields. Some ganglion cells receive input from both types of bipolar cells, as do some amacrine cells. Although the interactions of amacrine cells are limited to the inner plexiform layer, they synapse with all the cell types found there.

Reflecting the various interactions, there appear to be different subsets of amacrine cells: inhibitory cells that use glycine as a neurotransmitter and excitatory cells that use acetylcholine. Some of these appear to be involved in light adaptation of visual sensitivity independently of mechanisms present in the photoreceptors. Amacrine cells also modulate the time-course of a visual response. Some amacrine cells, like ganglion cells, generate action potentials, unlike photoreceptors, bipolar cells, and horizontal cells, which generate sustained and graded voltage potentials. The ganglion-cell layer consists of ganglion-cell bodies and a few amacrine cells. The ganglion cells send the final relay, turning the input they receive from bipolar and amacrine cells into action potentials that are then sent to the brain for further processing. It is impressive that more than half of all ganglion cells receive input solely from the foveal and parafoveal area, which makes up only about 5% of the retinal surface. There is an extreme bias toward central (e.g., fine) vision rather than peripheral (coarser) visual perception.

The number of bipolar cells is much smaller than the number of photoreceptor cells, and there is an even further reduction in the relative number of ganglion cells. In humans, there may be as many as 140 million rods and cones, but only 1 million ganglion cells. Each photoreceptor cell contacts a number of different neurons, and each neuron has several different synapses. The integrative abilities of the retinal neurons are probably indispensable for sorting out the signals.

Contrary to what might be expected, photoreceptor cells are actually depolarized in the dark and hyperpolarized in the light. In the on or dark state, glutamate is released by the photoreceptors at bipolar and horizon-

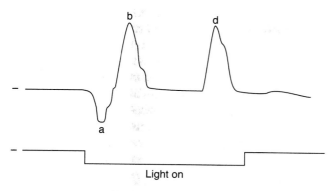

Fig. 5. Idealized electroretinogram (ERG) tracing. The a-wave indicates photoreceptor activity, the b-wave indicates activity in the inner nuclear layer, especially bipolar and Muller cells, and the d-wave indicates the off response of the inner nuclear layer.

tal-cell synapses. The horizontal cells are also on in the dark as a result. The on bipolar cells are inhibited by the photoreceptor cells' release of glutamate and are excited in the light, and the off bipolar cells are excited by glutamate and therefore are excited in the dark.

The electrical activity of the various retinal neurons can be measured by a noninvasive procedure known as and electroretinogram (ERG). The ERG is similar to the electrocardiogram (ECG) and electroencephalogram (EEG) in that it assesses the activity of large numbers of cells by measuring the changing potential difference between a corneal and reference electrode. Figure 5 depicts a highly idealized ERG tracing. The a-wave indicates photoreceptor activity, the b-wave indicates activity in the inner nuclear layer (especially bipolar and Müller cells), and the d-wave indicates the off response of the inner nuclear layer. Because different components of the ERG can be attributed to different cell types in the retina, it is clinically useful to identify possible retinal dysfunction and to narrow the diagnostic focus to specific cell types when looking for the source of visual difficulties.

5. THE OPTIC PATHWAYS

Axons of the ganglion cells collect in fine bundles that converge in a radiating pattern at the optic disc to form the optic nerve, connecting the eye to the brain. Because the optic disc contains no photoreceptors, it is insensitive to light, causing a small blind spot that is noticeable only on monocular vision. On, off, color, and movement-related signals are passed to the brain through a set of closely approximated parallel chan-

nels. The spatial relations of the visual field are maintained in the fibers that make up the optic nerves and optic radiations to the visual cortex. After passing through the optic foramina, the right and left optic nerves converge at the optic chiasm. At this point, nerve fibers originating in the nasal halves of the retina cross to the opposite side, and those from the temporal retinal halves continue uncrossed. As a result of this pattern, the entire right visual field (received by the left temporal and right nasal halves of the retinas) projects to the left hemisphere, and the left visual field (received by the right temporal and left nasal halves of the retinas) projects to the right hemisphere (Fig. 6). Beyond the optic chiasm, the optic fibers continue on to the thalamus as the optic tract.

Some fibers continue to the superior colliculus and the pretectal area of the midbrain, which actuate reflex responses of the eyes and body to visual stimuli and the pupillary light reflex, respectively. However, most of the optic tract fibers synapse on neurons in the lateral geniculate nucleus (LGN), consistent with its role as the most important subcortical region for further visual processing. The spatial relations of the retina and visual field continue to be maintained in the lateral geniculate body, creating a retinotopic map of the visual field. Inputs from the two eyes (that is, the nasal retina of the contralateral eye and the temporal retina of the ipsilateral eye) remain anatomically segregated in the LGN, with separate layers of LGN neurons receiving the inputs from each eye. The retinotopic maps of the binocular field from each eye are in register, with a small monocular segment representing the far periphery of the visual field of the contralateral eye that is also present (Fig. 7). Different classes of ganglion cells in each retina project fibers to three distinct cell layers in the LGN, giving a total of six layers in all.

Axons of the upper quadrants (receiving the lower visual fields) project to the medial laminae, and these cells project as the geniculostriate pathway or optic radiation to the cerebral cortex in the superior edge of the calcarine sulcus. Axons of the lower quadrants (receiving the upper visual fields) project to the lateral half of the lateral geniculate body, and these cells then project to the inferior lip of the calcarine sulcus. The cortical area that receives LGN input is known as the primary visual cortex (V1), striate cortex, or Brodmann's area 17.

The main target of LGN neurons is a band of cells in the middle of the cortex, known as layer IV. The input from the different LGN layers that subserve the

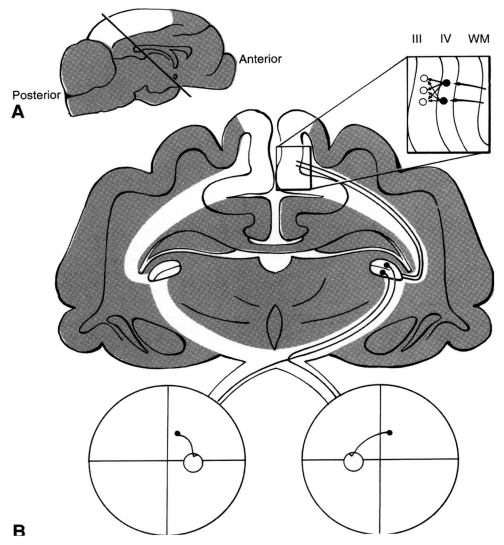

Fig. 6. Organization of the mammalian retinogeniculocortical projection. (**A**) Midsagittal view of a cat brain showing the location of the primary visual cortex (e.g., striate cortex or area 17). The line indicates a plane of section, illustrated in B, that reveals all the components of the ascending visual pathway. (**B**) The temporal retina of the left eye and the nasal retina of the right eye project axons through the optic nerve and optic tract to the LGN of the left dorsal thalamus. Inputs from the two eyes remain segregated in separate laminae at the level of this synaptic relay. The lateral geniculate cells project on to striate cortex through the optic radiations. These axons terminate mainly in layer IV, where inputs subserving the two eyes continue to be segregated. *(Inset)* The first site of major convergence of inputs from the two eyes is in the projection of layer IV cells onto cells in layer III. WM, white matter. (Modified from Baer MF, Cooper LN. Molecular mechanisms of synaptic modification in the visual cortex: interaction of theory and experiment. In Gluck M, Rumelhart D (eds.). Neuroscience and connectionist theory. Hillsdale, NJ: Lawrence Erlbaum Associates, 1990; 65.)

two eyes are not intermingled in layer IV. This was elegantly shown by Hubel and Weisel by transmission of radioactive proline injected into one eye to eye-specific dominance columns in layer IV of the striate cortex (Fig. 8). The proline was transmitted down the optic nerve into the LGN, where it spilled over through synaptic junctions to LGN neurons and was further transmitted down these neurons to layer IV. The

roughly 1 million ganglion cells in each eye feed information to a similar number of lateral geniculate neurons with little transformation in the receptive fields by this synaptic relay. Similarly, the layer IV neurons that receive synaptic input from the LGN are characterized by small, circular, monocular receptive fields. Cells of this layer feed information to cells in the more superficial cortical layers, especially layer III, in which

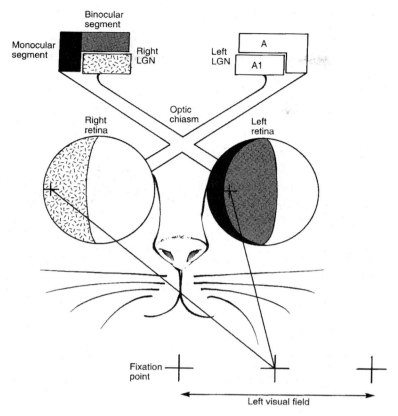

Fig. 7. The general organization of the lateral geniculate nucleus (LGN). Each eye projects to a separate cell layer in the lateral geniculate. In the cat, the principal layers are called A and A1. Layer A receives input from the nasal half of the contralateral retina, and layer A1 receives input from the temporal half of the ipsilateral retina. The retinotopic maps in the two layers of the lateral geniculate occur in perfect register, except for a lateral region of layer A called the monocular segment. Cells in the monocular segment are activated by visual stimuli in the far periphery that fall outside the binocular visual field and are viewed only by the contralateral eye.

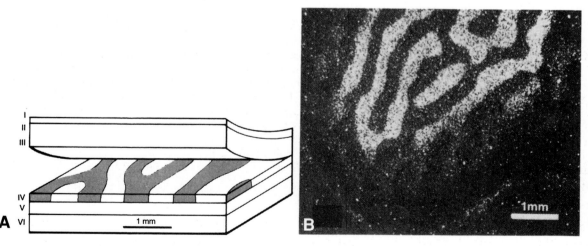

Fig. 8. **(A)** The organization of ocular-dominance columns in layer IV of the striate cortex of macaque monkeys. The distribution of geniculate afferents that subserve one eye is darkly shaded. In cross-section these eye-specific zones appear as columns of approx 0.5 mm width in layer IV. When the superficial layers are peeled back, allowing a view of the ocular-dominance columns in layer IV from above, these zones take on the appearance of zebra stripes. **(B)** Dark-field autoradiograph of a histologic section of layer IV viewed from above. Two weeks before sacrifice, this monkey received an injection of ^{3}H-proline into one eye. In the autoradiograph, the radioactive lateral geniculate terminals appear bright on a dark background. (From Wiesel TN. Postnatal development of the visual cortex and the influence of the environment. Nature 1982; 299:583.)

axons from different ocular-dominance columns project onto the same cells. Thus, most neurons in layer III are responsive to stimulation of both eyes, and the receptive fields mapped through the two eyes are matched to the same position in space. This convergence initiates the process of binocular vision, in which information from the two eyes is combined to form a single perception of visual space. Neurons from layer III then project to other cortical areas. The first significant elaboration of receptive fields occurs at the projection from layer IV to layer III. Layer III neurons have elongated receptive fields and are especially responsive to elongated, high-contrast bars or edges with the same orientation as the long axis of the receptive field, known as orientation selectivity. Thus, most cortical neurons respond poorly or not at all to changes in diffuse illumination of the retina. As a result of both excitatory and inhibitory intracortical connections, cortical neurons respond best to contrast borders.

From the striate cortex, there are additional projections to a surprisingly large number of other (extrastriate) visual areas of the cortex. For example, it is known that areas V_1 and V_2 integrate most of the visual information regarding color, movement, and form, and that other areas play some role in fine-tuning that information. The geniculo-cortical pathway is the most important for the conscious experience of vision in mammals. People with lesions of the striate cortex claim to be completely or almost completely blind. However, they are also partially able to identify or locate some objects, indicating that the retinotectal pathway is able to supply some type of vision, albeit subconsciously. These pathways are not independent of each other, because there is also a corticotectal path, that provides input from the cortex to the superior colliculi. In addition to these two pathways, there are several minor pathways that are not well-understood. These project to the ventral lateral geniculate (or pregeniculate) nuclei, tegmentum, and hypothalamus. This hypothalamic projection is probably involved in the synchronization of the circadian rhythm with the day/night cycle.

The cortex also receives input from the same cortical areas to which it projects, including the cortex of the opposite hemisphere through the corpus callosum. There are brainstem inputs originating in the locus ceruleus that use epinephrine as a neurotransmitter and the Raphe nuclei using serotonin as a neurotransmitter. Unlike LGN inputs, the axons from the brainstem project to a variety of cortical layers, and their fibers ramify widely. A similar organization is seen in the projection from the nucleus basalis of Meynert in the

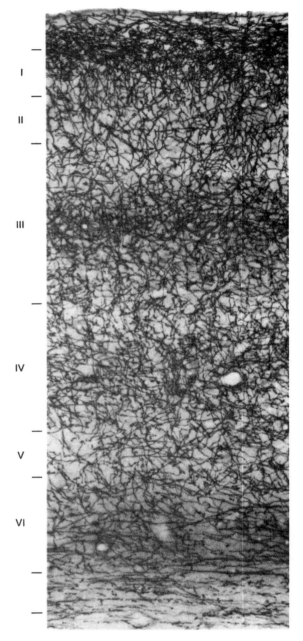

Fig. 9. Distribution of fibers that use the neurotransmitter acetylcholine in the cat striate cortex. Unlike the projection from the thalamus, this projection from the basal forebrain innervates all cortical layers. These cortical inputs modulate the activity patterns that arise from retinal stimulation and are believed to influence experience-dependent aspects of cortical development. (From Bear MF, Carnes KM, Ebner FF. And investigation of cholinergic circuitry in cat striate cortex using acetylcholinesterase histochemistry. J Comp Neurol 1985; 234:411.)

forebrain, which uses acetylcholine as a neurotransmitter (Fig. 9). Based on their anatomy and the effects of applying their neurotransmitters to cortical neurons, these inputs appear to function in modulating visual processing according to behavioral state.

6. CRITICAL PERIODS IN VISUAL SYSTEM DEVELOPMENT

A critical period of development may be defined as a period of time in which intercellular communication alters a cell's fate. The concept is usually credited to the experimental embryologist Hans Spemann, who—working around the turn of the twentieth century—showed that transplantation of a piece of early embryo from one location to another would often cause the "donor" tissue to take on the characteristics of the 'host,' but only if transplantation had taken place during a well-defined period. After the transplanted tissue had been induced to change its developmental fate, the outcome could not be reversed. The intercellular communication that altered the phenotype of the transplanted cells was shown to be mediated by contact and by chemical signals.

The term took on new significance with respect to brain development as a result of the work of Konrad Lorenz in the mid-1930s. Lorenz was interested in the process by which graylag goslings come to be socially attached to their mother. He discovered that, in the absence of the mother, the social attachment could occur instead to a wide variety of moving objects, including Lorenz himself. Once imprinted on a object, the goslings followed it and behaved toward it as they normally would their mother. The term "imprinting" was used by Lorenz to suggest that this first visual image was somehow permanently etched in the young bird's nervous system. Imprinting was also found to be limited to a finite time (e.g., the first two days after hatching), which Lorenz called the critical period for social attachment. Lorenz himself drew the analogy between this process of imprinting the external environment on the nervous system and the induction of tissue to change its developmental fate during critical periods of embryonic development.

This work had a tremendous impact in the field of developmental psychology. The terms "imprinting" and critical period conjure images (and generated heated debate) that changes in "behavioral phenotype" caused by early sensory experience were permanent and irreversible later in life, much like the determination of tissue phenotype during embryogenesis. Numerous studies extended the critical period concept to aspects of mammalian psychosocial development. The implication was that the fate of neurons and neural circuits in the brain depended on the experience of the animal during early postnatal life. It is not difficult to appreciate why research in this area took on political as well a scientific significance.

By necessity, the effects of experience on neuronal fate must be exercised by neural activity generated at sensory receptors and communicated by chemical synaptic transmission. The idea that synaptic activity can alter the fate of neuronal connectivity during central nervous system (CNS) development eventually received solid neurobiologic support from the study of mammalian-visual-system development, beginning with the experiments of Hubel and Wiesel that partly earned them the 1981 Nobel Prize in medicine. They found, using anatomic and neurophysiologic methods, that visual experience or lack thereof was an important determinant of the state of connectivity in the central visual pathways, and that this environmental influence was restricted to a finite period of early postnatal life. Because much work has been devoted to the analysis of experience-dependent plasticity of connections in this system, this is an excellent model system to illustrate the principles of critical periods in nervous-system development. Although the effects of synaptic transmission in the development of other systems (e.g., neuromuscular connections) and the effects of other types of intercellular communication (e.g., long-range hormonal signals) are not covered in detail here, the general principles of other critical periods are believed to be quite similar to those illustrated by visual-system development.

7. ADULT ORGANIZATION OF THE VISUAL PATHWAY FROM RETINA TO CORTEX

7.1. The Anatomical and Physiological Organization of the Visual Pathway Is Precise

The detailed structure and function of the visual system is covered earlier in this chapter. Certain aspects are reviewed and emphasized here to provide a perspective on what must be accomplished during development to ensure proper wiring and function of this sensory system. The central visual pathway begins with the projection of ganglion-cell axons from the retina into the optic nerve. In general, the ganglion cells that "view" the right visual hemifield project to the left hemisphere of the brain. Conversely, the ganglion cells that are responsive to visual stimuli in the left visual hemifield project to the right hemisphere. Because human eyes are situated frontally in the head, a significant fraction of each visual hemifield is viewed by both retinas. This region of space is the *binocular visual field*. Each retina must project to both hemispheres; ganglion cells in the nasal retina (e.g., the half closer to the nose) project across the midline to the contralateral hemisphere, and ganglion cells in the temporal retina project axons into the hemisphere of the ipsilateral side.

8. ACTIVITY-INDEPENDENT DEVELOPMENT OF ORDER IN THE VISUAL SYSTEM

The preceding discussion indicates that there is considerable precision in the connections of the mature visual pathway. There are several examples:

1. Only ganglion-cell axons from nasal retinas cross at the chiasm.
2. The mixed population of axons in the optic tract is sorted out at the lateral geniculate nucleus by eye and by retinotopic position.
3. The LGN axons project to a specific layer of cells in the cortex, and within this layer, they segregate again according to retinotopic position and by eye.
4. Layer IV cells make connections with cells in other layers that are appropriate for binocular vision and are specialized to enable detection of contrast borders.

Before addressing the question of the extent to which the establishment of these highly specific connections depends on activity during critical periods of development, it is important to recognize that activity often precedes experience during CNS development. Action potentials and chemical synaptic transmission occur in the visual pathway *in utero*, even before the development of the photoreceptors. Thus, the occurrence of a developmental process before visual input does not imply that it is independent of activity. One way to evaluate the dependence on activity is through the drug tetrodotoxin (TTX), which binds tightly to voltage-sensitive sodium channels and blocks action potentials. Thus, developmental processes that are insensitive to TTX are considered to occur independently of intercellular communication, and those that are sensitive are dependent on synaptic activity.

Development of long-range connections in the CNS can be categorized into three phases: pathway selection, target selection, and address selection. Examples of pathway selection include the decisions made by growing axons that originate in the nasal retina to cross the midline at the optic chiasm, and the decisions

made by LGN axons to project to the cortex through the optic radiation rather than to the spinal cord via the cerebral peduncle. Examples of target selection include the decision made by optic-tract axons to form connections with the LGN and not another part of the thalamus, and the decision made by LGN axons to innervate cortical layer IV instead of layer V. Examples of address selection are the sorting of inputs by retinotopic location in the LGN and cortex, the segregation of axons that subserve the two eyes in the LGN and layer IV of the cortex, and the convergence of retinotopically matched inputs from the two eyes onto layer III neurons.

Experimental evidence has now shown that pathway and target selection occur entirely in the absence of neural activity. Many aspects of address selection, such as the establishment of crude retinotopy, are also activity-independent. This does not indicate that these aspects of development occur independently of intercellular communication, because virtually all phases of visual-pathway development critically depend on communication by cell-cell contact and by gradients of diffusible chemicals. The process by which specific connections are established by differential chemical attraction or repulsion is termed "chemoaffinity."

The axons from the retina grow along the substrate provided by the extracellular matrix (ECM) of the ventral wall of the optic stalk. One glycoprotein in this matrix is laminin. The growing tips of the axons, called growth cones, express surface molecules called integrins that bind laminin, and this interaction promotes axonal elongation (Fig. 10). The ECM along the optic stalk forms a molecular highway on which retinal axons grow. The journey down this highway is aided by another mechanism that causes axons that are growing together to stick together, a process known as fasciculation. This stickiness is caused by the expression of specific cell-adhesion molecules on the surface of axonal membranes.

The ECM can be repulsive as well as attractive to growing axons, depending on the cell-surface receptors the axons express. Axons from the temporal retina grow toward the midline at the chiasm, but they encounter a signal there that causes them to veer sharply away. In contrast, nasal axons continue right across the midline and into the contralateral optic tract. These differences must be explained by differential expression of cell-surface molecules based on cell position in the retina. Such a nasal-temporal gradient in axon-surface markers is believed to be matched to

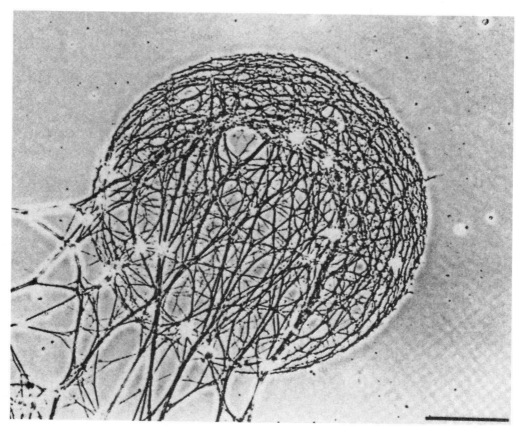

Fig. 10. Neurites that grow in a collagen-coated culture dish enter a region containing the extracellular matrix (ECM) protein laminin. On this preferred substrate, the neurites branch profusely but stay within the border of the circular laminin dot. The interplay of ECM and specific axon-surface molecules is believed to be crucial for pathway and target selection during visual-system development. (From Gunderson RW. Response of sensory neurites and growth cones to patterned substrata and fibronectin in vitro. Dev Biol 1987; 121:423.)

complementary gradients on the surfaces of cells in target structures, and this match gives rise to retinotopy.

When axons reach their target, they often encounter a new extracellular environment that retards further growth. These environmental signals can be the absence of specific glycoproteins in the ECM, such as the absence of laminin. Axonal growth also can be inhibited by diffusible signals released from target structures. In some systems, application of neurotransmitters can inhibit axonal growth, probably by raising calcium concentrations in the growth cone. There is evidence that diffusible factors can promote axon growth, and guide that growth to distant targets in a process known as chemotropism. The number and nature of the chemical signals that guide activity-independent pathway formation are currently being investigated.

Considerable order can develop in the visual system solely under the influence of these molecular mechanisms. The role of activity appears to be reserved for the final refinement of the patterns of connectivity, according to functional criteria.

9. ACTIVITY-DEPENDENT DEVELOPMENT OF ORDER IN THE VISUAL SYSTEM

Much of the organization of the visual pathway is specified without any contribution from neural activity and synaptic transmission. The retinal and lateral geniculate axons navigate down the appropriate paths and terminate in retinotopic order in the appropriate target structure. The main features of visual-system organization that depend on retinal activity are the segregation of axons in the LGN and cortex according to the eye that drives activity in them and the establish-

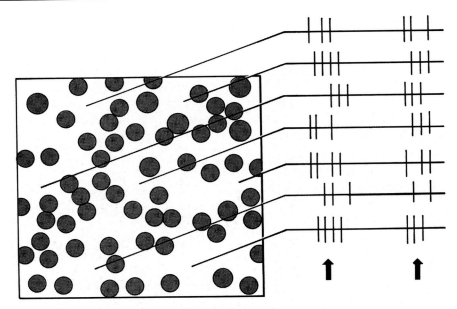

Fig. 11. Illustration of an experiment in which action-potential recordings were made from a whole-mount specimen of the fetal retina in vitro. Circles represent ganglion-cell outlines. Action potentials occur in spontaneous bursts (*arrows*) that are almost synchronous in widely separated regions of the retina. These local correlations in activity are believed to play a critical role in the sorting of retinal axons in the LGN. (Modified from Shatz CJ. The developing brain. Sci Am 1992; 267:61.)

ment and maintenance of connections in the visual cortex that generate binocular and stimulus-selective receptive fields. The eye-specific segregation in the LGN occurs entirely before birth, but many refinements of cortical circuitry occur postnatally, and are under the influence of the visual environment during infancy.

9.1. Segregation of Axons in the Lateral Geniculate Nucleus Is Influenced by Activity

The first axons to reach the LGN are usually those from the contralateral retina, and they disperse to occupy the entire nucleus. Somewhat later, the ipsilateral projection arrives and intermingles with the axons of the contralateral eye. Over the next several weeks, the axons from the two eyes segregate into the eye-specific domains that are characteristic of the adult nucleus. Intra-ocular injection of tetrodotoxin prevents this process of segregation, showing that it depends on activity generated in the retina. This raises the question of what the source of the activity is, and how it orchestrates segregation.

Because segregation occurs in utero, before the development of photoreceptors, it cannot be driven by photic stimulation. It appears that ganglion cells are spontaneously active during this period of fetal development. This activity is not random. Ganglion cells fire in quasisynchronous waves that spread across the retina (Fig. 11). The origin of the wave and its direction of propagation may be random, but during each wave the activity in a ganglion cell is highly correlated with the activity in its nearest neighbors. Because these waves are generated independently in the two retinas, the activity patterns arising in the two eyes are not correlated with one another.

Segregation is believed to depend on a process of synaptic stabilization in which only retinal terminals that are active at the same time as their postsynaptic LGN target neuron are retained, a model first proposed by Donald Hebb in the 1940s. Thus, the mnemonic: "neurons that fire together wire together," attributed to Sigrid Lowel and Wolf Singer. Connections that are modified according to this rule are said to employ *Hebb synapses*. According to the hypothesis, when a wave of retinal activity drives a postsynaptic LGN neuron, the active retinal inputs onto this neuron are consolidated. Because the activity from the two eyes does not occur in register, the inputs compete on a winner-takes-all basis until one input is retained and the other is eliminated, leading to complete segregation of the two inputs.

9.2. Segregation of Axons in Layer IV Is Influenced by Activity

Similar to the situation in the LGN, the afferents subserving the two eyes are initially intermingled in

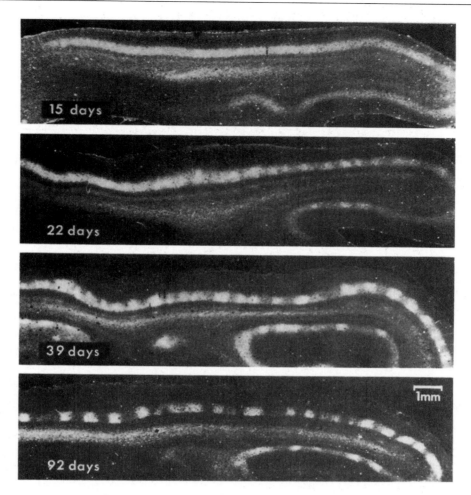

Fig. 12. Dark-field autoradiographs of the cat visual cortex cut in horizontal sections. In each case, one eye had been injected with ^{3}H-proline, and the animals were later sacrificed at the ages shown. At 15 d of age, the radioactivity is uniform in layer IV. Ocular-dominance columns segregate progressively over the next several weeks. (From LeVay S, Stryker MP. The development of ocular dominance in the cat. Soc Neurosci Symp 1979; 483.)

cortical layer IV and then segregate under the influence of activity (Fig. 12). To the extent that segregation occurs postnatally, the formation of ocular dominance columns can be affected by deprivation of normal-pattern vision. This is most dramatically demonstrated by *monocular deprivation*, in which the amount of light reaching the affected retina is only slightly decreased, but image formation is greatly impaired (e.g., experimentally by suturing the eyelid closed, or clinically by a unilateral congenital cataract). In experimental animals that have their eyes sutured shortly after birth and whose eyes remain sutured throughout the period of natural segregation, columns representing the open eye develop to be much wider than columns representing the closed eye (Fig. 13). If deprivation is begun later, after the period of natural segregation, anatomic effects on LGN axon

arbors are not observed in layer IV. Thus, a *critical period* exists for this type of plasticity.

Within this critical period, closing the previously open eye and opening the previously closed eye can reverse the anatomic effects of monocular deprivation. The shrunken ocular-dominance columns of the formerly closed eye expand and the expanded columns of the formerly open eye shrink. This suggests that within the critical period, even after ocular-dominance column segregation appears to be anatomically complete, the afferents subserving the two eyes exist in a dynamic equilibrium that can still be disrupted by deprivation. At the end of the critical period, the afferents apparently lose their capacity for growth and retraction.

One correlate of the change in cortical ocular-dominance columns during the critical period is a change in

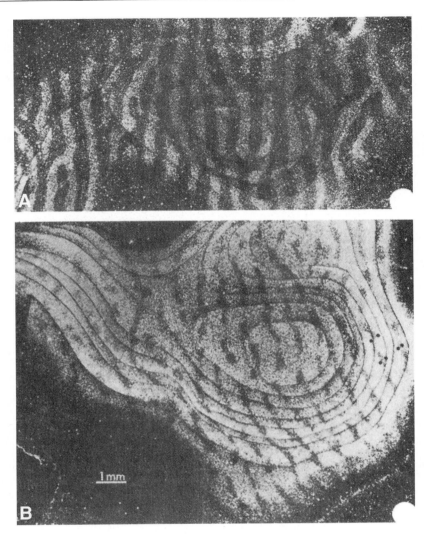

Fig. 13. Dark-field autoradiographs of tangential sections through layer IV of monkey striate cortex after injection of one eye with 3H-proline. **(A)** Normal monkey. **(B)** Monkey that had been monocularly deprived for 18 mo starting at 2 wk of age. The nondeprived eye had been injected, revealing expanded ocular-dominance columns in layer IV. (From Wiesel TN. Postnatal development of the visual cortex and the influence of the environment. Nature 1982; 299:583.)

the size of the neurons in the LGN that relay information to the visual cortex. LGN cells deprived of normal visual input are visibly shrunken. This change in soma size is believed to reflect the decreased axonal arbors of these cells in layer IV. Curiously, shrinkage is observed only in the segment of the LGN where both retinas are represented. Cells in the monocular segment are largely unaffected by deprivation. In addition, destruction of part of the central retina in the non-deprived eye results in a region of the LGN that is relatively free of the effects of binocular competition, showing much less shrinkage of LGN neurons (Fig. 14). These observations suggest that the loss of territory in layer IV by afferents deprived of normal

visual input is not caused by simple disuse, but rather by a more active process of binocular competition that requires pattern vision in the open eye. Evidently, the activity in the open eye actively promotes the synaptic disconnection of afferents that subserve the closed eye.

9.3. The Establishment and Maintenance of Binocular Connections Is Influenced by Visual Experience

The last connections to be specified during the development of the retinal-geniculate-striate pathway are those that subserve binocular vision. These are formed and modified under the influence of sensory experience during early postnatal life. Unlike the seg-

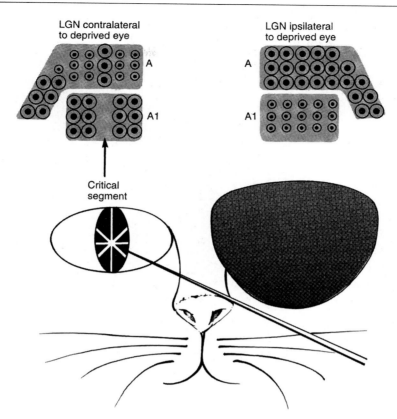

Fig. 14. Illustration of the critical segment in the experiment by RW Guillery, who found that cells in the monocular segment of the lateral geniculate layer A did not shrink like those in the binocular segment after monocular deprivation of the contralateral eye. To test the hypothesis that the shrinkage resulted from some competitive interaction of inputs arising from homotypic points in the two retinas, Guillery produced a lesion in the central region of the nondeprived retina. This removed the competition from the open eye in a critical segment of the lateral geniculate, and in this region, the cells in layer A did not shrink after monocular deprivation. Lateral-geniculate-cell size is believed to accurately reflect the extent of the axon arbor in cortical layer IV. These results supported the concept of binocular competition in the regulation of ocular-dominance columns in the visual cortex. (From Guillery RW. Binocular competition in the control of geniculate cell growth. Comp Neurol 1972; 144:117.)

regation of eye-specific domains, which evidently depends on asynchronous patterns of activity spontaneously generated by the two retinas, the establishment of binocular receptive fields depends instead on correlated patterns of activity that arise from the two eyes as a consequence of vision. For example, bringing the patterns of activity from the two eyes out of register by monocular deprivation that replaces pattern vision in one eye with "white noise" profoundly disrupts the binocular connections in the striate cortex. Neurons outside of layer IV, which normally have binocular receptive fields, respond only to stimulation of the non-deprived eye after even a brief period of monocular deprivation. This change in the binocular organization of the cortex is known as an *ocular dominance shift* (Fig. 15).

These effects of monocular deprivation are not merely a passive reflection of the anatomic changes in layer IV. An ocular-dominance shift occurs in response to monocular deprivation initiated well beyond the period of susceptibility of LGN-axon arborization. However, this form of plasticity is also limited to a critical period of postnatal life. Although ocular-dominance plasticity in the cat peaks at 1 mo of age and declines to very low levels by 3–4 mo of age (Fig. 16), it is estimated that in human children this plasticity extends to about 10 yr of age. These critical periods coincide with the times of greatest growth of the head and optical axes. Plasticity of binocular connections is probably required to maintain good binocular vision throughout this period of rapid growth. The hazard associated with this activity-dependent fine-tuning is that these connections are also highly susceptible to deprivation.

Strabismus, or misalignment of the two eyes, also disrupts cortical binocularity. Visually evoked patterns

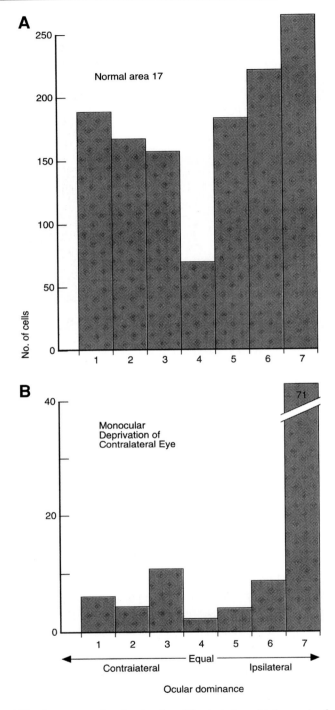

Fig. 15. The ocular-dominance shift after monocular deprivation. Illustrated are histograms of ocular-dominance data obtained from the striate cortex of (**A**) normal monkeys and (**B**) a monkey that had been monocularly deprived early in life. The bars show the number of neurons outside of layer IVc in each of the seven ocular-dominance categories. Cells in groups 1 and 7 are activated by stimulation of the left or right eye, respectively, but not both. Cells in group 4 are activated equally well by either eye. Cells in groups 2 and 3 and in groups 5 and 6 are binocularly activated, but they show a preference for the left or right eye, respectively. The histogram in A reveals that most neurons in the visual cortex of a normal animal are driven binocularly. The histogram in B shows that a period of monocular deprivation leaves few neurons responsive to the deprived eye. (Modified from Wiesel TN. Postnatal development of the visual cortex and the influence of the environment. Nature 1982; 299:583.)

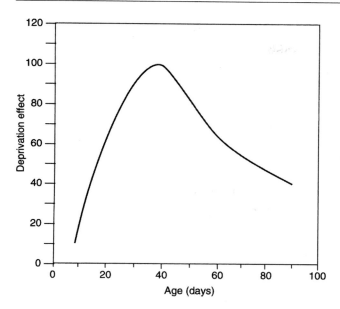

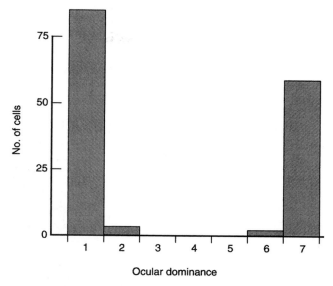

Fig. 16. Sensitivity of binocular connections in cat striate cortex to monocular deprivation at different postnatal ages. The deprivation effect is the percentage of neurons in area 17, whose responses are dominated by stimulation of the nondeprived eye. This critical period begins at about 3 wk of age and declines to low levels after 3 mo of age. (Modified from Dudek SM, Bear MF. A biochemical correlate of the critical period for synaptic modification in kitten visual cortex. Science 1989; 246:673.)

Fig. 17. Ocular-dominance histogram of cells recorded in the striate cortex of a 3-yr-old strabismic monkey, in which the lateral rectus muscle of the right eye was sectioned at 3 wk of age. Binocular cells are almost completely absent; the cells are driven exclusively by the right or the left eye. (Modified from Wiesel TN. Postnatal development of the visual cortex and the influence of the environment. Nature 1982; 299:583.)

of activity arrive at the cortex out of register, causing a total loss of binocular receptive fields although the two eyes retain equal representation in the cortex (Fig. 17). This is a clear demonstration that the disconnection of inputs from one eye occurs as the result of competition rather than disuse; the two eyes are equally active, but for each cell, a winner takes all. Strabismus, if produced early enough, can also sharpen the segregation of ocular-dominance columns in layer IV.

The changes in ocular dominance and binocularity after deprivation have clear behavioral consequences. An ocular-dominance shift after monocular deprivation leaves the individual (or test animal) visually impaired in the involved eye, and the loss of binocularity associated with strabismus completely eliminates stereoscopic depth perception. However, both of these effects can be reversed if they are corrected early enough in the critical period. The clinical lesson is that congenital cataracts or ocular misalignment must be corrected in early childhood, as soon as is surgically feasible, to avoid permanent visual disability.

9.4. The Development and Modification of Binocularity Is Influenced by Extraretinal Factors

With increasing age, there appear to be additional constraints on the forms of activity that can modify cortical circuits. Before birth, spontaneously occurring bursts of retinal activity are sufficient to orchestrate aspects of address selection in the LGN and cortex. After birth, an interaction with the visual environment is of critical importance. However, even visually driven retinal activity may be insufficient for modifications of binocularity during this critical period. Such modifications seem to require that the patient (or test animal) attend to visual stimuli and use vision to guide behavior. For example, modifications of binocularity after monocular stimulation do not occur in anesthetized animals, although cortical neurons respond briskly to visual stimulation under this condition. These and related observations have led to the proposal that synaptic plasticity in the cortex requires the release of extraretinal "enabling factors" that are linked to the behavioral state. There is some evidence to suggest that this release may occur in response to eye movements.

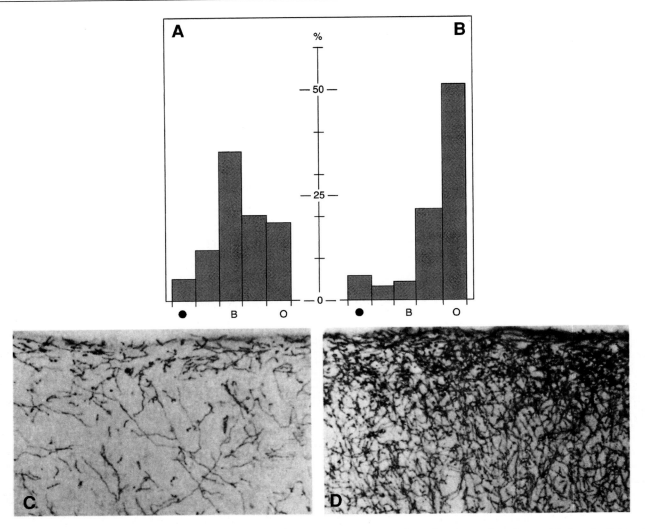

Fig. 18. Destruction of the modulatory noradrenergic and cholinergic inputs to the striate cortex interferes with the plasticity of binocular connections. **(A,B)** Percentages of cells in each of five ocular-dominance categories in striate cortex of monocularly deprived kittens. Open circles indicate the monocular open-eye group; *filled circles* indicate the monocular closed-eye group, and the *x*-axis B indicates the strictly binocular group. Data in **(A)** were obtained from the striate cortex ipsilateral to a unilateral transection of the cingulated bundle, a fiber tract that brings the modulatory inputs to the visual cortex. Data in **(B)** were obtained from the contralateral hemisphere where the modulatory inputs were intact. The ocular-dominance shift occurred only in the intact hemisphere. **(C,D)** Distribution of cholinergic axons in the striate cortex of a hemisphere with a lesion of the ascending modulatory fibers and of the contralateral hemisphere with these fibers intact, respectively. (From Bear MF, Singer W. Nature 1986; 320:172.)

Some data suggest that these enabling factors might be related to several modulatory systems converging at the level of the striate cortex, including the noradrenergic inputs from the locus coeruleus and the cholinergic inputs from the basal forebrain. These axonal projections have a trajectory that is distinct from the optic radiation from the LGN to the cortex. Surgical transection of these modulatory inputs in animal models substantially impairs ocular-dominance plasticity outside of cortical layer IV, although transmission in the retinal-geniculate-cortical pathway is apparently normal (Fig. 18). It is known that stimulation by acetylcholine and norepinephrine increase the excitability of cortical neurons, perhaps increasing the chance that they will generate action potentials in response to visual stimulation.

9.5. The Elementary Mechanisms of Synaptic Plasticity During the Critical Period May Involve NMDA Receptors

Much of the activity-dependent development of the visual system can be explained using Hebb synapses, particularly the development of binocular connections, in which afferents converging onto the same cell are consolidated only if they carry synchronous patterns of activity. The mechanisms by which consolidation of afferent connections is induced by synchronous firing derives from excitatory synaptic transmission. The transmitter at all of the modifiable synapses (e.g., retinogeniculate, geniculocortical, and corticocortical) is likely to be an amino acid, glutamate, or aspartate, and is known to recruit a family of postsynaptic receptors called excitatory amino acid receptors. These receptors may be divided into two broad categories known as metabotropic and ionotropic. The metabotropic receptors are linked by G proteins to intracellular second-messenger systems. The ionotropic receptors are ion channels that allow passage of positively charged ions into the postsynaptic cell. These receptors may be further divided into two categories named for compounds that act as selective agonists at these sites: the AMPA (a-amino-3-hydroxy-5-methyl-4-isoxazole propionic acid) receptor and the NMDA (N-methyl-D-aspartate) receptor. AMPA and NMDA receptors are co-localized at many synapses. Synaptic activation of the AMPA receptor activates a monovalent cation conductance that shows a linear current-voltage association with a reversal potential of approx 0 mV. Activation of this receptor by glutamate stimulates an inward (i.e., depolarizing) current whose amplitude diminishes as the postsynaptic membrane is depolarized because of decreased driving force.

The NMDA receptor has two unusual features that differentiate it from the AMPA receptor. First, the NMDA-receptor conductance is voltage-dependent because of the action of Mg^{2+} at the channel. At the resting-membrane potential, the inward current through the NMDA receptor is interrupted by the movement of Mg^{2+} ions into the channel, where they become lodged. However, as the membrane is depolarized, the Mg^{2+} block is displaced from the channel, and current is free to pass into the cell. Substantial current through the NMDA-receptor channel requires concurrent release of glutamate by the presynaptic terminal and depolarization of the postsynaptic membrane. The other distinguishing feature of this receptor is that the NMDA receptor channel conducts Ca^{2+} ions. The magnitude of the Ca^{2+} flux passing through the NMDA-receptor channel specifically signals the level of presynaptic and postsynaptic co-activation. It is believed that NMDA receptors in the cortex and LGN serve as Hebbian detectors of coincident presynaptic and postsynaptic activity and that Ca^{2+} entry through

the NMDA-receptor channel triggers the biochemical mechanisms that modify synaptic effectiveness. Hebbian enhancement of synaptic effectiveness has been shown experimentally in the connections from layer IV onto layer III neurons in the visual cortex.

Pairing low-frequency stimulation of layer IV with intracellular depolarization of a cell in layer III results in a *long-term potentiation* (LTP) of the conditioned synapses (Fig. 19). This long-term potentiation (LTP) is prevented by application of the drug 2-amino-5-phosphonovaleric acid (APV), an antagonist of the NMDA receptor. The theory that similar mechanisms contribute to naturally occurring synaptic remodeling is suggested by observations that application of APV in vivo can disrupt the natural segregation of eye-specific inputs in the LGN, binocular competition in layer IV, ocular-dominance domains after monocular deprivation, and the modification of binocular connections in the superficial layers under a number of experimental manipulations of visual experience (Fig. 20).

The strong activation of NMDA receptors that occurs when presynaptic and postsynaptic neurons fire together is believed to account partly for why they wire together during visual-system development. However, the NMDA-receptor does not function as a switch that is only "on" when input activity coincides with strong postsynaptic depolarization. Weak coincidences are signaled by lower levels of NMDA-receptor activation and les Ca^{2+} influx. Experiments suggest that the lower level of Ca^{2+} admitted under these conditions triggers an opposite form of synaptic plasticity, long-term depression (LTD), by which the effectiveness of the active synapses is decreased. The maintenance of a connection formed during development may depend on its success in evoking an NMDA receptor-mediated response beyond some threshold level. Failure to achieve this threshold leads to disconnection. Both processes depend on activity in the retinofugal pathway and on postsynaptic Ca^{2+} entry.

9.6. The Visual Cortex Is Plastic Beyond the Critical Period

In visual-system development, there are multiple critical periods. For example, the critical period for activity-dependent anatomic rearrangements of geniculate axonal arbors in layer IV ends much earlier than the critical period for the experience-dependent modification of binocular connections. It is important to understand that the primary visual cortex of the adult brain is not immutable simply because it has aged beyond the critical period for a particular develop-

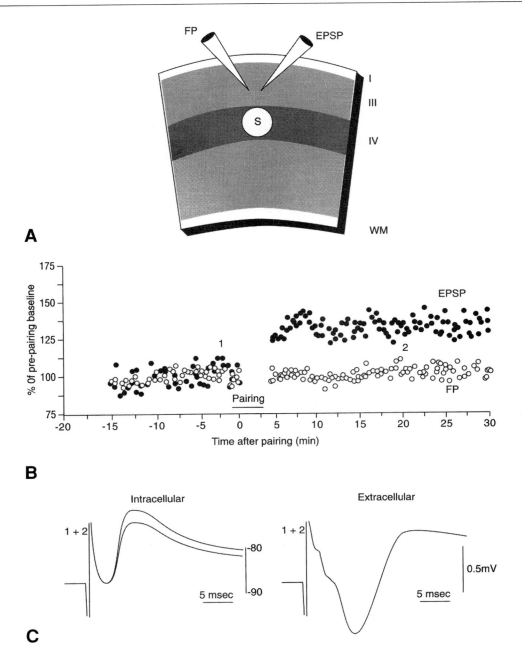

Fig. 19. Record of an experiment demonstrating Hebbian synaptic modification of the connections between layer IV and layer III in the rat visual cortex. (**A**) Layer IV was electrically stimulated (at the site marked [S]) every 30 s, and (**B,C**) the intracellular (EPSP) and extracellular synaptic responses in layer III were monitored. At the time indicated, the electrical stimuli to layer IV were paired with strong depolarization of the intracellularly recorded layer III neuron. As a consequence of this pairing, the intracellular response of the layer III neuron to the test stimulation of layer IV was potentiated. The extracellular response, which reflects the summed activity of a large population of synapses on many layer III neurons, is unchanged. FP, field potential.

mental process. Critical periods must be defined according to which type of intercellular interaction is being considered.

Modification of striate cortical circuits following a circumscribed lesion in the retina provides and example

of plasticity in the adult brain. The cortical neurons at the corresponding point in the retinotopic map initially fall silent, and are unresponsive to any type of visual stimulation. However, in a period of a few weeks, the same neurons again become visually

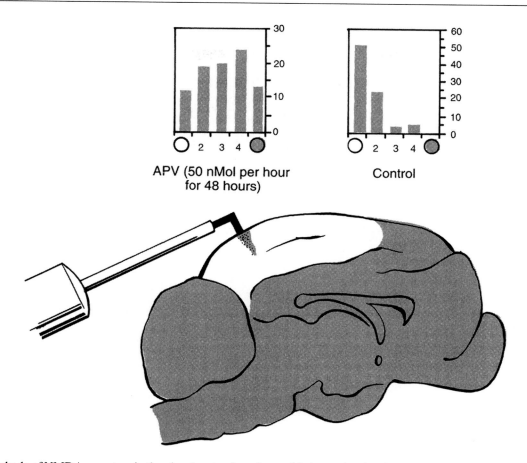

Fig. 20. Blockade of NMDA receptors in the visual cortex interferes with the ocular-dominance shift after monocular deprivation. Implanted small osmotic pumps delivered the NMDA-receptor antagonist 2-amino-5-phosphonovaleric acid (APV) directly to the visual cortex. At the same time as the infusion, the animal was monocularly deprived. No ocular-dominance shift was observed in the APV-treated cortex compared with controls. Conventions for these histograms are the same as used in Fig. 19. (Data from Bear MF, Kleinschmidt A, Gu Q, Singer W. Disruption of experience-dependent synaptic modifications in the striate cortex by infusion of an NMDA-receptor antagonist. J Neurosci 1990; 10:909.)

responsive, but to the region of retina surrounding the lesion. The retinal lesion causes a "filling in" of the cortical retinotopic map (Fig. 21). The anatomic substrate of this map plasticity is thought to be an adjustment in the effectiveness of horizontal projections that interconnect the layer III neurons in different parts of the retinotopic map. This demonstrates that cortical circuits can be modified by peripheral lesions well after the end of the critical period that is defined by the effects of monocular deprivation.

It is assumed that synaptic adjustments to more subtle changes in the sensory environment give the cortex a life-long capability to reorganize itself. The elementary mechanisms of synaptic plasticity, LTP and LTD, persist in the superficial layers of the adult striate cortex. It is likely that experience-dependent synaptic remodeling in the cortex is one mechanism that contributes to environmental adaptation, and possibly to learning and memory in the adult brain.

9.7. Why Do Critical Periods End?

Although plasticity of visual connections persists in the adult brain, the dynamic range over which this plasticity occurs decreases with increasing age. Early in development, gross rearrangements of axonal arbors are possible, but in the adult, the plasticity appears to be restricted to local changes in synaptic efficacy. The adequate stimulus for evoking a change also appears to be increasingly constrained as the brain matures. An obvious example is the fact that patching one eye causes a profound alteration in the binocular connections of the superficial layers during infancy, but by adolescence, this type of experience fails to cause a lasting alteration in cortical circuitry.

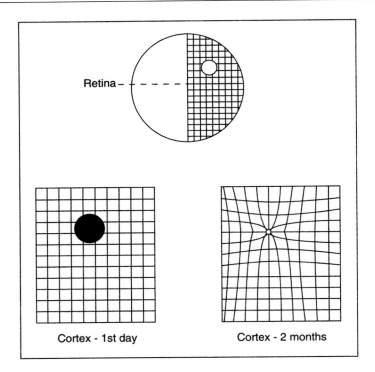

Fig. 21. Plasticity in the adult visual cortex. A lesion in the retina initially causes a patch of cortex to fall silent. However, these silent neurons later become responsive to stimulation of the surrounding areas of retina, causing the map to "fill in." (Modified from Barinaga M. The brain remaps its own contours. Science 1992; 258:216.)

There still is no satisfactory single explanation of why critical periods end. As more is learned about the elementary mechanisms of axonal path-finding and synaptic plasticity, insights will be gained about how these processes are regulated. However, it is already possible to identify some of the rate-limiting factors that govern activity-dependent plasticity in the developing visual pathway.

One common feature in the establishment of connectivity in the LGN and cortex is the initial activity-independent establishment of widespread "exuberant" connections that are sculpted by activity to achieve their final form during a critical period. One explanation for the end of a critical period of, for example, ocular-dominance-column formation in layer IV is that, once segregation is complete and the afferents no longer contact the same postsynaptic cells, the substrate for the winner-takes-all competition is lost (Fig. 22). According to this view, monocular deprivation, by removing a competing input, only "saves" the initially widespread open-eye axonal arbors from being retracted. If it is assumed that axons lose the ability to grow after they have invaded their target structure and established their initial pattern of con-

nectivity, the final state of connectivity is permanently "imprinted" after segregation (by loss of synapses and axon retraction) is complete.

This is unlikely to be the full explanation for the visual cortex, because reverse suture experiments have shown that ocular-dominance columns retain some capacity for re-expansion after segregation is anatomically complete. Another factor that limits the critical period in layer IV appears to be a loss of the capability for axonal elongation, which may be caused by changes in the ECM or surface glycoproteins expressed by the geniculate axons.

A third possible reason the critical period ends reflects changes in the elementary mechanisms of synaptic plasticity. There is evidence that some EAA receptors change during postnatal development. For example, it has been shown that EAA-stimulated phosphoinositide turnover, that is mediated by one of the metabotropic receptors peaks in the visual cortex when binocular connections are most susceptible to monocular deprivation, and then virtually disappears at the end of this critical period (Fig. 23). The effectiveness of NMDA receptors appears to be downregulated in layer IV at the same time as the end

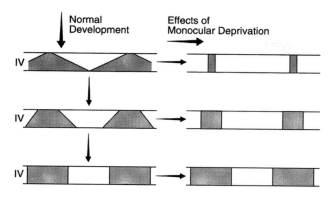

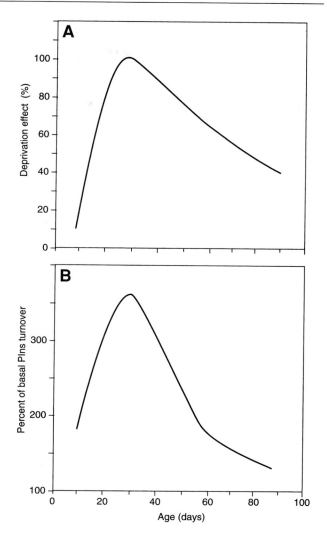

Fig. 22. Segregation of ocular-dominance columns in layer IV at three times during postnatal development and the effects of monocular deprivation initiated at these same times.

of the critical period for ocular-dominance column segregation. This change in effectiveness can be detected at the single-channel level, and may result from a developmental change in the NMDA-receptor subunit composition.

As development proceeds, certain types of activity may be filtered by successive synaptic relays until they no longer activate NMDA receptors or other elementary mechanisms sufficiently to trigger plasticity. The neuromodulators acetylcholine and norepinephrine facilitate synaptic plasticity in the superficial cortical layers, and may do this by enhancing polysynaptic intracortical transmission. A decline in the effectiveness of these neuromodulators or a change in the conditions under which they are released may contribute to the decline in plasticity. There is some evidence that supplementing the adult cortex with norepinephrine can restore some degree of modifiability. There is also evidence that intrinsic inhibitory circuitry is late to mature in the visual cortex. Consequently, patterns of activity that may have gained access to modifiable synapses in superficial layers early in postnatal development may be damped by inhibition in the adult.

Whatever the reason for the decline in synaptic plasticity at the end of the critical periods, it is clear that the duration of the critical periods is not always locked to a certain postnatal age. For example, rearing kittens in complete darkness appears to slow the critical period for modification of binocular connections (Fig. 24). Dark-rearing also slows segregation of ocular dominance columns and some of the changes in EAA-receptor properties. It seems that the duration of this critical period may be measured by the history of stimulation rather than by age.

Fig. 23. (A) Sensitivity of binocular connections in striate cortex to eyelid suture at different postnatal ages. (B) Phosphoinositide turnover stimulated by an excitatory amino acid in synaptoneurosomes prepared from kitten striate cortex at different postnatal ages. These data suggest that excitatory synaptic transmission during this critical period is characterized by unique patterns of second messenger activity. (Modified from Dudek SM, Bear MF. A biochemical correlate of the critical period for synaptic modification in the kitten visual cortex. Science 1989; 246:673.)

10. BASIS OF DISEASE STATES

10.1. Anatomic Lesions at Various Points in the Visual Pathways Produce Characteristic Patterns of Visual Field Loss

The complexity of the visual system provides diagnostic clues as to the causes of at least some visual deficits. Lesions at different locations along the optic

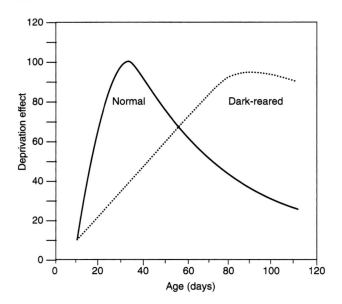

Fig. 24. Raising cats in complete darkness before visual experience with one eye open slows the critical period for the modification of binocular connections. (Data from Mower GC. The effect of dark rearing on the time course of the critical period in cat visual cortex. Dev Brain Res 1991; 58:151.)

pathways result in characteristic visual defects (Fig. 25). Lesions of a single retina or optic nerve anterior to the optic chiasm result in a visual defect limited to one eye. A complete lesion of one optic nerve results in blindness of the corresponding eye. The pupil of the blind eye constricts consensually when light stimulates the opposite retina, because each pretectum receives input and sends output fibers bilaterally. However, direct stimulation of the blind eye in a darkened room reveals an unreactive dilated pupil. This leads to an afferent pupillary defect or Marcus-Gunn pupil. Lesions that occur beyond the pretectum and superior colliculus do not affect the pupillary light reflex. Of course, bilateral lesions anterior to the chiasm affect both visual fields. This can occur symmetrically in diseases such as macular degeneration, which affects the macula, resulting in isolated central visual defects (called a central scotoma).

Lesions at or behind the optic chiasm give recognizable visual field deficits that affect both visual fields. Lesions that compress the optic chiasm (e.g., pituitary tumors) damage the crossing fibers preferentially, producing bitemporal hemianopia. Rarely, one or both lateral angles of the chiasm may be compressed, causing destruction of the noncrossing fibers and resultant nasal or binasal hemianopia.

Unilateral lesions of the optic pathways behind the chiasm (e.g., optic tract, lateral geniculate body, optic radiation, or visual cortex) result in a loss of the corresponding opposite field of vision, ranging from specific field defects to complete opposite-field loss, known as homonymous hemianopia. Occasionally, patterns of visual-field deficits can suggest a more precise localization of lesions along this pathway. The spatial relationships observed in the retina are maintained in the optic radiations. As the optic radiations sweep anteriorly and then posteriorly through the temporal lobe to form Meyer's loop, fibers from the inferior retina occupy the more anterior part of the path, and damage limited to this part of the optic radiation can cause a homonymous field defect limited to the superior quadrants (superior quadrantanopia). Conversely, injuries to the optic radiations in the parietal lobes can result in a homonymous field defect limited to the inferior quadrants (inferior quadrantanopia).

Occipital lesions often result from cerebrovascular accidents involving branches of the posterior cerebral artery. Because the tip of the occipital lobe, which is responsible for central vision, is supplied collaterally from the middle cerebral artery, central (e.g. macular) vision can be preserved, while the rest of the visual field is ablated. This causes a homonymous hemianopia with macular sparing.

Diseases of the visual system are not limited to gross morphologic damage. Many genetic disorders that affect vision have been described, affecting primarily affecting the rods, cones, or both, but it is only with the advent of molecular biology that the molecular basis

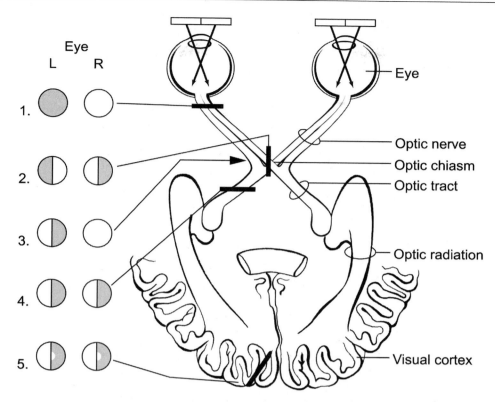

Fig. 25. Optic pathways in the brain and visual field defects that their lesions produce: total visual loss of the left eye; bitemporal hemianopsia; left nasal hemianopsia; right homonymous (contralateral) hemianopsia; right homonymous hemianopsia with macular sparing. At the optic chiasm, nerve fibers from the nasal retina cross to the other side of the brain, joining the opposite optic nerve to form the optic tract.

of these has been described. Two are considered here: blue cone monochromacy, which is a form of color blindness, and retinitis pigmentosa.

10.2. Loss of Color Vision Can Result from Genetic Lesions Causing Defects in the Color Pigments

An interesting ophthalmologic disease that has been elucidated at a molecular level is blue cone monochromacy (BCM). This is an X-linked form of color blindness in which only the short-wavelength-sensitive ("blue-sensitive") cones are present. Clinically, it is characterized by poor visual acuity, nystagmus, glare-induced visual loss, and severely limited color vision in males. In some families the retinas of affected individuals show progressive macular atrophy.

The highly similar red and green color pigment genes normally occur as a head-to-tail tandem array, with a red pigment gene followed by one or more green pigment genes. Most instances of BCM arise from unequal homologous recombination events that occur in this array during meiosis, resulting in the deletion

of all but a single remaining gene(in some cases, a red-green hybrid gene). Alternative, two genes may be present, one inactivated by a point mutation. Finally, deletions in a locus control region approx 4–18 kilobases upstream from the red pigment gene can result in inactivation of both genes. These molecular lesions leave the patient able to discriminate brightness using rod input. However, they have essentially absent color vision, since only one of the three cone types is present.

The elegant delineation of the pathophysiology of BCM is a classic example of the power of combining the techniques of molecular genetics with clinical acumen.

10.3. Retinitis Pigmentosa Can Result from Mutations in Highly Expressed Retinal Specific Genes

Retinitis pigmentosa (RP) is the clinical term used to describe a large, genetically and phenotypically heterogeneous group of visual disorders in which the rod photoreceptors degenerate, resulting in partial or total blindness. These are characterized by poor rod function and a progressive degeneration of the retina that begins at the mid periphery. RP has a variable age of onset and rate of progression, and affects approx 1 in every 2000–4000 persons worldwide.

For the purposes of clinical diagnosis, the classic symptoms of RP include night blindness (e.g., nyctalopia), alterations in the ERG, and the deposit of so-called "bone spicules" of pigment on the retinal surface, accounting for the name of the disease. RP shows genetic heterogeneity as well. Autosomal dominant (adRP), autosomal recessive, and X-linked forms of RP have been described

Lesions in multiple genes have been shown to cause RP. In 1989, Peter Humphries and colleagues established the linkage between one form of adRP and a marker on the long arm of chromosome 3 in a large Irish pedigree. The gene for human rod opsin had been previously shown to map to the long arm of chromosome 3. Using this knowledge, Dryja and his colleagues quickly identified a point mutation in the rhodopsin gene that could be identified as the defect in 17 of 148 unrelated adRP families. The specific change, a C to A transversion, resulted in the substitution of a histidine for a highly conserved proline at amino acid 23, in the amino-terminal region of the mature opsin moiety. In a mouse line that was transgenic for the P23H rhodopsin mutation (along with two others) the photoreceptors developed normally, but the light-sensitive outer segments never reached normal length. As the mice aged, their retinas showed a slow but progressive retinal degeneration with decreased light-evoked responses on ERG. Many other rhodopsin mutations have been described in patients with RP, accounting for about 15% of all RP cases. Identification of additional genes associated with RP has been carried out by a combination of linkage analysis and by systematically screening candidate genes for mutations in individuals who are affected by RP.

Currently, over 120 genes that cause inherited retinal diseases when mutated have been mapped in the human genome, and more than half of these have been identified and cloned, and the causative mutations characterized. The number of these genes is growing weekly, so that an updated summary is maintained on the RetNet web site. Twelve genes have been implicated in autosomal dominant RP, of which six have been cloned. Nineteen additional genes have been implicated in autosomal recessive RP, of which 14 have been cloned, and five genes have been implicated in X-linked RP, with two cloned. Current studies

are examining the precise molecular mechanisms whereby the mutant opsins give rise to the RP phenotype. Preliminary studies of some alleles indicate that these defective opsins are poorly transported to and incorporated into the membrane, and others result in a constitutively activated phototransduction cascade. However, the detailed pathophysiology leading to the relatively late onset of symptomatic RP has yet to be delineated. It seems likely that mutations in various photoreceptor-specific genes can have a direct effect on vision through changes in their function, and perhaps cause RP by damaging retinal cells sufficiently to induce apoptosis as a common final pathway of cellular death.

These candidate genes often encode phototransduction proteins or other proteins produced at high levels in the retina. In addition to rhodopsin, perhaps the most prominent retinal protein, mutations in peripherin, which stabilizes the discs in the rod outer-segment membranous discs cause RP. Other proteins that have been implicated in RP include rod cGMP-gated channel alpha subunit, arrestin, the alpha and beta subunits of cGMP phosphodiesterase, RPE-retinal G protein-coupled receptor (GPCR), cellular retinaldehyde-binding protein, and rod outer segment membrane protein 1. Interestingly, many of the genes associated with RP can, when mutated at a different amino acid or in some cases even with the same mutation, cause other retinal degenerations such as congenital stationary night blindness (rhodopsin), macular degeneration (peripherin), and others.

Mutations in rhodopsin, peripherin, and the other implicated proteins still account for a minority of RP cases, indicating that many more genes may be involved in other forms of the disorder. Probable candidates include genes encoding proteins involved in phototransduction specifically and genes that code for retinal housekeeping-type proteins. Several laboratories are actively looking for the genes and for lesions that may be linked to RP.

The clinical heterogeneity of RP, even among siblings carrying the same RP-causing mutation, is still not explained. Eventually, it is possible that such studies will lead to cures for selected cases of RP-induced blindness.

ACKNOWLEDGMENT

This chapter incorporates material from the chapter "Critical Periods in Visual System Development" authored by Dr. Mark F. Bear in the first edition of this work.

SELECTED READINGS

Albert DM, Jakobiec FA (eds). Principles and proctice of Ophthalmology. Philadelphia: W.B. Saunders Co., 2000.

Bornstein MH (ed). Sensitive periods in development: interdisciplinary perspectives. Hillsdale, NJ:Lawrence Erlhaum Associates, 1987.

Greenough WT, Juraska JM (eds). Developmental neuropsychobiology. Orlando: Academic Press, 1986.

Hubel DH. Eye, Brain, and Vision. New York: WH Freeman, 1988.

Kandel ER, Schwartz JH, Jessell TM (eds). Principles of neural science. New York: McGraw-Hill, 2000.

Landmesser LT (ed). The Assembly of the Nervous System. New York: Alan R Liss, 2001.

Lowel S, Singer W. Selection of intrinsic horizontal connections in the visual cortex by correlated neuronal activity. Science 1992; 255:209.

Nathans J. Rhodopsin: structure, function, and genetics. Biochemistry 1992; 31:4923.

Palczewski K, Benovic JL. G-protein-coupled receptor kinases. Trends Biochem Sci 1991; 16:387.

Rauschecker JP, Marler P (eds). Imprinting and cortical plasticity. Comparative aspects of sensitive periods. New York: John Wiley & Sons, 1987.

Shatz CJ. The developing brain. Sci Am 1992; 267:60.

Tessier-Lavigne M. Phototransduction and information processing in the retina. In Kandel ER, Schwartz JH, Jessell TM (eds). 1993; 401.

Wiesel TN. Postnatal development of the visual cortex and the influence of environment. Nature 1982; 299:583.

24 Audition

Tom C. T. Yin

Contents

1. INTRODUCTION

This chapter provides an introduction to the physiological mechanisms underlying audition. We first consider the physical properties of sound, then examine the processing of acoustic input by the peripheral auditory system, and then explore the central auditory system.

2. THE PHYSICAL NATURE OF SOUND

A few basic properties of sound must be understood before analyzing the auditory system. Physically, sound is a mechanical disturbance that is propagated through an elastic medium. This medium usually is air, but sound can also propagate through solids or liquids. Air molecules are in constant, random motion, thus, the large number of air molecules striking any given point in space produces a static pressure, which depends on conditions of the system, such as the density of gas and air temperature. With a sudden change in the position of some large object in the air, such as clapping hands or vibrating the cone of a loudspeaker, the mechanical disturbance causes a temporary increase in pressure locally with a corresponding decrease elsewhere (e.g., an increase on one side of the

speaker cone and a decrease on the other). The disturbance is propagated through the medium as the air molecules collide with each other and transfer energy to neighboring molecules. This variation in pressure as a function of time is known as a *sound wave*. It represents the characteristics of the population of molecules as a whole rather than any single air molecule, which moves back and forth randomly without necessarily propagating energy.

The velocity at which the wave travels depends on the density and elasticity of the medium. Sound travels about four times faster in water than in air. The strength of the sound wave is usually measured as the deviation in sound pressure from atmospheric pressure.

Most sound waves result from the vibrations of an object, and the simplest form of vibration is a sine wave, which produces a pure tone. Figure 1 shows a diagram of the instantaneous pressure and the spatial distribution of air molecules as a function of distance in the medium for a pure tone at one instant in time. It can be considered to be a snapshot of the sound wave at some moment. Because sound propagates through air at a constant velocity (340 m/s or taking about 30 μs to travel 1 cm), the abscissa in Fig. 1 could also be time; it would then depict the variation in pressure at a given point in the medium as a function of time. The time between peaks would then be the *period* of the tone.

The relationship between the wavelength λ, conduction velocity c, and frequency f expressed in cycles/

From: *Neuroscience in Medicine, 2nd ed.* (P. Michael Conn, ed.),
© 2003 Humana Press Inc., Totowa, NJ.

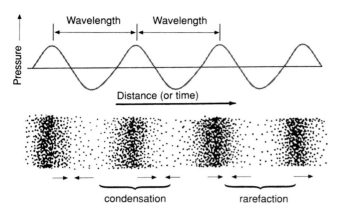

Fig. 1. Diagram of air molecules in response to sinusoidal sound vibrations. The rarefactions and condensations are shown.

second or hertz (Hz) and the period T of the sine wave is given by: $\lambda = c/f$, in which $f = 1/T$. For a 100-Hz pure tone, which is near the lower limit of human hearing, λ is 3.3 m; at 10,000 Hz, it is 3 cm. The musical note middle C has a frequency of 256 Hz. These variations in wavelength with frequency are important in discussions of the cues that are available for sound localization.

The sensitivity of the auditory system is quite remarkable. On the lower end, the faintest sound that can be detected by humans is generated by movements of the eardrum of approx $10^{-10}\,M$, which is in the range of diameters of air molecules. On the high end, sound pressures that are 10^6 larger begin to result in painful sensations. Because of this large dynamic range, the intensities of sounds are usually expressed in decibels (dB), which is a logarithmic unit of ratios. The arithmetic definition of a decibel is $dB = 20\log_{10}(P/P_{ref})$, in which P is the pressure of interest and P_{ref} is a reference pressure, which can be arbitrarily chosen. Usually, P_{ref} is chosen to be near the average normal threshold of hearing, and, when so chosen the decibels are denoted as dB sound pressure level (SPL). The dynamic range in humans is about $20\log_{10} 10^6 = 120$ dB.

The physical parameters of frequency and SPL correspond to the perceptual qualities of *pitch* and *loudness*, respectively. In audiology and speech analysis, any particular sound can be represented by a spectrogram that plots the SPL as the darkness of spots on a time-frequency axis, as shown in Fig. 2. A pure tone is represented by a single frequency that persists over time, a musical note generally has many harmonics, and speech consists of a complex mixture of frequencies that vary with time. A topic of considerable clinical interest is how the auditory system can encode a

complex sound, such as speech, and distinguish the subtle differences between similar sounds or the same sound uttered by different people that constitute daily human experience. We know very little about these questions.

3. THE PERIPHERAL AUDITORY SYSTEM

It is convenient to divide the ear into an outer, middle, and inner ear, as shown in Fig. 3, which depicts a cross-section of the human ear. A standard sequence of events leads to activation of auditory-nerve fibers in response to an acoustic stimulus. Sound waves enter the external ear and travel down the external auditory meatus to strike the tympanic membrane, or eardrum. Movements of the tympanic membrane are transferred by means of the ossicular chain to the oval window of the cochlea, and back-and-forth movements of the oval window cause a traveling wave to be set up in the fluid-filled cochlear ducts. The traveling wave causes deflections of the basilar membrane, which vibrates and activates the receptor cells, the hair cells in the organ of Corti (Figs. 3 and 4).

3.1. The Outer Ear Is Important for Collecting Sound Waves

The outer ear consists of the pinna, or external ear, and the external auditory meatus, or ear canal. This apparatus has important acoustic properties, because it accentuates or attenuates sounds of certain frequencies and those coming from particular directions. The degree to which the pinna can influence a sound wave depends on the wavelength of the sound and thus its frequency. If the wavelength is much longer than the dimensions of the pinna, as it is for low-frequency sounds, it appears to be transparent to the sound and produces no diffractive or reflective effects. Only high-frequency sounds of at least 5 kHz are greatly affected by the pinna. Because of the directional properties of the pinna, these transformations are important for localizing sounds, particularly those in the vertical plane. In humans, unlike most other mammals, there is virtually no control over the direction in which the pinna is pointing other than movements of the head.

3.2. The Middle Ear Acts as an Impedance Matching Device

The middle ear consists of the *tympanic membrane* and the three bony *ossicles* that conduct vibrations to the oval window: the *malleus, incus,* and *stapes* (e.g.,

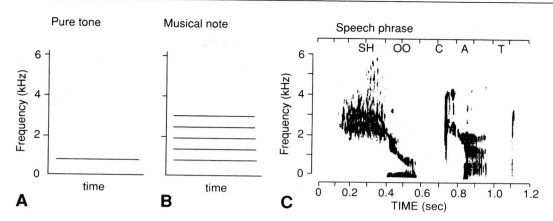

Fig. 2. Spectograms of (**A**) a pure tone of 800 Hz, (**B**) a musical note from a flute, and (**C**) a speech phrase (e.g., shoo cat). Darkness represents acoustic energy in the signal at the corresponding frequency. (Adapted from Kiang NYS. Stimulus representation in the discharge patterns of auditory neurons. In Tower DB (ed). The Nervous System (Vol 3): Human Communication and its Disorders. New York: Raven Press, 1975; 81.)

hammer, anvil, and stirrup). The middle ear is important in providing an *impedance matching*, or interface, for the airborne sound waves to transmit their energy to the fluid in the cochlea. If there were no middle ear, only 0.1% of the energy of a sound wave would be transmitted to the fluid in the cochlea. The middle ear reduces this energy loss, chiefly by the mechanical advantage resulting from the reduction in surface area from the large tympanic membrane to the small footplate of the stapes. The principle is the same as that used in hydraulic jacks, in which force is applied through a combination of a large and small cylinder connected by a pipe and filled with a fluid. A small amount of fluid pressure applied to the large cylinder results in large pressure on the small piston. The force on the tympanic membrane is equal to the pressure times the total area of the eardrum and, assuming negligible frictional losses in the transmission through the ossicles, it is equal to the force exerted at the stapes footplate on the oval window. Because the area of the stapes is much smaller than that of the tympanic membrane, there is a *pressure amplification* given by the ratio of these areas (approx 20:1).

Two other factors amplify the pressure at the stapes: a lever-arm action through the ossicular chain and a buckling factor that results from the conical shape of the tympanic membrane. The potential loss in energy transmission at the air–fluid boundary is reduced considerably, as is evident in the 20–30-dB hearing loss suffered by patients in whom the ossicular chain has been broken.

There are two important muscles in the middle ear: the tensor tympani and stapedius. Both muscles are attached to the ossicles. The stapedius muscle is innervated by motor neurons in the facial nucleus that run with cranial nerve VII, and the tensor tympani is innervated by motor neurons in the motor division of the trigeminal nucleus that travel in the V nerve. Contraction of these muscles increases the stiffness of the ossicular chain and can decrease the sound transmission by as much as 15–20 dB. Loud sounds cause the muscles to contract reflexively, a response that protects the ear from very loud sounds by reducing energy transmission.

3.3. The Inner Ear Contains the Mechanisms for Sensory Transduction

The inner ear is divided into three interconnected parts: the semicircular canals, the vestibule, and the cochlea, all of which are located in the temporal bone. Only the *cochlea* is considered here. The cochlea is the small, shell-shaped part of the bony labyrinth that contains the receptor organ of hearing. It resembles a tube that is coiled increasingly tightly on itself. One end of the tube is called the apex, and the opposite end, closest to the middle ear, is called the base. The fluid-filled spiral canal of the cochlea is divided along its length by a partition, the *basilar membrane*, which is attached to the bony walls of the cochlea. Cross-sections of the cochlea show that the canal is divided into three ducts: the scala vestibuli, scala tympani, and scala media (*see* Fig. 5).

The input to the cochlea is supplied by movements of the oval window by means of the stapes footplate. Because the fluid in the cochlea is incompressible, there must be some point where the pressure applied at

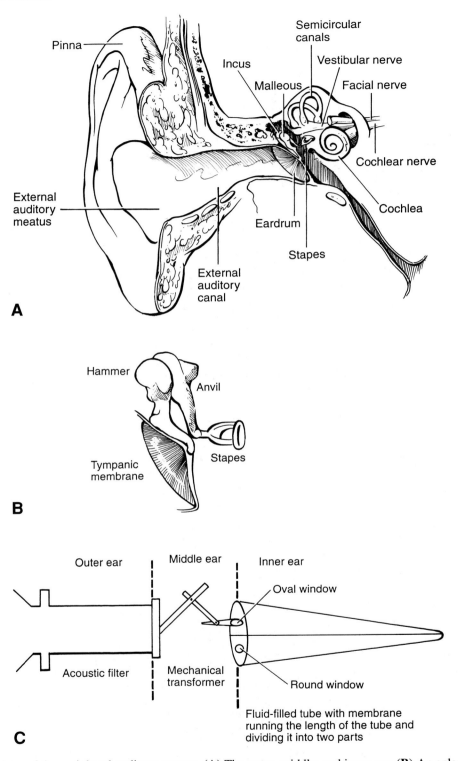

Fig. 3. Major divisions of the peripheral auditory system. (**A**) The outer, middle, and inner ear. (**B**) An enlarged version of the middle ear. (**C**) The mechanical analogs of the outer and middle ear.

the oval window, which is in the scala vestibuli, is transferred. This occurs at the *round window*, which is in scala tympani, through the helicotrema at the apex of the cochlea, where the scala vestibuli joins the scala tympani (*see* Fig. 4). As the pressure wave travels the length of the cochlea, it creates a pressure differential

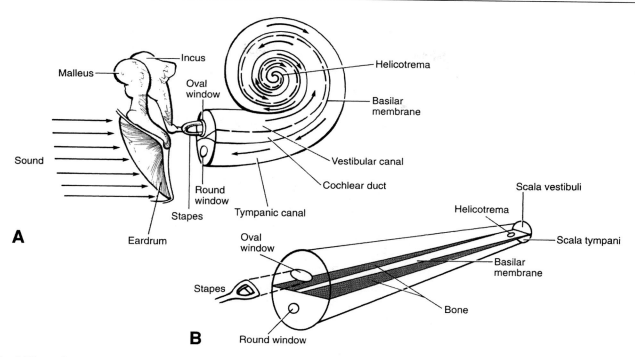

Fig. 4. The major structural features of the cochlea. (**A**) Coupling of the middle ear to the coiled cochlea through the oval and round windows. (**B**) The cochlea is shown uncoiled. The basilar membrane is narrow near the round window and wider near the heliocotrema, a taper opposite to the cross-sectional area of the cochlea.

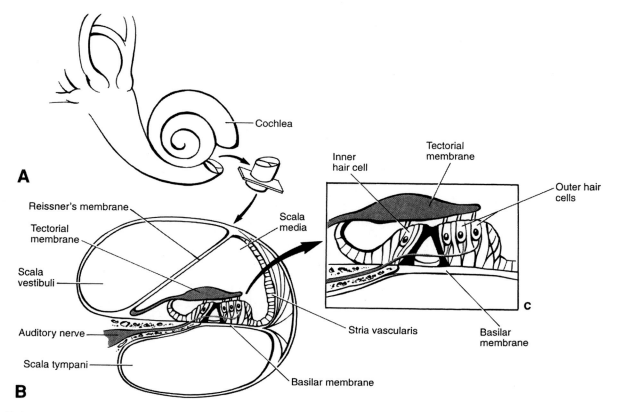

Fig. 5. Anatomic features of the cochlea. (**A**) The cochlea in relation to the vestibular channels (partially illustrated). (**B**) Cross-section of the cochlea showing the cochlear ducts (scala media, scala tympani, and scala vestibuli) as well as the placement of the basilar membrane, tectorial membrane, and auditory nerve. (**C**) The structures within the scala media.

across the basilar membrane (between the scala vestibuli and scala tympani) that sets the membrane in motion in the form of a traveling wave.

Within the scala media and attached to the basilar membrane is the receptor organ of hearing, the *organ of Corti* (Fig. 5). The organ of Corti is composed of numerous structures, and most of these are not considered here. Of special importance are the receptor cells, which are similar to the hair cells in the semicircular canals. The hairs are in contact with an auxiliary structure, the *tectorial membrane*. Sound waves that reach the inner ear set the basilar membrane and the organ of Corti into motion. This motion results in a shearing force between the tectorial membrane and the hairs of the hair cells. Displacement of the hairs results in transmitter release at the base of the hair cell, where fibers of cranial nerve VIII make synaptic contact. All information about the acoustic environment is carried to the central nervous system (CNS) by trains of all-or-none action potentials generated in primary afferent fibers.

The coding of acoustic information depends on the vibratory pattern of the basilar membrane. The basilar membrane is a relatively flaccid structure that increases in width and decreases in stiffness from its base to apex. Curiously, the change in the width of the basilar membrane is the opposite of the change in width of the cochlear duct as it coils from base to apex (*see* Fig. 4). The vibratory undulations generated in the cochlea by sound waves contain all the information about the acoustic environment that must be coded into neural information. A key factor in this process is the mechanical response to sound waves of the basilar membrane and organ of Corti. Most of the pioneering work on the vibratory patterns of the basilar membrane was done by Georg von Bekesy, who was awarded the Nobel Prize in 1960.

To understand the motion of the basilar membrane and how the frequency of a sound affects this movement, we first consider the responses to a sinusoidal stimulus (e.g., tone). Each point along the basilar membrane that is set in motion vibrates at the same frequency as the acoustic stimulus. However, the amplitude of membrane vibration varies with location along the length of the basilar membrane from base to apex, depending on the frequency of the sound. A wave motion is set up along the membrane as the fluids of the inner ear are driven by motion of the stapes. This wave motion on the basilar membrane is referred to as a *traveling wave* (Fig. 6).

Because the basilar membrane becomes wider and more flaccid as the distance from the base increases, the natural frequency of vibration (e.g., resonance) of the basilar membrane decreases toward the helicotrema. Because of this variation in stiffness, low and high frequencies cause maximal vibration amplitudes along the apex and base, of the basilar membrane respectively, (Fig. 7A). If two different frequencies are received by the cochlea simultaneously, they each create a maximal displacement at different points along the basilar membrane. This separation of a complex signal into different points of maximal displacement along the basilar memhrane, corresponding to the frequency of the sinusoids of which the complex signal is composed, means that the basilar membrane performs like a series of filters. The basal part of the basilar membrane responds maximally to high-frequency sounds, and the region of maximal displacement of low-frequency tones is in the apical portion (Fig. 7B); the basilar membrane is tonotopically organized.

The receptor cells are hair cells that line the length of the cochlea. In most mammals, there are three rows of *outer hair cells* and a single row of *inner hair cells*. The tops of the outer hair cells are embedded in the overlying tectorial membrane (*see* Fig. 5), but it is unknown whether the same is true of the inner hair cells. When the basilar membrane is set into motion by an acoustic stimulus, the basilar membrane and tectorial membranes do not move in unison, because they pivot about different points. The result is that a shearing force is applied to the cilia of the hair cells, which bends the cilia. Just as with the hair cells in the semicircular canals, this mechanical action results in a depolarization or hyperpolarization of the membrane potential of the cell, depending on the direction of movement. The afferent nerve fibers of cranial nerve VIII make chemical synapses onto the base of the hair cells, and depolarization of the hair cell increases the resting impulse discharge of the fiber. Hyperpolarization from movement in the opposite direction decreases the resting discharge level.

We do not understand the exact role of the two types of hair cells. A clue can be obtained from considering their innervation by auditory nerve fibers, because the pattern is quite different for the inner and outer hair cells. In the cat, there are about 50,000 auditory nerve fibers. Not all of these are afferent fibers; approx 5% are efferent fibers that have cell bodies in and around the superior olivary complex and convey information

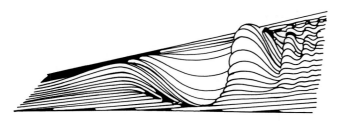

Fig. 6. Representation of a traveling wave at one instant in time. Cochlear base is at left, and the apex at right. Notice the rapid decline in amplitude just to the right of the region of maximal displacement amplitude. (Redrawn from Tonndorf J. Shearing motion in scala media of cochlear models. J Acoust Soc Am 1960; 32:238.)

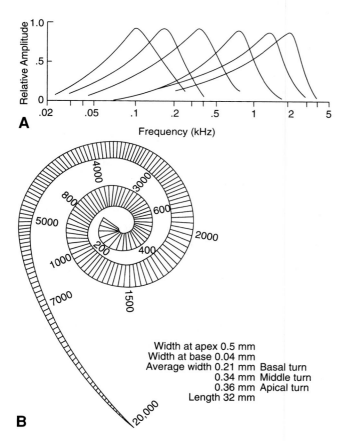

Width at apex 0.5 mm
Width at base 0.04 mm
Average width 0.21 mm Basal turn
0.34 mm Middle turn
0.36 mm Apical turn
Length 32 mm

Fig. 7. (A) Envelopes of traveling waves at seven different frequencies. (Redrawn from Bekesy G von. Experiments in hearing. New York: McGraw-Hill, 1960.) **(B)** Diagram of the human basilar membrane, showing the approximate positions of maximal displacement to tones of different frequencies and changes in width going from the base near the stapes and oval window to the apex near the helicotrema. The ratio of width to length is exaggerated to show the variation in width more clearly. (Redrawn from Stuhlman O. An Introduction to Biophysics. New York: Wiley, 1943.)

back to the cochlea. The precise nature of this efferent innervation of the cochlea is not well-understood. Of the remaining afferent fibers, about 95% terminate only on inner hair cells (Fig. 8) so that each inner hair cell is contacted by about 20 afferent fibers; these are the Type I afferents. The remaining Type II afferent fibers innervate the outer hair cells in a much more diffuse manner, typically crossing over to the rows of outer hair cells and traveling toward the base before innervating a number of outer hair cells in all three rows. It is reasonable to conclude that the inner hair cells are most important for conveying information about the vibrations in the cochlea to the CNS.

The exact role of the outer hair cells and the reason there should be three times as many have yet to be determined. Current speculations center on their role in efferent innervation and evidence for an active mechanism in the cochlea. Evidence for an active process comes from the surprising observation that the cochlea can emit sound spontaneously or in response to acoustic stimulation. The outer hair cells are motile, and can be made to contract when stimulated electrically. Furthermore, one hypothetical scenario is that the efferent system enables the CNS to contract the cilia of the outer hair cells, changing the micromechanical sensitivity of the basilar membrane to low-level stimuli. This remains an active area of research.

Because the eighth cranial-nerve afferent fibers are distributed along the entire length of the basilar membrane, a tone of one frequency will excite the afferents connected to the region that is undergoing suprathreshold vibration. The fact that a discrete population of fibers is activated by a pure tone and that this population changes when the stimulus frequency changes is the basis for the *place principle* of hearing. This principle states that the perceived pitch of a sound depends only on the particular population of nervous elements activated. The tonotopic organization of the array of auditory nerve terminals along the basilar membrane is maintained in all major areas of the central auditory system, but this tonotopic organization is probably not precise enough to explain a listener's ability to discriminate one frequency from another.

4. FREQUENCY TUNING AND TEMPORAL INFORMATION IS TRANSMITTED BY AUDITORY-NERVE FIBERS

There are several ways in which information about an acoustic stimulus is coded in the discharges of fibers

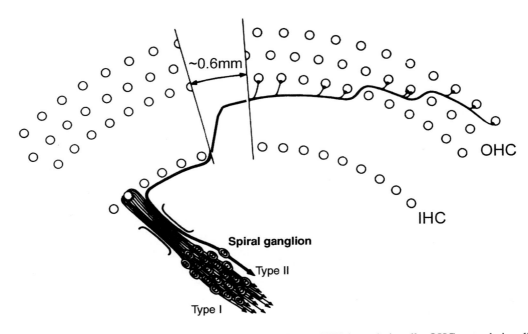

Fig. 8. Schematic view of cochlear innervation for afferent fibers in the cat. IHC, inner hair cells; OHC, outer hair cells. (Redrawn from Spoendlin H. Stuctural basis of peripheral frequency analysis. In Plomp R. Smoorenburg GF (eds). Frequency Analysis and Periodicity Detection in Hearing. The Netherlands: AW Sitjhoff, 1970; 2.)

of the auditory nerve. These results come from studies in which fine micropipet electrodes are used to record from single auditory-nerve fibers.

4.1. Tuning Properties

Auditory-nerve fibers are responsive only within a restricted range of frequencies and intensities. This frequency-intensity domain is known as the response area, which may be considered analogous to the receptive field in the visual and somatic sensory systems. A plot of the threshold sound intensity vs stimulus frequency is known as the *tuning curve* of the fiber (Fig. 9). The frequency of lowest threshold is designated as the best or characteristic frequency. Different fibers have different best frequencies, reflecting their connections along the basilar membrane. Fibers with high best frequencies are connected to basal regions of the cochlea, and fibers with low best frequencies are connected more toward the apical regions.

The CNS receives information about stimulus frequency in terms of which fibers are activated in accordance with the place principle of pitch perception. However, at even moderate intensity, the tuning curve is relatively broad, especially on the low-frequency side. If the place principle is the only mechanism that allows pitch identification by the CNS, we can assume

that all of the activity is ignored except at the peak or that the place principle operates only near the threshold of hearing. Because neither possibility seems reasonable, there must be other mechanisms for coding acoustic information. The *time principle* states that the acoustic waveform is encoded in the temporal discharge pattern of auditory nerve fibers.

4.2. Temporal Properties

Information about the frequency of low-frequency tones is conveyed to the CNS by another method. When the fiber discharges, it tends to do so around the same phase of the stimulus waveform, corresponding to movements of the basilar membrane that move the hair bundles of the hair cells in the excitatory direction (Fig. 10). This phenomenon is called *phase-locking*, and in mammals is observed only at frequencies below about 4000 Hz. This temporal coding of low-frequency sounds is important because the energy in speech signals is predominantly below 4000 Hz (*see* Fig. 2), and the changes in sound pressure resulting from complex sounds consisting of many low-frequency spectral components are encoded in the temporal discharge in a similar fashion. With phase-locking, the time interval between spikes tends to be a multiple of the period of the stimulating tone. No single fiber fires on every

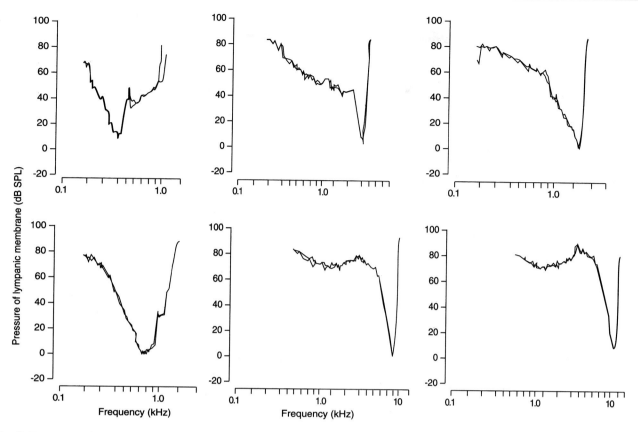

Fig. 9. Representative tuning curves (e.g., frequency threshold curves) of cat auditory-nerve fibers are shown for six different regions. In each panel, two fibers from the same animal of similar characteristic frequency and threshold are shown, indicating the constancy of tuning under such circumstances. (Redrawn from Liberman MC, Kiang NYS. Acoustic trauma in cats: cochlear pathology and auditory-nerve activity. Acta Otolaryngol (Suppl.) 1978; 358:1.)

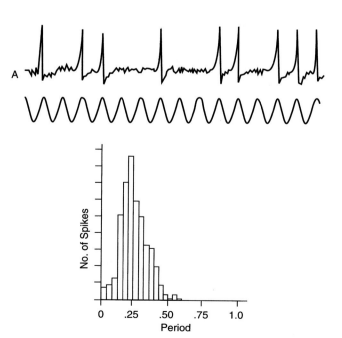

cycle of a tone, but if we consider an array of many fibers, the phenomenon known as volleying is revealed. In the total array of responding fibers, there are discharges in some fibers on each of the stimulus cycles. Information about the period (and thus the frequency) of a low-frequency tone is represented in the temporal rhythm of nerve impulses. The CNS uses these rhythms to encode speech sounds and to localize a sound source in space. Mechanisms by which the timing of neural volleys from the two ears is used in sound localization are described in the following sections.

Fig. 10. (*Left*) Representation of the phase-locked response of a single auditory-nerve fiber to a low-frequency tone. The period histogram below it shows the distribution of phase angles at which the nerve preferentially discharges.

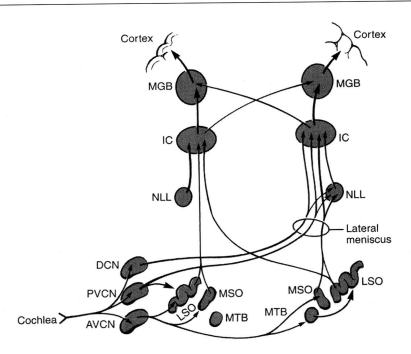

Fig. 11. The ascending (afferent) neuronal chain from the cochlea to the cortex: spiral ganglion, cochlear nucleus, superior olivary complex, inferior colliculus, and medial geniculate. Notice the many crossed pathways that allow interactions between the outputs of the two ears. AVCN, anteroventral cochlear nucleus; DCN, dorsal cochlear nucleus; IC, inferior colliculus; LSO, lateral superior olive; MGB, medial geniculate body; MSO, medial superior olive; MTB; medial nucleus of trapezoid body; NLL, nucleus of lateral lemniscus; PVCN, posteroventral cochlear nucleus.

5. THE CENTRAL AUDITORY SYSTEM

5.1. The Central Auditory Pathway Consists of Many Relay Nuclei

The central auditory pathway comprises a number of nuclear groups within the medulla, pons, midbrain, thalamus, and cerebral cortex. These cell groups are interconnected by fiber tracts that ascend from the cochlea to the auditory cortex (Fig. 11). These pathways carry information about the acoustic environment that reaches consciousness. A descending pathway carries information back to the cochlea, primarily to the outer hair cells, but we do not understand the function of these descending pathways. Other pathways that communicate acoustic reflexes that are activated by sound stimulation and involve various motor systems to move the head, eyes, and ears, which are not described here.

5.1.1. COCHLEAR NUCLEUS

The cochlear nucleus is composed of a complex of cell groups on the lateral surfaces of the medulla within which all auditory nerve fibers terminate. Entering auditory-nerve fibers bifurcate in an orderly way,

sending an ascending branch to innervate cells in the *anteroventral cochlear nucleus* (AVCN) and a descending branch to innervate neurons in the *posteroventral* (PVCN) and *dorsal cochlear nuclei* (DCN). The ascending auditory pathways coming out of the cochlear nucleus to the lower brainstem exhibit a bewildering combination of bilateral and unilateral connections. For example, the AVCN projects bilaterally to the medial superior olive, but only unilaterally to the ipsilateral lateral superior olive. From the medial superior olive, there is an ipsilateral projection to the inferior colliculus, but the lateral superior olive projects to the inferior colliculi of both sides. As we will see, these particular connections do make sense functionally because they are the basis for the representation of contralateral space in the auditory system.

5.1.2. SUPERIOR OLIVARY COMPLEX

The superior olivary complex lies in the tegmentum of the pons and consists of several subdivisions. One of the most significant aspects of the superior olivary complex is that it is the first point at which outputs from the two ears converge. Evidence shows that the various subdivisions of the superior olivary complex are involved in different aspects of the processing of the acoustic signal, especially for binaural processing. The superior olivary complex projects to the inferior colliculi of both sides by way of the lateral lemniscus and to the nuclei of the lateral lemniscus. The superior olivary complex also is the source of the efferent projection back to the cochlear hair cells.

5.1.3. INFERIOR COLLICULUS

The inferior colliculus comprises the caudal pair of protuberances that make up the roof of the midbrain. Although the superior colliculus is primarily visual in function, the inferior colliculus is an important auditory relay station. It receives input from the cochlear nuclear complex, superior olivary complex, nuclei of the lateral lemniscus, and inferior colliculus of the opposite side. All fibers ascending in the *lateral lemniscus* synapse in the inferior colliculus.

Many neurons in the inferior colliculus, like those in the superior olivary complex, are sensitive to extraordinarily small differences in the time of arrival of the stimulus at the two ears, or small differences in interaural intensity. The inferior colliculus is also tonotopically organized. Although the inferior colliculus sends its axons centrally only as far as the medial geniculate body, it receives an impressive descending projection from the auditory cortex. The output of the inferior colliculus travels by way of the brachium of the inferior colliculus to innervate the medial geniculate body of the thalamus on the same side, and there is a smaller contralateral projection.

5.1.4. MEDIAL GENICULATE BODY

The medial geniculate body represents the thalamic relay for auditory information. Its neurons project in an orderly fashion to the auditory areas of the cerebral cortex by way of the sublenticular portion of the internal capsule. The auditory cortex projects back on the medial geniculate body in a highly organized way. The medial geniculate body is also tonotopically organized.

5.1.5. AUDITORY CORTEX

The cortical auditory receiving areas in humans and other primates is located on the dorsal surface of the superior temporal lobe. In humans, it occupies one or more of the transverse gyri of Heschl in Brodmann's areas 41 and 42. The auditory cortex is not uniform in its cellular architecture. It consists of a primary receiving area which is tonotopically organized and which has a relatively uniform cellular structure throughout.

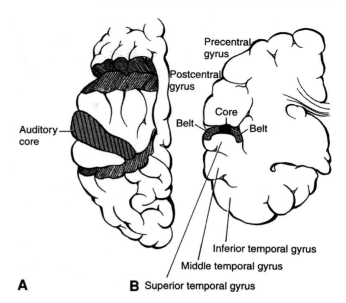

Fig. 12. The human auditory cortex in the first transverse gyrus of the temporal lobe. **(A)** The parietal lobe has been removed to reveal the superior temporal plane as seen from above. **(B)** A frontal section passes through the auditory cortex, showing the core area (A1) buried in the sylvian fissure, surrounded by a belt area of auditory association cortex. (Redrawn from Neff WD, Diamond IT, Casseday JH. Handbook of sensory physiology: auditory system: physiology (CNS): behavioral studies: psychoacoustics. Berlin: Springer-Verlag, 1975; 307.)

Several other auditory cortical fields can be identified surrounding the auditory core (Fig. 12). Each auditory cortical area has complex afferent and efferent connections with the thalamus, with nearby cortical fields, and with auditory areas in the opposite hemisphere. The functional significance of multiple cortical areas is unknown, although it has been suggested that each processes a different aspect of the acoustic stimulus.

5.2. Central Auditory Neurons Show Some Common General Properties

A microelectrode inserted into the auditory nerve or a central auditory nucleus records trains of action potentials that are evoked by sounds reaching the ears. This method has enabled study of the way in which acoustic information is encoded in trains of nerve spikes and in the transformations that take place in these spike trains at successive levels of the auditory system. Many of the response properties of auditory-nerve fibers are also observed in neurons throughout the auditory pathway. However, numerous transformations in the sound-evoked discharge take place at each successive synaptic station as the result of convergence of excitatory and inhibitory activity from various sources.

One obvious transformation is illustrated in Fig. 11. Notice that the projection from the cochlear nucleus to the superior olivary complex is bilateral, as is the projection from the superior olivary complex to the inferior colliculus. This means that, starting from the superior olivary complex, most auditory neurons respond to stimulation of either ear. The nature of binaural interactions is discussed later.

In general, most central auditory neurons have a best or characteristic frequency. Their response areas and tuning curves share similarities with those of auditory nerve fibers, but many differences are also apparent. One general property found in many central auditory neurons is the presence of *inhibitory sidebands* in the response area. Sidebands are presumably the result of inhibitory circuits that allow cells responding to a particular frequency to inhibit the responses of other cells that are tuned to neighboring frequencies. These sidebands limit the response areas of single cells to narrower frequency ranges, and are reminiscent of the center-surround receptive fields of visual neurons.

Another common characteristic of all the major auditory nuclei is a tonotopic organization. The distribution of best frequencies of single neurons can be studied systematically by microelectrode recording techniques. The resultant three-dimensional map is an orderly arrangement of best frequencies that is referred to as *tonotopic organization*. This organization is a reflection of the preservation of the orderly projection of eighth cranial-nerve fibers from the cochlea to the CNS. Because frequency representation is related to the spatial distribution of points of maximal displacement along the basilar membrane, this organization also can be referred to as cochleotopic. It can be viewed in much the same way as retinotopic organization in the visual system and somatotopic organization in the somatic sensory system.

5.3. The Information Is Transformed in the Cochlear Nucleus

The fibers of the cochlear nerve terminate in an orderly way within the three cochlear nucleus subdivisions, the AVCN, PVCN, and DCN, preserving the innervation pattern along the basilar membrane. The result is that each subdivision is tonotopically organized.

The morphology of the cells and auditory-nerve terminals within each subdivision determine the type of information that is relayed to higher auditory centers. Cells in the PVCN and DCN receive bouton endings from auditory-nerve fibers and from interneurons and higher centers. This neuronal network results in interactions of excitation and inhibition that are reflected in the complex discharge patterns of single neurons, which differ considerably from the incoming volleys in eighth cranial-nerve fibers. Some bushy cells in AVCN receive very specialized endings (e.g., *end bulbs of Held*) from just a few auditory nerve fibers. Figure 13 shows one of these end bulbs making contact with a "bushy cell" in the AVCN. Notice the unique morphology of the synaptic ending, which ensures that an action potential on the auditory nerve fiber is transmitted with great temporal fidelity to the AVCN. As a result, the activity of these bushy cells has been found to be similar to the activity in incoming auditory nerve fibers. In this case, the bushy cells serve as relay cells, with little transformation of the input. The end bulb synapse on bushy cells is an example of a unique specialization in the auditory system, which is believed to preserve timing information.

An important function of the bushy cells in the AVCN is to relay the precise low-frequency time information carried by auditory-nerve fibers. In fact, the convergence of a few end-bulb synapses on each bushy cells has been found to actually enhance the ability of bushy cell to encode the temporal information as compared to their auditory-nerve inputs. This time information is relayed primarily to the superior olivary complex, which is the first region in the brain in which outputs from the two ears converge. On the other extreme are cells in the DCN, which only respond to acoustic inputs with a single spike, or with some complex pattern of discharges that bear no simple relation to the acoustic stimulus. Some intrinsic circuitry in the DCN or the membrane properties of these cells are responsible for a different kind of transformation. We do not understand the reasons for all of these different transformations, and the only one addressed in this chapter is that of the bushy cell in the AVCN. Already at the first relay station, the auditory and visual systems manifest different processing schemes. Most of the lateral geniculate neuron cells relay the signals from the ganglion cells, but only a subset of the cochlear nucleus cells can be considered to be relay cells.

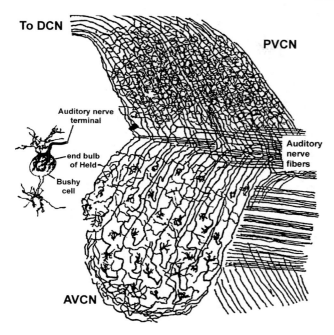

Fig. 13. Axons of the cochlear nerve entering ventral cochlear nuclei. Each axon branches to send an ascending branch to the anteroventral (AVCN) nucleus, which is characterized by specialized end bulbs and limited convergence from the cochlea, and a descending branch to the dorsal (DCN) and posteroventral (PVCN) nuclei. Notice the difference in the morphology of the terminals and the orderly, cochleotopic arrangement of fibers. (Adapted from Histologie du systeme nerveux (Vol 1). Madrid: Instituto Ramon y Cajal, 1909.)

5.4. Binaural Interactions Are Important for Sound Localization

In analyzing the anatomic connections of the central auditory system, it has been emphasized that some cells receive input from both ears. What are the advantages of having two ears instead of one? If one ear is plugged, it is clear that many acoustic tasks are not affected. It is still possible to understand speech, perceive music, and discriminate sounds of different pitch. However, certain tasks are much more difficult to perform with only one ear. Two tasks especially depend on binaural hearing: the ability to localize the source of sound and the ability to differentiate one sound from background noise. Psychophysical tests have demonstrated that localizing a sound source along the horizontal plane depends largely on the differences in the sound that reaches the two ears. Related to this is the ability to focus on a single sound source in noisy environment, which is commonly referred to as the

"cocktail party" phenomenon. The latter ability is a common complaint of patients suffering from presbycusis (e.g., progressive, bilateral, symmetric hearing loss in the elderly).

There are two important cues for sound localization: *interaural level differences* (ILDs) and *interaural time differences* (ITDs), as shown in Fig. 14. A listener employs one or both cues in localizing a sound source. For low-frequency tones (below about 1000 Hz), a listener relies on ITD cues for sound localization, and for higher-frequency tones, the listener relies on ILDs. This dichotomy between the cues used for localizing high- and low-frequency tones is known as the *duplex theory of sound localization*, which is valid only for pure tones. Corresponding to the duplex theory, the ability to localize pure tones is worst in the mid-frequency range, where neither cue is very effective and improves at both higher and lower frequencies. The localization of complex sounds, which contain both high and low frequencies, uses both mechanisms. Because fundamentally different processes are required for encoding ITDs and ILDs, this processing could be expected to use different anatomic structures and physiologic mechanisms. This is the case in the superior olivary complex: some cells are important for encoding ITDs, and others encode ILDs.

Acoustically, the ears can he regarded as a pair of holes that are separated by a spherical obstacle, the head. Sound on one side of the head reaches the farther ear some 30 μs later for each additional centimeter it must travel. If we assign a radius of about 20 cm to the spherical head, the maximal ITD is about 600 μs, though the actual maximal ITD in humans is about 800–900 μs. This maximal ITD occurs if the stimulus is located directly to one side; it is as far as possible from the opposite ear.

The ability of the auditory system to detect ITDs is remarkable. Under optimal conditions, the just noticeable difference in ITD in humans is 6 μs. This is accomplished in a nervous system that uses action potentials whose width and synaptic delays are over 100 times longer! Animals that are specialized for acoustic communication can do even better; bats can detect interaural arrival times of echoes of less than l μs. The preservation of timing information is clearly an important task for the central auditory system. How does the auditory system achieve this discrimination? The end bulbs of Held are one anatomic specialization for preserving timing information.

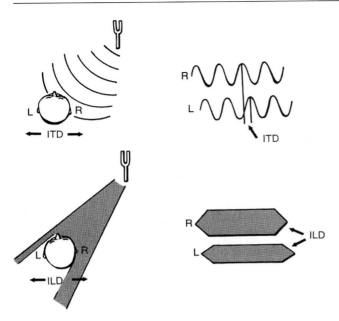

Fig. 14. The drawings illustrate interaural time differences (ΔT) for a low-frequency tone (*top*) and level differences (ΔL) for a high-frequency tone (*bottom*) when a sound source is off the midline. Those on the left are schematic diagrams of the physical situation; those on the right are the signals received at the right (R) and left (L) ears. For the high-frequency tone, only the envelope of the sine curve is shown.

ILDs are not so simple in behavior. The far ear lies in a sound shadow whose depth depends on the direction and wavelength of the sound. The head acts as an effective acoustic shadow only if the wavelength of the sound is smaller than the size of the head. The head can act as an effective acoustic shadow only at higher frequencies. For the size of human heads, interaural intensity differences are negligible at frequencies below about 1000 Hz, and may be as great as 20 dB at 10 kHz.

For several of the auditory nuclei, spatial maps of ITDs or ILDs have been described, creating neural maps of the acoustic environment. Such maps are fundamentally different from the topographic maps of the body and retinotopic maps of the visual world that are seen at all levels of the somatosensory and visual systems. Auditory space does not map onto the cochlea, which differentiates it from the sensory maps of somesthesia and vision that are direct projections of the sensory surface. The auditory map is said to be a *computational map*, because it must be derived from neuronal processing of the cues—the ITDs and IIDs—that produce the map.

Studies of the encoding of sound localization cues in the central auditory system have shown that, above the level of the superior olivary complex, the representation of auditory space is primarily of the contralateral sound field. Patients with lesions of the auditory cortex, for example, are unable to localize sounds originating from the contralateral sound field, without deficits in detection or discrimination of the sound. The auditory system derives a map of the contralateral field just as the visual and somatosensory maps in the CNS are of the contralateral visual field and body. The contralateral representation in the auditory system is derived from the particular way in which some fibers cross and others remain uncrossed in the ascending projection from the cochlear nucleus to the inferior colliculus. There is order behind the seemingly haphazard interconnections of the various auditory nuclei.

5.5. The Physiology of the Auditory System Is Reflected Clinically

5.5.1. BRAINSTEM AUDITORY EVOKED RESPONSE

One of the clinically important consequences of the preservation of temporal information by the peripheral and central auditory system is that it allows a record of the *brainstem auditory evoked potential* (BAEP). This record consists of complex, time-locked, electrical slow waves, which can be recorded from the scalp (e.g., non-invasively, like electroencephalographic patterns) of human subjects in response to a brief, abrupt sound, such as a click or tone burst (Fig. 15). These electrical potentials are extremely low in amplitude (some <1 μV) and are usually lost within the higher-amplitude spontaneous activity recorded on the electroencephalogram (EEG). However, by using computer signal-averaging techniques, it is possible to extract from the EEG a well-defined complex waveform whose peaks and troughs can be associated with activity in various parts of the auditory system.

Many recognized components of an auditory evoked potential have been somewhat arbitrarily divided into three epochs: early-, middle-, and long-latency components. The early components, defined as those that occur during the first 8 ms after stimulus onset, are believed to represent activation of the cochlea and auditory nuclei of the brainstem, and it is these early components that are clinically of interest. The middle and late components represent a mixture of activity in the brainstem and higher auditory centers and in the association cortex.

During the past few years, the early components have been employed in evaluating hearing loss and in

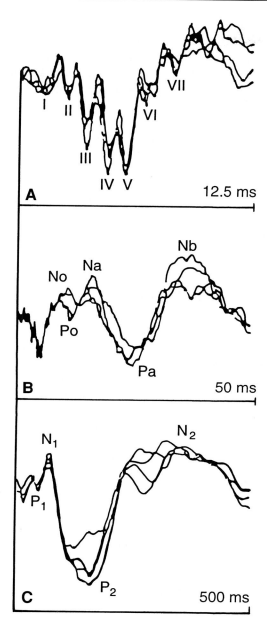

Fig. 15. Scalp-evoked potentials shown on three different time scales. (**A**) Auditory brain stem responses. (**B**) Middle components. (**C**) Late components. Electrodes are vertex to mastoid (positive up). Each trace shows the average of 1024 clicks (60 dB SL) delivered at 1/s to the right ear. Labels shown are commonly used for individual wave components. (Redrawn from Picton TW, Hillyard SA, Krausz HI, Galambos R. Human auditory evoked potentials, I: evaluation of components. Electroenceph Clin Neurophysiol 1974; 36;179.)

helping to diagnose trauma or disease involving the brainstem. This technique is proving to be important in assessing the hearing of persons unwilling (e.g., malingerers) or unable (e.g., newborns, the mentally retarded) to cooperate in routine audiometric testing.

The ability to identify the activity of specific auditory nuclei by the presence of characteristic waves of the BAEP is of great clinical value. Many of the children who had previously been believed to he "slow learners" or developmentally disabled were instead found to be suffering from hearing loss. The absence or degradation of acoustic input during the first few years, when the recognition and expression of speech is so critical, can cause permanent developmental damage, which can he prevented by restoring the acoustic experience.

The reason that such analysis can be done in the auditory system and not in the visual system, for example, is that the specialization within the auditory system to preserve timing information of the stimulus results in a synchronous activation of many cells at each of the early brain stem nuclei. This synchrony is able to be detected by computer averaging even when recording from the scalp of a subject.

5.5.2. CONDUCTIVE AND SENSORINEURAL DEAFNESS

Anything that interferes with the transmission of sound to the hearing apparatus or of the neural signal to the auditory cortex can produce deafness. There are two major categories of deafness: conductive and sensorineural deafness. *Conduction deafness* is caused by a malfunction in the transmission of sound through the middle ear. A common example, particularly in young children, is the buildup of fluid in the middle ear because of infection known as otitis media. Treatment with antibiotics has greatly reduced the incidence of conductive hearing loss from otitis media. In adults, otosclerosis is the most frequent cause of conduction deafness, in which there is overgrowth of the labyrinthine bone around the oval window, leading to fixation of the stapes. This condition can often be treated by surgical intervention to loosen or replace the stapes. Boosting the input to the ear with a hearing aid alleviates many cases of conduction deafness.

Sensorineural or *nerve deafness* is caused by damage to the cochlea, to the auditory nerve, or to the central auditory system. There are many causes of sensorineural deafness. The hair cells of the inner ear are especially susceptible to damage from prolonged exposure to loud sounds, antibiotics (such as streptomycin, kanamycin, or gentamicin), or rubella infection *in utero*. The most common type of hearing loss in the aged—presbycusis—is characterized by a progressive loss of high frequencies, which is probably caused by progressive changes in the cochlea. In the central auditory system, any damage to the pathways leading from the cochlear nucleus to the auditory cortex can result in deafness. Acoustic neuroma, a tumor that develops in the auditory nerve in the internal auditory meatus or at the the cerebellopontine angle, produces an ipsilateral deafness, tinnitus (e.g., sensation of ringing in the ears), or vestibular problems. Not much can be done about most cases of sensorineural deafness.

Because many cases of sensorineural deafness involve problems in the cochlea without involvement of the auditory nerve fibers or central connections, it may be possible to stimulate the auditory nerve fibers electrically. Much attention has been focused in recent years on the development of a cochlear prosthesis in which an electrode is implanted directly into the cochlea. Electrical stimulation of the cochlear implant can activate the still viable ends of auditory-nerve fibers, and some sense of hearing can be restored.

It is important to differentiate conductive from sensorineural deafness, because many types of conductive deafness can be treated. This is particularly important in young children during the critical time during which they are learning language. Two tests with tuning forks are helpful. They both rely on the fact that the middle ear can be bypassed when the sound is delivered directly to the bone. Air conduction usually is much more efficient than bone conduction, but in cases of conductive deafness, bone conduction becomes more efficient. Weber's test can be used when a patient complains of deafness in one ear. A vibrating tuning fork (usually 512 Hz) is applied to the forehead at the midline, and the resulting vibrations are conducted through the bone to each ear. Patients with conduction deafness report that the sound is heard louder in the deaf ear, presumably because bone conduction is equal in the two ears, but the deaf ear also hears no background noise from the air. Patients with sensorineural deafness cannot hear the sound even through bone conduction and report that it is louder in the normal ear. In *Rinne's test*, the tuning fork is applied to the mastoid process. As soon as the sound ceases, the fork is moved to just outside the auditory meatus. In a normal ear, the fork is heard again when the sound waves travel by air conduction, because it is

more efficient than bone conduction. In conduction deafness, the fork's vibration remains imperceptible when held next to the ear. In sensorineural deafness, the reverse is true, although the thresholds for air and bone conduction are increased.

5.5.3. Effects of Lesions in the Auditory Cortex

Lesions of the auditory cortex make up a special case of sensorineural deafness. Many behavioral experiments have been conducted using cats, and extensive damage to these areas has little effect on the animal's ability to discriminate between tones of different frequencies or intensities. The major effect appears to be on the animal's ability to localize the source of a sound in space and to discriminate between complex sound patterns.

There have been numerous reports in the literature on the effects of temporal-lobe damage in humans. Unfortunately, in only a few cases complete audiometric tests have been made and postmortem examination of the brain have been carried out. It is not surprising that conflicting reports have appeared on the effects of temporal-lobe damage on hearing in humans. However, several effects usually are detected in humans after auditory cortical damage. After the period following bilateral lesions of the auditory cortex, the pure tone hearing threshold appears to return to normal, and there is usually little or no change in threshold. There is also little or no change in discrimination of alterations in intensity or frequency. Deficiencies are detected more commonly for the discrimination of changes in the temporal order or sequence of sounds, their duration, or in the abiliy to localize sounds in space.

SELECTED READINGS

Gilkey RH, Anderson TR (eds). Binaural and Spatial Hearing in Real and Virtual Environments. Mahwah, NJ: Lawrence Erlbaum Assoc., 1997; 1–795

Popper AN, Fay RR (eds). The Mammalian Auditory Pathway: Neurophysiology. New York: Springer-Verlag, 1992: 1–43.

Webster DB, Popper AN, Fay RR (eds). The Mammalian Auditory Pathway: Neuroanatomy. New York: Springer-Verlag, 1992: 1–485.

25 The Vestibular System

Robert F. Spencer* and A. Tucker Gleason

CONTENTS

1. VESTIBULAR PATHWAYS

1.1. Vestibular Receptors in the Semicircular Canals and Otolith Organs Are Innervated by Neurons in Scarpa's Ganglion

The vestibular portion of the membranous labyrinth consists of three pairs of *semicircular canals*, the horizontal, anterior, and posterior, and two pairs of *otolith organs*, the *utricle* and the *saccule* (Fig. 1). Like the cochlea, these structures are filled with endolymph, which communicates with the cochlea through the ductus reuniens. The horizontal, anterior, and posterior semicircular canals are oriented nearly at right angles to one another, and the result is the representation of the three rotational dimensions of space. When the head is tilted approx 25° forward, the horizontal canal is in the horizontal plane, and the anterior and posterior canals, also known as the vertical canals, are in vertical planes. As for the otolith organs, the utricle is oriented almost horizontally, and the saccule is oriented almost vertically in the sagittal plane. The receptors for the vestibular system are hair cells that are morphologically similar to those in the organ of Corti in the cochlea. These receptors are located in the cristae ampullares of the semicircular canals and in the maculae of the utricle and saccule.

*Deceased.

From: *Neuroscience in Medicine, 2nd ed.* (P. Michael Conn, ed.), © 2003 Humana Press Inc., Totowa, NJ.

A *crista ampullaris* is located in the ampullated (or widened) end of each of the semicircular canals. The neurosensory epithelium of each crista ampullaris is composed of supporting cells and two types of hair cells. Projecting from each hair cell are *stereocilia* (40–110 per cell) and a single *kinocilium* (Fig. 2). The cilia are embedded in a gelatinous *cupula* that extends to the roof of the ampulla. The stereocilia for each hair cell have graded lengths that increase in the direction of the kinocilium. All hair cells in the crista ampullaris of a single canal are arranged in the same fashion, with all kinocilia in the same ampulla positioned on the same side of the hair cell. In the horizontal canals, the polarization of the kinocilia is toward the utricle (e.g, utriculopetal), and in the vertical canals, the polarization of the kinocilia is away from the utricle (e.g., utriculofugal). The hair cells in the cristae of the semicircular canals are stimulated by an appropriate *angular acceleration* of the head that causes relative movement of the endolymph, with a resulting deflection of the cilia.

The utricle and the saccule each contain a *macula* (Fig. 3). As in the cristae, the neurosensory epithelium of each of the maculae consists of hair cells and supporting cells, and the hair cells have bundles of stereocilia and a single kinocilium. These cells are embedded in an otolithic membrane, which is a gelatinous matrix containing *statoconia* (calcium carbonate crystals). The hair cells in the maculae of the utricle and saccule are stimulated by an appropriate *linear acceleration* of the head that produces deflection of the cilia by the

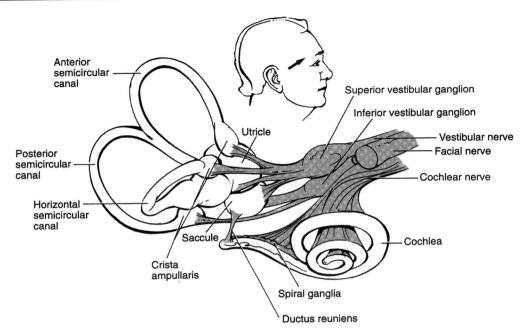

Fig. 1. Components of the membranous labyrinth: the three semicircular canals (e.g., horizontal, anterior, and posterior), the otolith organs (e.g., saccule and utricle), and the cochlea. The spiral-shaped cochlea winds around a central bony modiolus. Bipolar neurons in the spiral ganglion innervate hair cells in the organ of Corti, and their central processes form the cochlear nerve. Peripheral processes of bipolar neurons in the superior and inferior vestibular (Scarpa's) ganglia innervate hair cells in the cristae ampullares of the semicircular canals and the maculae of the saccule and utricle, and their central processes form the vestibular nerve. The *arrow* indicates the plane of the horizontal semicircular canal.

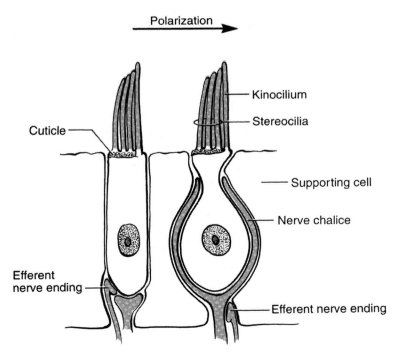

Fig. 2. Two principal types of hair cells in the cristae of the semicircular canals and the maculae of the otolith organs. Type I hair cells are goblet-shaped and are innervated by chalice-type nerve endings that arise from large-diameter axons of bipolar neurons in the vestibular (Scarpa's) ganglion. Type II hair cells are columnar and have simple nerve endings associated with small-diameter axons at the base of the cells. Vestibular efferent nerve endings establish synaptic connections with the primary afferent ending

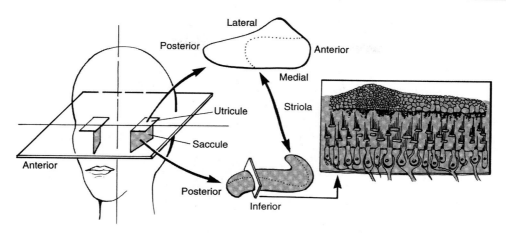

Fig. 3. Spatial orientation of the utricle and saccule. The maculae of the utricle and saccule are curved structures on which the hair cells are polarized in opposite directions in relation to the striola, which corresponds to the maximal thickness of the overlying layer of statoconia. In the macula of the utricle, which is oriented approximately parallel to the ground, the hair cells are polarized *toward* the striola on each side. In the macula of the saccule, which is oriented approximately perpendicular to the ground, the hair cells are polarized *away from* the striola. The shape of the maculae of the utricle and saccule and the polarizations of their respective hair cells effectively provide a means of responding to linear accelerations in three dimensions.

overlying statoconia. The orientation of the maculae of the utricle and saccule serves to represent linear acceleration vectors produced by gravity or by translation of the head.

The macula of the utricle is located on the floor of the utricle. When the head is upright, the macula is oriented almost parallel with the ground. The posterior end is horizontal, and the anterior end is elevated about 45° from the horizontal. As in the cristae of the semicircular canals, the hair cells in the utricular macula are polarized, but they have a different arrangement (Fig. 3). Half of the macula is stimulated by displacement of the statoconia in one direction, but the other half is inhibited, and the opposite is true for the opposite direction. The utricular macula is stimulated predominantly by linear forces near the horizontal plane, such as those encountered while accelerating or decelerating in a car.

The macula of the saccule is an elongated structure that lies perpendicular to the ground when the head is upright (Fig. 3). The vertical orientation of the saccular macula suggests that the cilia are deflected optimally by vertically directed linear forces of the head, such as those encountered while riding in an elevator.

The *hair cells* in the cristae of the semicircular canals and the maculae of the utricle and saccule are similar to those seen in the cochlea. There are two types of hair cells (Fig. 2). *Type I hair cells* are spherical or goblet-shaped cells (similar to inner hair cells in the cochlea), and are innervated by a large chalice-like afferent ending which encompasses most of the cell. These cells typically respond to strong stimulation. *Type II hair cells* are smaller and cylindrical (similar to outer hair cells in the cochlea), and afferent and efferent endings are distributed at the base of the cell. These cells are innervated by small-diameter afferent axons, and respond to weak stimulation. As in the cochlea, vestibular hair cells are activated or inhibited by deflection of the cilia. In the cristae, the cilia are displaced by movement of the cupula caused by the flow of endolymph through the canals as the head moves. In the maculae, changes in the position of the head produce a shearing effect of the statoconia on the cilia. In both cases, each hair cell is activated when its cilia are displaced toward the kinocilium, and is inhibited with displacement in the opposite direction.

The mechanism of activation of vestibular hair cells is the same as that described for cochlear hair cells.

(*Fig. 2. continued*) on type I hair cells and directly on the base of type II hair cells. Both types of hair cells have an array of stereocilia that are polarized according to increasing length in the direction of the kinocilium. In the crista ampullaris, the stereocilia and kinocilia are embedded in a gelatinous cupula, and in the macula, they contact the crystalline statoconia matrix. The structural and innervational differences between the two types of hair cells are correlated with differences in their physiological activity.

With deflection of the cilia toward the kinocilium, the hair cells are depolarized by an influx of K^+ from the surrounding endolymph, which activates voltage-sensitive Ca^{2+} channels. The influx of Ca^{2+} produces the release of a neurotransmitter, which causes activation of the primary vestibular afferent terminal. Because the hair cells normally have a small influx of K^+ at rest, deflection of the cilia in the opposite direction closes the cation channels, resulting in hyperpolarization of the cell and decreased neurotransmitter release.

The innervation of hair cells in the semicircular canals and the otolith organs is provided by *bipolar neurons* in the vestibular (Scarpa's) ganglion, which lies at the base of the internal auditory meatus. Peripheral processes from neurons in the superior division of the ganglion provide innervation for the anterior and horizontal semicircular canals as well as the macula of the utricle and part of the saccule. Bipolar neurons in the inferior division of the ganglion innervate hair cells in the posterior semicircular canal and most of the macula of the saccule. The central processes of these bipolar neurons form the superior and inferior branches of the vestibular portion of the vestibulocochlear, or eighth cranial nerve.

The information transmitted by vestibular nerve axons is related to head movement and head position, and is encoded in the frequency of discharge of primary vestibular axons. Topographic organization, like that in other sensory systems (e.g., somatotopic, retinotopic, or tonotopic), is not apparent in the vestibular system.

1.2. Central Vestibular Connections and Pathways Are Related to the Control of Gaze, Posture, and Balance

1.2.1. BRAINSTEM VESTIBULAR NUCLEI

The vestibular nerve courses through the cerebellopontine angle medial to the cochlear nerve, and enters the brainstem dorsally between the inferior cerebellar peduncle and the spinal trigeminal tract. Most vestibular fibers terminate in one or more of the brainstem vestibular nuclei (Fig. 4). These nuclei lie in the floor of the fourth ventricle and extend from a level rostral to the hypoglossal nucleus to slightly beyond the level of the abducens nucleus. The nuclei of the brainstem vestibular complex are arranged in two longitudinal columns: the lateral column consists of the inferior (i.e., spinal or descending) vestibular nucleus, the lateral vestibular nucleus of Deiters,

and the superior vestibular nucleus of Bechterew. The medial (e.g., triangular) vestibular nucleus of Schwalbe constitutes the medial cell column.

On entering the brainstem vestibular complex, most primary fibers bifurcate into ascending and descending rami. In general, primary vestibular fibers that innervate the cristae of the semicircular canals project predominantly to rostral portions of the brainstem vestibular complex, including the superior vestibular nucleus, ventral portions of the lateral vestibular nucleus, and rostral portions of the medial vestibular nucleus. The primary vestibular fibers that innervate the maculae of the otolith organs terminate in caudal portions of the medial and inferior brainstem vestibular nuclei.

Some primary vestibular fibers bypass the brainstem vestibular nuclei and ascend to the cerebellum through the *juxtarestiform body* (Fig. 5). Cells in all parts of the vestibular ganglion send mossy fiber projections to the ipsilateral *nodulus* and *uvula* of the cerebellar vermis.

1.2.2. SECOND-ORDER VESTIBULAR CONNECTIONS

Unlike the auditory system and most other sensory systems, the central connections of the vestibular system are related primarily to motor behaviors. These behaviors include compensatory movements in response to changes in head and body position as well as the ongoing maintenance of balance and posture. These functions are achieved by connections of the brainstem vestibular nuclei with motor neurons in the extra-ocular motor nuclei, the spinal cord, and the cerebellum.

1.2.2.1. Vestibulocerebellar Fibers. The cerebellum plays a major role in the integration of vestibular and visual information. In addition to first-order vestibular ganglion neurons, some neurons in the superior, medial, and inferior brainstem vestibular nuclei project their axons through the juxtarestiform body bilaterally to the nodulus, uvula, and flocculus of the cerebellar cortex and to the *fastigial nucleus* (Fig. 5). Reciprocal connections with the cerebellum are achieved by cerebellovestibular fibers from the fastigial nuclei of both sides and from Purkinje cells in the ipsilateral flocculus that course through the juxtarestiform body to terminate in all four brainstem vestibular nuclei. In this manner, the cerebellum exerts considerable influence throughout the vestibular complex, which may play an important role in recovery following loss of vestibular function from illness or injury.

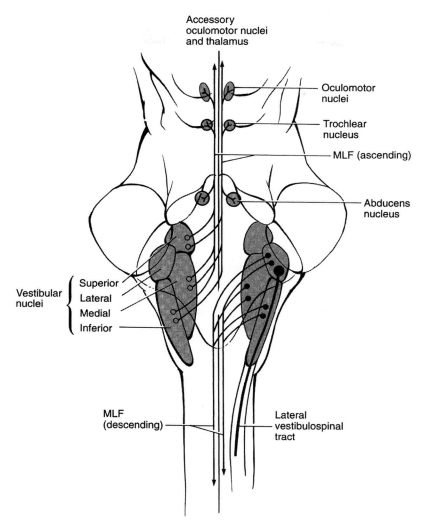

Accessory
oculomotor nuclei
and thalamus

Oculomotor
nuclei

Trochlear
nucleus

MLF (ascending)

Abducens
nucleus

Vestibular
nuclei

Superior

Lateral

Medial

Inferior

MLF
(descending)

Lateral
vestibulospinal
tract

Fig. 4. The ascending (*left*) and descending (*right*) vestibular pathways. Ipsilateral inhibitory and contralateral excitatory ascending projections from the vestibular nuclei course through the medial longitudinal fasciculus (MLF) and target motor neurons in the abducens, trochlear, and oculomotor nuclei. The ascending connections mediate the vestibulo–ocular reflex (VOR). Bilateral descending fibers in the MLF project primarily to motor neurons in the cervical spinal cord that innervate dorsal neck muscles, forming the basis for the vestibulo–collic reflex. The lateral vestibulospinal tract is formed from the lateral brainstem vestibular nuclei and descends ipsilaterally in the spinal cord, primarily targeting motor neurons that innervate axial extensor muscles that maintain posture.

1.2.2.2. Medial Longitudinal Fasciculus. The superior, medial, and inferior brainstem vestibular nuclei are the main sources of fibers that comprise the medial longitudinal fasciculus (MLF). Ascending fibers in the MLF from these nuclei project primarily to the oculomotor, trochlear, and abducens nuclei, which contain the motor neurons innervating the extra-ocular muscles, as well as to accessory oculomotor nuclei (Fig. 4).

The connections of second-order vestibular neurons with motor neurons in the extra-ocular motor nuclei are specific to the semicircular canal of origin and are related to the spatial orientation of the canals and their alignment with the pulling actions of the corresponding extra-ocular muscles (Fig. 6B). Excitatory second-order vestibular neurons that receive input from the posterior semicircular canal project to inferior rectus motor neurons in the oculomotor nucleus and superior oblique motor neurons in the trochlear nucleus. Bilateral activation of the posterior semicircular canals, which occurs when the head pitches up, results in downward eye movement. Excitatory sec-

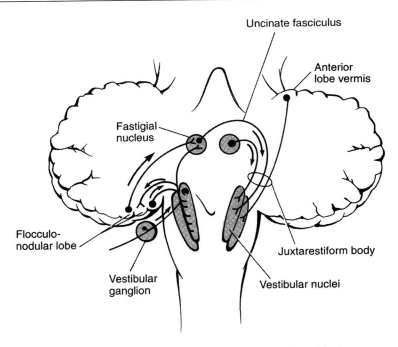

Fig. 5. Vestibulocerebellar and cerebellovestibular connections. First-order fibers from bipolar neurons in the vestibular ganglion and second-order fibers from neurons in the brainstem vestibular nuclei project to the flocculus, nodulus, and uvula of the cerebellar cortex (e.g., vestibulocerebellum) and to the fastigial nucleus by way of the juxtarestiform body. Purkinje cells in the cerebellar cortex project directly and indirectly by the fastigial nucleus to the brainstem vestibular nuclei through the juxtarestiform body. Purkinje cells in the vermis of the anterior lobe of the cerebellum (e.g., spinocerebellum) project directly through the juxtarestiform body to neurons in the lateral brainstem vestibular nucleus that are the cells of origin of the lateral vestibulospinal tract.

ond-order vestibular neurons that receive input from the anterior semicircular canal project to superior rectus and inferior oblique motor neurons in the oculomotor nucleus (Fig. 6C). Bilateral activation of the anterior semicircular canals, which occurs when the head pitches down, results in upward eye movement. Excitatory second-order vestibular neurons that receive input from the horizontal semicircular canal project directly to lateral rectus motor neurons in the abducens nucleus and indirectly to medial rectus motor neurons in the oculomotor nucleus by a relay neuron in the abducens nucleus, thereby controlling horizontal eye movements (Fig. 6D). Torsional eye movements, which occur in response to head roll, are produced by coactivation of the anterior and posterior semicircular canals on the same side (Fig. 6E).

In almost all cases, the motor neurons that innervate the antagonistic muscles are inhibited in the same canal-specific manner. Although transection of the MLF rostral to the abducens nucleus produces abnormalities in visually guided eye movements, labyrinthine stimulation still produces nystagmus. This finding is attributable to some fibers from the ventral lateral brainstem vestibular nucleus that course

uncrossed to the oculomotor nucleus through the ascending tract of Dieter's, which lies dorsolateral to the MLF in the pontine tegmentum. Some second-order vestibular fibers also may cross rostrally through an additional pathway in the ventral tegmentum.

Ascending second-order vestibular fibers in the MLF are involved with two general functions: maintained postural deviation of the eyes at rest, and postural adjustments of the eyes relative to the head and neck during movement. These postural adjustments are made in response to the combination of stimulation of the semicircular canals brought about by head rotation (e.g., angular acceleration) and proprioceptive impulses arising in the dorsal neck muscles that course through the spinovestibular tract. The proprioceptive input terminates in the inferior vestibular nucleus from which information is relayed to the motor nuclei of the extra-ocular muscles via the MLF. Vestibular connections with the oculomotor system form the basis of the vestibulo-ocular reflex (VOR).

The VOR is one example of vestibular function. The VOR is a compensatory eye movement that is an accurate reproduction of head movement, but in the opposite direction. The VOR functions to stabilize

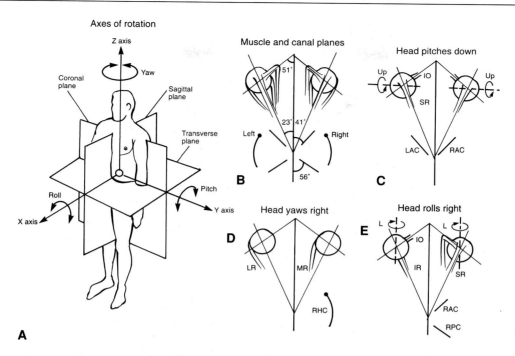

Fig. 6. Compensatory eye movements produced by movements of the head in the VOR. **(A)** The planes of reference and axes of rotation. **(B)** Angular relationship between the orientation of the semicircular canals and the pulling actions of the vertical extra-ocular muscles. The orientation of the anterior semicircular canal approximates the pulling action of the superior rectus muscle, and the orientation of the posterior semicircular canal approximates the pulling action of the superior oblique muscle. The orientation of the horizontal semicircular canal approximates the pulling actions of the lateral rectus and medial rectus muscles. **(C,D,E)** Activation of different pairs of extra-ocular muscles resulting from rotation in different axes. **(C)** When the head is pitched down, the anterior semicircular canals are excited bilaterally, producing a compensatory upward eye movement that results from activation of inferior oblique and superior rectus motor neurons. **(D)** A head turn to the right excites the right horizontal semicircular canal and inhibits the left horizontal semicircular canal, which produces a compensatory eye movement to the left resulting from activation of the left lateral rectus and right medial rectus muscles. **(E)** A roll movement to the right coactivates the anterior and posterior semicircular canals on the right side, producing a compensatory torsional eye movement achieved by activating the inferior oblique and inferior rectus muscles in the left eye and the superior oblique and superior rectus muscles in the right eye.

visual images on the retina despite movement of the observer, the object of visual regard, or both. These compensatory eye movements are always *conjugate*—both eyes moving simultaneously in the same direction (Fig. 6C–E).

Descending fibers in the MLF originate from the medial and inferior brainstem vestibular nuclei, and establish synaptic connections predominantly with motor neurons in the cervical spinal cord that innervate muscles of the neck and control movements of the head (Fig. 4). The descending limb of the MLF also is called the *medial vestibulospinal tract*, particularly with reference to fibers that project caudal to cervical levels. Some second-order vestibular neurons have axons that bifurcate and project to the extra-ocular motor nuclei and the cervical spinal cord.

1.2.2.3. Vestibular Commissural Connections.
The vestibular nuclei on both sides of the brainstem

are connected homotopically to the same nuclei on the contralateral side by direct and indirect excitatory and inhibitory commissural pathways. The direct commissural pathway courses through the dorsal tegmentum of the brainstem. Indirect connections use the vestibulocerebellar pathways and the *prepositus hypoglossi nucleus*, which is intimately related to the vestibular nuclei by extensive reciprocal connections. Vestibular commissural connections play a significant role in the phenomenon of *vestibular compensation*, which is a recovery of function from the deficits that are associated with peripheral lesions of the vestibular end organs or nerve.

1.2.2.4. Vestibular Efferent Connections.
Cholinergic neurons in the vicinity of the abducens nucleus project their axons into the vestibular nerve and establish efferent connections with the hair cells in the cristae of the semicircular canals and the maculae of the

otolith organs. Synaptic connections are made indirectly on type I hair cells via the primary afferent nerve endings and directly with the cell bodies of type II hair cells (Fig. 2). Little is known about the function of the vestibular efferent pathway. Because the synaptic connection of vestibular efferent neurons with vestibular hair cells is reminiscent of those established by efferent olivocochlear neurons with hair cells in the cochlea, it seems likely that the vestibular efferent pathway is capable of modulating the activity of the hair cells during movements of the head.

1.2.2.5. Vestibular-Thalamic-Cortical Pathway.
Some second-order fibers that project to the oculomotor and trochlear nuclei and the accessory oculomotor nuclei continue rostrally to terminate in the *ventral posterior inferior nucleus* of the thalamus, which is located in the vicinity of the ventral posterior somatosensory relay nuclei. The ventral posterior inferior nucleus projects to a distinct region of the postcentral gyrus, coextensive with Brodmann's area 3a. This region is believed to be responsible for complex position and movement perception, possibly by integrating vestibular information with proprioceptive information from joint afferents and group I muscle afferents.

1.2.2.6. Lateral Vestibulospinal Tract.
The lateral vestibulospinal tract arises from neurons that are located in the lateral vestibular nucleus (Fig. 4). Only the ventral portion of the lateral vestibular nucleus receives direct primary vestibular input from the semicircular canals. The dorsal region of the nucleus has connections with the vermis of the anterior lobe of the cerebellum, which is the site of termination of the dorsal spinocerebellar tract. The projection from the anterior cerebellar vermis to the lateral vestibular nucleus is somatotopically organized so that cervical regions are represented rostral and lumbar regions are represented caudal in the nucleus. The lateral vestibulospinal tract descends *uncrossed* in the anterior funiculus of the spinal cord and establishes *excitatory* synaptic connections with motor neurons in lamina IX, primarily at the cervical and lumbar levels of the spinal cord. The lateral vestibulospinal tract is involved in the regulation of posture by influencing motor neurons that primarily innervate axial *extensor muscles*.

These vestibulospinal fibers are necessary for the development of decerebrate rigidity induced by the rostral midbrain (e.g., intercollicular) transection, which interrupts descending rubrospinal fibers that control flexor muscles. The rigidity is abolished by destruction of the lateral vestibular nucleus or by interruption of the lateral vestibulospinal tract. Decerebrate rigidity is strictly an antigravity reaction that is characterized by tremendously increased tone in the antigravity muscles, apparently caused by an increased rate of firing of muscle spindles by gamma motor neurons. The increased firing rate of muscle-spindle afferents activates alpha motor neurons, which increase muscle tone.

2. NYSTAGMUS

Nystagmus is a rhythmic, oscillatory, involuntary movement that occurs in one or both eyes in any or all fields of gaze. Nystagmus is always pathologic if it occurs in the absence of stimulation, or is prolonged following stimulation. It may be induced in normal persons by two different methods: rotation, or caloric stimulation of the external auditory canals.

Postrotatory nystagmus is the result of angular acceleration produced by several seconds of rotation followed by a sudden stop. The fast phase of postrotatory nystagmus (e.g., the direction for which the nystagmus is named) is toward the side opposite to the direction of rotation. The slow phase (e.g., the active component) is in the same direction as rotation. When the head is rotated, the initial inertia of the endolymph in the semicircular canals deflects the cupula in one direction (Fig. 7A) producing *per-rotatory nystagmus* with the fast phase in the same direction as rotation. If the rotation is continued in the same direction, the endolymph eventually attains the same velocity of rotation as the canal and stimulation ceases (Fig. 7B). When the rotation suddenly stops, the inertia of the endolymph continues its flow, with a renewed stimulation of the vestibular cupula, but in the opposite direction (Fig. 7C). Stimulation of the vestibular receptors gives rise to potentials transmitted to the vestibular nuclei, which are then relayed through the MLF to the appropriate motor nuclei of the extra-ocular muscles, initiating a conjugate eye movement. Following rotation, if the person is asked to touch a certain point with the eyes closed, the arm deviates in the opposite direction of the nystagmus (e.g., past pointing). There is also a tendency to fall in this direction. The direction of past pointing and the tendency to fall are in accord with the fact that the slow phase of the nystagmus is the active component.

Caloric nystagmus depends on the production of convection currents in the endolymph of the semicircular canals by extreme temperature stimulation.

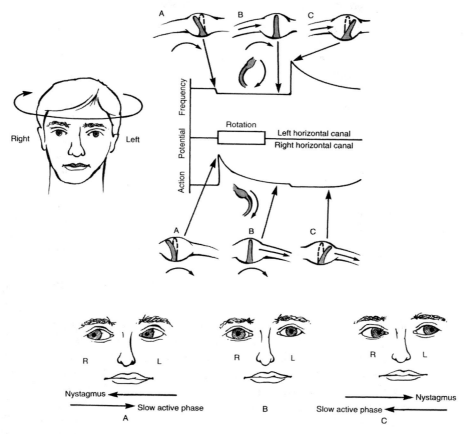

Fig. 7. Principles of rotatory nystagmus during rotation to the right. **(A)** At the start of rotation, as the head and horizontal semicircular canals begin to move, the endolymph remains stationary and effectively causes excitation of the right horizontal semicircular canal, inhibition of the left horizontal semicircular canal, and nystagmus to the right (e.g., in the direction of rotation). **(B)** During rotation, the head, semicircular canals, and endolymph are moving at the same velocity, and the eyes remain stationary. **(C)** Immediately after stopping rotation, the head and the semicircular canals are stationary, but the endolymph continues to flow in the direction of rotation to the right, resulting in excitation of the left horizontal semicircular canal, inhibition of the right horizontal semicircular canal, and nystagmus to the left (e.g., in the opposite direction of rotation).

Because the horizontal semicircular canal is the most likely to respond to caloric stimulation of the external auditory canal, the person either lies supine with the head elevated 30° or sits erect with the head tilted backward 60°. These positions bring the horizontal canal into a vertical position, where it is maximally influenced by convection currents set up in the endolymph as a result of caloric stimulation. Irrigating the ear canal with cool water (30°C) lowers the temperature of the prominence of the horizontal canal, condensing the endolymph and inducing a circulating motion of the endolymph. This results in inhibition of the hair cells. The induced endolymph flow causes the eyes to deviate slowly toward the side of the irrigated ear (e.g., slow phase of the nystagmus), and then return quickly in the opposite direction (e.g., fast phase of the nystagmus). If the ear is irrigated with warm water (40°), the endolymph expands, and the resulting circulation of endolymph produces the reverse; the nystagmus slow phase is directed away from the irrigated ear, and the fast phase is directed toward the irrigated side.

3. VESTIBULAR ASSESSMENT

The principles of rotary and caloric nystagmus are utilized in the evaluation of individuals who present with dizziness and balance disorders. The tests of vestibular function seen most often in clinical practice include rotary chair testing and electronystagmography (ENG). These tests provide information regarding the origin (e.g., peripheral vs central) and extent (e.g., bilateral or unilateral) of vestibular deficit by making use of vestibular pathways related to the control of gaze. Dynamic posturography, a more recently developed procedure, examines the relative contributions of vestibular, visual, and proprioceptive input in the control and maintenance of balance and posture.

Rotary chair testing consists of eye-movement recordings made either electrographically, via the cornea-retinal potential, or videographically during and after rotational stimulation. The rotational stimulation can be either sinusoidal (e.g., to and fro) or sustained in one direction, resulting in the production of the VOR and nystagmus, which are utilized to determine overall vestibular responsiveness and symmetry.

The ENG battery is comprised of tests of ocular motility, positional maneuvers of the head and body, and caloric stimulation. Eye-movement recordings are made for visual targets stimulating saccadic, tracking, eccentric gaze, and optokinetic eye movements, and abnormalities generally suggest a central deficit. The positional subtests evaluate the effects of gravitational forces in sitting, supine, right lateral, left lateral, and head-hanging positions. The presence of nystagmus in positional tests can be indicative of either central or peripheral abnormality. The slow phase of nystagmus resulting from caloric irrigation of the external auditory canals is evaluated for symmetry and direction in order to distinguish unilateral or bilateral weakness of peripheral vestibular function.

In dynamic posturography, the center of mass of the person is inferred from reaction-force measurements made by a force plate incorporated into the surface upon which the person stands during the evaluation. The person attempts to maintain quiet stance as visual and proprioceptive cues that contribute to balance and posture are systematically manipulated in order to determine the sensory integration of vestibular, visual, and proprioceptive input, or as these cues are suddenly and unexpectedly perturbed in order to evaluate movement coordination during challenges of balance maintenance.

SELECTED READINGS

Annikko M. Functional morphology of the vestibular system. In Jahn AF, Santos-Sacchi J (eds). Physiology of the Ear. New York: Raven Press, 1988; 457.

Gresty MA, Bronstein AM, Brandt T, Dieterich M. Neurology of otolith function. Brain 1992; 115:647.

Markham CH. Vestibular control of muscular tone and posture. Can J Neurol Sci 1987; 14:493.

Peterson BW, Richmond FJ. The control of head movements. New York: Oxford University Press, 1988; 322.

Shepard NT, Telian SA. Practical Management of the Balance Disorder Patient. San Diego: Singular Publishing Group, 1996.

Uemura T, Cohen B. Effects of vestibular nuclei lesions on vestibulo-ocular reflexes and posture in monkeys. Acta Otolaryngol Suppl 1973; 315:5.

Waespe W. The physiology and pathophysiology of the vestibuloocular system. In Hofferberth B, Brune GG, Sitzer G, Weger HD (eds). Vascular Brainstem Diseases. Basel: Karger, 1990; 37.

Wilson VJ, Jones MG. Mammalian Vestibular Physiology. New York: Plenum Press, 1979; 365.

26 The Gustatory System

David V. Smith, Steven J. St. John, and John D. Boughter, Jr.

1. INTRODUCTION

The term *taste* is used to refer to the complex of sensations known as *flavor perception*, which includes afferent information from the olfactory, gustatory, and trigeminal systems. More strictly defined, taste refers to the sensations arising from stimulation of the gustatory receptors located within the oropharyngeal mucosa. Throughout this chapter, the terms *taste* and *gustation* are used interchangeably to refer to the gustatory system.

The sense of taste provides a gateway for monitoring and controlling the ingestion of food. It responds to chemical substances in the oral cavity, and helps to regulate the interaction between ingestive behavior and the internal milieu. Taste information arises from stimulation by chemicals dissolved in saliva, which initiate the activation of receptor mechanisms located on specially modified epithelial cells distributed throughout the oral mucosa. Taste transduction initiates depolarization of these receptor cells, which make synaptic contact with first-order fibers of one of several cranial nerves. These fibers project to the medulla and into the nucleus of the solitary tract (NST), where second-order projections arise to connect to the pons or thalamus, depending on the species studied. Pontine neurons project to the thalamus and to various areas of the limbic forebrain involved in food and fluid regulation. Thalamic cells connect to the gustatory cortex.

The various populations of taste buds on the anterior and posterior tongue, palate, and laryngeal mucosa have somewhat different sensitivities and project in a topographic, overlapping manner throughout the taste pathway. Cells at all levels of the gustatory system are typically responsive to stimuli that represent different taste qualities. Various neuron types can be identified on the basis of their profiles of sensitivity, and taste quality appears to be represented by the pattern of activity evoked across these neuron types. In addition to its role in the perception of salty, sweet, sour, and bitter sensations, taste input is important in regulating several visceral reflexes involved in ingestive and digestive functions.

2. GUSTATORY SYSTEM ANATOMY

2.1. Taste Receptor Cells Are Situated Within Taste Buds

Taste is mediated through chemical stimulation of gustatory receptor cells, which are located within taste buds distributed throughout the oral, pharyngeal, and laryngeal mucosa. Taste buds on the tongue are contained within distinct papillae; those in other areas are distributed across the surface of the epithelium. At the ultrastructural level, at least two types of cells can be identified within the taste bud (Fig. 1). They are

From: *Neuroscience in Medicine, 2nd ed.* (P. Michael Conn, ed.),
© 2003 Humana Press Inc., Totowa, NJ.

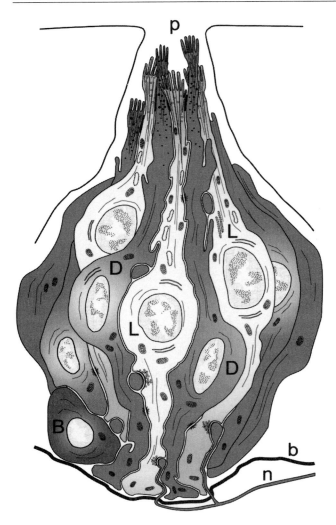

Fig. 1. Mammalian taste bud. This barrel-shaped structure contains different cell types, including basal cells (B), dark cells (D), and light cells (L). These epithelial-receptor cells make synaptic contact with distal processes (n) of cranial nerves VII, IX, or X, which penetrate the basement membrane (b) to enter the basal portion of the taste bud. Cell bodies of the peripheral nerve fibers lie within the cranial nerve ganglia. The microvilli of the taste cells project into an opening in the epithelium, the taste pore (p), where they make contact with gustatory stimuli. The apical processes of the taste cells are joined by tight junctions, which restrict most taste stimuli to the apical membrane.

called *dark cells* and *light cells*, based on their relative densities in electron micrographs and on several other ultrastructural characteristics. These two cell types are also distinguishable by their expression of a number of immunocytochemical markers such as the neural-cell adhesion molecule (NCAM), the gustatory G protein, α-gustducin, the human blood group A and Lewis[b]

antigens, and serotonin, all of which are expressed exclusively on subsets of light cells, and the human blood group H antigen, which is expressed only on dark cells. Any of a number of cell-surface molecules could play a role in the structural integrity of the taste bud or in the mediation of axon-taste cell recognition during cell turnover. Of the 50–100 cells in each taste bud, approximately two-thirds of them are dark cells and one-third are light cells. Within a taste bud, the cells are arranged in a concentric columnar fashion, with their apical microvilli projecting toward a pore that opens through the epithelium into the oral cavity (Fig. 1); gustatory stimuli interact with receptors and ion channels on these microvilli. Tight junctions between these apical processes restrict the access of most taste stimuli to the apical receptor-cell membrane. The base of the taste bud is penetrated by terminal branches of the afferent nerve, which make synaptic contact with the receptor cells. A single nerve fiber may innervate cells in more than one taste bud, each of which is innervated by several different afferent fibers.

2.2. The Turnover and Replacement of Taste Cells Is a Continuous Process

Taste-receptor cells arise continually from an underlying population of basal epithelial cells. It is not entirely clear, primarily because the cells are in a constant state of turnover, whether the cell types identifiable on structural grounds are different cell types or a single type at different stages of maturation. It is known, however, that more than one cell lineage contributes to cells within the taste bud, and that dark and light cells turn over at different rates. The lifespan of a dark cell in a fungiform papilla of the rat is approx 10 d; light cells appear to live for a longer time. The afferent nerve maintains a trophic influence over the taste buds, which degenerate if the nerve supply is removed.

Although the innervation by gustatory-nerve fibers is necessary to maintain the structural integrity of the taste bud, the gustatory sensitivities of the receptor cells are determined by the epithelium itself. A classic experiment in which the glossopharyngeal nerve (e.g., cranial-nerve IX) and the chorda tympani nerve were transected and cross-anastomosed demonstrated that, when the ninth cranial nerve was rerouted to the anterior tongue, its fibers responded like those of the chorda tympani and vice versa, demonstrating that the receptor phenotype is a property of the target epithelium rather than the innervating nerve. Recent experiments have shown that immunocytochemical differences between taste cells on the anterior and posterior tongue are also determined by the epithelium from which they derive and are not influenced by the innervating nerve. The several branches of a chorda tympani axon that innervate different fungiform papillae have been shown to have similar profiles of sensitivity. Combined with the fact that the sensitivity of a given receptor field appears to be determined by the epithelium, this suggests that during cell turnover the nerve fibers are guided to make contact with particular types of receptor cells.

2.3. Taste Buds Are Distributed in Distinct Subpopulations and Are Innervated by Several Cranial Nerves

Taste buds are found on the anterior portion of the tongue in fungiform papillae and in circumvallate and foliate papillae on the posterior tongue. There are also taste buds on the soft palate, pharynx, epiglottis, and upper third of the esophagus. The distribution of taste buds on the human tongue and within the oral cavity is shown schematically in Fig. 2. In humans, the 200–300 fungiform papillae on the anterior portion of the tongue contain approx 1600 taste buds, although there is considerable variation among persons. The 8–12 circumvallate papillae contain about 230 taste buds each, for a total of almost 3000 taste buds, and the foliate papillae have about 1300 taste buds. Although taste buds have been described on the soft palate of human adults only in biopsy material and only in very small numbers, a few studies have reported that human infants have about 2600 taste buds in the pharynx and larynx and on the soft palate. On the tongue of adult rhesus monkeys (e.g., fungiform, circumvallate, and foliate papillae), there are approx 8000 to 10,000 taste buds, which are maintained well into old age. Most electrophysiological studies of taste have involved stimulation of the fungiform papillae on the anterior portion of the tongue, although most taste buds in all mammalian species studied are located in other areas.

Taste receptors are innervated by branches of the seventh (i.e., facial), ninth (i.e., glossopharyngeal), and tenth (i.e., vagus) cranial nerves. These special visceral afferent fibers project centrally into the rostral pole of the NST, which is the rostral-most extension of the visceral afferent column in the medulla. Taste buds in the fungiform papillae on the anterior portion of the tongue are innervated by the chorda tympani branch of

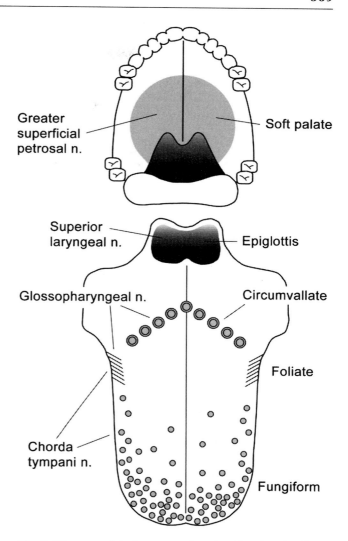

Fig. 2. Diagram of the human oral cavity, showing the distribution of various taste-bud populations, which are found on the anterior tongue (e.g., fungiform papillae), posterior tongue (e.g., circumvallate and foliate papillae), the soft palate, and the laryngeal surface of the epiglottis. These taste buds are innervated by several branches of cranial nerves VII (facial nerve, chorda tympani and greater superficial petrosal branches), IX (glossopharyngeal nerve, lingual-tonsillar branch), and X (vagus nerve: superior laryngeal branch).

the facial nerve, and those on the soft palate are innervated by its greater superficial petrosal branch. The cell bodies of these fibers are located in the geniculate ganglion and project to the most rostral extension of the NST. Circumvallate and most foliate taste buds are supplied by the lingual-tonsillar branch of the glossopharyngeal nerve, although the most rostral foliate taste buds are innervated by the chorda tympani nerve. Afferent fibers of the glossopharyngeal nerve project

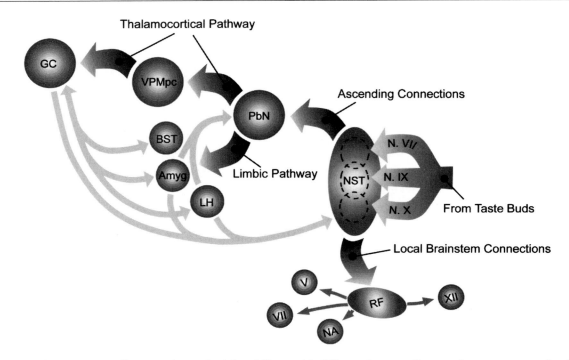

Fig. 3. Mammalian gustatory afferent pathway. Peripheral fibers with different degrees of responsiveness to taste stimuli project into the NST. Fibers of cranial nerves VII, IX, and X project in an organized, overlapping termination within the rostral portion of the NST. Second-order cells project into the parabrachial nuclei (PbN) of the pons, from which a classic *thalamocortical pathway* proceeds to the parvicellular division of the ventroposteromedial nucleus (VPMpc) of the thalamus and then to the gustatory cortex, located within the agranular insular cortex of rodents. Another projection, the *limbic pathway*, arises from the PbN to connect to areas of the ventral forebrain involved in the control of feeding and in autonomic regulation, including the lateral hypothalamus (LH), the bed nucleus of the stria terminalis (BST), and the central nucleus of the amygdala. Cells of the NST also make local reflex connections through the reticular formation (RF) with cranial motor nuclei (trigeminal, V; facial, VII; nucleus ambiguous, NA; hypoglossal, XII) that control muscles involved in facial expression, licking, chewing, and swallowing. In primates, cells of the NST bypass the PbN and project directly to the thalamus (not shown). Many of the forebrain targets of the gustatory system send descending projections back to the brainstem nuclei (PbN and NST).

through the inferior glossopharyngeal (i.e., petrosal) ganglion to the NST just caudal to, but overlapping with, the facial nerve termination. The pharyngeal branch of the glossopharyngeal nerve innervates taste buds in the nasopharynx. Taste buds on the epiglottis, aryepiglottal folds, and esophagus are innervated by the internal portion of the superior laryngeal nerve, which is a branch of the vagus nerve. Afferent fibers of the superior laryngeal nerve project by means of their cell bodies in the inferior vagal (i.e., nodose) ganglion to the NST caudal to, but overlapping with, the glossopharyngeal-nerve termination.

2.4. There Are Both Thalamocortical and Limbic Forebrain Projections of Gustatory Afferent Information

Secondary gustatory fibers arise from the NST to project rostrally more or less parallel to the projection of general visceral sensation, which arises from the

more caudal aspects of the solitary nucleus. In most mammalian species, there is a second-order projection into the parabrachial nuclei (PbN) in the pons, from which third-order fibers arise to project ipsilaterally through a classic sensory path to the parvicellular division of the ventroposteromedial nucleus (VPMpc) of the thalamus and then to the agranular insular cortex (Fig. 3).

In addition to the thalamocortical projection, fibers travel from the pons, along with other visceral afferent fibers, along a limbic pathway into areas of the ventral forebrain involved in feeding and autonomic regulation, including the lateral hypothalamus, the central nucleus of the amygdala, and the bed nucleus of the stria terminalis (Fig. 3). In the monkey, taste fibers bypass the pontine relay and project ipsilaterally through the central tegmental tract directly to the VPMpc in the thalamus. The VPMpc projects in the primate to the insular and opercular cortex and to area

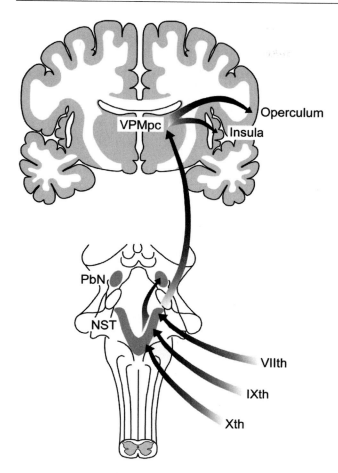

Fig. 4. Drawing of the probable gustatory afferent pathway in humans. Fibers of cranial nerves VII, IX, and X project into the NST, from which there is a direct projection to the parvicellular division of the ventroposteromedial nucleus (VPMpc) of the ipsilateral thalamus. From the thalamus, fibers project into the insular cortex and frontal operculum. Visceral afferent fibers from the caudal NST project to the parabrachial nuclei (PbN), which also receives gustatory projections in nonprimates. In addition to this classic sensory projection, there are numerous subcortical projections of the gustatory nuclei in a variety of species (*see* Fig. 3).

3b on the lateral convexity of the precentral gyrus. What may be a secondary cortical area, receiving input from the anterior insula, is found within the posterior orbitofrontal cortex. None of these cortical areas are purely gustatory, because they all contain neurons that are responsive to other sensory modalities such as touch and temperature. There are few studies of the anatomy of these projections in humans, although a careful review of the clinical literature suggests that the human gustatory system is very similar to that of the Old World monkey. A schematic of the probable gustatory projections in humans is shown in Fig. 4.

3. TASTE PHYSIOLOGY

3.1. Taste Receptors Are Coupled to Several Transduction Mechanisms

The mechanisms of taste transduction are receiving a good deal of attention. Although the nature of gustatory transduction is not fully understood, a coherent story is beginning to emerge from physiological and molecular studies of amphibian and mammalian-receptor cells (Fig. 5). Ionic stimuli such as salts and acids exert their effects on taste-receptor cells by directly interacting with ion channels. Sodium chloride (NaCl) produces a relatively pure salty taste in humans. Na^+ ions depolarize taste-receptor cells by inward movement through passive sodium channels located on their apical membranes. These channels, like similar sodium channels of the kidney, can be blocked with the diuretic compound amiloride. NaCl also produces a response in taste-receptor cells that is not blocked by amiloride. This mechanism may involve the ability of cations to diffuse through tight junctions between receptor cells in an anion-dependent fashion—through a paracellular pathway. The transduction of nonsodium salts, such as potassium chloride (KCl) or ammonium chloride (NH_4Cl), which are characterized by multiple taste qualities, is not completely understood. Human studies show that the saltiness of a wide array of salts is eliminated by adaptation to NaCl, implicating at least one common mechanism among sodium and nonsodium salts. It is likely that at least part of the transduction of nonsodium salts may involve the paracellular pathway implicated in the non-amiloride-sensitive transduction of Na^+ ions. Sour taste is produced by acids (H^+); protons also permeate amiloride-sensitive sodium channels, and some mammalian taste buds express a proton-gated cation channel that may be involved in acid sensing. In amphibians, voltage-dependent K^+ channels restricted to the apical membrane of the taste-receptor cell are blocked by acidic stimuli, causing direct depolarization of the cell, but there is no evidence for this mechanism in mammalian cells.

Transduction of sweet and bitter stimuli appears to primarily involve specific membrane receptors linked to second-messenger systems. Families of putative taste receptors for bitter and sweet taste have been recently cloned; there may be as many as 40–80 receptor proteins for bitter substances. These receptors are G-protein-coupled and activate several different second-messenger pathways, ultimately leading to an

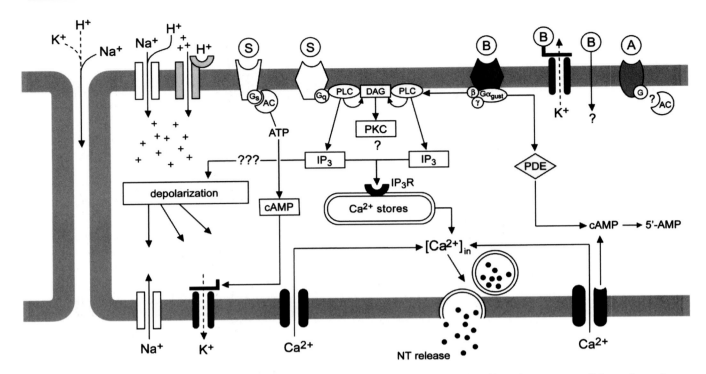

Fig. 5. Taste transduction mechanisms. Sodium salt transduction involves the passage of Na^+ into the receptor cell through passive, amiloride-blockable ion channels on the apical membrane (top of figure); protons (H^+) can also penetrate this pathway. In addition, Na^+—and probably other cations (such as K^+) and protons—can pass through the tight junctions between cells in the taste bud to enter basolateral (*bottom of figure*) ion channels. Both of these mechanisms lead to direct depolarization of the taste-receptor cell. Transduction of the taste of acids in amphibians involves H^+ blockage of voltage-dependent K^+ channels on the apical membrane of the taste-receptor cell (not depicted); in mammals H^+ has been shown to gate an apical ion channel, which allows entry of cations. The transduction of sweet tasting stimuli (S) involves membrane-bound G-protein-coupled receptors (GPCRs) on the apical membrane that bind to sugars and artificial sweeteners. Sugar transduction involves receptor-mediated stimulation of adenylate cyclase (AC), which leads to closing of K^+ channels on the basolateral membrane by a cAMP-dependent phosphorylation. Artificial sweeteners appear to couple to an IP_3 pathway, leading to release of Ca^{+2} from intracellular stores. Bitter substances (B) bind to a family of GPCRs, some of which couple to α-gustducin and lead to opening of a cyclic nucleotide-gated ion channel; others appear to engage an IP_3 pathway. Amino acids (A), such as glutamate, stimulate via a type of metabotropic glutamate receptor, although the intracellular pathway for this mechanism is unknown. All of these mechanisms result in elevated intracellular Ca^{+2} and subsequent release of neurotransmitter onto terminals of the afferent nerve.

increase in intracellular calcium, and neurotransmitter release (Fig. 5). Additionally, some bitter compounds are lipophilic and may directly permeate the taste-receptor cell to interact with one or more second messengers; other bitter stimuli are known to directly block K^+ channels. Sugars and artificial sweeteners use separate transduction pathways, but either pathway ultimately results in a block of basolateral K^+ channels leading to depolarization. The receptor for the amino acid glutamate (which produces the "umami taste") is a type of metabotropic glutamate receptor, although its intracellular pathways are still unknown. Recent studies also indicate the existence of a taste-transduction mechanism for dietary fat: Essential fatty acids directly inhibit delayed rectifying K^+ channels in taste

receptor cells, leading to depolarization. *In situ* patch-clamp recording of the responses of gustatory-receptor cells indicate that most taste cells in mammals are broadly sensitive to stimuli representing different taste qualities, suggesting that several of these transduction mechanisms may exist within a single taste-receptor cell.

3.2. The Neural Representation of Taste Quality Is a Complex Phenomenon

The perception of saltiness, sweetness, sourness, or bitterness emerges from neural activity within the central nervous system (CNS). The way in which this information is represented in neural activity has been the subject of considerable debate. Many physiology

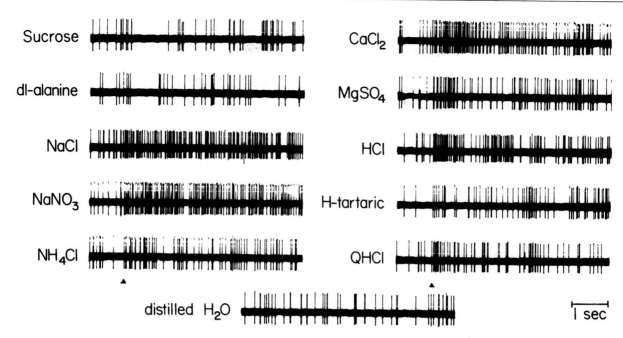

Fig. 6. Responses of a neuron in the NST of the hamster to several taste stimuli applied to the fungiform papillae. The triangles indicate the onset of the response, of which about 5 s is shown, preceded by about 1 s of response to distilled water. The concentrations of the stimuli are those that produce a half-maximal response to these chemicals in the hamster's chorda tympani nerve. This cell shows an excitatory response to all of these stimuli except sucrose and DL-alanine, which inhibit ongoing activity. (Smith DV, Travers JB, Van Buskirk, RL. Brain Res Bull 1979;4:359.)

textbooks show a diagram of the human tongue that suggests that saltiness and sweetness are appreciated at the tip, sour on the sides, and bitter on the back of the tongue. Although there are slight differences in the absolute threshold for different taste qualities in different regions of the human tongue and palate, all taste qualities (e.g., salty, sour, sweet, or bitter) can be perceived by stimulation of each of the oral taste-bud populations. However, physiological studies of rodents suggest some fairly striking differences between the various taste-bud populations in their response to different tastants. Fibers of the seventh cranial nerve are much more responsive to sweet and salty stimuli, and those of the ninth cranial nerve are relatively more responsive to sour and bitter substances. These differences may relate to different functional roles for the separate taste-bud populations.

Most of what is known about the neurophysiology of the mammalian gustatory pathway has been derived from studies of chorda tympani nerve fibers that innervate taste buds on the anterior portion of the tongue, or central neurons that receive information from these receptors. Like individual receptor cells, single fibers in the chorda tympani nerve typically respond to more than one taste quality. Individual second- and third-

order gustatory neurons in the NST and parabrachial nuclei that respond to anterior tongue stimulation are similarly broadly tuned across taste qualities. Fibers of the glossopharyngeal nerve are also broadly responsive. Despite this broad tuning, individual gustatory fibers appear to fall into functional groups, which can be identified by their "best" stimulus. Among taste-responsive cells of the peripheral and central nervous system, there are distinct groups of "tuning curves," each responding best to one of the four taste qualities. Attempts to understand the neural processing of taste quality information have relied heavily on this best-stimulus classification (e.g., sucrose-best, NaCl-best), which assumes the existence of four basic taste qualities: salty, sour, sweet, and bitter.

Inputs from the separate peripheral taste fields project into the NST, where the cells receive converging input from separate peripheral fields, and are even more broadly tuned than peripheral fibers. The response of a broadly tuned cell in the hamster NST is shown in Fig. 6. Of the four prototypical stimuli, the cell illustrated responds best to hydrochloric acid (HCl), but it also responds to NaCl and quinine-HCl (QHCl); it is inhibited by sucrose. Other salts and acids are excitatory for this cell, and DL-alanine, which tastes sweet to humans and is similar to sucrose in hamster behavioral studies, inhibits the cell. Further increases in the breadth of tuning have been shown in the third-order cells of the PbN.

Because taste fibers in peripheral gustatory nerves and cells in central taste nuclei are broadly tuned across stimulus qualities and are also modulated by stimulus concentration, the activity in any one cell cannot unambiguously signal either quality or intensity. Thus, the neural representation of taste quality involves a comparison of activity across taste neurons. The across-neuron pattern theory of quality coding was first suggested when it was apparent from the earliest recordings from peripheral taste nerve fibers that these afferent neurons lacked stimulus specificity. The mean responses of three classes of neurons in the hamster parabrachial nuclei to an array of 18 taste stimuli are shown in Fig. 7A. Neurons in each of three best-stimulus categories are broadly responsive to stimuli that vary widely in taste quality. For example, the sucrose (S)-best neurons respond well to all the sweet-tasting stimuli (shaded), but they also respond well to sodium nitrate (NaNO$_3$), magnesium chloride (MgCl$_2$), calcium chloride (CaCl$_2$), and urea, among other stimuli. Thus, any one neuron group does not distinguish among many stimuli of different quality. However, these broadly tuned neurons as a population can represent taste quality by their relative patterns of activity, as shown in Fig. 7B. Here, across an array of PbN neurons, the two sodium salts, NaCl and NaNO$_3$, have highly correlated patterns of neuronal activity, whereas neither of these stimuli produces a pattern similar to that produced by sucrose. NaCl and NaNO$_3$ are behaviorally alike to hamsters, and are easily discriminated from sucrose.

Similarities and differences in across-neuron patterns of activity, such as those shown in Fig. 7, can be quantified by calculating the correlations among the responses evoked by a series of chemical stimuli across a sample of taste neurons. These correlations can then be subjected to a multivariate analysis to create a "taste space," which represents the neurophysiological similarities and dissimilarities among the responses to the stimuli across the neuronal population. An across-neuron taste space generated from the responses of cells in the hamster PbN to several stimuli is shown in Fig. 8.

The positions of the stimuli in this space reflect similarities and differences in the population response of the gustatory system to these compounds. Stimuli with similar tastes (to hamsters) are grouped together,

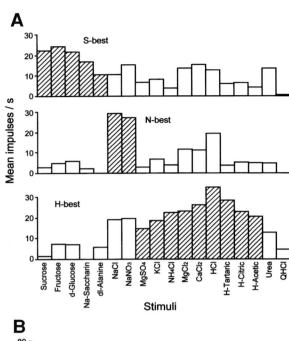

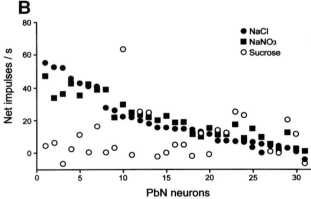

Fig. 7. Broad tuning of gustatory neurons and its relationship to patterns of neuronal activity. (**A**) Mean responses of each of three neuron classes in the hamster PbN to 18 stimuli. The sweet-tasting stimuli are shaded in the profile for the sucrose (S)-best cells, the sodium salts are shaded in the profile for the NaCl (N)-best neurons, and the nonsodium salts and acids are shaded in the response profile for the HCl (H)-best neurons. (Modified from Smith DV, Van Buskirk RL, Travers JB, Bieber, SL J Neurophysiol 1983;50,541.) (**B**) Patterns of activity generated across the hamster PbN neurons depicted in A by two sodium salts (*filled symbols*) and by sucrose (*open symbols*). The across-neuron patterns evoked by NaCl and NaNO$_3$ correlated +0.94, whereas that to sucrose was not correlated with the pattern evoked by either sodium salt (e.g., $r = -0.09$ with NaCl). Stimuli with similar taste produce highly similar responses across the entire population of taste-responsive neurons.

and those with different tastes are separated within this space. The similarities and differences in the patterns of activity evoked by these stimuli provide a basis for

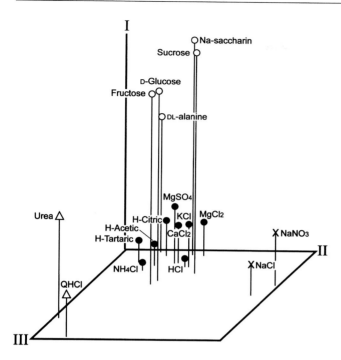

Fig. 8. Three-dimensional "taste space," showing the similarities and differences in the across-neuron patterns evoked by 18 stimuli delivered to the anterior tongue of the hamster. This space was derived from multidimensional scaling of the across-neuron correlations among these stimuli recorded from neurons in the PbN of the hamster. The proximity of stimuli within this space indicates a high degree of correlation between the across-neuron patterns elicited by these compounds. Four groups of stimuli are indicated by different symbols: sweeteners, sodium salts, nonsodium salts and acids, and bitter-tasting stimuli. Stimuli with similar taste produce highly correlated patterns of activity. (Modified from Smith DV, Van Buskirk RL, Travers JB, Bieber SL J Neurophysiol 1983;30:541.)

their discrimination. By relating the responses of the various neuron types (e.g., sucrose-best, NaCl-best) to these across-neuron patterns, it has been shown that a comparison of activity across neuron types is necessary for the neural discrimination between stimuli of different taste quality.

Apart from the issue of quality-coding mechanisms is the interesting question of how any kind of code for quality is maintained in the face of the constant turnover of receptor cells. Because the receptor expression is determined by the epithelium, the gustatory nerve fibers must recognize and make contact with the appropriate receptor cells during turnover to maintain a constant sensory code. Another alternative is that the synaptic organization of the medullary relay could be continually altered to maintain a constant representa-

tion of a changing periphery. Whatever the mechanism, the representation of taste quality in gustatory nerve fibers and central neurons must somehow remain constant during the continual turnover of taste receptor cells and their reinnervation by fibers of the peripheral nerve. Because the taste-system is composed of broadly tuned and redundant elements, it may be particularly suited to representing information during continual receptor replacement; the contribution of any small number of cells at any given point in time is much less important than the overall pattern of activity.

3.3. Taste-Mediated Behavior Requires the Interplay of Many Neural Systems

Although taste physiologists have focused largely on the role of gustatory afferent fibers and central neurons in taste quality perception, there are several taste-mediated behaviors, ranging from tongue movements to salivation to oral-mediated preabsorptive insulin release, that have their neuronal substrate within the brainstem. Input from the various gustatory nerves contributes differentially to these diverse taste-mediated behaviors. Some of the relationships between gustatory input and taste-mediated behavior are summarized in the diagram of Fig. 9.

Taste may be viewed as the oral component of a visceral afferent system, which includes gustatory, respiratory, cardiovascular, and gastrointestinal functions. The functional contribution of the taste nerves seems to be organized in a rostral to caudal continuum, with ingestive substrates more rostral and protective components more caudal. For example, facial-nerve fibers are responsive primarily to preferred stimuli such as sucrose and NaCl; ninth nerve fibers are most sensitive to aversive stimuli such as HCl and QHCl; and vagal-nerve fibers respond to stimuli that deviate from the normal pH and ionic milieu of the larynx (Fig. 9).

The output of sucrose-sensitive neurons of the NST ascends to the forebrain to generate the perception of sweetness (*see* Fig. 9). These cells also provide input to the motor system that drives the ingestive components of feeding behavior, including (in rodents) rhythmic mouth movements, tongue protrusions, lateral tongue protrusions, salivary secretion, preabsorptive insulin release, and swallowing. Similarly, quinine-sensitive cells of the NST send ascending projections to the forebrain to give rise to sensations of bitterness (*see* Fig. 9), but they also provide input to motor systems that drive protective behaviors such as gaping, chin rubbing, forelimb flailing, locomotion, and fluid

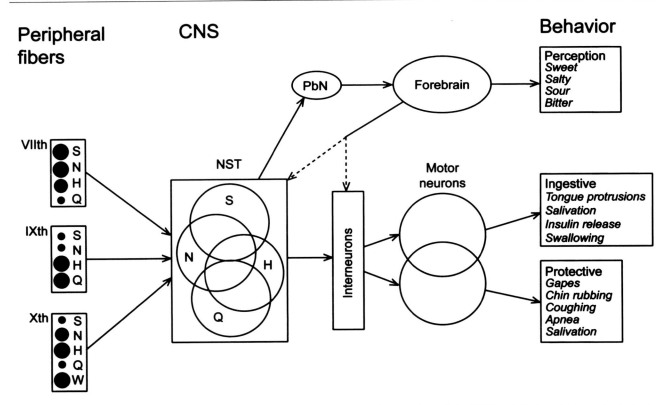

Fig. 9. Chemosensory inputs of three cranial nerves to the taste-responsive portion of the NST and their putative roles in taste-mediated behaviors. The size of the filled circles for each of the peripheral nerves (i.e., VIIth, IXth, Xth) depicts the relative responsiveness of these nerves to sucrose (S), NaCl (N), HCl (H), quinine hydrochloride (Q), and water (W). The sensitivities of NST cells are largely overlapping, with each cell type somewhat responsive to two or three of the basic stimuli, although sucrose and QHCl stimulate few of the same NST cells. Output from the NST ascends in the classic taste pathway to produce perceptions of sweetness, saltiness, sourness, and bitterness and to contribute to hedonic tone (not depicted). Local reflex circuits within the brainstem control the ingestive and protective responses evoked by taste stimulation. Behavioral data suggest that the ingestive and protective responses can be triggered in parallel, depending on the quality of the stimulus. (Smith DV, Frank ME. Sensory coding by peripheral taste fibers. In Simon SA, Roper SD (eds). Mechanisms of taste transduction. Boca Raton, FL: CRC Press, 1993:295.)

rejection. Sucrose and quinine produce different patterns of ingestive and protective taste reactivity, and a combination of these behaviors can be triggered by mixtures of sucrose and quinine.

Although there are regional differences in taste sensitivity, as noted here, all taste qualities are represented throughout the oral cavity. However, some researchers suspect that the various regions of the oral cavity contribute differentially to taste-mediated behaviors. Nerve-transection studies in rodents, for example, show that aversive reflexes (such as gapes) are mediated predominantly by input from the glossopharyngeal nerve. Transection of the ninth nerve, however, does not alter ingestive responses (such as tongue protrusions). Although damage to the glossopharyngeal nerve does not diminish a rat's ability to discrimi-

nate taste stimuli (even if the stimuli are naturally aversive), transection of the facial nerve typically has severe consequences for discrimination behavior. In rats, discrimination between NaCl and KCl or between KCl and quinine is completely disrupted by seventh-nerve axotomy. These data suggest that taste input from the seventh nerve is crucial for discrimination based on taste quality, whereas input from the ninth nerve is more important for reflexive oromotor behavior.

Chemoreceptive fibers of the tenth cranial nerve are more involved in visceral functions than in taste-quality perception. The superior laryngeal nerve is involved in swallowing, airway protection, and several other visceral reflexes. Respiratory apnea is produced by laryngeal stimulation with water, and chemosensory fibers of the rat superior laryngeal nerve mediate diuresis in response to stimulation of the laryngeal mucosa with water. In addition to its role in controlling ingestive behavior, taste triggers several metabolic responses, including salivary, gastric, and pancreatic secretions. Thus, taste buds may have a number of roles related to gustatory-visceral regulation, depending on their peripheral distribution and innervation.

In summary, taste input guides a variety of behavioral, perceptual, and autonomic responses. Undoubtedly, separate (and possibly overlapping) neural circuits process taste information for these different functions. For example, the thalamocortical pathway may be more important for identification of a taste stimulus, the limbic pathway for evaluating the pleasantness of a taste, and the brainstem connections for cephalic-phase reflexes such as salivation or insulin release. Input from the three cranial nerves that innervate the various taste buds may contribute more to some neural circuits than others. For now, however, the precise functional roles of different neuronal populations in the peripheral and central gustatory system are largely unknown and remain an area of active research.

3.4. Brainstem Taste Activity Is Modulated by Descending Pathways

Responses of brainstem cells to gustatory stimulation are subject to several modulatory influences. For example, glucose, insulin, and pancreatic glucagon, when systemically administered, alter the responses of cells in the rat NST to tongue stimulation with glucose. Conditioned taste-aversion learning shifts the patterns of response to taste stimuli recorded from the rat NST. The precise mechanisms underlying these effects are unknown. There are direct descending projections from gustatory areas of the ventral forebrain to both PbN and NST (see Fig. 3). Inputs from the gustatory cortex, the central nucleus of the amygdala, and the lateral hypothalamus have all been shown to both excite and inhibit the activity of cells of the rostral NST; inhibitory responses produced by cortical activation are blocked by the $GABA_A$-receptor-antagonist bicuculline.

Recent studies have begun to reveal mechanisms of synaptic transmission within the gustatory region of the NST. Electrophysiological recordings from cells in the rostral NST from both rats and hamsters have shown that gamma-amino butyric acid (GABA) produces inhibition of activity in these cells, which is mediated predominantly by the $GABA_A$-receptor subtype. These studies show that the gustatory portion of the NST is under the influence of a tonic GABAergic inhibitory network. One of the roles of GABA is to regulate the breadth of tuning of these cells, which respond to more taste stimuli when GABA activity is blocked by bicuculline.

The responses of cells in the gustatory zone of the NST can be blocked by glutamate antagonists. Excitatory postsynaptic potentials (EPSPs) recorded from rat NST cells in vitro in response to electrical stimulation of the solitary tract are reduced by both CNQX and APV, antagonists to the AMPA-kainate and NMDA glutamate receptors, respectively. Both of these agents also reversibly block or reduce the responses to chemical stimulation of the anterior tongue in hamster NST cells recorded in vivo. All cells responsive to taste stimulation are blocked by CNQX, regardless of their profiles of sensitivity; there is no evidence that the neurotransmitter is different for cells of different types (e.g., sucrose- vs NaCl-best). Therefore, it is very likely that glutamate acts as a neurotransmitter between gustatory afferent fibers and taste-responsive cells in the NST.

Evidence also indicates that taste-responsive cells in the NST are excited by substance P (SP) and inhibited by met-enkephalin (Met-ENK). Immunocytochemical studies have shown that SP- and enkephalin-containing neurons are present within the gustatory zone of the NST, and SP-containing fibers enter this nucleus from a number of still unknown sources. In vitro experiments on rat brainstem slices have shown that bath application of SP excites a number of cells in the gustatory zone of the NST. A role for these SP-responsive NST cells in gustatory processing has been demonstrated in the hamster NST in vivo, where responses to anterior tongue stimulation with NaCl or sucrose are enhanced by local microinjection of SP. In vivo experiments also show that a subset of taste-responsive neurons in the NST is inhibited by met-ENK.

SELECTED READINGS

Erickson RP. Stimulus coding in topographic and non-topographic afferent modalities: on the significance of the activity of individual sensory neurons. Psychol Rev 1968; 75:447–465.

Erickson RP. The "across-fiber pattern" theory: an organizing principle for molar neural function. In Neff WD (ed). *Contributions to Sensory Physiology, Vol 6.* New York: Academic Press, 1982, 79–110.

Farbman AI. Renewal of taste bud cells in rat circumvallate papillae. Cell Tiss Kinetics 1980; 13:349–357.

Frank ME. An analysis of hamster afferent taste nerve response functions. J Gen Physiol 1973; 61:588–618.

Frank ME, Bieber SL, Smith DV. The organization of taste sensibilities in hamster chorda tympani nerve fibers. J Gen Physiol 1988; 91:861–896.

Gilbertson TA, Boughter JA Jr, Zhang H, Smith DV. Distribution of gustatory sensitivities in rat taste cells: whole-cell responses to apical chemical stimulation. J Neurosci 2001; 21:4931–4941.

Gilbertson TA, Damak S, Margolskee RF. The molecular physiology of taste transduction. Curr Opin Neurobiol 2000b; 10:519–527.

Herness MS, Gilbertson TA. Cellular mechanisms of taste transduction. Ann Rev Physiol 1999; 61:873–900.

Lindemann, B. Taste reception. Physiol Rev 1996; 76:719–766.

Murray RG. Ultrastructure of taste receptors. In Beidler LM (ed). Handbook of Sensory Physiology Vol. IV Chemical Senses Part 2 Taste. Berlin: Springer-Verlag, 1971, 31–50.

Norgren R. The gustatory system. In Paxinos G (ed). The Human Nervous System. New York: Academic Press, 1995, 845–861.

Pfaffmann C. Gustatory nerve impulses in rat, cat and rabbit. J Neurophysiol 1955; 18:429–440.

Pritchard T. The primate gustatory system. In Getchell TV, Doty RL, Bartoshuk LM, Snow Jr JB (eds). Smell and Taste in Health and Disease. New York: Raven, 1991, 109–125.

Smith DV, Margolskee RF. Making sense of taste. Sci Amer 2000; 284:32–39.

Smith DV, St. John SJ. Neural coding of gustatory information. Curr Opin Neurobiol 1999; 9:427–435.

Smith DV, Van Buskirk RL, Travers JB, Bieber SL. Coding of taste stimuli by hamster brainstem neurons. J Neurophysiol 1983; 50: 541–558

27 The Olfactory System

Michael T. Shipley, Matthew Ennis, and Adam C. Puche

CONTENTS

1. INTRODUCTION

Transduction of olfactory information occurs when odorant molecules contact the dendrites of olfactory-receptor neurons (ORNs). These neurons reside in the olfactory epithelium, a specialized region of the dorsal nasal cavity. ORN axons project through the lamina propria underlying the olfactory epithelium, and into the glomerular layer of the olfactory bulb. This projection forms the olfactory nerve, or cranial nerve I. Within glomeruli, ORN axons synapse onto the apical dendrites of mitral and tufted cells, which are the output neurons of the olfactory bulb. In turn, axons from these cells project to the primary olfactory cortex, through the lateral olfactory tract. The primary olfactory cortex comprises several brain regions, including the anterior olfactory nucleus, the piriform cortex, parts of the amygdala, and the entorhinal cortex. These areas, in turn, are interconnected with many areas of the brain, including the neocortex, hippocampus, mediodorsal thalamus, preoptic area, hypothalamus, and other parts of the limbic system. Through these connections, the olfactory system influences a wide range of behaviors and physiological functions, including reproduction, social behavior and communication (e.g., scent marking), food finding and selec-

tion, and maternal behavior, in addition to regulating neuroendocrine functions.

Compared to vision, audition, touch, and even taste, our understanding of olfactory-system function lags behind. A major reason for this is that we are only beginning to understand how odors are "coded" by primary olfactory neurons in the nasal epithelium and by activity patterns in the olfactory bulb. Recent advances in molecular biology, membrane biophysics, and imaging of neural function promise to rapidly close this critical gap. A second reason for the slow progress in olfaction has been the lack of a critical mass of researchers in this field. This is changing; there have been significant advances in olfaction since the previous edition, and there are likely to be major advances in our understanding during the next decade. This chapter focuses on the anatomy and circuit organization of the olfactory system, as these have been relatively well-characterized. In addition, it summarizes recent advances in the molecular biology and activity imaging of olfactory function.

Although there are many gaps in our knowledge, there are also many features of the olfactory system that make it a very interesting object of study. (i) it is the only sensory system that is essentially cortical from the first synaptic relay in the brain. Other sensory systems involve several layers of subcortical synaptic processing before information reaches the cortex. In the olfactory system, the primary sensory nerve end-

From: *Neuroscience in Medicine, 2nd ed.* (P. Michael Conn, ed.),
© 2003 Humana Press Inc., Totowa, NJ.

ings synaptically terminate in the olfactory bulb—itself a cortical structure that derives embryoliogically from the telencephalon, the same tissue that also gives rise to the neocortex. Thus, neural mechanisms of cortical sensory processing are directly accessible in the olfactory system. (ii) ORNs are the only neurons in the mature mammalian nervous system that regenerate continually throughout life, and following disease or injury. The newly formed neurons successfully reconnect with the brain to restore sensory function. Thus, the olfactory system holds important clues to such puzzles as why the human brain cannot repair itself after damage and how growing axons find their appropriate postsynaptic targets. Recent clinical interest has focused upon this area with the discovery that specialized glia from the olfactory system are beneficial to restoring a damaged spinal cord in lower mammals. A better understanding of the olfactory system may therefore provide important information about basic processes common to other sensory and integrative systems in the brain.

2. THE OLFACTORY EPITHELIUM

2.1. The Sense of Smell Is Mediated Through the Stimulation of Olfactory Receptor Neurons (ORNs) by Volatile Chemicals

ORNs are contained in a neuroepithelium, which is located in the dorsocaudal nasal vault, along the upper portion of the nasal septum, the cribriform plate region, and the medial wall of the superior turbinate. Afferent information from these receptors is carried along their axons to the olfactory bulbs through the olfactory nerve—the first cranial nerve. In order to stimulate the olfactory receptors, airborne molecules must enter the nasal cavity, where they are subjected to relatively turbulent air currents. The duration, volume, and velocity of a sniff are important determinants of an odor's stimulating effectiveness. Although these parameters differ markedly among individuals, they are quite constant for any one person. Once airborne volatiles reach the olfactory epithelium, they must pass through the layer of mucus that covers the olfactory epithelium. The relative partitioning of the odor between air and mucus thus also determines the stimulating effectiveness of an odor. Macromolecule odorant-binding proteins are present in the mucus and may function in the mucus to bind odorants and present

them to receptors. Similarly, these macromolecules may be required to remove odorants from the receptors and or chemically inactivate odorants.

The ORNs lie in a pseudostratified columnar epithelium, which is thicker than the surrounding respiratory epithelium of the nasal cavity (Fig. 1). This epithelium rests on a vascular lamina propria. Within the epithelium are the bipolar ORNs, supporting cells (sustentacular cells), microvillar cells, and basal cells. Bowman's glands lie within the underlying lamina propria. Unlike taste-receptor cells, which are modified epithelial cells (see Chapter 26), olfactory receptors are true neurons. Their cell bodies lie in the basal two-thirds of the epithelium, and their apical dendrites extend to the surface. At the peripheral tip of the dendrite, the process swells slightly to form the olfactory knob, from which several cilia extend into the mucous layer. Although human cilia do not appear to be motile, in some vertebrate species ciliary length and motility have been related to receptor age and development. Substantial evidence suggests that the cilia are the primary sites of chemosensory transduction. Basal to the ORN cell body, an unmyelinated axon arises and joins small bundles of other ORN axons. These axons penetrate the basal lamina, at which point the bundles become ensheathed by specialized Schwann cells, the ensheathing cell. These bundles join others to make up the 15–20 fascicles (fila olfactoria) of the olfactory nerve, which pass through the cribriform plate to synapse in the olfactory bulb.

The supporting cells of the olfactory epithelium separate and partially wrap the ORNs. In humans and some other vertebrates, their apical surface, is covered with microvilli, which project along with the olfactory cilia into the mucous layer. A third cell type, the microvillar cells, present at about one-tenth the number of the ORNs in humans, have microvilli on their apical surface that project into the mucous layer. Their basal end tapers into a cytoplasmic extension that appears to enter the lamina propria. It is not known whether this projection is an axon, although the ultrastructural appearance of the microvillar cells appears to be neuronal. Deep to the ORNs, sustentacular and microvillar cells are the basal cells; globose basal and horizontal cells. These cells sit on the basement membrane and are stem cells for the replacement of the ORNs, which in the mouse have a lifespan of approx 40 d. It is unclear which—or whether both—basal cell types act as stem cells. Within the lamina propria are

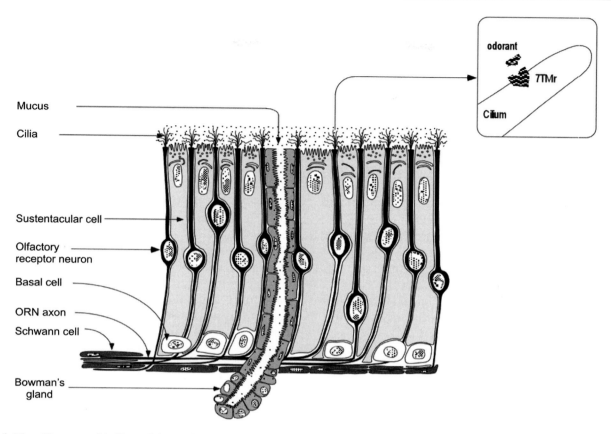

Fig. 1. The olfactory epithelium. Schematic illustration of the olfactory epithelium showing the major cell types. *Inset* shows the location of 7-TM odorant receptors on cilia of ORNs. Additional details of the receptors, transduction pathways, and channels presumed to mediate odorant transduction are shown in Fig. 2.

the secretory Bowman's glands, which provide a serous component to the mucous layer covering the olfactory epithelium.

ORNs and their axons contain olfactory marker protein (OMP), which is unique to olfactory neurons and is present in a number of mammalian species, including humans. OMP appears to be expressed in all ORNs, and accounts for approx 1% of the total protein content of these cells. The exact role of OMP is poorly understood, but recent evidence suggests that if this molecule is absent, olfactory signal transduction is slightly impaired.

In addition to input from the olfactory epithelium, some chemical stimuli give rise to activity in the trigeminal system through the stimulation of nerve endings in the nasal and oral cavities. The burning or irritation arising from stimuli such as ammonia or hot peppers interacts with olfactory and gustatory input in what has been termed the "common chemical sense."

Fibers in each of the three branches of the fifth cranial nerve carry information about intranasal or intraoral chemical irritation. These sensations usually remain intact in patients who complain of taste or smell dysfunction, and can be useful in the assessment of the malingering patient.

2.2. The Function of the ORNs Has Been Studied by a Number of Physiological Methods

In one of the earliest, a surface electrode placed on the olfactory epithelium was used to record a slow, monophasic negative field potential (termed the electroolfactogram, or EOG) in response to odorant stimulation. The EOG is believed to be the summated generator potentials from a large number of ORNs. It has also been possible to record spike-discharge activity from individual ORNs and to use calcium-sensitive dyes to image calcium transients evoked by odor stimulation. The ability of ORN cilia to respond to odorants was also confirmed by imaging calcium transients in ORNs when only the cilia was exposed to an odor plume. These approaches suggest that ORNs are typically responsive to several odors. Although a given cell responds better to some odors than to others, attempts to classify the receptors into groups on the basis of their profiles of sensitivity have been unsuccessful. Some experiments suggest that different regions of the olfactory epithelium give maximal responses to different odorants, as though the nose and mucosa were somehow operating like a chromatograph, separating odors on the basis of their physical and chemical properties. The measurement of radioactive odorants delivered to the nose suggests that different odors result in distinctive spatiotemporal patterns of sorption across the olfactory mucosa. Nevertheless, there is no general agreement about the way in which quality is coded by the olfactory system.

2.3. A Large Multigene Family Encodes Odorant Receptors

It is widely accepted that electrical signals are generated in ORNs when odorants bind to specific membrane receptors located on their cilia. Classically, the existence of olfactory receptors as discrete, specific molecules was largely a theoretical construct advanced to explain the initial step in the transduction process. However, the existence of olfactory receptors was strongly supported by the 1991 discovery of a very large multi-gene family expressed by ORNs. This family consists of as many as one thousand separate genes in mammals, which represents almost 2–3% of the genome. In humans, approximately two-thirds of these genes have become pseudo-genes, which are genes that have undergone evolutionary mutations that insert stop codons into the reading frame of the gene, rendering them nonfunctional. Members of this odorant-receptor-gene family have a high degree of base-sequence homology with other genes that encode seven transmembrane (7-TM)-receptor molecules that function as receptors for neurotransmitters. These odorant-receptor gene transcripts (mRNAs) appear to be preferentially expressed in ORNs and other chemosensory cells such as vomeronasal neurons. In mammals, each ORN appears to express only a single member of this gene family, and ORNs expressing the same odorant-receptor gene (ORG) are widely dispersed in one of four broad expression zones within the epithelium. Significantly, these genes do not appear

to be expressed by any other neurons or any other tissues, although there are reports of the presence of some of these genes in sperm cells. The evidence for these genes functioning as odorant receptors comes mainly from two sources. When several of these genes were heterologously expressed in cell lines along with the appropriate signal-transduction molecules, the transfected cells responded to specific odorants (e.g., transfection with the I7 ORG conferred a strong response to octanol on the cells with weaker responses to related molecules). In a second approach, a specific ORG was expressed in a large number of ORNs in the mouse. The "extra" ORG expressed in these cells dramatically enhanced the response to specific odorants. Although it remains to be formally demonstrated that all of the ~1000 odorant-receptor genes have molecular specificity for odor molecules in the environment, these initial findings strongly support the role of this gene family in odorant detection. Studies on additional members of this large gene family should make it possible to determine whether receptors are broadly or narrowly "tuned" for different odors at the molecular level, perhaps corresponding to the response range of individual ORNs. In addition, it may be possible to learn if the receptors expressed by different ORNs are under strict genetic control or whether epigenetic factors (e.g., cell–cell interactions; odor experience) can regulate the receptor types expressed by individual ORNs.

2.4. Mechanisms of Olfactory Signal Transduction

The transduction mechanisms used by ORNs have been the focus of intense investigation since the previous edition of this book. These studies indicate that the 7-TM odorant receptors activate an olfactory specific G-protein (G_{olf}). Activation of these G-proteins stimulates adenylate cyclase type III, resulting in an increase in cAMP production (Fig. 2). Initial patch-clamp studies on excised patches of olfactory cilia demonstrated the expression of a cyclic nucleotide-gated, cation-permeable channel. This olfactory cyclic nucleotide channel (OCNC) was recently cloned, and together with the G_{olf} G-protein, is a critical element of the odor-transduction cascade. Binding of intracellular cyclic nucleotides opens the OCNC channel, allowing the influx of calcium, and thus, elevated cyclic adenosine monophosphate (cAMP) levels are transduced into alterations in the membrane potential. Sufficient membrane depolarization leads to the gen-

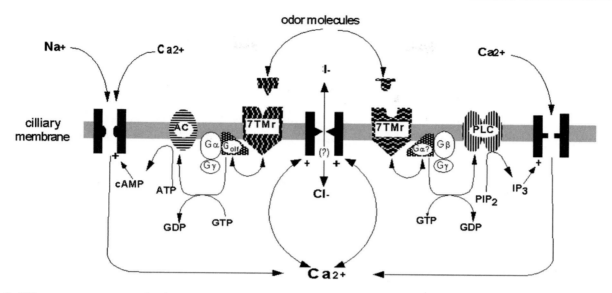

Fig. 2. Olfactory receptor-transduction mechanisms. Current evidence suggests that odor molecules bind to specific odorant-receptor proteins located in the cilia of ORNs. These 7-TM receptors are coupled to G-proteins that activate either adenylate cyclase III (AC) to generate cyclic AMP (cAMP) or putatively phospholipase C (PLC) to generate phosphatidyl inositol (IP_3). These second messengers in turn open channels that admit calcium (CA^{2+}) and/or sodium (Na^+) into the cilium. These ions lead to membrane depolarization and modulate intracellular free Ca^{2+} levels, both of which lead to the generation of action potentials that are conducted along ORN axons to the olfactory bulb.

eration of action potentials that are conducted along ORN axons to the olfactory bulb. In invertebrates, there is compelling evidence for inositol triphosphate (IP_3) as well as cAMP as second messengers; however, the use of IP_3 by mammalian ORNs is still controversial.

2.5. The Olfactory System Has the Unique Capacity to "Replace" Itself

ORNs are constantly undergoing turnover throughout life. Cutting the olfactory nerve results in retrograde degeneration of ORNs, which are subsequently reconstituted from a stem-cell population in the basal epithelium. These new ORNs mature and send axons to the olfactory bulb, where they form new synaptic connections. The olfactory epithelium may have the capacity to replace ORNs because these cells, which are directly exposed to airborne molecules, are vulnerable to injury from environmental factors. The regenerative capacity of the olfactory epithelium allows recovery of function following damage to the olfactory nerve, toxic exposure, viral infection, and other conditions that injure the olfactory receptor sheet. The ability of the adult epithelium to generate new neurons and the ability of these neurons to grow axons that re-establish functional synaptic connections with

target cells in the olfactory bulb, are unique among all mammalian neural structures. Understanding the mechanisms that allow this remarkable neural replacement to take place may eventually provide therapies for promoting repair in other parts of the brain. Indeed, recent studies indicate that it may be possible to use the ensheathing cells that surround the olfactory nerve as therapeutic agents for axon regrowth in models of spinal cord injury.

2.6. The Olfactory Nerve Is a Portal for the Entry of Foreign Substances Into the Brain

ORNs, situated in the nasal cavity, are exposed to airborne substances including viruses, industrial pollutants, and toxins. There is evidence that some viruses and other substances can be incorporated into ORNs and transported along their axons to the olfactory bulb. In experimental animal studies, it has been demonstrated that some of these substances escape from ORN synaptic terminals, and are incorporated into neurons and axons within the olfactory bulb. These substances are then further disseminated to other parts of the brain by anterograde or retrograde axonal transport. Thus, the olfactory nerve is a potential conduit for the entry and spread of foreign substances into the brain. It has been suggested that some forms of Alzheimer's and other degenerative diseases could be the result of viruses, metals, or silicates entering the brain from the olfactory epithelium.

2.7. There Is a Second, Parallel Olfactory System

In many species there is a second olfactory organ in the nasal cavity, the vomeronasal organ (VNO), located at the base of the midline nasal septum. The VNO contains receptor neurons that are morphologically similar to ORNs, but express a different family of odorant-receptor genes that share only low homology with those present in the main olfactory epithelium. This vomeronasal-receptor family consists of 100–200 separate genes. VNO-receptor neurons (vORNs) are generally believed to be preferentially sensitive to nonvolatile odorants, including relatively large proteins. In many species, vORNs respond to "pheromones," molecules emitted by conspecifics (members of the same species), with high specificity and selectivity. These pheromones often signal the gender and/or reproductive status of the sender, and can affect unconscious physiological processes in the recipient such as fertility cycles or puberty onset. In species with a VNO, the axons of vORNs project to a specialized structure at the dorsocaudal end of the "main" olfactory bulb (MOB) called, the accessory olfactory bulb (AOB). The structure and neuronal-cell types of the AOB are remarkably similar to those of the MOB; however, the axons of AOB mitral and tufted cells project to sites in the brain that are contiguous but non-overlapping with the projections of mitral and tufted cells from the MOB. This anatomical organization has given rise to the concept of two parallel olfactory systems—the main and accessory olfactory systems. Lesions of the VNO or the AOB cause significant impairment of reproductive behaviors and gonadosteroid function.

The VNO appears to be present in most human fetuses, but persists to adulthood in only some individuals. To date, studies have not revealed whether humans have a "functional" accessory olfactory system, as there is also no histologically recognizable AOB. The central structures that receive AOB innervation in mammals with VNOs are present in humans, and these structures also play important roles in human reproductive behavior and endocrine function. Thus, an important question is whether odors play any role in human sexual and endocrine functions, and if

so, what are the anatomical substrates for olfactory modulation of these functions. It is possible that ORNs specialized to transduce vORN-specific odorants exist but are not anatomically segregated from ORNs in humans. To date, only one 7-TM-receptor molecule specific to the vORN class of receptor genes has been cloned from human tissue, and at the chromosomal level most members of this gene family are nonfunctional pseudo-genes, suggesting that this class of receptors has a dramatically reduced function in humans.

3. THE OLFACTORY BULB

The olfactory bulb is the first site of olfactory information processing. The olfactory bulb is an oval structure that lies on the ventral surface of each frontal lobe and dorsal to the cribriform plate of the ethmoid bone. The olfactory bulb is arranged in layers, from superficial to deep: the olfactory-nerve layer (ONL), the glomerular layer (GL), the external plexiform layer (EPL), the mitral-cell layer (MCL), the internal plexiform layer (IPL) and the granule-cell layer (GCL) (Figs. 3,4,5).

There are two major neuronal groups in the olfactory bulb—second-order neurons—the mitral and tufted cells—and interneurons—the juxtaglomerular and granule cells. Axons of the mitral/tufted cells constitute the primary output pathway of the olfactory bulb, the lateral olfactory tract (LOT). Juxtaglomerular and granule cells are interneurons that modulate the activity of the mitral and tufted cells, and thus function to regulate the transfer of information from olfactory-nerve inputs to mitral/tufted outputs from the olfactory bulb. This regulation is organized into two distinct and largely separate levels—juxtaglomerular cells acting on mitral/tufted-cell apical dendrites in the glomerular layer, and granule cells acting on mitral/tufted-cell lateral dendrites in the external plexiform layer.

3.1. The "Unit Glomerulus"

ORN axons terminate exclusively in the glomeruli. Glomeruli are spheroid structures composed of a cellular shell surrounding a core that is rich in neuropil. Neuroanatomical tract-tracing studies conducted over several decades indicated that each point within the bulb receives input from ORN neurons that are widely scattered in the olfactory epithelium. Histochemical studies with cell surface markers showed that subpopulations of ORN axons sort out and terminate in regionally specific patterns that are highly consistent across

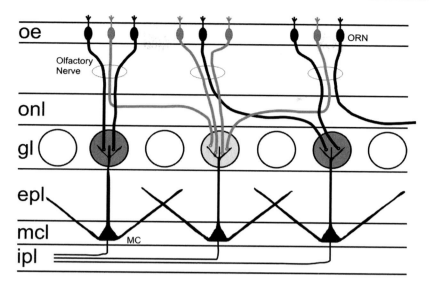

Fig. 3. Convergence of axons from ORNs expressing the same receptor gene. The axons from ORNs expressing the same odorant-receptor gene converge and terminate in only two or a few glomeruli. This is schematically displayed with the lighter axons representing one group of ORNs and the black axons representing ORNs expressing different receptors. The gray axons sort at the surface of the bulb to converge to a single target. oe, olfactory epithelium; onl, olfactory nerve fiber layer; gl, glomerular layer; epl, external plexiform layer; mcl, mitral cell layer; ipl, internal plexiform layer; ORN, olfactory receptor neuron; MC, mitral cell.

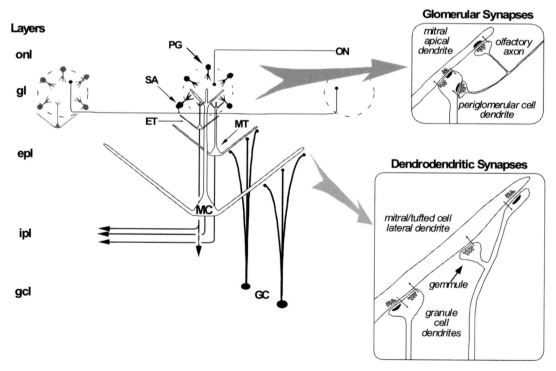

Fig. 4. The basic circuitry of the olfactory bulb. Axons of ORNs form the olfactory nerve (ON). These axons terminate in the glomeruli onto mitral (MC) and tufted cells (external tufted cell, ET; middle tufted cell, MT) and onto juxtaglomerular neurons including periglomerular cells (PG), ET cells, and short axon cells (SA). There are one-way and reciprocal synapses between the apical dendritic branches of mitral and tufted cells and the dendrites of juxtaglomerular neurons (*upper inset*, glomerular synapses). The lateral dendrites of mitral and tufted cells form one-way and reciprocal synapses with the apical dendrites of granule cells (GC; *lower inset*, dendrodendritic synapses).

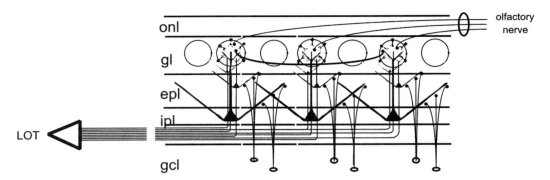

Fig. 5. The lateral olfactory tract. The axons of mitral and tufted cells collect at the caudal end of the olfactory bulb to form the lateral olfactory tract (LOT). These axons project throughout the olfactory cortex (*see* text and Figs. 5,6).

animals. More recently, transgenic mice in which ORNs expressing a particular ORG coordinately expresses β-galactosidase or green fluorescent protein (GFP) were constructed. These mice demonstrated that the axons from ORNs expressing the same ORG (e.g., an ORN cohort) converge and terminate in only two (or a few) glomeruli. Each glomerulus appears to be the result of homogeneous convergence of ORNs with the same odorant specificity. The convergence of ORN cohorts has only been directly demonstrated for small number (approx 20) of the 1000 potential receptor genes, and whether the general pattern of one ORN cohort projecting to one or a few glomeruli holds for all genes has not yet been determined.

Over the last several years, intense interest has focused on visualizing the activation of glomeruli when animals are exposed to specific odor cues. A variety of approaches, including 2-deoxyglucose incorporation, calcium-sensitive dyes, intrinsic imaging, and fMRI, indicate that specific odor molecules activate specific sets of glomeruli within the bulb. Different glomerular activation patterns are elicited by stimulation with different odorant molecules, but are generally bilateral and consistent between animals. Thus, the glomeruli represent a spatial map of the activity of ORNs to odor stimuli. The neural computational problem in the identification of odors thus becomes not how the brain recognizes odors, but how the brain recognizes patterns of glomerular activity elicited by different odors.

3.2. The Glomerular Layer

Glomeruli are the first site of synaptic integration in the olfactory pathway. The cellular shell surrounding glomeruli contains glial cells as well as several classes of juxtaglomerular neurons, including periglomerular

cells, external tufted cells, and short axon cells. However, the majority of cells in the glomerular layer consist of periglomerular cells and external tufted cells. The apical dendrites of mitral and tufted cells and the dendrites of periglomerular cells richly invest the glomerular core, and these dendrites are heavily targeted by ORN axons. ORNs utilize glutamate as their primary neurotransmitter, which acts on α-amino-3-hydroxy-5-methyl-4-isoxazole propionic acid (AMPA)/ kainate and *N*-methyl-D-aspartate (NMDA) receptors located on the dendrites of the olfactory-bulb target cells. Mitral and tufted cells (M/T cells) have a single apical dendrite that extends from the cell body through the EPL to ramify within a single glomerulus. In addition to olfactory nerve terminals, M/T cell apical dendrites are synaptically contacted by the dendrites of periglomerular cells, via dendrodendritic synapses. The predominant action of periglomerular neurons is likely to be inhibitory, either to M/T cells and/or to olfactory nerve terminals. Release of the inhibitory neurotransmitter GABA from these cells can inhibit M/T cell dendrites, or can act to presynaptically suppress the excitability of olfactory nerve terminals via GABA$_B$ receptors expressed on the terminal. Dopamine is a second inhibitory transmitter expressed by numerous juxtaglomerular neurons; release of this transmitter also acts to presynaptically suppress the olfactory nerve terminals via the dopamine D2 receptor. Since juxtaglomerular neurons can project processes over a distance corresponding to approx 2–3 glomeruli in any direction, lateral inhibitory circuits can act over a region comprising as many as 4–9 glomeruli. In addition to local circuits, juxtaglomerular neurons and/or the apical processes of M/T cells can be influenced by the axons of neurons from other parts of the brain (via the so-called centrifugal afferents).

Cholinergic axons from the basal forebrain terminate in glomeruli, as do serotonergic axons from the midbrain raphe. Thus, olfactory information transmitted from the olfactory nerve to the output neurons of the olfactory bulb—the M/T cell—is influenced by both the actions of local inhibitory circuits and by long-range centrifugal modulatory systems. The purpose of this modulation is unclear, but is believed to increase the signal to noise ratio in the system.

3.3. External Plexiform Layer

M/T cells have 4–6 lateral dendrites extending for considerable distances (1–2 mm in the mouse) through the EPL, deep to the glomerular layer. These dendrites are a primary target for the apical dendrites of the GABAergic granule cells, whose cell body resides in the mitral and granule cell layers. These granule cell apical dendrites form dendrodendritic inhibitory synapses onto the lateral dendrites of the M/T cells, which in turn form reciprocal dendrodendritic excitatory glutamatergic synapses back onto dendrites of the granule cells. These dendrodendritic synapses probably function to provide lateral inhibition or a temporal filter in the processing of olfactory information from the primary olfactory neuron to the output of the M/T cells.

3.4. Granule Cell Layer

Granule cells are small interneurons that project a spiny dendrite radially into the EPL. As indicated, this dendrite forms reciprocal dendrodendritic contacts with the lateral dendrites of M/T cells in the EPL. In addition to the dendrodendritic contacts, granule cells are heavily targeted by excitatory synaptic inputs from ipsi- and contralateral olfactory cortical structures via the centrifugal afferents. Excitatory inputs onto the granule cell induce the release of GABA onto the M/T cell lateral dendrites, thus inhibiting the M/T cells. The cortical regions targeting granule cells are the very structures that are targeted by the M/T cells. Therefore, output from the olfactory bulb can cause a massive negative feedback to the output M/T cells via the centrifugal afferents and granule cell circuit. The functional significance of this circuitry is not fully understood, but it would appear that the coding of olfactory information involves feedback mechanisms in which the output of the bulb at any moment is fed back to the bulb to modify its subsequent outputs. In addition to these olfactory cortical inputs, granule cells are also selectively targeted by norepinephrine containing terminals from the locus coeruleus. The soma of some granule cells are also coupled by gap junctions, which could serve to electrically couple clusters of granule cells so that synaptic activation of one cell leads to the activation of other cells in the cluster. This arrangement could "amplify" or "synchronize" granule-cell inhibition of M/T lateral dendrites.

Because the two classes of M/T cell dendrites ramify in two distinct layers of the bulb they are regulated by different interneurons—M/T apical dendrites are regulated by juxtaglomerular cells, and granule cells regulate M/T lateral dendrites. As a result, the input–output functions of the olfactory bulb are critically determined by neural signals that influence juxtaglomerular and granule cells as well as signals that directly influence M/T cells.

3.5. Convergence in the Olfactory Bulb

In the rabbit there are ~50,000,000 olfactory receptors and ~2000 glomeruli; thus, each glomerulus receives ~25,000 olfactory axons. As there are ~25 mitral cells associated with each glomerulus, the average number of ORN axons terminating on each mitral cell is approx 1000. Thus, the sensory input to mitral cells is highly convergent. There is little evidence examining whether the mitral cells associated with a single glomerulus project to common targets in olfactory cortex; thus, it is difficult to draw conclusions about convergence to higher processing areas.

3.6. Cellular Responses to Odor Stimulation

There have been very few electrophysiological studies of the responses of olfactory bulb neurons to odors in vivo. The few published studies indicate that mitral-cell responses to odors are typically complex: during odor exposure, single-unit recordings show that mitral cells may be initially excited and then inhibited, inhibited and then excited, or may exhibit more complex responses. The character of these responses can alter with odor concentration. Potentially, individual units may more reliably discriminate between odors if unit activity is recorded in relation to an artificial sniff cycle. Recent studies have also emphasized the necessity of testing the response of each cell over a range of odor concentrations. Testing with several odors, each at several different concentrations, showed that a significant number of cells respond differently to at least two odors at all odor concentrations. Similar results in the salamander led to the concept of "concentration tuning" of the mitral cell: individual cells appeared to

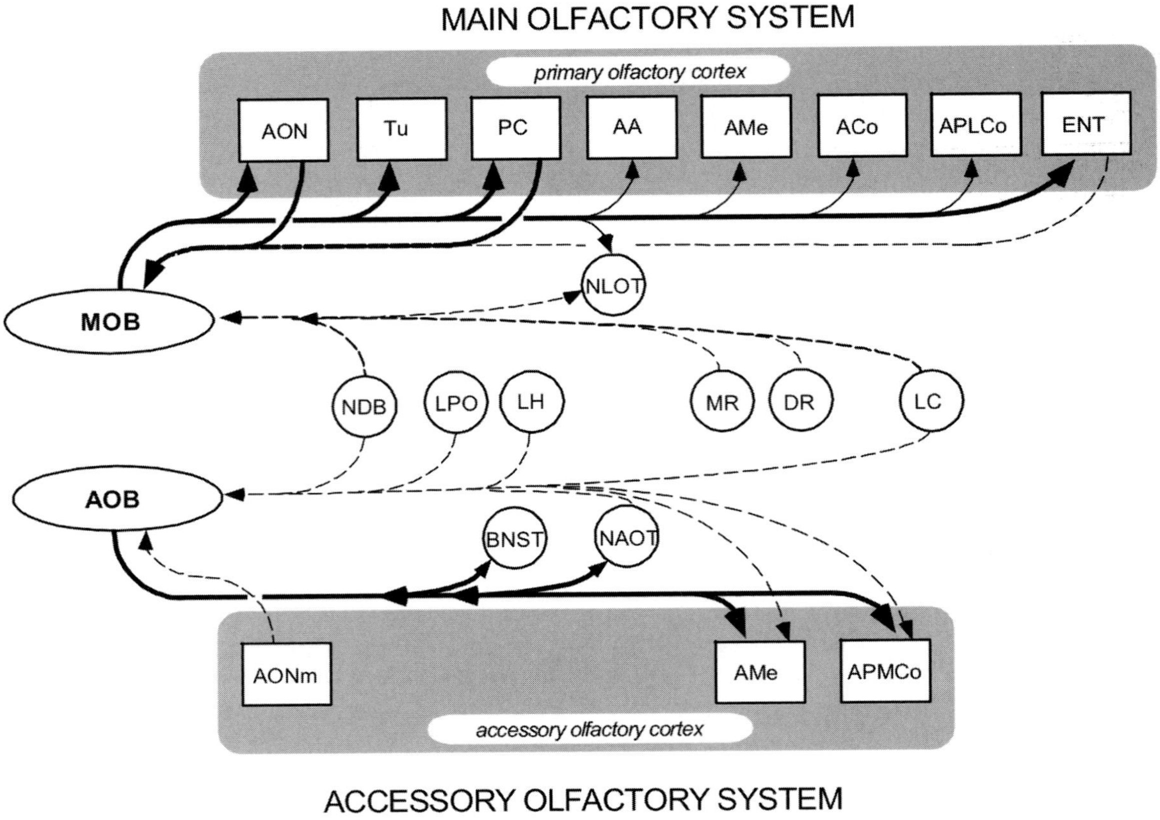

MAIN OLFACTORY SYSTEM

Fig. 6. Major connections of the main and accessory olfactory systems. Connections of the main (MOB) and accessory (AOB) bulbs with cortical (*gray panels*) and subcortical (*circles*) structures. Relative strengths of connections are represented by *line thickness*. Output projections of MOB and AOB shown by *solid lines*, and the reciprocal and centrifugal projections to MOB and AOB are shown by *dashed lines*. Cortical areas comprising the primary and accessory olfactory cortex are indicated by *squares*. AA, anterior amygdala; AOB, accessory olfactory bulb; ACo, anterior cortical amygdaloid nucleus; AMe, medial amygdaloid nucleus; AON, anterior olfactory nucleus (m, medial division); APLCo, posterolateral cortical amygdaloid nucleus; APMCo, posterolmedial cortical amygdaloid nucleus; BNST, bed nucleus of the stria terminalis; DR, dorsal raphe nucleus; ENT, entorhinal cortex; LH, lateral hypothalamus; LC, locus coeruleus; LPO, lateral preoptic area; MOB, main olfactory bulb; MR, median raphe; NAOT, nucleus of the accessory olfactory tract; NLOT, nucleus of the lateral olfactory tract; NDB, nucleus of the diagonal band; PC, piriform cortex; Tu, olfactory tubercle.

respond best to a particular concentration of each odorant. However, because ORNs adapt rapidly to continuous exposure to the same odor, it is difficult to obtain consistent repeated measures of bulb neurons to the same odor. Additionally, most electrophysiological studies of bulb neurons have been done in anesthetized animals, and most anesthetics profoundly alter the firing characteristics of these cells.

Clearly, our understanding of the neural correlates of odor perception lag far behind our knowledge of the stimulus-response characteristics of neurons in other sensory systems. It may be that odor quality and concentration are not uniquely represented by single neurons, but rather by populations or ensembles of cells.

Analysis of this possibility will require the use of experimental techniques that allow simultaneous measures of large numbers of cells during the presentation of odors.

4. THE PRIMARY OLFACTORY CORTEX

4.1. Anterior Olfactory Nucleus

The olfactory bulb is connected to the base of the temporal lobe by a stalk of tissue called the olfactory peduncle. In most infra-primate species, the peduncle consists of a population of neurons, the anterior olfactory nucleus (AON), and two major tracts of fibers—the LOT and the anterior limb of the anterior

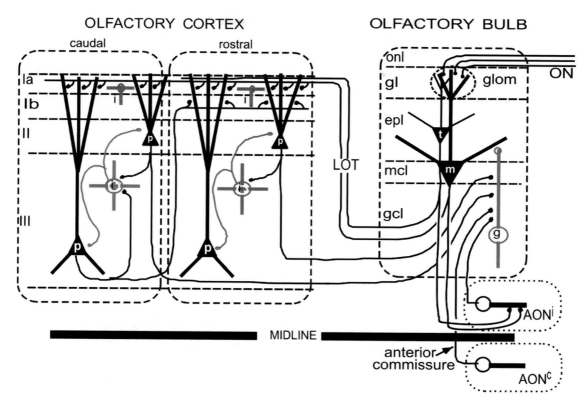

Fig. 7. Basic olfactory network. Schematic of the networks linking the olfactory bulb and primary olfactory cortex. Olfactory nerve axons (ON) terminate in the glomeruli (glom) onto mitral (m) and tufted (t) cells that project via the lateral olfactory tract (LOT) to layer Ia of primary olfactory cortex to terminate on the dendrites of layer II–III pyramidal (p) cells. Layer II–III pyramidal cells in rostral olfactory cortex project to layer Ib in caudal olfactory cortex and *vice versa*. Olfactory cortical pyramidal cells send reciprocal projections back to the olfactory bulb. Thus olfactory-bulb output is continuously modified by feedback from areas it targets. Inhibitory interneurons in olfactory bulb and olfactory cortex (shown in gray) modulate network function. Neurons in the ipsilateral (AONi) and contralateral anterior olfactory nuclei (AON) link olfactory-network function in the two hemispheres via the anterior commissure.

commissure (Figs. 6,7). Although historically referred to as a "nucleus," the AON is now considered a cortical structure, with several subdivisions distinguished on the basis of cellular architecture and connectional patterns. A substantial number of AON neurons are pyramidal cells whose apical dendrites extend toward the pial surface of the AON. The major afferents to AON arise from the ipsilateral bulb and the contralateral AON. In addition, the AON also receives afferents from more caudal primary olfactory cortical structures and from a variety of cortical and subcortical structures associated with the limbic system. The major efferents of the AON are to: (i) the *ipsilateral* bulb and olfactory cortex, and (ii) the *contralateral* bulb and AON. Our understanding of the functional significance of the AON is still rudimentary. Clearly, the major interbul-bar connections of the AON impli-

cate this structure in the interhemispheric processing of olfactory information. There is evidence that binasal mechanisms may function in spatial localization of odors, and the AON system would be suspected to play a significant role in such mechanisms. There is also evidence from animal studies that the AON plays a key role in the interhemispheric transfer of olfactory memories.

4.2. Primary Olfactory Cortex

Beginning at the caudal limits of the AON, the cortex of the basal temporal lobe expands in the caudal direction, forming a pear shaped structure, the piriform lobe. The rostral part of this structure contains the piriform cortex, the major cortical component of the primary olfactory cortex. Further caudally, the medial part of this cortex overlies the amygdaloid complex; this part of the piriform cortex is referred to as the periamygdaloid cortex. Further caudally and medially, the piriform–periamygdaloid cortex gives way gradually to the parahippocampal cortex, and then to the hippocampus. Thus, there is a continuous expanse of gradually changing cortical architecture that leads from the olfactory bulb, the AON, piriform, periamygdaloid, entorhinal, and subicular cortices that leads directly into the fields of the hippocampus. This orderly anatomical arrangement is one reason that early anatomists referred to the olfactory cortex, parahippocampus, and hippocampus as the "rhinencephalon," believing that the entire expanse of cortex constituted the "smell brain." This view was tempered by subsequent research showing that the projections of the olfactory bulb directly innervate only the AON, piriform, periamygdaloid, and lateral entorhinal cortices. Thus, most of the parahippocampal region and the hippocampus are now considered to be part of the "limbic system." Notwithstanding this considerable loss of cortical real estate, the olfactory system can still claim to be the sensory system with the most direct access to the hippocampus, because there are direct projections of the olfactory bulb and piriform cortex to the entorhinal cortex, and the entorhinal cortex is the major source of afferent input to the hippocampus.

Together, the piriform, periamygdaloid, and parts of the entorhinal cortex are often referred to as the "primary olfactory cortex" (POC), as they are all directly targeted by synaptic inputs from the olfactory bulb. The rostral parts of POC receive terminals from both tufted and mitral cells. The caudal parts of the piriform, the periamygdaloid and lateral entorhinal cortex, receive terminals primarily or exclusively from mitral cells. In all parts of the POC, the olfactory-bulb projection terminates in the superficial half of layer I, designated layer Ia. As for the olfactory bulb and AON, there is little evidence for point-to-point topography in the projections of the olfactory bulb to the POC. This further reinforces the idea that point-to-point topography does not play a significant role in the central representation of odor space, and has led several researchers in the field to suggest that processing of olfactory information in the olfactory cortex can be best understood by considering the olfactory cortex as a content addressable, distributed neural network. In this view, the functioning of a network is inherent in the organization of its microcircuits, the patterns of connection between input and output of the circuits do

not matter as much as the ability of the circuitry to form associative (memory) linkages with no (obviously) discernible spatial patterns of anatomical connectivity.

4.3. The Connections of the POC Are Well Characterized

These connections can be divided into four classes: (i) *intrinsic* or *local*—short connections between neurons in different layers of POC; (ii) *associative*—connections with different parts of the POC, (iii) *extrinsic*—connections with other structures; and (iv) *modulatory inputs*—afferents that terminate in POC as part of a broader innervation of other cortical and subcortical neural systems.

4.3.1. INTRINSIC OR LOCAL CONNECTIONS

The POC has two principal layers of pyramidal neurons, layers II and III, which comprise several morphological classes, as well as several classes of non-pyramidal neurons. There are extensive translaminar or local connections among POC neurons. Layer II neurons give off axon collaterals to deeper layer III pyramidal cells, and there are local inhibitory interneurons in layers I and II that are contacted both by olfactory bulb terminals and by local collaterals of pyramidal cells. Deeper pyramidal cells also give rise to extensive local collaterals that may synapse with local interneurons or with more superficial pyramidal cells. Thus, there are extensive translaminar connections from superficial to deeper layers and vice versa. In addition, there are several classes of GABAergic and neuropeptide-containing neurons in POC, and although the connection of these neurons is unknown, many of them have the appearance of local interneurons.

4.3.2. ASSOCIATION CONNECTIONS

Cortico–cortical projections within POC are extensive, and exhibit some degree of laminar and regional organization. Axons from pyramidal cells of layer IIb are primarily directed at more caudal sites in the POC; cells in layer III project predominantly to rostral parts of the POC. Commissural fibers to the contralateral POC arise from layer IIb of the anterior parts of POC. The ipsilateral and commissural association projections of POC terminate in a highly laminar fashion in layer Ib, immediately below the zone that contains the inputs from the olfactory bulb; a lighter projection terminates in layer III. POC projections back to AON also terminate in layer Ib, below the bulb recipient zone. Neurons in layers IIb and III send a dense projection back to the olfactory bulb; as noted previously, this feedback pathway terminates primarily in the granule cell layer.

4.3.3. EXTRINSIC CONNECTIONS

The major extrinsic connections of the POC are its reciprocal connections with the olfactory bulb and AON and its efferent projections to various nonolfactory cortical–subcortical targets. These are discussed in the following section.

4.3.4. MODULATORY INPUTS

The POC also receives subcortical modulatory inputs from the locus coeruleus (norepinephrine), midbrain raphe nuclei (serotonergic) and magnocellular basal forebrain—the nucleus of the diagonal band—(cholinergic, and a small number GABAergic) and from the ventral tegmental area (dopaminergic).

4.4. POC Impacts on a Diversity of Brain Structures

Two classes of POC outputs have already been discussed—the feedback projection to the olfactory bulb and the association connections between the rostral and caudal olfactory cortex. A third class of outputs is treated separately because it represents the projections of POC to brain regions not generally included in the olfactory system *per se*, although their receipt of inputs from POC obviously implicates these POC targets in olfactory function. The extrinsic outputs of the piriform cortex are both to cortical and subcortical structures.

4.4.1. NEOCORTICAL PROJECTIONS

The olfactory-bulb projection to the POC extends dorsally beyond the cytoarchitectural limits of the POC into the ventral parts of the granular insular and perirhinal cortices. There are also direct projections from the POC to insular and orbital cortex. Insular and orbital cortexes are the primary cortical targets of ascending pathways arising in the nucleus of the solitary tract (NTS) in the medulla, and appear to contain the primary cortical representations for both gustatory and visceral sensation. Thus, olfactory projections to the insular and orbital cortex may be sites that integrate olfactory and gustatory signals to generate the integrated perception of flavor. These same cortical areas also have descending projections to the hypothalamus and back to the NTS; these corticofugal projections influence visceral-autonomic and possibly gustatory functions. Therefore, this circuitry could also allow olfactory modulation of autonomic function. Neurons in these cortical areas in primates respond to odors with a higher degree of selectivity than neurons in either the olfactory bulb or the POC. Thus, these neocortical sites may play a role in the discrimination of different odors.

4.4.2. SUBCORTICAL PROJECTIONS

(i) Hypothalamus: The heaviest and most direct projections to the hypothalamus arise from neurons in the deepest layers of the piriform cortex and the anterior olfactory nucleus. These projections terminate most heavily in the lateral hypothalamic area. Olfactory recipient parts of the cortical and medial amygdaloid nuclei also project to medial and anterior parts of the hypothalamus. (ii) Thalamus: There is a strong projection from the POC to the magnocellular, medial part of the mediodorsal thalamic nucleus and the submedial nucleus (nucleus gelatinosa). These thalamic nuclei project to the orbital cortex and the frontal lobes.

5. OLFACTION AND BEHAVIOR

5.1. Olfaction Has an Important Impact on Behavior

Complete removal of both olfactory bulbs eliminates the ability to detect or discriminate odors. This is not particularly surprising because the bulb is the sole target of ORNs, and following "bulbectomy," ORNs degenerate. What is somewhat surprising is that following removal of all but 10% of the olfactory bulbs, experimental animals can detect and discriminate odors. This suggests that odors are not represented in discrete sites in the olfactory bulb; otherwise animals with 90% of the bulb removed should be unable to detect some odors. Contrasting with this conclusion are functional imaging experiments showing that discrete sites in the bulb have increased glomerular activity following exposure of the animal to some odorant molecules. However, other odorant molecules show a more distributed pattern of glomerular activation across broad regions of the bulb. It is likely that lesion of a large area of the bulb would render the animal anosmic to certain specific odorant molecules, and leave residual responsiveness to other molecules. Most environmental odors are combinatorial mixes of separate odorant molecules that together give the perception of the odor (e.g., coffee contains as many as 900 different volatile molecules). The question of how the olfactory system resolves these highly complex odorant mixtures is presently unresolved.

Olfaction is a critical sensory system for many behaviors. For many animals, odors play an absolutely essential role in reproductive and maternal behaviors. Experimental studies have shown that bulbectomized males of some mammalian species will not mate with receptive females. In other species, olfactory cues are not absolutely essential, but mating behavior is reduced by damage to the olfactory system. In females, olfactory bulb lesions severely impair gonadal steroid function.

In humans, a developmental disorder known as Kallmann's syndrome is caused by impaired migration of certain neurons from the developing olfactory epithelium into the brain. One of the neuron types that fails to enter the brain contains the neuropeptide GnRH. Normally, GnRH cells migrate from the epithelium to the hypothalamus and preoptic area during fetal development; many of these cells generate axons that terminate in the median eminence (ME) where they release GnRH. The GnRH acts on cells in the pituitary, causing the release of the hormone leutinizing hormone (LH) into circulation. LH is necessary for the proper development of reproductive organs at puberty. In Kallmann's syndrome, the GnRH cells do not enter the brain, and Kallman's patients have gonadal atrophy. The genetic defect that prevents the normal migration of GnRH cells into the brain often also prevents ORN axons from reaching the olfactory bulb. As a result, the olfactory system fails to develop and these individuals are anosmic—e.g., they are unable to smell.

In some species, odors also signal identity and social status. For example, if a pregnant female mouse is exposed to the odor of the urine of a strange male, she aborts. There is also evidence that the hormonal status of some animals influences their ability to detect certain odors. Female sheep, for example, become unusually sensitive to odors of their own lambs at parturition.

In humans, odors do not appear to have such profound effects on behavior and endocrine function, although there have been relatively few experimental studies of this subject. It should not be concluded, however, that, olfaction is unimportant in humans. A casual glance at the ledger sheets of the food, beverage (remember that the perception of "flavor" is more olfaction than taste) and fragrance industries leaves little doubt about the importance of olfaction and taste to the quality of our lives!

5.2. Why Do We Still Not Understand Olfaction?

There is considerable information about the anatomy, transduction molecules, and classical electrophysiology of the olfactory system. Unfortunately, this body of knowledge gives little indication how the system works to allow us to detect and recognize odors, or how odors are able to influence behavior and endocrine function. Thus, in comparison to other sensory systems, our knowledge of the integrative properties of the olfactory system is very rudimentary. Because it is the primary output target of the olfactory bulb, it has been tempting to think that the olfactory cortex is involved in some kind of hierarchical or higher-order stimulus feature extraction. This expectation is based upon analogy with the organization of the other major sensory systems, where it has been possible to infer how neurons, at successive levels from the periphery through subcortical relays to the primary sensory cortex, transform inputs to extract different features of the sensory signal. In the case of the olfactory system, this prevailing "sensory systems paradigm" has provided little insight into the neural operations that lead to the perception of odor qualities or the features of odors that modify behavior. It is reasonable, therefore, to wonder why the paradigm that has worked so well in understanding relationships between sensory stimuli and the neural mechanisms that encode stimulus features in other sensory systems has fallen so short in the olfactory system.

Nonetheless, there have been repeated efforts to understand olfactory anatomy and physiology by comparison with other sensory systems. Almost every decade, someone attempts to make the olfactory bulb like the retina. The similarity between the alternating layers of neuron types with intervening plexuses of synaptic integration in the retina and the olfactory bulb make it irresistibly tempting to try to understand the circuitry of the bulb in terms of the retina. This analogy is maintained only as long as one ignores equally compelling and fundamental differences between the retina and the bulb. Chief among these is the existence of massive feedback inputs to the olfactory bulb and the total absence of centrifugal inputs to the retina in mammals (in some nonmammalian vertebrates, there is a midbrain nucleus that projects to the retina, but this feature is lacking in mammals). The retina transduces light, processes the neural responses via networks of intrinsic neurons, and then conducts the output to the geniculostriate or collicular systems. In the olfactory bulb system, the *outputs* of the bulb are paralleled at every step by massive *feedback* pathways that modulate populations of bulbar interneurons, which in turn directly regulate the output neurons. In this sense, the bulb is not so much a *relay* to higher olfactory structures as the first stage in a circuit that feeds back upon itself at every stage of synaptic transfer. From this perspective, attempts to analogize the olfactory bulb with the retina may be misleading because the functional status of bulb neurons at any moment reflects activity not only in sensory afferents and interneurons, but also the activity in feedback pathways from AON and olfactory cortex. As AON and POC are the predominant output targets of the bulb, it follows that olfactory-bulb neurons are continuously modulated by

signals that represent transformations of their own output. The retina does not work this way. The output of ganglion cells is modulated by intra-retinal processing, but not by operations performed in the output targets of the retina. Future progress in understanding the functions of the olfactory system, therefore, may depend in large measure on our ability to develop new paradigms of neural network operation because traditional paradigms lack the power necessary to encompass the complexity of olfactory circuits. This may be a useful and important endeavor, because the "classical sensory paradigm" has probably outlived its utility and is not adequate to model the neural operations that underlie cognitive functions. The olfactory system is an inherently cortical sensory system. Thus, the eventual understanding of olfactory-network operations may provide new insights for the analysis of higher cortical functions.

28   Sleep, Dreams, and States of Consciousness

Robert W. McCarley

Contents

1. INTRODUCTION AND ORGANIZATION OF SLEEP–WAKEFULNESS

An understanding of the brain basis of consciousness is one of the oldest dreams of neuroscientists and physicians. Although a knowledge of its subtleties is at a very early stage, we are now beginning to understand some of the basic mechanisms that control the changes of consciousness associated with sleep and wakefulness.

1.1. The EEG Is an Important, but Limited Tool for the Study of States of Consciousness

We begin with a brief review of the biological basis of the electroencephalogram (EEG) and evoked potentials (EPs). When activity is synchronous, neurons in the cerebral cortex generate electrical signals

From: *Neuroscience in Medicine, 2nd ed.* (P. Michael Conn, ed.), © 2003 Humana Press Inc., Totowa, NJ.

strong enough to be detected through the skull by sensors (electrodes) placed on the scalp. These small (microvolt) electrical signals are amplified and filtered to produce EEG recordings. Although the EEG is a crude method of analyzing brain activity (similar to figuring out what is happening in a football game by putting microphones outside the stadium), it has proven to be a remarkably useful tool for studying the basic structure of sleep in humans.

Figure 1 illustrates, for one cortical neuron, the source of currents underlying the EEG. The influx of positive ions into the soma of the neuron (following a depolarizing postsynaptic potential) generates a current "sink," since, by convention, current is composed of positive ion flow. The apical dendrites of this cortical neuron, in contrast, act as a "source" of positive ions and current flow. This current flow pattern of a source in the dendrites and a sink in the soma creates a *dipole*, literally a "two pole" with the positive pole (source) in the dendrites and the negative pole (sink) in the soma. In cerebral structures with a regular lami-

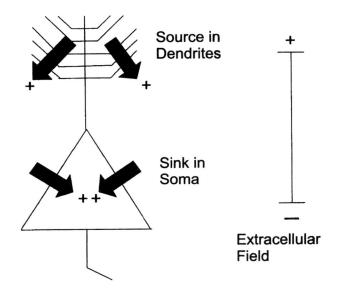

Fig. 1. Example of a cortical neuronal "dipole" occurring with a depolarizing postsynaptic potential on the soma of a pyramidal neuron. This pattern of current flow, repeated over many thousands of cortical neurons, is likely the main generator source for EEG and evoked potential waves (EP) (*see* text).

nar structure such as the cerebral cortex, this simple dipole model repeated over many constituent neurons provides a reasonable first approximation of how positive EEG waves are generated. In the case of a hyperpolarizing postsynaptic potential in the soma, the dipole polarity would be reversed, with the source (positive pole) in the soma and sink in the dendrites (it will be recalled that membrane hyperpolarization arises as the consequence of a net efflux of positive ions). Most of the components of the EEG arise from the currents generated by postsynaptic potentials, as described in our example, and not from the currents generated by action potentials. Action potentials are generally too brief and too asynchronous to summate and produce a signal that is detectable from the scalp. (Some of the very short latency (<10 ms) brainstem auditory, EP components are derived from synchronous volleys of action potentials, and are an important exception to this rule.) EPs may be considered as EEG waves that occur following a sensory stimulus. Since they are time-locked to the stimulus, they may be averaged to improve the signal-to-noise ratio; this is important because the biological EP signals recorded from the scalp are typically only a few μv in amplitude.

Many investigators are currently exploring the utility of modeling "equivalent dipoles" as a representation of the average amplitude and polarity of EEG and

EPs arising within a cerebral region, such as the sensory receiving areas of the cortex. Practical constraints to localizing the source of EP and EEG include the use of scalp recordings and the consequent "smearing" of current flow as the boundaries between zones of different conductivities are traversed. For example, the brain and its extracellular fluid are a much better conductor than the scalp. Studies have applied an experimental approach to the question of the accuracy of source localization possible with electrical signals. Using patients who had deep electrodes implanted to locate the seizure source prior to surgery, a low-level signal was passed through two deep electrodes (a true dipole source), and then it was determined how closely the signal source within the brain could be localized from scalp electrode recordings. For this single source, brain localization was found to be accurate to within about 1 cm. However, as the number of sources increases, as is usually the case in brain processing, the ability to localize them becomes less.

The EEG is perhaps most useful in its roles in detecting the presence of seizure activity and in pinpointing changes in alertness and sleep stages. a major topic of this chapter. The EEG is described in terms of the amplitude of its waves and their frequency. As shown in Table 1, EEG frequencies are grouped into bands which range from the very low frequencies (delta, 0.5–4 Hz) to the very fast (beta, 14–32 Hz, and gamma). As a general rule, the delta EEG frequencies are associated with states of consciousness with little complex processing, such as nonREM sleep, and those with higher frequencies are associated with more complex processing, as occurs in wakefulness and rapid eye movement (REM) sleep (dream sleep).

The *alpha rhythm* has a frequency range of 8–14 Hz, and is best recorded over the occipital scalp region. It occurs during wakefulness, often appearing upon eye closure and disappearing with eye opening. Depth recordings in animals indicate that alpha-rhythm frequencies may also be present in the visual thalamus (lateral geniculate body, pulvinar), and the cortical component appears to be generated in relatively small cortical areas that act as epicenters. Unfortunately, there are still no definitive studies of the genesis of this rhythm, although the interaction of cortico–cortical and thalamo–cortical neurons has been postulated. Origins of the delta waves are discussed below.

The high-voltage, slow-wave activity in cortex during nonREM sleep—termed EEG synchronization—contrasts sharply with the low-voltage fast-pat-

Table 1
EEG Frequency Bands

Name	Frequency range in Hz
Delta	0.5–4
Theta	4–8
Alpha	8–14
Beta	14–32
Gamma (*see* text)	20–60+

tern—often termed *activated*—characteristic of both waking and REM sleep and consisting of frequencies in the beta range and higher. A term often used to describe the EEG of wakefulness and REM sleep is "desynchronized," meaning that the slow waves of nonREM sleep are not visible.

1.1.1. GAMMA ACTIVITY

It should be noted that recent work indicates that high-frequency ("gamma") synchronized waves may be present in waking and REM sleep, although these are of low amplitude. As the term is currently used, gamma frequencies are centered on about 40 Hz, and range from about 20–60 Hz, and even higher. Table 1 shows a frequency overlap of gamma and beta. This arose because, although, the beta-frequency band was originally designated in a largely arbitrary, ad hoc manner, the current concept of gamma-frequency activity is based on considerable basic and clinical neuroscience work. Thus, the use of gamma frequency has come to supplant the term of "beta activity." Gamma activity may index synchronous activity of the cortical-cell columns involved in neural processing, and recent work in cognitive neuroscience suggests that rapid EEG activity in the gamma band (20–60 Hz) increases during—and may be involved in—the formation of percepts and memory, linguistic processing, and other behavioral and perceptual functions, including associative learning. Furthermore, recent work from the author's laboratory indicates that gamma activity may be deficient in schizophrenia.

1.2. Sleep Is Organized Into a Definite Structure

One-third of our lives is spent in sleep. No other single behavior occupies so much of our time, yet few other behaviors have been so mysterious. We now know that there are two main states of sleep, REM

sleep, typically associated with a high level of brain neuronal activity and the distinctive conscious state of dreaming, and nonREM sleep, typically associated with a low level of neuronal activity and nonvisual, ruminative thinking. A typical study of sleep includes records of the EEG, of eye movements (the electro-oculogram or EOG), and of muscle tone (the electromyogram or EMG). This ensemble of records is known as a *polysomnogram,* and the recording process is known as *polysomnography.* These key records enable us to describe the main stages of sleep. As sleep onset approaches, the low-amplitude, fast-frequency EEG of alert wakefulness, often with alpha present (Fig. 2A), yields to Stage 1 sleep, a brief transitional phase between wakefulness and "true" sleep. This stage is often called "descending Stage 1" because it is a prelude to deeper sleep stages and it is characterized by low-voltage (amplitude), relatively fast-frequency EEG patterns and slow, rolling eye movements. During Stage 2 sleep, there are episodic bursts of rhythmic, 14–16 Hz waveforms in the EEG, known as *sleep spindles,* interspersed with occasional short-duration, high-amplitude "K complexes," so named because of their morphologic resemblance to this letter. During Stage 2, the EEG slows still further. Stages 3 and 4 are defined, respectively, by a lesser and greater occurrence of high-amplitude, slow (0.5–4 Hz) waveforms known as *delta waves.* The low-voltage, fast EEG pattern of REM sleep is in marked contrast to delta sleep, and resembles the nonalpha EEG pattern of active wakefulness and Stage 1 descending (Fig. 2A). REM sleep is further characterized by the presence of bursts of REM (hence the name), and by the loss of muscle tone in certain major muscle groups of the limbs, trunk, and neck. Often, the nonREM sleep stages are lumped together and simply termed "nonREM sleep." (Researchers working with animals often use the term "slow-wave sleep" for "nonREM sleep," and this term sometimes occurs in the studies with humans, although, properly speaking, stages 1 and 2 do not have slow waves.) Table 2 summarizes the major differences between waking, nonREM, and REM sleep in a polysomnographic recording.

There is a fairly predictable pattern of shifting between one sleep state and another during a typical night's sleep (Fig. 2B). As the night begins, there is a stepwise descent from wakefulness to Stage 1 through to Stage 4 sleep, followed by a more abrupt ascent back toward Stage 1. However, in place of Stage 1, the first REM sleep episode usually occurs at this transi-

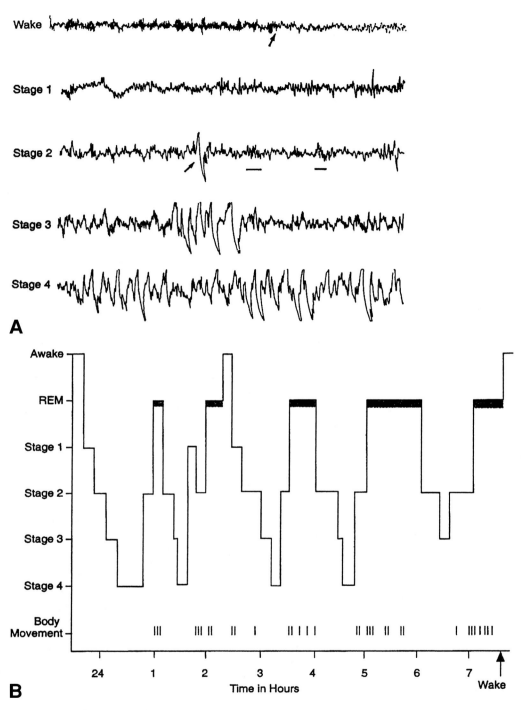

Fig. 2. (A) Shows the EEG patterns associated with wakefulness and the stages of sleep and (B) shows the time-course of sleep stages over a night's sleep in a healthy young man. During wakefulness there is a low-voltage, fast-EEG pattern, often with alpha waves, as shown here. At the arrow there is a transition to "Stage 1" sleep, with loss of the alpha rhythm, and the presence of a low-voltage, fast EEG. As sleep deepens, the EEG frequency slows more and more. Stage 2 is characterized by the presence of K complexes (*arrow*) and sleep spindles (*underlined*). During stage 3 delta waves (0.5–4 Hz) appear and in stage 4 they are present more than 50% of the time. During REM sleep (*black bars*) the EEG pattern returns to a low-voltage, fast pattern. The percentage of time spent in REM sleep increases with successive sleep cycles and the percentage of stages 3 and 4 decreases. (EEG segments recorded from C3, except from O2 in waking, in order to show the alpha rhythm most clearly. Figure adapted from Carskadon and Dement, 1989.)

Table 2
Polysomnographic Definition of Wakefulness, NonREM and REM Sleep

State	EEG amplitude and main frequencies	Rapid eye movement (EOG)	Muscle tone (EMG)
Waking	Low-voltage, fast	+	+
NonREM Sleep	High-voltage, slow	−	−
REM sleep	Low-voltage, fast	+	−

tion point, about 70–90 min after sleep onset. The first REM sleep episode in humans is short. After the first REM sleep episode, the sleep cycle repeats itself with the appearance of nonREM sleep and then, about 90 min after the start of the first REM period, another REM sleep episode occurs. This rhythmic cycling persists throughout the night. The REM sleep cycle length is 90 min in humans, and the duration of each REM sleep episode after the first is approx 30 min. Over the course of the night, delta-wave activity tends to diminish and nonREM sleep has waves of higher frequencies and lower amplitude. As Fig. 2B indicates, body movements during sleep tend to cluster just before and during REM sleep. In general, the ease of arousal from sleep parallels the ordering of the sleep stages; REM and Stage I are the easiest for arousal, and Stage 4 is the most difficult.

2. SLEEP HAS DISTINCTIVE ONTOGENETIC AND PHYLOGENETIC FEATURES

Periods of immobility and "rest" are present in many lower animals, including insects and lizards. Because of the absence of a cortical brain structure like that of humans, it is difficult to say whether the absence of slow waves in these animals means they are not having the equivalent of human nonREM sleep, or whether this is present but expressed in a different form that is not detectable with EEG recordings. Recent work in molecular biology suggests that the evaluation of changes in gene expression in activity periods vs rest periods, as well as adenosine pharmacology may help to evaluate similarities/differences in lower and higher animals during quiescence and nonREM sleep. REM sleep occurs in all mammals, except for egg-laying mammals (monotremes), such as the echidna (spiny anteater). Birds have very brief bouts of REM sleep. REM sleep cycles vary in duration according to the size of the animal; elephants have the longest cycle and smaller animals have shorter cycles. For example,

the cat has a sleep cycle of approx 22 min, and the rat cycle is about 12 min.

In utero, mammals spend a large percentage of time in REM sleep, ranging from 50–80% of a 24-h day. Animals born with immature nervous systems have a much higher percentage of REM sleep at birth than the adults of the same species. For example, sleep in the human newborn occupies two-thirds of the time, with REM sleep occupying one-half of the total sleep time, or about one-third of the entire 24-h period (Fig. 3A). In infants born 10 wk prematurely, the percentage of REM sleep in the total sleep time reaches 80%. The percentage of REM sleep declines rapidly in early childhood, so that by approximately age 10 the adult percentage of REM sleep is reached—20–25% of total sleep time. Obviously, the predominance of REM sleep in the young suggests an important function in promoting nervous-system growth and development. Also in favor of this functional theory is the fact that the absolute amount of REM sleep is greater at birth in animals that are born immature (altricial) than those that are born more mature (precocial).

Stage 4, defined by the presence of delta EEG frequencies, is minimally present in the newborn but increases over the first years of life, reaching a maximum at about age 10 and declining thereafter (Fig. 3B). The time-course of delta-wave intensity over the first three decades of life is fit by a particular probability distribution (gamma distribution) and approximately the same time course obtains for synaptic density and positron emission tomography (PET) measurements of metabolic rate in the human frontal cortex. It has been suggested by Feinberg and colleagues that the correlated reduction in these three variables may reflect a pruning of redundant cortical synapses that is a key factor in cognitive maturation, allowing greater specialization and sustained problem-solving.

A frequent question asked of physicians is how much sleep is needed. As previously discussed, the answer partly depends on the age of the individual. A

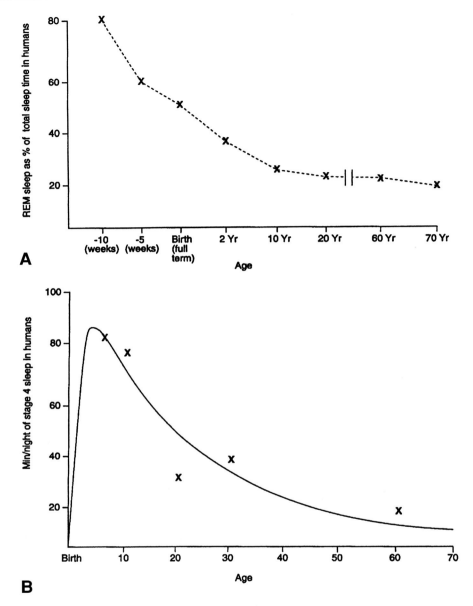

Fig. 3. (A) REM sleep as a percentage of total sleep time in infants born 10 (-10W) and 5 wk prematurely, at full-term birth **(B)**, and in children and adults at the indicated years of age. Note the dramatic decline of REM sleep during early life and the long plateau during maturity, with a decline observed only in the 7th decade. **(B)** Stage 4 (delta) sleep minutes as a function of age. There is little delta wave activity at birth, presumably reflecting cortical immaturity. Delta-wave activity peaks at about age 3–5, and declines exponentially thereafter. (Figures adapted from Fineberg, 1969.)

good general rule is that enough sleep is needed to prevent daytime drowsiness. Each individual seems to have a particular "set-point" of need. In adults, the modal value of sleep need appears close to the traditional 8 h, but there is considerable individual variation. If someone functions and feels well on less sleep, there is little need for concern.

3. SLEEP ONSET AND SLEEPINESS ARE DETERMINED BY CIRCADIAN TIME OF DAY AND BY PRIOR WAKEFULNESS

3.1. Circadian Factors in Sleepiness

In adult humans, the period of maximal sleepiness occurs at the time of the circadian low point of the temperature rhythm (Fig. 4). (Circadian means about a day, "circa" = "about," and the circadian temperature rhythm of humans can be considered as a sine-wave function with a minimum that occurs from 4–7 a.m. in subjects with a normal daytime activity schedule.) It is no accident that accidents are most frequent at the time near circadian temperature minima, since this is the time of maximal sleepiness. Per vehicle mile, the risk for truck accidents is greatest at this time. The nuclear-reactor incidents at both Chernobyl and Three Mile Island also occurred in the early morning hours. There is a secondary peak of sleepiness that occurs at about 3 PM (Fig. 4), corresponding to a favored time for naps. The main functional consequence of deprivation of sleep seems to be the presence of "microsleeps"— very brief episodes of sleep during which sensory input from the outside is diminished and cognitive function is markedly altered. As every parent knows, human newborns do not have a strong circadian modulation of sleep, and some species, such as the cat, do not have much circadian modulation even as adults.

3.2. The Second Factor Determining Sleepiness Is the Extent of Prior Wakefulness

Mathematical models of sleep propensity have been developed that emphasize circadian control and also by Borbély and colleagues, who emphasize the extent of prior wakefulness. Borbély and colleagues model postulates that the intensity and amplitude of delta-wave activity (as measured by power spectral analysis) indexes the level of sleep factor(s) and slow-wave sleep drive. In this model, the time-course of delta activity during the night, a declining exponential, reflects the dissipation of the sleep factor(s). These workers did not identify the underlying sleep factor(s), but adenosine and other candidate factors are next discussed.

4. SLOW-WAVE SLEEP FACTORS

4.1. Adenosine: A Mediator of the Sleep-Inducing Effects of Prolonged Wakefulness

A growing body of evidence supports the role of purine nucleoside adenosine as a mediator of the sleepiness that follows prolonged wakefulness. Common-sense evidence for the role of adenosine in sleepiness comes from the nearly universal use of coffee and tea to increase alertness, since these beverages contain

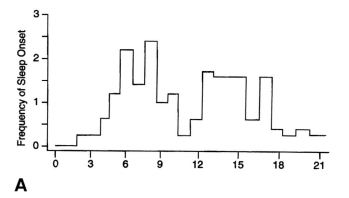

A

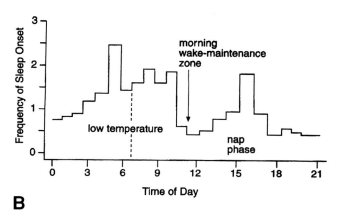

B

Fig. 4. Circadian control of sleepiness and sleep onset. (**A**) Sleepiness at various clock times for subjects on a constant routine. Sleepiness was measured by Carskadon as frequency of unintended microsleeps in subjects instructed to stay awake, with a frequency of 1 indicating the average across all measurements. Note the major peak about 6 AM, at the presumptive time of circadian temperature minimum, and a secondary peak about 3 PM, a favored time for a nap. (**B**) Sleep propensity measured as the number of self-selected-bedtimes/sleep onsets in subjects in whom temperature was continuously monitored indicates average across all measurements. Note that, as in the top panel, the maximum number of sleep onsets occur near the temperature minimum, and a secondary peak occurs at a circadian phase corresponding to about 3 PM. These subjects were maintained without circadian cues, and showed decoupling of the activity and the temperature rhythms ("internal desynchronization") that are otherwise synchronized by external circadian cues, such as dawn and dusk. The sleep onsets were converted to approximate times of day by assuming a temperature minimum at 6:30 AM. (Figure adapted from Strogatz, 1986.)

the adenosine-receptor antagonists caffeine and theophylline. The author and colleagues have advanced the hypothesis that, because of the metabolic demands during prolonged wakefulness, adenosine accumu-

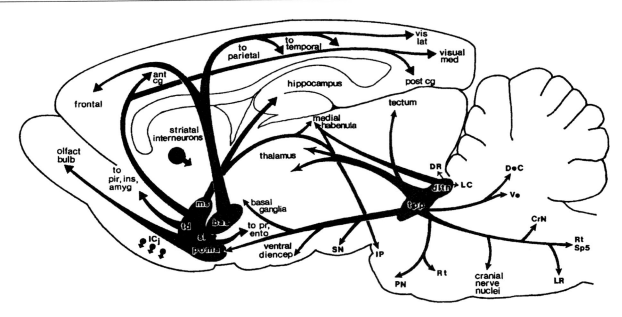

Fig. 5. Schematic of cholinergic systems and their projections in the rat. The clustered group of cholinergic nuclei in the basal forebrain form a center important for control of wakefulness and an activated EEG. These include: ms, medial septal nucleus; bas, nucleus basalis; si, substantia innominata; poma, preoptic magnocellular field; and td, diagonal band nuclei. Note that projections from this group encompass almost the entire extent of the neocortex. In the brainstem, the cholinergic nuclei are tpp, pedunculopontine tegmental nucleus (abbreviated in text as PPT) and dltn, laterodorsal tegmental nucleus (abbreviated in text as LDT). The section on REM sleep discusses these nuclei in detail. (Reproduced with permission from Cooper, Bloom, and Roth. The Biochemical Basis of Neuropharmacology, 7th ed, Oxford University Press, 1996.)

lates selectively in the basal forebrain and promotes the transition from wakefulness to slow-wave sleep (SWS) by inhibiting basal forebrain neurons that are important in the maintenance of wakefulness, as measured by an activated EEG.

Many studies have indicated that the basal forebrain contains both cholinergic and noncholinergic neurons that are important in the maintenance of wakefulness (*see* Fig. 5; cholinergic neurons use the neurotransmitter acetylcholine). There is strong evidence that adenosine acts to suppress the activity of these neurons and thus promotes sleep. In vivo work in animals has demonstrated that microdialysis perfusion of adenosine in the basal forebrain zones of cholinergic neurons produced a strong reduction in wakefulness and in the activated EEG. This finding implicates this region as a specifically important site of adenosine action. Key evidence that adenosine fulfilled criteria for a sleep factor mediating sleep following prolonged wakefulness was the finding that, in the basal forebrain, extracellular adenosine progressively accumulated with each succeeding hour of wakefulness (*see* Fig. 6). Moreover, increasing basal forebrain adenosine concentrations to approximately the level

that occurs during sleep deprivation by a nucleoside-transport blocker mimicked the effect of sleep deprivation on both the EEG power spectrum and behavioral state distribution: wakefulness was decreased, and there were increases in nonREM sleep. As predicted, microdialysis application of the specific A1-receptor antagonist cyclopentyltheophylline (CPT) in the basal forebrain produced the opposite effects on behavioral state, increasing wakefulness and decreasing SWS and REM. Data from combined unit recording and microdialysis studies have shown that basal forebrain neurons selectively active in wakefulness, compared with SWS, have discharge activity suppressed by both adenosine and the A1-specific agonist cyclohexyladenosine (CHA), and discharge activity is increased by the A1-receptor antagonist, CPT.

How is the extracellular concentration of adenosine regulated? The author's current hypothesis is that regulation of extracellular concentration of adenosine depends first on metabolism, with increased metabolism leading to reduced high-energy phosphate stores and thus to increased adenosine which, through an equilibrative transporter, leads to increases in extracellular adenosine (*see* schematic description in

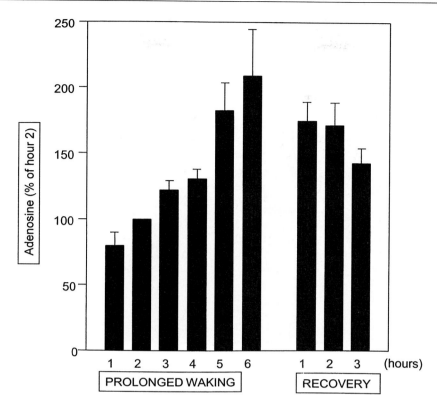

Fig. 6. Mean basal forebrain extracellular adenosine values by hour during 6 h of prolonged wakefulness and in the subsequent 3 h of spontaneous recovery sleep. Microdialysis values in the 6 cats are normalized relative to the second hour of deprivation. (Adapted from Porkka-Heiskanen et al., 1997.)

Fig. 7A). The increased extracellular adenosine then inhibits those basal forebrain neurons important in the promotion of wakefulness/cortical activation (Fig. 7B). Extracellular adenosine may also be increased by the release of adenosine 5' triphosphate (ATP) as a co-transmitter and its breakdown, by 5' ectonucleo-tidases, to adenosine. Support for an adenosine-metabolism-link hypothesis comes from the fact that EEG arousal is known to diminish as a function of the duration of prior wakefulness and also with brain hyper-thermia—both associated with increased brain metabolism—as well as recent data indicating glyco-gen depletion during wakefulness and restoration dur-ing non-REM sleep.

Does adenosine exert its effects in localized brain region(s) or globally? Measurements in multiple brain areas in the cat showed sustained adenosine accumu-lation during prolonged wakefulness (6 h) occurred only in the basal forebrain and to a lesser extent in the cerebral cortex, but adenosine concentrations did not increase elsewhere during prolonged wakefulness, even in regions important in behavioral state control

(Fig. 7C). These data suggest the presence of brain region-specific differences in AD transporters and/or degradation. These differences become evident with prolonged wakefulness, although AD concentrations were higher in all brain sites sampled during the natu-rally occurring (and shorter-duration) episodes of wakefulness in freely moving and behaving animals.

4.1.1. Adenosine and Sleep Debt

With continuing sleep restriction, such as to 5 h per night in humans, the cumulative and long-term changes in alertness and cognitive performance that occur are often termed "sleep debt." Recent data from the author's laboratory indicate that sleep deprivation may alter transcriptional activity in the basal forebrain via an adenosine-induced induction of the transcriptional factor, nuclear factor kappa B (NF-κB), which is known to bind to the promotor region of the adenosine A1 receptor. Data suggest that this adenosine- and sleep deprivation-induced NF-κB may lead to an overexpression of adenosine A1 receptors, thus increasing the sensitivity to adenosine and provid-

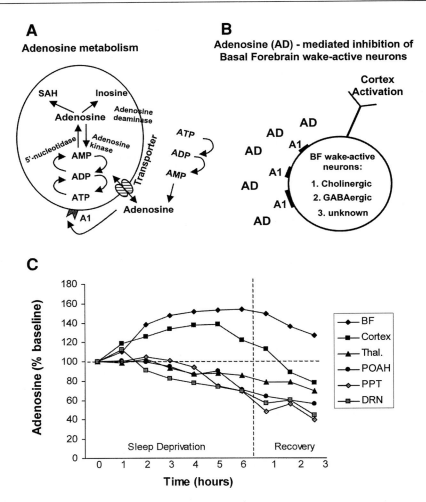

Fig. 7. (A) Schematic of main intra- and extracellular metabolic pathways of adenosine. The intracellular pathway from ATP (adenosine 5'-triphosphate) to ADP (adenosine diphosphate) to AMP (adenosine monosphate) to Adenosine is respectively regulated by the enzymes ATP-ase, ADP-ase and 5'-nucleotidase and extracellularly by the respective ecto-enzymes. Adenosine kinase converts adenosine to AMP, and adenosine deaminase converts adenosine to inosine. The third enzyme to metabolize adenosine is S-adenosylhomocysteine hydrolase, which converts adenosine to S-adenosylhomocysteine (SAH). Adenosine concentration between the intra- and extracellular spaces is equilibrated by nucleoside transporters. **(B)**. Schematic of Adenosine's effects on cells in the basal forebrain. Extracellular adenosine (AD) acts on the A1 adenosine-receptor subtype to inhibit neurons promoting EEG activation and wakefulness. **(C)** Adenosine concentrations in different brain areas during sleep deprivation and recovery sleep. Cats were kept awake for 6 h using gentle handling/playing (hours 1 to 6) and then allowed to sleep for 3 h (hours 7 to 9). Prior to the beginning of the sleep deprivation, samples were collected to obtain baseline wakefulness values for each probe (predeprivation value = hour 0 = 100%). Two patterns are evident in the sleep deprivationinduced changes in adenosine; in the basal forebrain (BF) and cortex, adenosine levels could be seen to rise during the sleep deprivation, whereas in the other 4 areas adenosine levels were either stable or declined slowly during the 6 h of sleep deprivation. By the second hour of sleep deprivation, adenosine values were significantly higher in the BF than all other brain areas but cortex (Ctx), which was lower in hour 6. During recovery, sleep adenosine concentrations were significantly higher in the BF than in all other areas. Abbreviations: DRN, dorsal raphe nucleus; POA, prepoptic hypothalamic area; PPT, pedunculopontine tegmental area.

ing a possible mechanism for the production of "sleep debt."

4.1.2. ACTIVE NonREM SLEEP-PROMOTING MECHANISMS

Electrophysiological recordings of basal forebrain/anterior hypothalamic neurons indicate that some are selectively active during nonREM sleep, and may rep-

resent an active sleep-promoting mechanism. Studies by Sherin and colleagues used the immediate early gene protein product cFos to detect neurons in the ventrolateral preoptic area that were selectively active during nonREM sleep. Immunohistochemistry suggested that these neurons were GABAergic, and anatomical studies indicated projections to wakefulness-promoting histaminergic neurons in the posterior hypothalamus and to brainstem nuclei that were important in EEG arousal. Many current studies are investigating the interaction of these neurons with other systems that are important in sleep.

4.1.3. OTHER HUMORAL FACTORS

There is also evidence supporting a role for interleukin-1 (IL-1), tumor necrosis factor (TNF), and growth hormone releasing hormone (GHRH) as part of the humoral mechanisms regulating physiological sleep. Their injection enhances nonREM sleep, whereas their inhibition reduces spontaneous sleep and sleep rebound after sleep deprivation. Changes in their mRNA levels and changes in their protein levels in the brain are consistent within their proposed role in sleep regulation, as are results from transgenic and mutant animals. However, they appear to be involved in the regulation of propensity to sleep over longer time periods than the actions of adenosine. Notably, IL-1 is a cytokine that is produced in response to infections. In this case, it increases nonREM sleep, and also produces hyperthermia. Hyperthermia itself may increase nonREM sleep, but blocking the hyperthermic effects of IL-1 does not block the nonREM sleep-inducing effects. The argument that IL-1 is important in the hypersomnia associated with infections is thus strong.

Hayaishi and colleagues have reported that injections of prostaglandin D2 into the third ventricle and the ependemal surface of the ventral forebrain reliably produces slow-wave sleep. They have proposed that it is a natural sleep-regulatory factor. Interestingly, Hayaishi and colleagues have found that at least some of the sleep-inducing effects of prostaglandin could be mediated by changes in extracellular adenosine, and Krueger and colleagues have suggested a model in which some of the effects of IL-1 may be mediated by adenosine. Thus, the possibility exists that adenosine might be a "final common factor" for other sleep factors.

5. CONTROL OF EEG SYNCHRONIZATION AND DESYNCHRONIZATION

The high-voltage, slow-wave activity in the cortex that occurs during most nonREM sleep—termed EEG synchronization—contrasts sharply with the low-voltage, fast pattern—termed desynchronized or activated—characteristic of both waking and REM sleep and consisting of frequencies in the beta range (approx 14–32 Hz). We have already discussed the basal-forebrain component of this activating system. As shown in Fig. 5, there are also important brainstem components of the cholinergic-activating system. This is

likely a major component of the "Ascending Reticular Activating System," a concept that arose from the work of Moruzzi and Magoun before methods were available for the labeling of neurons utilizing specific neurotransmitters. The brainstem cholinergic nuclei at the pons–midbrain junction are termed the laterodorsal and pedunculopontine tegmental nuclei (LDT/PPT). There is also extensive anatomical evidence that these cholinergic neurons project to thalamic nuclei that are important in EEG desynchronization and synchronization. Both in vivo and in vitro neurophysiological studies have indicated that the target neurons in the thalamus respond to cholinergic agonists in a way that is consistent with EEG activation, as detailed below. Cholinergic systems are not the exclusive brainstem substrate of EEG desynchronization. Brainstem reticular neuronal projections to thalamus, likely utilizing excitatory amino acid (EAA) neurotransmission, as well as noradrenergic projections from the locus coeruleus and serotonergic projections from the dorsal raphe nucleus also play important roles in EEG desynchronization. Wakefulness appears to be too important to be left to maintenance by one neurotransmitter system.

5.1. Sleep Spindles

Spindles occur during stage two of human sleep and in the light slow-wave sleep phase of animals. They are composed of waves of approx 14–16 Hz frequency; the wave amplitudes waxes and then wanes over the spindle duration of 1–2 s. Wave frequency varies between species, and is higher in primates. Spindles are relatively well-understood at the cellular level. Studies by Steriade and colleagues indicate that spindle waves arise as the result of interactions between spindle pacemaker GABAergic thalamic nucleus reticularis (RE) neurons and thalamocortical neurons. Spindle waves are blocked by cholinergic brainstem–thalamus projections, which act to hyperpolarize the RE neurons. The forebrain nucleus basalis also provides cholinergic and hyperpolarizing GABAergic input to RE that assists brainstem input in disrupting the spindles.

5.2. Delta EEG Activity

The cellular basis of delta waves (0.5–4 Hz) originating in thalamo-cortical neurons is sketched in Fig. 8. This sketch portrays intracellularly recorded events in a thalamocortical neuron during delta-wave generation, and is based on both in vivo and in vitro recordings by McCormick and by Steriade and their colleagues. The basic concept is that a hyperpolarized

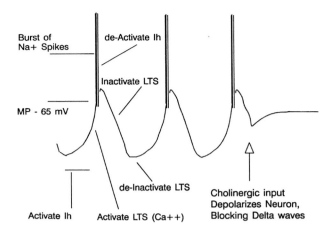

Fig. 8. Schematic of mechanisms proposed for generation of delta waves by thalamocortical neurons, which, without exogenous input, show a spontaneous membrane potential and action-potential oscillation in the delta frequency and, it is hypothesized, drive the cortical delta rhythm. Oscillation occurs because of the following interplay of intrinsic membrane currents: When the membrane potential is hyperpolarized, (−80 mV) a particular cation current, called Ih (I = symbol for current, h = hyperpolarized), is activated. This inward flow of positive ions depolarizes the membrane to the point where the low-threshold spike (LTS), is activated. The inrush of calcium ions in the LTS further depolarizes the neuron to the point where the firing threshold of the sodium action potential is crossed, and action potentials are produced. Ih is turned off or "deactivated" at depolarized potentials. The LTS current is automatically turned off by another process called "inactivation." The membrane then returns to its baseline, hyperpolarized level where the LTS calcium current is "de-inactivated" or rendered ready for activation. The cycle then repeats itself. Delta oscillations are halted by exogenous, depolarizing input, such as the cholinergic input illustrated. (This figure and the mechanisms described are based on the in vitro data of McCormick and Pape and the in vivo data of Steriade and colleagues.)

membrane potential permits the occurrence of delta waves in thalamocortical circuits. Any factors that depolarize the membrane will block delta waves. During waking, input from the cholinergic forebrain nucleus basalis is important for the suppression of slow-wave activity, as shown by lesion studies. Brainstem norepinephrinergic and serotonergic projections may disrupt delta activity in waking, although they are inactive during REM sleep. During REM sleep, cholinergic input from the brainstem is a major factor leading to membrane depolarization, with reticular formation input, likely utilizing EAA neurotransmission, which also plays an important role. This membrane depolarization leads to suppression of delta-wave activity. Thus, delta waves that occur dur-

ing sleep may be seen to represent thalamocortical oscillations that occur in the absence of activating inputs. From the perspective of the cellular physiologist, the relative intensity of cortical desynchronization correlates well with the intensity of cholinergic input to the thalamus; conversely, the relative intensity of cortical synchronization, including delta waves, correlates well with the relative absence of cholinergic activity. The identification of desynchronizing processes in sleep with ascending brainstem cholinergic and reticular activation means that the increasing intensity of EEG desynchronization preceding REM sleep is related to the increasing level of activity of REM-related cholinergic and reticular activity that precedes this state.

5.3. Slow-Wave Sleep at the Cellular Level in the Thalamus: The "Burst Mode" of Relay Cell-Discharge is Responsible for the Failure of Information Transmission

Extracellular recordings by the author and Benoit demonstrated that dorsal-lateral-geniculate-relay neurons discharged in stereotyped bursts during nonREM sleep, but not during waking or REM. Subsequent in vivo (Steriade and colleagues) and in vitro investigations (McCormick and colleagues) indicate the bursting in thalamocortical neurons occurs when the membrane is hyperpolarized, as illustrated in Fig. 8 in association with the delta EEG rhythm. This hyperpolarization removes the inactivation of particular Ca^{2+} channels and enables the production of a "calcium spike" (e.g., an inrush of depolarizing calcium ions) when a small depolarization occurs. This depolarizing calcium spike is termed a "low-threshold spike" (LTS) to distinguish it from other calcium currents with different triggering thresholds. The LTS depolarizes the neuron enough to reach the threshold for fast sodium action potentials, and a burst of these action potentials rides on the LTS. However, the production of a LTS limits the following frequency of relay neurons and thus blocks rapid information transmission.

6. REM SLEEP PHYSIOLOGY AND RELEVANT BRAIN ANATOMY

6.1. Overview and Summary

It is important to note that there are two distinctly different types of discharge patterns in brainstem cholinergic neurons. One type has a maximal discharge rate in activated EEG states of both REM and non-REM sleep, and has been discussed extensively in

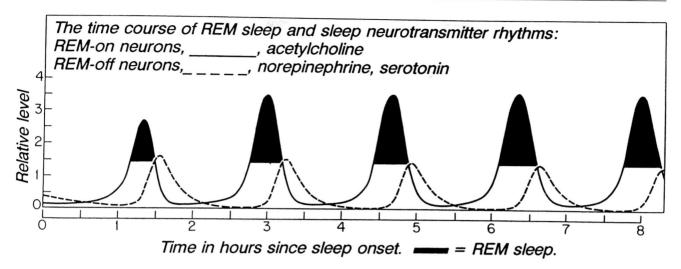

Fig. 9. Schematic of a night's course of REM sleep in humans, showing that the occurrence and intensity of REM sleep as dependent upon the activity of populations of "REM-on" (= REM promoting neurons), indicated by the *solid line*. As the REM-promoting neuronal activity reaches a certain threshold, the full set of REM signs occurs (*black areas under curve* indicate REM sleep). Note, however that, unlike the steplike EEG diagnosis of sleep in Fig. 2, the underlying neuronal activity is a continuous function. The neurotransmitter acetylcholine is believed to be important in REM sleep production, acting to excite populations of brainstem RF neurons to produce the set of REM signs. Other neuronal populations that utilize the monoamine neurotransmitters serotonin and norepinephrine are likely to be REM-suppressive; the time-course of their activity is sketched by the *dotted line*. (These curves mimic actual time-courses of neuronal activity, as recorded in animals, and were generated by a mathematical model of REM sleep, the limit cycle reciprocal interaction model of McCarley and Massaquoi.)

conjunction with non-REM sleep. However, another type has maximal activity during REM sleep, but is relatively silent during both wakefulness and non-REM sleep. This type of cholinergic neuron, termed a "REM-on" neuron, is believed to be important in the generation of the state of REM sleep. Fig. 9 schematizes the time-course of discharge activity of the "REM-on" neurons. Activity in this group of neurons recruits activity in effector neurons located in the brainstem reticular formation (RF) to produce REM sleep phenomena. Neurons in the locus coeruleus that utilize norepinephrine and neurons in the dorsal raphe that utilize serotonin have an opposite time-course, becoming selectively inactive during REM (Fig. 10 sketches the location of these nuclei). They act to suppress REM sleep-promoting activity.

6.2. Transection Studies Show that the Brainstem Contains the Neural Machinery of the REM Sleep Rhythm

As illustrated in Fig. 10, a transection made just above the junction of the pons and midbrain produces a state in which periodic occurrence of REM sleep can be found in recordings made in the isolated brainstem and, in contrast, recordings in the isolated forebrain

show no sign of REM sleep. These lesion studies by Jouvet and colleagues in France established the importance of the brainstem in REM sleep.

6.3. Brainstem RF Neurons Are Important as Effectors in the Production of the Physiological Events of REM Sleep

The cardinal signs of REM sleep in lower animals, as in humans, are muscle atonia, EEG desynchronization (low-voltage fast-pattern), and REMs. EEG depth recordings in animals show another important component of REM sleep, the *PGO waves*, so named because they are recorded from the pons, the lateral geniculate nucleus (LGN), and the occipital cortex. They are visible in the recording from the cat LGN in Fig. 11. (The depth recordings necessary to establish their presence in humans have not been done.) PGO waves arise in the pons, and are then transmitted to the thalamic lateral geniculate nucleus (LGN) and to the visual occipital cortex. PGO waves represent an important mode of brainstem activation of the forebrain during REM sleep, and are also present in nonvisual thalamic nuclei.

Most of the physiological events of REM sleep have effector neurons located in the brainstem RF, with

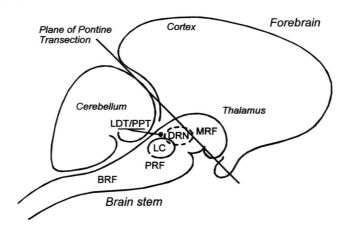

Fig. 10. Schematic of a sagittal section of a mammalian brain (cat) showing the location of nuclei that are especially important for sleep. BRF, PRF, and MRF, bulbar, pontine, and mesencephalic reticular formation; LDT/PPT, laterodorsal and pedunculopontine tegmental nuclei, the principal site of cholinergic (acetylcholine-containing) neurons important for REM sleep and EEG desynchronization. LC, locus coeruleus, where most norepinephrine-containing neurons are located; DRN, dorsal raphe nucleus, the site of many serotonin-containing neurons. The oblique line is the plane of transection that preserves REM sleep signs caudal to the transection but abolishes them rostral to the transection (Adapted from McCarley, 1989.)

many important neurons concentrated in the pontine reticular formation (PRF). Thus PRF neuronal recordings are of special interest for information on the mechanisms of production of these events. Intracellular recordings of PRF neurons (Fig. 11) show that these neurons have relatively hyperpolarized membrane potentials and generate almost no action potentials during nonREM sleep. As illustrated in Fig. 11, PRF neurons begin to depolarize even before the occurrence of the first EEG sign of the approach of REM sleep, the PGO waves that begin 30–60 s before the onset of the remainder of the polysomnographic signs of REM sleep. As PRF neuronal depolarization proceeds and the threshold for action-potential production is reached, these neurons begin to discharge (generate action potentials). Their discharge rate increases as REM sleep is approached, and the high level of discharge is maintained throughout REM sleep, because of the maintenance of a membrane depolarization.

Throughout the entire REM sleep episode, almost the entire population of PRF neurons remains depolarized. The resultant increased action-potential activity leads to the production of those REM sleep physiological signs, which have their physiological bases in PRF neurons. Fig. 12 provides a schematic overview of REM sleep as arising from increases in excitability and discharge activity of the various populations of RF neurons that are important as effectors of REM sleep phenomenona. PRF neurons are important for: (i) the REMs (the generator for saccades is in PRF); (ii) the PGO waves (a different group of neurons); and (iii) a

group of dorsolateral PRF neurons controls the muscle atonia of REM sleep (these neurons become active just before the onset of muscle atonia). Neurons in midbrain reticular formation (MRF, *see* anatomical schematic in Fig. 10) are especially important for EEG desynchronization, for the low-voltage fast EEG pattern. As mentioned previously, these neurons were originally described Moruzzi and Magoun as making up the ascending reticular activating system (ARAS), the set of brainstem neurons that are important for EEG desynchronization. Subsequent work has expanded this original ARAS concept to include cholinergic and monaminergic neurons. Neurons in the bulbar RF are important for muscle atonia.

6.4. Cholinergic Mechanisms Are Important for REM Sleep

Extensive work has led to an appreciation of the importance of the neurotransmitter acetylcholine for REM sleep, and to a reasonably detailed knowledge of the nature of the anatomy and physiology of the cholinergic influences on REM sleep. The essential points are outlined here:

1. Injection of compounds that are acetylcholine agonists into the PRF produces a REM-like state that very closely mimics natural REM sleep. The latency to onset and duration are dose-dependent. Muscarinic receptors appear to be especially critical, and nicotinic receptors are of lesser importance.
2. There are naturally occurring cholinergic projections to effector neurons in the brainstem reticular

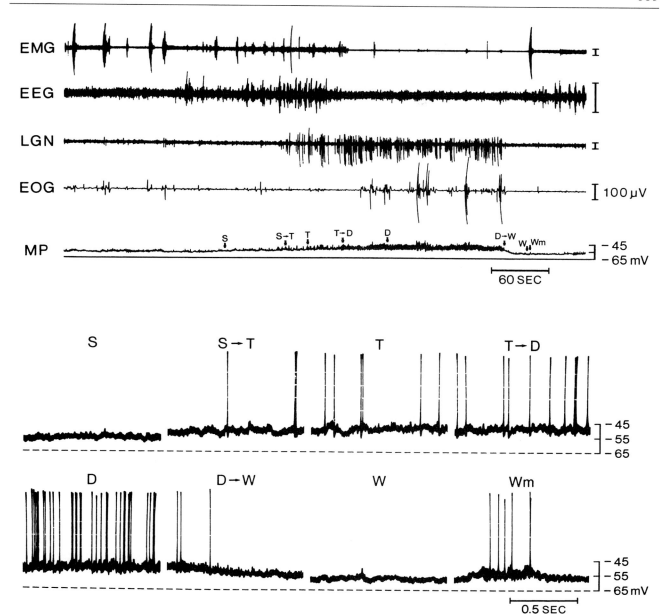

Fig. 11. REM sleep in the EEG and at the brainstem cellular level. (*Top panel*) Continuous polysomnographic record of waking, nonREM sleep, REM sleep, and return to waking in the cat. Waking is indicated by EMG activity, low-voltage, fast EEG, eye movements (EOG); nonREM sleep (here abbreviated as S, for slow-wave sleep) shows high-voltage, slow waves in the EEG; the transition to REM sleep (REM sleep is here abbreviated by D, for desynchronized sleep) is heralded by the onset of spiky waves in the LGN EEG recording (PGO waves), and with the occurrence of REM sleep there is muscle atonia, low-voltage, fast-EEG, PGO waves, and REMs. The bottom trace is of the membrane potential (MP) of an intracellularly recorded PRF neuron with the action potentials filtered out; note the membrane potential depolarization that begins before and remains present throughout REM sleep. The *bottom panel* shows samples of the oscilloscope record of the intracellular recording and the occurrence of action potentials and postsynaptic potentials at the times indicated on the MP tracing. (S, slow-wave sleep or nonREM sleep); S→T, beginning of transition to REM sleep, as indicated by PGO waves; T, transition, T→D onset of REM sleep, D, REM sleep, D→W, transition to waking, Wm, waking with body movement and action potentials in the neuron.) (Data from Ito and McCarley.)

formation. These arise in the two nuclei at the pons–midbrain junction (Fig. 13): the laterodorsal tegmental nucleus (LDT) and the pedunculopontine tegmental nucleus (PPT).

3. In vitro studies in the PRF slice preparation show that a majority (80%) of RF neurons are excited by cholinergic agonists, with muscarinic effects being especially pronounced. In vitro studies in

REM Sleep State Control Schematic

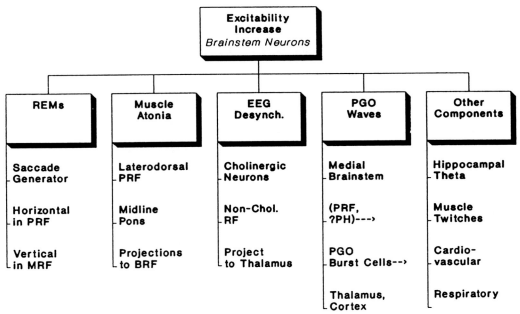

Excitability Increase Brainstem Neurons				
REMs	**Muscle Atonia**	**EEG Desynch.**	**PGO Waves**	**Other Components**
Saccade Generator	Laterodorsal PRF	Cholinergic Neurons	Medial Brainstem	Hippocampal Theta
Horizontal in PRF	Midline Pons	Non-Chol. RF	(PRF, ?PH)---›	Muscle Twitches
Vertical in MRF	Projections to BRF	Project to Thalamus	PGO Burst Cells--›	Cardio-vascular
			Thalamus, Cortex	Respiratory

Fig. 12. Schematic of REM sleep control. Increasing the excitability (activity) of brainstem neuronal pools subserving each of the major components of the state causes the occurrence of this component. For example, the neuronal pool important for the REMs is suggested to be the brainstem saccade-generating system whose main machinery is in paramedian PRF. Although vertical saccades are fewer in REM, their presence suggests similar involvement of the mesencephalic RF. Information under the other system components sketches the major features of the anatomy and projections of neuronal pools important for muscle atonia, EEG desynchronization, PGO waves, and the last part of the diagram lists other components of REM sleep.

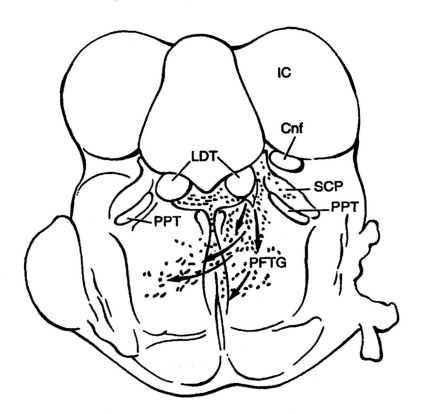

the PRF slice preparation show that the increased excitability and membrane depolarization produced by cholinergic agonists is a direct effect, since it persists when synaptic input has been abolished by addition of tetrodotoxin (TTX), which blocks sodium-dependent action potentials.

4. Experiments lesioning the LDT/PPT nuclei confirm their importance in producing REM sleep phenomena. Destruction of the cell bodies of LDT/PPT neurons by local injections of excitatory amino acids (EAAs) leads to a marked reduction of REM sleep.

5. Work by McCarley, Sakai, Steriade, and their colleagues have shown that a group of LDT/PPT neurons discharges selectively in REM sleep, and the onset of activity begins before the onset of REM sleep. This LDT/PPT discharge pattern and the presence of excitatory projections to the PRF suggest that these cholinergic neurons may be important in producing the depolarization of reticular-effector neurons for REM sleep events. The group of LDT/PPT and RF neurons that become active in REM sleep are often referred to as *REM-on neurons*.

6. Cholinergic neurons are important in the production of the-low voltage, fast (LVF) EEG pattern (representing "cortical activation") in both REM sleep and waking. As shown by Steriade and colleagues, a different group of cholinergic neurons in LDT/PPT is active during this LVF pattern in both REM and waking. As described, this cholinergic system is especially important in generating the LVF-EEG pattern, often called the "activated EEG." Projections from midbrain reticular neurons and aminergic neurons, especially those in the locus coeruleus, also play a role in forebrain activation. Together, these neuronal groups form "the ascending reticular activating system." Evidence that multiple systems are involved in EEG desynchronization comes from the inability of

lesions of any single one of these systems to disrupt EEG desynchronization on a permanent basis.

6.4.1. PEPTIDES

The reader should be aware that many peptides are colocalized with the neurotransmitter acetylcholine in LDT/PPT neurons; this colocalization likely also means they are coreleased with acetylcholine, and may modify responsiveness to acetylcholine, as well as having independent actions. The peptide substance P is found in about 40% of LDT/PPT neurons and, overall, more than fifteen different colocalized peptides have been described. The role of these peptides in modulating acetylcholine activity that is relevant to wakefulness and sleep remains to be elucidated, but it should be emphasized that the colocalized peptide VIP has been reported by several different investigators to enhance REM sleep when it is injected intraventricularly.

6.5. REM-Off Neurons Suppress REM Sleep Phenomena

As illustrated in Fig. 9, REM-on neurons are those neurons that become active in REM sleep compared with slow-wave sleep and waking, and presumably have a protagonist role in the production of REM sleep phenomena. Neurons with an opposite discharge time-course that become inactive in REM sleep are known as *REM-off neurons*. REM-off neurons are most active in waking, have discharge activity that declines in slow-wave sleep, and are virtually silent in REM until they resume discharge near the end of the REM sleep episode. This inverse pattern of activity to REM-on neurons and to REM sleep phenomena such as PGO waves has led to the hypothesis that these neurons may be REM-suppressive and interact with REM-on neurons in control of the REM sleep cycle. This concept is indirectly supported by production of REM sleep from cooling (inactivating) the nuclei where REM-off neurons are found and by some in vivo pharmacological studies. In vitro data have provided direct support for the inhibition of cholinergic LDT neurons by serotonin, and in vivo unit recording and microdialysis experiments have shown it is the REM-on neurons whose activity is suppressed by serotonin (5-HT). The following classes of neurons are REM-off (*see* Fig. 10 for anatomy): *Norepinephrine-containing neurons* that are principally located in the locus coeruleus, called the "blue spot" because of its appearance in the unstained brain. *Serotonin-containing neurons* are located the *raphe system* of the brainstem, the mid-

Fig. 13. (*Opposite page*) Coronal section of the brainstem at the pons-midbrain junction, showing the location of the acetylcholine-containing neurons most important for REM sleep in LDT/PPT (laterodorsal tegmental nucleus/pedunculopontine tegmental nucleus), and a schematic of projections of LDT to PRF. (PFTG is an abbreviation of one component of PRF). IC, inferior colliculus; Cnf, cuneiform nucleus; scp, superior cerebellar peduncle. (Figure adapted from Mitani et al., 1988.)

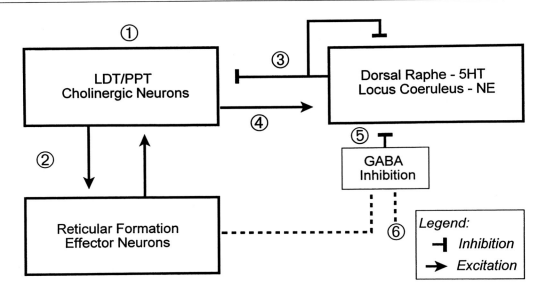

Fig. 14. Structural model of REM sleep control. *See* text for discussion.

line collection of neurons that extends from the bulb to the midbrain, with higher concentrations of serotonin-containing neurons in the more rostral neurons.* *Histamine-containing neurons* are located in the posterior hypothalamus, and are REM-off. This system has been conceptualized as one of the wakefulness-promoting systems, in agreement with drowsiness as a common side effect of antihistamines. However, transection studies indicate that the histaminergic neurons are not essential for the REM sleep oscillation. A mathematical and structural model of the occurrence of REM sleep based on interaction of REM-off and REM-on neurons, originally proposed by McCarley and Hobson and revised by McCarley and Massaquoi, rather accurately predicts the timing and percentage of REM sleep during a night of human sleep and its variation with the circadian temperature rhythm, and is the basis for Fig. 9. Fig. 14 and its legend sketches discusses the interaction of groups of neurons proposed to generate the REM sleep. The area of most intense current investigation is examining why raphe and locus coeruleus activity declines over the sleep cycle and become nearly absent in REM sleep. One explanation is that the discharge activity of locus coeruleus/dorsal raphe nucleus (LC/DRN) neurons diminishes

as a result of feedback inhibition from the recurrent inhibitory collaterals that are present in both LC and DRN neurons (illustrated as #3, Fig. 14). This recurrent inhibition acts at 5-HT$_{1A}$ receptors in DRN and at α_2 receptors in LC. However, although the evidence for recurrent inhibition is strong, there is currently no direct evidence for second-messenger-mediated inhibitory effects, needed because of the long duration of the inhibition. Another, and nonexclusive possibility, illustrated as #5, Fig. 14, is that GABAergic input, active during REM, inhibits DRN and LC neurons. GABA levels, as measured with in vivo microdialysis, are significantly increased in REM sleep compared with waking at both DRN and LC sites. The interrupted line in Fig. 14 from the RF to the GABAergic neurons indicates the uncertainty about the exact source of increased GABA in DRN/LC. Recent data suggest that this may come from GABAergic neurons outside these nuclei, since microiontophoresis of GABA-A antagonist bicuculline restores tonic DRN discharge during REM sleep and retrograde labeling shows GABAergic (GAD-positive) neurons from widely dispersed areas project to the DRN. These areas include hypothalamus (the most dense projection), the substantia nigra reticular part, the ventral tegmental

---

*Before it was known that serotonin-containing neurons in the dorsal raphe had maximal discharge activity in waking, slowed discharge during non-REM sleep, and virtually ceased discharge in REM sleep, it was proposed that serotonin neurotransmission might induce REM sleep. This theory, proposed by Jouvet and others, was based on very indirect evidence. With the present knowledge of the REM-off nature of dorsal raphe neurons, there is now no solid evidence for this theory. Unfortunately, this theory is still stated as fact in some textbooks, although it is now nearly 20 yr out of date!

area, the ventral pontine periaqueductal gray, and the rostral oral pontine reticular nucleus and other brainstem regions, including the parabrachial region and prepositus hypoglossi. However, unit recordings in these areas have yet to identify neurons with the proper time-course of activity to produce, through inhibition, the observed state-related decrease in DRN activity in nonREM sleep and the virtual silence in REM sleep.

7. OREXIN, NARCOLEPSY, AND THE CONTROL OF SLEEP AND WAKEFULNESS

One exciting recent development is the discovery of the important role of lateral hypothalamic neurons containing the neuropeptide orexin (alternatively known as hypocretin) in behavioral-state regulation and narcolepsy/cateplexy (*see* anatomical schematic in Fig. 15). Narcolepsy is a chronic sleep disorder that is characterized by excessive daytime sleepiness, fragmented sleep, and other symptoms that are indicative of abnormal REM sleep expression. These latter symptoms include cataplexy, hypnogogic hallucinations, sleep-onset REM periods, and sleep paralysis. Cataplexy consists of sudden attacks of bilateral atonia, especially in anti-gravity muscles, frequently with consequent collapse; these attacks are often provoked by emotion or excitement. Hypnogogic hallucinations consist of hallucinations upon falling asleep. Work by Mignot and colleagues indicated an abnormality in the gene for the orexin type II receptor was the basis of canine inherited narcolepsy, whereas Yanagisawa and colleagues found that orexin II-receptor knockout mice (–/–) have increased REM sleep, sleep-onset REM periods and also cataplexy-like episodes entered directly from states of active movement (*see* Fig. 15). Recent confirmation in man of orexin's importance has been provided by evidence that narcoleptic humans often have undetectable levels of orexin in CSF and by a human postmortem study that found the number of orexin neurons reduced by 90%. Orexins may play a neuromodulatory role in several neuroendocrine/homeostatic functions, such as food intake, body-temperature regulation, and blood-pressure regulation, as well as in the control of wakefulness and sleep.

7.1. The Orexin System

The orexins likely function as neurotransmitters, since they are localized in synaptic vesicles and had neuroexcitatory effects on hypothalamic neurons.

Orexin/hypocretin was identified by two independent groups. De Lecea and colleagues identified two related peptides from mRNA from hypothalamic tissue, which they named hypocretin-1 and -2. Sakurai and colleagues identified these same two peptides, which they termed orexin-A (=hypocretin-1) and orexin-B (=hypocretin-2) in a systematic biochemical search to find endogenous peptide ligands that would bind to G protein-coupled cell-surface receptors that had no previously known ligand (orphan receptors). Orexin-A and -B are neuropeptides of 33 and 28 amino acids, respectively; they are derived from a single precursor protein.

Immunohistochemical studies reveal a distribution of orexin projections that is remarkable for the targeting of a number of distinct brain regions known to be involved in the regulation of sleep and wakefulness, including both brainstem and forebrain systems. Orexin projections to the forebrain include the cholinergic basal forebrain (*see* Fig. 5) and the histaminergic tuberomammillary nucleus (TMN). Brainstem targets include the pontine and medullary brainstem RF, the cholinergic mesopontine tegmental nuclei (LDT/PPT), the locus coeruleus, and the dorsal raphe nucleus (*see* brainstem schematic in Fig. 10.).

Two orexin receptors have been identified. Orexin-A is a high-affinity ligand for the orexin-receptor type I (orexin-I), whose affinity for orexin-B is 1–2 orders of magnitude lower. The orexin-receptor type II (orexin-II) exhibits equally high affinity for both peptides. There are currently no ligands sufficiently specific for orexin I and II receptors to define their distribution. Of the brain regions involved in state control, only the dorsal raphe nucleus and the locus coeruleus appear to show a predominance of mRNA for type I receptors.

7.2. Orexin and the Control of REM-Related Phenomena

The knockout and canine narcolepsy data suggested that an absence of orexin or a defective orexin II receptor will produce cataplexy. Which brain region(s) might mediate this effect? In the absence of an effective antagonist to orexin receptors, the author's laboratory decided to use anti-sense oligodeoxynucleotides (ODN) against the mRNA for orexin type II receptors, thereby producing a "reversible knockout" or "knockdown" of the type II orexin receptor. Spatial specificity was obtained by microdialysis perfusion of orexin type II receptor anti-sense in the rat PRF just ventral to the LC (but presumably not affecting the LC, which has predominantly type I receptors). This treatment, as predicted, increased REM sleep two- to

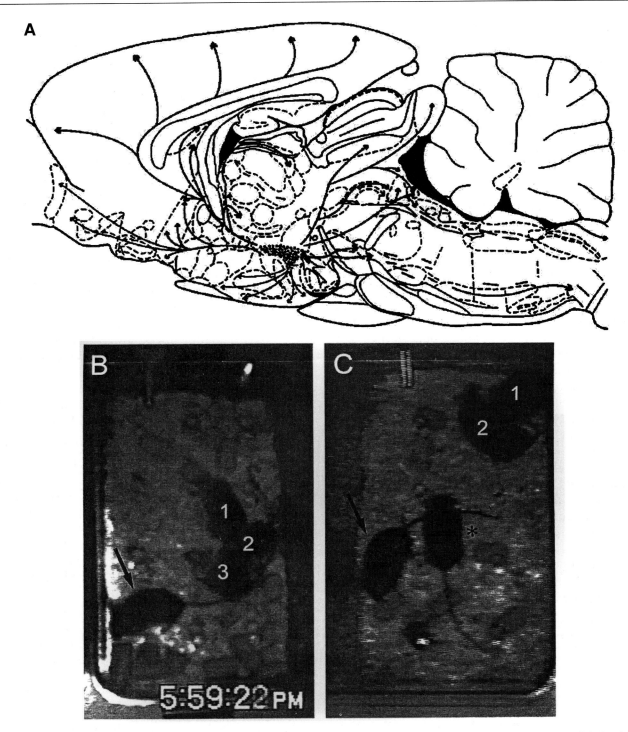

Fig. 15. (A) Schematic sagittal section drawing of location of orexin-containing neurons (*dots* in hypothalamus) and their widely distributed projection pathways in the rat brain. (Modified from Fig. 14 of Peyron et al., 1998.) **(B)** Digitally captured infrared video image of orexin knockout mice at 4 wk of age. Note that one mouse (*arrow*) has completely fallen onto his side in a cataplexy episode (confirmed in other mice by EEG). The film shows the fuzziness (motion artifact) associated with body movement in behaving acting littermates designated 1 to 3. **(C)** Digitally captured infrared video image of orexin-knockout mice at 4 wk of age. Note that one mouse has fallen completely onto his side (*arrow*), and the another is collapsed onto his ventral surface (*asterisk*). Littermates designated 1 and 2 are quietly sleeping in their usual corner of the cage. In both **(B)** and **(C)**, the dark (active) phase onset was at 5:30 PM and **(C)** was recorded at 8:26 PM. ([B] and [C] reproduced with permission from Fig. 3 in Chemelli et al., 1999; a video of these episodes is available at http://www.cell.com/cgi/content/full/98/4/437/DC1.)

threefold during both the light period (quiescent phase) and the dark period (active phase). Furthermore, this manipulation produced increases in behavioral cataplexy, suggesting that the REM sleep and narcolepsy-related role of orexin is mediated via the action of orexin in the brainstem nuclei that control the expression of REM sleep signs.

7.3. Orexin and the Control of Wakefulness

Orexin A has been shown to excite the noradrenergic neurons of the locus coeruleus, providing at least one documented mechanism by which orexin can promote wakefulness and suppress REM sleep. However, orexin is not always excitatory, and orexin exerts a variety of effects at the cellular level, both presynaptic and postsynaptic. The net effect of these actions on a particular brain circuit system physiology and consequent behavioral effects needs to be determined at the systems level for each brain region. The author's laboratory has recently found that microdialysis perfusion of orexin into the cholinergic basal forebrain of the rat produced a dose-dependent enhancement of wakefulness, and the highest dose produced more than a five-fold increase in wakefulness.

It is not yet certain whether orexin release is a function of the circadian cycle and/or a function of the behavioral state, but initial data from a number of groups favor a model of circadian control of release. At the present time, the field of orexin research is characterized by intense activity. Orexin is particularly interesting to the sleep researcher and clinician because it affects both REM sleep and wakefulness, and is probably closely linked to the human sleep disorder of narcolepsy.

8. MOLECULAR BIOLOGY OF SLEEP

An early round of studies focused on immediate early genes (IEG), such as c-fos, and found that in a number of species, the expression of IEG is very low or absent during nonREM sleep but, as a rule, is very high when the animal is spontaneously awake or sleep-deprived. One notable exception is c-fos expression in the ventral preoptic area, where some cells express c-fos as a function of the time asleep. Recently, other techniques have been used to obtain more specific indicators of which genes might be differentially expressed, including differential display and cDNA microarray technology. Interestingly, Tononi et al. reported that only a small subset (<0.01%) of genes have their expression altered during the sleep cycle, and an even smaller subset is affected by long-term

sleep deprivation. Wakefulness expression of IEG seems to be under the control of the locus coeruleus. The mRNA transcripts of genes affected by wakefulness and sleep fall into three main groups: (i) genes resident in mitochondria, probably reflecting changes in energy demand during wakefulness and relatively short-term (3 h in the rat) sleep deprivation; (ii) IEG and genes for transcription factors, perhaps related to plasticity; and (iii) a heterogeneous group of other genes, including growth factors brain-derived neurotrophic factor (BDNF) and bone morphogenetic protein (BMP). This latter group showed more expression after long term sleep deprivation (8 h in the rat), a pattern not seen in the first two groups. There is increasing interest in rest-activity cycles in lower animals, such as Drosophila, in which an analysis of genetic expression is simpler than in higher organisms. Obviously, the molecular biology of sleep is in a phase of rapid advancement of knowledge, and its integration with the considerable body of information on sleep mechanisms appears to be an important future pathway for progress.

9. THE FORM OF DREAMS AND THE BIOLOGY OF REM SLEEP

REM sleep is strongly associated with dreaming. In experiments that involve awakenings at random intervals throughout the night, 80% of all such randomly elicited dream reports have been found to occur in REM sleep. Those dreams that do occur in nonREM sleep have been found to be less vivid and intense than REM sleep dreams, suggesting they may represent a preREM state in which brainstem neuronal activity is approximating that of REM sleep, but the EEG has not yet changed.

Dreams have a long history of interest, both in popular culture and in psychiatry. Sigmund Freud, writing before the presence of the biological state of REM sleep was known, suggested that dreams represented a symbolic disguise of an unacceptable unconscious wish (e.g., sexual or aggressive wishes); the purpose of the disguise was to prevent the disruption of sleep that would occur with consciousness of the undisguised wish. Today, the activation of the neural systems responsible for REM sleep would seem to be a more accurate and simple explanation for the instigation of the dream state that is linked to the cyclic appearance of REM sleep. There remains the question, however, of why dreams have their own distinctive characteristics, and why they differ from waking consciousness. One obvious hypothesis is that the con-

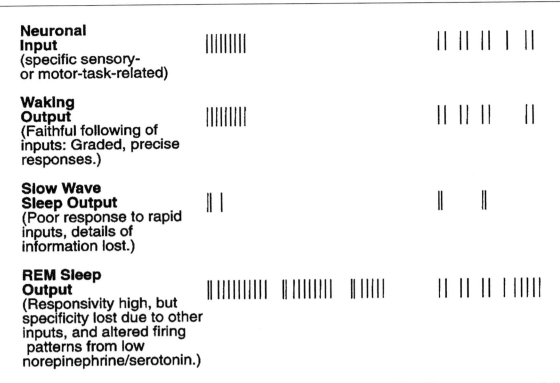

Fig. 16. Schematic of cortical neuronal processing during various behavioral states. The spikes represent neuronal discharge.

scious states are different because the brain states differ. Fig. 16 schematizes the "input-output" relationships in a cortical neuron during the various states of consciousness. This schematic is based on inferences from in vivo recordings in animal and in vitro experiments examining firing patterns as a function of membrane potential. This schematic suggests obvious differences in processing during the different behavioral states.

The *activation-synthesis hypothesis* proposed by Hobson and McCarley suggests that many of the characteristic formal features of dreams are isomorphic with (e.g., "parallel") distinctive features of the physiology of REM sleep. Formal features indicate universal aspects of dreams, distinct from the dream content that is particular to an individual. As an example of a formal feature of a dream, consider the presence of motor activity in dreams. At the physiological level it is known that motor systems, both at the motor cortex and at the brainstem level, are activated during REM sleep episodes. Parallel to the motor-system activation at the physiological level is the finding that movement in dreams is extremely common; almost one-third of all verbs in dreams indicate movement, and 80% of dreams have some occurrence of leg movement (a movement that was easily and reliably scored in dream reports).

Similarly, there is activation of sensory systems during REM sleep. The visual system is intensely activated in REM, and all dreams have visual experiences (and indeed these are one of the defining features of a dream). An important source of visual-system activation during REM sleep is from the PGO waves. The activation synthesis theory suggests that this intense activation of visual and other sensory systems are the substrate for dream sensory experiences. Supporting this theory is the rather frequent occurrence of dreams with intense "vestibular sensations"—about 9% of all REM sleep dreams—e.g., dreams of flying, floating, falling, soaring, or tumbling, easily related to the vestibular-system functions of sensing position of the body in space and changes of position. The presence of dreams with vestibular sensations was highly atypical of the daytime sensory experience of the subjects whose dream reports were examined, and is thus incompatible with any dream theory linked to a simple "recall" of previous experiences. Rather, the dream experience may reflect the intense REM sleep vestibular-system activation, followed by its elaboration and synthesis into dream content. The final product, the dream, thus represents the synthesis of both the brainstem-induced motor and sensory activation with the particular memories and personality characteristics of the dreamer.

Lesion-induced release of REM sleep motor activity supports: (i) the presence of neural commands for patterned motor activity in REM sleep, and (ii) a direct correspondence of the motor-system commands and the subjective content of the dream. Activation of motor systems in REM can be observed in cats with a lesion of the muscle atonia zone of the PRF and a subsequent *REM sleep without atonia*, a state in which motor activity is released but all of the other signs of REM sleep are present. The failure of muscle atonia is also observed in a human disorder reported by Schenck and Mahowald, known as *REM sleep behavior disorder*. In individuals with this disorder, the muscle activity observed has been found always to parallel the dreamed activity. This close linkage between the physiology and psychology of REM sleep and dreams supports the activation-synthesis hypothesis.

When the activation-synthesis hypothesis was first proposed, it aroused considerable controversy, perhaps because it seemed to threaten psychological interpretation of dreams. Although this theory clearly places instigation of the dream state as a concomitant of a basic biological rhythm, there appears, to be more than ample room for addition of personal characteristics in the process of synthesis of brainstem-instigated activation. For example, interpretations of Rorschach cards are rich sources of information on personality, although the images on the cards themselves were certainly not generated by psychologically meaningful mechanisms.

Finally, it should be noted that as more is learned about forebrain processing during REM sleep, a more complete and complex theory will emerge. Recent neuroimaging studies in both man and cat have indicated activation of the limbic system, with little activation of the prefrontal cortex. These data suggest a biological basis of activation of memories and emotions in REM sleep, and perhaps also a mechanism of their linkage, as well as the absence of prefrontal activation being reflected in the absence of a sense of control over one's activities in the dream. Also, as described in the next section on REM sleep function, many current theories postulate a role for this state in memory processing, and dreams may come by their unusual character as a result of the complex associations that are culled from memory during the REM sleep state.

10. FUNCTION(S) OF NONREM AND REM SLEEP

There is little question about the importance of sleep to the organism. Perhaps the most dramatic evidence is the work of Rechtschaffen, showing that rats die after 2–3 wk of total sleep deprivation and after about 5 wk of selective REM sleep deprivation. These numbers may be compared with the 16 d of survival with total food deprivation. Other factors arguing for the importance of sleep is its ubiquity among higher organisms, its evolutionary persistence, although it is maladaptive with respect to other key functions (food gathering, and nurturing young), and its homeostatic regulation. As to the exact nature of its function(s), there are many theories but most have relatively little solid supporting data. Here, we summarize some of the most plausible functional theories for each sleep phase.

10.1. NonREM Sleep: A Time for Rest and Recovery?

10.1.1. REST THEORY

Neuronal recordings and brain metabolic studies indicate the presence of rest on the neural level as well as the behavioral level during nonREM sleep. The data on adenosine provides rather strong support for nonREM sleep as a time of restoration of energy stores that are consumed during wakefulness.

10.1.2. BEHAVIORAL IMMOBILIZATION OR "OUT OF HARM'S WAY"

This theory suggests that sleep evolved as a way of arresting behavior at a time when it may not be advantageous, such as night activity in animals with poor night vision and vulnerability to predators.

10.1.3. CONSOLIDATION OF LEARNING

Recent data suggest that at least some of the plastic changes associated with learning of events occurring during wakefulness takes place during nonREM sleep; it is speculated that the inrush of calcium during delta waves is mechanistically related to these plastic changes.

10.2. REM Sleep: Does Its Activity Promote Growth and Development?

The following theories are not mutually exclusive. Indeed, it seems a cogent argument that a complex behavioral state such as REM sleep may have multiple functions, and as for wakefulness, it may not be meaningful to speak of "the" function of REM sleep.

10.2.1. PROMOTION OF GROWTH AND DEVELOPMENT OF THE NERVOUS SYSTEM

The abundance of this metabolically and neurally active state in the young argues for this hypothesis.

Recent work has also indicated that REM-like activity in the brainstem may alter the activity of "immediate early gene" systems, such as c-fos, thereby suggesting a mechanism by which REM activity may affect DNA transcription and thus effect developmental and structural changes. Along this line of reasoning, the French scientist Jouvet has suggested that the stereotyped motor command patterns of REM sleep are useful in promoting epigenetic development of these circuits.

10.2.2. A "Circuit Exercise/Maintenance Function" in the Adult

It is postulated that maintenance of neural circuits requires use, and that with increasing diversity of behaviors possible in more advanced animals, REM sleep serves as a "fail safe" mode for ensuring activation and consequent maintenance of sensorimotor circuits. Crick and Mitchison suggested that the REM sleep activity involves removal of unwanted, "parasitic" modes of neural-circuit processing.

10.2.3. Memory Processing

Memories may be consolidated and/or processed during sleep. Hippocampal neurons that encode spatial location and are activated during wakefulness are preferentially activated in subsequent REM periods compared to the nonwakefulness-activated neurons; the inference is that "memories" are being related to other brain information.

ACKNOWLEDGMENTS

Work supported by awards from the Department of Veterans Affairs, Medical Research Service and NIMH (R37 MH39,683 R01 MH62522, and R01 MH40,799). Portions of this chapter are adapted from McCarley RW, Greene RW, Rainnie D, Portas CM. Brain stem neuromodulation and REM sleep. Sem Neurosciences 1995; 7:341–354. McCarley RW. Neurophysiology of sleep: basic mechanisms underlying control of wakefulness and sleep. In Chokroverty S (ed). Sleep Disorders Medicine, 2nd ed. Boston: Butterworth-Heinemann, 1999; 21–50. McCarley RW. Human electrophysiology: cellular mechanisms and control of wakefulness and sleep. In Yudofsky S, and Hales RE, (ed). Handbook of Neuropsychiatry, 4th ed. New York: American Psychiatric Press, 2001; In press.

INTERNET

Available as a free download (.pdf format, 3.8 MB) is the following excellent collection of summary articles by leading workers in the field; this is suitable for students wishing to explore the field further. Some individual articles in this collection are also cited below.
The Regulation of Sleep. Borbély AA, Hayaishi O, Sejnowski TJ, Altman JS (eds). Strasbourg, France, Human Frontier Science Program, 2000 http://www.hfsp.org/scientific_activities/scientific_activities_workshop8.htm

SELECTED READINGS

Borbély AA. 1982, A two process model of sleep regulation. Human Neurobiol 1982; 1:195–204.

Chemelli RM, Willie JT, Sinton CM, Elmquist JK, Scammell T, Lee C, et al. Narcolepsy in orexin knockout mice: molecular genetics of sleep regulation. Cell 1999; 98:437–451.

Chokroverty S. (ed). Sleep Disorders Medicine, 2nd ed. Boston: Butterworth-Heinemann, 1999.

Hayaishi O. Regulation of sleep by prostaglandin D2 and adenosine. In Borbély AA, Hayaishi O, Sejnowski TJ, Altman JS (eds). The Regulation of Sleep. Strasbourg: Human Frontier Science Program, 2000; 97–102. http://www.hfsp.org/scientific_activities/scientific_activities_workshop8.htm

Hobson JA, McCarley RW. The brain as a dream state generator: an activation_synthesis hypothesis of the dream process. Am J Psychiatry 1977; 134:1335–1348.

Jouvet M. What does a cat dream about? Trends Neurosci 1979; 2:15–16.

Krueger JM. Cytokines and growth factors in sleep regulation. In Borbély AA, Hayaishi O, Sejnowski TJ, Altman JS (eds). The Regulation of Sleep. Strasbourg: Human Frontier Science Program, 2000; 122–130. http://www.hfsp.org/scientific_activities/scientific_activities_workshop8.htm

Kryger MH, Roth T, Dement WC. Principles and Practices of Sleep Medicine, 3rd ed. New York: Saunders, 2000.

Lin L, Faraco J, Li R, Kadotani H, Rogers W, Lin X, et al. The sleep disorder canine narcolepsy is caused by a mutation in the hypocretin (orexin) receptor 2 gene. Cell 1999; 98:365–376.

Maquet PAA. Functional neuroanatomy of normal human sleep. In Borbély AA, Hayaishi O, Sejnowski TJ, Altman JS (eds). The Regulation of Sleep. Strasbourg: Human Frontier Science Program, 2000; 86–93. http://www.hfsp.org/scientific_activities/scientific_activities_workshop8.htm

McCarley RW, Strecker RE, Thakkar MM, Porkka-Heiskanen T. Adenosine and 5-HT as regulators of behavioural state. In Edited by Borbély AA, Hayaishi O, Sejnowski TJ, Altman JS (eds). The Regulation of Sleep. Strasbourg: Human Frontier Science Program, 2000; 103–112.

McCarley RW, Greene RW, Rainnie D, Portas CM. Brain stem neuromodulation and REM sleep. Seminars in the Neurosciences 1995; 7:341–354.

Moruzzi G, Magoun HW. Brain stem reticular formation and activation of the EEG, Electroenceph Clin Neurophysiol 1949; 1:455–473.

Nitz D, Siegel JM. GABA release in the locus coeruleus as a function of sleep/wake state. Neuroscience 1997; 78:795–801.

Porkka-Heiskanen T, Strecker RE, Thakkar M, Bjørkum AA, Greene RW, McCarley RW. Adenosine: a mediator of the sleep-inducing effects of prolonged wakefulness. Science 1997; 276:1265–1268.

Sherin JE, Shiromani PJ, McCarley RW, Saper CB. Activation of ventrolateral preoptic neurons during sleep. Science 1996; 271:216–219.

Steriade M, McCarley RW. Brainstem Control of Wakefulness and Sleep. New York: Plenum Press, 1990.

Steriade M, Curró Dossi R, Nuñez A. Network modulation of a slow intrinsic oscillation of cat thalamocortical neurons implicated in sleep delta waves: cortically induced synchronization and brainstem cholinergic suppression. J Neurosci 1991;11: 3200–3217.

Thakkar M, Strecker RE, McCarley RW. Behavioral state control through differential serotonergic inhibition in the mesopontine cholinergic nuclei: a simultaneous unit recording and microdialysis study, J Neurosci 1998; 18:5490–5497.

Thannickal TC, Moore RY, Nienhuis R, Ramanathan L, Gulyani S, Aldrich M, et al. Reduced number of hypocretin neurons in human narcolepsy. Neuron 2000; 27:469–474.

Tononi G, Cirelli C, Shaw PJ. Molecular correlates of sleep, the awake state and sleep deprivation. In Borbély AA, Hayaishi O, Sejnowski TJ, Altman JS (eds). The Regulation of Sleep. Strasbourg, France: Human Frontier Science Program, 2000. http://www.hfsp.org/scientific_activities/scientific_activities_workshop8.htm

29 Higher Brain Functions

Daniel Tranel

CONTENTS

1. INTRODUCTION

Higher brain functions are the operations of the brain that stand at the pinnacle of evolution and are largely unique to humans. Verbal communication, the ability to "think in the future," and the capacity to hold multiple tracks of complex information "on-line" at the same time, are examples of higher mental functions that are subserved by various structures in the brain. The higher-order capacities of the human brain can be captured under the terms "cognition" and "behavior." *Cognition* is composed of intellectual function, memory, speech and language, complex perception, orientation, attention, judgment, planning, and decision-making. *Behavior* is the manifestation of these cognitive functions. Behavior is guided by another facet of higher brain function—namely, *personality*, which describes the psychological make-up, traits, and response styles that typify a person's behaviors across a range of situations and circumstances.

From: *Neuroscience in Medicine, 2nd ed.* (P. Michael Conn, ed.), © 2003 Humana Press Inc., Totowa, NJ.

Most neuroscientists have come to view *brain functions* as synonymous with *mind functions*, although we do not yet know all, or even many, of the details of how mental operations are served by neural machinery. In fact, it remains to be seen whether we will ever be able to explain all human behavior in neural terms, and some might even consider this a ludicrous potentiality. Nonetheless, breakthroughs in neuroscience over the past few decades have provided more and more compelling evidence indicating that brain facts and mind facts are one and the same. One basic premise behind the ideas presented in this chapter is that there are orderly, predictable relationships between neural operations and cognitive/behavioral capacities.

2. BRAIN AND BEHAVIOR ASSOCIATIONS

2.1. History

The systematic study of brain-behavior relationships can be traced back to a number of landmark observations, beginning nearly a century and a half ago. In the 1860s, the surgeon and physical anthropologist Paul Broca reported on a patient who developed an inability to produce speech following damage to the left front part of the brain. The discovery led to the suggestion—at the time quite startling, but something now accepted as a basic principle of neuropsychology—that humans speak with the left side of the brain. Some ten years later, the neuropsychiatrist Carl Wernicke reported a complementary finding: damage to the posterior part of the left hemisphere rendered patients unable to comprehend speech, yet left speech production relatively unaffected. And in this same general era, John Harlow reported on the case of Phineas Gage, a young man who developed a bizarre and striking impairment in personality and social conduct following an accident in which an iron bar was propelled through the front part of his brain, destroying the prefrontal cortex bilaterally.

Other historical developments were also centered around key case studies. In 1957, Scoville and Milner reported on the patient who came to be known as HM, who developed severe and permanent anterograde amnesia (learning impairment) following bilateral resection of the mesial temporal lobes, performed to control intractable epilepsy. Neuropsychological studies of HM yielded a number of key breakthroughs in the understanding of the neural basis of memory, and focused attention on the role of the mesial temporal region—especially the hippocampus—in memory. And shortly after the middle of the twentieth century, studies by Roger Sperry, in collaboration with Joseph Bogen and Michael Gazzaniga, sparked interest in the dramatic differences between the two hemispheres of the brain. These investigators studied "split-brain" patients, who had undergone separation of the two hemispheres for control of seizures. Specifically, the *corpus callosum*, the large bundle of fibers that connects the left and right hemispheres, was surgically cut, so that the left and right hemispheres were no longer in communication. Careful studies of these patients revealed that the two hemispheres retained two more or less separate modes of consciousness, one in the left hemisphere that was language-based and operated in sequential, analytical style, and one in the right hemisphere that was spatially based and operated in gestalt, holistic style. Modern cognitive neuroscience has confirmed many of these earlier findings.

In the past few decades, my colleagues and I have described a number of additional important cases. For example, we have described a modern-day "Phineas Gage"-type patient, known as EVR, who developed a profound impairment in social conduct and personality following bilateral damage to the ventromedial prefrontal cortex. Another patient, known as Boswell, developed one of the most severe amnesic syndromes that has ever been reported, following bilateral damage to both the mesial and lateral sectors of the temporal lobes. Boswell cannot learn any new declarative information, and he cannot recall anything more than a few shreds of information from his past. And the patient known as SM cannot recognize emotional facial expressions, or learn new associations between salient events and strong emotional responses, because of bilateral damage to the amygdala. We have conducted numerous investigations of these and many other brain-damaged patients over the past few decades, paving the way for many new breakthroughs in cognitive neuroscience.

2.2. Lateral Specialization: Left vs Right

The pioneering discoveries of Broca and Wernicke, and the pathbreaking work of Sperry and colleagues, led to the establishment of what has become one of the most robust principles in neuropsychology—namely, that humans have left-hemisphere specialization for language. This principle applies to nearly all right-handed persons (about 99%), and to the majority of left-handed people (about 70%). Moreover, this principle holds regardless of the mode of sensory input—verbal material apprehended through the visual (as in reading) or auditory (as in hearing spoken language) modalities is processed by the left hemisphere; and it holds regardless of the mode of output—both spoken speech and written language production are subserved by left-hemisphere structures.

For many years in the early history of neuropsychology, the right hemisphere was believed to be the "silent" or "minor" hemisphere, because it did not participate to great extent in language. Thus, in early conceptualizations of the differences between the left and right hemispheres, the prevailing notion was that the left hemisphere was the major or *dominant* side, and the right hemisphere was the minor or *nondominant* side. This attitude reflected an emphasis on language—because language is a highly observable and uniquely human capacity, it received the most attention from neurologists and neuropsychologists, and was considered the quintessential human faculty. For many decades, the right hemisphere was believed to contribute little to higher-level cognitive function-

Table 1
Functional Dichotomies of Left and Right Hemispheric Dominance

Left side	Right side
Verbal	Nonverbal
Serial	Parallel
Analytic	Holistic
Controlled	Creative
Logical	Pictorial
Propositional	Appositional
Rational	Intuitive
Social	Physical

Adapted from Benton (1991).

ing. Lesions to the right hemisphere typically did not produce language disturbances, and it was often concluded that the patient had lost little in the way of higher-order functions after right-sided brain injury. We know that this is far from true—although the right hemisphere has an entirely different type of specializtion, it has cognitive and behavioral capacities that are every bit as important as those of the left hemisphere.

As the field evolved, it became clear that each hemisphere was dedicated to certain cognitive capacities, and the notion of "dominance" gave way to the idea of "specialization" (in fact, one rarely encounters the terms "dominant/nondominant" or "major/minor" any more, in reference to the two cerebral hemispheres). That is, each hemisphere was specialized for certain types of cognitive functions (Table 1). As noted, early work had already established the role of the left hemisphere in language function, and subsequent investigations confirmed this conclusion. By contrast, the right hemisphere is specialized for *nonverbal processing*, and it handles information such as complex visual patterns (e.g., faces and geographical routes) or auditory signals (e.g., music) that are not coded in verbal form. The right side of the brain is also specialized for the mapping of emotions—patterns of bodily sensations that are linked to feelings such as happiness, anger, and fear. Another right-hemisphere capacity concerns the perception of our bodies in space, in intrapersonal and extrapersonal terms. For example, an understanding of where our limbs are in relation to our trunk and where our body is in relation to the space around us is under the purview of the right hemisphere.

2.3. Longitudinal Specialization: Anterior vs Posterior

Another useful organizational principle for understanding brain–behavior relationships is an *anterior* and *posterior* distinction. The major demarcation points are the *Rolandic (central) sulcus*, which is the major fissure separating the frontal lobes (anteriorly) from the parietal lobes (posteriorly), and the *Sylvian fissure*, which forms a boundary between the temporal lobes (inferiorly) and the frontal and parietal lobes (superiorly). These landmarks and the major lobes of the brain are illustrated in Fig. 1.

As a general principle, the posterior regions of the brain are dedicated to *perception*—the apprehension and intake of information from the world outside. (The "world outside" actually refers to two domains: the world that is outside our bodies and brains, and the world that is outside our brains but inside our bodies. The latter, the *soma*, comprises the smooth muscle, the viscera, and other bodily structures innervated by the central nervous system [CNS]). The primary sensory cortices for vision, audition, and tactile perception are in the posterior sectors of the brain, in the occipital, temporal, and parietal regions, respectively.

By contrast, anterior brain regions generally comprise effector systems that are specialized for the execution of behavior. For example, the primary motor cortices are located in the strip of cortex immediately anterior to the Rolandic sulcus (area 4). The motor area for speech, known as *Broca's area*, is in the left frontal operculum (areas 44 and 45). The right-hemisphere counterpart of Broca's area, in the right frontal operculum, is important for executing stresses and intonations that infuse speech with emotional meaning, such as prosody. A variety of "executive functions,"—judgment and decision-making, and the capacity to construct and implement various plans of action—are associated with structures in the frontal lobes. Thus, it is a useful heuristic to consider the anterior part of the brain as comprising a variety of effector systems, and the posterior part as comprising a variety of perceptual systems.

3. THE OCCIPITAL LOBES
3.1. Primary Visual Vortex

The occipital lobes are situated in the posterior part of the hemispheres, and they can be subdivided into the primary visual cortex and visual association cortices (Fig. 2). The primary visual cortices are composed

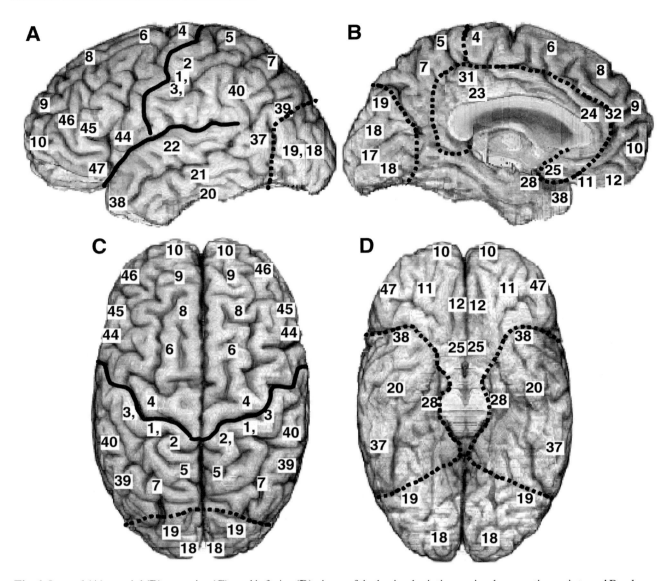

Fig. 1. Lateral (**A**), mesial (**B**), superior (**C**), and inferior (**D**) views of the brain, depicting major demarcation points and Brodmann areas (numbers). The left hemisphere is shown in the lateral (**A**) and mesial (**B**) views; the mappings would be the same on the right hemisphere. In the superior perspective (**C**), the left hemisphere is on the left, and the right hemisphere is on the right; the sides are reversed in the inferior perspective (**D**). The Rolandic (central) sulcus runs in a roughly vertical fashion from the top of the brain (just behind area 4) down to an intersection with the Sylvian fissure, just behind area 44. The Sylvian fissure (lateral sulcus) runs in a roughly horizontal fashion, just above area 22. The main lobes of the brain are demarcated: the frontal lobe is anterior to the Rolandic sulcus and superior to the Sylvian fissure; the parietal lobe is posterior to the Rolandic sulcus and superior to the Sylvian fissure; the occipital lobe is behind the dotted line that separates areas 37 and 39 from areas 19 and 18; the temporal lobe is below the Sylvian fissure. Also, a region commonly referred to as the "limbic lobe" includes the cingulate gyrus (areas 24 and 23), and areas 25, 26, 27, and 28.

of area 17, located primarily in the region directly above and below the calcarine fissure in the mesial aspect of the hemispheres. This region is dedicated to *form vision*, and damage here produces blindness in the corresponding visual field. The system is wired in a crossed fashion, in both the vertical and horizontal dimensions. Thus, visual information from the hemispace to the right of the vertical meridian is perceived with the left visual cortex, and information from the left hemispace is perceived with the right visual cortex. Similarly, information from the visual space above the horizontal meridian reaches the visual cortex below

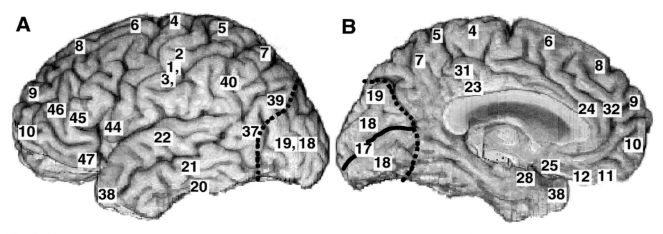

Fig. 2. The major subdivisions of the occipital lobes, mapped on lateral (**A**) and mesial (**B**) views of the left hemisphere (the mappings would be the same in the right hemisphere). The calcarine fissure is a major landmark, separating the ventral (inferior) visual system from the dorsal (superior) visual system. The primary visual cortex is formed by the superior and inferior banks of the calcarine region, in area 17. Areas 18 and 19 make up the visual-association cortices.

the calcarine fissure, and information from the visual space below the midline reaches cortex above the calcarine fissure.

Other features of the visual world are processed in or near the primary visual cortices. The processing of color, for example, is strongly linked to the lingual gyrus, immediately below the primary visual cortex on the inferior bank of the calcarine sulcus. *Depth perception* (e.g., stereopsis) and *motion perception* are associated with cortices in and near the superior component of the primary visual region, in an area known as the cuneus.

3.2. Visual Association Cortices

The visual-association cortices include areas 18 and 19 on the lateral and mesial aspects of the hemispheres. Area 37, and the posterior parts of areas 20 and 21 in the inferior and ventral banks of the temporal lobes, are also dedicated primarily to the processing of visual information. The visual-association cortices, which communicate with the primary visual cortex posteriorly and with more anterior regions in the temporal and parietal lobes through a series of extensive feedforward and feedback connections, are specialized for progressively higher-order aspects of visual processing.

3.3. The Ventral and Dorsal Visual Systems

Visual-system characteristics can be conceptualized along anatomic and functional lines that comprise two distinct subsystems: a ventral system and a dorsal system. These are referred to as the "what" and "where" systems, respectively. Consistent with its dedication to the "what" aspects of stimuli, the ventral system processes primarily featural information such as shape, color, and texture. For example, the ability to perceive and assign meaning to orthographic symbols (e.g., reading) is associated with the region of the cortex, and white matter in the lower part of the visual-association cortex in the left hemisphere. In the right hemisphere, the ventral visual-association cortices are specialized for the registration and decoding of nonverbal patterns, such as the holistic perception and recognition of faces. The ventral occipitotemporal cortices are also important for retrieving conceptual knowledge regarding various concrete entities—e.g., recognition of animals, fruits/vegetables, tools/utensils, musical instruments, and other categories. Recent studies have demonstrated remarkable specialization within these systems. For example, recognition of animals is subserved by a system that includes cortices in the right mesial occipital/ventral temporal region and the left mesial occipital region, and recognition of tools/utensils is subserved by a system that includes cortices in the left occipital-temporal-parietal junction.

The dorsal or "where" system processes primarily the features of motion, depth, and the position of stimuli in space. Thus, superior parts of the visual-association cortices are important for deriving meaningful information from motion and depth. The anterior part of this region, which overlaps with the posterior part of the superior parietal region, is specialized for visuospatial capacities that relate to the placement of external stimuli in space and to the tracking of those stimuli when they are in motion. This region is also important for the accurate mental assemblage of extrapersonal space and the subsequent placement and location of oneself in that space. For example, the ability to know where your body is in relation to the chair on which you are sitting and to guide your arm down to a book to turn the page depends on association cortices in the upper parts of the occipital and posterior parietal regions. The upper part of the visual system is important for attending to multiple visual elements concurrently. When watching a politician who is delivering a speech from center stage, flanked on both sides by other dignitaries, we may be aware of the speech giver and the person just to the left of the podium who is having trouble staying awake. The capacity to do this is known as simultaneous visual perception.

4. THE TEMPORAL LOBES

The temporal lobes can be subdivided into three sectors, according to the type of specialization the regions have for different cognitive operations (Fig. 3).

4.1. Superior Sector: Primary Auditory Cortex and Auditory-Association Cortices

Heschl's gyrus (areas 41 and 42), which is buried in the depths of the Sylvian fissure in the posterior aspect of the temporal lobes (Fig. 3), constitutes the primary auditory cortex that is crucial for basic perception of auditory information. The system is relatively crossed, so that auditory information from the right ear is sent primarily to the left Heschl's gyrus, and information from the left ear is sent primarily to right Heschl's gyrus. However, this decussation is incomplete, and a significant amount of information is perceived ipsilaterally (e.g., by the primary auditory cortex on the same side as the ear). Interestingly, information can be "forced" into more complete crossing using a special paradigm known as *dichotic listening*. In this task, auditory information is presented to each ear simultaneously. If the information varies sufficiently between the left and right ears (e.g., if the word "science" is input to the left ear and the word "professor" is input to the right ear), the auditory system will be driven in such a way that the subject will perceive the word "science" with the right auditory cortex and the word professor with the left auditory cortex. When verbal material is presented in dichotic listening paradigms, the right ear (e.g., left brain) shows a relative advantage (e.g., perceives information first and more

strongly) over the left ear. By contrast, if nonverbal material is presented (e.g., music), the left ear (right brain) shows a relative advantage over the right ear. This pattern is in keeping with the overall verbal-left, nonverbal-right hemispheric specialization.

The posterior third of the superior temporal gyrus (posterior area 22) contains important auditory-association cortices (Fig. 3). On the left, this region comprises the heart of what is known as *Wernicke's area*, specialized for decoding aural verbal information, such as deciphering the meaning of speech input. The right side is specialized for nonspeech auditory information, such as environmental sounds, musical melodies, timbre, and prosody. In general, the left auditory-association cortices are specialized for the perception and decoding of *temporal* components of auditory information—information pertaining to timing, the sequential aspects of auditory signals, the pace of information delivery (e.g., cadence), and the duration of signals and intervals between sounds. The right auditory-association cortices are specialized for *spectral* information—the pitch (e.g., fundamental frequency) of signals and their spectral complexity (e.g., harmonic structures).

4.2. Lateral and Inferior Sector

The lateral and inferior parts of the temporal lobe are comprised by areas 37, 20, 21, and 38 on the lateral and inferior aspects of the hemisphere (Fig. 3). The posterior parts of the second, third, and fourth temporal gyri formed by areas 37, 20, and 21, are strongly linked to the higher-order decoding of visual information. As alluded to here in the discussion of the ventral occipital region, the cortices in the ventral occipital and posterior inferotemporal regions are critical for face recognition, and for visual recognition of other entities such as animals, fruits/vegetables, and tools/utensils. On the left side, the more anterior parts of the inferotemporal region are specialized for the retrieval of lexical items that denote various entities, including common nouns such as the names of animals and fruits/vegetables. Progressively more anterior parts of the system on the left are concerned with progressively more unique items, and in the temporal polar region (area 38), there is a specialization for the retrieval of proper nouns—unique lexical entries that denote items that constitute a class of one (such as names of people and places). Actually, new evidence has suggested that these regions contain important intermediary units that broker between the retrieval of conceptual knowledge (knowing what things are) and the retrieval of names

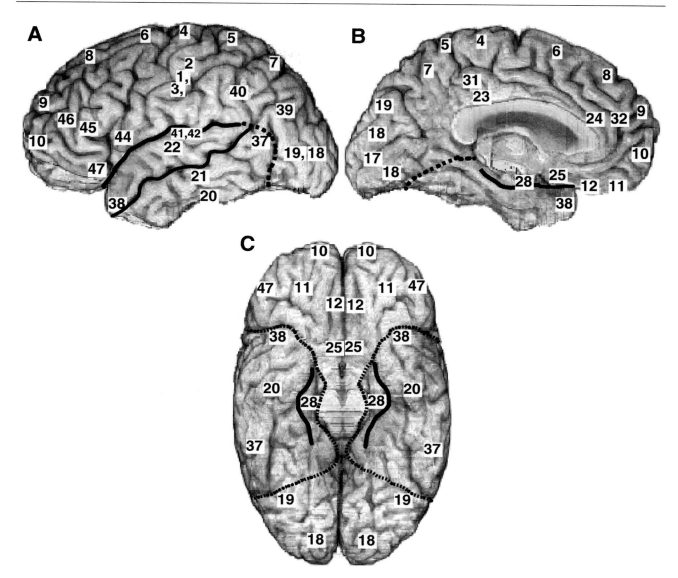

Fig. 3. Three major subdivisions of the temporal lobes are depicted on lateral (**A**) and mesial (**B**) views of the left hemisphere (the mappings would be the same in the right hemisphere). An inferior view of these regions is shown in (**C**) (*where the left hemisphere is on the right*). The temporal lobes are bounded overall by the Sylvian fissure superiorly, and by the junction with the parietal and occipital lobes posteriorly (*dotted line* in **A**). The primary auditory cortices (areas 41 and 42) are buried in the depths of the Sylvian fissure; the auditory-association cortices in the posterior superior temporal gyrus (area 22) surround this region. The lateral/inferior sector is made up of areas 21, 20, 37, and 38. The mesial sector is made up of area 28 and other limbic structures (hippocampus, amygdala) in the mesial part of the temporal lobes (**B** and **C**).

(knowing what things are called). The intermediary units do not contain the words themselves; rather, the word assembly is performed by language-related structures in the perisylvian region. The properties of these intermediary units are only recently beginning to be understood, but new evidence hints at some very intriguing design characteristics. For example, it appears that the intermediary units for retrieving animal names are the same whether one is retrieving names from seeing pictures of animals, or retrieving names from hearing the characteristic sounds of those animals. So, for instance, the "broker" unit for retrieving the name "rooster" is the same whether one sees a picture of a rooster, or whether one hears a cock-a-doodle-doo. Another interesting feature is that in the left temporal polar region, the specialization appears to be for unique names, rather than for names of persons per se. Thus, the temporal pole is specialized for proper nouns, whether these are for persons or for places—the key is that the name refers to a unique entity.

The inferior and anterior temporal sectors in the right hemisphere play an important role in the retrieval of nonverbal information from retrograde memory—the retrieval of knowledge that was acquired prior to the onset of a brain injury. This stands in distinction to the learning of new information, which depends on mesial temporal structures. Remarkably, patients with damage to anterior lateral and ventral temporal structures, but not to mesial structures, can develop a pattern of amnesia that involves severe disruption of retrograde memory, but nearly complete sparing of anterograde memory—the patients can learn new information, but they cannot retrieve information from their past. The right anterior temporal region works in conjunction with structures in the prefrontal sector to subserve retrieval of knowledge related to one's autobiography.

Structures in the right anterior temporal region appear to play an important role in the *recognition* of unique entities—e.g., familiar persons and landmarks—in a manner akin to the role of the left anterior temporal region in retrieving names for such entities. Thus, when the right temporal pole is damaged, patients develop impairments in the retrieval of conceptual knowledge for familiar persons. This finding has been corroborated by functional imaging studies, which have demonstrated activation of this region when subjects are identifying familiar persons and landmarks. These results are also consistent with the importance of anterior and lateral aspects of the right temporal lobe in the retrieval of retrograde memories. Together with interconnected right prefrontal cortices, the right anterolateral temporal region is probably of critical importance for the retrieval of unique, factual memories.

4.3. Mesial Sector

The mesial temporal lobe is comprised by the amygdala, hippocampus, entorhinal and perirhinal cortices, and the anterior portion of parahippocampal gyrus not occupied by the entorhinal cortex (Fig. 3). These structures play a crucial role in memory, especially learning of new information (anterograde memory). In the following section, a brief summary of the roles of the hippocampal complex and amygdala is presented.

4.3.1. Hippocampal Complex

The hippocampus and the adjacent entorhinal and perirhinal cortices are referred to as the *hippocampal complex*. The components of the hippocampal complex are highly interconnected by means of recurrent neuroanatomical circuits. In turn, the hippocampal complex is extensively interconnected with higher-order association cortices located in the temporal lobe. Those cortices receive signals from the association cortices of all sensory modalities, and also receive feedback projections from the hippocampus. Structures in the hippocampal complex thus have access to, and influence over, signals from virtually the entire brain. Anatomically, the system is in a position to create integrated records of various aspects of memory experiences, including visual, auditory, and somatosensory information. In a general sense, the principal function of the hippocampal complex is the acquisition of new factual knowledge. There are two hippocampal complexes, one in the left hemisphere and one in the right. Anatomically, the two are roughly equivalent, but there are major differences in their functional roles. Specifically, the two hippocampal complexes are specialized for different types of material in a manner that parallels the overall functional arrangement of the brain, namely, left-verbal and right-nonverbal.

The landmark report by Scoville and Milner described how patient HM became severely amnesic following bilateral mesial temporal-lobe resection for control of intractable seizures. This observation established the mesial aspect of the temporal lobes, and the hippocampus in particular, as unequivocally linked to memory—specifically, to the acquisition of new information, such as *anterograde memory*. Also, research has established a fairly reliable relationship between the extent of damage to the hippocampal system, and the degree of amnesia with which a patient is left. More extensive mesial temporal damage, involving the peripheral cortex and parahippocampal gyrus in addition to the hippocampal region and entorhinal cortex, usually produces a proportionate increase in the severity of amnesia.

With respect to the nature of the amnesia associated with hippocampal damage, several relationships have been firmly estalished. First, there is a consistent relationship between the side of the lesion and the type of learning impairment. Specifically, damage to the left hippocampal system produces an amnesic syndrome that affects verbal material (such as spoken words or written material), but spares nonverbal material; conversely, damage to the right hippocampal system affects nonverbal material (such as complex visual and auditory patterns), but spares verbal material. For example, after damage to the left hippocampus, a paitent may lose the ability to learn new names, but remain capable of learning new faces and spatial arrangements. By contrast, damage to the right hippocampal system frequently impairs the ability to learn new geographical routes.

A second point is that the hippocampal system does not appear to play a role in the learning of perceptuomotor skills and other knowledge known as *nondeclarative memory*. Patient HM, for example, can learn new perceptuomotor skills, although he has no recall of the situation in which the learning of those skills took place. We have reported similar findings in other patients with bilateral mesial temporal-lobe damage. In fact, not only can such patients acquire perceptuomotor skills at a normal level, but they can retain those skills for many years after the initial learning, despite the fact that they cannot recall the circumstances of the learning situation. Thus, the role of the hippocampus in memory is principally for acquiring declarative knowledge—facts, faces, names, and other information that can be "declared" and brought into the mind's eye.

Finally, the hippocampus and related mesial temporal structures do not appear to be crucial for the retrieval of previously learned information *(retrograde memory)*. As noted previously, other structures in anterior and lateral temporal cortices appear to be the critical repositories of retrograde memory. By contrast, the hippocampal system, although it is crucial for the acquisition of information, does not seem to be necessary for the retrieval of information, once that information has been consolidated and stored. In short, the hippocampal system plays a time-limited role in memory—it is critical for acquisition, but not for long-term storage and retrieval.

4.3.2. AMYGDALA

The amygdala plays an intriguing role in memory. Recent studies have shown that the amygdala is important for the acquisition and expression of *emotional memory*, but not for neutral memory. Specifically, the amygdala contributes critically to the potentiation of memory traces for emotional stimuli during their

acquisition and consolidation into long-term declarative memory. These findings are in accord with other evidence indicating that that amygdala is important for the recognition of emotion in facial expressions, especially fear, and in the processing of other information that has emotional significance. Also, it has been shown that the amygdala is important for classical conditioning of autonomic responses. One study found that a patient with circumscribed bilateral amygdala damage was able to acquire declarative knowledge normally, but was impaired in acquiring conditioned autonomic responses. A patient with circumscribed bilateral hippocampal damage (but with intact amygdala) showed the opposite pattern. These findings have led to the idea that the amgydala is important for processing stimuli that communicate emotional significance in social situations; specifically, the amygdala may orchestrate patterns of neural activation in disparate sectors of the brain that would encode both the intrinsic, physical features of stimuli (e.g., shape, position in space), and the value that certain stimuli have to the organism, especially emotional significance.

5. THE PARIETAL LOBES

The parietal lobes, situated posterior to the Rolandic sulcus and superior to the sylvian fissure, comprise a heterogenous collection of primary sensory and association cortices (Fig. 4). Basic somatosensory perception, including perception of touch, vibration, and temperature, takes place in the strip of cortex formed by the postcentral gyrus (areas 3, 1, and 2). A secondary somatosensory area (SII) is in the inferior parietal operculum, and this region may play an important role in higher-order tactile perception (e.g., recognition of objects from touch). In the right hemisphere, SII is important for the mapping and interpretation of emotional states. The inferior parietal lobule, which includes areas 40 and 39, is closely linked to the auditory modality, and is strongly connected to nearby auditory-association cortices in the temporal lobe. The superior parietal lobule, made up of areas 7 and 5, is linked to the visual modality and is strongly connected to visual-association cortices in the occipital lobe. However, the region formed by the transition zone between the occipital, temporal, and parietal cortices on the lateral aspect of the hemisphere is highly heteromodal, and is specialized for polymodal sensory integration, such as integration of visual, auditory, and somatosensory signals.

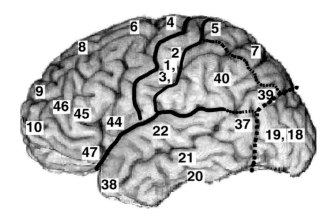

Fig. 4. The major subdivisions of the parietal lobe are depicted on a lateral view of the left hemisphere (the mappings would be the same in the right hemisphere). The primary somatosensory cortex is made up of areas 3, 1, and 2. The superior parietal lobule includes areas 5 and 7. The inferior parietal lobule is made up of areas 40 (supramarginal gyrus) and 39 (angular gyrus).

On the left, the inferior parietal lobule is involved in language functions. The ability to repeat verbatim words, digits, or sentences, for example, depends on intact parietal opercular cortices and underlying white matter. This function requires accurate perception of auditory information, the retrieval of matching information from one's store of acoustic records, and the triggering of anterior motor cortices to produce the information. Inferior parietal cortices on the right side play a significant role in self-perception, the placement of a person's body in space, and in the mapping of physical and emotional states. The ability to direct attention to the external and internal milieu, for example, depends critically on right inferior parietal cortices. The right parietal region is also crucial for many aspects of visuospatial processing, such as perceiving and deciphering complex spatial patterns and comprehending and manipulating spatial knowledge (e.g., planning how to pack a large amount of luggage into your car trunk). Visuoconstructional skills, e.g., drawing complex figures, or architecture-type endeavors, are also related to the right parietal region.

6. THE FRONTAL LOBES

The frontal lobes comprise a vast expanse of cortex and white matter anterior to the Rolandic sulcus (Fig. 5). The frontal lobes make up nearly one-half of the entire cerebral mantle, and they represent the high-est level of neural evolution. The cognitive operations mediated by the frontal lobes, such as foresight, complex decision-making, and social conduct, stand at the zenith of evolution of mental processes. The frontal lobes can be subdivided into several functional units that have distinctive behavioral correlates (Fig. 5). Four major subdivisions are reviewed here.

6.1. Motor and Premotor Region

Immediately anterior to the Rolandic sulcus is the strip of motor cortex (area 4) that mediates basic motor activity of all parts of the body. Anterior to this is area 6, which together with area 44 comprises the premotor region. The cortex in area 6 also participates integrally in motor behavior, as a sort of motor "association" cortex—it is involved with the planning and initiation of motor behaviors. The premotor region has access to complex information from all major sensory modalities, and it participates in the formation of a plan for motor activity in response to particular stimulus configurations, and provides the "impetus" to set the plan into action.

The frontal operculum includes areas 44, 45, and 47. On the left side, areas 44 and 45 of this region constitute *Broca's area*, which is the main speech-output center; that is, the region responsible for motor aspects of linguistic expression. In the right hemisphere, the frontal opercular region plays a role in expressive prosody—the infusion of speech with various intonations that add emotional coloring to the content.

6.2. Dorsolateral Prefrontal Region

The dorsolateral prefrontal region is composed of the cortices and white matter formed by the lateral expanses of areas 8, 9, 46, and 10 (Fig. 5). This region plays an important role in many types of higher-order intellectual behavior. Recent investigations, especially those using new functional neuroimaging techniques such as positron emission tomography (PET) and functional magnetic resonance imaging (fMRI), have provided some consistent clues regarding the functions of the dorsolateral prefrontal region, and some of the most notable findings are summarized here.

Various types of high-level intellectual abilities appear to depend on the dorsolateral prefrontal region. Examples include mental operations that require the retrieval and manipulation of information, especially when there is a demand for creativity and originality. To the extent that such operations involve verbal

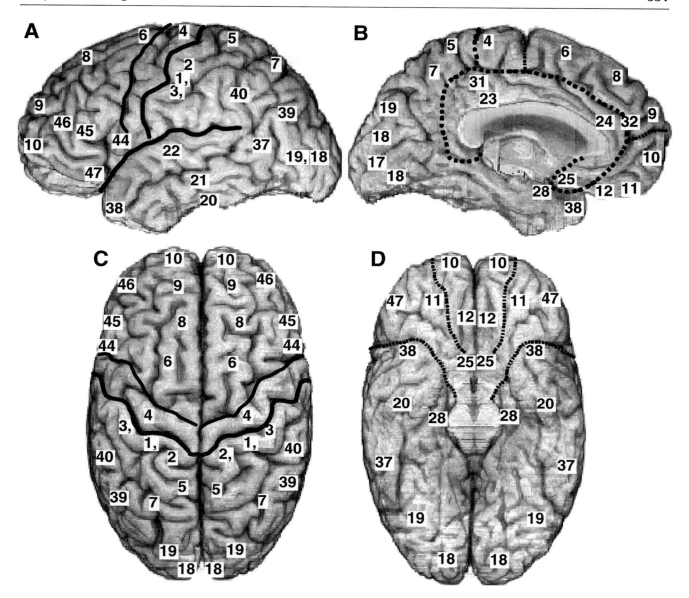

Fig. 5. The major subdivisions of the frontal lobes are depicted on lateral (**A**) and mesial (**B**) views of the left hemisphere (the mappings would be the same in the right hemisphere). Superior (**C**) and inferior (**D**) mappings are also depicted; in (**C**). the left hemisphere is on the left, and in (**D**), the left hemisphere is on the right. The primary motor cortex is formed by area 4. The premotor region includes areas 6 and 44. In the left hemisphere, areas 44 and 45 make up Broca's area. The large expanse of cortex comprised primarily by the lateral aspects of areas 8, 9, 46, and 10, forms the dorsolateral prefrontal region. The superior mesial prefrontal region is formed by the mesial aspects of areas 6, 8, 9, and the upper part of area 32. The ventromedial prefrontal region is made up of areas 12, 11, 25, and the lower mesial parts of areas 32 and 10.

material and the use of language symbols, the left dorsolateral region has the dominant role. When operations depend on and require the use of nonverbal information, the right dorsolateral region takes the lead. Consider the following two neuropsychological tasks, which are analogous in their demand for creative, flexible mental production, but which vary in the use of verbal vs nonverbal mediation. In one, known as *verbal fluency*, a person is required to generate as many words as possible that begin with a particular letter of the alphabet (e.g., *f*) within a specified time limit. In the other task, known as *design fluency*, the person is asked to generate as many unique geometric designs as possible within a particular time constraint. Both tasks require retrieval, manipulation, and execution in a manner that depends critically on flexible, creative thought processes, and the dorsolateral prefrontal region is an important neural substrate for the performance of tasks such as these.

Another important function subserved by the dorsolateral prefrontal region is *working memory*. Working memory refers to a brief window of mental processing—on the order of a minute or two—during which a limited amount of information is held in a sort of mental scratchpad, and operations can be performed on it. Working memory is used to bridge temporal gaps, so that we can perform operations on material that is being held "in-mind" but is no longer existent in our perceptual space. For example, when we look up a phone number and run it through our minds a couple of times, and then cross the room to the telephone and dial the number, the ability to keep the number in mind during the time it takes to cross the room and dial the number is an example of working memory. The two hemispheres are specialized for working memory in a manner that parallels overall hemispheric specialization—the left dorsolateral region is dominant for verbal working memory (e.g., remembering a list of grocery store items) and the right dorsolateral region is dominant for spatial working memory (e.g., remembering a geographical route after asking for directions in a strange town).

The dorsolateral prefrontal region is also associated with the capacities of judging the *recency* and *frequency* of events. For example, consider the following question, which calls for a *recency* judgment: "When was the last time you talked to your father on the telephone?" The answer may be anywhere from a few minutes ago up to many years ago, and to find the answer, your brain will engage a memory search that requires complex and simultaneous activations of various interrelated memories. Now consider a judgment of *frequency*: "How many times did the temperature go above 100 degrees last summer?" Again, answering such a question requires a complex activation and search of memory that depends on dorsolateral prefrontal structures. And as with many other brain-behavior relationships, there appears to be some hemispheric specialization for recency and frequency judgments, and the left dorsolateral prefrontal region is more important for verbally coded information, and the right is more important for visuospatial information. The dorsolateral prefrontal sector has also been linked to other types of "cognitive estimations" that

require rough approximations rather than retrieval of rote knowledge, such as guessing the average number of publications that full professors have, or the average number of weeks that a hit song stays in the "Top Forty."

6.3. Superior Mesial Prefrontal Region

On the mesial surface of the cerebral hemispheres, there is a region of the frontal lobes composed of the supplementary motor area (SMA; mesial area 6) and the mesial parts of areas 8, 9, and 32 (Fig. 5). Together with the anterior part of the cingulate gyrus (e.g., area 24), this region is closely linked to emotional behavior and to basic drive states associated with motivation and arousal. The SMA plays a crucial role in motivating the execution of motor behaviors. Without the input of the SMA, a person may never get past the stage of intention to act. The same principle applies to speech production—the SMA plays an important role in the basic drive to produce speech, and when the SMA is dysfunctional, patients tend to remain mute, although they retain the basic capacity for speaking.

The superior mesial prefrontal region is also important for a variety of emotional and motivational behaviors. For example, this region participates in behaviors that include elements of obsessiveness, compulsiveness, anxiety, and introversion or extroversion. The maintenance of an adaptive and optimal state of arousal and alertness is linked to this region. Having one's surveillance systems "set" in a way that maximizes the relation between energy expenditure and the detection of important external and internal events is a function that is linked to the superior mesial prefrontal region. A sense of how long to persevere on a particular line of goal-directed behavior or when to desist and seek an alternate track is another example. The spontaneous, automatic selection and implementation of an appropriate emotional response to a particular stimulus configuration is linked to the superior mesial prefrontal region and anterior cingulate. Examples include having a humorous response to a good joke, having a feeling of sorrow when told of a sad event, or having a response of empathy while watching a child endure a painful social learning experience.

In a related vein, recent studies have linked the anterior cingulate region to a set of functions that have to do with *response selection* and *conflict resolution*. For example, when confronted with situations that call for selecting the best course of action from among several closely matched alternatives, the brain shows increased activity in the anterior cingulate region. Similarly, when trying to decide between two conflicting response options, each of which carries with it certain rewards and punishments, the anterior cingulate comes into play in a critical fashion.

6.4. Ventromedial Prefrontal Region

The ventromedial prefrontal region includes the orbital frontal cortex, formed by areas 11 and 12, and nearby regions in the ventral and lower mesial aspects of the frontal lobes, including parts of areas 25, 32, and the mesial aspect of areas 10 and 9 (Fig. 5). The ventromedial prefrontal region comprises a functional unit that plays a key role in judgment, planning, and decision-making, and in a wide range of behaviors that can be grouped under the heading of social conduct. The mediation of these functions is conducted partly through the use of emotional states as guideposts for behavior, so that we use our emotions and feelings, both consciously and unnconsciously, to help make complex decisions in a way that is in our best long-term interests. These emotional guideposts have been termed "somatic markers."

Social conduct, when executed in such a way as to maximize one's personal gain in the short and long term, and in the overall best interests of society in general, depends on the rapid selection of appropriate courses of action, often in highly ambiguous situations. Such selection requires several component processes, including bringing on-line a range of viable potential courses of action, the assignment to each of these a degree of likelihood in terms of its short-term and long-term consequences for reward or punishment, and consideration of the implications of such courses of action in the context of the person's current position in the world. This type of decision-making process is intimately linked to the ventromedial prefrontal region. Damage to the ventromedial prefrontal region produces severe disturbances in social contact, yet spared most basic components of cognition.

Anatomically, the ventromedial prefrontal cortices are well-situated for these functions. They receive signals from a large range of neural structures engaged by perception, including external information from vision, audition, and olfaction, and internal somatic information from skeletal and visceral states. In turn, the ventromedial prefrontal cortices are a source of projections from frontal regions toward central autonomic control structure. Also, the ventromedial cortices receive and reciprocate projections from hip-

pocampus and amygdala. Thus, the ventromedial cortices are in a position to form conjunctive records of concurrent signals hailing from external and internal stimuli, and they can also activate somatic effectors.

The ventromedial prefrontal region also appears to play a role in *prospective memory*, which refers to the capacity of "remembering in the future." There are numerous everyday situations that require this capacity—e.g., when we must remember to place a phone call at a certain time of day, or remember to keep a preset appointment. The manner in which the brain actually mediates this function remains largely unknown, but it may utilize a mechanism whereby a "somatic marker" can be affixed to a particular stimulus array in such a way that when that array (or parts thereof) becomes extant in perceptual space, the marker is triggered, which in turn triggers a "feeling to act,"—e.g., a reminder that we are supposed to execute a particular task.

7. SUBCORTICAL STRUCTURES

Many subcortical structures participate in various aspects of higher-order cognition and behavior, although subcortical structures are not, usually, as directly linked to such functions as the cerebral cortex. Such structures include the basal ganglia, thalamus, cerebellum, and brainstem nuclei. Two of these—the basal ganglia and thalamus—are reviewed here.

7.1. Basal Ganglia

The basal ganglia are a collection of gray matter nuclei deep in the brain, comprised mostly by the *striatum*, which includes the caudate nucleus and the putamen, and the *pallidum*, which includes the globus pallidus. The striatum and pallidum play basic roles in motor behavior, particularly in the automatic execution of highly learned motor patterns. For example, the kinds of motor behaviors that are called into play when a person rides a bicycle, skates, or skis, depend on the basal ganglia.

In addition to their role in automatic motor behaviors, the striatum and pallidum also make important contributions to some aspects of higher-order cognition and behavior. The left caudate nucleus, especially the region known as the "head" of the caudate, plays an important role in language function, paralleling to some extent the roles played by interconnected cortical regions in the perisylvian region of the left hemisphere. The left putamen has a role in speech articulation—specifically, in the implementation of strings of phonemes in the motor system in a smooth, seamless manner that allows fluent, canonical articulation. On the right side, the striatum plays an important role in prosody. It is also involved in various visuospatial functions, including visual perception and visual construction, in a manner generally analogous to the cortical regions of the right hemisphere.

The striatum and pallidum are important for the acquisition of information that falls under the designation of nondeclarative knowledge. In contrast to declarative knowledge (the learning of which is mediated by mesial temporal structures, as discussed earlier), nondeclarative knowledge cannot be brought to mind for conscious inspection, and instead, typically depends on a motor output in order to be instantiated. For example, the learning of perceptuomotor skills such as typing, playing the guitar, hitting a golf ball, or ice skating, depends on the basal ganglia. The learning of "habits" (e.g., a tendency to respond automatically and consistently to a particular stimulus configuration) is also probably linked to the basal ganglia. In addition, there is evidence that the learning of "gut-level" likes or dislikes for certain stimuli may depend on the striatum.

7.2. Thalamus

The thalamus plays a critical role in the transmission of motor and sensory information from lower subcortical systems to various regions of the cortex. Evidence also supports a role for the thalamus in higher-order cognition and behavior, especially in attention, memory, and language. The thalamus contains the reticular nuclei, which have an important role in the network of neural structures responsible for arousal and attention. The capacity to direct attention to a particular stimulus and to attend to it sufficiently to allow the selection of an appropriate response are linked to basic arousal and attentional mechanisms mediated in part by the reticular nuclei.

The thalamus has a left-right specialization that mirrors that of the cortex. Structures in the left thalamus are geared more for verbal material, and structures in the right thalamus are geared more for nonverbal, spatial material. The left anterior thalamus plays a role in language that is related to comprehension and production aspects of linguistic function. The anterior part of the thalamus, which contains important pathways that link the thalamus to the hippocampus and amygdala (especially the mammillothalamic tract and the ventroamygdalofugal pathway), has been

linked to material-specific learning capacities; the left is important for verbal information, and the right is important for nonverbal information. There are midline thalamic nuclei, including the medial dorsal nucleus, which have an important role in memory. In general, the thalamus is more important for anterograde memory than for retrograde memory, and for learning declarative types of knowledge as opposed to nondeclarative types of knowledge.

8. CONCLUDING REMARKS

The past two decades have witnessed an unparalleled growth in our understanding of how higher cognitive and behavioral functions are subserved by different brain structures. This expansion owes much to the power of new imaging techniques, beginning with the structural methods that arrived in the 1970s (CT) and 1980s (MRI), and continuing with the functional methods that have begun to dominate the recent literature (PET, fMRI). These tools have provided powerful windows into the operation of the human brain and mind, and have led to many new discoveries regarding brain-behavior relationships. At the same time, the development of sophisticated neuropsychological experimentation has allowed the design of elegant experiments that can isolate the basic constituents of various mental processes. And no less important are concurrent advances on the theoretical front, which have provided explanatory and predictive frameworks that have helped shape some of the most interesting questions in cognitive neuroscience, and have helped fuel the rapid explosion of new studies in this area.

One would be remiss not to sound a cautionary note here: the exciting new advances in cognitive neuroscience and in the understanding of brain-behavior relationships can lure the naïve student down a path of "neophrenology." Here, the notion that most or even all mental functions can be assigned to discrete brain regions is not only acceptable, but is seen as the main objective of modern cognitive neuroscience. The fact is that for virtually any cognitive or behavioral function that one can imagine, the degree of variance accounted for by neuroanatomy is still far short of 100%; in most cases, in fact, it is more on the order of 10–30%, at best. This leaves a huge amount of room for many other factors, including those that have to do with individual differences, learning history, and the interaction of cognition and personality. This is not to say that science will never be able to account for more than it does now, insofar as brain-behavior relationships are concerned, but it is to say that we must remain cautious and critical in our evaluation of the new explosion of studies that claim to have localized various functions to a particular brain region.

SELECTED READINGS

Adolphs R, Tranel D, Damasio AR. The human amygdala in social judgment. Nature 1998; 393:470–474.

Adolphs R, Tranel D, Damasio H, Damasio AR. Impaired recognition of emotion in facial expressions following bilateral damage to the human amygdala. Nature 1994; 372:669–672.

Anderson SW, Bechara A, Damasio H, Tranel D, Damasio AR. Impairment of social and moral behavior related to early damage in the human prefrontal cortex. Nat Neurosci 1999; 2: 1032–1037.

Baddeley AD. Working memory. Science 1992; 255:566–569.

Bauer RM. Agnosia. In Heilman, KM, Valenstein E. (eds). Clinl Neuropsychol, 3rd ed. New York:Oxford University Press, 1993; 215–278.

Bechara A, Damasio H, Tranel D, Damasio AR. Deciding advantageously before knowing the advantageous strategy. Science 1997; 275:1293–1295.

Bechara A, Tranel D, Damasio H. Characterization of the decision-making deficit of patients with ventromedial prefrontal cortex lesions. Brain 2000; 123:2189–2202.

Benton AL. Neuropsychology: Past, present, and future. In Boller F, Grafman J. (eds). Handbook of Neuropsychology, Vol. 1. Amsterdam:Elsevier, 1988; 1–27.

Benton AL. The Hecaen-Zangwill legacy: Hemispheric dominance examined. Neuropsychol Rev 1991; 2:267–280.

Benton A, Tranel D. Historical notes on reorganization of function and neuroplasticity. In H.S. Levin & J. Grafman (eds). Cerebral Reorganization of Function After Brain Damage. New York: Oxford University Press, 2000; 3–23.

Cabeza R, Nyberg L. Imaging cognition II: an empirical review of 275 PET and fMRI studies. J Cogn Neurosci 2000; 12:1–47.

Damasio AR. Time-locked multiregional retroactivation: a systems-level proposal for the neural substrates of recall and recognition. Cognition 1989; 33:25–62.

Damasio AR. Descartes' Error: Emotion, Reason, and the Human Brain. New York:Grossett/Putnam, 1994.

Damasio AR. The Feeling of What Happens. New York:Harcourt Brace, 1999.

Damasio AR, Tranel D. Nouns and verbs are retrieved with differently distributed neural systems. Oric Natl Acad Sci 1993; 90:4957–4960.

Damasio AR, Tranel D, Rizzo M. Disorders of complex visual processing. In Mesulam MM (ed). Principles of Behavioral and Cognitive Neurology, 2nd ed. New York:Oxford University Press, 2000; 332–372.

Damasio H, Damasio AR. The lesion method in behavioral neurology and neuropsychology. In Feinberg TE, Farah MJ (eds). Behavioral Neurology and Neuropsychology. New York: McGraw-Hill, 1997; 69-82.

Damasio H, Grabowski TJ, Tranel D, Hichwa RD, Damasio AR. A neural basis for lexical retrieval. Nature 1996; 380:499–505.

Denburg NL,Tranel D. Accallculia and disturbances of the body schema. In Heilman KM, Valenstein E. (eds). Clinical Neurop-

sychology, Fourth Edition. New York:Oxford University Press, 2003; 161–184.

Geschwind N. Disconnexion syndromes in animals and man. Brain 1965; 88:237–294,585–644.

Harlow JM. Recovery from the passage of an iron bar through the head. Publications of the Massachusetts Medical Society 1868; 2:327–347.

Heilman KM, Watson RT, Valenstein E. Neglect and related disorders. In Heilman KM, Valenstein E (eds). Clinical Neuropsychology, 3rd ed. New York:Oxford University Press, 1993; 279–336.

Kopelman MD. The neuropsychology of remote memory. In Boller F, Grafman J. (eds). Handbook of Neuropsychology, Vol. 8. Amsterdam:Elsevier, 1992; 215–238.

Levin HS, Eisenberg HM, Benton AL. (eds). Frontal Lobe Function and Dysfunction. New York:Oxford University Press, 1991.

Lezak MD. Neuropsychological Assessment, 3rd ed. New York: Oxford University Press, 1995.

Martin A, Haxby JV, Lalonde FM, Wiggs CL, Ungerleider LG. Discrete cortical regions associated with knowledge of color and knowledge of action. Science 1995; 270,102–105.

Milner B. Disorders of learning and memory after temporal lobe lesions in man. Clinical Neurosurgery 1972; 19,421–446.

Newcombe F, Ratcliff G. Disorders of visuospatial analysis. In Boller F, Grafman J. (eds). Handbook of Neuropsychology, Vol. 2. Amsterdam:Elsevier, 1989; 333–356.

Scoville WB, Milner B. Loss of recent memory after bilateral hippocampal lesions. J Neurol Neurosurg Psychiatry 1957; 20:11–21.

Smith EE, Jonides J, Koeppe RA. Dissociating verbal and spatial working memory using PET. Cerebral Cortex 1996; 6:11–20.

Sperry RW. The great cerebral commissure. Sci Am 1968; 210: 42–52.

Squire LR. Memory and hippocampus: A synthesis from findings with rats, monkeys, and humans. Psychol Rev 1992; 99:195–231.

Stuss DT, Benson DF. The Frontal Lobes. New York:Raven Press, 1986.

Teuber H-L. Alteration of perception and memory in man: reflections on methods. In Weiskrantz L. (ed). Analysis of Behavioral Change. New York:Harper & Row, 1968; 274–328.

Thompson RFL. The neurobiology of learning and memory. Science 1986; 233:941–947.

Tranel D, Anderson S. Syndromes of aphasia. In Fabbro, F. (ed). Concise Encyclopedia of Language Pathology. Oxford, England:Elsevier Science Limited, 1999; 305–319.

Tranel D, Bechara A, Damasio AR. Decision making and the somatic marker hypothesis. In Gazzaniga MS (ed). The New Cognitive Neurosciences. Cambridge,MA:The MIT Press, 2000; 1047–1061.

Tranel D, Damasio AR. The covert learning of affective valence does not require structures in hippocampal system or amygdala. J Cog Neurosci 1993; 5:79–88.

Tranel D, Damasio AR. Neuropsychology and behavioral neurology. In Cacioppo JT, Tassinary LG, Berntson GG (eds). Handbook of Psychophysiology. Cambridge, MA:Cambridge University Press, 2000; 119–141.

Tranel D, Damasio AR, Damasio H, Brandt JP. Sensorimotor skill learning in amnesia: additional evidence for the neural basis of nondeclarative memory. Learning and Memory, 1994; 1: 165–179.

Tranel D, Damasio H, Damasio AR. Double dissociation between overt and covert face recognition. J Cogn Neurosci 1995; 7:425–432.

Tranel D, Damasio H, Damasio AR. A neural basis for the retrieval of conceptual knowledge. Neuropsychologia 1997; 35: 1319–1327.

Tranel D, Damasio H, Damasio AR. Amnesia caused by herpes simplex encephalitis, infarctions in basal forebrain, and anoxia/ischemia. In Boller F, Grafman J (eds). Handbook of Neuropsychology, 2nd ed, Volume 2 (Cermak l, Section Editor). Amsterdam: Elsevier Science, 2000; 85–110.

Van Hoesen GW. The parahippocampal gyrus. Trend Neurosci 1982; 5:345–350.

The Aphasias and Other Disorders of Language

Gregory Cooper and Robert L. Rodnitzky

Language is the mechanism by which communication is achieved through the use of specific sounds or symbols. In the clinical realm, it is extremely important to differentiate this process from that of *speech*, the coordinated motor mechanism which allows the utterance of sound. Either language or speech can be abnormal with total preservation of the other, although in some clinical circumstances, both are involved simultaneously. Conceptual abnormalities of production or understanding of spoken language are referred to as *aphasia*, and mechanical abnormalities in the motor production of speech are known as *dysarthria* or *anarthria*.

APHASIA

Aphasic Disorders Are Usually Caused by Lesions of the Left Hemisphere

Language dominance is located in the left hemisphere in approx 95% of right-handed persons and in approx 66% of those people who are left-handed. Because most of the population is right-handed, a useful clinical principle is that the left hemisphere must be considered dominant in all persons until proven otherwise. In some circumstances, it is critical to determine the hemisphere in which language dominance resides with absolute certainty. For example, in patients undergoing surgical removal of a brain tumor or surgical excision of a portion of the temporal lobe as a treatment for epilepsy, the surgeon must know whether cortical structures in the hemisphere being operated on can be ablated without fear of inducing aphasia. Several techniques can be used to determine hemisphere dominance for language. Positron emission tomography (PET) can be used to identify the cortical areas activated during speech, although its accuracy is still questioned. The most widely used and time-honored technique involves the injection of an anesthetizing drug, first into the carotid artery that perfuses the right hemisphere and then into the carotid-artey system that perfuses the left hemisphere of the brain. The drug produces transient aphasia when injected into the artery perfusing the dominant hemisphere, but it has no effect when injected into the nondominant side.

Several Forms of Brain Pathology Can Cause Aphasia

Damage to the speech area of the dominant hemisphere may be caused by stroke, tumor, infection, trauma, or neurodegenerative conditions. Generally, the more rapid the development of the damage (e.g., sudden stroke), the more sever the aphasia. The extent of the damage is also related the severity of language dysfunction. Regardless of the form of brain pathology, the age of the affected person may be a modifying factor. Dominant hemisphere pathology acquired in infancy or childhood does not usually cause aphasia, reflecting the plasticity of the brain at that age.

Several Facets of Language Must Be Assessed in Evaluating an Aphasic Disorder

Suspicion of an aphasic disorder usually develops as the examiner is listening to a patient's ordinary conversational or *propositional speech*. There may be abnormalities in the rhythm and inflection of speech (e.g. *dysprosody*), in the use of proper word sequence or connecting words (e.g., *agrammatism*), in naming objects (e.g., *anomia*), or in repetition. In addition, words or sounds may be incorrectly substituted (e.g., *paraphasias*). The substitution of an incorrect sound (e.g., "spoot" for spoon) is known as a *phonemic paraphasia*. The substitution of a work related in meaning (e.g., fork for spoon) is known as a verbal paraphasia. When the substitution in a word is so severs as to render it unrecognizable (e.g., "sporaker" for spoon) it is referred to as a neologism. A person whose language is characterized by agrammatic speech, containing many neologisms and rendering it virtually incomprehensible, is said to have *jargon aphasia.*

Aphasia Can Be Divided into Fluent and Nonfluent Types

Nonfluent aphasia typically results from dysfunction of the anterior portion of the speech area. Broca's aphasia, resulting from a lesion of the posterior portion of the inferior frontal gyrus, is the classic example of a nonfluent aphasia. In this condition, speech is hesitant and effortful, and the affected person appears frustrated. Connecting words such as articles and conjunctions are omitted, resulting in agrammatic and telegraphic speech, but the retention of appropriate nouns and verbs preserves meaning. Instead of "I want to see the doctor, " the nonfluent, Broca aphasic may utter "want, see, doctor." In this form of aphasia, comprehension of language is largely intact. Because of the proximity of Broca's area to the motor cortex, most Broca aphasics also suffer from significant weakness on the right side of the body.

Fluent aphasia is characterized by a normal or increased output of words. Prosody and construction are often normal, but speech contains many paraphasic errors. This form of aphasia is typically caused by a lesion in the posterior speech area. A lesion of the posterior third of the superior temporal gyrus gives rise to Wernicke's aphasia, the classic aphasia of the nonfluent type. In this aphasia, comprehension of language is distinctly impaired. Unlike Broca aphasics, who are frustrated by their language impairment, Wernicke aphasics show little awareness of their deficit, but after a time can become paranoid an agitated, perhaps related in part to an inability to communicate their needs and to a verbal isolation caused by impaired comprehension. Unlike Broca's aphasia, there is typically no weakness associated with Wernicke's aphasia, because the causative lesion is usually far removed from the motor cortex. In fact, these patients may have an isolated aphasia without other associated neurologic signs or symptoms. For these reasons, patients with a Wernicke's aphasia have occasionally been misdiagnosed as having a psychiatric illness.

Repetition Is Usually Abnormal in Aphasia Caused by Lesions in the Perisylvian Region

Broca and Wernicke aphasics manifest abnormalities of repetition. This tends to be true of any aphasia resulting from a lesion involving perisylvian structures. Aphasias resulting from lesion distant from this region are characterized by intact repetition and are known as the transcortical aphasias. A lesion just anterior or superior to Broca's area results in language dysfunction similar to Broca aphasia with the exception that repetition is intact. This is known as a *motor transcortical aphasia*. Similarly, a lesion just posterior to Wernicke's area results in a fluent aphasia with intact repetition known as a *sensory transcortical aphasia*. Persons for whom impaired repetition is the predominant abnormality are said to have *conduction aphasia*. The lesion is considered to be in one of the two loci, the supra marginal gyrus or the area encompassing the primary auditory cortices, insula, and underlying white matter, especially the arcuate fasciculus.

DISORDERS OF WRITTEN LANGUAGE

Impaired production and comprehension of written words is another common form of language disturbance. Impairment in production of written language is called *agraphia*. Agraphia almost always accompanies aphasia of spoken language. The writing abnormality may take the form of misspelling, agrammatism, or imperfectly constituted letters and words. Agraphia is such a common accompaniment of aphasia that its absence in a patient apparently afflicted with aphasia raises serious doubt about the diagnosis. Isolated agraphia without other disorders of language sometimes occurs when the dominant angular gyrus is damaged.

Abnormal comprehension of written words is called *alexia*. Acquired alexia, typically associated with agraphia, may result from lesions in a variety of locations, but damage to the dominant parietal lobe has traditionally been believed to be the most common cause of this combination of deficits. *Alexia without agraphia* is a distinct and relatively common syndrome. It results from infarction of the dominant (typically left) occipital lobe and the splenium of the corpus callosum. In this circumstance, visual-language information is prevented from gaining access to the language areas of the left hemisphere from the left occipital lobe, which is infarcted, and from the intact right occipital lobe, which has been disconnected from the dominant hemisphere by destruction of the splenium of the corpus callosum. Because the language areas are spared, agraphia is conspicuously absent in this syndrome. Prominent loss of vision in the right half of the visual field is a usual accompaniment of this syndrome because of the involvement of the primary visual cortex on the left.

Developmental dyslexia refers to impaired development of reading and writing skills relative to that expected, based on overall intelligence. Typically, it becomes apparent in the school-age child. Intellectual functions often are not impaired, but affected children are sometimes mistakenly believed to be mentally dull until the specific isolated language dysfunction is discovered. Although there are no gross abnormalities

of the brain in these persons, postmortem and MRI studies have shown that developmental dyslexics often exhibit subtle structural abnormalities. For example, they may lack the expected interhemispheric asymmetry in a portion of the temporal lobe known as the planum temporale. In normal persons, this structure is usually larger in the dominant hemisphere. Abnormal architecture and cell clusters of the cerebral cortex (e.g., cortical dysplasia and ectopias) have been identified in these persons, suggesting that there may have been failure of normal neuronal migration or excessive neuronal death during fetal development.

SELECTED READINGS

Damasio AR. Aphasia. N Engl J Med 1992; 326:531.
Ramsey JM. The biology of developmental dyslexia. JAMA 1992; 268:912.

30 Neuroimmunology

An Overview

Michael D. Lumpkin

CONTENTS

1. INTRODUCTION

The term neuroimmunology means different things to different biomedical scientists and clinicians. This newly evolving and broad discipline includes the study of secreted immune-cell products known as *cytokines*, *lymphokines*, *monokines*, and *chemokines* and their presence and actions in the central and peripheral nervous systems. Another area of study is that in which the *nerve supply and nervous system regulation of lymphoid organs* such as the spleen and thymus gland are considered. A third connotation of this word involves the investigation of how *neuroendocrine* substances of the hypothalamic-pituitary unit regulate the proliferation and activities of *monocytes, macrophages, lymphocytes,* and *glial cells* (considered to be the "macrophages of the brain"). A fourth implication of neuroimmunology is recognition of the fact that immune cells can produce neuroendocrine peptides such adrenocorticotropic hormone (ACTH) and luteinizing hormone-releasing hormone (LHRH). A fifth important aspect of neuroimmunology involves the ability of the body to produce *antibodies* that can attack *cholinergic receptors* at the neuromuscular junction, and

From: *Neuroscience in Medicine, 2nd ed.* (P. Michael Conn, ed.),
© 2003 Humana Press Inc., Totowa, NJ.

the *myelin* components of the white matter of nervous tissue. A common theme throughout all of these approaches to the understanding of neuroimmunology is that there is *bidirectional* communication between the cells of the nervous system and the immune system. In some instances, neurons communicate with the immune cells (and vice versa) by way of endocrine messengers interposed between these other two systems. An example of this is when a stressful event causes the cytokine interleukin-1 (IL-1) to be produced by either activated monocytes, glial cells, or neurons residing in or traveling through the *hypothalamus* of the brain. The IL-1, in turn, causes certain hypothalamic neurons to release *corticotropin-releasing factor (CRF)*, which then stimulates adrenocorticotropic hormone (ACTH) secretion from the anterior pituitary gland. The ACTH next stimulates the production of cortisol by the adrenal gland, and this glucocorticoid then suppresses further proliferation and cytokine secretion by monocytes, lymphocytes, and glial cells. The cortisol also exerts a classical *negative-feedback* action on both the CRF neurons and the pituitary corticotrope that manufactures ACTH in order to reduce their increased levels of secretion. Thus, the "bidirectional communication" occurs between these three great systems of the body (Fig. 1).

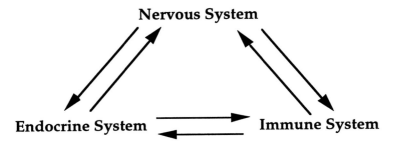

Fig. 1. Bidirectional communication occurs among components of the nervous, endocrine, and immune systems. Neuroimmunomodulation occurs throughout the organism by means of these interactions and feedback loops, and a stimulus to any one of these systems inevitably involves the others in the resultant reactions.

2. INNERVATION OF LYMPHOID ORGANS

Some of the original concepts about neuroimmunology have come from the work of Dr. David Felten. He and others have shown that *noradrenergic* nerve fibers originating from the postganglionic sympathetic nervous system innervate the thymus gland, spleen, lymph nodes, and intestinal Peyer's patches. These norepinephrine-containing nerve fibers have been seen in contact with thymocytes, B lymphocytes, and macrophages. Further, both alpha and beta adrenergic receptors have been found on the surfaces of these immune cells. In general, activation of the sympathetic nervous system or administration of epinephrine produces leukocytosis, lymphopenia, and suppression of natural-killer (NK)-cell activity. In other words, activation of catecholaminergic beta receptors on lymphocytes inhibits their proliferation and results in a suppressed immune response. The role of catecholamines in suppressing lymphocyte activity has led some to believe that this is one explanation for why prolonged stress, which activates the sympathetic nervous system, leads to greater susceptibility to disease, infections, and cancer in human patients. For instance, it has been shown that the stress of foot shock, cold-exposure, maternal deprivation, or fear may cause thymus-gland involution, decreased lymphocyte proliferation and cytotoxicity, and diminished antibody production. Conversely, it was found that sympathetic denervation of immune organs causes proliferation of lymph node, spleen, and bone-marrow cells, as well as antigen-stimulated immunoglobulin production. Interestingly, the use of mind-body medicine stress-reduction techniques such as meditation, imagery, biofeedback, and breath control can also reduce sympathetic outflow from the central nervous system (CNS) to the immune organs. These relaxation methods, when employed by stressed individuals such as medical students, *have* been shown to increase the number of CD4 T-lymphocytes and NK-cell activity, thus improving the students' immune status.

Dr. Felten's laboratory has also been instrumental in showing that a number of peptides found in autonomic nerves that innervate the thymus, spleen, and lymph nodes, are also regulators of cells of the immune system. In particular, *vasoactive intestinal peptide (VIP), neuropeptide Y (NPY), and substance P (SP)* have been observed in nerve fibers that make contact with thymocytes, lymphocytes, and macrophages found in the thymus gland and spleen.

Not unexpectedly, the receptors for these peptides have been observed on lymphoid cells. The most studied of these nerve-ending peptides is VIP and its lymphoid receptor. When VIP is released from these nerve endings, it may act to inhibit the proliferation of lymphocytes, inhibit NK-cell activity, and alter antibody production.

Some peptidergic nerve fibers that innervate lymphoid organs will produce the peptide *substance P*. In keeping with its known pro-inflammatory action and its role in mediating pain responses via peripheral nerves, activation of receptors by substance P stimulates lymphocyte proliferation and the release of pain mediators such as histamine and leukotrienes from mast cells. The peptide *somatostatin* (SS), which is found both in the brain and peripheral nerves and is mostly inhibitory to all types of cellular activity, can block the release of substance P from peripheral-nerve endings.

The peptide NPY has been found in the same nerve fibers and terminals that contain norepinephrine and that innervate the thymus, spleen, and lymph nodes. It is likely that NPY and norepinephrine are cosecreted and act in a synergistic fashion to suppress lymphocyte proliferation and cytokine release, in keeping with the general idea of sympathetic-nervous-system inhibition of immune function.

Another example of the commonality between the brain and the immune system is the fact that other neuropeptides and their receptors are found in both locations. This would include CRF, ACTH, enkephalins, beta-endorphin, vasopressin, oxytocin (OT), and neurotensin. It is useful to note that most of these neuropeptides are also released during episodes of physical or psychological stress. Further, these peptides are mostly inhibitory to immune-cell proliferation and function. Thus, the suggestion has been made that these peptides may mediate the suppression of the immune system, and the subsequent susceptibility to disease and infection that often follows periods of prolonged stress in an individual.

3. CYTOKINES IN THE NERVOUS SYSTEM

It is well-known that immune-system cells produce and secrete soluble mediators known as cytokines whose original defined role was to modify the proliferation and activity of other cells of the immune system. However, it is now appreciated that activated immune cells, including monocytes, lymphocytes, and macrophages, can breach the blood–brain barrier and establish themselves as a presence in the brain, where they may release their specific cytokines into the cerebrovasculature, the cerebrospinal fluid (CSF) and the parenchyma of the CNS. In addition, microglial cells, and to a lesser extent, astroglial cells of the brain secrete the cytokines interleukin-1, 2, 4, and 6 and tumor necrosis factor α (TNF-α). Accordingly, the receptors for IL-1, 2, and 6 have also been identified in the brain. Most provocative is the recent finding that IL-1 is also produced by neurons, particularly in the hypothalamic and hippocampal neuronal populations that are involved in stress and homeostatic responses. Likewise, IL-1 receptors have also been identified in the hypothalamus and hippocampus.

Physical stressors such as trauma, infection, and inflammation of brain tissue, as well as psychological stressors, stimulate the production of cytokines such as IL-1 by glial cells and neurons. IL-1, IL-6, and TNF, when so manufactured by brain cells for prolonged periods in pathological states, can produce anorexia, fever, sleep induction, dementia, and even neuronal death. During invasion of the brain by the human immunodeficiency virus (HIV) and in patients with Alzheimer's disease, the levels of IL-1 are increased, and contribute to the behavioral disturbances observed in these patients. However, the brain has apparently developed a protective mechanism against the persistent presence of pathologically elevated IL-1 levels,

since such situations also lead to the subsequent production of an *endogenous IL-1 receptor antagonist* that is homologous to the structure of IL-1 and competes for the same receptor in order to dampen further IL-1 activity. The IL-1-receptor-antagonist has no known inherent activity of its own except to occupy the IL-1 receptor and block its activation by IL-1.

Although sustained high levels of cytokines in the brain produce deleterious effects on neuronal function, normal physiological oscillations in brain cytokines in response to acute changes in homeostatic activity or intermittent stressors are beneficial to the organism. The presence of physiological concentrations of IL-1, IL-2, and IL-6 in the hypothalamus appears to regulate certain neuroendocrine axes. For instance, IL-1 produced in or injected into the brains of experimental animals increases the expression of CRF mRNA and synthesis and release of its neuropeptide product. This in turn causes the secretion of ACTH from the anterior pituitary gland. The ACTH then binds to its receptors on the cortex of the adrenal gland, leading to the increased secretion of glucocorticoids such as cortisol. This corticosteroid provides a classical negative-feedback signal back to the neurons, glia, and monocytes/macrophages that provided the elevated levels of CRF-stimulating cytokines. Elevated cortisol levels then decrease the secretion of cytokines from glial cells and neurons and reduce the proliferation and secretion of cytokines from monocytes and lymphocytes. More specifically, cortisol inhibits the production of IL-1, IL-2, IL-2 receptors, gamma-interferon, and immunoglobulin production. In this fashion, the increased activities of immune cells and neuroendocrine cells in response to physical or emotional stressors are prevented from running amok. This is important during a stress-induced cortisol-release period, when it may be necessary to suppress inflammatory responses during a "fight or flight" situation. Stated differently, cortisol downregulates IL-1, IL-2, IL-6, and CRF secretion, thereby maintaining homeostatic concentrations of cytokines and hormones in the body, specifically in response to acute stress.

Another beneficial effect of IL-1 may occur after nervous-tissue injury. This positive influence derives from IL-1's ability to stimulate the synthesis and secretion of nerve-growth factor (NGF). NGF acts as a neutrophic growth factor that promotes both the healing and the regeneration of certain types of nerve cells.

IL-1 and its related cytokines also exert effects on other neuropeptides of the brain. IL-1 can act both directly on other releasing factor systems and through the stimulation of CRF, the neurons of which make synaptic contact with growth hormone-releasing hormone (GHRH), luteinizing hormone-releasing hormone (LHRH), and thyrotropin-releasing hormone (TRH) nerve cells. In each case, the master stress hormone CRF, when activated, will inhibit these other neuroendocrine axes and stimulate adrenal cortical production of glucocorticoids. In the short term, the organism benefits from increasing cortisol levels. The cortisol will ensure that blood glucose concentrations are maintained for the increased stress-induced demands on the brain, heart, and skeletal muscle. The cortisol will also enhance catecholamine production by the adrenal medulla, thereby sustaining the blood pressure and blood flow to critical tissues. Thus, the stress hormone system is turned on and other hormonal systems for growth, reproduction, and metabolism are turned off to spare resources for the stress response. Further indicative of the integrated nature of the stress response, the stimulation of CRF elements in the hypothalamus also stimulate sympathetic outflow from the brain to visceral and immune organs. This further suppresses immune-system activity. IL-1 alone and/or through CRF neuronal mediation acts in the hypothalamus to increase somatostatin (SS) synthesis and secretion, and in a coordinated fashion it also inhibits the release of GHRH. The overall result of this action is to reduce growth-hormone (GH) secretion from the anterior pituitary. This mechanism may contribute to the protein wasting syndrome in adult patients with HIV infection of the brain, and to the failure of somatic growth in children suffering from acquired immunodeficiency syndrome (AIDS). The reason for this, of course, is that GH is anabolic for protein synthesis in muscle and connective tissue and stimulates the growth of both long bones and soft tissues in children. Thus, an IL-1-induced GH deficiency could explain the failure to thrive and the negative nitrogen-balance that are characteristic of AIDS patients.

IL-1 in the hypothalamus also inhibits the secretion of LHRH and TRH. Sustained increases in IL-1 that may be encountered during prolonged stressful situations can lead to amenorrhea in women and decreased spermatogenesis accompanied by lowered testosterone levels in men, the outcomes being decreased libido and reproductive failure. Hormonally, this deficit is considered to be the cessation of the normal pulsatile secretion of luteinizing hormone (LH) and follicle-stimulating hormone (FSH) from the pituitary gland. Without sufficient stimulation of the gonads by LH and FSH, both sex-steroid synthesis and germ-cell production will fail.

Both IL-1 and TNF-alpha suppress thyroid function directly at the level of the thyroid gland and through the inhibition of TRH production by the hypothalamus. Inflammation and sepsis decrease thyroid-stimulating hormone (TSH) secretion from the pituitary because IL-1 from both peripheral and central sources inhibits TRH secretion, and TNF alpha lowers the hypothalamic mRNA content of TRH. These actions result in lowered plasma-thyroid-hormone levels, leading to a reduced metabolic rate and perhaps aggravating the fatigue and lethargy caused by the action of IL-1 and TNF directly on the brain, particularly in AIDS patients.

Specific CRF-receptor antagonists that could be administered to patients with disorders related to chronic stress are currently in therapeutic development. Such therapeutic agents would have the potential to enhance immune function in chronically ill patients by relieving CRF- and cortisol-induced suppression of immune cell activity.

4. THE PRESENCE OF NEUROENDOCRINE PEPTIDES IN IMMUNE CELLS

Another recent development in the field of neuroimmunology is the discovery by Dr. Edwin Blalock and colleagues that neuroendocrine peptides are produced by immunocompetent cells. For instance, B lymphocytes contain ACTH and enkephalins, and their secretion can be stimulated by CRF and inhibited by glucocorticoids. The T cells synthesize growth hormone, TSH, LH, and FSH. Monocytes are a source of prolactin, VIP, and SS. As a general rule, when a "pituitary" hormone is found in a cell of the immune system, the corresponding releasing-factor peptide is also found there, and usually has the ability to stimulate the secretion of its "target" hormone from a particular type of immune cell. An example of this is the presence of GHRH in lymphocytes that may be secreted locally among other lymphocytes and act on GHRH receptors on the lymphocyte-cell membrane, thereby eliciting the *local* secretion of growth hormone by similar cell types. The same is true for TRH/TSH and LHRH/LH, which have been located in immune cells. However, such mechanisms of local control are controversial and are not extensively studied at this time. It is important to note that although the secretion of neuropeptides by monocytes and lymphocytes may provide significant levels of paracrine and autocrine regulation among immune cells, there is little evidence to suggest that lymphocyte-derived releasing-factor peptides or pituitary hormones exert actions on peripheral endocrine glands. The extremely small quantities of neuropeptides that are secreted by lymphocytes essentially preclude them from playing major roles as circulating hormones with peripheral endocrine glands as their targets.

5. NEUROIMMUNOMODULATION BY NEUROENDOCRINE PEPTIDES

Once the presence of various neuroendocrine peptides in and among the immune-cell population has been established, it is useful to understand how they affect the immunoregulatory activities of these cells. In the inhibitory category, ACTH suppresses macrophage activation and the synthesis of antibodies by B cells. Gonadotropins decrease the activity of T cells and NK cells. SS and VIP inhibit T-cell proliferation and the inflammatory cascade. These actions are somewhat opposed by growth hormone and prolactin (which are homologous in their structures) because these peptides can stimulate lymphocyte proliferation and antibody synthesis, and oppose the inhibitory effects of glucocorticoids on lymphocyte proliferation and cytokine production. Furthermore, growth hormone and prolactin stimulate the growth and activity of the thymus gland and lymphoid cells Growth hormone also functions as a macrophage-activating factor, and prolactin enhances the tumoricidal activity of macrophages and the synthesis of interferon-gamma. TSH enhances antibody synthesis, and beta-endorphin stimulates the activity of T, B, and NK cells.

6. AUTOIMMUNITY AND NEUROIMMUNOLOGY

Perhaps the best example of autoimmunity in human neurologic disorders is that of myasthenia gravis, in which autoantibodies attack acetylcholine receptors, rendering them unresponsive to the acetylcholine secreted into the synaptic cleft. Two mechanisms involved in this loss of receptor responsiveness include complement-mediated lysis and downregulation of the acetylcholine receptor secondary to crosslinking of receptors. The precipitating event in the origin of myasthenia gravis is not understood. However, it is possible that T cells of the thymus gland may mediate this type of autoimmune response. (*See*

Chapter 31 for a more detailed review of this autoimmune disorder.)

Another example of derangements in normal neuroimmunological function is that represented by the chronic inflammatory, neural-disease multiple sclerosis (MS). In this disease, there is demyelination of CNS neurons with the subsequent loss of neuronal function. T-cell-mediated immunity is the principal mechanism in which autoimmunization to myelin antigens results from actual immunization with myelin components or infection with crossreactive viruses or viral proteins. Antibodies to myelin basic protein and other myelin breakdown products appear in CSF and plasma. This condition also results in an elevation of other nonantibody products in blood and CSF. The activation of lymphocytes and macrophages in MS increases levels of interferon-gamma and prostaglandin E_2. Interestingly, and consistent with previous information in this chapter, the activated immune cells in MS patients secrete elevated levels of ACTH, prolactin, beta-endorphin, and substance P. However, at this time, the roles of these peptides and hormones on the clinical state of the MS patient are unknown.

SELECTED READINGS

Reichlin S. Mechanisms of disease. Neuroendocrine-immune interaction. N Engl J Med 1993; 329:1246–1253.

Blalock JE. A molecular basis for bidirectional communication between the immune and neuroendocrine systems. Physiol Rev 1989; 69:1–32.

Lumpkin MD. Cytokine regulation of hypothalamic and pituitary hormone secretion. In Foa PP, (ed). Humoral Factors in the Regulation of Tissue Growth: Blood, Blood Vessels, Skeletal System, and Teeth. Endocrinology and Metabolism 5. New York: Springer-Verlag, 1993, 139–159.

Scarborough DE. Cytokine modulation of pituitary hormone secretion. Ann NY Acad Sci 1990; O'Dorisio MS, Panesai A, (eds). Vol. 594, 169–187.

Advances in Neuroimmunology. Ann NY Acad Sci 1988; Raine CS, (ed). Vol. 540.

Hubbard JR, Workman EA, (eds). Handbook of Stress Medicine: An Organ System Approach, Boca Raton, FL: CRC Press, 1998.

Reichlin S. Neuroendocrinology. In Wilson J, Foster D, Knonenberg H, Larsen P, (eds). Williams Textbook of Endocrinology, Philadelphia: WB Saunders Co., 1998, 229–232.

Peisen JN, McDonnell KJ, Mulroney SE, Lumpkin MD. Endotoxin-induced suppression of the somatotropic axis is mediated by interleukin-1 beta and corticotropin releasing factor in the juvenile rat. Endocrinology 1995; 136:3378–3390.

Mulroney SE, McDonnell KJ, Pert CB, Ruff MR, Resch Z, Samson WK, Lumpkin MD. HIV gp 120 inhibits the somatotropic axis: a possible GH-releasing hormone receptor mechanism for the pathogenesis of AIDS wasting. Proc Natl Acad Sci USA 1998; 95:1927–1932.

31 Nervous System
Immune System Interactions

Sonia L. Carlson

Contents

Introduction
Interactions of the Nervous and Immune Systems in the Periphery
Immune Interactions Within the CNS
Inflammatory Responses in the CNS During Trauma or Disease
Conclusion
Selected Readings

Clinical Correlation: **Myasthenia Gravis**
Gregory Cooper and Robert L. Rodnitzky

Acetylcholine Receptors in Myasthenia Gravis
Treatment
Selected Reading

1. INTRODUCTION

It was once believed that the nervous system and immune system were separate and independent systems, each with their own regulatory systems. However, it is now clear, that these systems overlap and communicate extensively on a continuous basis, both as a part of normal function and in disease and trauma. It has been clearly shown that these two systems share common receptors and ligands for hormones, neurotransmitters, and cytokines that form the basis for this communication. In addition, as discussed here, the central nervous system (CNS) is not exclusively "immunoprivileged", although it does have the capacity to limit the activation of an inflammatory response under many circumstances.

2. INTERACTIONS OF THE NERVOUS AND IMMUNE SYSTEMS IN THE PERIPHERY

2.1. Innervation of Lymphoid Tissue

Peripheral lymphoid tissues receive extensive innervation by nerve fibers, particularly from the sympathetic nervous system. Prominent innervation by neuropeptides has also been documented. All lymphoid tissues, including primary (bone marrow, thymus) as well as secondary lymphoid tissues (spleen, lymph nodes, and gut-associated lymphoid tissue) have been found to be innervated by nervous system fibers. Innervation of lymphoid tissues by the sympathetic nervous system has been the most extensively characterized. In tissues such as spleen, this innervation is found as a plexus surrounding the vasculature, entering with the splenic artery and continuing in a subcapsular plexus. Fibers also extend into the trabeculae and enter the white-pulp areas in association with

From: *Neuroscience in Medicine, 2nd ed.* (P. Michael Conn, ed.),
© 2003 Humana Press Inc., Totowa, NJ.

the central arterioles, where branches extend into the parenchyma in close proximity with lymphocytes (Fig. 1). In general, this innervation is most prominent in T-cell zones of the tissues (periarteriolar lymphatic sheath) and in the marginal zone that is heavily populated by macrophages. Much more sparse innervation is found in B-cell zones and follicles. A similar pattern is found in lymph nodes where the subcapsular and medullary regions are innervated, with fibers extending into the T-cell zones of the cortex. Little innervation is found in the B-cell follicles. In the medulla, the nerve fibers are found in association with both vascular and lymphatic channels. Innervation has also been documented in other lymphoid tissues such as the bone marrow, thymus, and gut-associated lymphoid tissues, which is discussed extensively in the suggested readings.

Neuropeptides have also been found to innervate the primary and secondary lymphoid tissues. These include neuropeptide Y (NPY), substance P, calcitonin gene-related peptide (CGRP), vasoactive intestinal peptide (VIP), somatostatin (SS), and opiate peptides. Peptides such as NPY often appear to be co-localized with the noradrenergic sympathetic innervation. VIP is found in similar compartments, but not co-localized with the noradrenergic fibers. The neuropeptides substance P and CGRP are often co-localized; they can be found along the vasculature, but also extend into the parenchyma. Their distribution is somewhat different than the sympathetic innervation. Although substance P and CGRP are generally associated with sensory systems, it is not clear whether they serve a sensory function in the lymphoid tissues. Catecholamines and neuropeptides have been shown to modulate the vasculature of lymphoid tissues by affecting vasodilation and adhesion-molecule expression. This could affect leukocyte trafficking and retention within the lymphoid tissues. They also have clear effects on lymphocyte and macrophage function that are distinct from their effects on blood flow and leukocyte trafficking. Thus, there are numerous actions through which neural innervation can modulate localized inflammatory responses.

Receptors for catecholamines as well as numerous neuropeptides have been proven to be present on the various subsets of leukocytes. Thus, cells of the immune system are capable of responding to stimulation by neurotransmitters released by nerves that innervate lymphoid tissues. Denervation and agonist/antagonist treatment paradigms have shown that modulating the level of catecholamines and neuropep-

tides can significantly alter a variety of responses from the immune system, including cytokine production, lymphocyte proliferation, antibody production, cytotoxic functions, and lymphocyte trafficking to lymphoid tissues and sites of inflammation. Unfortunately, it is difficult to generalize about the role of lymphoid-tissue innervation because interpretation of the literature is complicated by the fact that the response found is affected by the combination of cell types included in the analysis and the time-points examined. However, the interaction should probably be viewed as one in which the neural input modulates the extent of an inflammatory response as opposed to controlling or regulating it. Under normal circumstances, it may provide some of the feedback that prevents overstimulation of the immune response so that the response remains specific and is terminated at the appropriate time. The innervation of lymphoid tissue is also important in mediating the effects of the CNS on peripheral immune function, and is an important factor in the effect of chronic stress on immune function.

2.2. Neuroendocrine Interactions with the Peripheral Immune System

In addition to direct neural input to lymphoid tissues, the CNS can modulate immune function though outflow from the neuroendocrine system. The effect of hypothalamo-pituitary-adrenal axis—where physiologic stimuli such as stress can rapidly signal an increase in ACTH and glucocorticoid production, which in turn can stimulate cells of the immune system that possess glucocorticoid receptors—is especially well-documented. It was originally believed that stress was inhibitory to immune function because glucocorticoids can be immunosuppressive. Several studies have shown that stress is not universally inhibitory, as some levels of stress have been found to positively affect certain measures of immune function. Prolonged or repeated extreme or inescapable stress, however, has been shown to be associated with reduced immune responses. The effect of stress is not mediated entirely through effects on glucocorticoids, but also through the outflow from the sympathetic nervous system, which modulates activity of the sympathetic innervation of lymphoid tissues and the release of epinephrine from the adrenals. A review of the literature may allow a few generalizations to be made concerning the effects of stress on lymphocyte distribution and function: acute stress, which is par-

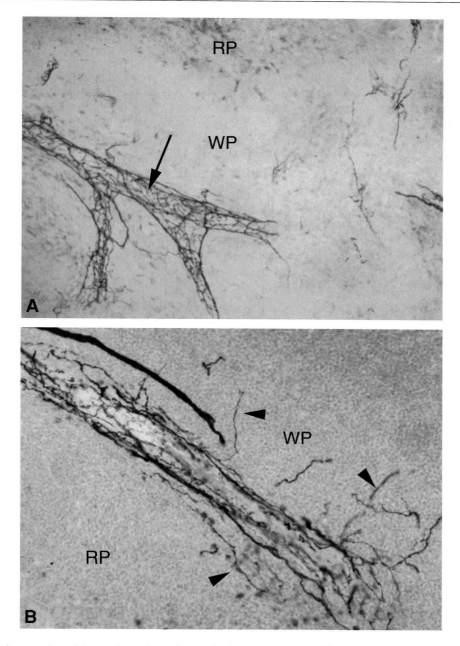

Fig. 1. Sympathetic innervation of the murine spleen. Sympathetic nervous system fibers were revealed using an antibody against tyrosine hydroxylase, the rate-limiting enzyme in the synthesis of catecholamines. (**A**) Robust innervation is found surrounding the central artery (*arrow*) of the white pulp (WP), an area heavily populated with T-cells and B-cell nodules. Little innervation is found in the red pulp (RP). (**B**) A higher-magnification view of an area of murine spleen shows that individual nerve fibers (*arrow heads*) can be found in the midst of lymphocytes in the periarteriolar lymphatic sheath (PALS) of the white pulp. This region is heavily populated with T-cells; B-cell nodules have little innervation. The tissue has been counterstained with methyl green; thus, the lymphocyte nuclei can be faintly seen in the white pulp.

ticularly associated with the rapid release of catecholamines, can stimulate a rapid (within minutes) release of leukocytes into the general circulation. As glucocorticoid levels are increased over the next few hours, the increase in leukocytes is reversed as the leukocytes redistribute to tissues such as skin and lymph nodes, resulting in a decrease in circulating leukocytes. The number of leukocytes in the blood is not a direct indicator of immune function, however, as specific immune responses are occurring at localized tissue sites. In terms of immune function, acute stress has often been shown to enhance humoral and cell-mediated immunity, whereas chronic or repeated severe stress can result in immunosuppression. Thus, numerous factors determine the ultimate outcome of stress on immunity. In addition to the ACTH-glucocorticoid axis, many other hormones of the neuroendocrine system have been shown to interact with cells of the immune system, including growth hormone, thyroid hormones, β-endorphin, luteinizing hormone-releasing hormone (LHRH), prolactin, SS, corticotrophin-releasing hormone (CRH), and others. Receptors for numerous neuroendocrine hormones have been found on leukocytes, and there is some evidence of neuroendocrine hormone production by leukocytes, although the levels are generally very low.

In summary, there are two major outflow systems from the CNS that can communicate with and modulate responses from the immune system: the neuroendocrine system and the peripheral outflow through the sympathetic nervous system. There is extensive evidence that these systems are in constant communication, and act together in normal homeostasis. However, extreme perturbations can be associated with maladaptive responses and compromised immune function.

2.3. Immune Signaling to the CNS

In contrast to CNS outflow that communicates with and modulates the peripheral immune system, products of the immune system can signal the CNS in several ways. Presumably, this is to alert the CNS to inflammatory events occurring in the periphery as part of a system to maintain homeostasis or to coordinate a CNS response to the immune activation. It has been long recognized that peripheral activation of the immune system results in a host of "sickness behaviors" that are initiated at the level of the CNS. These sickness behaviors include induction of fever, increased sleep (particularly slow-wave sleep or SWS), hyperalgesia, stimulation of the ACTH-glucocorticoid axis and of the sympathetic nervous system. One of the most important cytokines in mediating these effects is interleukin 1 (IL-1). Cytokines such as IL-1 produced in the periphery can signal the CNS through different pathways. The first means is through direct stimulation of the CNS from blood-borne cytokines. Cytokines are too large to enter the CNS through passive diffusion; however, there is evidence for active transport of

cytokines across the blood–brain barrier, although the levels transported by this means are relatively small. The transport can occur at endothelial cells of the brain and spinal cord and the choroid plexus. Cytokines shown to have a saturable transport into the CNS include IL-1, IL-6, and tumor necrosis factor (TNF-α). Another route of communication is at the circumventricular organs (CVOs), areas of the brain that lack a blood-brain barrier. The uptake of cytokines is facilitated through transport mechanisms, so that levels of cytokine are elevated over what is found at other CNS sites. Cytokines at CVOs do not directly diffuse into deeper CNS structures, however, because of the cells at the CVO–brain interface. Subsequent signaling into the CNS is in part through the production of prostaglandins in response to the cytokine. Prostaglandins are lipophilic, and thus can diffuse into the CNS parenchyma and stimulate neurons or induce cytokine production by various cells within the CNS. This, in turn, can stimulate endocrine and autonomic centers to initiate the sickness response.

Another pathway for peripheral cytokines to stimulate the CNS is through vagal-nerve afferents that synapse in the nucleus solitarius and the area prostrema (AP), areas that are the first to become activated following peripheral administration of IL-1 or lipopolysaccharide (LPS). LPS is derived from the cell walls of Gram-negative bacteria, and is a potent stimulator of macrophages. This mechanism is most likely to be important in signaling the brain in response to localized inflammation in tissues innervated by vagal afferents, including the lung and viscera of the gut. It has been shown that cutting the vagus nerve at a subdiaphragmatic level results in loss of many of the sickness behaviors and responses in the hypothalamus and preoptic area that are initiated after injection of IL-1 or LPS into the gut. Many details of the signaling via this route still must be established; however, there is evidence that locally produced IL-1 can either directly stimulate vagal afferents or the paraganglion cells that could subsequently stimulate the vagus.

In conclusion, there appear to be two major routes for peripheral cytokines to stimulate the CNS that can initiate sickness behaviors. First, there is evidence for direct signaling of the CNS at the level of the vasculature or at the CVOs that is from blood-borne cytokines. Secondly, localized production of cytokines in the abdominal or thoracic viscera can alert the CNS to an infection through vagal afferents. Thus, there is communication with the CNS of inflammatory events in the periphery that allow a coordinated response to deal with the infection.

3. IMMUNE INTERACTIONS WITHIN THE CNS

Although it is commonly believed that the CNS is an immune-privileged site, it is now apparent that this is more likely the result of a relative lack of the immune-related molecules and costimulatory signals that would allow normal immune responses to occur within the CNS, as opposed to a complete lack of leukocyte trafficking through the CNS. The existence of tight junctions between endothelial cells in the capillaries of the brain does highly regulate which molecules cross the blood–brain barrier, thus limiting access of cells and molecules to the CNS. Another means of protection is the tissue environment that exists within the CNS that tends to prevent the activation of an immune response. As part of the regulatory system that helps to control and direct immune responses, the cells of the immune system cannot be stimulated in isolation, but instead require a series of cellular interactions and the development of a cascade of events to allow a full immune response to occur. Among the molecules that are expressed by all cells that help to identify self are the major histocompatability complex (MHC) antigens, in particular, MHC class I. Expression of this molecule is extremely limited within the CNS under normal circumstances. Foreign antigens are recognized by cells of the immune system in association with MHC molecules, which in turn signals the immune system to initiate a response. The lack of MHC expression blocks some of the basic signaling that is required to initiate the process of an immune response. In addition, cells such as the microglia of the CNS normally express limited amounts of MHC class II that is also important in antigen presentation and initiation of inflammatory responses. It is likely that the nervous system developed a means to protect itself from spurious inflammatory responses and "remodeling" resulting from inflammation or phagocytosis that would have harmful effects on a system that must maintain consistent connections. However, this protection is at the expense of repair mechanisms that exist in the periphery.

Another method that limits inflammatory responses to antigens within the CNS is the relative lack of lymphatic drainage from the CNS to lymph nodes. In peripheral tissues, the generation of an effective immune response is partly caused by the drainage of antigens to the draining lymph nodes, where interactions are optimized to allow the appropriate cells to interact and initiate a full response. In the CNS, there are no classic lymphatic channels to drain directly into regional lymph nodes. However, antigens can ultimately reach these lymph nodes, through the drainage of the interstitial fluid of the brain into the cerebrospinal fluid (CSF), which subsequently drains into the venous system at the arachnoid villi. In addition, some CSF drains along some of the cranial nerves and spinal nerve roots to lymphatics, thus providing a more direct method for proteins from the CNS to reach regional lymph nodes. There is evidence to suggest that this can result in the generation of a non-inflammatory humoral immune response.

Additional evidence for the relative protection of inflammatory responses within the CNS comes from studies that involve transplantation of cells or tissue into the CNS. Even with minor MHC incompatibility, the transplants are often not rejected. However, if the peripheral immune system is exposed to the same tissue, an inflammatory response is generated that results in the production of cytotoxic T-cells. These activated cells are subsequently able to cross the intact blood-brain barrier and stimulate rejection of the transplant. Thus, activated T-cells are able to migrate into the CNS. It is likely that there is a continuous surveillance of the CNS by cells such as activated T-cells, but under normal circumstances there are few stimuli within the CNS to further activate these cells or to promote the generation of an inflammatory response.

3.1. Microglia Within the CNS

Microglia are considered by many to be the macrophages of the CNS. Microglia are widely dispersed throughout the brain and spinal cord, and are present in both the gray matter and white matter. Microglia are normally highly ramified, with a relatively small cell body and highly branched, thin cellular processes. Under normal conditions, microglia appear to be resting cells with a relatively small amount of perinuclear cytoplasm or organelles. The morphology of microglia is affected by the local microenvironment in various regions of the CNS, and the morphology can be strikingly different. Microglia within gray and white matter have a ramified morphology, although the pattern of the processes can be distinct in different regions. Microglia in the gray matter have processes that are ramified in all directions, whereas white-matter

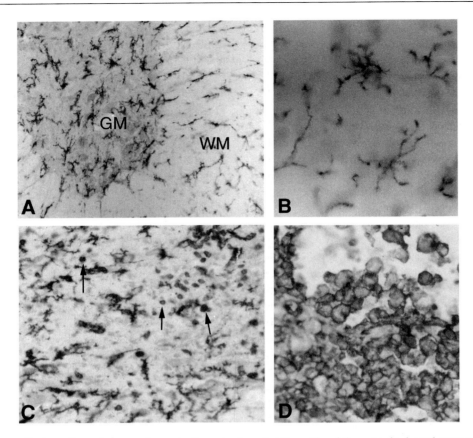

Fig. 2. Morphology of microglia and macrophages in the spinal cord. Microglia of the rat spinal cord were visualized with the OX-42 antibody that recognizes the C3b complement receptor. (**A**) Microglia of the gray matter (GM) have a more stellate pattern compared to the more linear pattern of microglia of the white matter (WM). (**B**) A higher-magnification view of normal gray-matter microglia reveals that they have numerous fine processes extending from the cell body. (**C**) Microglia become activated after traumatic injury to the spinal cord. This view taken 24 h post-injury shows that many microglia have become activated, and have begun to retract their processes so that they appear thicker and more blunt. Some microglia or macrophages have a round phagocytic morphology (*arrows*). (**D**) 1 wk post-injury, the macrophages/microglia have engulfed much tissue debris, and have become greatly enlarged.

microglia often have processes that are arranged in a more linear fashion (Fig. 2A). In contrast, microglia in the CVOs are more compact with short processes, suggesting a more activated morphology in these regions that lack a blood-brain barrier. There also are regional differences in microglial density, with high densities present within areas such as the substantia nigra, ventral pallidum, and olfactory tubercle. Microglia show very slow turnover, with a small amount of proliferation within the normal CNS. Through the use of cellular labeling and chimera studies, there also is evidence for small amounts of renewal through migration of macrophages into the CNS, although this is a slow process. Although there is little proliferation of microglia within the normal CNS, the capacity to proliferate is increased following injury or trauma.

In addition to the resident microglia within the CNS, macrophages are also found in the perivascular spaces in the CNS. These cells lack the highly ramified morphology of the microglia, and are found to be associated with the vasculature and the basement membrane that surrounds the CNS vessels. These cells show greater turnover than microglia, as new macrophages from the blood can enter this space. Macrophages are also normally found in other areas of the CNS including the choroid plexus, the leptomininges, and on the walls of the cerebral ventricles.

3.2. Function of CNS Microglia and Macrophages

As stated previously, cells of the CNS express very low levels of molecules that normally would be required to initiate an immune response. In keeping with this, resting microglia express little or no MHC class I and few express MHC class II. Thus, they do not appear to be acting as antigen-presenting cells on a continuous basis. It is not clear whether resting microglia are playing a functional role during times of normal homeostasis within the tissue. However, microglia are extremely sensitive to perturbations in the local environment, and thus can respond rapidly to toxic stimuli or to trauma. Microglia can rapidly change from the resting state, where they exhibit the morphology noted previously with an extensive arbor of fine processes, to an activated state that can take on a range of forms (Fig. 2C,D). The initial response involves upregulation of a number of cell-surface markers, including the MHC molecules, complement receptors, CD4, and others. In addition, the morphology of the microglia changes as the fine processes are retracted, resulting in a more hypertrophied cell body and thicker, more blunt processes (Fig. 2C). With sufficient activating stimuli, microglia can become fully activated and achieve what is often referred to as a phagocytic morphology, in which the cells become rounded and cannot be distinguished from peripheral macrophages (Fig. 2C,D). Indeed, in areas of trauma and breakdown of the blood–brain barrier, it is not possible to fully discern which cells are activated microglia vs macrophages that have entered the tissue from the vasculature. The nature of the stimulus affects the macrophage response that is elicited. Differences in the magnitude and timing of the response can differ, depending on whether the scenario includes an intact vs a breached blood–brain barrier, and if the neurons or glia in the area are undergoing cell death.

There is much debate as to whether the activation and recruitment of microglia and macrophages to sites of injury are beneficial, or contribute to further damage. Clearance of tissue debris following injury or myelin from areas undergoing Wallerian degeneration is crucial for the process of repair and regeneration. There is much evidence, however, that the rate of macrophage recruitment into these sites is slower than what occurs in the periphery, and the functional ability of macrophages and microglia to phagocytose and remove the debris is considerably slower within the CNS. Thus, there appear to be inhibitory molecules present in the CNS that reduce these aspects of macrophage/microglial function that is ultimately detrimental to regeneration. Myelin contains molecules that are inhibitory to axonal regeneration; thus, prolonged

presence of myelin and other tissue debris is believed to underlie part of the relative inability of the CNS to recover from injury to the same extent as is found in peripheral nerves.

In contrast, the chronic activation of microglia is believed to underlie some of the damage that can occur in the CNS during certain neurodegenerative diseases. Microglia are capable of producing numerous cytokines, including IL-1 and TNFα, which are associated with promoting inflammation. These cytokines can act on endothelial cells to induce edema and leakiness of the blood–brain barrier, thus allowing greater access of cells and molecules into the CNS that normally would be tightly regulated. These cytokines also can induce the expression of adhesion molecules that promote the influx of inflammatory cells and promote the upregulated expression of molecules such as MHC and complement receptors that are utilized in promoting an inflammatory response. In conjunction with this, pro-inflammatory cytokines can induce the activation of macrophages and microglia so that they can release damaging mediators such as reactive oxygen species (ROS), nitric oxide, and damaging enzymes. Microglia can also be a source of potent proinflammatory bioactive lipids such as platelet-activating factor (PAF) that have many actions that are similar to the pro-inflammatory cytokines. In addition, PAF has been shown to be toxic to neurons, and may be one of the molecules released by activated macrophages and microglia during diseases such as AIDS dimentia that cause damage to neurons.

One interpretation regarding microglia of the CNS is that the role they play is dependent on the cellular cues present in the particular microenvironment and on the extent to which they become activated. Much experimental evidence suggests that microglia can have a positive role in promoting wound healing and regeneration through the release of trophic factors when they are activated, but not to the extent that they have achieved the phagocytic morphology. In this latter state, they are capable of producing an oxidative burst, and of releasing degradative enzymes that can contribute to tissue damage. It is also possible that endogenous microglia may play a different role than peripheral macrophages that are recruited into a site of damage. A better understanding of the positive and negative effects of these cells awaits a more complete characterization of the products produced by these cells in various activation states, and in the context of different pathologies within the CNS.

3.3. Other Cells Within the CNS that Can Participate in Inflammatory Responses

Microglia are not the only cells of the CNS that can be part of an inflammatory cascade. Cells such as the endothelial cells and astrocytes also play an important role. Endothelial cells provide much more than a barrier function between the blood and the brain. They are responsive to substances in the blood and to injury or trauma so that they can release pro-inflammatory substances (cytokines and bioactive lipids such as PAF and prostaglandins). These substances in turn can upregulate adhesion molecules (e.g., ICAM-1, integrins and selectins) expression by endothelial cells that helps direct migration of leukocytes into a site of injury or inflammation. Pro-inflammatory molecules also promote alterations in the tight junctions between endothelial cells after injury, or during an inflammatory response resulting in edema and more ready access of large molecules and inflammatory cells into the CNS. Endothelial cells, along with microglia, astrocytes, and other cells, can also release chemokines that act to actively direct leukocytes to follow the chemokine gradient into the tissue. Thus, endothelial cells play a dynamic role in the cascade of events that allows immune responses in the CNS to develop.

Astrocytes have been shown to produce cytokines and to respond to cytokines in the environment. Astrocytes have been shown to secrete numerous cytokines, including IL-1, IL-6, IL-8, TNF-α, IFNγ, and TGFβ, among others. In turn, they can respond to many of these same cytokines, suggesting a possible autocrine loop. Cytokine activation of astrocytes can lead to a variety of responses, including effects on astrocyte growth and maturation, release of nitric oxide, and further production of cytokines. Astrocytes can also be induced to express adhesion molecules and MHC molecules, thus providing other means to participate in inflammation. The expression of MHC molecules by astrocytes and endothelial cells allows these cells to act in antigen presentation to T-cells, although they are unlikely to be as important as microglia for this function. Cytokine stimulation has also been linked to production of nerve-growth factor (NGF) by astrocytes. The physical apposition of astrocytic end feet to ependymal cells and to capillaries allows a role in regulation of the entry of substances or cells into the CNS. Thus, astrocytes are now known to be involved in a wide range of functions, some of which interact directly in the immune system.

4. INFLAMMATORY RESPONSES IN THE CNS DURING TRAUMA OR DISEASE

The generation of an inflammatory response, including the recruitment of leukocytes, is dependent on the type of injury. Degeneration of a nucleus within the CNS in response to peripheral axotomy may result in local activation of microglia, but may not induce the recruitment of other leukocytes, such as neutrophils or peripheral macrophages. In direct trauma to the CNS, however, a robust inflammatory response is elicited that involves a full cascade of events that is not unlike what occurs in the periphery. This includes edema, rapid production of cytokines (particularly TNF, IL-1, and IL-6), upregulation of adhesion molecules on endothelial cells, and production of chemotactic agents. The chemotactic agents, or chemokines, help to direct which leukocytes enter and in what sequence because there are different classes of chemokines that are specific for neutrophils, macrophages, and lymphocytes. The timing of chemokine production generally correlates well with the influx of different subsets of leukocytes into the injured tissue. Although there is debate on the positive vs the negative effects of leukocyte influx into the damaged CNS, there is considerable evidence that the early, robust influx of neutrophils and macrophages following traumatic injury can contribute to secondary-injury mechanisms that expand the lesion beyond the original injury site.

The first leukocytes to enter the CNS following ischemia, traumatic cortical damage, or spinal cord injury are neutrophils. These cells represent the first-line, nonspecific arm of the immune system that enters the tissue rapidly, with a peak from 4–24 h following injury. Ischemia has been shown to cause a rapid influx of neutrophils into CNS tissue; thus, the amount of ischemia may modulate the rate of the neutrophil response. Neutrophil accumulation in the tissue is even greater in ischemia/reperfusion in which blood flow is re-established because the blood supply can bring new neutrophils to the damaged tissue. This in turn is associated with even greater tissue damage. Neutrophil and other leukocyte influx is specifically directed into inflammatory sites by pro-inflammatory mediators produced by the damaged tissue. These mediators include cytokines such as interleukin-1 (IL-1), tumor necrosis factor α (TNFα) and bioactive lipids, including PAF and LTB4. These mediators stimulate a rapid increase in the expression of adhesion molecules on endothelial cells of postcapillary venules, which are then recognized by their counter-receptors on neutrophils. Selectin adhesion molecules mediate the initial adhesion of neutrophils in the blood to endothelial cells. Subsequent higher-affinity interactions of neutrophil integrins LFA-1 (CD11a/CD18) and Mac-1 (CD11b/CD18) with endothelial-cell ICAM-1 are essential for neutrophil transmigration across the endothelial barrier to enter the inflamed tissue. Endothelial ICAM-1 expression has been shown to increase rapidly after ischemia and trauma and to correlate temporally with the influx of neutrophils and the appearance of activated microglia and macrophages. Studies that use antibodies to block adhesion molecules have been shown to decrease neutrophil migration into CNS inflammatory sites following ischemia or spinal cord injury, which has been correlated with reduced lesion size. Such studies give support to the hypothesis that the robust influx of neutrophils into sites of CNS injury can contribute the tissue damage through the release of ROS and degradative enzymes that accompanies neutrophil activation. Such events also occur in the periphery, but these tissues are generally able to repair more readily than the CNS. These events can cause more permanent injury in the CNS, where axonal sprouting and regeneration are relatively inhibited compared to the peripheral nervous system.

The activation of microglia and the recruitment of macrophages into a damaged area of the CNS is delayed by a period of few hours to days as compared to neutrophil influx. Significant presence of activated microglia/macrophages can be seen within 24 h, but the number of cells and amount of activation continues to increase for several days. Macrophages can be found in the tissue for several months following injury, particularly in areas of Wallerian degeneration that occur over a prolonged time-course. As discussed previously, a great deal of controversy surrounds the issue of whether the presence of activated microglia and macrophages contributes to further damage or to tissue repair. The answer is likely a combination of both, depending on the type of injury and the amount of cellular activation that occurs.

Lymphocytes, particularly T cells, also can enter the CNS using adhesion-molecule interactions for extravasation across the endothelial cell barrier. In particular, interaction of the adhesion molecule VLA-4 on T-cells with VCAM-1 on endothelial cells is important for this process. T-cell entry into the CNS has been particularly associated with viral infections

of the CNS and autoimmune processes. The most widely studied autoimmune disease of the CNS is multiple sclerosis (MS). The rodent model used extensively for this disease is experimental allergic encephalomyelitis (EAE), which is associated with $CD4^+$ T-cell attack within the CNS. Studies have shown that activated or memory T-cells are particularly able to cross into the parenchyma of the CNS. Their retention in the tissue is dependent on them interacting with their specific antigen. Without that interaction, the T-cells appear to migrate out of the tissue again. Lymphocytic infiltrates found in this model are composed of T-cells that are specific for various myelin peptide antigens and with antibody-producing B-cells, along with some macrophages. The presence of lymphocytes is associated with areas of demyelination that result in loss of neural function. The initiating stimulus for MS and EAE is still not definitively known; however, there is support for a role played by an inflammatory response in the CNS (perhaps viral), allowing activated microglia to present myelin peptides to specific T-cells. When paired with a peripheral inflammatory event that provides the cytokines and costimulatory signals needed for full T-cell activation, T-cell trafficking to the CNS and subsequent autoimmune damage to CNS myelin and oligodendrocytes can occur.

CONCLUSION

This chapter has shown that the CNS and the immune system are in constant communication. Under normal circumstances, this would help with the overall maintenance of homeostasis, as the nervous system and immune system work together in dealing with infections and damage. As shown schematically in Fig. 3, the major outflow systems from the CNS to the peripheral immune system is through direct neural and neuroendocrine systems. Hypothalamic connections to the spinal cord modulate outflow to the lymphoid tissues and sites of inflammation through the sympathetic nervous system and neuropeptide systems. Modulation of lymphoid innervation has been shown to have major effects on inflammatory responses. In addition, hypothalamic stimulation of the pituitary and neuroendocrine system modulates the release of neuroendocrine hormones that can modulate immune function. In particular, stress, inflammation, or CNS cytokine-stimulated release of ACTH and glucocorticoids can strongly influence immune function. In turn, peripheral immune activation and release of cytokines

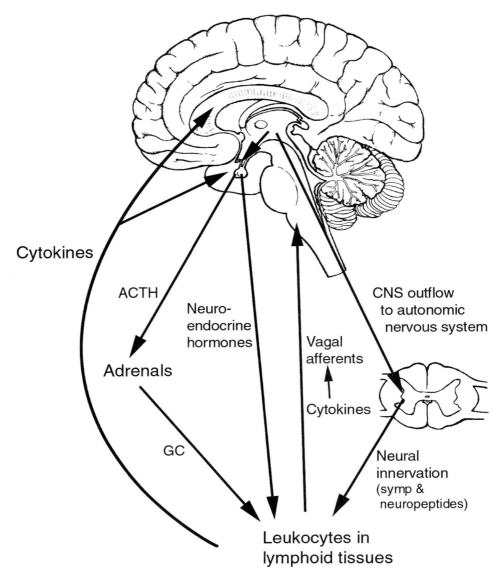

Fig. 3. Schematic of nervous system—immune system interactions. There are numerous routes of communication between the nervous and immune systems. Outflow from the CNS is predominantly through the neuroendocrine system, and through connections to sympathetic or neuropeptide innervation of lymphoid tissues. The hypothalamic connections to the pituitary can stimulate the release of various neuroendocrine hormones that can influence the immune system. In addition, inflammatory stimuli or stress can stimulate the release of ACTH, which in turn stimulates production of glucocorticoids (GC) from the adrenals, which can then influence the immune system in numerous ways. Hypothalamic output to the sympathetic preganglionics in the thoracic spinal cord or to other neuropeptide systems has also been shown to have a profound effect on immune function. Peripheral inflammatory responses can signal the CNS through blood-borne cytokines that are detected in CVOs or taken up through specific transporter systems. In addition, localized cytokines can stimulate afferents in the vagus nerve that can signal the brainstem and hypothalamus. Both routes can induce sickness behaviors that are mediated at the level of the CNS. The CNS itself can also produce cytokines that mediate inflammatory responses within the CNS, or that affect efferent signals to the peripheral immune system.

can signal the CNS either directly or through vagal afferents. This in turn can stimulate prostaglandin and cytokine production in the CNS and initiate sickness behaviors in response to immune activation. Under normal circumstances, the coordinated response of the nervous and immune systems efficiently deal with infection and disease. Under certain conditions, however, inflammatory events in the CNS or alterations in the peripheral neural/neuroendocrine input to the immune system can become the basis of disease. Much has yet to be learned of the normal role of neural-immune interactions and of the processes that could be effective targets in developing therapies for disease.

SELECTED READINGS

Ader R, Felten DL, Cohen N. (eds). Psychoneuroimmunology, 3rd ed. Academic Press, San Diego, 2001.

Antel J, Bernbaum G, Hartung HP. (eds). Clinical Neuroimmunology. Malden, MA: Blackwell Science, 1998.

Keane RW, Hickey WF. (eds). Immunology of the Nervous System. New York: Oxford University Press, 1997.

Martino G, Adorini L. (eds). From Basic Immunology to Immune-Mediated Demyelination. New York; Milano: Springer, 1999.

Martino G, Furlan R, Brambilla E, Bergami A, Ruffini F, Gironi M, et al. Cytokines and immunity in multiple sclerosis: the dual signal hypothesis. J Neuroimmunol 2000; 109:3–9.

Ransohoff R, Benveniste E. (eds) Cytokines and the CNS. Boca Raton: CRC Press, 1996.

Rolak L, Harati Y. (eds) Neuroimmunology for the Clinician. Boston: Butterworth-Heinmann, 1997.

Rothwell NJ. (ed). Cytokines in the Nervous System. Austin: RG Landes, 1996.

Scharrer B, Smith EM, Stefano GB. (eds). Neuropeptides and Immunoregulation. Berlin; New York: Springer-Verlag, 1994.

Myasthenia Gravis

Gregory Cooper and Robert L. Rodnitzky

Myasthenia gravis is the most common disorder of neuromuscular transmission. Patients experience weakness, with abnormally rapid fatigue of the muscles that move the extremities, face, eyelids, and eyes and the muscles required for swallowing and respiration. Involvement of these last two groups of muscles can be fatal if severe and untreated. Myasthenia is an autoimmune condition in which there is antibody-mediated alteration of the postsynaptic membrane of the neuromuscular junction and destruction of acetylcholine receptors. Although its clinical manifestations are protean, there are several useful serologic, pharmacologic, and electrophysiologic means of confirming the diagnosis.

ACETYLCHOLINE RECEPTORS IN MYASTHENIA GRAVIS

The Discovery of α-Bungarotoxin Began the Modern Understanding of the Acetylcholine Receptor

The discovery that a Taiwanese poisonous snake's toxin, α-bungarotoxin, selectively binds to the nicotinic acetylcholine receptor at the neuromuscular junction provided a scientific tool that significantly enhanced efforts to understand the physioanatomic basis of myasthenia gravis. Using radioactive α-bungarotoxin to label acetylcholine receptors, it was confirmed that their numbers are significantly reduced in myasthenic patients. It was demonstrated that inoculation of laboratory animals with acetylcholine-receptor protein resulted in the development of an experimental form of myasthenia gravis, strongly suggesting an autoimmune basis for the illness. Antibodies against acetylcholine receptors can be demonstrated in most human patients with myasthenia gravis, and their presence is a useful means of confirming the diagnosis.

Antibodies Can Affect Acetylcholine-Receptor Functions in Several Ways

Several types of antibodies can be found in myasthenic patients. Approximately 90% of myasthenic patients with generalized weakness harbor one or more types of acetylcholine-receptor antibody. The most commonly found antibody binds to the acetylcholine receptor but does not block its receptive sites. The acetylcholine receptor has five constituent subunits arrayed around a central ion channel. The acetylcholine and α-bungarotoxin-binding sites are separate, but they are both located on the two α-subunits of the receptor. Antibodies that do block the acetylcholine-receptive site are found in a much smaller percentage of patients, but are often associated with more severe disease. Collectively, these abnormal antibodies accelerate the degradation of receptors by enhancing the normal process of endocytosis, and they impair the function of the remaining receptor by blocking their active sites and promoting a complement-mediated alteration of the architecture of the postjunctional membrane. The latter process includes widening of the synaptic cleft and smoothing of the normally infolded architecture of the postsynaptic membrane, with a resultant loss of receptor containing surface area.

The specificity of circulating acetylcholine-receptor antibodies for myasthenia gravis is high. False-positive results have been recorded for few persons without myasthenia gravis, such as those who received snake venom as a form of therapy, patients with tumors of the thymus, and those who received the drug penicillamine.

Epidemiology and Diagnosis

Myasthenia gravis occurs most often in young women and older men, peaking in the second and third decades in women and the sixth and seventh decades in men.

Neonatal myasthenia gravis is a transient condition resulting from transplacental transfer of acetylcholine-receptor antibodies from a myasthenic mother to her infant. As the antibodies are cleared by the affected infant, the myasthenic symptoms gradually resolve. This phenomenon confirms the importance of circulating antibodies in the pathogenesis of myasthenia gravis.

Weakness and Easy Fatigability Are the Clinical Hallmarks of Myasthenia Gravis

Virtually any muscle in the body can become weakened in myasthenia gravis. Often, the first muscles to become involved are those responsible for movement of the eye or eyelid. Affected patients complain of diplopia and eyelid ptosis. Ocular symptoms are the presenting sign of myasthenia gravis in more than 50% of patients, and ultimately affect more than 90% of patients. In a few patients, the symptoms remain confined to the eyes, resulting in the syndrome of ocular myasthenia gravis.

Appendicular, bulbar, and respiratory muscles are also commonly involved. In the arms and legs, proximal muscles tend to be involved more severely, resulting in difficulty arising from a chair, climbing stairs, or raising the arms over the head. Bulbar-muscle involvement results in symptoms such as difficulty in swallowing, nasal regurgitation of ingested fluids, and a characteristic nasal quality of the voice. Weakness of the facial muscles results in an inability to grimace, pucker the lips, or whistle. Involvement of respiratory muscles severely limits the volume of air that can be maximally moved in and out of the lungs.

One feature of myasthenic weakness that differentiates it from weakness caused by most other conditions is extreme and early muscle fatigability. Patients who ascend stairs may notice that the first few steps can be accomplished without difficulty, but that the next several steps become progressively more difficult.

Serologic, Pharmacologic, and Electrophysiologic Testing Can Help Confirm the Diagnosis

The usefulness of assaying acetylcholine receptor-antibodies was previously discussed. Acetylcholine-receptor antibodies can be demonstrated in only 90% of myasthenic patients with generalized weakness, and other tests may be needed to confirm the diagnosis.

Pharmacologic testing involves the use of cholinesterase-inhibiting drugs. These agents improve myasthenic symptoms by preventing the normal hydrolysis and inactivation of elaborated acetylcholine in the neuromuscular synaptic cleft. The duration of the effect of elaborated acetylcholine is prolonged, allowing an increased number of interactions with the remaining acetylcholine receptors and some repair of neuromuscular transmission. Edrophonium (Tensilon) is a rapid and short-acting cholinesterase-inhibiting agent that results in a brief but striking improvement in myasthenic symptoms. After injecting it intravenously, marked improvement in symptoms can be demonstrated within minutes, which is helpful in confirming the diagnosis.

Electrophysiologic testing for myasthenia gravis consists of measuring the amplitude of a muscle's response to repetitive stimulation of its nerve. In normal persons,

the amplitude of the muscle response remains constant during repetitive nerve stimulation at three cycles per second. In myasthenia gravis, the muscle response to stimulation at this frequency becomes progressively smaller, mirroring the fatigue experienced after repetitive limb movements. Typically, this *decremental response* can only be demonstrated in clinically weak muscles.

TREATMENT

With therapy, myasthenia gravis is seldom a fatal disorder. Cholinesterase inhibitors are useful in testing and in treating myasthenia gravis. Administered in proper amounts, they produce a mild improvement in muscle strength. If given in excessive amounts, they can produce side effects related to overstimulation of muscarinic acetylcholine receptors, including excessive salivation and tearing, diarrhea, and slowing of the heart rate. A similar cholinergic stimulation of muscle may paradoxically lead to increased weakness, presumably resulting from continuous end-plate depolarization. In its most extreme form, a cholinergic crisis develops, in which there is marked weakness of the respiratory muscles.

Because cholinesterase inhibitors are only mildly effective, most severely myasthenic patients require immunotherapy. This approach, along with improved ventilatory support, has reduced the mortality rate for generalized myasthenia from the 40–70% reported before 1960 to less than 10% in 1994. One of the earliest immunologic therapies used for myasthenia gravis was removal of the thymus. In most myasthenia gravis patients, the thymus is microscopically hyperplastic, and in 20% of these patients, a tumor of the gland (e.g., thymoma) develops. Many myasthenic patients are improved after removal of the thymus, probably because of the gland's role in promoting and sustaining an autoimmune attack on acetylcholine receptors. The finding of acetylcholine receptor protein in the thymus supports this idea.

Immunosuppressive drugs, such as corticosteroids and azathioprine, are extremely effective in inhibiting the aberrant immune response underlying myasthenia gravis. Often, as the patient improves on these therapies, there is a corresponding drop in the titer of anti-

bodies to the acetylcholine receptor. A more direct way to lower this antibody titer is through the use of plasmapheresis. In this process, the patient's plasma, which contains the abnormal antibody, is removed and replaced with a plasma substitute. This procedure effectively lowers the titer of abnormal antibodies and can result in remarkable improvement until more antibody is produced. Intravenous immunoglobulin (IVIg) has also been used effectively.

SELECTED READING

Massey JM. Acquired myasthenia gravis. Neurologic Clinics 1997; 15:577–595.

32 Degeneration, Regeneration, and Plasticity in the Nervous System

Paul J. Reier and Margaret J. Velardo

CONTENTS

1. INTRODUCTION

The exquisitely organized pathways and neural circuits discussed elsewhere in this textbook mediate precisely coordinated neurophysiological interactions that subserve a range of sensory, motor, cognitive, and autonomic modalities. These elaborate cellular interactions are the product of a dynamic series of developmental mechanisms involving neurogenesis and the formation of neuronal projections and synaptic networks via orchestrated neuritic outgrowth, postsynaptic target recognition, and synaptogenesis. The disruption of this intricate functional architecture by such catastrophic insults as brain or spinal cord injury—as well as neurodegenerative, demyelinative, and other diseases—can result in devastating disabilities with profound socioeconomic consequences at virtually every stage of an individual's lifetime. The immediate question thus arises: to what degree can functional outcomes be improved? To address this issue, the present chapter explores principles underlying neural-tissue reactions to trauma and how these differ relative to peripheral nervous system (PNS) vs central nervous system (CNS) pathologies. The discussion will then turn to intrinsic repair mechanisms and potential therapeutic interventions designed to rescue tissue at risk or promote regeneration and neuronal replacement. For illustrative purposes, much of the emphasis will be on neuronal changes after blunt damage to the CNS or severance of nerve fibers in the PNS. However, many of the cellular dynamics associated with trauma can be exhibited in other neuropathological states.

From: *Neuroscience in Medicine, 2nd ed.* (P. Michael Conn, ed.),
© 2003 Humana Press Inc., Totowa, NJ.

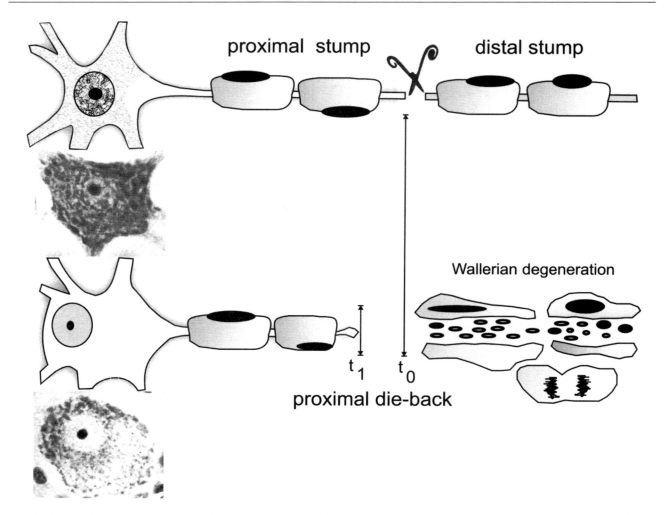

Fig. 1. An illustration of early neuronal responses to nerve injury. The *upper diagram* depicts axonal transection of an intact neuron. Axotomy results in the formation of two axonal compartments—the proximal and distal stumps—relative to the site of injury. The lower drawing shows axonal degeneration (e.g., anterograde or Wallerian degeneration) in the distal stump. In addition, proximal die-back is indicated by the distance between the original transection site (t_0) and the subsequent leading edge of the proximal stump (t_1). The *photomicrograph inserts* complement the drawings showing with cresyl violet staining the transition from a normal neuronal soma with clusters of Nissl substance to a swollen (*lower micrograph*) cell body with a displaced and more lightly stained nucleus and absence of prominent Nissl bodies.

2. NERVE-CELL RESPONSES TO AXONAL DAMAGE: GENERAL PRINCIPLES

2.1. Changes That Occur at the Level of the Axon

When nerve fibers in the CNS or PNS are either severed or simply compressed (e.g., *axotomy*), they are then essentially divided into two cytoplasmic compartments. The portion of the axon that remains in continuity with the cell body is referred to as the *proximal segment*, and the region isolated from the neuronal soma is called the *distal segment* or stump (Fig. 1). The metabolic maintenance and integrity of

the axon is dependent on the cell body through antero-grade axonal transport. For this reason, interruption of axonal continuity invariably leads to the progressive degeneration of the distal segment—a phenomenon referred to as *Wallerian* or *anterograde degeneration* (Figs.1,2).

After transection of a nerve fiber, axoplasm leaks from the proximal and distal segments until healing of the cut ends occurs by fusion of the axonal membrane, and the cut ends often retract and leave an intervening gap (Fig. 1). In addition to the abnormal accumulation of axonal organelles (Fig. 2), the hallmark feature of Wallerian degeneration is the dissolution of cytoskeletal

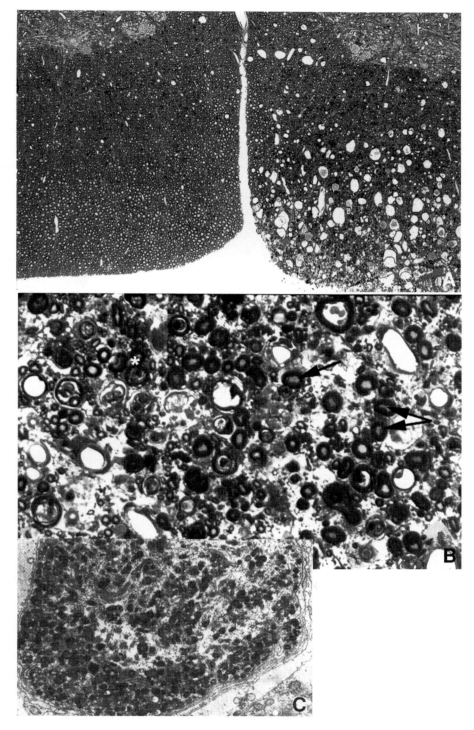

Fig. 2. Histological (*plastic sections stained with toluidine blue*) and ultrastructural views of Wallerian degeneration. (**A**) Shows a cross-sectional view of ventral white matter in an adult rat spinal cord that had undergone a prior hemisection. The histological section was obtained at a level caudal to the level of injury. Since neurons giving rise to these myelinated axons are located at suprasegmental levels, the region of the spinal cord shown is "distal" to the injury. Note the extensive fiber swelling and overall disruption of white matter on the side of the lesion (*right*). (**B**) Is a higher-magnification view of the damaged white matter showing various stages of myelin breakdown as evidenced by large vacuoles or dark patches of debris within macrophages (*). Some axons are still recognizable as donut-like figures with darkly stained cores (*arrows*). (**C**) Is an electron micrograph of one such degenerating axon in which large accumulations of abnormal mitochondria and lysosomes are seen.

components—microtubules and neurofilaments—in the distal stump. The latter is caused by injury-associated influxes of calcium that lead to the activation of calcium-dependent proteases. This has been suggested by studies of protracted anterograde degeneration in a strain of mutant mice, which have been found to have deficiencies in such protease activity. Degradation of the cytoskeleton probably contributes directly to axonal fragmentation and collapse. Axonal degeneration can also progress in a retrograde direction (Fig. 1), but such *proximal axonal die-back* is usually limited in distance, and is not believed to extend beyond the first node of Ranvier or level at which the first axonal collateral emerges prior to the site of axonal injury. However, if the lesion occurs close to the cell body, retrograde axonal degeneration can then advance to the soma and thus result in *retrograde neuronal degeneration* (*see* below).

In addition to axonal breakdown, Wallerian degeneration also entails the demise of the surrounding myelin sheath (Figs. 1,2). Such myelin pathology secondary to nerve injury implies an intimate dependency of the myelin-producing glial cell (e.g., Schwann cell in the PNS and oligodendrocyte in the CNS) on axonal structural and/or functional integrity. In some respects, this principle is an extension of development, during which the axon dictates whether myelin is formed and the ultimate thickness of the sheath to be established.

A concomitant loss of the axonal terminals (e.g., *terminal degeneration*) is also associated with anterograde degeneration. Axonal damage results in a loss of synaptic transmission, which can occur even before the first visible anatomical signs of terminal disruption. For example, damage to axons from motoneurons results in neuromuscular junction breakdown and phagocytosis of debris by Schwann cells over the course of a few days post-axotomy. Transmission at the neuromuscular junction ceases within a few hours of nerve damage, and the actual time-course of transmission failure correlates with the length of the distal stump preserved.

2.2. Neuronal Cell Body Alterations Are Exhibited After Axotomy

The consequences of axonal damage are not limited to the distal stump, and either positive or negative effects are exhibited at the level of the cell soma in terms of metabolic, molecular, cytological, and neurophysiological changes. The neuronal-cell-body response can thus be characterized on one hand by anabolic changes that lead to the neuron's capacity to survive. Alternatively, axotomy may lead to regressive somal changes that could cascade into molecular events directed at neuronal death (e.g., programmed cell death [PCD], or apoptosis). The neuronal-cell-body response is usually unpredictable and depends on many variables, including the age of the subject at the time of injury, the distance of the lesion from the cell body, species differences, the nature and severity of the lesion, extent of axonal collateralization between the site of axotomy and the cell body, the functional type of cells involved, and PNS or CNS location of the axotomized neuronal populations. For this reason, it cannot be generalized how any given neuronal population will respond to axotomy.

2.2.1. CHROMATOLYSIS

A phenomenon known as *chromatolysis* is often highlighted in textbook discussions about axotomy because it provides a classical visualization of one type of neuronal-cell-body response. Chromatolysis is characterized by histological changes that include: cytoplasmic vacuolation, nucleolar enlargement, displacement of the nucleus from a central to an eccentric or peripheral somal location beneath the cell membrane, and swelling of the cell body (Fig. 1). A prominent feature of chromatolysis is the dissolution of Nissl substance, as demonstrated by decreased cytoplasmic staining and granularity. The ultrastructural correlate is the fragmentation of rough endoplasmic reticulum (ER) with a concomitant increase in the density of free polyribosomes. The cytological changes associated with chromatolysis are consistent with elevated RNA metabolism and protein synthesis. Some neurons thus exhibit a shift toward the biosynthesis of structural proteins, materials associated with axonal transport, membrane lipids, and many other growth-associated proteins (GAPs). A reduction in the synthesis of constituents that are more typically involved in neurotransmitter metabolism, for example, is consistent with the loss of neuronal excitability after axotomy. It should be noted that chromatolysis *is not a universal neuronal response*, but one that is exhibited only by certain neuronal populations, and this can be subject to many variables. Therefore, no generalizations should be made about the functional significance of this specific cell-body response or the fates of injured neurons based on whether or not they exhibit chromatolysis after injury.

Although many hypotheses have been advanced, the axotomy-related signal(s) that trigger(s) metabolic changes in the cell soma are still unknown. However, it appears, that retrograde axonal transport may play a partial role in delivering some form of molecular message from the site of axonal injury to the cell body. Alternatively, the absence of certain molecules that would be normally derived from target structures can likewise prompt neuronal biosynthetic changes as a matter of deprivation. In experiments in which retrograde transport was blocked without axotomy, the same type of responses were detected in the cell body that would appear because of axonal interruption. A classic example of this principle is the interrupted retrograde transport of target-derived trophic factors.

2.2.2. Other Neuronal Reactions That Occur at the Level of the Cell Body

In contrast with neurons that have some regenerative capacity, cells that cannot restore synaptic connections with suitable targets ultimately show reduced cell-body size, and persist in that state or die. Such changes in an axotomized neuron are referred to as *retrograde cell-death or atrophy*, respectively (Fig. 3A,B). For example, after experimental lesions that interrupt ascending dorsal spinocerebellar axons, neurons in the dorsal nucleus of Clarke, which give rise to these fibers (*see* Chapter 9), undergo degeneration over time (Fig. 4). In other cases, death can occur in neuronal populations that are uninjured but are synaptically associated with damaged neurons. For instance, axotomy can lead to a phenomenon referred to as *anterograde* (orthograde) *transneuronal* or *transsynaptic degeneration*. As the result of Wallerian degeneration, postsynaptic neurons become at least partially deafferented. Under certain circumstances, such a reduction in presynaptic inputs can then precipitate an eventual degeneration of the target cell (Fig. 3C). An analogous situation also can be seen with regard to peripheral nonneural target structures such as muscle, where denervation atrophy usually ensues peripheral-nerve injury (Fig. 5). A frequently cited example of anterograde transneuronal degeneration is the lateral geniculate nucleus (LGN) of the thalamus, in which the postsynaptic cells are deafferented following damage to the optic nerves. Conversely, neurons that synapse on to axotomized cells can die by virtue of *retrograde transneuronal* or transsynaptic degeneration (Fig. 3D). These transsynaptic phenomena are not limited to degeneration, but may likewise

entail survival of shrunken or atrophic cells—a condition known as *transsynaptic neuronal atrophy*. An inportant corollary of these secondary degenerative responses to axotomy is that similar principles apply to many neurodegenerative diseases. For instance, the loss of certain neuronal populations that are the primary targets of a particular neurological disorder could lead to more widespread cell degeneration elsewhere in the nervous system as a result of deafferentation (e.g., orthograde transneuronal degeneration) or the loss postsynaptic of targets (e.g., retrograde transneuronal degeneration).

2.2.3. Neuronal Fates Can Be Defined by Changes in Nutritive Support

These illustrations of primary and anterograde or retrograde trans-synaptic neuronal degeneration underscore the important concept of *neurotrophism*. This principle refers to the establishment of sustaining molecular interactions between either neurons or neurons and their peripheral target structures. For instance, denervation neuromuscular atrophy (Fig. 5) can be caused by a loss of muscle activity as part of a lower motor neuron phenomenon or an absence of neuronal "nutritive" or trophic support. In similar ways, diminished synaptic drive or neurotrophic support, which are not mutually exclusive, can account for orthograde transneuronal degeneration or atrophy. Alternatively, the death of an axotomized cell can contribute to neurotrophic imbalances that affect cells that project to it, thereby leading to retrograde transneuronal degeneration or atrophy.

Trophic substances that are derived from the target cell are normally conveyed to the cell body of the presynaptic element by retrograde axonal transport. This principle also applies to retrograde degeneration of axotomized neurons, which are no longer in contact with their targets (e.g., sources of trophic support) because of axonal interruption and failure to reestablish such connections. However, retrograde degeneration may be curtailed by trophically effective inputs from other cells onto the injured neuron, and sustaining inputs may prevent anterograde and retrograde transneuronal degeneration (Fig. 3E). The axotomized cell, for example, may have numerous collaterals emerging from the proximal axon segment. Projections to other targets that represent alternative sources of neurotrophic substances may thus be preserved. These could support the survival of a damaged cell, although it may still exhibit some degree of atrophy,

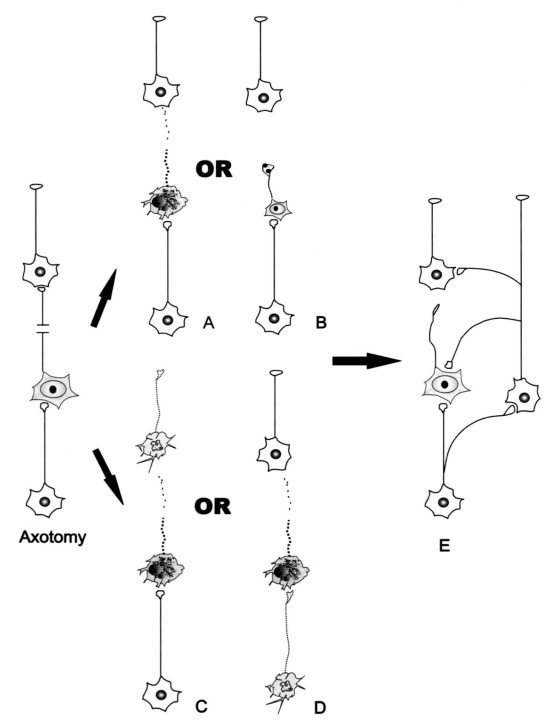

Fig. 3. Several basic neuronal responses to injury are illustrated in this diagram (*see* text). Three neurons are shown on the *left*, with the middle cell depicted as having been axotomized. (**A**) The progressive demise of a neuron after axonal interruption is referred to as retrograde cell death. (**B**) In other nonregenerative circumstances, the injured neuron survives, but undergoes a retrograde atrophy. (**C**) Wallerian degeneration and resulting deafferentation of postsynaptic neurons can result in anterograde transsynaptic or transneuronal cell death. (**D**) Conversely, death of the axotomized neuron can lead to a retrograde transneuronal degeneration of neurons originally presynaptic to the injured neuron. (**E**) Rescue of neurons that can be directly or indirectly affected by axotomy may occur in a variety of ways. One that is illustrated is by virtue of trophically sustaining inputs from uninjured cells that project onto the vulnerable neurons or by way of projections from cells that are at risk of neuronal death or atrophy.

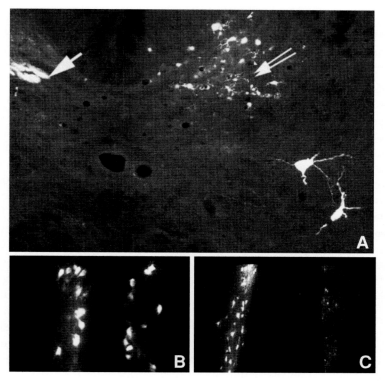

Fig. 4. Shown is an example of *retrograde cell death* in the dorsal nucleus of Clarke (e.g., neurons that give rise to dorsal spinocerebellar axons) (*upper half* of [**A**]) of the adult rat spinal cord (*transverse histological section*). This histological section was obtained at the L_1 spinal level several weeks after a right-sided hemisection of the spinal cord was made at T_{11}. Prior to that procedure, neurons projecting to the cerebellum were prelabeled by retrograde transport of a fluorescent dye that was injected into appropriate regions of the cerebellum. The tissue sections were then viewed and photographed by fluorescence microscopy. At the *upper left* of (**A**), a small cluster of spinocerebellar neurons (*single arrow*) is seen on the uninjured side of the spinal cord, whereas only fluorescent debris in small cells with ramified processes (*double arrows*) can be seen in the same region on the injured *right side* (*see also* Fig. 16). (**B,C**) illustrate the progressive loss of the axotomized spinocerebellar neurons in longitudinal sections of the spinal cord (*caudal to the hemisection*) that were obtained several weeks after axotomy. The intact side is seen on the *left* in both micrographs; gradual disappearance of the prelabeled injured neurons on the *right* can be seen.

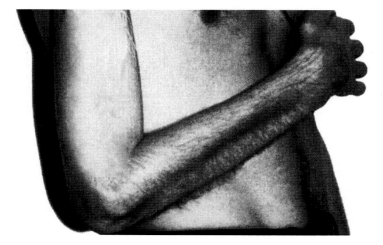

Fig. 5. Prominent muscular atrophy is seen in this individual's forearm following peripheral-nerve injury at the level of the brachial plexus and suboptimal regeneration. Although the ability to flex the arm has recovered, the overall degree of functional recovery is minimal. This illustrates an example of the absence of trophic interaction between nerve and muscle. (Illustration kindly provided by Dr. Susan E. Mackinnon, Washington University School of Medicine and Barnes-Jewish Hospital.)

```
┌─────────────────────────────────────────┐
│        GROWTH FACTORS WITH              │
│        NEUROTROPHIC ACTIVITY            │
├─────────────────────────────────────────┤
│                                         │
│       Nerve Growth Factor (NGF)         │
│ Brain Derived Neurotrophic Factor (BDNF)│
│ Glial Derived Neurotrophic Factor (GDNF)│
│     Leukemia Inhibitory Factor (LIF)    │
│  Ciliary Neuronotrophic Factor (CNTF)   │
│ Platelet Derived Growth Factor (PDGF)   │
│    Insulin-like Growth Factor (IGF)     │
│    Epidermal Growth Factor (EGF)        │
│    Fibroblast Growth Factor (FGF)       │
│ Transforming Growth Factor-alpha (TGFa) │
│ Transforming Growth Factor-beta (TGFb)  │
│  Neurotrophic Factors –3,4,5 (NT-3,4,5) │
│                                         │
└─────────────────────────────────────────┘
```

Box 1.

depending on the extent of collateralization and amount of target-derived trophic support available.

2.3. Neurotrophic Factors Represent Families of Molecules With Diverse Functions: A Basic Orientation

Box 1 presents a partial listing of neurotrophic factors, which are a subclass of molecules (hormones and proteins) that play important roles in the developing and adult nervous system. These functions include influences on cell differentiation, survival, and growth. Some of these factors (e.g., fibroblast growth factors, FGF) also can stimulate cellular proliferation involving neural-stem and progenitor-cell populations, as well as neuroglial elements. The first tangible demonstration of the presence of growth factors in the nervous system dates back to research conducted over 60 yrs ago, which ultimately set the stage for subsequent identification of FGF activity in the brain. Long before this time, neurotrophism was already being conceptually interpreted from experimental findings. Classic studies in neuroembryology showed, for example, that enhancement of target tissue availability in embryos of various species could decrease the extent of naturally occurring neuronal cell death, thereby suggesting a mechanism for the developmental rescue of neurons that were otherwise destined to die.

It was not until the 1950s that growth-factor biology was accepted as a "grassroots" concept in the neurosciences. This largely resulted from Nobel Prize-winning experiments that led to the identification of nerve-growth factor (NGF). NGF is only one member of the neurotrophin family of molecules that also includes brain-derived neurotrophic factor (BDNF), and neurotrophins NT-3 and NT-4/5 (see Box 1). In a series of elegant experiments, it was shown that certain target tissues elaborate NGF, which in turn is critical to the survival of sensory (e.g., dorsal-root ganglion cells) and sympathetic neurons (Fig. 6). In addition to neuronal survival, NGF also was shown to have stimulatory effects on nerve-fiber outgrowth (Fig. 6).

Relative to the present discussion of degeneration and regeneration, NGF has been shown to have a profound effect on certain neuronal populations in the adult CNS following axotomy. One illustration involves septohippocampal cholinergic projections. The hippocampus contains high levels of NGF. Transection of the fimbria or fornix results in the interruption of the septohippocampal projection, after which approximately one-half of the cholinergic neurons in the septum either die or exhibit severe atrophy and loss of their cholinergic phenotype (Fig. 7). The fate of these vulnerable cells, however, can be reversed by the infusion of exogenous NGF. Because these basal forebrain cells appear to degenerate in Alzheimer's disease, findings of this nature have suggested provocative therapeutic possibilities involving NGF delivery to rescue these neurons, as discussed at the end of this chapter. Similarly, another factor, glial cell-derived neurotrophic factor (GDNF) can rescue dopamine-producing neurons in the substantia nigra after experimental lesions, and this has implications for the eventual treatment of Parkinson's disease.

In general, neurotrophic factors exert very specific effects after binding with their appropriate receptors. The actions of neurotrophic molecules can also differ in terms of whether they are being produced and released by cells in the developing or adult nervous system. By binding with specific receptors, neurotrophic factors trigger intracellular signaling pathways, and these neurotrophic factors can then be retrogradely transported back to the cell body via ligand-receptor complexes or second-messenger molecules. It can thus be seen that axonal transection interrupts this target-to-cell body flow of trophic factor and can thereby place neurons at risk of imminent cell death as a result of an interrupted neurotrophic supply. As its designation implies, GDNF exemplifies that trophic support can also be derived in a paracrine fashion from surrounding glia in addition to target-derived and autocrine routes.

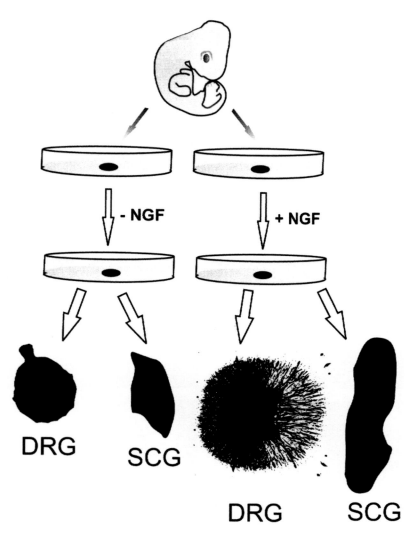

Fig. 6. A schematic illustrating two experimental examples of neurotrophic action using NGF as the model neurotrophic factor. Dorsal root (DRG) and superior cervical ganglia (SCG) are dissected from the embryo (such as the rat, mouse, or chicken) and then grown in tissue culture in either the presence or absence of NGF. In the case of the DRG example, NGF stimulates extensive fiber outgrowth as seen on the right, thereby demonstrating the neurite-promoting action of this factor. The SCG diagrams provide an example of NGF's effect on neuronal survival and growth, as exhibited by the larger size of the treated SCG explant.

3. PERIPHERAL NERVE INJURY AND REGENERATION

3.1. Neural Regeneration Is Synonymous With the Regrowth of Damaged Axons

When used in reference to the nervous system, the term "regeneration" has a meaning that is distinct from that applied to most other parts of the body, where cell proliferation leads to large-scale self-repair (such as liver regeneration). In contrast, mature neurons do not divide, and are thus incapable of replacing themselves. Consequently, trauma or disease leading to extensive neuronal death has the poorest prognosis for functional recovery. However, when only axons are severed (e.g., *axotomy*), neurons can survive, and some axotomized neurons will support the regrowth of damaged nerve fibers. *Neural regeneration* thus commonly refers to the reconstitution of severed axons (as well as dendrites), and the subsequent restoration of projections and synaptic interactions.

3.2. Neurons That Survive Axonal Damage in the PNS Can Exhibit Robust Regrowth of Damaged Axons

Neurons located exclusively within the PNS or those that send axons from the CNS into peripheral

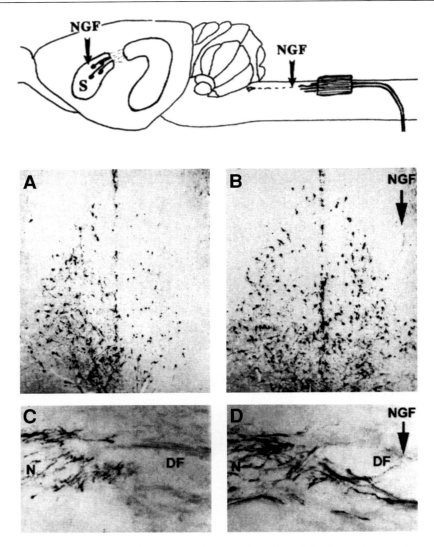

Fig. 7. Nerve-growth factor (NGF) has been used to prevent degeneration of basal forebrain cholinergic neurons, including those of the septum (S) after traumatic lesions and to promote regeneration of sensory axons after spinal cord injury, most often in rodent models. **(A)** Chronic treatment with control solutions does not prevent the disappearance of ChAT-positive (cholinergic) neurons after a lesion on one side of the brain, but **(B)** NGF does. **(C)** Sensory axons that have grown vigorously across a peripheral nerve bridge (N) do no reenter the dorsal funiculus (DF) white matter of the spinal cord, as it is nonsupportive. **(D)** After NGF infusion, many sensory fibers can extend into that white matter tract over millimeters, responding to the chemoattractant properties of NGF. (Figure kindly provided by Dr. Theo Hagg, University of Louisville.)

nerves (e.g., motoneurons) have the innate capacity to support axonal regrowth, even for long distances. The onset of regeneration does not occur immediately after axotomy, and the length of delay depends on variables such as the severity of the injury or the proximity of the lesion to the cell body. An important consideration is that robust regeneration is not necessarily synonymous with functional recovery. Instead, the degree and quality of functional return via regeneration is highly dependent on the ability of axons to reconnect with their proper targets.

3.3. Cellular Dynamics Proximal to the Site of Injury and at the Lesion Site

3.3.1. Regeneration is Initiated by the Formation of Nerve-Growth Cones That Possess Selective Preferences for Some Tissue Constituents and Not Others

At the preserved end of the proximal nerve segment, the spherical axonal end-bulbs appearing after injury exhibit morphological changes that lead to the formation of growth cones (Figs. 6,8,9). Growth cones are highly specialized motile structures that move in an amoeboid-like, crawling fashion by extending and retracting cytoplasmic finger-like extensions (e.g., filopodia) or flattened veil-like projections (e.g., lamellipodia). Aside from its mobility, the growth cone has the remarkable capacity to sense and respond to cues in the surrounding tissue milieu. Growth cones thus have affinities for some molecules, and are either repulsed or growth-arrested by others. As growth cones advance, they extend their delicate filopodia, which have receptors for various tissue-associated ligands. Once they contact favorable or growth-promoting permissive substrates, the filopodia attach, and this leads to a traction-generating mechanism within the growth cone itself to allow it to continue moving forward. Alternatively, if filopodia encounter non-permissive tissue environments, their initial attachment is unstable, they retract, and the growth cone is arrested in its advance or turns in the direction of those filopodia that have found more favorable substrates.

The mechanisms of growth-cone advance closely parallel those that underlie mobility in other cell and tissue types. Simply stated, the movement of growth cones has been associated with actin polymerization-depolymerization and myosin II-dependent contractile processes. Actin is intimately involved in the extension of filopodia (Fig. 8), whereas myosin II appears to underlie the traction-based movement of growth cones. Guidance cues appear to influence growth-cone trajectories by modulating the rate and location of actin polymerization via intracellular signaling mechanisms that appear to be mediated by transient elevations of intracellular calcium.

As this discussion has indicated, growth cones have selective chemoaffinities for molecules that attract them and induce them to form stable attachments. Proteins that lure growth cones are called neuro*tropic*. Although this term has a meaning different from neuro*trophic*, it is interesting to note that in some cases a neurotrophic factor also can exhibit neurotropic properties (Figs. 7C,D). For example, tissue-culture experiments have shown that neurites can be attracted to minute deposits of NGF at distances from their growth cones. Other molecules that have neurite-growth-promoting properties include a variety of extracellular (ECM) matrix molecules—most notably laminin and fibronectin—and various cell-adhesion molecules. Many of these molecules bind with receptors on the growth cone (e.g., integrins), which can then activate calcium-ion influx, thereby affecting stability of growth-cone attachments and directionality.

In addition to these molecular interactions, growth cones are highly responsive to physical aspects of their surrounding environment. As seen in tissue culture, growth cones can either be diverted by certain types of physical terrains or induced to grow on them.

The important point to consider in this thumbnail overview of growth-cone biology is that these structures are very dynamic, and they have the ability to sample various cellular environments and possess inherent sensitivities to different molecules that are critical to the overall success of regeneration. Thus, in addition to the injured neuron's intrinsic ability to initiate a growth response following axotomy, regeneration also is highly dependent on how the growing tip of a regenerating nerve fiber interacts with different molecular, physiological, and physical cues as it navigates toward a functionally appropriate destination.

3.3.2. DIFFERENT CELLULAR SETTINGS IN NERVE CRUSH VS TRANSECTION SITES CAN EITHER FACILITATE OR IMPEDE AXONAL OUTGROWTH

The cellular composition and geometric orientation at the site of nerve damage influences the ultimate success of regeneration by affecting how these variables can differentially affect growth-cone behavior. In the PNS, the most important cell types to consider are Schwann cells, invading macrophages, and connective-tissue elements, which together play significant roles during the immediate aftermath of nerve injury. Once growth cones emerge from the proximal nerve stumps, they must encounter the cellular and molecular microenvironment of the lesion site. The cellular composition and organization of the injury site can exhibit considerable variability depending on whether nerve damage was inflicted by crush or transection. A nerve crush, in which the integrity of surrounding epi- and perineurial connective tissue sheaths are preserved, yields the most favorable setting for unimpeded regeneration and end-organ reinnervation. This is because of a lack of scar tissue and preservation of the internal architecture of the endoneurial fascicles.

The setting of a nerve crush stands in stark contrast with what growth cones must encounter following nerve transection, when the resulting gap between the retracted cut ends is usually a very incompatible environment for directed fiber outgrowth. Proliferating cells from the proximal and distal stump endoneurium and epineurium, as well as surrounding non-neural tissues, infiltrate the wound site and form scars, which in some cases can be so dense that the nerve ends

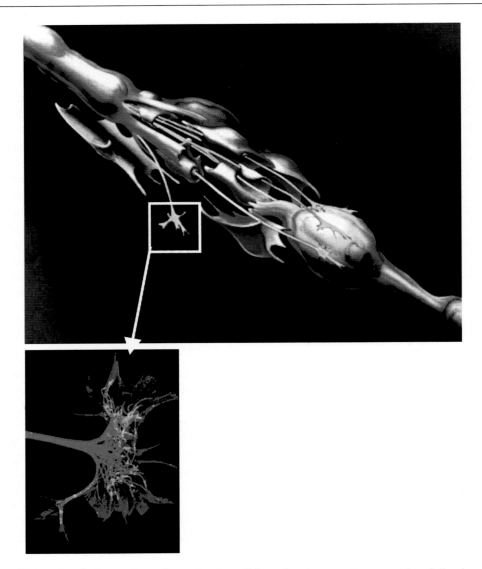

Fig. 8. The *upper illustration* depicts a three-dimensional rendition of early axonal regeneration following peripheral-nerve damage. Growth cones (e.g., *boxed profile*) are seen extending into the lesion gap (*blue profiles* representing connective tissue elements), and some make contact with Schwann cells (*red profiles*) in the distal stump. (Drawing kindly provided by Dr. Susan E. Mackinnon, Washington University School of Medicine and Barnes-Jewish Hospital). At the *lower left*, an axonal growth cone of an embryonic chick sensory neuron is shown. The growth cone is doubly stained with an antibody against tubulin (*green*), which labels microtubules, and rhodamine-phalloidin to label actin filaments red. The bundle of axonal microtubules (*green*) splays apart in the growth cone, and individual microtubules extend forward to interact with actin filament bundles and networks. These interactions between actin filaments and microtubules are important in determining directions of axonal growth and branching (*see* text). A small axonal sprout has formed at the lower left margin of the growth cone. (Figure generously provided by Paul C Letourneau, PhD, University of Minnesota.)

become blindly embedded in fibrotic tissue consisting of fibroblasts and dense collagen. In other cases, axons can wander, and may never make contact with the distal nerve stump. As the distance of the lesion gap increases, the chances of regenerating fibers reaching the distal nerve stump become progressively less, thereby negating the potential for any useful recovery.

Scarring at the wound site can likewise promote the development of highly disorganized bulbous enlargements at the cut edge of the proximal nerve stump. Such swollen structures contain a tangled meshwork of profusely branched regenerated nerve fibers, Schwann cells, fibroblasts, and collagenous matrices that collectively constitute a posttraumatic *neuroma*.

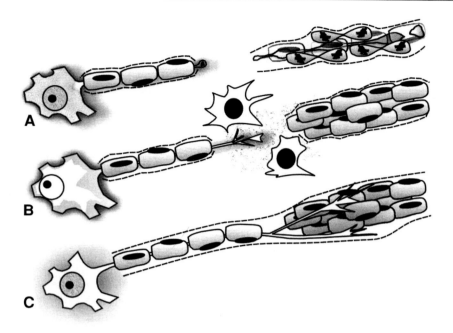

Fig. 9. Features associated with axotomy and regeneration. (**A**) Wallerian degeneration distal to axotomy with the proliferation of Schwann cells. The distal axonal segment can assume a beaded appearance during the course of axonal breakdown. At the proximal cut end, the axon assumes a bulbous profile. (**B**) An early stage of axonal outgrowth with development of the growth-cone profile extending into the connective tissue matrix of the lesion gap. Distal to the lesion, Schwann cells are aligned in longitudinal columns within an investing basal lamina (*dashed line*). (**C**) More advanced stage of regeneration, in which the growth cone has traversed the lesion gap and is growing close to the Schwann-cell tubes formed during the course of Wallerian degeneration.

The neuroma can severely impede further regeneration, and even more importantly, can be a source of painful stimuli. This is related to the close approximation of fine-caliber fibers that are incompletely isolated from each other by Schwann-cell cytoplasmic processes. In normal peripheral nerves, several unmyelinated fibers can be surrounded by a single Schwann cell, but each fiber is isolated within a trough of Schwann cytoplasm. Unmyelinated axons in a neuroma can be bundled together, as seen during early stages of peripheral-nerve development. This close approximation of fibers enables the spread of electrical current from one fiber to another. Such *ephaptic transmission* to sensory fibers can evoke disordered sensory phenomena, including pain.

3.4. Cellular Responses and Regenerative Dynamics Distal to a Nerve Injury

3.4.1. SCHWANN CELLS PROVIDE AN ESSENTIAL PERMISSIVE SUBSTRATE FOR AXONAL ELONGATION AND ARE RESPONSIBLE FOR MYELINATION OF REGENERATED AXONS

Within the first 24 h after injury, Schwann cells start to divide and reach a peak of proliferative activity by the end of the first week. Schwann-cell proliferation is typically confined within the basement membrane that originally invests each myelinated axon or group of unmyelinated fibers. Accordingly, Schwann cells and their progeny are aligned in linear arrays that are parallel to the initial trajectory of the axons they had surrounded (Fig. 9A). This results in the formation of long, linear columns of cells that in conjunction with other Schwann cell attributes can yield a favorable setting for nerve regeneration. In addition to what occurs in the distal nerve stump, when a nerve is severed, Schwann-cell proliferation at the cut ends of the distal and proximal stumps can infiltrate the lesion gap. This can result in a restoration of Schwann-cell continuity between the proximal and distal cut ends that can greatly aid in subsequent axonal regeneration. How extensively Schwann cells migrating from the proximal and distal ends meet depends on the length of the gap and degree of scarring. However, the distribution of Schwann cells at a crush site is virtually identical to that seen more distal to the lesion.

Unless otherwise hindered by adverse conditions in the lesion site, regenerating neurites reach the distal stump by as little as 3–5 d after injury, where they encounter a terrain of linearly oriented Schwann cells that were orphaned by axonal degeneration. Schwann cells have long been considered to have a significant role in peripheral-nerve regeneration. Each Schwann-cell tube is enclosed within a common basal lamina (Fig. 9B,C), and growth cones adhere closely to the inner surface of the Schwann-cell basal lamina because of their affinity for laminin, which is a major constituent. Besides this extracellular matrix protein, the Schwann cell surface also has growth-promoting, cell adhesion and recognition molecules. In general, the distal stump shows dramatic changes in gene expression involving an upregulation of neurotrophic factors, neural-adhesion molecules, cytokines, and other factors and related receptors.

Schwann cells are a source of some neurotrophic factors such as NGF. After the loss of axonal contact caused by Wallerian degeneration, Schwann cells begin to express a specific class of NGF receptors on their surfaces. At the same time, NGF synthesis and release is upregulated in these cells. By an autocrine mechanism, the newly synthesized NGF binds to receptors on Schwann cells. Meanwhile, regenerating axons express another specific class of NGF receptor that binds and retains the NGF released from the Schwann-cell receptors. This mechanism of receptor-mediated intercellular transfer of NGF subsequently leads to the stimulation of NGF-sensitive neurons. The observations pertaining to NGF provide a model for other important underlying neurotrophic factors and associated mechanisms that are operable during PNS regeneration.

Another important postnerve-injury feature is the removal of cellular debris, and the rate at which this occurs seems to influence the extent of neural regeneration. In the PNS, myelin debris resulting from Wallerian degeneration is scavenged primarily by activated macrophages, which gain access to the degenerating nerve stump through an increase in capillary permeability. In addition to debris removal, macrophages appear to play other significant roles in wound healing by producing growth factors, and certain cytokines that have neurite-growth-promoting effects. Inflammation is frequently an essential prerequisite for tissue healing, and a robust macrophage response during Wallerian degeneration in the PNS has been implicated in tissue remodeling and the establishment of an environment that can support axonal regrowth. Activated macrophages also function as secretory cells and release apolipoprotein E, which

may be important for regeneration and remyelination after nerve injury.

Once axonal contact is re-established during regeneration, Schwann cells begin to remyelinate axons in a manner analogous to peripheral myelination during development, and there is a progressive increase in the number of myelinated axons in the distal stump (Fig.10B,C; *see* also Fig.17B). There are, however, some functionally relevant morphological differences in regenerated vs. normal axons. In contrast with intact, adult axons, the myelin internodes (e.g., myelinated segments between successive nodes of Ranvier) are shorter and undergo persistent remodeling for a year or more. In addition, regenerated axons are usually of much smaller diameter with thinner myelin sheaths (Fig.10A,C) than the parent axon, and may persist as such throughout the course of regeneration. Consequently, regenerated nerves can exhibit markedly altered conduction properties.

3.4.2. Neuronal and Target Viability Are Dependent on the Rate of Axonal Elongation

The total time for regeneration to be completed entails an initial proximal stump delay, lesion delay, distal stump growth phase, and functional recovery period. The rate of axonal regeneration is influenced by a variety of factors, including the age of the patient, the location and type of injury, and the duration that the distal stump is denervated before the arrival of regenerating fibers. Generally, nerve regeneration progresses 3–4 mm/d after crush and approx 2–3 mm/d after transection injury. In humans, it has been commonly held that axonal regrowth proceeds at a relatively constant rate of one mm/d, but it has been shown that there is a diminishing rate over time, which is a function of the growing tip's distance from the cell body. Biologically, the importance of time relates to interactions between the nerve and target tissue—muscle in particular. Following denervation, as noted previously, affected muscles can become atrophic because of the loss of neurotrophic support and disuse (Fig. 5). Therefore, if the injury is a considerable distance from the target, then even under optimal, natural conditions, the chance of reinnervating viable muscle becomes increasingly remote. Since damaged neurons are dependent upon target-derived trophic support, their viability or capacity to remain in a growth mode is vitally dependent on how quickly fibers can reach their targets. If there is very protracted or limited regrowth into the distal stump, caused by extensive scarring at the lesion, then eventually the remaining

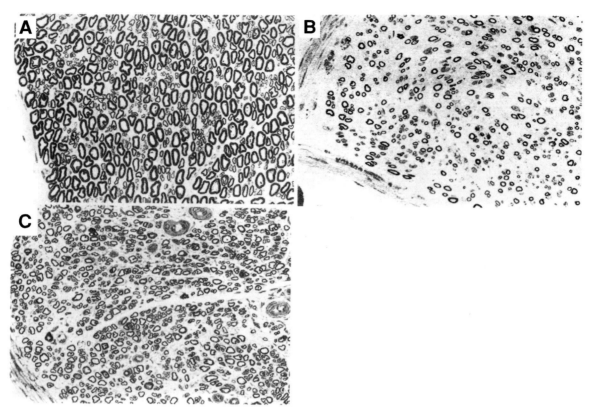

Fig. 10. (**A**) shows a cross-section of a normal peripheral nerve in which many myelinated profiles are seen. (**B**) shows an intermediate time-point during regeneration of the same peripheral nerve. Note the initial difference in the number of myelinated fibers and their smaller caliber. At a more advanced stage of regeneration (**C**), the number of myelinated axons is much greater; however, their diameters remain smaller than normal.

Schwann-cell tubes begin to decrease in number and the nerve stumps become increasingly collagenous, thereby losing many growth-promoting qualities.

3.4.3. The Fascicular Geometry of the Distal Nerve Stump Presents a Complicated Pathway for Growing Axons

Although Schwann-cell tubes provide a compatible cellular superhighway for axon regrowth, this matrix does not guarantee that fibers will reach appropriate target sites. Even at a macroscopic level, the multi-fascicular nature of a peripheral nerve, as described previously, is readily apparent (Fig. 11A). From a three-dimensional perspective (Fig. 11B), these fascicles establish a complex interconnecting landscape, and any disruption of this geometry can readily cause regenerating axons to become misdirected. Because of this, the potentially different outcomes of crush vs transection injuries become more understandable. In the latter case, one surgical approach in the case of short gaps is to suture the proximal and distal cut ends

together in such a way that perineurial fascicles are appropriately matched as much as possible, but even this approach has its limitations. Therefore, the closer the lesion is to its original sites of innervation, the greater the probability of achieving significant functional return. Overall, the functional outcome of PNS regeneration is usually not as much a question of the vigor of axonal elongation as it is an issue of axonal guidance and targeting accuracy.

3.5. Summary

This review of degeneration and regeneration in the PNS highlights several basic aspects of successful nerve regrowth that will serve as a basis for later discussions of the injured CNS. As shown in Box 2, the essential prerequisites of optimal regeneration fall under two main headings—intrinsic and extrinsic. The former refers to properties inherent to the neuron itself, whereas the latter addresses cellular environmental influences surrounding the injured neuron, especially at the level of the growth cones and regen-

---

BASIC REQUIREMENTS FOR OPTIMAL NERVE REGENERATION

Intrinsic or Native Properties of the Neuron

- Neurons that have been injured must have the metabolic capacity to initiate and maintain regrowth of damaged axons over long distances.

Extrinsic Conditions

- Regenerating axons should be able to encounter a surrounding cellular environment that is compatible (actively or passively) with fiber outgrowth.

- Ideally, the cellular terrain should provide cues (chemical, physiological, etc.) that can help guide axons to their correct targets.

- Regenerating axons should be able to respond to these cues and ultimately establish functional relationships with appropriate targets.

Box 2.

erating neurites. Thus, under optimal conditions, regeneration in the PNS can hold promise for useful functional outcomes because neurons can muster the metabolic energy to initiate and sustain an active regrowth of damaged axons through various alterations in gene expression. Furthermore, the growth cones of the newly formed neurites are exposed to a cellular and molecular milieu that, in the absence of severe scar formation and other limiting factors, is actively and passively fully compatible with fiber elongation.

4. CENTRAL NERVOUS SYSTEM INJURY: BASIC NEUROPATHOLOGY HALLMARKS

4.1. Injury to the CNS Can Lead to Neuronal and Glial Cell Death Through a Variety of Mechanisms

Extensive cell death within one or more neuronal populations can occur as a result of aging, disease, or trauma. Therefore, it is important to define the mechanisms that contribute to cell death, in terms of both minimizing degeneration and developing methods by which to encourage cellular and functional repair.

There are a number of triggers or initiators of cell death in the nervous system. The best known of these include, but are not limited to: i) direct traumatic dam-

age; ii) secondary damage (which is the aftermath of multiple pathophysiological events post-trauma); iii) withdrawal of neurotrophic support; iv) excitotoxicity, v) increased oxidative stress; vi) metabolic stress; and vii) environmental stressors such as toxins or infectious agents. The cellular response of nervous tissue to these insults can vary, and depends on many factors, including the nature and location of the injury or disease and the genetic background of the organism, as well as the maturity of the nervous system. However, despite the variety of triggers and their modulation by genetic and epigenetic factors, the subsequent biochemical processes that result in cell death are highly conserved.

4.1.1. DIRECT DAMAGE TO THE CELL BODY HAS IMMEDIATE AND DEVASTATING CONSEQUENCES

Neural cells can be damaged directly or indirectly. In the majority of cases, direct damage to the CNS initiates forces that cause vascular rupture and devastating physical insult to neurons, white-matter tracts, neuroglia, and other supporting cells. The immediate, collective outcome of this mechanical disruption is irreversible tissue destruction and death, known as *primary injury*. Although trauma is the most common cause of primary injury, other perpetrators of cellular harm (such as toxins) can act directly on nervous tissue

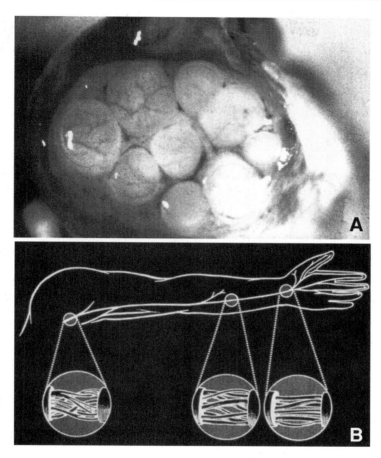

Fig. 11. The complex three-dimensional geometry of a peripheral nerve is shown macroscopically (**A**) and as a diagrammatic reconstruction (**B**). *See* text for details. (Illustrations provided by Dr. Susan E Mackinnon, Washington University School of Medicine and Barnes-Jewish Hospital.)

to primarily injure or kill cells without apparent physical trauma.

4.2. Indirect Neural Cell Damage Can Result from a Host of Pathophysiological Reactions to Insult Leading to Secondary Injury

Damage to the PNS or CNS also can adversely affect the survival of neuronal and glial populations that did not sustain direct insult. This phenomenon, termed *secondary injury*, results in tissue deterioration and cell death that becomes superimposed upon the primary injury, and can develop over a period of hours or weeks after primary tissue damage. The underlying principle of secondary injury is that damaging agents or biochemical mediators are released because of the original insult, and these byproducts of tissue damage participate in destructive reactions that create further tissue demise. Secondary damage becomes ongoing because these biochemical mediators set into action

complex, interacting and destructive feedback mechanisms. These can initiate a cascade of biochemical and pathophysiological signaling processes that can cause damage or death by themselves, or can result in the further release of damage-inducing mediators.

Many of these agents of secondary tissue damage are normally occurring cellular processes or products, which become injurious when: i) the reactions are exaggerated; ii) normal cellular safeguards are overwhelmed as a result of trauma or disease; or iii) the agents act upon previously compromised cells. As a result, cellular regulation of these pathways is lost, leading to destructive feedback cascade reactions. Experimental evidence indicates that these secondary pathophysiological processes include membrane damage, systemic and local vascular effects, inflammation, electrolyte imbalances, altered energy metabolism, neurotransmitter toxicity, and a plethora of biochemical changes leading to oxidative stress. Increasing evidence implicates these processes in widely varied CNS conditions ranging from head trauma to spinal cord injury, stroke, and some neurodegenerative diseases. For example, after spinal cord injury, considerable devastation of gray matter occurs at various distances that are rostral and caudal to the site of injury (e.g., lesion epicenter) (Fig. 12; *see also* Fig. 20). This occurs because of the disruption of blood flow and the integrity of the blood–brain barrier, inflammation, ischemia, hypoxia, edema, and many biochemical, enzymatic, and ionic alterations. Similar conditions exist after stroke and some types of head injury and may occur at less dramatic levels in neurodegenerative disease.

4.3. Necrosis and Apoptosis Are Opposite Ends of a Cell-Death Continuum

To appreciate how cells die because of nervous-system trauma or disease, the contrast must be understood between the two classically defined types of cell death, *necrosis* and *apoptosis* (Fig. 13). The form of cell death that occurs from primary injury is usually necrosis. Necrotic cell death is characterized by a loss of ionic homeostasis. Dying cells—typically in apposition to each other—have leaky membranes, and both the cell and its organelles swell and then fragment. In the process, intracellular contents spill and damage surrounding tissues, often creating an inflammatory reaction.

In contrast, apoptosis is a process by which a cell undergoes an intrinsically programmed transition from an intact, metabolically active state to cellular breakdown, with the formation of a number of membrane-bound fragments. These fragments or apoptotic bodies contain intact cellular organelles and masses of condensed DNA that are usually quickly phagocytosed by macrophages or neighboring cells. This often occurs without lysis of organelles or spillage of intracellular contents and without an accompanying inflammatory response. Apoptotic cells are found singly or in small groups, and are reduced in volume. One characteristic feature of apoptotic cell death is that cellular DNA is cleaved at internucleosomal linkages; therefore, the sizes of the resultant fragments are multiples of nucleosomal length, (e.g., 180 basepairs). These fragments give a "laddered" appearance when separated by agarose gel electrophoresis, and this is characteristic of apoptotic cell death. This form of cellular suicide may advance through the programmed stages very quickly, or over a protracted time-course.

Apoptosis is believed to be the main form of death that occurs from secondary injury.

Apoptosis of neural cells occurs as a result of highly orchestrated biochemical reactions that cleave structural and nuclear proteins in an orderly, stepwise fashion. These proteolytic reactions are catalyzed by a family of aspartyl proteases known as caspases. Normally, a balance of anti- and pro-apoptotic forces exists in the cell that is achieved by tight regulation of classes of proteins that promote or suppress neuronal apoptosis. Cell death is initiated when this balance is disrupted. The pro-apoptotic group of proteins includes the caspases, FAS, Bax and Bad, PAR-4 and *p53*. Proteins that are anti-apoptotic in nature include Bcl-2, Bcl-X, IAPs (inhibitors of apoptosis), and multiple, common cellular proteins such as antioxidants.

4.4. Apoptosis Is Not Restricted to Neurons Alone

Both neurons and glia can be affected by primary and secondary injury processes, and therefore, multiple nervous-system-cell types can undergo apoptosis. This is a critical point because of the interdependency of nervous-system cells. For example, experimental spinal cord lesions entail an initial, and, delayed wave of oligodendroglial cell death in white-matter tracts near and distant to the site of injury. Since oligodendrocytes produce myelin, post-traumatic loss of these cells could explain the persistence of spared but denuded nerve fibers. These demyelinated axons may compromise action-potential propagation and account for the functional deficits seen after injury. Furthermore, since astrocytes provide proper pH, glucose, and clearance of neurotransmitters for neurons, their death would disrupt local homeostasis and have profound effects on neuronal survival and function. Other glial cells, such as microglia, are believed to enhance regenerative processes at specific times post-injury, and to contribute to degeneration at other times or in disease processes. Thus, it is possible that the inappropriately timed death of microglia could impact regeneration and plasticity.

4.5. Multiple Pathophysiological Processes Combine to Create Secondary Injury

In summary, there are three important concepts to consider regarding cell death in the nervous system. First, cells die by both necrosis and apoptosis after injury and in neurodegenerative disease states. Second, in the nervous system, as opposed to other organ

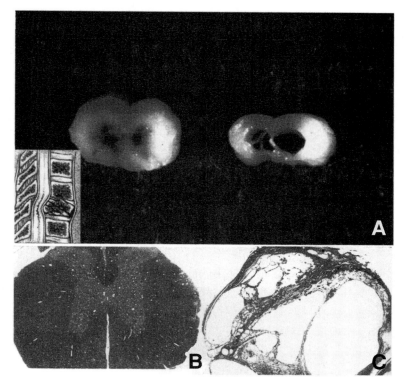

Fig. 12. Secondary tissue damage following spinal cord injury. The inset depicts damage of the spine causing trauma to the spinal cord with subsequent compression and hemorrhaging. Macroscopically (**A**) gray-matter damage is indicated by a central zone of hemorrhages early after spinal cord injury (*left*). Subsequently, tissue progressively degenerates and often leaves in its wake large cysts surrounded by varying degrees of spared white matter depending on the nature and severity of the injury (*left*). Histologically, the dramatic nature of this progressive loss of tissue and cyst formation can be readily appreciated (**C**) when compared to the appearance of a normal spinal cord (**B**).

systems, there may be a continuum between the two types of cell death so that the morphological and biochemical distinctions between the types of cell death may not always be straightforward. Third, either apoptosis or necrosis may be triggered directly by some biochemical mediators of secondary injury, or indirectly, as a result of secondary pathophysiological processes that may act in concert with each other rather than singular stimuli for cell death.

4.5.1. Oxidative Stress is a Major Cause of Neurodegeneration and a Pervasive Component of Secondary Injury

The *"free radical"* or oxidative stress theory of cellular injury has its theoretical basis in the "oxygen paradox," whereby aerobic life forms need oxygen to burn carbon and hydrogen for energy, but as part of this vital act of oxidation, *reactive oxygen species* (ROS) are produced directly or indirectly as toxic byproducts. These extremely reactive chemical moieties contain one or more unpaired electrons, and, therefore are potent oxidizers of proteins, lipids, and DNA. The process of ROS-catalyzed oxidation can irreversibly damage these cellular constituents or overwhelm repair mechanisms, with resultant cellular injury or death. This is termed *"oxidative stress."* Because of the toxicity of these ROS, and their prevalence in normal cellular reactions, several antioxidant detoxification systems have evolved in mammals. These include enzymes such as catalase, glutathione peroxidase, superoxide dismutase and antioxidants such as vitamins E and C. In the normal cell, the balance between pro-oxidant and anti-oxidant species must be maintained for cellular health, but in oxidative stress, this balance is perturbed.

Under ordinary circumstances, the nervous system is especially susceptible to oxidative stress because of its high lipid content and because gray matter has a higher metabolic rate than most tissues. Neuronal cytoplasm, axons, dendrites, and synaptic boutons pos-

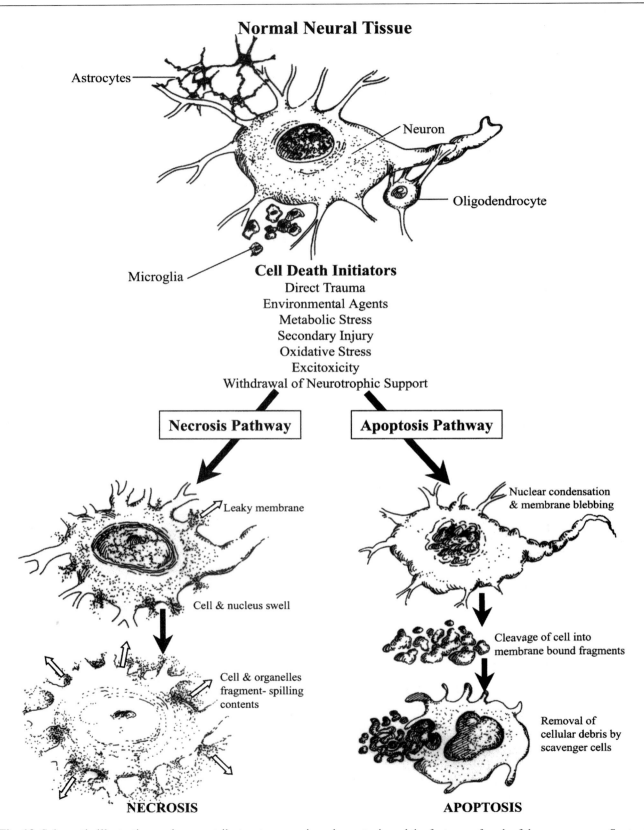

Fig. 13. Schematic illustrating various contributors to necrosis and apoptosis and the features of each of these processes. *See* text for details.

sess a large number of mitochondria. Therefore, a greater number of ROS are generated in the nervous system relative to its size in comparison to other organs. In addition, by their nature, many routine reactions in neural tissue produce free radicals. Enzymatic reactions such as the monoamine oxidase (MAO) catalyzed production of dopamine, epinephrine, and norepinephrine produce hydrogen peroxide (H_2O_2) as byproducts. The degradation of serotonin produces ROS. The neurotransmitters, glutamate, and aspartate yield ROS upon stimulation of their respective receptors. Another neurotransmitter, nitric oxide, is itself an ROS that is produced from l-arginine by the nitric-oxide synthase reaction.

The excessive production of oxygen radicals and lipid peroxides directly or indirectly during the acute phases of nervous-system trauma and ischemia has been repeatedly demonstrated. This is superimposed upon the abundant ROS that are already present in the uninjured state. Oxygen free radicals are generated from a variety of sources in the stressed or injured CNS, such as the arachidonic acid and eicosanoid cascades, excitotoxic reactions (glutamate and quinolinate), catecholamine oxidation, mitochondrial leaks, oxidation of extravasated hemoglobin, infiltrating neutrophils, activated microglia, nitric oxide, and various cytokines and growth factors. The release of heme after the hemorrhage accompanying neural trauma, significantly contributes to ROS production. The injury or neurodegenerative disease states themselves can compromise antioxidant defenses by reducing the number of viable neural cells that are available to produce antioxidants and by depleting the intracellular pool of antioxidants in individual cells.

How does increased production of free radicals harm the nervous system? Oxidative stress results in lipid peroxidation, the injurious reaction that involves free-radical attack on the double bonds of polyunsaturated fatty acids that comprise membrane phosholipids forming lipid peroxides within cell membranes and organelles. Membrane lipid peroxidation is an injurious free-radical-mediated biochemical reaction in which lipid peroxides are formed within cell membranes and organelles that can modify membrane structure, fluidity, and permeability. These oxidized lipids alter the cell structure of mitochondrial membranes and thus directly affect calcium compartmentalization, electron transport, and energy production. Membrane destruction is also accompanied by the loss of membrane-bound ionic pumps, transporters, and receptors, and this compromises tissue ionic homeo-stasis, cellular signaling, glucose uptake, and neurotransmitter clearance. Furthermore, ROS can destroy the structural integrity of protein and DNA molecules in all areas of the cell, thereby disrupting enzyme-mediated catalytic reactions and DNA repair and replication. Thus, oxidative stress can affect every major cellular function.

4.5.2. Disruption of Ionic Homeostasis Leads to Immediate Cellular Stress and Death

Malfunction of Ca^{2+} and Na^+/K^+-ATPase ionic pumps results in altered gradients of sodium, potassium, and other ions, and is a major factor in tissue destruction. Because of physical damage to membranes and transporters and sustained depolarization, injury causes large shifts of sodium from the extracellular to intracellular compartment and from the surrounding tissues and blood to the extracellular milieu. These ionic shifts are followed by massive edema at the injury site caused by cellular swelling, expansion of the potential extracellular space, and loss of the blood–brain barrier and vascular integrity. Swelling of the neuronal-cell body, promoted by the influx of Na^+ and water, is one of the primary cytological hallmarks of neuronal damage (e.g., chromatolysis) and when these fluxes are extreme, cell death occurs immediately from loss of osmotic regulation. At best, these fluid and electrolyte shifts stress the cytoarchitecture of the cell, alter its bioenergetic state and drastically decrease its ability to conduct electrical impulses, thus weakening its ability to withstand the other biochemical insults occurring after injury.

4.5.3. Alterations in Calcium Regulation and Signaling Are Primary Modalities of Cell Death

Although sodium and potassium fluxes mediate cell death directly by disruption of intracellular and extracellular fluid and electrolyte balance, alterations in cellular calcium concentrations cause death by more complicated and interacting intracellular signaling pathways. In disease or injury states, calcium compartmentalization can be dysregulated by calcium entry via voltage-sensitive calcium channels, reversal of the sodium-calcium-exchange pump, through membrane damage and ROS, and via excitotoxic mechanisms. Increased intracellular calcium has profoundly injurious effects. It induces phospholipases that affect the integrity and physiology of cellular membranes and protein kinases that alter signaling and gene expression. Apoptosis-inducing proteases and endonucleases are calcium-sensitive, and some proteins, such as calpain, cleave cellular structural proteins, thus degrading the neuronal cytoskeleton and disrupting axoplasmic transport. Increased intracellular calcium also leads to increased production of damaging ROS as by-products of eicosanoid production, activation of nitric oxide synthase, and mitochondrial reactions. The entrance of calcium into the mitochondrion through an ROS-induced transition pore disrupts mitochondrial energy production. This "multiplier effect" of calcium signaling pathways makes disruption of calcium homeostasis the most deleterious pathophysiological event of secondary injury. Similarly, increasing evidence indicates that the same is true of neurodegenerative diseases.

4.5.4. Excessive Activation of Glutamate Receptors Produces Excitotoxic Injury and Death

Trauma and certain disease states can induce widespread, massive neuronal depolarization leading to an excessive release of excitatory amino acid (EAA) neurotransmitters, such as glutamate or aspartate, which become concentrated at synaptic sites. This situation is exacerbated by traumatic disruption of glutamate-containing vesicles and reversal or malfunction of glutamate reuptake transporters. EAA-associated secondary neuronal death, known as "excitotoxicity," follows because of excessive activation of EAA receptors.

Current evidence suggests that activation of all three classes of glutamate neurotransmitter receptors (e.g., N-methyl-D-aspartate [NMDAR], α-amino-3-hydroxyl-5-methyl-4-isosoxazole-propionic acid and kainic acid [AMPA/kainate R], and metabotropic [mGLUR]), can contribute to excitotoxic processes. Each class of glutamate receptor contributes to the process in its unique way, but receptor-class cross-communication and synergy also occurs. For example, activation of any of the receptor categories can contribute in some way to calcium perturbations, mitochondrial dysfunction, and calcium activation of caspases and proteases. Many, but not all, of these processes are calcium-mediated. Calcium can enter cells directly through NMDA receptors and through special subtypes of AMPA/kainate receptors comprised of calcium-permissive subunits. mGLUR activation can alter intracellular calcium compartmentalization via phospholipase C-activated second messengers. Excessive entry of sodium through AMPA/kainate receptors can also occur and may lead to osmotically induced cell

death, and repetitive firing of this receptor class is necessary for the opening of NMDA receptors.

Excitotoxicity is believed to be a major driving force in trauma-induced injury and in some neuro-degenerative diseases such as amyotrophic lateral sclerosis. The pathways set into play by their role in calcium dysregulation augment ROS levels and may induce cytokines or transcription factors that initiate or participate in inflammatory and apoptotic cascade reactions. Nitric oxide can be produced by mGLUR activation, and reacts with peroxides to form peroxynitrate anions that are extremely toxic to cells. Arachidonic acid in conjunction with ROS enhances release of glutamate and inhibits its reuptake by neuronal and glial transporters leading to a feedback cycle of overstimulation of glutamate receptors. In this way, either acutely or chronically, excessive activation of glutamate receptors could perturb multiple cellular functions.

4.5.5. Cellular and Chemical Inflammatory Responses to Disease and Injury

The role of macrophages—one class of immune cell involved in injury—is discussed later in this chapter. However, it is well-established that many other immune cells, such as T lymphocytes, are also activated by CNS trauma, and that inflammation plays a key role in both degeneration and regeneration in the CNS. For these reasons, it is important to consider that many lipid and vascular mediators are released after trauma, and possess significant inflammatory potential. Pro-inflammatory vascular mediators, such as platelet-activating factor (PAF), prostaglandins, leukotrienes, thromboxane, and kinins are secreted immediately after injury, and can act upon leucocytes, platelets, endothelial cells, microglia, and astrocytes. Similarly, immune-system modulators such as cytokines and chemokines show immediate response patterns following injury that are characteristic to the specific category. In addition, activation of the nuclear factor-kappa B (NF-κB) family of transcription factors occurs after trauma and in disease. NF-κB is known to regulate the activation of several inflammatory genes, including tumor necrosis factor-α (TNF-α), interleukin-1β (IL-1β), and inducible nitric oxide synthase (NOS). Other immune modulators show characteristic patterns of elevation in injury and disease states. These patterns of immunomodulator regulation suggest that these substances play an important role in the recruitment of immune cells, the initiation and propagation of secondary injury, and in neurodegenerative conditions.

4.6. CNS Injury Activates a Variety of Cell Types

4.6.1. ASTROGLIAL REACTIVITY IS A COMMON CELLULAR RESPONSE TO CNS INJURY THAT IS ESSENTIALLY DIRECTED AT A FORM OF WOUND HEALING

In the case of a laceration, where the interior of the CNS is breached, astrocytes respond by reinstating a glial limiting membrane along the externalized regions of the CNS neural parenchyma (Fig. 14). The process of glial encapsulation and repartitioning of CNS from non-CNS tissue elements after injury can result in the development of dense astroglial scars—a process known as *gliosis* or *astrogliosis*. In many ways, this is similar to fibroblasts and other cells that form scars over a skin wound. Eventually, this glial capsule, which can be one or more layers thick, walls off the interior of CNS tissue from a dense, collagenous mesodermal matrix that fills the lesion analogous to the gap in a transected peripheral nerve. Some evidence suggests that the presence of connective tissue-related cells and molecules may actually stimulate this astroglial walling-off process.

Astrocytic reactivity, characterized by hypertrophy of the cell and its processes and varying degrees of proliferation, also occurs along damaged white-matter tracts, and in gray matter as an aftermath to Wallerian degeneration. In degenerated white matter, a dense astrocytic meshwork is formed over time that most notably consists of enlarged and intertwining hypertrophic astroglial processes (Figs. 14B,15). Similarly, astrocytes exhibit considerable reactivity in regions of gray matter after fiber and terminal degeneration and in response to primary or secondary neuronal death, but this usually does not develop into the extensive three-dimensional astroglial scars seen in the sites of lesions and in degenerated white matter. In general, astrogliosis appears to play a major role in filling voids in white and gray matter caused by the degeneration of cells and processes.

4.6.2. MICROGLIAL ACTIVATION ALSO ENSUES IN CNS INJURY, AND CELLULAR DEBRIS REMOVAL IS ONE MAJOR FUNCTION

During Wallerian degeneration in the PNS, macrophages are quickly recruited, and the removal of myelin and other forms of cellular debris is completed within a period of days. In contrast, myelin clearance is much slower in the injured CNS extending for even several months or more. The difference has been attributed to failure of activated peripheral macrophages to gain access into the CNS because of the blood-brain barrier. Debris removal in the brain and spinal cord is thus left to microglia, which—like astrocytes, exhibit reactivity or *microgliosis*. Microgliosis is characterized by cellular changes, including altered morphology, increases in cell size and number, and modifications in gene expression, particularly with regard to cytokines and trophic factors. Like astrocytes, microglia are known to have the capacity to synthesize a variety of pro-inflammatory cytokines that mediate chemotaxis, extravasation, and activation of leukocytes. Microglia can also transform into brain macrophages (Fig. 16 *insert*). Both astrogliosis and microgliosis run almost in tandem, although in several circumstances that have been studied, the microglial response appears to be a forerunner of the astrocytic reaction. Astro- and microglial activation usually occurs very soon after axotomy, and often well in advance of any overt signs of Wallerian degeneration *per se*. Furthermore, these glial responses are highly restricted. In the case of two adjacent white-matter tracts—one damaged, the other intact—only the former will exhibit signs of astro- and microgliosis (Fig. 16). This indicates that the signaling mechanisms involved are spatially limited.

5. CNS NEURONS EXPRESS INTRINSIC GROWTH CAPACITIES UNDER CERTAIN CONDITIONS

In terms of neuronal and glial responses, the events following CNS injury that have been described here are central to a basic appreciation of the biological setting that can affect the restoration of motor, sensory, cognitive, or autonomic modalities. With regard to neurons that survive injury, the CNS is in sharp contrast with the PNS regarding intrinsic (e.g., neuronal) and extrinsic (e.g., the surrounding cellular environment) factors that define the success or failure of axonal regrowth. Most notably, it is well-established that nerve fibers intrinsic to the CNS show an outgrowth after injury that can only extend for approx 0.5 mm. Regeneration then comes to a halt, and the newly formed sprouts die back or become stationary terminal enlargements. This transient regrowth of axons within

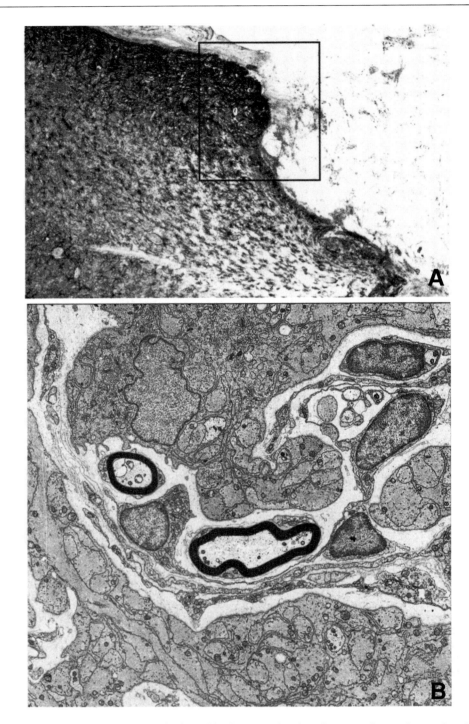

Fig. 14. In (**A**) a longitudinal section of the rat spinal cord is shown at the site of an experimental resection. The *darkly stained profiles* are astrocytes, which undergo striking changes in size and apparent number near the wound site as they attempt to wall off the interior of the breached spinal cord from non-CNS elements in the wound site. The *boxed area* illustrates a region of gliosis that is seen at the ultrastructural level in (**B**). Many compactly clustered circular and longitudinal profiles of astrocytic processes are seen along the irregular edge of the damaged spinal cord. Two axons are seen in the *center of the figure* that are myelinated by Schwann cells. These fibers are in the connective tissue matrix which the astrocytes are essentially "walling off," and nuclei of connective-tissue elements can also be seen in this region. Axons rarely are seen among the densely packed astroglial processes. (Fig. 14A kindly provided by Dr. Larry Eng, Stanford University.)

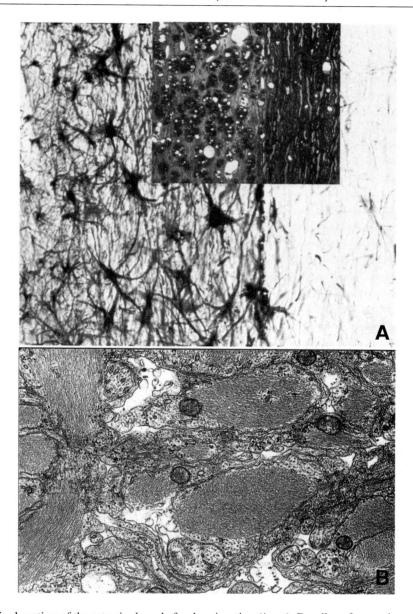

Fig. 15. (A) A longitudinal section of the rat spinal cord after hemisection (*inset*). Bundles of normal, myelinated axons are seen in white matter on the intact side of the spinal cord (*right*), but on the lesioned side (*left*), advanced degeneration is apparent and is indicated by macrophages and myelin debris (*darkly stained profiles*). The section was obtained caudal to the level of injury. Astroglial pathology resulting from the same type of surgical preparation is illustrated in (**A**) using an antibody staining technique directed at a cytoskeletal protein constituent of astrocytes. Notice the extensive astroglial reactivity in white matter on the lesioned side of the cord (*right*). (**B**) An ultrastructural view of white-matter gliosis showing numerous filament-laden large glial profiles.

the CNS has led to the long-held view of *abortive regeneration*, and it is inferred from this that most neurons confined to the brain, spinal cord, and retina lack the intrinsic metabolic ability to sustain regeneration. It has come to be recognized, however, that limited neuronal-growth dynamics are not the sole explanation for regenerative failure.

In an elegant study by Drs. Sam David and Albert Aguayo at Montreal General Hospital in 1985, evidence was obtained that led to major restructuring of basic scientific and clinical views of the potential for regeneration in the CNS. In this set of experiments, the investigators introduced one end of an autologous peripheral-nerve segment into the midthoracic spinal

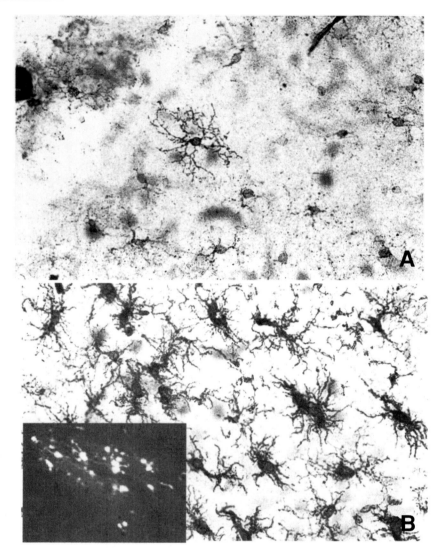

Fig 16. Microgliosis. (**A**) Resting, ramified (e.g., process-bearing) microglia are seen in the normal CNS, which under pathological conditions (**B**) increase in number and exhibit hyperramification as reactive microglia. *(Inset)* A high power view of the region of spinocerebellar retrograde cell death in Fig. 4. The label used to mark these neurons prior to the spinal hemisection has leached out of the dying neurons and have been phagocytosed by microglia that play a role in debris removal after CNS injury. (Fig. 16A and B were kindly provided by Dr. WJ Streit, University of Florida McKnight Brain Institute.)

cord region of an experimental rat and inserted the other end of the nerve graft into the medulla (Fig. 17). An axon-free bridge (recall that Wallerian degeneration is in progress), consisting of Schwann cells and other peripheral-nerve-tissue elements, was made that extended several mm from end to end. Subsequently, neuroanatomical tracing methods were used to determine whether axons had grown into the peripheral-nerve bridge and if so, to identify the cells from which such axons originated and their destination after leaving the peripheral-nerve grafts. The results of that

study and subsequent approaches using Schwan cells (Fig. 17B) showed that neurons intrinsic to the CNS could extend fibers into these bridges and that these axons could then traverse the length of the grafts. Such peripheral/central nervous system grafting experiments have been instrumental in reversing previous theories by demonstrating that neurons in the brain, spinal cord, or retina have an inherent capacity to sustain long-distance axonal elongation, even after previous injury. In some cases, the elongation of axons exceeded the distances originally exhibited by compa-

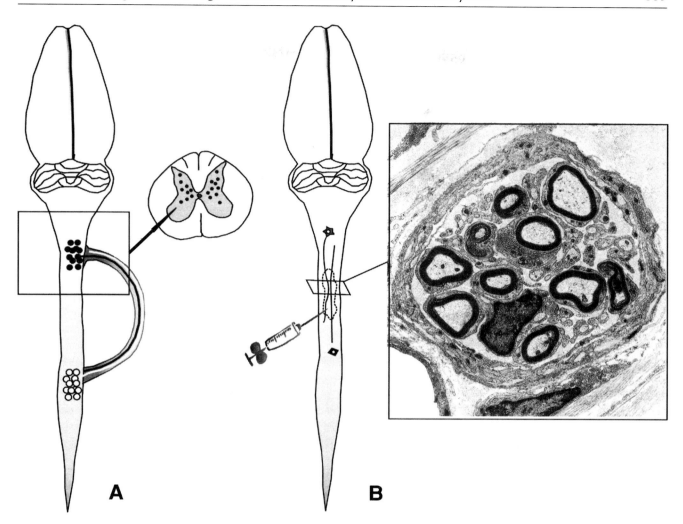

Fig. 17. Two examples of peripheral (PNS) to central nervous system (CNS) grafting experiments that have illustrated the intrinsic capacity of CNS neurons to initiate and sustain axonal growth over substantial distances when the CNS cellular microenvironment is replaced by that of the PNS. (**A**) A peripheral nerve bridge formed between the lower medulla/upper cervical spinal cord and upper lumbar spinal cord. Neuroanatomical tracing subsequently showed axons extending through such grafts. Neurons from which the axons in peripheral nerve grafts arose were demonstrated by a retrograde tracing method (*filled and unfilled circles*), and their distribution in spinal gray matter is illustrated by the accompanying transverse section of the spinal cord (*arrow*). (**B**) Schwann cells that were grown in tissue culture are injected into the rat spinal cord, where they form an intraspinal SC bridge in the completely transected, adult rat thoracic cord. Several weeks after transplantation, numerous fibers have regenerated into the bridge as seen in the accompanying electron micrograph. Such profiles are very similar to what is seen during peripheral-nerve regeneration, as described and illustrated above. (The electron micrograph was kindly provided by Drs. Henglin Yan and Mary Bartlett Bunge, The Miami Project to Cure Paralysis, University of Miami School of Medicine.)

rable neuronal populations during development. In addition to revealing such remarkable growth potential, some studies indicate that certain functional synaptic connections can be re-established in the mature CNS through peripheral/central nervous system grafts. Therefore, some degree of appropriate target recognition and functional re-innervation can occur, even in the mature CNS, when regeneration is induced.

6. A BALANCE BETWEEN INTRINSIC AND EXTRINSIC FACTORS GOVERNING AXONAL REGENERATION

A corollary to the demonstration of regenerative potential in the injured CNS with peripheral-nerve grafts is that such a capacity can only be seen when the CNS cellular environment is replaced by a milieu of peripheral-nervous-system tissue elements. Thus, regeneration in the CNS can be elicited when a nonpermissive tissue terrain is substituted by a permissive one. This principle becomes more apparent when centrally derived axons growing through these peripheral-nervous-system grafts begin exiting at the opposite end. Invariably, fibers stop elongating soon after their growth cones re-establish contact with CNS tissue. For many years, researchers have held the notion that a major limitation to regeneration in the CNS was the absence of cells (e.g., Schwann cells) that could facilitate axonal regrowth via a permissive milieu involving the elaboration of neurotrophic and neurotropic factors. Several other nonpermissive environmental conditions have now been identified that center on the inhibitory effects of astroglial scars and CNS white matter. Inadequate inflammatory responses, coupled with protracted debris removal, have also been implicated.

As a prelude to the following discussion, it should be emphasized that the problem of regenerative failure in the CNS is a complex one, and there are no hard and fast rules. Accordingly, regenerative failure is not always caused exclusively by the presence of any one or more nonpermissive tissue environments; it also can be coupled with modest growth responses exhibited by different populations of injured neurons. In fact, several studies have shown that the administration of certain neurotrophic factors can significantly enhance the vigor of axonal elongation in the presence of cellular environments, which otherwise would be major obstacles.

6.1. Astroglial Scarring Can Impede Axonal Outgrowth

Astrogliosis, as described previously, is a hallmark feature of CNS injury that has long been considered to be one impediment to CNS regeneration. There are several examples of the inhibitory effects of reactive astrocytes on growing axons. To provide some perspective, one illustration involves dorsal-root axons, which after injury, regenerate and advance vigorously within the peripheral-nervous-system compartment of an injured spinal sensory root. Then, as they reach the spinal cord-dorsal root entry zone, these axons either terminate as large bulbous enlargements or synapse-like structures, assume random growth patterns, or are deflected back toward the spinal ganglion of origin (Fig. 18). This region, also known as the peripheral/central nervous system transition zone, is character-

ized by a progressive shift from a peripheral-nervous-system cellular environment to a CNS tissue terrain. The altered axonal growth pattern at this interface appears to be associated with the presence of enlarged astrocytic processes that are interspersed with Schwann cells and endoneurial connective tissue.

Because of the complex network of enlarged and intertwined cytoplasmic processes that characterize astroglial scars, (Figs. 14,15) one is left with the impression that such scars are physical obstacles to growing axons. However, specific biosynthetic properties of reactive astrocytes may have a more direct relationship to glial inhibition of axonal elongation. Several well-defined chemorepellant or growth-inhibitory molecules, some of which are major extracellular matrix (ECM) constituents, have been identified as being produced by reactive astrocytes.

6.2. White Matter-Associated Inhibition

Experimental evidence also indicates that several proteins associated with myelin and myelin-producing oligodendrocytes may contribute to growth cone collapse and overall regenerative failure in the CNS. Early experiments showed that when axons growing in tissue culture encounter substrates that are white matter-like, the neurites stop growing (Fig. 19). For that matter, in some cases neuritic outgrowth can be impaired by oligodendrocytes and CNS myelin even when potent stimulators of neuritic elongation, such as neurotrophic factors, are readily accessible. However, if the same cultures have peripheral-nervous-system-coated substrates as well, then the neurites will preferentially extend toward the PNS rather than CNS surfaces. One of the myelin-associated proteins that can squelch axonal outgrowth is referred to as Nogo-A, and various experiments have shown that its inhibitory effect can be circumvented by neutralizing this protein with a specific antibody. From a histological perspective, it is not surprising that some myelin-associated inhibitors of axonal outgrowth are associated with glial scar formation because evolving astrogliotic regions often have large, interspersed accumulations of myelin debris even long after injury (Fig. 15, *insert*). Despite many lines of compelling evidence, there are some contrasting observations suggesting that under certain experimental conditions myelin-inhibition does not apply to all neuronal populations to the same degree. Again, this may be reflective of the critical balance between intrinsic and extrinsic controls of axonal regeneration.

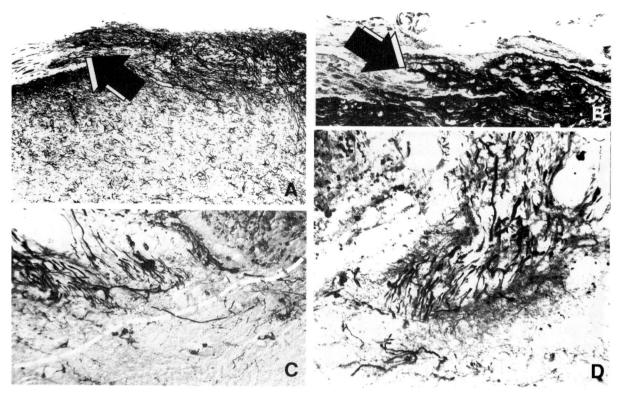

Fig. 18. Damage to central processes of dorsal-root ganglion cells leads to a striking degree of astrogliosis at the dorsal-root entry zone (DREZ, *arrow*), as seen from this comparison of normal (**A**) and (**B**) reactive DREZs in the adult rat spinal cord. This glial reactivity and associated expression of nonpermissive ECM molecules is thought to be at least partially responsible for the failure of regenerating dorsal root fibers to re-enter the spinal cord. As shown below (**C,D**), such axons approach the PNS–CNS transition zone, where they either turn back on themselves or form terminal endbulbs. Similar observations can be made in the case of CNS lesions.

6.3. Slow Removal of Cellular Debris

As discussed previously, monocyte recruitment from the blood and macrophage activity in the CNS do not evolve as quickly in the CNS as in the PNS after injury. There is some indication that this may be related to an absence of induction of the complement system since complement attracts and activates macrophages in the PNS. The persistence of myelin-related axonal growth inhibitors and repellant molecules represents a logical result of inefficient debris removal in the injured CNS. However, the lack of activated macrophages in the damaged CNS has other implications. For example, although post-injury inflammation can have deleterious effects on neuronal survival, activated macrophages are also known to produce various cytokines that can lead to the expression of neurotrophic factors and other neurite-promoting molecules that are conducive to axonal growth. Once again, this principle is exemplified by experiments that

involve regeneration of dorsal-root fibers after rhizotomy. While phagocytic activity is robust within the peripheral-nervous-system milieu of the central roots, it is initially quiescent at the peripheral/central nervous system transition zone and further centrally. However, if activated macrophages are introduced, then regeneration through the otherwise impenetrable dorsal-root entry zone is substantially facilitated.

7. THE INJURED CNS HAS SOME INTRINSIC POTENTIAL FOR SELF-REPAIR: CONCEPT OF NEUROPLASTICITY

7.1. Denervation Can Be a Growth Stimulus for Axonal Growth from Uninjured Neurons

Before proceeding further with a discussion of potential interventions for promoting regeneration in the CNS, it is important to note that there are many examples of compensatory phenomena in the dam-

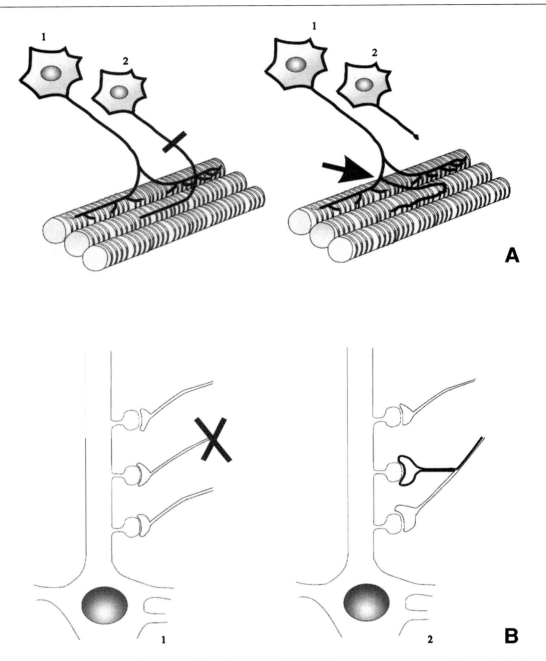

Fig. 19. Collateral or terminal sprouting in the (**A**) peripheral and (**B**) CNS. Axotomy of a neuron (2) results in the emergence of a new collateral (*arrow*) from the uninjured cell (1). The new axonal outgrowth reinnervates the postsynaptic region originally occupied by the presynaptic terminal of neuron 2. In the CNS (**B**), a neuron has three separate sources of axonal input on neighboring dendritic spines. After one input is eliminated by a lesion (1), reactive synaptogenesis occurs (2), whereby a new synapse is made with the denervated spine by short-range outgrowth of a collateral axonal process from a neighboring uninjured axon.

aged brain and spinal cord that demonstrate some biological potential for spontaneous functional recovery in the CNS. Collectively, this is referred to as *functional neuroplasticity*, which can include various mechanisms involving anatomical reorganization, neurophysiology, neuropharmacology, and other modalities as well. Experiments first performed over 50 yrs ago demonstrated the principle of *collateral*

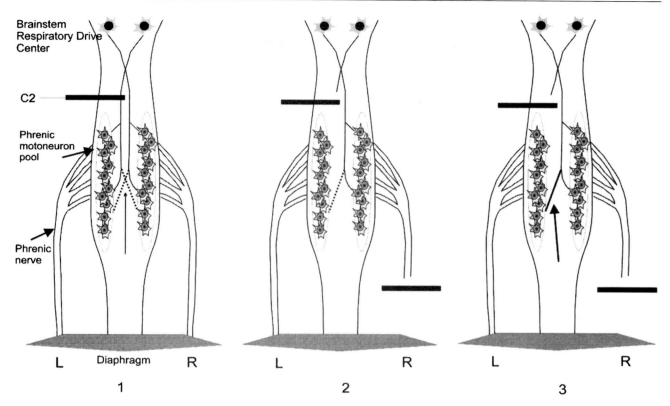

Box 3. An illustration of functional neuroplasticity in the spinal cord involving brainstem inspiratory drive to the phrenic motoneuron pool in the adult rodent spinal cord. (**1**) The normal organization of this system involves descending bulbospinal pathways from respiratory premotor neurons in the brainstem which project directly (i.e., monosynaptically) onto spinal phrenic motoneurons at C3-C5. Also present are midline collaterals from these descending pathways which cross at the level of the phrenic nucleus (*dashed lines, arrow*). These collaterals are normally nonfunctional. (**2**) A unilateral lesion (*left-sided* in this example) of the spinal cord at C2 interrupts the bulbospinal fibers thereby denervating the phrenic motoneurons and thus causing a hemiparalysis of the ipsilateral diaphragm. (**3**) Under certain conditions involving respiratory stress (e.g., asphyxic challenge due to a contralateral phrenic nerve transection [i.e., phrenicotomy]), the otherwise physiologically latent midline collaterals from the intact bulbospinal pathway on the right side of the spinal cord can sprout and become functional such that they will provide some inspiratory drive to the original denervated phrenic motoneurons on the left side of the cord. Some diaphragm function ipsilateral to the original hemilesion is thus restored. This example of neuroplasticity involving the activation and other functionally relevant morphological changes associated with a previously "silent" population of fibers is referred to as the *crossed phrenic phenomenon* (*see* text for additional details).

sprouting by showing that when some nerve fibers to a muscle are transected, neighboring intact fibers projecting to the same muscle begin to extend accessory neuritic branches, and subsequently innervate the partially deafferented muscle (Fig. 19A). The same principle was later extended to the CNS in studies documenting that denervation of a neuronal target can lead to the sprouting of adjacent fiber systems and the formation of new synapses onto the denervated cell (Fig. 19B). This type of growth offers an explanation of cellular events that can be associated with restored normal functions, the emergence of inappropriate functions, or the development of compensatory behaviors. Collateral sprouting does not take place over long distances, and it is generated by previously uninjured cells. Such forms of axonal growth thus have little significance in terms of regeneration *per se*.

7.2. Functional Plasticity Occurs in the Injured Brain and Spinal Cord and Is Often Activity-Dependent

Many examples of functional neuroplasticity in the CNS, most extend beyond the scope of this chapter. However, one relevant illustration to provide an immediate frame of reference is the *crossed phrenic phenomenon*. As described in Box 3, this is an example

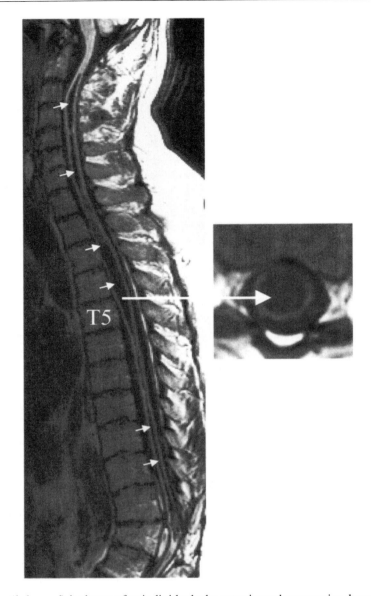

Fig. 20. A sagittal MR image (*left panel*) is shown of an individual who experienced progressive degeneration of spinal cord tissue over the course of 30 yr following an initial spinal injury at T_{12} (*see* text for more details). A continuous cystic cavitation (*arrows*) is seen extending to the level of C_2. A transverse MRI taken at T_5 is highlighted to the right, showing a large cyst and a thin rim of surrounding white matter. Extensive gray-matter loss is also suggested at mid-cervical levels (e.g., region of phrenic motoneurons), however, no respiratory compromise or severe upper-extremity motor abnormalities were noted other than a gradual weakening of strength.

of short-range sprouting with accompanying activation of previously silent circuits that can lead to functional recovery in a pool of neurons previously silenced because of an interruption of descending fiber projections and resulting denervation. Although the type of combined injuries that were required to show the existence of this phenomenon are not ones encountered clinically, there are examples of high cervical injuries in animals and humans that result in varying degrees of spontaneous recovery of diaphragm function that may be mediated by a crossed phrenic phenomenon-like mechanism.

Ironically, some of the more striking examples of neuroplasticity is derived from neuropathology. In Parkinson's disease, for instance, approx 80% of the dopaminergic neuronal population of the substantia nigra can degenerate before the first motor signs and symptoms are detected. Figure 20 depicts an even more remarkable example of this principle. Shown is an magnetic resonance (MR) image of an individual who had a spinal cord injury at T_{12}, which resulted in severe lower-extremity weakness and partial paralysis. This person eventually regained significant ambulatory capabilities with the assistance of bracing and a cane or walker. Approximately 30 yrs after the initial injury, this individual began experiencing upper-extremity weakness as well as greater ambulatory difficulty. However, there was no evidence of abnormal sensory manifestations such as allodynia, or deteriorated upper-extremity function. Routine pulmonary function testing also showed that performance was within normal limits. Surprisingly, subsequent MR examination showed extensive degeneration of the spinal cord from the original level of injury at T_{12} to C_1–C_2. This is an example of a slowly progressing secondary degeneration of spinal cord tissue that occurs in a small subset of individuals who previously sustained a spinal cord injury. These examples illustrate the idea that very devastating, slowly evolving pathologies do not lead to the immediate and extensive functional losses that would accompany acute traumatic injuries with comparable degrees of large-scale necrosis and apoptosis. This basic tenet of neuropathology can only be explained by the fact that dramatic levels of cellular reorganization and functional compensation must be simultaneously superimposed on the degenerative process.

Although it is generally believed that cortical plasticity is more vigorously exhibited in the developing nervous system, studies have shown that a similar capacity also exists in the mature brain. Neurophysiological, neuroanatomical, and various imaging approaches, including functional MRI, have provided a large body of evidence that points toward experience- or activity-dependent modifications in receptive-field properties, cellular functional organization and domains, and synaptic efficacy even in the adult CNS. Therefore, the mature nervous system is more mutable than once believed and maps of the motor and sensory cortices are now known to be more labile and capable of extensive modifications based on environment and behavioral experiences. Denervation of specific limb regions can result in the corresponding cortical area of representation being remapped to represent adjacent unaffected regions of that limb. This principle also extends to auditory, visual, and motor areas among other cortical regions. For example, motor learning—especially when it involves training in new tasks requiring fine and repetitive motor skills, can produce predictable alterations in movement-related representations in the motor cortex.

Many instances of cortical reorganization and adaptive plasticity are seen in studies of human stroke patients and experimental animal models of brain attack. In adult subhuman primates with focal ischemic lesions, it has been shown that subtotal damage restricted to a finite representation of a hand can extend to further loss of hand representation in the adjacent, undamaged cortex, as well as changes in other more remote cortical areas. These changes relate to functional/anatomical maps as well as to underlying cellular modifications in the arborizations of dendrites and changes in the distributions of different types of synaptic profiles.

7.3. Synaptic Reorganization and the Reacquisition of Certain Functions Can Be Modulated by Training

This newly discovered appreciation of cortical neuroplasticity that can be expressed under different circumstances has formed an important new basis and rationale for neurorehabilitative medicine. In the example of focal ischemic damage in the monkey just described, ensuing alterations in adjacent cortical regions could be prevented by retraining skilled hand (affected) use, and such training led to behavioral improvements. These findings have suggested that forced use of an affected upper extremity in human subjects may promote motor recovery by modulating reorganization in neighboring regions of undamaged cortex, thereby underscoring the concept of activity-dependent plasticity. Similar approaches may ultimately prove useful for cerebral palsy and other brain disorders. Rehabilitative training approaches are showing recovery of walking patterns in some individuals who have been paralyzed by spinal cord injury. Coupled with these observations, when spared fiber systems have assumed functions of damaged tracts, these findings raise the intriguing possibility of some neurological deficits being more reversible than previously believed. Neuroplasticity-based rehabilitation will undoubtedly serve as an adjunct to a broad spectrum of novel therapeutic approaches being investigated for treating brain and spinal cord disease or trauma, as discussed in the following section.

8. POTENTIAL INTERVENTIONS TO PROMOTE CNS REGENERATION ARE BASED ON CELLULAR RESPONSES TO INJURY AND DISEASE

The purpose of this comprehensive overview of the many neural and non-neural responses to neuronal damage is to provide a basis for understanding the rationale for the bold interventions now being investigated as possible treatments to promote regeneration and functional recovery in the CNS. To facilitate the regenerative potential of the CNS, therapeutic strategies must be directed at specific aspects of neuronal injury at the level of the cell body, lesion site, in regions of Wallerian degeneration, and at denervated target sites. These therapies must promote neuronal survival and stimulate intrinsic genetic programs for the initiation and maintenance of axonal outgrowth. Other approaches must render the cellular environment more permissive to axonal elongation. At the same time, re-establishment of connectivity must be facilitated through methods to encourage anatomical and functional plasticity as growth cones advance near prospective target sites and establish new synapses. Finally, in the event of neuronal cell death, efforts will be required to replace lost cells.

It is self-evident that the most effective therapeutic approaches will rely on a combination of these treatment modalities. Furthermore, as the previous discussion on neuroplasticity suggests, orchestrated rehabilitative approaches are likely to be at the core of most combinatorial treatments in the future. The remainder of this chapter is a summary of experimental strategies and related technologies that currently appear to offer promise for promoting regeneration in the CNS by enhancing neuronal survival, strengthening neuronal regenerative responses, improving the cellular environment at and distal to the site of axotomy, promoting remyelination, and replacing cells that have died.

8.1. Injured Neurons at Risk of Atrophy or Imminent Apoptosis Can Be Rescued

Understandably, optimization of regeneration and functional outcomes in the CNS is critically dependent upon maximizing the survival of neurons that are at risk of apoptotic death. In theory, this should be achievable in the case of traumatic injury by using pharmacological or *neuroprotective* approaches directed at key biochemical, neurochemical, and molecular mechanisms associated with secondary tissue damage, as previously discussed. By attenuating second-

ary events, the rescue of cells could translate into less severe neurological deficits and improved functional outcomes in many disorders. For example, administration of the steroid methylprednisolone within a few hours after spinal trauma has had significant neuroprotective effects. This is attributed to the antioxidant action of this compound, which minimizes lipid peroxidation and membrane lysis that otherwise lead to neuronal and glial cell death.

Additional pharmacological interventions are focused at the excitotoxic component of the secondary neuronal responses occurring as part of certain neurodegenerative diseases (e.g., Huntington's disease) or as the sequelae to spinal cord or brain injury, stroke, hypoglycemia, and hypoxia. Certain competitive and noncompetitive glutamate-receptor antagonists have shown therapeutic promise in blocking the binding of excitatory amino acids and reducing cellular toxicity after CNS injury.

Other ways in which neuronal rescue can be achieved involve the use of neurotrophic factors or the activation of antiapoptic genes to prevent cell death or neuronal atrophy. One approach to this involves the introduction of genes that encode for specific molecules into cell lines that are subsequently grafted into the CNS. For example, genetically engineered cells that express NGF have been shown in experimental models to contribute to an enhanced survival and axonal regeneration by NGF-responsive septal neurons that would otherwise die after axotomy. Novel genes also have been introduced directly into CNS neurons *in situ* (Fig. 21) by way of benign viral platforms. Using this approach, transduced cells can contribute to their own rescue in an autocrine fashion, or to the survival of surrounding neurons by way of a paracrine mechanism.

8.2. The Regenerative Potential of CNS Neurons Can Be Enhanced

The molecular foundation of neuronal growth is becoming rapidly defined with the advent of new technologies such as differential gene expression and proteomics. The knowledge gained from these techniques will elucidate appropriate molecules for such strategies as gene delivery. Some of these may influence the synthesis and transport of cytoskeletal elements involved in axonal structure and growth cone mobility, as discussed earlier. One molecule of particular interest has been a growth-associated protein (GAP-43), which is produced by neurons during development and mature neurons that are capable of

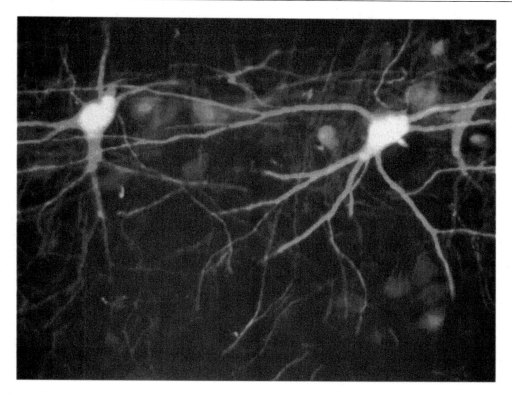

Fig. 21. This micrograph provides an example of the application of in vivo gene delivery. An injection was made into the rat spinal cord of a benign virus (adeno-associated virus), which was constructed to carry a novel gene that encodes for the synthesis of a nonmammalian protein, which emits an intense green signal under fluorescence microscopy. In this illustration, two of many transduced spinal neurons are shown, thus illustrating how it may be possible to alter regenerative properties of neurons through the introduction of genes that could stimulate synthesis of growth-promoting molecules.

sustaining renewed growth after nerve damage. GAP-43 is conveyed from the cell body to the axon by fast axoplasmic transport, and represents one of the more abundant constituents of the growing tips of regenerating axons. With recent technical advances in gene profiling such as DNA microarrays, it is likely that many more molecules will be identified that play important roles in initiating and maintaining nerve regeneration. Also, neurotrophic factors may play vital roles in gene delivery, as some investigations already suggest, because of their ability to trigger regeneration-friendly metabolic responses through intracellular signalling pathways.

8.3. CNS Lesions Can Be Bridged and Neurotrophic Factors Provided Locally

As PNS-to-CNS grafting experiments have illustrated, a variety of neuronal types in the adult brain and spinal cord can regenerate axons for long distances when presented with an appropriate tissue substratum. Neurons in the brain and spinal cord also appear capable of making new connections with appropriate targets when presented with favorable growth conditions. So, another focus of therapeutic development is aimed at improving the cellular microenvironment at the lesion site. This involves providing a compatible cellular substratum with appropriate neurotrophic factors, extracellular matrix proteins, and cell adhesion molecules. Some cells, such as Schwann cells, are capable of providing such cocktails in themselves (Fig. 17B), and experiments with Schwann Cells have provided insight for other cell-based strategies to circumvent the nonpermissive nature of the CNS. This includes grafting genetically modified cells that can secrete molecules which favor axonal growth. Some other investigations raise the possibility for developing artificial polymeric matrices containing molecules that can nurture axonal regeneration. It is important to consider that the success of any bridging method will be dependent on the elements used and the inhibitory nature of the scar matrix at the borders of the lesion, as well as the nonpermissive nature of the CNS at more distant levels.

8.4. Options Are Beginning to Emerge for Improving the Cellular Milieu Away from the Injury Site

Once axons traverse a lesion site, they must navigate through an unfriendly CNS cell environment to reach their original or alternative postsynaptic sites. There is increasing information about the identity and nature of nonpermissive molecules, such as those associated with white matter, and strategies are being developed for clinical application that are designed to immunologically neutralize these molecules with specific antibodies that may entail simple vaccination schemes. Similarly, specific guidance molecules and other growth-promoting substances may be used to stimulate regeneration in the same way that would be required for some combined therapies for bridging lesions.

Improving the cellular environment also means expediting the removal of cellular debris that may be depots of inhibitory molecules. Controlled enhancement of macrophage activation in the CNS and phagocytosis of myelin debris could be beneficial. One approach, now being tested in clinical trials, involves grafting of activated peripheral macrophages into the injured spinal cord. Similarly, there is some evidence that grafts of cultured microglia may have a stimulatory effect on axonal regeneration. Recently, several chemokines and cytokines also have been identified that appear to control the postinjury immune response associated with rapid removal of myelin debris in the CNS. These types of basic science findings are paving the way for the development of rational cellular and pharmacological therapies.

8.5. Interactive Training and Related Approaches Can Be Employed to Make New Connections Work

In some laboratory experiments, it has been shown that although central axons do not extend very far after exiting from Schwann-cell bridges, they can make occasional, functionally appropriate connections with postsynaptic neurons in the immediate vicinity of the peripheral-nervous-system-graft-CNS interface. This and other lines of evidence suggest that some target recognition is possible even in the chronically injured CNS. Point-to-point accurate connectivity, however, is more likely to be the exception than the rule until the molecular foundations of axonal pathfinding and target recognition are more fully understood. Furthermore, even when some useful synapses are re-estab-

lished, the efficacy of those connections may need to be reinforced, since they will probably be suboptimal in number.

It is more likely that novel projections and circuits will be formed as more and more regeneration is encouraged. These new connections will require reprogramming to be functional. In that case, it is possible that such unique circuitries could be an engineered form of neuroplasticity. In order to optimize functional outcomes achieved by any therapeutic strategy, activity-dependent mechanisms will need to be invoked by either interactive training (e.g., programmed rehabilitation) or neuropharmacological stimulation. Computer-assisted prosthetics and similar facilitative devices, which are currently being used in lieu of volitional function, also can be envisioned as vital components of the overall therapeutic puzzle that is now being pieced together.

9. CAN CELLS THAT DIE BECAUSE OF NECROSIS OR APOPTOSIS BE REPLACED?

Regardless of the efficacy of neuroprotection, it is inevitable that some significant cell loss will be experienced. In the case of trauma, nothing can stop tissue necrosis at the site of injury, and some secondary tissue damage seems unavoidable even under optimal circumstances. For many years, the inability to replace dying cells represented an insurmountable biological obstacle to CNS repair. When coupled with the intrinsic and extrinsic limitations to regeneration, this failure contributed to a pervading sense of clinical pessimism that is now being gradually reversed. Cell replacement is now a more feasible objective in many neuropathological conditions, and may be accomplished through transplantation approaches involving cells from various sources including embryonic- and adult-derived neural and nonneural stem cells. Some speculation is now being expressed that cellular replacement could someday be facilitated through endogenous mechanisms involving resident populations of neural stem or progenitor cells.

9.1. Neuroplasticity in the CNS May Also Eventually Involve Neuronal Replacement and Self-Repair Via Endogenous Stem Cells and Trophic Factor Expression

Neurons are postmitotic cells, and thus are unable to generate new progeny. In medical neuroscience,

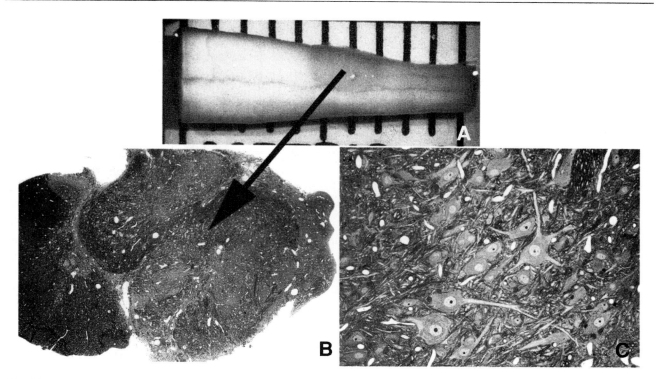

Fig. 22. Transplantation of cells from various sources, including stem cells from adult neural and non-neural structures, may provide one component of future therapies for promoting repair of the CNS. The potential of such cell-replacement strategies has been suggested by years of experimental fetal CNS tissue transplantation experiments. One example is the reconstruction of lesions in the adult rat spinal cord. (**A**) A macroscopic view of a fixed spinal specimen in which a graft of embryonic rat spinal cord was placed into a hemisection cavity. Four months later, a large transplant can be seen in what otherwise would have been a cavity such as illustrated in Fig. 14. (**B**) A transverse histological section through the graft site in (**A**) shows a large transplant (*arrow*) fused with the intact half of the host spinal cord on the left half of the micrograph. (**C**) At higher magnification, the graft in (**B**) contains a normal complement of neurons and glia and is well-vascularized.

one tenet has been that humans are born with a full complement of neurons that are irreplaceable if lost or damaged. It is now recognized that cell populations exist in the developing and adult CNS that have neural stem- or progenitor-like characteristics and can give rise to new neurons and glia. For example, neurogenesis has been demonstrated throughout life in the hippocampus and olfactory bulbs of several species. In addition, some evidence indicates that apoptosis in some regions of the mammalian neocortex can induce neurogenesis to the extent that replacement neurons repopulate areas of tissue destruction in a layer- and region-specific manner, and can re-establish appropriate corticothalamic projections. These neural stem cells may even be multipotential, as suggested by data showing that under certain conditions these cells can convert to hematopoietic elements.

Neurons are not the only cells in the CNS at risk of death. For example, oligodendrocytes are lost in the demyelinating disease multiple sclerosis (MS), as well as in many cases of blunt trauma, as noted previously. For many years, the potential for endogenous replacement of these cells was vigorously debated. However, considerable evidence now indicates that oligodendroglial progenitor cells are present in the adult brain and spinal cord, and are capable of giving rise to new oligodendrocytes.

In light of previous discussions of activity-dependent plasticity, it is interesting that correlations have been found between the level of new neuron production in the brain and certain environmental and behavioral variables. In fact, physical activity has been linked to neurogenesis in the mature hippocampus, which as noted previously, also appears to be associated with functional recovery from injury. The occurrence of neurogenesis in the adult brain and its enhancement by activity adds to the strong evidence for activity-dependent induction of neurotrophic factors and increased synaptic efficacy. The role of activity in neurogenesis further underscores the important role of rehabilitation in optimizing recovery from CNS injury or disease. In addition, these findings set the stage for a radical change in how scientists and clinicians view prospects for long-range improvements in clinical outcomes in CNS disorders.

9.2. Neuronal and Oligodendroglial Replacement Can Be Achieved With Neural and Nonneural Cellular Grafts

In view of the presence of endogenous neural stem cells, an ideal strategy for repair in many CNS disorders would focus on fostering intrinsic cellular replacement. Many issues must be resolved, however, before this can become a reality. For example, little is currently known as to how to recruit and mobilize endogenous stem-cell populations in sufficient numbers. An immediate alternative is to replace degenerated neurons and oligodendrocytes via transplantation of cells. Many years of extensive research involving transplants of fetal CNS tissue has provided an important experimental template for this approach at both the basic science and clinical levels. Although fetal grafts are unlikely to be the therapy of choice for the future, such tissue has provided a clear indication that it is possible to replace discrete populations of dying or dysfunctional neurons in the CNS of newborn, juvenile, and adult recipients (Fig. 22). Neuroanatomical methods have demonstrated that axonal projections can develop between host and donor tissues. Host neurons also are capable of forming some afferent and efferent synaptic interactions with grafted embryonic cells. These connections can contribute to the development of functional neural circuitries, as demonstrated electrophysiologically in several regions of the mature CNS. Many examples of behavioral recovery also have been reported for several experimental models of neurological disease and trauma.

Although discussions of some bench-to-bedside translation of the fetal-tissue transplantation experience in Parkinson's disease have drawn attention to potential adverse effects, these concerns can be resolved. Many efforts are underway to identify other sources of donor tissue. The potential alternatives encompass a range of neural and non-neural cell types. Among some of the more promising sources of cells are those that can be found in the adult. These include neural stem cells in the adult CNS that can be even harvested from cadaveric brains within defined postmortem intervals. Although it is too early to predict, the possibility exists that someday cells for neural

replacement can be derived from a patient's own tissues (e.g., autografts) which could even represent nonneural cells that can be stimulated to transdifferentiate into neurons or glia. The availability of techniques to harvest such cells would circumvent a variety of logistical issues (e.g., long-term immunosuppression), not to mention ethical and legal debates over the use of cells from human embryonic and fetal sources.

10. EPILOGUE

In this chapter, we have attempted to provide a comprehensive overview of various basic principles related to neural-tissue damage and regeneration. Several diverse neuronal responses to axotomy and blunt trauma have been described. For those neurons that can survive injury, the capacity to regenerate effectively is dependent upon several intrinsic and extrinsic variables. In the PNS, achieving a high degree of functional improvement after peripheral-nerve injuries is feasible, though not always achieved. Nevertheless, the PNS satisfies many of the basic prerequisites for regeneration. The issue of ultimate functional recovery is not purely a matter of the possible vigor and robustness of the regenerative response, but is also a question of guidance and targeting. Intrinsically, neurons that project axons to the periphery can metabolically exhibit considerable ability to initiate and maintain axonal regrowth over long distances. Unfortunately, this is not the case for CNS injury. However, it is encouraging that some neurons in the brain, spinal cord, and retina are capable of exhibiting robust regenerative responses when the cellular environment is rendered permissive. The multidimensional nature of various neuronal and extraneuronal variables that can dictate the success or failure of regeneration, and what has been learned about these factors presents a variety of therapeutic targets. These options include strategies aimed at the cellular, molecular, pharmacological, and neurorehabilitative levels using a variety of sophisticated approaches, including gene therapy. Such therapies are not mutually exclusive, and CNS repair will undoubtedly require interventions that utilize more than one modality, much like a designer therapy.

With regard to neuronal death in association with injury or disease, viable options have begun to emerge that can overcome another major obstacle to functional repair of the CNS. Whereas once large-scale neuronal replacement was considered a fantasy, the reality of this approach now seems both rational and within reach. Although there is a great deal of enthusiasm for using cellular strategies and cell types, there are many issues to be resolved as scientists and clinicians learn more about effective reconstruction of neural circuitries. The notion of "self repair" is sparked by advances in our appreciation for neuroplasticity and techniques to encourage anatomically and functionally compensatory changes, including interactive training. In assessing future prospects, it is important to remember that the objective is not a matter of restoring normal functions, as much as it is an issue of achieving useful changes, no matter how large or small they may be. The recovery of even crude volitional movements or restored sensation can be meaningful to an individual's quality of life, and in turn can signal important progress. Although the challenges are formidable, progress made in the last two decades has begun to shape dramatic new visions and approaches in the treatment of a broad spectrum of debilitating neuro-

logical disorders that has captured the imagination of even the most conservative scientists and clinicians.

SELECTED READINGS

Ingoglia NA, Murray M (eds). Axonal Regeneration in the CNS. New York: Marcel Dekker, Inc., 2001.

Leist M, Nicotera P. Calcium and cell death. In Koliatsos V, Ratan R (eds). Cell Death and Diseases of the Nervous System. New Jersey: Humana Press, 1999; 69.

Martin LJ. Neuronal cell death in nervous system development, disease, and injury. Int J Mol Med 2001; 7:455.

Raper JA, Tessier-Lavigne M. Growth cones and axon pathfinding. In Zigmond MJ, Bloom FE, Landis SC, Roberts JL, Squire LR (eds). Fundamental Neuroscience. San Diego: Academic Press, 1999; 519.

Tuszynski ME, Kordower J (eds). CNS Regeneration: Basic and Clinical Advances. San Diego: Academic Press, 1999.

Velardo MJ, Reier PJ, Anderson DK. Spinal cord injury. In Crockard A, Hayward R, Hoff JT (eds). Neurosurgery: The Scientific Basis of Clinical Practice. Oxford: Blackwell Science, 2000; 499.

Index

A

Abducens nerve,
  anatomy, 242
  nucleus, 247
  oculomotor system, 280, 281, 290
Accessory nerve, anatomy, 242, 249
Acetylcholine,
  cholinergic neurons,
    anatomy and function, 462
    neurochemistry, 462–464
  co-transmitters, 459
  degradation, 463, 464
  sexual behavior control, 341
  synthesis, 463
Acetylcholine receptor, *see* Nicotinic acetylcholine
    receptor
ACTH, *see* Adrenocorticotropin
Actin, cytoskeletal polymers, 10, 11
Action potential,
  all-or-none characteristics, 45, 83
  components, 43, 44
  definition, 43
  energy requirements, 47
  ion movements, 44, 45
  myelin enhancement, 46
  postsynaptic potential modulation, 75
  propagation, 45
  shapes and functions, 48
  speed, 46
  summation, 77
AD, *see* Alzheimer's disease
Adenosine, sleep role, 601–604
Adrenergic receptors,
  α-adrenergic receptors, 101, 102
  β-adrenergic receptors, 102, 103
  types, overview, 89, 101
Adrenocorticotropin (ACTH),
  fight-or-flight response, 335
  localization in hypothalamus, 316, 317
  neuroimmunology, 644, 645, 648
  processing, 316
  sequence, 309
Agouti-gene-related peptide (AGRP),
  appetite control, 337, 338
  sequence, 339

Agraphia, features, 638
AGRP, *see* Agouti-gene-related peptide
AICAs, *see* Anterior inferior cerebellar arteries
Alexia, features, 638
Alzheimer's disease (AD),
  dementia, 367, 368
  memory loss, 368
  neurofibrillary tangles, 356
  symptoms, 367
Alzheimer's disease, limbic system abnormalities,
    386, 386
γ-Aminobutyric acid (GABA),
  co-transmitters, 459
  degradation, 476, 477
  energy-producing shunt, 476
  gustation role, 577
  REM-off neuron suppression of REM sleep
    phenomena, 612
  synthesis, 475, 476
γ-Aminobutyric acid (GABA) receptor,
  chloride conductance, 62
  structure, 59, 62, 93, 106
  types, 82, 106
G-protein-coupled receptors (GPCRs),
  cholera toxin inhibition, 97
  G-protein complex, 96
  olfactory signal transduction, 582, 583
  peptide receptors, 108, 109
  phototransduction, 514
  signal transduction, 97
  structure, 90, 94, 95
  thalamus, 409
  types, 96
Amygdala,
  affective behavior role, 384
  higher brain functions, 629
  regions, 375
Angiography, overview, 130
Angiotensin II,
  drinking behavior control, 339, 340
  functions, 319, 483
  localization in hypothalamus, 319, 320
  processing, 319
  processing, 482
Anterior cerebral artery,